The Sports Medicine Physician

Sérgio Rocha Piedade • Andreas B. Imhoff
Mark Clatworthy • Moises Cohen
João Espregueira-Mendes
Editors

The Sports Medicine Physician

Springer

Editors
Sérgio Rocha Piedade
Orthopedics and Traumatology
State University
of Campinas – UNICAMP
Campinas / Sao Paulo
Brazil

Mark Clatworthy
Ascot Hospital
Auckland
New Zealand

João Espregueira-Mendes
Espregueira-Mendes Sports Centre
Clínica do Dragão
Porto
Portugal

Andreas B. Imhoff
Orthopaedic Sports Medicine
University of Munich (TUM)
München, Bayern
Germany

Moises Cohen
Department of Orthopedics &
Traumatology
Federal University of São Paulo
Vila Clementino - São Paulo
São Paulo
Brazil

ISBN 978-3-030-10432-0 ISBN 978-3-030-10433-7 (eBook)
https://doi.org/10.1007/978-3-030-10433-7

This Springer imprint is published by the registered company Springer Nature Switzerland AG
The registered company address is: Gewerbestrasse 11, 6330 Cham, Switzerland

Preface

Throughout our life, we are driven toward our dreams; we define paths and strategies and fight for them to become true; we are all moved by challenges. Since ancient times, strife, conquest, and defeat are part of human nature; and this explains why sports are so amazing to practice, watch, and support.

Sports offer us magic moments in which we vent our anxieties and disappointments, share dreams and emotions, and also learn to win and lose. Moreover, sports play a fundamental role in health and education, as they make us aware of the importance of healthy habits, teamwork, and respect for others.

Sports are not only related to recreational and professional competitions, but they are also a tool to reach a quality lifestyle. It strengthens the importance of sports medicine in the management of the effects of physical, recreational, or competitive activity on people. The broad spectrum of sports medicine area accounts to sports practice principles, overtraining injuries, neurological disorders, sports trauma, special clinical conditions, different scenarios in sports (indoor and winter), sports footwear, biologics in sports injuries, major events in sports, and PROMs in sports. Moreover, it allows us to navigate throughout all life phases: childhood, adolescence, adult life, and, the "most experienced of all," old age.

The Sports Medicine Physician book has involved professionals of sports medicine area and orthopedic surgeons from over 20 countries in the world. This book has 50 chapters organized in 10 parts covering different aspects and domains in sports medicine.

Like any huge project, there is a great Team involved. I would like to thank the ISAKOS President Mark Safran and Former President Philippe Neyret, ISAKOS Board, Andreas B. Imhoff, Mark Clatworthy, Moises Cohen, Joao Espregueira-Mendes, Mark R. Hutchinson, Committee members, and all health professionals that have accepted to work in this book, sharing their academic and clinical knowledge as well as experience in sports medicine. Thanks to all of you, my Team, Ge, Cezar, Mariana and Ana Karina Piedade, and Magda S. Kimoto, for supporting me in this amazing project.

Sports make us better, stronger, and true because, in sports, we learn the importance of teamwork.

Campinas, Sao Paulo, Brazil — Sérgio Rocha Piedade

Contents

Part I Sports Practice Principles

1 Multidisciplinary Sport Medicine Team 3
Francesco Della Villa, Stefano Della Villa, and João Espregueira Mendes

2 Pre-participation Evaluation in Sports Practice 13
Sérgio Rocha Piedade, Daniel Miranda Ferreira, Mario Ferreti Filho, Rodrigo Kallas Zogiab, Ivan Córcoles Martínez, Vitaliy Zayats, and Philippe Neyret

3 Biomechanics of Musculoskeletal Injuries 27
Alan Getgood, Yuichi Hoshino, Philip P. Roessler, Ryosuke Kuroroda, and Sérgio Rocha Piedade

4 Physiological Demands in Sports Practice 37
Ana Sousa, João Ribeiro, and Pedro Figueiredo

5 Sports Activity at Childhood and Adolescence 45
Anderson Marques de Moraes, Vagner Roberto Bergamo, and Gil Guerra-Júnior

6 Physical Activity at Adulthood and Old Age 59
Sérgio Rocha Piedade, Mauro Mitsuo Inada, Gerson Muraro Laurito, Diego Navarro e Paiva, Gustavo Pereira Fraga, Rodrigo Goncalves Pagnano, Andre luis Lugnani de Andrade, and Tulio Pereira Cardoso

7 Oriented Warm-Up 71
Karina Mayumi Hatano

8 Nutrition and Hydration 85
Daniéla Oliveira Magro

9 Sports Rehabilitation 99
Knut Beitzel, Daniel Berthold, and Manuel Klose

10 The Role of a Strength and Conditioning Coach 107
Telmo Sousa

11 **Sport Injury Primary and Secondary Prevention** 121
Rogério Pereira, Renato Andrade, Alexandre Rebelo-Marques, and João Espregueira-Mendes

12 **Return to Play (RTP)** 149
Alexandre Rebelo-Marques, Renato Andrade, Rogério Pereira, and João Espregueira-Mendes

Part II Overtraining Injuries

13 **Treatment of Achilles Tendinopathies** 173
Jon Karlsson, Annelie Brorsson, Unnur Jónsdóttir, and Karin Grävare Silbernagel

14 **Muscle Injuries** 187
Gian Luigi Canata, Valentina Casale, Marco Davico, and Simone Lapi

15 **Stress Fractures** 197
Timothy L. Miller and Christopher C. Kaeding

16 **Shin Pain** 211
Sérgio Rocha Piedade, Luis António Mendes, Leonardo Manoel Carvalho, Ramon Medeiros Fagundes dos Santos, Luis Carlos Marques, and Daniel Miranda Ferreira

17 **Groin Injuries** 223
Per Hölmich, Lasse Ishøi, Andreas Serner, and Kristian Thorborg

Part III Neurological Disorders

18 **Epilepsy and Seizures** 235
Jorge Roberto Pagura and Rudá Alessi

19 **Spine Injuries** 241
Elcio Landim, Paulo Tadeu Maia Cavali, Marcelo Italo Risso Neto, and Mauricio Coelho Lima

Part IV Sports Trauma

20 **Facial Trauma** 261
Sérgio Rocha Piedade, Leonardo Manoel Carvalho, Luis António Mendes, Milton Possedente, and Daniel Miranda Ferreira

21 **Thoracic** 275
Ivan Felizardo Contrera Toro and Ricardo Kalaf Mussi

22 Abdomen 289
Rui Pedro Borlido Escaleira

23 Shoulder: The Thrower's Shoulder 307
Lukas N. Muench, Andreas B. Imhoff, and Sebastian Siebenlist

24 Sports Trauma: Elbow 317
Sebastian Siebenlist, Lucca Lacheta, Christine L. Redmond, and Gregory I. Bain

25 Sports Trauma: Wrist and Hand 331
Margaret W. M. Fok, Christine L. Redmond, and Gregory I. Bain

26 Sports Trauma: The Hip 347
Molly C. Meadows and Marc R. Safran

27 Traumatic Knee Injuries 357
Steffen Sauer and Mark Clatworthy

28 Sports Trauma: Ankle and Foot 375
Bruno Silva Pereira and C. Niek van Dijk

Part V Special Conditions

29 Female Athlete Triad and RED-S 395
Samantha Tayne, Melody Hrubes, Mark R. Hutchinson, and Margo Mountjoy

30 Sudden Cardiac Arrest 413
Clea Simone S. S. Colombo, Michael Papadakis, and Nabil Ghorayeb

31 Concussion 429
Natalie Sherry and Michael W. Collins

32 Doping 439
Maria João Cascais

33 Dermatological Injuries 447
Margarida Gonçalo and Luis Santiago

34 Oral Health 459
Silvia Maria Rocha Piedade Damasceno, Marly Kimie Sonohara Gonzalez, Renata Bastos Del Hoyo Fernandes, and Vera Lucia Gramuglia

35 Traveling Management 471
Steven R. Joseph

36 Sports Under Extreme Conditions 481
Helge Krusemark and Annika Hackemann

37 Sports After Knee Arthroplasty . . . 489
Bujar Shabani, Dafina Bytyqi, Cécile Batailler, Elvire Servien, and Sébastien Lustig

38 Ringside Medicine . . . 497
Joseph John Estwanik

Part VI Different Scenarios in Sports

39 Indoor Sports . . . 517
Alex Behar, Mark R. Hutchinson, Aimee Bobko, Benjamin Mayo, Garrett Schartzman, Erwin Secretov, Matthew Steffes, and Samantha Tayne

40 Outdoor Sports: Winter . . . 553
R. Kyle Martin, Mitchell I. Kennedy, J. P. Begly, Rob LaPrade, and Lars Engebretsen

Part VII Sports Equipment

41 Sports Footwear: Problems and Advances . . . 571
Marcelo Pires Prado and Guilherme Honda Saito

Part VIII Biologics in Sports Injuries

42 Biologic Treatment in Tendon and Muscle Injuries . . . 581
Moises Cohen, Gustavo Gonçalves Arliani, and Camila Cohen Kaleka

43 Biologic Treatment of Ligament Injuries by the Sports Physician . . . 591
Jonas Pogorzelski, Mitchell Kennedy, and Robert F. LaPrade

44 Biological Treatment in Cartilage Injuries . . . 599
Elizaveta Kon, Berardo Di Matteo, Francesco Iacono, Filippo Vandenbulcke, Nicolò Danilo Vitale, and Maurilio Marcacci

Part IX Major Events in Sports

45 Olympic Games: Special Considerations—Medical Care for Olympians . . . 617
David J. Pohl, Garrett Schwartzman, Mark R. Hutchinson, William Moreau, Roald Bahr, Robert McCormack, Juan-Manuel Alonzo, Andre Pedrenelli, and Roberto Nahon

46 Paralympic Sport . . . 631
Yetsa A. Tuakli-Wosornu, Fiona Doolan, and Jan Lexell

47 FIFA World Cup 641
Andre Pedrinelli and Caio Senise Drolshagen

48 Extreme Sports 657
Torrey Parry, Empryss Tolliver, and Scott C. Faucett

49 Judo, Brazilian Jiu-Jitsu, Wrestling, and Mixed Martial Arts 671
John A. Bergfeld, Jonathan Gelber, Scott A. Lynch, Peter H. Seidenberg, and Sérgio Rocha Piedade

Part X PROMs

50 PROMs in Sports Medicine 685
Sérgio Rocha Piedade, Mario Ferreti Filho, Daniel Miranda Ferreira, Daniel A. Slullitel, Sarthak Patnaik, Gonzalo Samitier, and Nicola Maffulli

Part I

Sports Practice Principles

1 Multidisciplinary Sport Medicine Team

Francesco Della Villa, Stefano Della Villa, and João Espregueira Mendes

1.1 Outline

The Sports Medicine care, either in a Sport team setting or in a Sports rehabilitation one, should be always based on a team effort. A patient- or athlete-centered approach, with different contributing professional figures, is warranted to maximize health and functional outcomes of our patients, either in primary prevention or rehabilitation setting. The central role of the caregiver team is highlighted in this first chapter in which we wish to present our experience in the basic principles of both playing in and managing a team around the patient in a Sports Medicine setting.

> A proper team, with a high performance culture is key for successful Sports Medicine practice.

1.2 The Crucial Principles

In building a Sport Medicine team, we'd like to share few important concepts at the beginning of this chapter: "No one professional nowadays can handle by his own the complexity of a sport rehabilitation path or injury prevention and training program." This concept is very easy and applies both to primary and secondary prevention of Sport injuries. If you play in team, your odds of winning (achieving good outcomes) are much higher. A proper team, with a high-performance culture, is warranted to carry on a successful Sport Medicine practice. With high-performance culture, we mean the ability to give your maximal effort in the day-by-day activity, helping the patient to reach the maximal possible functional recovery.

F. D. Villa (✉)
Education and Research Department, Isokinetic Medical Group—FIFA Medical Centre of Excellence, Bologna, Italy
e-mail: f.dellavilla@isokinetic.com

S. D. Villa
Educational and Research Department, Isokinetic Medical Group—FIFA Medical Centre of Excellence, Bologna, Italy
e-mail: s.dellavilla@isokinetic.com

J. E. Mendes
Clínica do Dragão—Espregueira-Mendes Sports Centre, FIFA Medical Centre of Excellence, FC Porto Stadium, Porto, Portugal

Orthopaedic Department, Minho University, Minho, Portugal

Publication Committee of the International Society of Arthroscopy, Knee Surgery and Orthopaedic Sports Medicine (ISAKOS), San Ramon, CA, USA

Patellofemoral Foundation, Farmington, CT, USA

FIFA MCE, Porto, Portugal

Porto University, Porto, Portugal

European Society of Sports Traumatology, Knee Surgery and Arthroscopy (ESSKA) 2012-2014, Bologna, Italy
e-mail: jem@espregueira.com

S. Rocha Piedade et al. (eds.), *The Sports Medicine Physician*,
https://doi.org/10.1007/978-3-030-10433-7_1

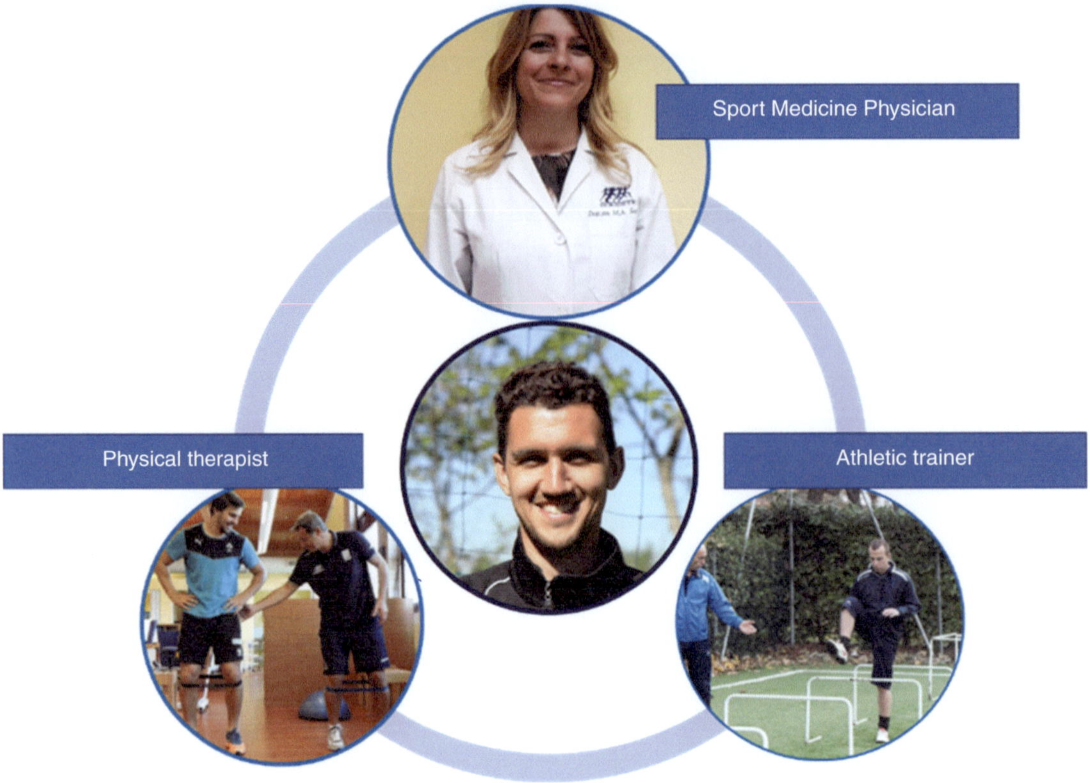

Fig. 1.1 Proper team. Sport Medicine physician, a physical therapist, and an athletic trainer. A patient-first approach is warranted as he/she needs to be guided in the recovery process

In our vision, considering Sport rehabilitation as a model of practice, you will need at least (1) *a Sport Medicine physician*, (2) *a physical therapist*, and (3) *an athletic trainer* to face a correct rehabilitation program (Fig. 1.1).

The Sports Medicine team should always adopt a patient-centered approach. The patient is the leading actor in every functional recovery path. The program must be tailored on his and her needs. Stated that, apart the professional figures listed above, the team can be larger. Chiropractors, specialists in nutrition, and sport psychologists can cover specific areas of functional recovery, optimizing specific areas of concern (Fig. 1.2).

Second point, you need to give the team the possibility to do a great job. Proper facilities are another important issue. If you wish to deliver an updated service, you will need also appropriate facilities to do this. For example, we strongly believe in different environments to give progressive stimuli during functional recovery, the use of *pools*, *gyms*, and *sports field* is key to optimize loading. The adoption of an on-field rehabilitation (OFR) setting is crucial to really complete the recovery path of a competitive athlete (Fig. 1.3).

Third and last general point, the team should follow an appropriate method. In our experience the method should be based on (1) a leader of the group, (2) an appropriate communication model, and (3) a proper and updated clinical method (Fig. 1.4).

First, besides shared decisionmaking, the team must be lead properly. The figure of the leader is always important and crucial in giving a precise tactical and strategic direction to the group, both in the day-by-day activity and in key decisionmaking. In organizing a rehabilitation service, we introduced the so-called concept of the *case manager*. The case manager is the doctor in charge of the patient, from the beginning to the end of functional recovery. He is also in charge of

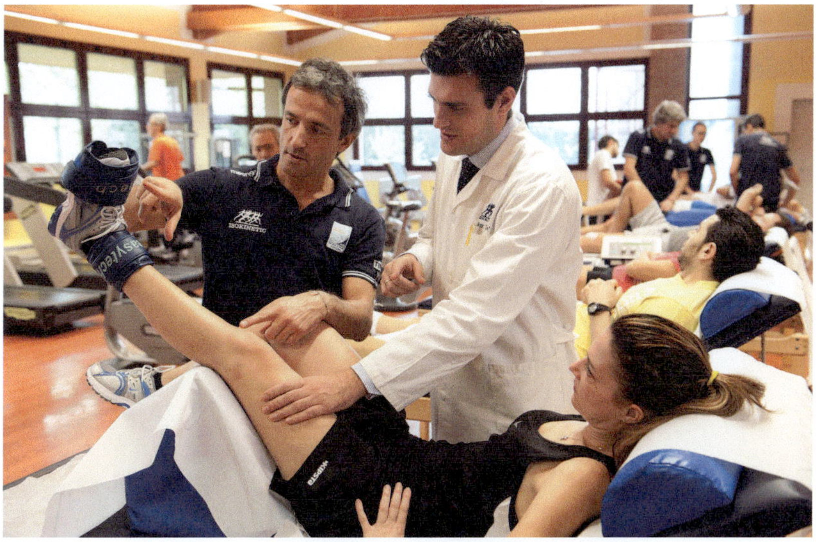

Fig. 1.2 Patient-centered approach. A Sport Medicine physician talking with the physical therapist and the patient during a gym rehabilitation session. High-quality communication, also based on nonformal meeting, is key to control the recovery process

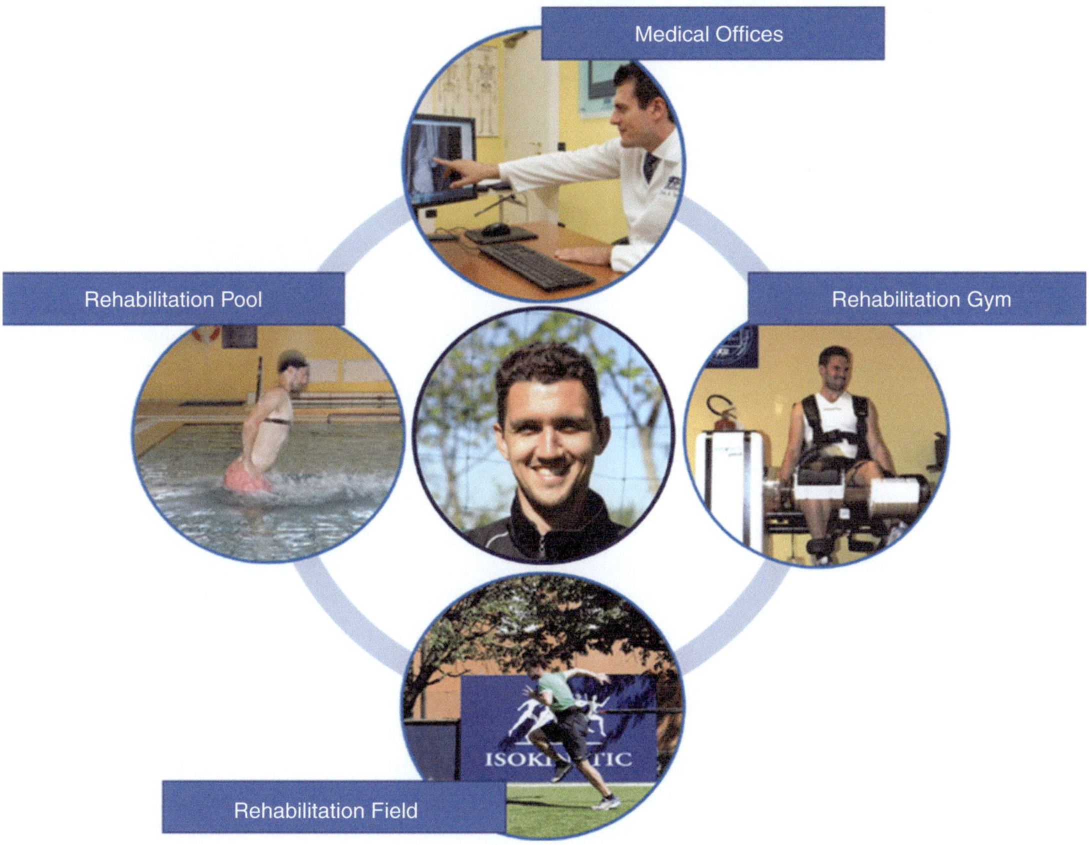

Fig. 1.3 Proper facilities. Different environments are crucial to customize treatments and allow a complete functional recovery

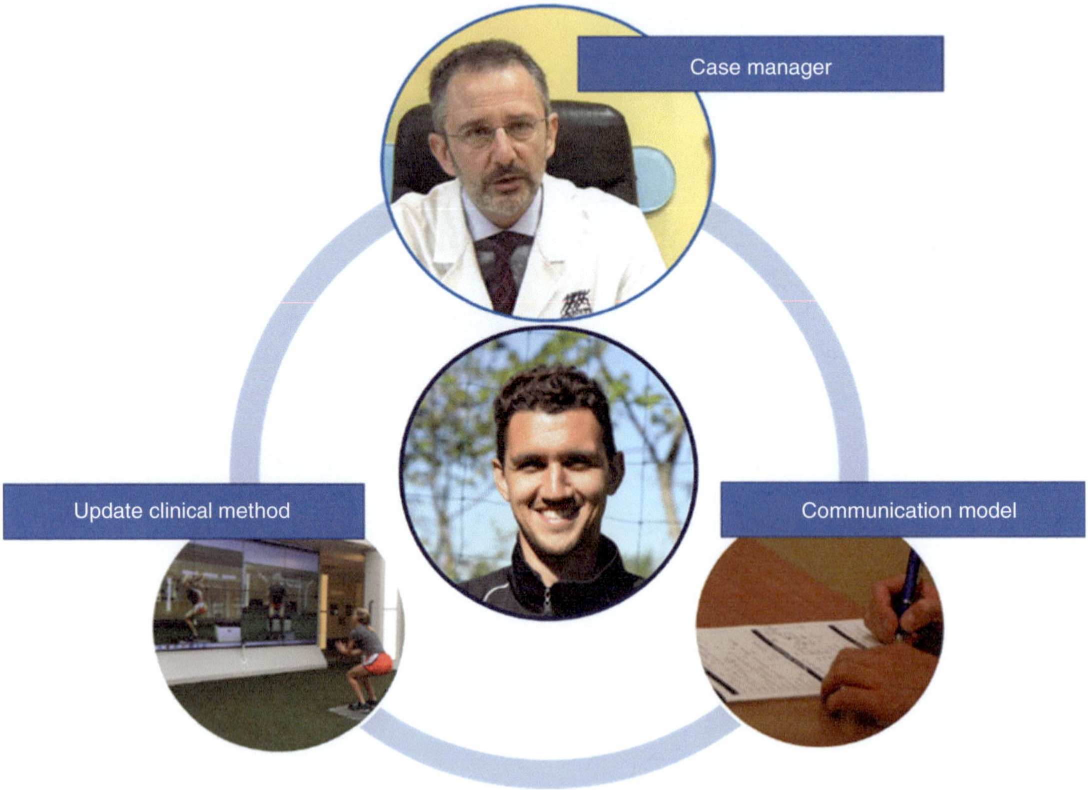

Fig. 1.4 Proper method. These three aspects are of paramount importance in the organization of teamwork

coordinating the team around the patient and communicating with patient environment. Such a figure is warranted in every recovery process.

A *continuous and effective communication* is warranted within the caregivers' team. Having a communication model (e.g., digital clinical records) and periodically (daily if necessary) meetings are the milestones of a well-organized service. Formal and informal communication is key to strengthen the relationship between the different players. The more you communicate within the team, the more you can maximize patient or athlete's perception of the recovery path and minimization of the risk of misleading information to the patient.

Adopting a proper and updated clinical method is the last aspect to be underlined. Statements like "I am doing like this because we have always done in this way" are no longer acceptable in the modern Sport Medicine landscape. Updated practice based on evidence-based recommendation has now to be imbedded in the practice. Considering again a rehabilitation perspective, we strongly believe in criteria-based, rather than time-based, rehabilitation protocols. In respect of the ACL-injured athletes, this statement is not based merely on a personal perspective but on the evidence that certain criteria should be met in order to RTP safely [1]. Current clinical guidelines are also recommending such an approach [2, 3]. Translating medical innovations inside this paradigm is not easy as new does not always mean effective. It is recommended to apply innovations that guarantee a reasonable optimization of functional outcomes, helping the patients and athletes to do better. For this reason, tracking patient's outcome is always wise to evaluate recent addictions.

1.3 We Are Doctors: Health and Performance Considerations

Another factor we need to consider is the existing relation between health, functional outcome, and performance. In the Sport Medicine scenario, our patients are athletes, and they need to perform, sometimes at elite level, at their best. Either working in a Sport team or in Sports rehabilitation facility, we need to prepare them to a sustainable performance. Winning in Sports is a key aspect, but, as doctors, we need to take care about the health of our athletes and patients, finding the correct balance for a sustainable (for the athlete) performance and short- and long-term outcomes. A good example of this concept is a possible existing relationship between the application of injury prevention and winning in football: the lower the injury rate, the higher the team success [4]. Another good example is the functional outcomes after anterior cruciate ligament reconstruction (ACLR). The patient faces two main outcomes; on one side there is the return to play at pre-injury level, and on the other side there is the second ACL injury risk. Again, we need to prepare the patient to perform again, minimizing the physical deficit related to the injury and surgery while reducing, as much as we can, the risk factors for the second injury. The goal of any sportsman or sportswoman is competing at their desired levels with a minimal risk of injury. The Sport Medicine team should help them to achieve this goal. When an injury happens, there should be a correct strategy to face it. As injuries are part of Sports, it is appropriate to speak about injury reduction strategies, as complete prevention is not possible.

1.4 The Case Manager Concept

In the first section of this chapter, we introduce the concept of the case manager. We would like to underline the importance of such a figure in the recovery process after Sport injuries. In the clinical practice, often, the patients see different professional's figures, in different places, potentially giving conflictual, sometimes opposite, suggestions. This is a common story that our patient faces every day. This situation is confusing and nonoptimal for the patient. To minimize the risk of this scenario, we introduced the concept of the case manager. The case manager (same Sport Medicine physician following the patient) oversees the patient through his or her whole recovery process. When surgery is needed, the case manager is in charge of cross talking with the surgeon and the surgical team. We really believe that surgery and rehabilitation are part of the same path; there is no stand-alone in this process (Fig. 1.5).

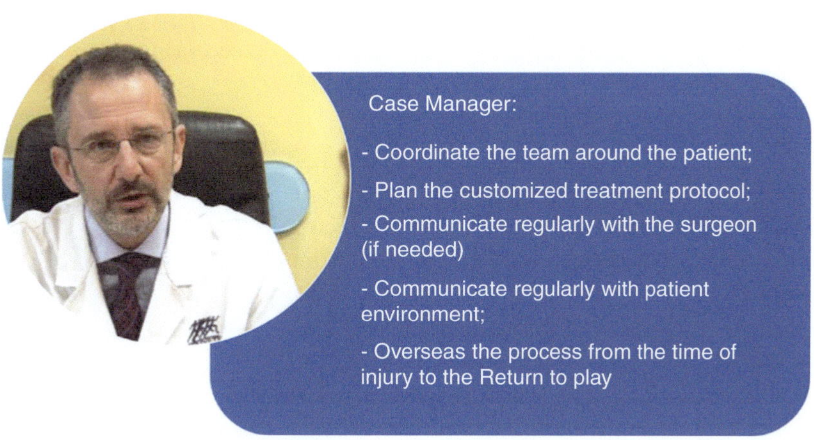

Fig. 1.5 The case manager. The physician should be the key figure for the patient. A reference point to guide the recovery process

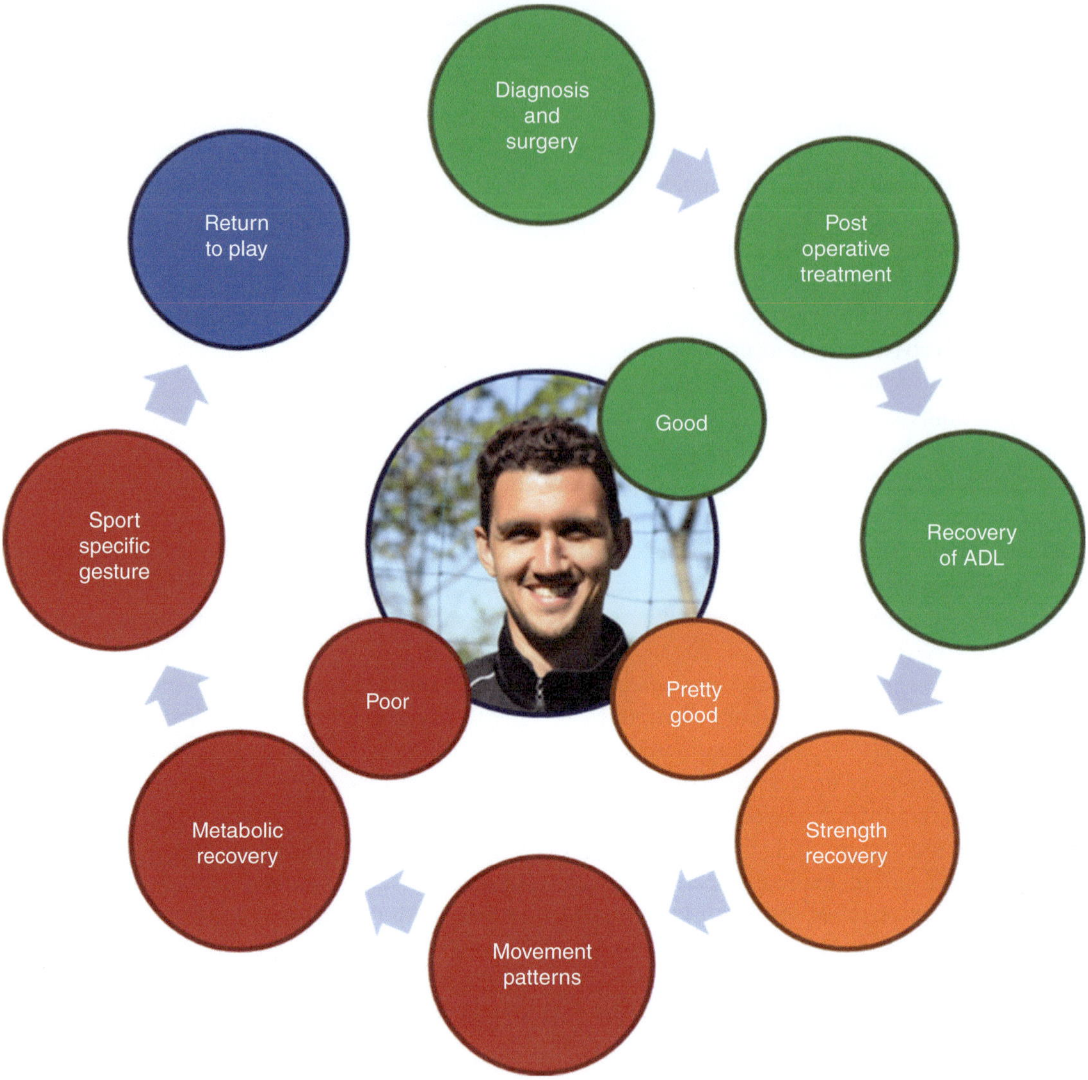
Diagnosis and surgery
Post operative treatment
Recovery of ADL
Strength recovery
Movement patterns
Metabolic recovery
Sport specific gesture
Return to play
Good
Pretty good
Poor

Fig. 1.6 The injury to recovery process. Many steps and obstacles must be overcome to reach a successful RTP. As a community we have a very good control of the first phases, but we generally lack in control over the last steps. This deficit has to be solved

Either with conservative or surgical patients, there is a clear need of taking and maintaining a precise direction in every recovery path, and the patient will benefit from this approach.

We also believe that the same Sport Medicine team should follow the patient from the time of injury to the time of official return to play. The injury to recovery process is tough for the athlete, and we should have a perfect control of the whole path. Taking the example of a major injury (Fig. 1.6) requiring surgery, it is not enough to do half of the way to the top.

> The same Sport Medicine team should follow the patient from the time of injury to RTP.

Generally, we have a good control of the first steps (including diagnosis, surgery, and postoperative treatment). It is a pretty good control of the strengthening phase, but we lack in control of the last crucial phases, when the patient is generally left alone, in the grey area before returning to play. We need to focus also the last part of the recovery process. To reach this goal, we need to challenge our physicians' mind and change our point of view.

1.5 Changing the Status Quo: Return-to-Play Philosophy

To change the status quo, we need to challenge our vision of Sports injuries as doctors. As clinician our focus is on the lesion, on the injured site. We want to fix it as soon as we can. This is right, but we also need to focus the athlete's functioning at 360°, shifting the focus from the injured site to the athlete (Fig. 1.7).

Focusing the return to play from the very first day allows the team to establish a comprehensive (and not reductionistic) return-to-play strategy. Once focusing the RTP, we have the opportunity to highlight some crucial, and often overlooked, aspects especially focusing our focus on end-stage rehabilitation concepts:

- *Criteria-based return-to-play progression*
- *Movement patterns treatment and motor learning techniques*
- *On-field rehabilitation and optimization of the acute on chronic workload*

1.5.1 Criteria-Based Return-to-Play Progression

The common sense, supported by emerging evidence, is that rehabilitation after major knee injuries should be criteria based rather than time based [5, 6]. Criteria-based protocols have been suggested also for muscle injuries [7]. With this

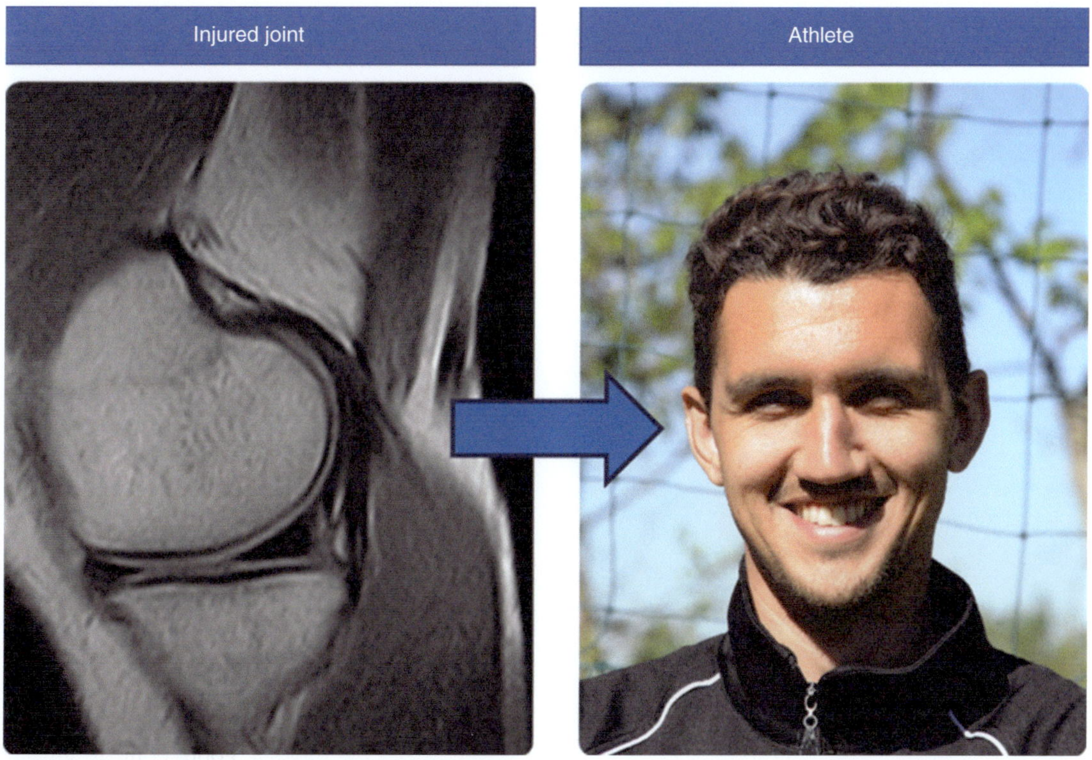

Fig. 1.7 Shift the focus. Shifting the focus on athlete at 360° allows the team to consider other key factors in the rehabilitation process

kind of approach, certain criteria or pitfalls have to be reached in order to progress in the recovery process. In this way a comprehensive and really customized program may be carried out for every patient. This approach has been recently demonstrated to reduce the risk of second ACL injury after ACLR [1]. The same approach can be applied to every recovery process.

1.5.2 Movement Pattern Treatment and Motor Learning Techniques

The comprehension of biomechanical and neurophysiological factors is affecting deeply the way of considering the whole recovery process after lower limb injuries (Fig. 1.8). Clinical, user-friendly, qualitative movement analysis test has been proposed [8–10] and should be part, together with targeted neuromuscular training, of the return-to-sport process after lower limb injuries. On the other hand, feedback techniques have been developed to enhance motor learning, helping the patient to optimize his or her movement patterns [11].

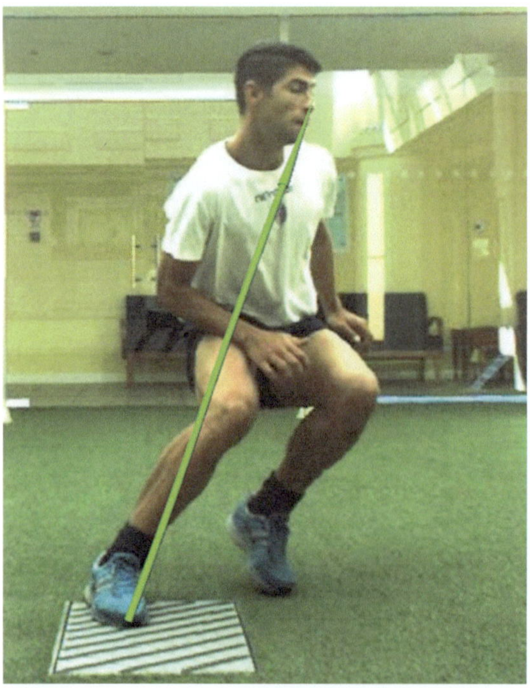

Fig. 1.8 Risky movement patterns, with dynamic knee valgus loading, are frequently present at the time of return to play, especially in young patients

Although the greater amount of research on this aspect is related to RTP after ACLR, there is a growing body of evidence and common sense that the dynamic control of the entire kinetic chain is a key aspect also for other kinds of patients [12].

There needs to be an increased focus on biomechanical and movement pattern aspects after injuries. However, this consideration has to be coupled with an underlined importance of the previous and concomitant work on knee and hip strength. It is nonsense to work on complex movement patterns if the patient has not recovered isolated strength yet; for this reason a battery of tests, instead of a single-dimension assessment, is warranted.

1.5.3 On-Field Rehabilitation and Optimization of the Acute on Chronic Workload

The completion of a stepwise OFR program has been previously presented and correlated to successful outcomes after major knee injuries [13–15]. The OFR program is key to fill the gap between standard rehabilitation and return to play. As stated above, the patient is often left alone. This situation is potentially threatening all the previous efforts, as a nonoptimal management of the RTP phase may be dangerous. At this time, the patient generally starts loading more the injured joint. The key aspects of OFR are (1) *movement quality in high speed and unpredictable movements*, (2) *complete aerobic and anaerobic reconditioning*, (3) *optimal progression of patient workload*, and (4) *sport-specific gesture recovery.*

The transition between the rehabilitation environment and the training fields has to be as smooth as possible. Measuring workloads progressively, with real-time feedback, can help in targeting the desired amount of load.

> End-stage functional recovery is as important as early stage rehabilitation.

The objective of this chapter is not covering technical aspects but instead giving an inspiration of some new area of potential clinical application in nowadays Sport Medicine.

1.6 Conclusions

Providing a Sport Medicine practice should be always based on a team effort. Proper facilities and proper logistic and clinical organizations are other important points not to be overlooked. A team of caregivers covering from the beginning to the end of the rehabilitation process is warranted in conjunction to an increased attention to the last part of the process. As Sport Medicine is a young and active branch of medicine, the Sport Medicine team should embrace new addictions in practice, always considering the clinical benefit for the patients.

References

1. Kyritsis P, Bahr R, Landreau P, Miladi R, Witvrouw E. Likelihood of ACL graft rupture: not meeting six clinical discharge criteria before return to sport is associated with a four times greater risk of rupture. Br J Sports Med. 2016;50(15):946–51. https://doi.org/10.1136/bjsports-2015-095908.
2. Davies GJ, McCarty E, Provencher M, Manske RC. ACL return to sport guidelines and criteria. Curr Rev Muscoskelet Med. 2017;10(3):307–14. https://doi.org/10.1007/s12178-017-9420-9.
3. Van Melick N, Van Cingel REH, Brooijmans F, Neeter C, Van Tienen T, Hullegie W, Der Sanden MWGN. Evidence-based clinical practice update: practice guidelines for anterior cruciate ligament rehabilitation based on a systematic review and multidisciplinary consensus. Br J Sports Med. 2016;50(24):1506–15. https://doi.org/10.1136/bjsports-2015-095898.
4. Eirale C, Tol JL, Farooq A, Smiley F, Chalabi H. Low injury rate strongly correlates with team success in Qatari professional football. Br J Sports Med. 2013;47(12):807–8. https://doi.org/10.1136/bjsports-2012-091040.
5. Adams D, Logerstedt D, Hunter-Giordano A, Axe MJ, Snyder-Mackler L. Current concepts for anterior cruciate ligament reconstruction: a criterion-based rehabilitation progression. J Orthop Sports Phys Ther. 2013;42(7):601–14. https://doi.org/10.2519/jospt.2012.3871.
6. Myer GD, Paterno MV, Ford KR, Quatman CE, Hewett TE. Rehabilitation after anterior cruciate ligament reconstruction: criteria-based progression through the return-to-sport phase. J Orthop Sports Phys Ther. 2006;36(6):385–402.
7. Heiderscheit BC, et al. Hamstring strain injuries: recommendations for diagnosis, rehabilitation, and injury prevention. J Orthop Sports Phys Ther. 2010;40(2):67–81.
8. Padua DA, DiStefano LJ, Beutler AI, De La Motte SJ, DiStefano MJ, Marshall SW. The landing error scoring system as a screening tool for an anterior cruciate ligament injury-prevention program in elite-youth soccer athletes. J Athl Train. 2015;50(6):589–95. https://doi.org/10.4085/1062-6050-50.1.10.
9. Garrison JC, Shanley E, Thigpen C, Geary R, Osler M, Delgiorno J. The reliability of the vail sport test™ as a measure of physical performance following anterior cruciate ligament reconstruction. Int J Sports Phys Ther. 2012;7(1):20–30.
10. Myer GD, Ford KR, Hewett TE. Tuck jump assessment for reducing anterior cruciate ligament injury risk. Athl Ther Today. 2008;13(5):39–44.
11. Benjaminse A, Gokeler A, Dowling AV, Faigenbaum A, Ford KR, Hewett TE, et al. Optimization of the anterior cruciate ligament injury prevention paradigm: novel feedback techniques to enhance motor learning and reduce injury risk. J Orthop Sports Phys Ther. 2015;45(3):170–82. https://doi.org/10.2519/jospt.2015.4986.
12. King E, Franklyn-Miller A, Richter C, O'Reilly E, Doolan M, Moran K, et al. Clinical and biomechanical outcomes of rehabilitation targeting intersegmental control in athletic groin pain: prospective cohort of 205 patients. Br J Sports Med. 2018. https://doi.org/10.1136/bjsports-2016-097089.
13. Della Villa S, Boldrini L, Ricci M, Danelon F, Snyder-Mackler L, Nanni G, Roi GS. Clinical outcomes and return-to-sports participation of 50 soccer players after anterior cruciate ligament reconstruction through a sport-specific rehabilitation protocol. Sports Health. 2012;4(1):17–24. https://doi.org/10.1177/1941738111417564.
14. Della Villa S, et al. Does intensive rehabilitation permit early return to sport without compromising the clinical outcome after arthroscopic autologous chondrocyte implantation in highly competitive athletes? Am J Sports Med. 2010;38(1):68–77.
15. Della Villa F, Ricci M, Perdisa F, Filardo G, Gamberini J, Caminati D, Della Villa S. Anterior cruciate ligament reconstruction and rehabilitation: predictors of functional outcome. Joints. 2016;3(4):179–85.

2 Pre-participation Evaluation in Sports Practice

Sérgio Rocha Piedade, Daniel Miranda Ferreira, Mario Ferreti Filho, Rodrigo Kallas Zogiab, Ivan Córcoles Martínez, Vitaliy Zayats, and Philippe Neyret

2.1 Background

Since ancient times, sports practice is well-recognized as a health-promoting activity as it has an effect act on our biological reserve, positively impacting the musculoskeletal, cardiovascular, and immunological systems, athletes' self-esteem and confidence, and improving their social integration [1–4]. This apart, participating in sports activities pushes people to compete and face challenges and also strengthens the desire to work as a team.

S. R. Piedade (✉) · R. K. Zogiab
Department of Orthopedics and Traumatology, State University of Campinas—UNICAMP, Exercise and Sports Medicine, Campinas, SP, Brazil
e-mail: piedade@fcm.unicamp.br

D. M. Ferreira
Department of Radiology, State University of Campinas—UNICAMP, Exercise and Sports Medicine, Campinas, SP, Brazil

M. F. Filho
Department of Orthopedics and Traumatology, UNIFESP, Sao Paulo, Brazil

I. C. Martínez
Hospital Universitario Joan XXII de Tarragona, Cataluña, Spain

V. Zayats
Trauma and Orthopedic Department, Pavlov First St. Petersburg State Medical University, Petersburg, Russia

P. Neyret
University Lyon 1, Lyon, France

However, sports practice is not an injury-free activity because it involves aspects of the modality of practiced sports, athletes' biological, and physical conditions. The intensity of physical demands is particular to each sports modality, varying according to its dynamic (soccer, basketball, volleyball, tennis, cricket, MMA, judo, surf), field, and environmental conditions where the sport is practised (indoor, outdoor) [5–8]. Within this context, the rules of the sport should be adjusted and improved whenever necessary such as the implementation of protective measures (helmets, mouth guards, gloves), time of the dispute, and rest intervals during the games, resulting in fairer dispute and contributing to decreasing the athlete's exposure to injuries [9–13].

However, the athletes' clinical and physical conditions are influenced by their age, gender, presence of chronic diseases (diabetes, hypertension, heart disease), overweight, previous injuries, neurological disorders, psychological distress, and handicaps. All these conditions do not necessarily preclude sports practice, but they must be identified and appropriately treated to define the best approach before starting sports practice and allowing the athlete to perform his/her activities within a safe zone, minimizing exposure to clinical adverse effects [14–17].

Unfortunately, sudden cardiac arrest, one of the most overwhelming events in sports practice, could signal the first clinical presentation of an underlying cardiovascular disease. Without a

S. Rocha Piedade et al. (eds.), *The Sports Medicine Physician*,
https://doi.org/10.1007/978-3-030-10433-7_2

doubt, this dramatic and stressful clinical event could happen in a sports physician's practice and may cause traumatic effects to the sports community (athletes, coaches, fitness instructors, and sports fans) as it could touch young individuals in the prime of their lives [18–25].

In this context, pre-participation evaluation (PPE) is considered the cornerstone of sports injury prevention as it plays a vital role to assess athlete's overall health, recognizing health problems, and defining medical strategies and recommendations to achieve and maintain the athletes' "wellness" [26–28]. The PPE main goals are to previously identify:

- Clinical conditions that may be life-threating and impose relative or formal contraindication to sports practice
- Prior injuries that can be treated and appropriately rehabilitated before starting sports activities
- Clinical comorbidities and handicaps that predispose to illness and injury, recognizing high-risk individuals for sports practice
- Also, to assess fitness for a specific sport

Although PPE presents a valuable tool to monitor the athletes' health during their lifetime in sports, offering numerous benefits to their health care, this approach is not well-standardized worldwide. An example of that is seen in Europe, where PPE rules and strategies are not similar among the countries [29]. In France, a general clinical assessment is well-accepted such as PPE for amateur athletes, but, for competitive athletes, a more rigorous health control to certify the absence of contraindications to sports practice is required. For more than 35 years, the Italian government has regulated and established PPE as mandatory for competitive athletes, while, in the Netherlands, citizens are regularly evaluated [29].

According to the modality of sports, PPE should pay particular attention to clinical aspects which are commonly associated with specific sports injuries**.** **In contact sports** such as rugby, martial arts, football, and ice hockey, the spine is exposed to high-energy trauma that potentializes the occurrence of **concussion, facial trauma, spinal cord injury due to the dynamics of these sports** [30–32]. Transient quadriplegia is a sports injury commonly seen in American football and contact sports. This injury results from axial trauma with flexion/extension of the athlete's head with underlying cervical spinal canal stenosis, a structural disorder that should be investigated and ruled out in these athletes during PPE.

In athletes of wilderness watersports, one of the concerns is that the athlete's breath holding and buoyancy capacities are limited to their physical status that decreases when exposed to cold water condition due to muscle overload in an attempt to control body temperature and avoid the occurrence of hypothermia [33]. In these athletes, PPE can focus on assessing acute and chronic clinical conditions that could impair the athlete's ability to swim.

In endurance sports, In endurance sports, weight-classified sports and aesthetic sports, there is a close relationship with pathogenic weight control behaviors, clinically manifested by disordered eating, the decrease of bone mass density, and menstrual dysfunction in females. As this pathological condition impacts negatively on athletes' performance, the PPE should take it into account [33, 34]. Therefore, all these points reinforce the importance of PPE to athletes' health care.

This chapter **presents** and discusses elements involved in PPE and particularities related to different athletes' population according to their gender, age (childhood and adolescence, adulthood and old age), and level of sports practice (recreational, disabled, and professional athletes).

2.2 Pre-participation Evaluation

A well-structured PPE should be based on athletes' medical and sports injury history and their family's medical history. It is considered the first step to screen and identify possible cardiovascular injuries related to sudden death. This strategy is a useful tool to map populations of athletes and tailor PPE regardless of their age, gender, modality of sports, and level of sports practice. In general, PPE has the same structure and design for every athlete, but it should be tailored

for each athlete according to their age, gender, clinical condition, handicap, as well as the level of sports practice (recreational, amateur, and professional) reported.

2.3 Periodization of PPE

In clinical practice, it is recommended that PPE be applied 6–8 weeks before starting sports practice because it allows enough time to rehabilitate injuries, identify, and manage any medical disorders properly, minimizing the risk of exposing athletes to injury.

PPE applied to athletes, recreational or professional, before starting a new program of sports practice is advisable, an important step to minimize the athlete's exposure to adverse clinical events such as a sudden cardiac arrest. Although, PPE is a dynamic issue, its advancements involve costs which should be justified by the cost-benefit. It presents excellent sensitivity, specificity, and effectiveness in reducing adverse effects and mortality [33–36]. However, its implementation also depends on national/regional settings to achieve the most accurate physical examination.

As discussed above, PPE may contribute to injury prevention and evaluation of prior clinical conditions that may predispose the athlete to illness or injuries as well as to the identification of conditions that do not present overt symptoms, reinforcing PPE periodization. In clinical practice, the sports physician's decision-making takes into consideration the questions listed below:

- Is there a formal risk to the athlete?
- Can the athlete:
  - Under medical treatment compete safely?
  - Participate in another sports activity?
  - Be cleared for certain sports?
- Could this problem affect other athletes?

PPE involves anamnesis, an athlete's general health history and sports injuries report and also the family health history [33–36]. These data are useful as they guide the physical assessment as well as laboratory and radiological exams needed to evaluate the athlete's physical health properly and, at the same time, rule out adverse clinical conditions to sports practice.

2.4 Anamnesis

The PPE anamnesis has a three-key point structure namely: the athlete's general health, sports injuries, and family health history. All these elements are a sensitive tool to analyze the athlete's health status and screen for potential clinical problems or deficits that can impair the athlete's performance or expose him/her to injury or illness. Moreover, it is helpful to carry out the physical assessment according to the reported data. Before starting PPE application, the sports medicine physician should try to offer a comfortable environment so that the athletes feel more confident to reply to questions. The physician should start talking and asking the athletes informally about their motivation to sports practice, sports/quality of life, and health concerns:

- How motivated are you to play sports?
- Do you feel in good shape to practise sports?
- Have you been sleeping well?
- Do you have any concerns about healthy eating?
- Do you have any complaints when playing sports?

2.4.1 Athlete's General Health History

It comprises of the data of complaints or clinical problems related to body systems, psychological status, exertional symptoms, dietary, oral health, social behavior, infectious diseases, hospitalizations, and surgical procedures. A point to be reinforced is the role of oral health assessment in monitoring nutritional deficiency and also systematic diseases that could affect athletes' performance. Table 2.1 summarizes some of the relevant points.

Table 2.1 Points to be assessed during an athlete's general health exam

Skin	
	Dermatitis, allergies (triggered by food, insects, medicines), infections (bacteria, virus), acne (wrestlers)
Psychological distress or disorders	
	Anxiety, depression, OCD, eating disorders, anorexia, REDS
Oral	
	Gingivitis, tooth loss, tooth pain, herpex simplex
Gastrointestinal disorders	
	Gastritis, hepatitis, abdominal tenderness or masses
Neurological	
	Mental status, suspicious of sports-related concussion, confusion or memory loss after a head trauma
Cardiovascular	
	Palpitations or irregular heartbeat, exertional chest pain, syncope, shortness of breath, and fatigue on exertion
Urinary	
	Calculus, infections, nephritis, kidney agenesis
Respiratory	
	Chronic respiratory problems (asthma, bk) or acute (infections, pneumonia), exercise-induced bronchospasm
Musculoskeletal	
	Arthrosis, ligament injury, fracture, muscle injury, sprain, patellofemoral dislocation, hernia, rheumatologic diseases, miopathy
Medication for chronic diseases	
	Beta blocker, diuretic, antidepressive, steroids, anti-inflammatory drugs
Prior surgeries	
	Fracture, ligament reconstruction, arthrodesis, heart revascularization
Endocrinological	
	Diabetes, hyperparathyroidism, hypercholesterolemia
Hospitalization/previous surgeries	
	Fracture, ligament reconstruction, arthrodesis, heart heart revascularization, prothesis
Special clinical signs in females	
	Menstrual dysfunction, amenorrhea or oligomenorrhea, osteoporosis (young female)

2.4.2 Athlete's Sports Injury and Clinical Complaints Related to Sports Practice

Recording the athlete's prior injuries, their surgical and rehabilitation treatments after sports trauma, and the reports on the regular use of protective equipment in sports practice allows a better understanding of athlete's health status and physical condition. In this context, sprains, fractures, ligament injuries, hernia, cervical and head trauma, chest pain, fatigue, and difficulty breathing during high-intensity exercises should be carefully investigated by the sports physician [37].

2.4.3 Family Medical History

Considering that people from the same family have many aspects in common such as genetics, environment, and life style, the athlete's family medical history has a vital role in PPE. It allows tracking health information about the athlete's close relatives and helps to identify chronic diseases that could impact the athlete's health when practicing sports like a cardiovascular diseases such as cardiovascular disease (hypertension, myocardiopathy), diabetes, asthma and exercise-induced bronchospasm, gastrointestinal disorders, hematological disorders, neurological diseases, eating disorders, psychiatric disorders and, cancer that could impact the athlete's health when practising sports.

2.5 Musculoskeletal Screening

A physical examination plays an essential role on the PPE process. It allows the screening and evaluation of muscle and joint function regarding balance and motion range symmetry as well as the level of muscle force between limbs [37–39]. Moreover, a physical examination can reveal clues and identify previous or even unknown injuries besides muscle weakness, stretching deficit, uni- or bilateral joint motion restriction, limb discrepancy or malalignment, collagene disease (such as Marfan from low expression (hiperlaxity) to server) which could present clinical disorders that will expose the athlete to injuries.

2.6 Starting the Physical Examination

2.6.1 Inspection

The athlete is asked to wear underwear and no shirt for a GENERAL view of their body. Starting with the athlete's gait, the sports physician seeks to identify any changes in gait such as limping. Then, with the athlete in standing position, the skin is screened for lesions and scars and also if the spine is aligned.

2.6.2 Oral Health Assessment

The athlete is requested to open their mouth by placing two folded fingers (index and middle) at the distal interphalangeal joints of the mouth which allows the physician to check any restricted motion of TMDs (temporomandibular disorders). Besides that, the oral health status is checked regarding the status and color of the lips, mucosas, and teeth conditions (integrity, biofilm stagnation (bacterial plaque), the presence of calculus (tartar), dental loss, and also tooth wear (indirect signs of anxiety, depression, or stress that could commonly be associated with bruxism). **The oral health exam is vital to assess** the athletes' oral hygiene and its maintenance (periodical exams) as well as to identify clues of systemic diseases that impact the athletes' performance.

2.6.3 Dynamic Physical Evaluation

It should be emphasized that the physical examination is guided by the anamnesis (athletes' general health history, athletes' sports injuries and clinical complaints related to sports practice, and also their family medical history). In clinical practice, the physical exam starts with the spine motion and then goes on to upper limbs and finishes with lower limbs; the most common clinical tests performed in this evaluation are presented in Fig. 2.1. However, it should be emphasized that the **physical** assessment is carried out according to the reported data in the anamnesis (athlete's general health history, sports injuries, clinical complaints related to sports practice, and also their family medical history).

2.7 Regarding PPE in Different Age Groups

2.7.1 In Childhood and Adolescence

In many countries and regions due to the economic conditions, sports participation is a huge opportunity for children and adolescents to change their lives and also have access to health. Thus, PPE plays an essential role in it. Sports practice during childhood and adolescence is considered an important factor associated with health in adulthood and old age, and, therefore, it is vital to public health actions [40–42]. Consequently, millions of children and adolescents are involved in organized sports worldwide every year. However, it should be taken into account that this population involves individuals that are developing their biological patterns as well as social behaviors that will manifest during the rest of their lives. It should be kept in mind that the bone and joint maturation is a high energy process that involves biomechanical changes of the living tissues. In childhood, a bone is defined as an immature structure which is weaker (less mineralized) and ductile, while during adolescence it starts becoming more mineralized, conferring a stiff and brittle characteristic to it, until bone maturation takes places (Fig. 2.2). In this context, individuals younger than 18 years old should be followed closely due to the huge and rapid body changes occurring in childhood and adolescence. Therefore, childhood involves biological and clinical patterns that make these athletes different from adult athletes, and, therefore, children cannot be considered as "small adults".

In children and adolescents starting regular physical exercises and sports practice, PPE is helpful to screen unfavorable athletes' clinical conditions to some modalities of sports. For instance, in contact sports, the athletes are submitted to high-energy trauma as well as physical demands (Fig. 2.3).

An example of that is a young patient with a medical health history of rhinitis or recurrent sinusitis willing to practice swimming. This condition does not necessarily exclude its practice but allows the sports physician to identify the problem previously and treat the athlete adequately before letting him practise water sports.

Regarding the psychological aspects, a young athlete can became stressed due to training, competiting, and also their parents' unconscious behavior of projecting their own personal desire to be champion on their sons and daughters. All these aspects may impact a young athlete's social behavior, and, therefore, alcohol, smoking, and also drug addiction should be carefully investigated. Thus, it is recommended that the athlete's parents or guardian be present at PPE to confirm

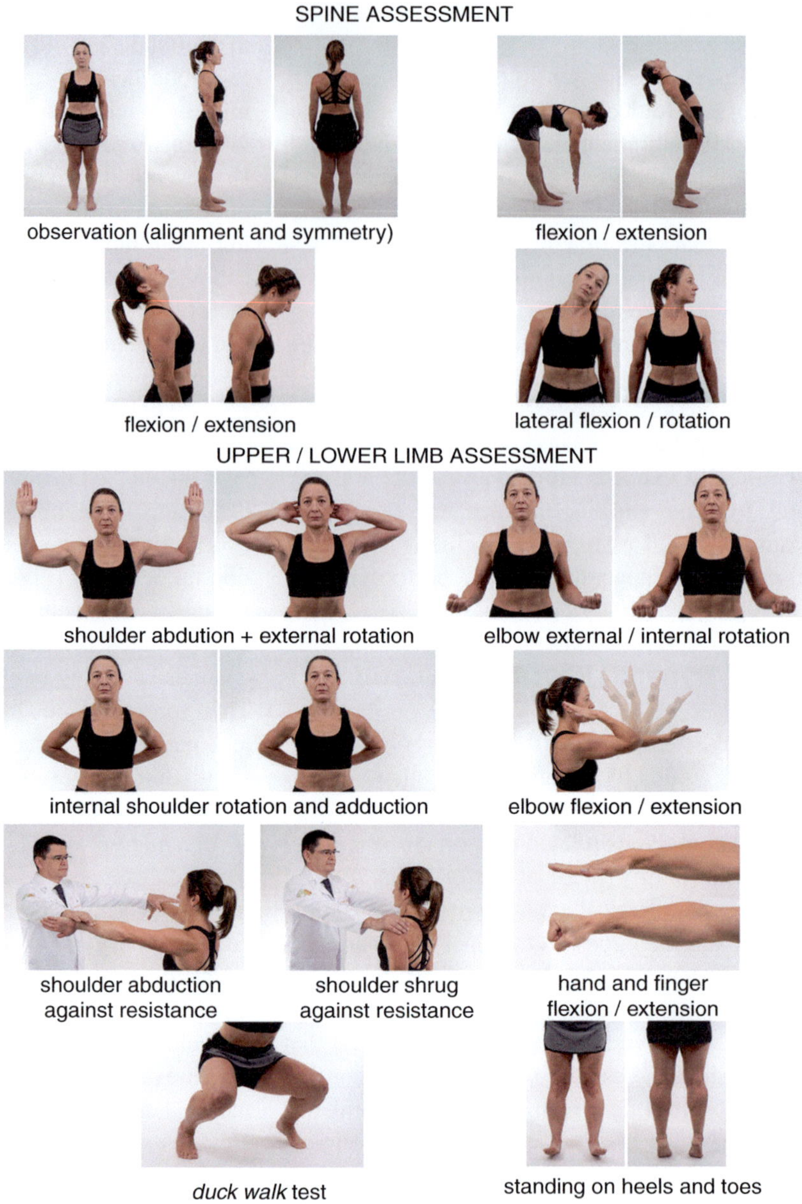
SPINE ASSESSMENT
observation (alignment and symmetry)
flexion / extension
flexion / extension
lateral flexion / rotation
UPPER / LOWER LIMB ASSESSMENT
shoulder abdution + external rotation
elbow external / internal rotation
internal shoulder rotation and adduction
elbow flexion / extension
shoulder abduction against resistance
shoulder shrug against resistance
hand and finger flexion / extension
duck walk test
standing on heels and toes

Fig. 2.1 Dynamic physical evaluation

and add details of the athlete and family medical history [27–29].

As stated before, the periodicity of PPE is essential as it can identify the initial stages of energy deficiency in sports (REDs), a clinical problem that affects both men and women and involves low energy availability (involving eating disorders or not), low bone mineral density, and menstrual dysfunction and, therefore, should be carefully investigated [43, 44].

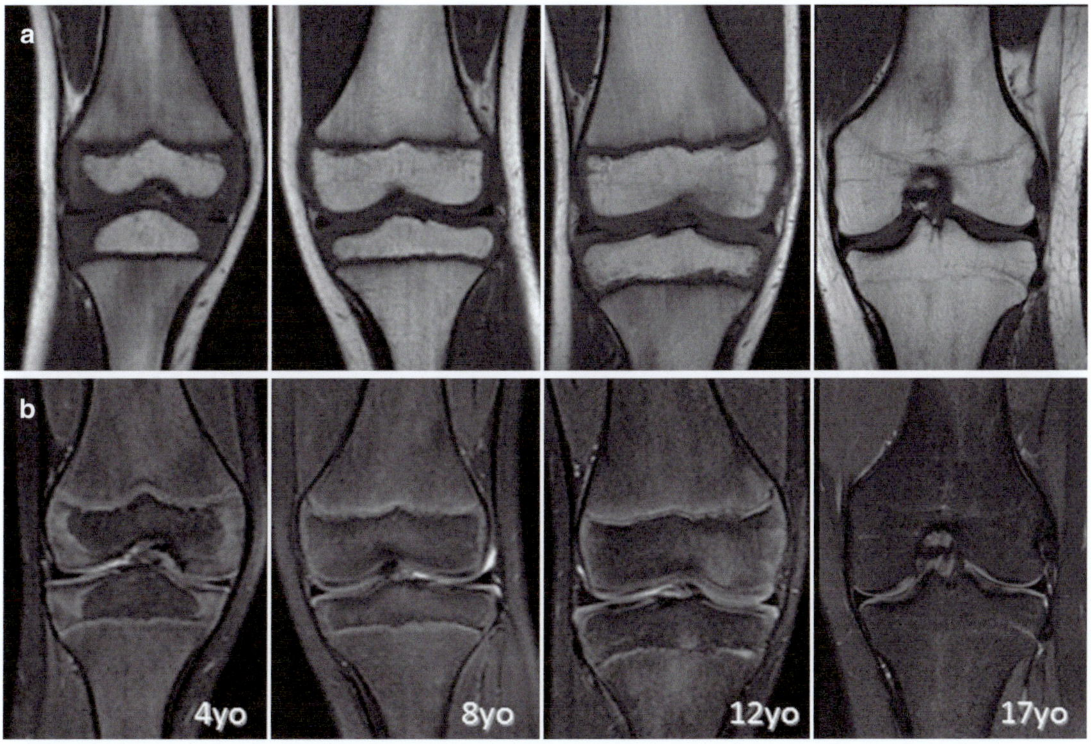

Fig. 2.2 Coronal T1 (**a**) and T2 fat sat (**b**) weighted of normal MRI views of the knee in young patients aged 4, 8, 12, and 17 years old

Fig. 2.3 Female rugby athletes

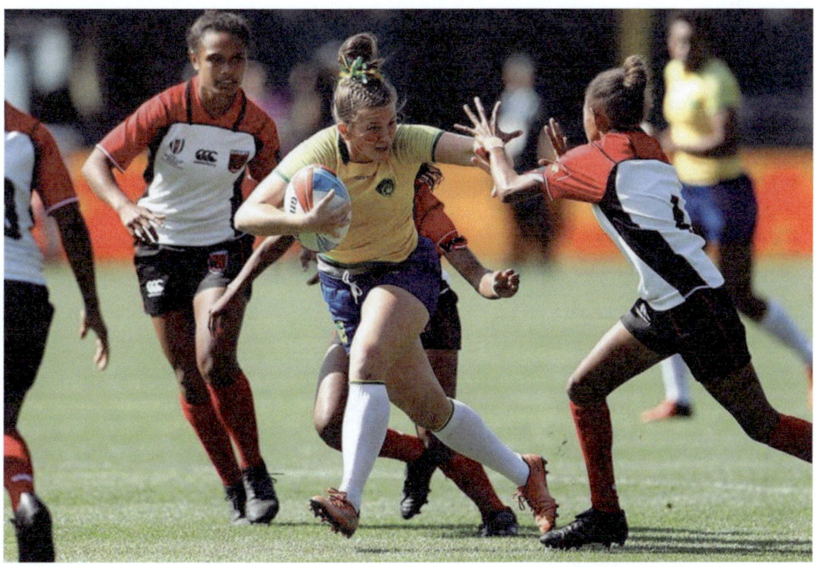

In general, the physical assessment in child and adolescent athletes focuses on the symmetry of lower-and-upper-limb joint movement strength, according to the modality of sports and its physical demands on the joints and muscles. In child and adolescent athletes, laboratory tests and radiological evaluation are requested, depending on the specific clinical disorder reported during the anamnesis or suspected in the physical assessment.

2.7.2 Adulthood and Old Age

Data from the World Health Organization has shown an increase in life expectancy in recent decades. In 2016 the average life expectancy at birth was 72 years. The global average life expectancy increased by 5.5 years between 2000 and 2016, the fastest increase since the 1960s [45]. Adulthood and old age are periods of life in which degenerative and chronic diseases begin to manifest (Fig. 2.4). Figure 2.3 compares the radiological patterns of a normal knee joint to a medial degenerative one.

According to a person's social habits, obesity, hypertension, diabetes, hypercholesterolemia, arthrosis, and cardiovascular diseases will take place. With the increasing ageing of the population, many people have begun to take up physical activity on a voluntary basis for a better quality of life and health benefits in the treatment and prevention of various diseases [46–50].

The population aged 35 years and older, so-called "masters" athletes, represents a challenge for health-care providers who are asked to make decisions regarding assessments of cardiovascular risk associated with different types of physical activity. Currently, there are no validated tools to help physicians assess the risk of physical activity in master athletes because most tools are geared towards screening younger participants [51]. Ageing athletes are exposed to exercise-induced cardiovascular events related to undiagnosed coronary artery disease, which is the primary cause of sudden cardiac death in masters' athletes [52].

The American Heart Association (AHA) and the American College of Sports Medicine (ACSM) developed the American Heart Association/American College of Sports Medicine Pre-participation Questionnaire (AAPQ) to enable cost-effective screening for cardiovascular risk among individuals who desire to initiate a fitness program [53]. If a subject responds positively to any of the statements regarding cardiac history or symptoms, or to two or more of the statements regarding risk factors, a recommendation is made for a pre-participation evaluation.

The 2001 Masters Athletics Working Group developed pre-participation guidelines for those who desire to participate in more competitive sporting events [54]:

- Stress test for men aged >40 years and women aged >50 years who also have one of the following conditions: hypercholesterolemia, systemic hypertension, current or recent cigarette smoking, diabetes mellitus, or history of myocardial infarction or sudden cardiac death in a first-degree relative aged <60 years
- Stress testing for all athletes aged ≥65 years
- Electrocardiogram (ECG) for all athletes male and female aged >40 years

Self-administered surveys such as the Physical Activity Readiness Questionnaire for Everyone (PAR-Q+) [55], the European Association of Cardiovascular Prevention and Rehabilitation (EACPR) recommendations [56], and the Framingham Risk Score (FRS) can be used in pre-participation screening of masters athletes [57].

Although some imaging tests that have sensitivity approaching close to 100% would be ideal to ascertain the prevalence of cardiovascular disease (Fig. 2.5), they are not performed routinely in PPE. The main reasons are that the current evidence for incorporating cardiac imaging into pre-participation screening is insufficient, expensive, potentially radioactive, and not indicated for testing generally healthy asymptomatic low-risk patients [58].

The optimal method to screen masters athletes requires continued study to decrease the number of false-positive with available and cost-effective screening tools to identify potentially at-risk individuals.

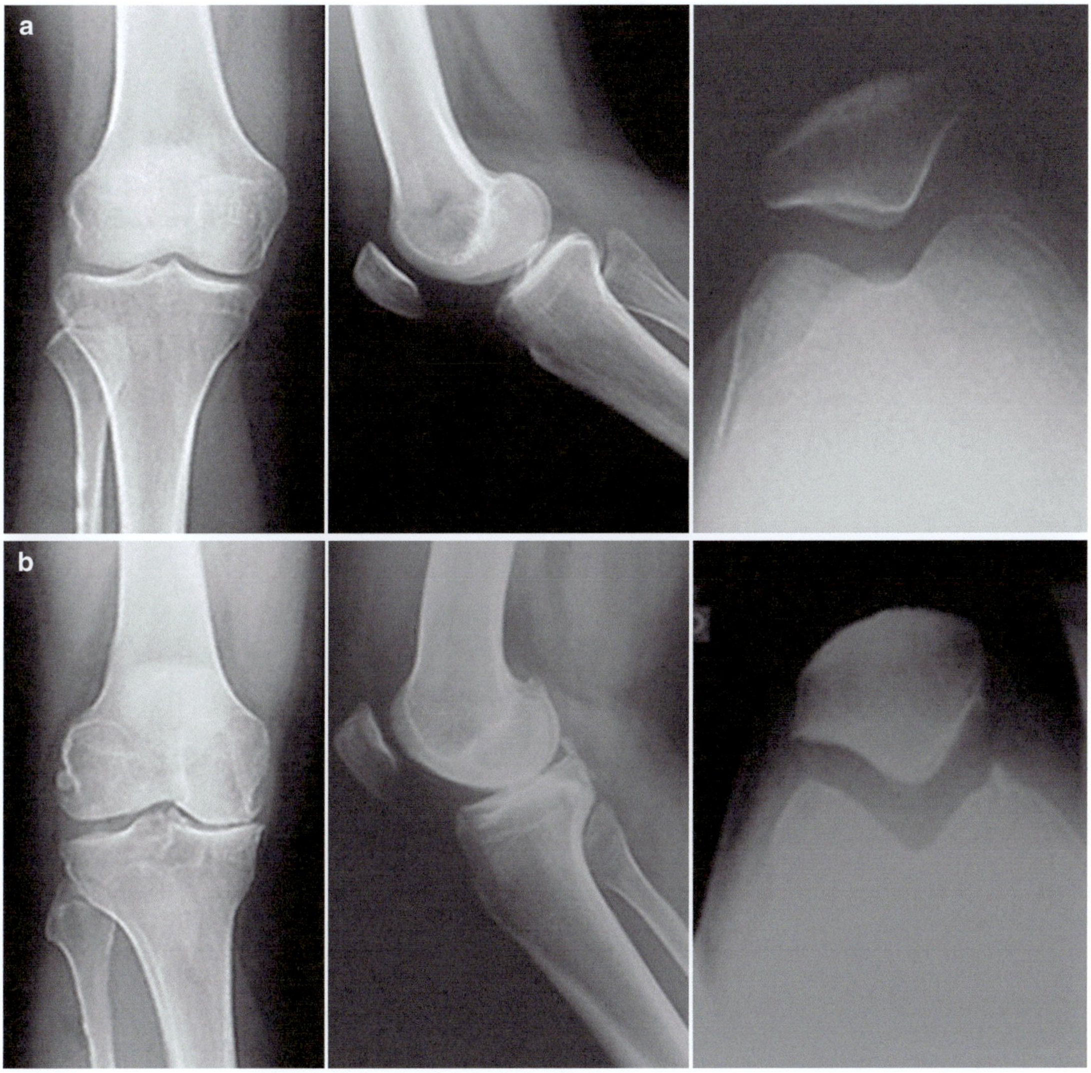

Fig. 2.4 Anteroposterior, lateral, and axial X-ray views of the knee (**a**) in the healthy knee of a 20-year-old patient. (**b**) Osteodegenerative changes (narrow of medial articular space, subchondral sclerosis, and femorotibial and femoropatellar osteophytes) in a 65-year-old patient

2.7.3 Disabled Athletes

Disabled athletes are a particular group of individuals that have functional impairment that could vary according to its cause. Considering that sports practice requires significant physical demands, disabled athletes should be subcategorized and also classified according to the type of physical handicap [59]. This allows the classification of athletes according to their functional impairment, establishes fair competition, and also minimizes the risk of athletes' injury in sports practice and competition events. In this context, the main reasons for functional impairment are summarized in Table 2.2.

In clinical practice, the ten most common physical impairments reported in disabled athletes are listed in Table 2.3. They serve as one of the parameters adopted to classify the athletes' functional level. However, it should be emphasized that the disabled athletes' classification remains a dynamic process. Each year, the technological advancement in the sports medicine

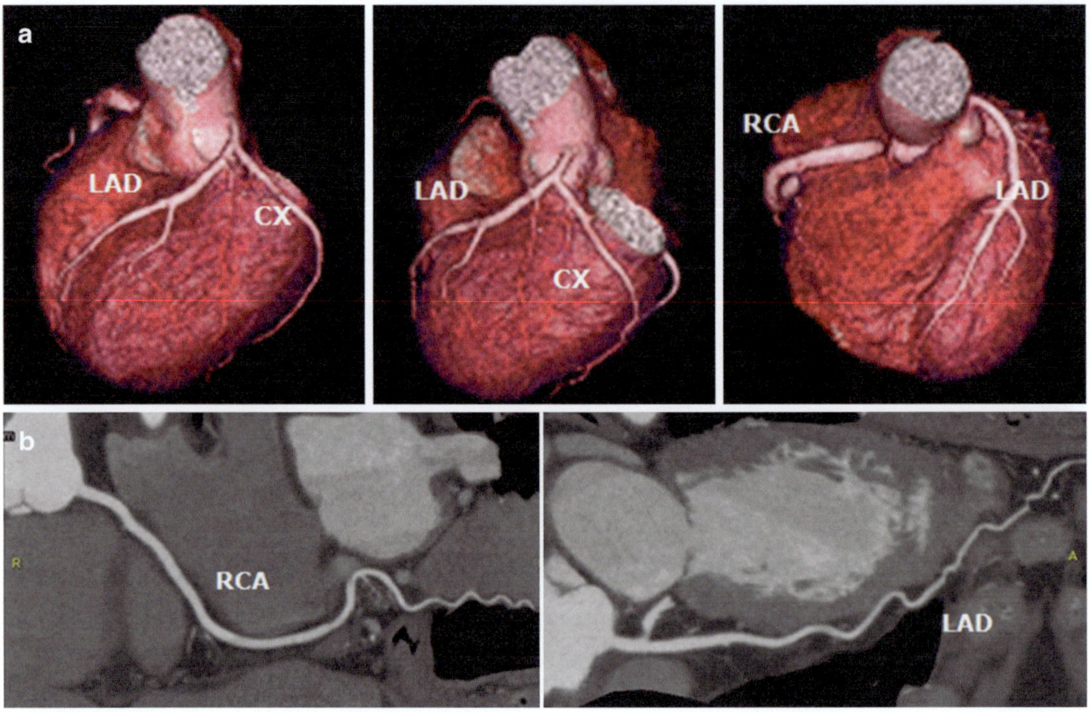

Fig. 2.5 Normal CT coronary angiography with no atheromatous plaques (**a**). Three-dimensional volume rendering technique and (**b**) maximum intensity projection technique. *RCA* right coronary artery, *LAD* left anterior descending, and *CX* circumflex artery

Table 2.2 Main reasons for functional impairment in disabled athletes

Spinal cord injury	Amputations
Cerebral palsy	Collagenosis
Muscular dystrophy	Limb malformation
Myelomeningocele	Acquired injuries due to traumas
Poliomyelitis	Blindness and low vision

Table 2.3 Most common physical impairments reported in clinical practice

Severely affected muscle power	Hypertonia
Impaired passive range of motion	Ataxia
Total or partial limb loss	Athetosis
Limb length discrepancy	Visual impairment
Short	Intellectual impairment

[a]Athletes with intellectual disability as well as youngsters with learning disabilities should be more explicitly instructed before starting regular sports practice

area has caused improvements in medical evaluation and diagnosis and consequently has promoted update on disabled athletes' functional classification for the Paralympics [60].

2.7.4 Elite Athletes

In general, in professional sports, the modality of sports and its dynamic (contact and noncontact sports) involve different physical demands. In this context, PPE focus should take into account the athlete's position in the field and its inherent risk, psychological and physical maturity, as well level of competition.

Elite athletes work under an elevated level of physical and psychological stress due to their level of competition, financial interests, and injuries. Therefore, in high-performance athletes of long running, cycling, endurance sports, football, basketball, volleyball, and MMA, PPE should involve a careful cardiological screening with a specialist, including an electrocardiogram at rest, laboratory tests for levels of glycemia, and cholesterol and triglyceride levels. The heart structure and function adapted to physical activity are screened by a Doppler echocardiogram, while an ergometric and cardiopulmonary test should be performed until exhaustion or stopped if the athlete presents adverse clinical signs or symptoms during the exam.

Table 2.4 Laboratory exams commonly performed by Premier League soccer teams before athletes' admission and clinical follow-up

Complete blood count (CBC)
Coagulation tests
Activated partial thromboplastin time
Prothrombin time and international normalized ratio (INR)
Platelet count
Bleeding time
Glucose
Kidney tests
Blood urea nitrogen, creatinine
Liver tests
Alkaline phosphatase (ALP) Alanine aminotransferase (ALT) Aspartate aminotransferase (AST) Creatine phosphokinase (CPK) Lactate dehydrogenase (LDH)
Serology
Hepatitis A, B, and C Chagas disease serology HIV serology
Lipid profile
Total cholesterol, HDL, LDL, and triglycerides
Hormones
Thyroid profile: thyroid-stimulating hormone (TSH), T3, T4 Total and free testosterone Dehydroepiandrosterone Dihydrotestosterone Uric acid
Rheumatoid factor
C-reactive protein Antinuclear factor (ANF)
Urinalysis

Moreover, creatinine, urine, and blood count should be demanded to evaluate the kidney function status. Contagious diseases are a common concern in sports practice, and, therefore, screening is recommended for hepatitis, AIDS, medical history of transfusion, tattoos, and risky social behavior related to drugs, alcohol, smoking, and sex. Table 2.4 presents the most common lab tests performed by the Premier League soccer team in Brazil.

2.8 Radiological Evaluation

Regarding the musculoskeletal evaluation, the athlete's medical history of sports injuries will guide the required radiological exams. In general, X-rays, IRM, and ultrasound are performed to evaluate the joints related to previous injuries or athlete's complaints; however, due to the substantial investment on the elite athletes, additional radiological evaluation can be required. In Brazil, most of the professional soccer teams submit their soccer players routinely to the following radiological exams of the lower limbs:

- Weight-bearing, anteroposterior knee view, lateral view at 30°, and patellar axial view at 30°.
- IRM and spine anteroposterior and lateral weight-bearing view.
- IRM is mandatory for athletes that have been submitted to the surgical procedure of the knee and ankle.

In elite and professional sports, radiological evaluation plays an essential role on the athletes' pre-evaluation before concluding the athletes' team acquisition.

Take-Home Messages

- A sudden cardiac arrest could signal the first clinical presentation of *an underlying cardiovascular disease*.
- The athletes could differ in age, sex, intellectual level, and physical impairment, and, therefore, PPE focus should be tailored to that end.
- Disabled athletes are a particular group of individuals that have functional impairment that could vary according to its cause.
- The three-key point structure of PPE anamnesis is valuable in defining the strategy of physical assessment.
- Some modalities of sports have a close relationship with specific sports injuries (contact sports and spinal cord injuries).
- The oral health exam assesses the athletes' oral hygiene and its maintenance (periodical exams) and could also identify clues of systemic diseases that impact on the athletes' performance.
- PPE should be applied 6–8 weeks before starting sports practice as it allows enough time to rehabilitate, identify, and manage injuries.
- Although PPE has a vital role in promoting a safe enviroment for sports practice, PPE rules and strategies are not standardized among countries.

References

1. Troy KL, Mancuso ME, Butler TA, Johnson JE. Exercise early and often: effects of physical activity and exercise on women's bone health. Int J Environ Res Public Health. 2018;15(5).
2. Warburton DER, Bredin SSD. Health benefits of physical activity: a systematic review of current systematic reviews. Curr Opin Cardiol. 2017;32(5):541–56.
3. Shanahan DF, Franco L, Lin BB, Gaston KJ, Fuller RA. The benefits of natural environments for physical activity. Sports Med. 2016;46(7):989–95.
4. Russo CR. The effects of exercise on bone. Basic concepts and implications for the prevention of fractures. Clin Cases Miner Bone Metab. 2009;6(3):223–8.
5. Bianchi FP, Veneziani V, Cantalice MA, Notarnicola A, Tafuri S. Epidemiology of injuries among Italian footballers: the role of the playing field. Inj Prev 2018;0:1–6.
6. Reissig J, Bitterman A, Lee S. Common foot and ankle injuries: what not to miss and how best to manage. J Am Osteopath Assoc. 2017;117(2):98–104.
7. Black AM, Eliason PH, Patton DA, Emery CA. Epidemiology of facial injuries in sport. Clin Sports Med. 2017;36(2):237–55.
8. Micieli JA, Easterbrook M. Eye and orbital injuries in sports. Clin Sports Med. 2017;36(2):299–314.
9. Scoggin JF 3rd, Brusovanik G, Izuka BH, et al. Assessment of injuries during Brazilian Jiu-Jitsu competition. Orthop J Sports Med. 2014;2:2325967114522184.
10. Cierna D, Lystad RP. Epidemiology of competition injuries in youth karate athletes: a prospective cohort study. Br J Sports Med. 2017;51:1285–8.
11. Cierna D, Barrientos M, Agrasar C, et al. Epidemiology of injuries in juniors participating in top-level karate competition: a prospective cohort study. Br J Sports Med. 2018;52:730–4.
12. Jones NS. Competitive diving principles and injuries. Curr Sports Med Rep. 2017;16(5):351–6.
13. Westermann RW, Giblin M, Vaske A, Grosso K, Wolf BR. Evaluation of men's and women's gymnastics injuries: a 10-year observational study. Sports Health. 2015;7(2):161–5.
14. Durstine JL, Gordon B, Wang Z, Luo X. Chronic disease and the link to physical activity. J Sport Health Sci. 2013;2:3e11.
15. Dinas PC, Koutedakis Y, Flouris AD. Effects of exercise and physical activity on depression. Ir J Med Sci. 2011;180(2):319–25.
16. Sigal RJ, Kenny GP, Wasserman DH, Castaneda-Sceppa C, White RD. Physical activity/exercise and type 2 diabetes: a consensus statement from the American Diabetes Association. Diabetes Care. 2006;29:1433e8.
17. Moore GE. The role of exercise prescription in chronic disease. Br J Sports Med. 2004;38(1):6–7.
18. Musso P, Carballo S. Current practice for the prevention of sudden death in young athletes. Rev Med Suisse. 2018;14(623):1849–53.
19. Dennis M, Elder A, Semsarian C, Orchard J, Brouwer I, Puranik R. A 10-year review of sudden death during sporting activities. Heart Rhythm. 2018;15(10):1477–83.
20. Adamczak DM, Oko-Sarnowska Z. Sudden cardiac death in hypertrophic cardiomyopathy. Cardiol Rev. 2018;26(3):145–51.
21. Wasfy MM, Hutter AM, Weiner RB. Sudden cardiac death in athletes. Methodist Debakey Cardiovasc J. 2016;12(2):76–80.
22. Carre F. Sport's related sudden death. Presse Med. 2014;43(7–8):831–9.
23. Marijon E, Tafflet M, Celermajer DS, Dumas F, Perier MC, Mustafic H, Toussaint JF, et al. Sports-related sudden death in the general population. Circulation. 2011;124(6):672–81.
24. Solberg EE, Gjertsen F, Haugstad E, Kolsrud L. Sudden death in sports among young adults in Norway. Eur J Cardiovasc Prev Rehabil. 2010;17(3):337–41.
25. Corrado D, Basso C, Rizzoli G, Schiavon M, Thiene G. Does sports activity enhance the risk of sudden death in adolescents and young adults? J Am Coll Cardiol. 2003;42(11):1959–63.
26. Lehman PJ, Carl RL. The preparticipation physical evaluation. Pediatr Ann. 2017;46(3):e85–92.
27. Mirabelli MH, Devine MJ, Singh J, Mendoza M. The pre-participation sports evaluation. Am Fam Physician. 2015;92(5):371–6.
28. Sanders B, Blackburn TA, Boucher B. Preparticipation screening—the sports physical therapy perspective. Int J Sports Phys Ther. 2013;8(2):180–93.
29. Galanti G, Stefani L, Liverani L, Gensini GF. Pre-participation assessment in young athletes: a state affair. Intern Emerg Med. 2012;7(5):403–5.
30. Schroeder GD, Vaccaro AR. Cervical spine injuries in the athlete. J Am Acad Orthop Surg. 2016;24(9):e122–33.
31. Al-Shaaibi K, Kariyattil R. Delayed transient post-traumatic quadriplegia. Oman Med J. 2015;30(2):135–7.
32. Aebli N, Wicki AG, Rüegg TB, Petrou N, Eisenlohr H, Krebs J. The Torg-Pavlov ratio for the prediction of acute spinal cord injury after a minor trauma to the cervical spine. Spine J. 2013;13(6):605–12.
33. Nathanson AT, Young JM, Young C. Pre-participation medical evaluation for adventure and wilderness watersports. Wilderness Environ Med. 2015;26(4 Suppl):S55–62.
34. Leischik R, Dworrak B, Foshag P, Strauss M, Spelsberg N, Littwitz H, Horlitz M. Pre-participation and follow-up screening of athletes for endurance sport. J Clin Med Res. 2015;7(6):385–92.
35. Sharma S, Merghani A, Gati S. Cardiac screening of young athletes prior to participation in sports: difficulties in detecting the fatally flawed among the fabulously fit. JAMA Intern Med. 2015;175(1):125–7.
36. Caswell SV, Cortes N, Chabolla M, Ambegaonkar JP, Caswell AM, Brenner JS. State-specific differences in school sports preparticipation physical evaluation policies. Pediatrics. 2015;135(1):26–32.

37. Zychowicz ME. Pre-participation physical evaluations for athletes. Nurse Pract. 2012;37(11):41–5.
38. Baptista CA, Foronda A, Baptista Lde P. Competitive sports for children and adolescents: should an electrocardiogram be required in the pre-participation physical examination? Arq Bras Cardiol. 2009;93(2):188–95.
39. Greydanus DE, Patel DR, Luckstead EF, Pratt HD. Value of sports pre-participation examination in health care for adolescents. Med Sci Monit. 2004;10(9):RA204–14.
40. Mitchell JH, Haskell W, Snell P, Van Camp SP. Task Force 8: classification of sports. J Am Coll Cardiol. 2005;45(8):1364–7.
41. Booth FW, Roberts CK, Laye MJ. Lack of exercise is a major cause of chronic diseases. Compr Physiol. 2012;2(2):1143–211.
42. Ross R, Janssen I. Physical activity, total and regional obesity: dose–response considerations. Med Sci Sports Exerc. 2001;33:S521–7.
43. Viner RT, Harris M, Berning JR, et al. Energy availability and dietary patterns of adult male and female competitive cyclists with lower than expected bone mineral density. Int J Sport Nutr Exerc Metab. 2015;25:594–602.
44. Mountjoy M, Sundgot-Borgen J, Burke L, et al. The IOC consensus statement: beyond the female athlete triad—relative energy deficiency in sport (RED-S). Br J Sports Med. 2014;48:491–7.
45. http://www.who.int/gho/mortality_burden_disease/life_tables/situation_trends_text/en/.
46. Iliffe S, Kendrick D, Morris R, Masud T, Gage H, Skelton D, Dinan S, Bowling A, Griffin M, Haworth D, Swanwick G, Carpenter H, Kumar A, Stevens Z, Gawler S, Barlow C, Cook J, Belcher C. Multicentre cluster randomised trial comparing a community group exercise programme and home-based exercise with usual care for people aged 65 years and over in primary care. Health Technol Assess. 2014;18(49):vii–xxvii, 1–105.
47. Leyk D, Sievert A. The effect of training on performance and health in middle age. Herz. 2012;37:493–8.
48. Lee DC, Pate RR, Lavie CJ, et al. Leisure-time running reduces all-cause and cardiovascular mortality risk. J Am Coll Cardiol. 2014;64:472–81.
49. Wannamethee SG, Shaper AG, Walker M. Changes in physical activity, mortality, and incidence of coronary heart disease in older men. Lancet. 1998;351:1603–8.
50. Leon AS, Connett J, Jacobs DR Jr, et al. Leisure-time physical activity levels and risk of coronary heart disease and death. The multiple risk factor intervention trial. JAMA. 1987;258:2388–95.
51. Corrado D, Basso C, Pavei A, Michieli P, Schiavon M, Thiene G. Trends in sudden cardiovascular death in young competitive athletes after implementation of a preparticipation screening program. JAMA. 2006;296(13):1593–601.
52. Kim JH, Malhotra R, Chiampas G, d'Hemecourt P, Troyanos C, Cianca J, Smith RN, Wang TJ, Roberts WO, Thompson PD, Baggish AL. Race Associated Cardiac Arrest Event Registry (RACER) Study Group. Cardiac arrest during long-distance running races. N Engl J Med. 2012;366(2):130–40.
53. Balady GJ, Chaitman B, Driscoll D, Foster C, Froelicher E, Gordon N, Pate R, Rippe J, Bazzarre T. Recommendations for cardiovascular screening, staffing, and emergency policies at health/fitness facilities. Circulation. 1998;97(22):2283–93.
54. Maron BJ, Araújo CG, Thompson PD, Fletcher GF, de Luna AB, Fleg JL, Pelliccia A, Balady GJ, Furlanello F, Van Camp SP, Elosua R, Chaitman BR, Bazzarre TL, World Heart Federation, International Federation of Sports Medicine, American Heart Association Committee on Exercise, Cardiac Rehabilitation, and Prevention. Recommendations for preparticipation screening and the assessment of cardiovascular disease in masters athletes: an advisory for healthcare professionals from the working groups of the World Heart Federation, the International Federation of Sports Medicine, and the American Heart Association Committee on Exercise, Cardiac Rehabilitation, and Prevention. Circulation. 2001;103(2):327–34.
55. Warburton DER, Jamnik VK, Bredin SSD, Gledhill N. PAR-Q+ research collaboration the physical activity readiness questionnaire (PAR-Q+) and electronic physical activity readiness medical examination (ePARmed-X+). Health Fitness J Can. 2011;4(2):3–23.
56. Borjesson M, Urhausen A, Kouidi E, et al. Cardiovascular evaluation of middle-aged/senior individuals engaged in leisure-time sport activities: position stand from the sections of exercise physiology and sports cardiology of the European Association of Cardiovascular Prevention and Rehabilitation. Eur J Cardiovasc Prev Rehabil. 2011;18:446–58.
57. Anderson TJ, Grégoire J, Hegele RA. 2012 update of the Canadian cardiovascular society guidelines for the diagnosis and treatment of dyslipidemia for the prevention of cardiovascular disease in the adult. Can J Cardiol. 2013;29:151–67. https://doi.org/10.1016/j.cjca.2012.11.032.
58. Morrison BN, McKinney J, Isserow S, Lithwick D, Taunton J, Nazzari H, De Souza AM, Heilbron B, Cater C, MacDonald M, Hives BA, Warburton DER. Assessment of cardiovascular risk and preparticipation screening protocols in masters athletes: the Masters Athlete Screening Study (MASS): a cross-sectional study. BMJ Open Sport Exerc Med. 2018;4(1):e000370. Published online 2018 Aug 9.
59. Blauwet CA, et al. Risk of injuries in paralympic track and field differs by impairment and event discipline: a prospective cohort study at the London 2012 paralympic games. Am J Sports Med. 2016;44(6):1455–62.
60. Bertoli S, Battezzati A, Merati G, et al. Nutritional status and dietary patterns in disabled people. Nutr Metab Cardiovasc Dis. 2006;16(2):100–12.

3 Biomechanics of Musculoskeletal Injuries

Alan Getgood, Yuichi Hoshino, Philip P. Roessler, Ryosuke Kuroroda, and Sérgio Rocha Piedade

3.1 Introduction

Musculoskeletal injury is one of the most common reasons for days off work and reduced activity with approximately 126.6 million patients affected in the United States on an annual basis (Source: American Academy of Orthopaedic Surgeons, 2016). This has a significant impact on work-related productivity, quality of life, and health expenditure in corresponding health-care systems.

While there are many modalities available to treat MSK injury of varying kinds, one of the most effective methods of treatment is injury prevention. In an effort to address these injuries, it is of paramount importance to understand the biomechanical principals behind the injury, to enable an effective treatment or prevention strategy to be implemented.

This chapter will focus on providing an overview of the pertinent biomechanical principals behind MSK injury. An overview of tissue-specific biomechanical properties will also be provided, with these terms and principals then illustrated in sport-specific injury scenarios and mechanisms.

3.2 Biomechanical Principals Relating to MSK Injury

When considering the mechanism of injury, it is important to understand the forces acting on the body and how they may affect the different tissues. The term ***kinematics*** describes the motion of body segments, while ***kinetics*** deals with a description of the forces that produce the specific motions [1].

When considering sports injuries, there are a number of simple units of measurement that must be taken into consideration to determine the magnitude of force acting on individuals. One such key measure is ***mass***. Mass is a measure of ***inertia***, being the property of an object to resist the changes in motion that affect it. A running back in American football, for example, must

A. Getgood (✉)
Fowler Kennedy Sports Medicine Clinic/Department of Surgery, Western University, London, ON, Canada
e-mail: alan.getgood@uwo.ca

Y. Hoshino
Department of Orthopaedic Surgery, Jichi Medical University, Tochigi, Japan

P. P. Roessler
Fowler Kennedy Sports Medicine Clinic, Western University, London, ON, Canada
e-mail: proessle@uwo.ca

R. Kuroroda
Department of Orthopaedic Surgery, Kobe University Graduate School of Medicine, Kobe, Japan
e-mail: kurodar@med.kobe-u.ac.jp

S. R. Piedade
Department of Orthopedics and Traumatology, State University of Campinas—UNICAMP, Exercise and Sports Medicine, Campinas, SP, Brazil
e-mail: piedade@fcm.unicamp.br

S. Rocha Piedade et al. (eds.), *The Sports Medicine Physician*,
https://doi.org/10.1007/978-3-030-10433-7_3

overcome inertia to start running; but his mass will also make it more challenging for him to be stopped. ***Weight***, on the other hand, is the force of gravity acting on an object.

In dynamic situations such as sports, ***Newton's laws of motion*** is important to understand, when considering how forces are acting on objects and, of course, participants or subjects in a game [2].

- ***Newton's first law*** states that a body continues in a state of rest, or of uniform motion in a straight line, unless it is compelled to change that state by forces impressed upon in.
- ***Newton's second law*** tells us that the change in motion of an object is proportional to the force impressed and is made in the direction of the straight line in which it is impressed. This law essentially describes acceleration, which is derived from length, time, and mass.
- ***Newton's third law*** of motion states that to every action, there is an equal and opposite reaction. This means that when the running back collides with the linebacker, the force of impact will be felt similarly on both players.

Stress and strain: ***Stress*** is defined as the force applied to an object divided by the cross-sectional area of the surface onto which the force is applied. There are three principal stresses that act on a body [2]:

1. ***Tension***—Tensile stress is that which occurs as a result of force that pulls apart molecules that bond the structure together. A lateral blow to the knee in soccer will result in tensile stress being applied to the medial collateral ligament (MCL), often resulting in a tear of that structure.
2. ***Compression***—Compressive stress is the axial stress that occurs when a load pushes or squashes molecules together. Take the example of the lateral blow to the knee. Tension is applied to the medial side, but a compressive stress may be experienced in the lateral tibiofemoral compartment that may result in a bone bruise or osteochondral injury.
3. ***Shear***—While tension and compression act in the axial plane, shear stress occurs as a result of forces acting perpendicular to this plane. Again, with the example of the above knee injury, shear stress observed in the lateral compartment may result in abnormal lateral meniscal loading and can result in a meniscal tear.

The majority of sports injuries do not occur as a result of simple uniaxial forces applied to the body. There are often combined loads such as the simultaneous compression and tension that is applied to a long bone when landing a ski jump. In the event of a ski catching an edge, the leg may have a torsional load applied to it; that is a load that acts about the long axis of the bone in rotation, due to the large lever arm and subsequent rotational moment applied by the ski. This may result in a spiral fracture of the tibia or femur [3].

When external forces are applied to a body, deformations occur. ***Strain*** is the quantification of the deformation of a material. When tensile or compressive forces are applied to an object, ***linear strain*** occurs due to the change in the object's length. This can be described in terms of the percentage of length change in relation to its original length [2].

Staying with the example of the MCL injury, a tensile force is applied to the medial aspect of the knee, secondary to the direct lateral blow. The tensile force exerts a linear stress to the MCL which in turn will cause a change in length of the tissue—also known as strain. The close relationship between stress and strain explains the behavior of a material or, in this instance, the MCL, under load.

The relationship of stress and strain can be illustrated via the ***stress-strain curve*** (Fig. 3.1). In the initial linear portion, there is a direct correlation between stress and strain. This is known as ***elastic behavior***, where the material returns to its original dimensions following removal of the applied load. The steeper the line, the stiffer the material, with the slope of the stress-strain curve representing the ***elastic (Young's) modulus*** of the material [2].

With continued applied load, the relationship will eventually not be directly proportional or linear; at this point it reaches the material ***yield***

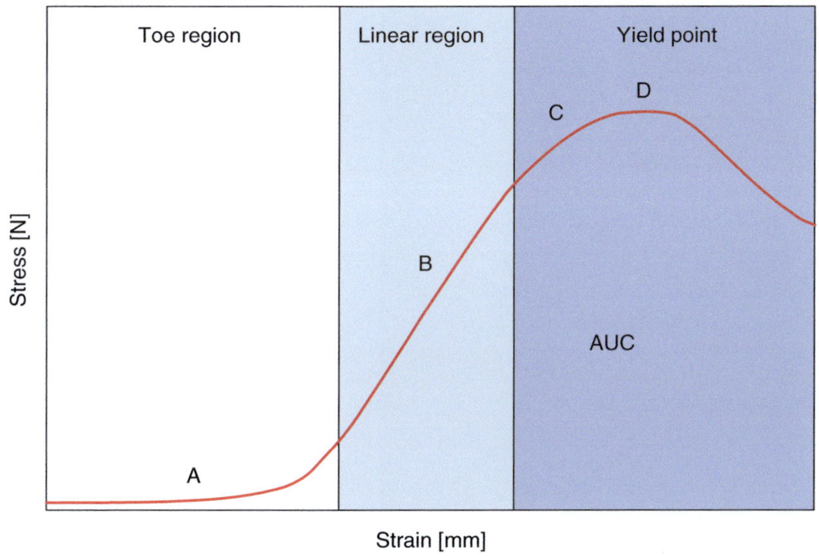

Fig. 3.1 The sinusoidal curve of the biomechanical behavior of the ligament submitted to the uniaxial tensile load. In the segment A of the diagram (toe region), lower force/stress followed by higher strain is observed, reflecting the crimp and nonuniform pattern of the fibers as they elongate. In B (linear region), a progressive stretching of fibers characterized by linear and elastic behavior is verified. The point C is the transition between the elastic limit and plastic region (yield point) and the maximum strength of the material, while the tissue damage (irreversible or permanent deformation) is present in D. The involved energy of rupture in the process is calculated by the area under the curve (AUC)

point and enters the ***plastic region***. In this region, the material no longer returns to its original dimensions and displays ***plastic deformation***. Once the material starts to continue to display increased strain with no further stress applied, it reaches its ***ultimate strength***, with the ***failure strength*** encountered on discontinuity or breakage of the material. For the MCL, a grade II MCL strain will result in a degree of plastic deformation and discontinuity of some of its fibers, with some remaining intact. Therefore, a complete MCL injury may not be observed [4, 5].

The degree of injury that is observed with an applied load is related to the ***viscoelastic behavior*** of musculoskeletal tissues. These material properties, and the way forces are applied to the material, will determine the nature and the severity of the injury [4].

Viscoelasticity: Musculoskeletal tissues, such as the bone, muscle, tendon, and ligament, are known as viscoelastic materials, and their biomechanical behavior is time-dependent, which results from a complex interaction between molecules of proteoglycans, water, collagen, and other components [1, 6]. Abrahams states that viscoelastic tissues work as a combined elastic solid and viscous fluid [7]. The elastic component presents a proportional deformation to the applied force, while the response of the viscous component is time-dependent. In certain conditions, one of these mechanical responses becomes more prevalent than the other, depending on the physical demand. Otherwise, their mechanical behavior has geometrical and structure specificity, as their anatomical site qualifies them mechanically.

Different viscoelastic materials behave differently depending on how quickly load is applied to them. Cortical bone, for example, is stronger and stiffer if a load is applied quickly, whereas it is weaker if applied slowly. This phenomenon of ***strain rate*** can help explain why avulsion fractures occur (Fig. 3.2). In the scenario of an eversion ankle injury, load applied quickly across the joint will more likely result in a deltoid ligament tear, whereas, if it is applied slowly, an avulsion of the tip of the medial malleolus may occur.

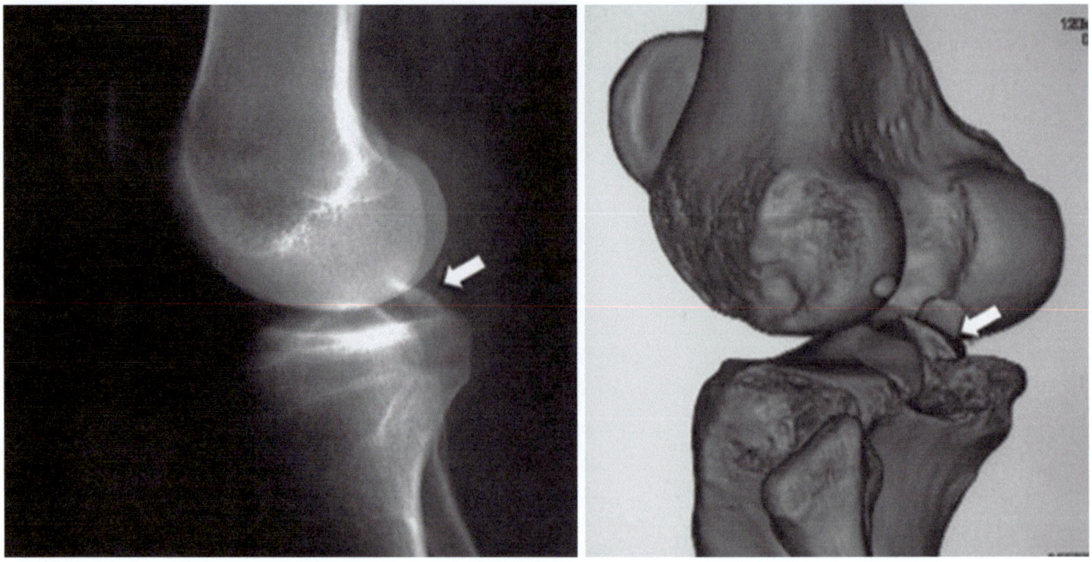

Fig. 3.2 PCL tibial avulsion fracture of the left knee in a 22-year-old BMX athlete

Understanding these principles of how load is applied to the body during sport may help understand the mechanism of injury, the injury pattern, and the methods to prevent injury. We will now look at specific tissues and how they have adapted to respond to these external loads.

3.3 Biomechanical Principals of Specific MSK Tissues

Tendons and ligaments: Tendons and ligaments are made up of bands of collagen fibers organized in parallel along their long axis. Both are extremely specialized structures, specifically adapted to bear tensile forces across joints. However, the variations of the ultrastructure pattern of ligament fibers (wavy pattern, called crimping) and their orientation allow them to resist higher levels of strain compared to tendons [4].

When applying tension to the ligament, elongation takes place, and more ligament fibers are recruited. The fibers become gradually uncrimped and oriented in a parallel fashion toward the applied force [1, 8]. As mechanical stress continues, the ligament gradually stiffens until it reaches its ultimate strength and fails. Figure 3.1 illustrates the nonlinear mechanical response (sinusoidal curve), which is a characteristic of the ligament when stressed at different levels of strain.

Bone: Bones are harder and stronger than cartilage, because their structure combines hard mineral (hydroxyapatite carbonate) and flexible collagen, without being brittle. Bones are ductile structures, which are able to adapt their mechanical response according to the direction of the applied force (***anisotropy***). A remarkable example is that bones can resist 30% more load applied through their longitudinal axis compared to their transversal axis (15 MPa and 12 MPa, respectively). Moreover, they have the ability of remodeling and will adapt their structural density to the mechanical environment and are highly specialized in supporting load, mainly in compression. In the elastic phase, the bone can deform up to 0.75%, and, with the deformation of 2–4%, a fracture often occurs. During the plastic deformation phase, the bone can absorb six times more energy before a fracture during the elastic period [9, 10].

During the human biological development, the biomechanical properties of the bone differ according to age. Compared to the immature bone of children, the adult bone is stiffer (more mineralized) and more brittle, while in children it is weaker (less mineralized) and ductile, which is a point to consider when developing a regimen of sports training for children [10].

In sports, athletes perform high-demand physical activities at different levels of speed in short periods, exposing them to direct and indirect loads. Take the example again of the running back colliding with the linebacker. Both players have adapted their bodies to be able to withstand with levels of external load. In some circumstances, the energy of the associated trauma overpowers the bones' ability to withstand the applied load, depending on its direction of application, and thus a fracture may occur.

Frequently, low-energy traumas are linear and do not promote large displacements, while higher-energy traumas will promote significant fracture comminution and dislocation and, subsequently, a substantial associated soft tissue damage. Therefore, the magnitude, duration, direction, and rate of the applying load play a critical role in defining the fracture pattern [9, 10].

A fracture occurs in the weakest plane of the bone, where there is a maximum of shear and tensile stress. According to the loading mode, different configurations of fractures could be produced; for example, a torsional load causes a spiral fracture, while compressive load leads to oblique fractures and combinations of bending and compressive forces result in transverse fractures or a so-called "butterfly" fragment [8] (Fig. 3.3).

Stress fractures: In sport, stress fractures can result from abnormal loads to the bone and can also occur due to muscle fatigue [11]. They frequently occur in individuals who are not adequately prepared for vigorous physical exercises and also in high-performance athletes of sports in which repetitive impact actions are performed, such as volleyball, athletics, and distance running. Dancers may also be subject to this type of injury. From a biomechanical point of view, it can be concluded that in these clinical situations, it is observed that constant load or strain, close to the physiological limit of tissue, could cause plastic deformation and consequently fracture. Besides that, osteoporosis (elderly athletes), preexisting metabolic bone disease (hyperparathyroidism, adrenal disorders), bone neoplasms, drug and alcohol use, vitamin D deficiency, and steroids could predispose to stress fracture (Fig. 3.4).

Muscle: Muscle injuries represent one of the most common clinical problems that cause suspension of sports activity for athletes. Skeletal muscle is the largest tissue in the body, accounting for 40–45% of body weight. Indirect (intrinsic) muscle injuries, also called stretching, and direct injury (extrinsic) are quite common in sports and recreational activities and are produced by direct and indirect trauma. Delayed-onset muscle soreness (DOMS) pain is another muscle problem that occurs with extreme exertion.

It is the mechanism of traumatic injury of the muscle where the ***direct force*** can produce

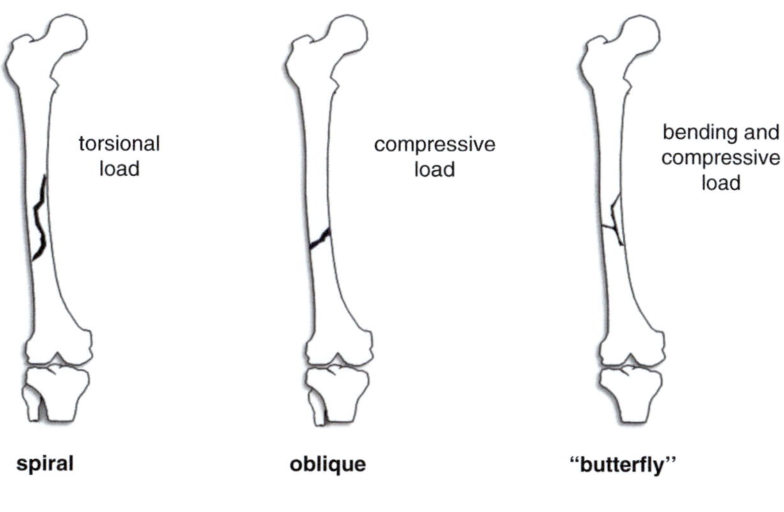

Fig. 3.3 Examples of fracture patterns according to the applied load

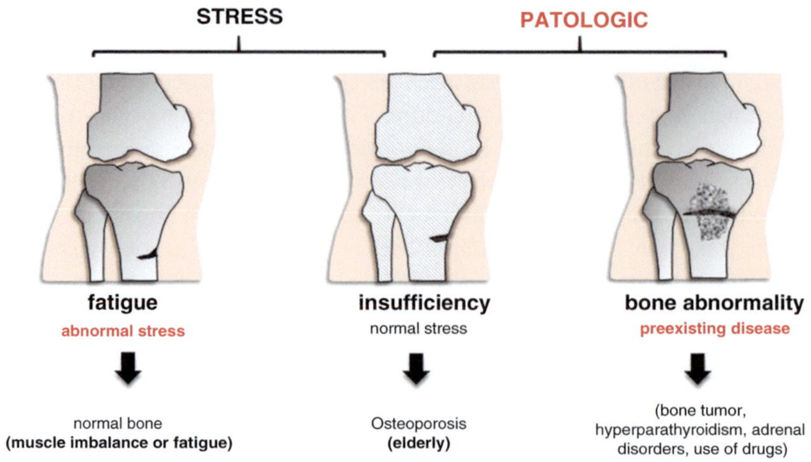

Fig. 3.4 Mechanism of stress fracture according to the quality of bone and mechanical stress (Source: adapted from Greenspan A, editor. Orthopedic Imaging: A Practical Approach. 4th ed. Philadelphia (PA): Lippincott Williams & Wilkins, c2004. Chapter 4, Radiologic Evaluation of Trauma, Figure 4.27, p. 57)

superficial injury, called muscular contusion (bruise), or deeply, characterizing more extensive muscular injury. Bleeding within the muscle can create increased pressure, cell necrosis, and inflammation. Moreover, heterotopic ossification may occur, which can be a major issue for athlete, eventually also leading to disability to continue sporting activity.

Muscle **activation** produces force within the muscle. During a concentric contraction, the resistance load is lower than the force generated by the muscle, and hence it shortens.

On the other hand, if the resistive force is higher than the force generated by the muscle, the muscle is elongated, and an eccentric contraction takes place. This type of muscle contraction is particularly vital in absorbing energy and protecting the joints, as in the case of the landing of the heel, where the quadriceps muscle contracts, protecting the knee. Loss of eccentric quadriceps strength in the postoperative phase of anterior cruciate ligament (ACL) reconstruction can result in a stiff knee landing with an inability to absorb load, predisposing athletes to a higher risk of ACL reinjury. ***Indirect muscle injury*** results from eccentric muscle contraction, which presents a clinical situation where the physiological limit of muscle elongation is exceeded and muscle fiber rupture occurs. These mechanisms usually are loads or velocity dependent [12].

3.4 Sports-Specific Injury Mechanisms

Mechanical factors that cause a musculoskeletal injury can be divided into both extrinsic (from factors outside the body) and intrinsic (from factors within the body) [13]. The primary extrinsic factor is physical contacts either between athletes or with other objects including the ground, shoes, or orthotic equipment. These additional extrinsic factors can aggravate mechanical stresses on musculoskeletal structures. Intrinsic factors include muscle strength and imbalance, body size, flexibility, anatomic alignment, and morphology.

In order to estimate the relative risk of an injury to the athlete, the frequency and magnitude of the physical contacts in each sport should be recognized. Categorization of sports established by the American Academy of Pediatrics Council on Sports Medicine and Fitness (Table 3.1) is most commonly used and quite useful for sports physicians [14]. Contact sports (e.g., soccer and basketball) include those where athletes routinely make contact with each other or with static objects, and some of them are classified as collision sports where the players' hits are made with great force. Limited-contact sports (e.g., baseball and handball) involve infrequent contact between athletes or between athletes and static objects. Non-contact sports (e.g., golf and swimming) are those where physical contact is

Table 3.1 Sports classification based on contact (Proposed by the American Academy of Pediatrics Council on Sports Medicine and Fitness)

Contact	Limited contact	Non-contact
Basketball	Adventure racing	Badminton
Cheerleading	Baseball	Bodybuilding
Diving	Bicycling	Bowling
Extreme sports	Canoeing or kayaking (white water)	Canoeing or kayaking (flat water)
Field hockey	Fencing	Crew or rowing
Gymnastics	Field events	Curling
Martial arts—sparring	High jump	Dance
Judo	Pole vault	Field events
Jujitsu	Floor hockey	Discus
Karate	Flag or touch football	Javelin
Kung-Fu	Handball	Slot-put
Taekwondo	Horseback riding	Golf
Rodeo	Martial arts—forms	Orienteering
Skiing, downhill	Racquetball	Power lifting
Ski jumping	Skating	Race walking
Snowboarding	Ice	Riflery
Soccer	In-line	Rope jumping
Team handball	Roller	Running
Ultimate Frisbee	Skiing	Sailing
Water polo	Cross-country	Scuba diving
Wrestling	Water	Swimming
Collision sports	Skateboarding	Table tennis
American football	Softball	Tennis
Boxing	Squash	Track
Ice hockey	Volleyball	
Lacrosse	Weight lifting	
Roller derby	Windsurfing or surfing	
Rugby football		

rare and mostly unexpected. Typical injuries and their mechanisms in each category of sports are illustrated in this section.

Collision sports: Physical contact with great force, or simply collision, is the main characteristic of collision sports and the primary reason for a high prevalence of musculoskeletal injuries. In collisions, energy is transferred from one body to another. In blocking and tackling, for example, transfer of energy between bodies can result in injury when the energy transferred exceeds the tolerance of the involved tissues (e.g., bones, tendons, ligaments). It is reported that American football has the highest injury rates at both the high school [15] and collegiate [16] levels. Thus, collision sports have undoubtedly the highest risk of injuries among all categories.

Acute traumatic fracture by applying a single high-magnitude load to the bone is one of the typical injuries. Such a fracture happens when the force exceeds over the bone's ability to resist it. Traumatic fractures are often seen in player-to-player contact, and the highest rate of fractures was reported as being more than 10% in American football according to the epidemiological study of high school athletes [17].

Contusion is also common in collision and contact sports, since it occurs when a direct blow or repeated blows from other players or a blunt object strike part of the body, crushing underlying muscle fibers and connective tissue. It consists of 20-30% of all the injuries in rugby players [18], whereas basketball, a contact sport, has fewer contusions, e.g., 15.3% on the professional league level [19]. However, most of these injuries are minor and heal quickly, without taking the athlete away from competition. But, once deep tissue is damaged, it may keep the athlete out of sports for months.

Contact sports: Musculoskeletal injuries in contact sports commonly occur by direct contact with another player. In basketball, player-to-player contact accounted for 79.8% of contact injuries and 34.9% of all injuries [20]. The most common injury is lateral ankle sprain, accounting for 13.2% of all injuries on the professional league level [19]. Lateral ankle sprains occur by landing on another player's foot and/or out of balance due to contact with other players, while most of the player's attention is paid to the ball and the rim above his/her head. Forceful ankle plantar flexion and inversion may damage the lateral ligaments of the ankle. Considering that the greatest number of injuries occurred within the three-point line [20], the amount of playing time spent is the key (greater exposure), and the increased player-to-player contact due to higher player concentration could be a major reason for high prevalence of lateral ankle sprains in basketball. Much attention has focused on prevention of ankle inversion injuries in basketball. The design of the shoes has been adapted subsequently to protect the ankle, and many players also tape their ankles or additionally wear braces. However, the persisting high frequency of ankle injuries suggests that more clinical and biomechanical research is necessary to improve protective shoe and ankle equipment.

Limited contact sports: Although the frequency and magnitude of contacts are fewer and smaller in limited contact sports compared to collision or contact sports, injuries in limited contact sports still mainly result from direct physical contact.

Fractures of the hand are quite characteristic of baseball and softball and are frequent causes for surgery [17] and subsequent disqualification from the game [21]. Rare but quite strong force is applied when the high-speed ball hits the player's hand at the time of batting or catching. Hand fractures can significantly limit sport participation [22], since most of the players have to utilize their hands independent of the sport practiced.

Non-contact sports: Musculoskeletal injuries in non-contact sports are mostly caused by repetitive or extreme force that is generated by athletes' own exertion.

Muscle strain is a quite common injury which refers to damage of a musculotendinous unit (or muscle-tendon complex). Acute muscular strain can result from overstretching an inactive muscle or dynamically overloading an active muscle either in concentric (active shortening) or eccentric (active lengthening) action. The leg or groin muscles, such as quadriceps and hamstring muscles, are most frequently affected. Hamstring muscle strain is more often seen in track athletes than in any other sports according to the report of NCAA athletes [23].

Fractures typically occur by applying a single great external force directly to the bone. But bones may also fracture in response to repeated low-magnitude loads, which results in what has been described as a stress fracture previously [11]. The magnitude of forces is less than the maximum tolerated by the bone, but applied repetitively, causing a disruption in the bone. The incidence of stress fractures in the general athletic population is approximately 1%; however, the incidence may be as high as 15% in certain populations at risk, such as runners [24]. Also, track and field athletes have a higher incidence of stress fractures than participants of contact sports, such as football, soccer, or basketball [25]. Furthermore, stress fractures are generally more difficult to be diagnosed and treated than traumatic fractures.

The categorization of sports indicates the comparative likelihood that participation in different sports will result in acute traumatic injuries from blows to the body. On the other hand, overuse injuries are also typical in athletes and mostly not related to contact or collision but to repetitive microtraumas. Furthermore, overuse injuries generally are not acute. Therefore, the applied categorization might be insufficient to adequately attribute relative risks of such overuse injuries. Further assessment of sports participation in terms of duration and intensity should be considered here.

Additionally, the prevalence of the injury can be differing among field positions, especially in team sports. For example, shoulder injury rates are much higher in flanker and five-eighths than in halfbacks in rugby [26]. Besides the field position, physicians might also consider the level of competition, the maturity of the competitors, the relative physical size, and the availability of effective protective equipment for further biomechanical assessment of musculoskeletal injury.

In summary, musculoskeletal injuries occur as a result of forces that are applied to the body. Understanding these forces and how they interact with individual MSK tissues is extremely important when treating sports injuries. Injury mechanisms can be specific to individual sports, and the sports categorization based on the contact level is useful to estimate the relative risk of musculoskeletal injuries.

References

1. Fung Y-C. The meaning of constitutive equation. In: Fung Y-C, editor. Biomechanics. New York City: Springer; 1993. p. 23–65.
2. McGinnis PM. Biomechanics of sport and exercise. 3rd ed. Champaign: Human Kinetics; 2013.
3. Bartlett R, Bussey M. Sports biomechanics. 2nd ed. London: Routledge Taylor & Francis; 2012.
4. Woo SL. Mechanical properties of tendons and ligaments. I. Quasi-static and nonlinear viscoelastic properties. Biorheology. 1982;19:385–96.

5. Woo SL, Gomez MA, Woo YK, Akeson WH. Mechanical properties of tendons and ligaments. II. The relationships of immobilization and exercise on tissue remodeling. Biorheology. 1982;19:397–408.
6. Cabaud HE. Biomechanics of the anterior cruciate ligament. Clin Orthop Relat Res. 1983;172:26–31.
7. Abrahams M. Mechanical behaviour of tendon in vitro. A preliminary report. Med Biol Eng. 1967;5:433–43.
8. Cordey J. Introduction: basic concepts and definitions in mechanics. Injury. 2000;31(Suppl 2):S-B1–13.
9. Harkess JW, Ramsey WC, Harkess JW. Principles of fractures and dislocation. In: Rockwood CA, Green DP, Heckaman JD, Bucholz RW, editors. Rockwood and Greens's fractures in adults. Philadelphia: Lippincott Williams & Wilkins; 1996. p. 3–120.
10. Wu Z, Ovaert TC, Niebur GL. Viscoelastic properties of human cortical bone tissue depend on gender and elastic modulus. J Orthop Res. 2012;30:693–9.
11. Bolin D, Kemper A, Brolinson PG. Current concepts in the evaluation and management of stress fractures. Curr Sports Med Rep. 2005;4:295–300.
12. Rehorn MR, Schroer AK, Blemker SS. The passive properties of muscle fibers are velocity dependent. J Biomech. 2014;47:687–93.
13. Taimela S, Kujala UM, Osterman K. Intrinsic risk factors and athletic injuries. Sports Med. 1990;9:205–15.
14. Rice SG. American Academy of Pediatrics Council on Sports Medicine and Fitness. Medical conditions affecting sports participation. Pediatrics. 2008;121:841–8.
15. Rechel JA, Yard EE, Comstock RD. An epidemiologic comparison of high school sports injuries sustained in practice and competition. J Athl Train. 2008;43:197–204.
16. Yang J, Tibbetts AS, Covassin T, Cheng G, Nayar S, Heiden E. Epidemiology of overuse and acute injuries among competitive collegiate athletes. J Athl Train. 2012;47:198–204.
17. Swenson DM, Yard EE, Collins CL, Fields SK, Comstock RD. Epidemiology of US high school sports-related fractures, 2005-2009. Clin J Sport Med. 2010;20:293–9.
18. Hoskins W, Pollard H, Hough K, Tully C. Injury in rugby league. J Sci Med Sport. 2006;9:46–56.
19. Drakos MC, Domb B, Starkey C, Callahan L, Allen AA. Injury in the national basketball association: a 17-year overview. Sports Health. 2010;2:284–90.
20. Meeuwisse WH, Sellmer R, Hagel BE. Rates and risks of injury during intercollegiate basketball. Am J Sports Med. 2003;31:379–85.
21. Tirabassi J, Brou L, Khodaee M, Lefort R, Fields SK, Comstock RD. Epidemiology of high school sports-related injuries resulting in medical disqualification: 2005-2006 through 2013-2014 academic years. Am J Sports Med. 2016;44:2925–32.
22. Messina DF, Farney WC, DeLee JC. The incidence of injury in Texas high school basketball. A prospective study among male and female athletes. Am J Sports Med. 1999;27:294–9.
23. Dalton SL, Kerr ZY, Dompier TP. Epidemiology of hamstring strains in 25 NCAA sports in the 2009-2010 to 2013-2014 academic years. Am J Sports Med. 2015;43:2671–9.
24. Greaser MC. Foot and ankle stress fractures in athletes. Orthop Clin North Am. 2016;47:809–22.
25. Hame SL, LaFemina JM, McAllister DR, Schaadt GW, Dorey FJ. Fractures in the collegiate athlete. Am J Sports Med. 2004;32:446–51.
26. Sundaram A, Bokor DJ, Davidson AS. Rugby Union on-field position and its relationship to shoulder injury leading to anterior reconstruction for instability. J Sci Med Sport. 2011;14:111–4.

4 Physiological Demands in Sports Practice

Ana Sousa, João Ribeiro, and Pedro Figueiredo

4.1 Energy Transfer During Exercise

Humans obtain energy either by consuming plants or by eating animals that feed on plants. The macronutrients—carbohydrates, fats, and proteins—from these ingested foods are ultimately broken down to release the stored energy. This energy can be used in different processes, such as building muscle mass, repairing muscle damage, active transport of many substances across cell membranes (e.g., sodium and potassium), and, for the epitome of mechanical energy, muscle action and, consequently, human movement. However, for all these processes to occur, the chemical energy released must be stored in the form of adenosine triphosphate (ATP). This molecule forms from a molecule of adenine and ribose (called adenosine) linked to three phosphates, each consisting of phosphorus and oxygen atoms. The bonds that link the two phosphates represent high-energy bonds because they release considerable useful energy (approximately 7.3 Kcal per molecule of ATP). In the specific case of muscle contraction, the myosin head contains a binding site for the molecule of ATP. The adenosine triphosphatase (ATPase), located here, splits the ATP to yield adenosine diphosphate (ADP), inorganic phosphate (Pi), and, mostly important, energy. Therefore, by releasing energy when broken down, ATP is the chemical energy source of the mechanical muscle contraction process.

However, cells can store only limited amounts of ATP (80-100 g at any time under normal resting conditions), which implies that they must be constantly generating new ATP to provide energy for all cellular ATP-dependent mechanisms, including muscle contraction. In this way, cells can generate ATP throughout three metabolic pathways—ATP-CP, glycolytic, and oxidative systems—as might expected, depending on exercise intensity. Energy transfer can increase about fourfold in the transition from rest to light exercise but can be higher than 100-fold within the supramaximal exercise. From the three energy metabolic pathways, the first two can be

A. Sousa (✉)
Research Centre for Sports, Exercise and Human Development, CIDESD, Vila Real, Portugal

University Institute of Maia, ISMAI, Maia, Portugal

J. Ribeiro
Research Centre for Sports, Exercise and Human Development, CIDESD, Vila Real, Portugal

University Institute of Maia, ISMAI, Maia, Portugal

Department of Performance Optimization, Sporting Clube de Braga, SAD, Braga, Portugal

P. Figueiredo
Research Centre for Sports, Exercise and Human Development, CIDESD, Vila Real, Portugal

University Institute of Maia, ISMAI, Maia, Portugal

Portugal Football School, Portuguese Football Federation, Oeiras, Portugal

S. Rocha Piedade et al. (eds.), *The Sports Medicine Physician*,
https://doi.org/10.1007/978-3-030-10433-7_4

developed in the absence of oxygen, and therefore, and jointly termed anaerobic metabolism. The last system, because it requires the presence of oxygen, is generally termed aerobic metabolism, which comprises both carbohydrates and fat oxidation.

4.1.1 Immediate Energy: ATP-PCr System

To overcome the ATP storage's limitation, cells contain another high-energy phosphate compound—phosphocreatine (PCr, sometimes called creatine phosphate). PCr share a similar characteristic to ATP, as a large amount of free energy is released. Some of this energy for ATP resynthesis comes directly from the anaerobic splitting of PCr into Pi and creatine (catalyzed by the enzyme creatine kinase—ck). This pathway comprises simply the donation of one molecule of Pi to ADP to form ATP (cf. Fig. 4.1).

In contrast to ATP, the energy released from the breakdown of PCr is not directly used for cellular work, and therefore, is essentially used to maintain a constant regeneration of ATP. Cells store approximately four to six times more PCr than ATP, and approximately 90% of PCr's hydrolysis occurs in the cytosol. The main regulating factors of this system are the concentrations of ADP, Pi, and ATP. Therefore, following the principle of negative feedback, when concentrations of ADP and Pi are elevated, creatine kinase activity is enhanced to synthesized ATP and vice versa. Another possibility to simply produce ATP comes from the adenylate kinase reaction, in which two ADP molecules are used to produce one molecule of ATP and AMP.

During the first seconds of supramaximal exercise (e.g., sprinting, c.f. Fig. 4.2), within the muscular cell, the need for higher concentrations of ATP is extremely high, and this is maintained, at a relatively constant level, mainly due to PCr breakdown. Consequently, PCr concentration declines as it is used to resynthesize ATP. However, beyond ~14 s of exercise, both ATP and PCr concentrations are insufficient to fulfill the energy requirements for muscle contraction, and therefore, muscles must rely on other energy processes.

4.1.2 Short-Term Energy: Glycolytic System

After the immediate source of energy for muscle contraction (ATP and PCr) have reached exhaustion, the next process, more complex than the ATP-PCr system, begins to take action within the cytosol. This is concerned with the breakdown of carbohydrate in the form of glucose or glycogen. In a series of 10-12 enzymatic reactions, the former is broken down to produce two molecules of pyruvate (glycolysis) and four molecules of ATP, but the initial process is ATP-dependent (two molecules), which means that the final balance is two molecules of ATP. In contrast, glycogen's breaking down (glycogenolysis) to pyruvate only

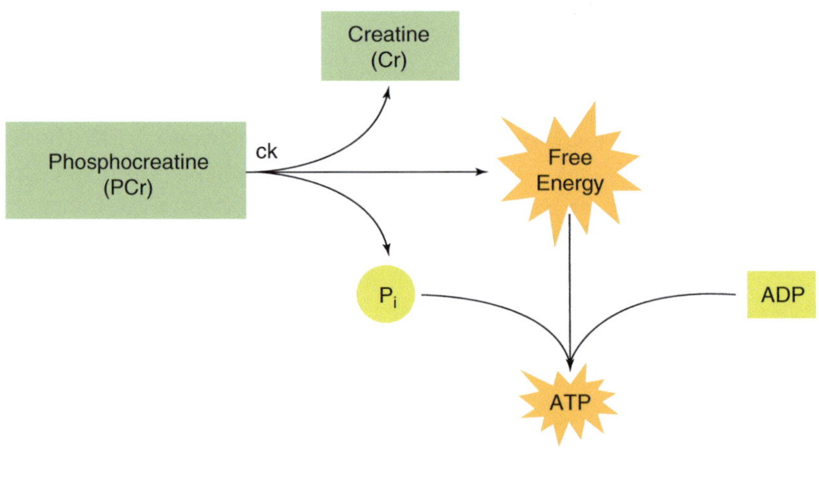

Fig. 4.1 In the ATP-PCr system, the energy liberated from the hydrolysis of phosphocreatine (PCr) is used to synthesized adenosine triphosphate (ATP) via the binding of inorganic phosphate (Pi) to adenosine phosphate (ADP)

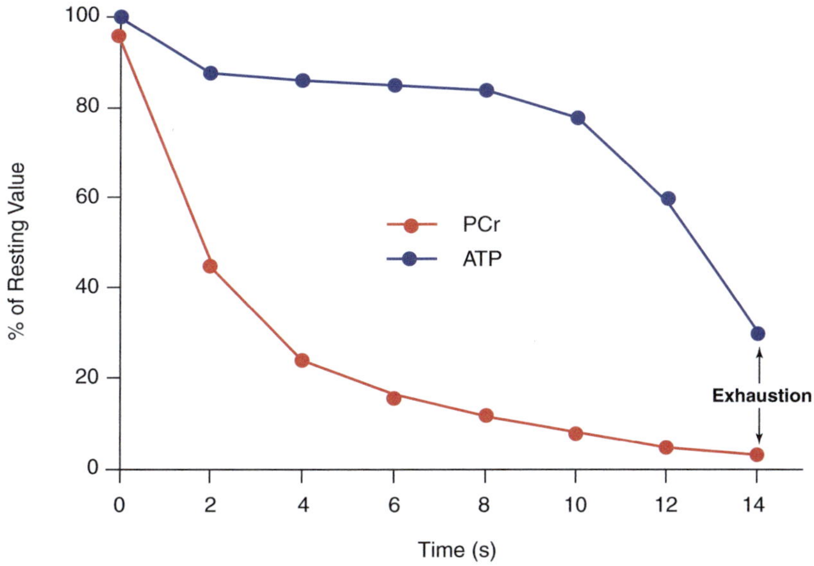

Fig. 4.2 The energy released from the breakdown of phosphocreatine (PCr) is used to synthesize ATP during 14 s of supramaximal exercise (sprinting), preventing the ATP level from decreasing in the first 10 s of exercise. However, at exhaustion (~14 s) both ATP and PCr levels are low, and if the exercise goes beyond, energy for continual ATP resynthesis must be originate from less-rapid catabolism of the stored macronutrients

consumes one ATP molecule, and therefore, the final balance is more attractive (three ATP). Ultimately, pyruvic acid is then converted to lactic acid. However, in both cases, the amount of energy produced is relatively small, and the available capacity of this system is ~1 min (cf. Fig. 4.3a). Despite the amount of ATP produced being scarce, the combined actions of both ATP-PCr and glycolytic systems allow the muscles to generate force when oxygen availability is low. However, if sufficient oxygen is available to the muscle cell during glycolysis, the oxidative system begins to assume the preponderance in energy production.

4.1.3 Long-Term Energy: Oxidative System

As stated above, the oxidative system begins to gain preponderance when intense exercise continues beyond the first minute of exercise. However, more than 2 h of intense exercise can deplete the glycogen stores, so, for events lasting longer than this, fats (lipids) are the likeliest source of energy. Regardless of the energy source used, oxidation starts in the mitochondria once acetyl coenzyme-A (acetyl Co-A) is formed, initiating a complex series of chemical reactions that will allow its complete oxidation throughout the Krebs cycle (also known as a citric acid cycle or tricyclic acid cycle; cf. Fig. 4.3b). Like stated for the ATP-PCr energetic pathway, the Krebs cycle is regulated by negative feedback, and additionally, because glycolytic pathway feeds it, both are upregulated by ADP and Pi and downregulated by ATP.

The Krebs cycle process will end up with the production of CO_2 and two molecules of ATP. Moreover, the several hydrogen ions here released, together with the hydrogen ions released in the previous chemical reactions, cannot remain in the system. Otherwise, the cell milieu would become too acidic. Therefore, these ions combined with two coenzymes, in its reduced form (nicotinamide adenine dinucleotide: NADH, and flavin adenine dinucleotide: $FADH_2$), will carry the hydrogen atoms (electrons—e^-) to the electron transport chain into the inner mitochondrial membrane (cf. Fig. 4.3c). This e^- will pass from complex to complex along this chain (with the final acceptor being O_2, forming consequently H_2O), and the energy that is released will be used to pump the hydrogen ions from the matrix to the mitochondrial outer membrane. Following the concentration gradient, these hydrogen ions move back across the membrane through an enzyme called ATP synthase, and, transferring energy to ADP, ATP is formed. The amount of ATP

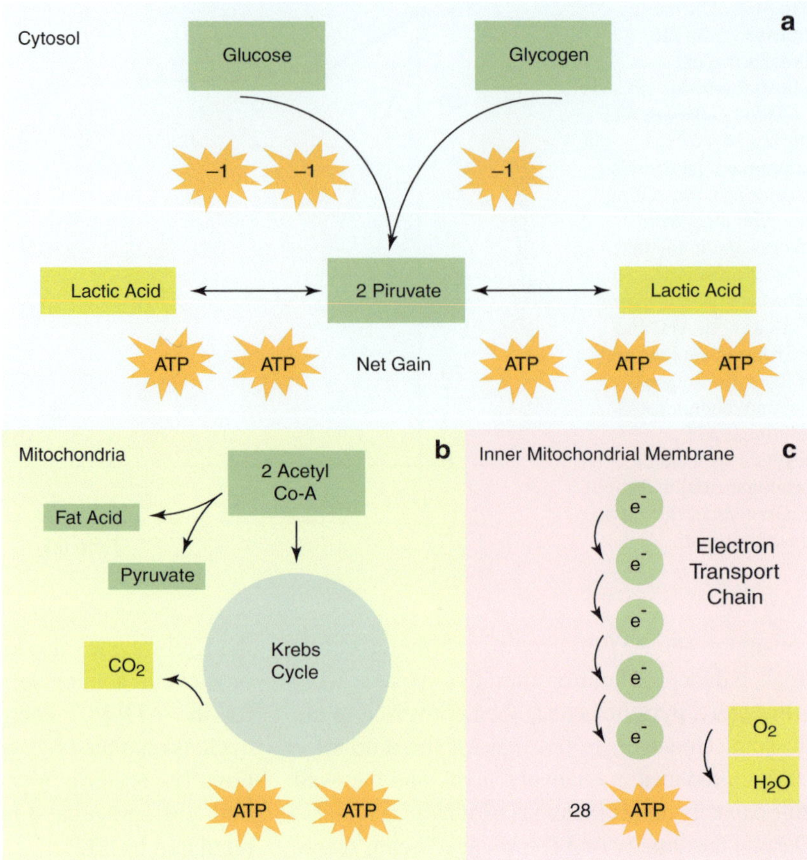

Fig. 4.3 The production of ATP starts in glycolysis (breakdown of glucose) or glycogenolysis with the production of pyruvate (**a**), which is further catalyzed into acetyl coenzyme A (which may also result from fat acid) to enter the Krebs cycle (**b**). The hydrogen ions released in this latter are carried to the electron transport chain where a large amount of ATP is formed (**c**)

formed is dependent on the coenzymes NADH and $FADH_2$ (every transported pair of e^- yields three molecules of ATP, respectively). Already counting with the energy required to pump the hydrogen ions throughout the membrane, the net energy gain is 28 ATP. Notwithstanding, the oxidation of fat contributes to an important energy input to the system, as its available capacity is unlimited. Therefore, to be used for energy, the free fatty acid must be converted into acetyl Co-A (a process called β-oxidation), and then, the Krebs cycle and electron transport chain pathways occur as described previously.

4.1.4 Energy Spectrum of Exercise

Identifying the predominant source(s) of energy required for an activity provides the basis for an effective exercise training prescription and, consequently, enhancement (cf. Fig. 4.4). Throughout the years, different suggestions have been presented, depending on the methods used to calculate the relative contribution of each energy pathway; however, analysis of the current literature suggests that all physical activities derive some energy from each of the three energy-supplying processes.

At one extreme, within very high-intensity efforts lasting ~14 s, the intramuscular high-energy phosphates supply almost all the energy for exercise performance and that in the first ~10 s of exercise, approximately 75-85% of the decline in PCr occurs [1, 2]. Examples of these efforts are weightlifter's performances and 100 m track-field running. In these cases, the rate of energy release is critical to success in the maintenance of high-power outputs during a short period of times. However, the capacity to produce that energy is extremely low (Fig. 4.5). When maximal efforts, lasting until ~1 min, are performed, ~60% of the

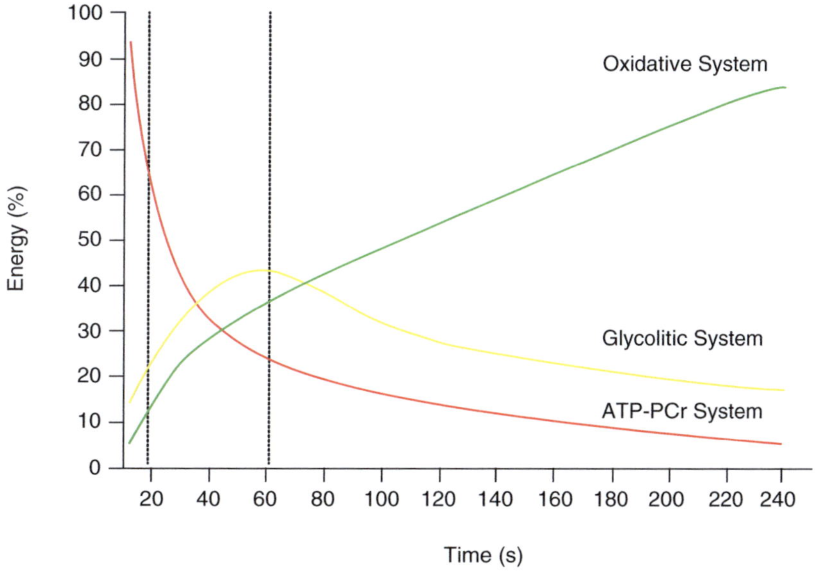

Fig. 4.4 The interaction and the relative contribution of the energy systems throughout different durations of single bouts of maximal exercise until exhaustion

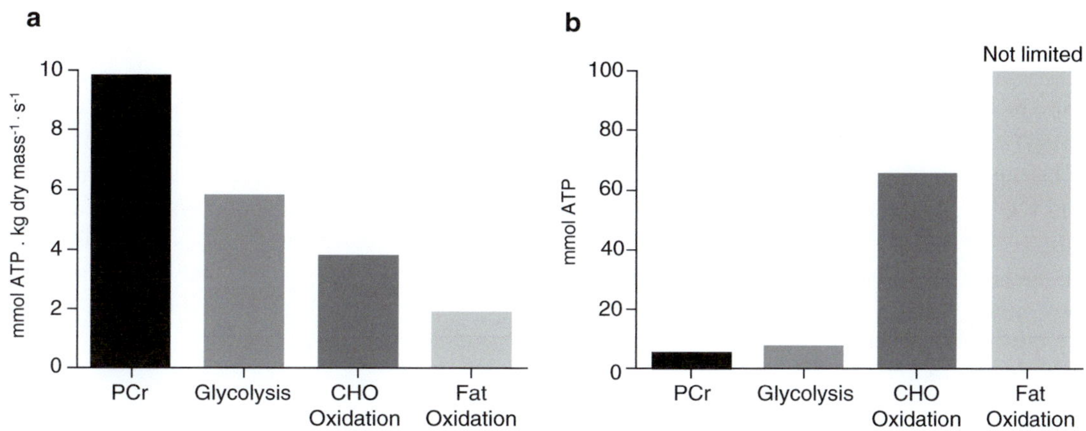

Fig. 4.5 The inverse relationship among the different energy systems regarding the maximal rate (power of the system) at which ATP can be synthesized (**a**) and the amount (capacity of the system) of ATP that can be produced (**b**)

total energy is derived from anaerobic sources, where the majority of this comes from the glycolytic pathway [2]. Examples of this effort is the 400-m run and the 100-m swim. Initial attempts suggested that the crossover point from anaerobic sources to predominantly aerobic energy supply occurred around 100 s [3], 120 s [4], or between 2 and 3 min [5]. Current knowledge suggests that a maximal effort of about 75 s derives equal energy from both the aerobic and anaerobic energy systems (cf. Gastin [6] for more details), from which, the oxidative system predominates—e.g., 800 m run and 200 m swim. The importance of the anaerobic energy supply diminishes, and consequently the aerobic energy supply increases as exercise distance/time increases and, consequently, exercise intensity decreases.

4.2 Measurement of Human Energy Expenditure

The measurement of human metabolism can involve direct calorimetry as well as indirect calorimetry. In direct calorimetry (first described by Zuntz and Hagemann), energy expenditure is measured through the body's heat production, as only ~40% of the energy liberated during the metabolism of glucose and fats is used to produce ATP and the remaining 60% is converted to heat. Therefore, measuring the body's heat production (traditionally in a specific closed chamber) allows assessing the energy production. However, these chambers are expensive to construct and operate, generating results in a slower pace, and consequently, the indirect calorimetry method is widely used.

As discussed previously, oxidative metabolism utilizes O_2 and produces CO_2 and water (cf. Fig. 4.3b, c). Considering that the rate of O_2 and CO_2 exchanged in the lungs equals the rate of their usage by the body tissues, indirect calorimetry assesses energy expenditure by measuring respiratory gases. These have traditionally been assessed to study the energetics of many individual sports since the beginning of the twentieth century. Trying to describe the changes in different cardiorespiratory parameters during light or heavy cycling exercise, Krogh and Lindhard [7] were pioneers as providing the first description of oxygen uptake (VO_2) time course at the onset of constant-work-rate exercise. A decade later, Hill and Lupton [8] proposed the concept of maximal oxygen uptake (VO_{2max}) during exercise in humans, and by using a specific bag (rubber-lined canvas bag invented by Douglas in 1911 for collecting expired air), they provided the impetus for later studies. Although the Douglas bag method was considered as the gold standard for gas exchange measurements, the need for faster and more efficient techniques led to the development of other gas analysis systems (the 1950s and 1960s), such as pneumotachography, mass spectrometers, infrared CO_2 analyzers and polarographic, thermal conductivity, and paramagnetic O_2 sensors [9]. Later in the 1970s, gas-analyzing systems used a computerized metabolic system fitted with mixing chambers (e.g., Sensormedics 2900 oximeter, USA) measuring mixed dead space and alveolar gases (representative of the mixed expired gas) [10]. It was now that the formal real-time breath-by-breath (B × B) measurement of pulmonary gas exchange during exercise started (cf. Ward [9] for more details). Over recent years, the need to evaluate the subjects in ecological conditions (especially athletes in different modes of exercise) and technological advances has resulted in a portable, lightweight, telemetric, and automated metabolic gas analysis systems (cf. MacFarlane [11] for more details). The first significant commercial development of truly portable and telemetric metabolic system occurred in 1989—Cosmed K2, Italy [12]—and until today, the portable metabolic gas analysis remains the gold standard for most field studies on energy expenditure (Fig. 4.6).

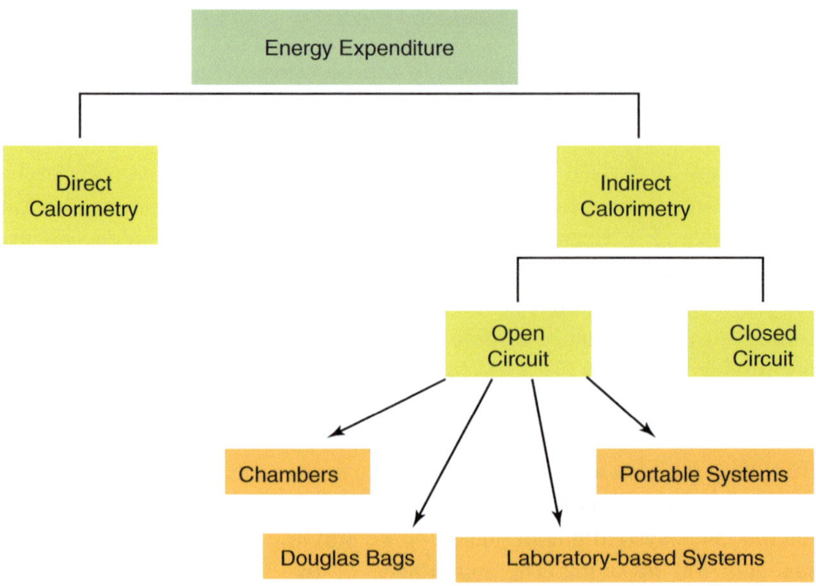

Fig. 4.6 A methodological overview of the methods used to estimate energy expenditure

4.3 Physiological Assessment for Athletes

Although it is not an aim of this chapter to discuss the importance of field testing, logistically it is somehow difficult to get an athlete or team of athletes to be tested in laboratory, despite accurate assessment of an athlete's aerobic function may be optimal during laboratory conditions, which led to the design of valid and reliable field tests. These tests are popular within coaches, athletes, and sports scientists due to their simplicity, time efficiency, and lack of equipment required and often produce a measure that relates to a specific physiological state, for example, velocity at maximal oxygen uptake or maximal aerobic speed. Both these concepts can be understood as the minimum speed at which VO_{2max}. In fact, VO_{2max} reveals itself as an important physiological parameter, expressing the subjects' maximal metabolic aerobic performance, being one of the primary areas of interest in training and performance diagnosis [13].

A variety of incremental exercise test protocols, either continuous or discontinuous, have been proposed in the last decades to measure VO_{2max} within laboratory conditions [14], with the most classical protocol for VO_{2max} testing being the incremental intermittent Astrand-type test [15]. Alongside this, several field tests have been developed to access the aerobic capacity, as time and distance trials (1-mile, 1600 m), the University of Montreal Track Test, the 20-m shuttle run test, the Yo-Yo Intermittent Recovery tests, and the 30–15 intermittent fitness test, to name a few, which can be used for individual or team sports. These tests (performed either in laboratory or field conditions) are traditionally used, as well, for the assessment of another submaximal cardiorespiratory parameter—anaerobic threshold.

During incremental exercise, O_2 uptake increases in proportion to the growing work rate to fuel aerobic muscle contraction until a point where aerobic metabolism alone cannot supply the energy needed and, consequently, the contribution from anaerobic metabolism becomes meaningful. The work rate, or O_2 consumption, just below that point at which metabolic acidosis and associated changes in gas exchange occur is described as the anaerobic threshold [16]. Above this specific boundary, ventilation exceeds its proportionality with a work rate that is in excess of O_2 consumption but matching CO_2 production. So, the anaerobic threshold is commonly described by reference either to (1) a metabolic change in blood lactate concentration, the anaerobic metabolic threshold, or (2) ventilatory gas exchange data, when the exercise intensity associated with anaerobic threshold exceeded due to a nonlinear increase in ventilatory data—the ventilatory anaerobic threshold. Hence, for the determination of the anaerobic threshold during exercise, basically two different methods are used: direct invasive measurement of blood lactate (obtained from capillary samples) or noninvasive measurement of the ventilatory and gas exchange response [17–19].

Considering the outcome of the tests used (either laboratory or field ones), speed or time and distance corresponding to these specific physiological boundaries—VO_{2max} and anaerobic threshold, as a measure of external work, can be easily applied in a practical setting, for prescribing exercise intensities, monitoring training adaptations, and subsequently enhancing performance [20].

References

1. Lakomy HA. Physiology and biochemistry of sprinting. In: Hawley JA, editor. Running: handbook of sports medicine and science. Oxford: Blackwell Science; 2000. p. 1–13.
2. Maughan RJ, Gleeson M, Greenhaff PL. Biochemistry of exercise and training. Oxford: Oxford University Press; 1997.
3. Bouchard C, Taylor AW, Simoneau J, Dulac S. Testing anaerobic power and capacity. In: MacDougall JD, Wenger HA, Green HJ, editors. Physiological testing of the high-performance athlete. Champaign: Human Kinetics; 1991.
4. Astrand P, Rodahl K. Textbook of work physiology. New York: McGraw-Hill; 1970.
5. Lamb DR. Basic principles for improving sport performance. GSSI Sports Science Exchange. 1995;8(2):1–6.

6. Gastin PB. Energy system interaction and relative contribution during maximal exercise. Sports Med. 2001;31(10):725–41.
7. Krogh A, Lindhard J. The regulation of respiration and circulation during the initial stages of muscular work. J Physiol. 1913;47:112–36.
8. Hill A, Lupton H. The oxygen consumption during running. J Physiol. 1922;56:32–3.
9. Ward S. Open-circuit respirometry: real-time, laboratory-based systems. Eur J Appl Physiol. 2018;118(5):875–98.
10. Sousa A, Figueiredo P, Pendergast D, Kjendlie P, Vilas-Boas J, Fernandes R. Critical evaluation of oxygen uptake assessment in swimming. Int J Sports Physiol Perform. 2014;9:190–202.
11. MacFarlane DJ. Open-circuit respirometry: a historical review of portable gas analysis systems. Eur J Appl Physiol. 2018;117(12):2369–86.
12. Dal Monte A, Faina M, Leonardi L, Todaro A, Guidl G, Petrelli G. Il consumo massimo di ossígeno in telemetría. Riv Cult Sport. 1989;15:35–44.
13. Levine BD. VO2max: what do we know, and what do we still need to know? J Physiol. 2008;586:25–34.
14. Bentley DJ, Newell J, Bishop D. Incremental exercise test design and analysis. Implications for performance diagnostics in endurance athletes. Sports Med. 2007;37:575–86.
15. Astrand PO, Rodahl K, Dahl HA, Strømme SB. Textbook of work physiology. Physiological bases of exercise. 4th ed. Champaign: Human Kinetics; 2003.
16. Wasserman K, Whipp BJ, Koyal SN, Beaver WL. Anaerobic threshold and respiratory gas exchange during exercise. J Appl Physiol. 1973;35:236–43.
17. Hollmann W. 42 years ago—development of the concepts of ventilatory and lactate threshold. Sports Med. 2001;31(5):315–20.
18. Binder RK, Wonisch M, Corra U, Cohen-Solal A, Vanhees L, Saner H, et al. Methodological approach to the first and second lactate threshold in incremental cardiopulmonary exercise testing. Eur J Cardiovasc Prev Rehabil. 2008;15(6):726–34.
19. Faude O, Kindermann W, Meyer T. Lactate threshold concepts: how valid are they? Sports Med. 2009;39(6):469–90.
20. Beneke R, Leithauser RM, Ochentel O. Blood lactate diagnostics in exercise testing and training. Int J Sports Physiol Perform. 2011;6(1):8–24.

Sports Activity at Childhood and Adolescence

5

Anderson Marques de Moraes,
Vagner Roberto Bergamo, and Gil Guerra-Júnior

5.1 Introduction

The international literature contains many studies concerning the technical and biological profiles of athletes. However, these studies neither cover athletes who participate in team sports nor assess the changes in physical characteristics of athletes during the growth process. Most studies have focused on elite adult athletes.

A. M. de Moraes
Faculdade Educação Física (FEF), Pontifícia Universidade Católica de Campinas (PUC-Campinas), São Paulo, Brazil

Laboratório de Crescimento e Desenvolvimento, Centro de Investigação em Pediatria (CIPED), São Paulo, Brazil

Faculdade de Ciências Médicas (FCM), Universidade Estadual de Campinas (UNICAMP), Campinas, São Paulo, Brazil
e-mail: anderson.moraes@puc-campinas.edu.br

V. R. Bergamo
Faculdade Educação Física, PUC-Campinas, Campinas, São Paulo, Brazil
e-mail: bergamo@puc-campinas.edu.br

G. Guerra-Júnior (✉)
Departamento de Pediatria, FCM, UNICAMP, São Paulo, Brazil

Laboratório de Crescimento e Desenvolvimento, CIPED, FCM, UNICAMP, Campinas, São Paulo, Brazil
e-mail: gilguer@fcm.unicamp.br

The key is not only to identify the biological profile of experienced athletes but also to follow the development process of young athletes because specific choices, solely based on physical abilities, are related to short-term results.

The physical changes that occur during the growth process and are accompanied by critical behavioral transformations deserve greater attention in the case of young athletes.

Thus, professionals working with children and young athletes must monitor changes during different developmental stages and design appropriate training programs for these athletes during the growth process to yield effective results while considering not only physical but also cognitive and social skills.

When studies employ a more comprehensive approach, the perspective on athlete development is broadened. Thus, learners and/or youths should be observed regarding their transformations in this period of life, biological age, coordination, cognitive skills, and psychological and social characteristics. It is unwise to indicate who is or will be an athlete of excellence in a specific sport based on a single criterion. The procedure of making specific (early) choices diminishes the importance of the environment and its multiple effects on the long-term development process in children. Therefore, the physical changes that occur at this stage and that are accompanied by critical behavioral transformations deserve greater attention during the development of young athletes.

S. Rocha Piedade et al. (eds.), *The Sports Medicine Physician*,
https://doi.org/10.1007/978-3-030-10433-7_5

According to Rowland [1], another factor that should be considered is the difficulty in understanding physiological responses to exercise in the case of children and young athletes, in addition to difficulties in establishing relationships between variables during the growth process. This is problematic and may induce errors in the development of future athletes because most teachers and coaches neither respect biological individuality nor assign due preparation time for technical development, especially considering that competitions are organized based on age groups.

Thus, training/competition programs must be designed according to the stage of biological maturation of athletes and not according to their chronological age. Training and competition models for young athletes should differ according to the level of growth and development and learning stage.

Another mistake is the wide variety of early competition models focused on training specialization, which promote early specialization while favoring young athletes who physically mature earlier and who, therefore, fail to develop essential skills (multi-faceted development).

This chapter aims to show readers the importance of using biological maturation to detect the key developmental stages of physical skills for appropriately shaping young athletes. For this reason, the relationship between the development of physical skills and the key training phases was used considering the development of general, neural, and reproductive systems.

5.2 Growth and Development Assessment and Prediction Methods

Pediatric physiology is dynamic, and children cannot simply be regarded as adults in miniature. (Rowland, 2005)

Growth is related to the quantitative changes that increase the total body dimensions or the dimensions of parts of the body as a function of time, whereas development refers to the quantitative and qualitative transformations that occur in the biological and behavioral context related to the improvement of the systems that contribute to the function of the organism [2].

Conversely, biological maturation simply refers to developmental progress toward a complete state of morphological, physiological, and psychological maturity that is necessarily affected by genetic and environmental factors. Possible differences between individuals of the same sex may reflect different degrees of biological maturity [3].

These transformations occur in an orderly and sequential manner, albeit at varying speeds according to the individual. The transformations can be classified as normal, early (fast), or late (slow) [2]. Furthermore, although growth and maturation are genetically regulated, environmental factors, which may positively or negatively affect development, must not be disregarded. Furthermore, sports training is among these multiple (external) factors.

Chronological age and biological age are not necessarily correlated with the physiological and somatic changes caused by puberty. Thus, when professionals evaluate the general development and sports skills of adolescents, they should consider different developmental areas, including somatic, neurological, cognitive, and psychosocial functions, in an integrated and interdependent manner. Therefore, individuals must be classified according to their biological age because individuals of the same chronological age differ with respect to growth rate. Those with a faster rate of maturation have an advantage in sports performance over individuals with normal or slower maturation rates. Therefore, classifying an individual as a talented sportsperson before the maturation process is completed can be a major mistake.

For example, physical tests may be problematic because children of the same age do not necessarily have the same growth rate and, most often, children with early maturation (often children born in the first school semester) are selected for competitive sports through the relative age effect (RAE), leading children of the same age who were born in the second school semester to be disregarded. This initial advantage does not necessarily ensure future success because surveys on adult athlete success have indicated that the most successful athletes in different sports were born in the second school semester [4].

Regarding childhood stages, height increases fast in the first stage of childhood before a gradual deceleration. In this phase, children are not involved in sports training. In the second stage of childhood, height increases slowly and regularly, and athletic training begins. During adolescence, growth rate increases again as a result of puberty, and during this period training occurs more intensively and may impact growth [5]. Thus, adolescence is a crucial period for linear growth, and sports training during this period can contribute positively or negatively to some physiological processes, including growth [6].

It should be noted that childhood is characterized by the prepubertal stage, whereas adolescence covers the pubertal and postpubertal stages. Puberty is defined by physical growth, the development of secondary sexual characteristics, and the maturation of psychosocial skills. Furthermore, the onset and rate of progression of pubertal changes varies among adolescents, albeit predictably and gradually (Fig. 5.1). Peak height velocity (PHV) occurs in this phase and is an indicator of the maximum development in different ages depending on the rhythms of maturation of its underlying functional systems. The optimal age to start training is mostly assessed based on this factor [7]. During adolescence, sex differences also become more evident and may significantly affect participation in sports [8].

In this period, the effects of maturation must be analyzed both when classifying sports in childhood and adolescence and when conducting research studies. All prospective studies on physiological processes in children should analyze maturity in some manner. The equitable classification of sports participants in this phase remains a key but unresolved issue [9]. Thus, acquiring knowledge of differences in biological maturation between boys and girls of the same chronological age requires the use of a precise measure of maturational level in sports involving children and adolescents. Biological maturity status and time are commonly assessed using methods such as skeletal age, pubertal stage, age of menarche, percentage of adult height, and age at PHV [2, 10].

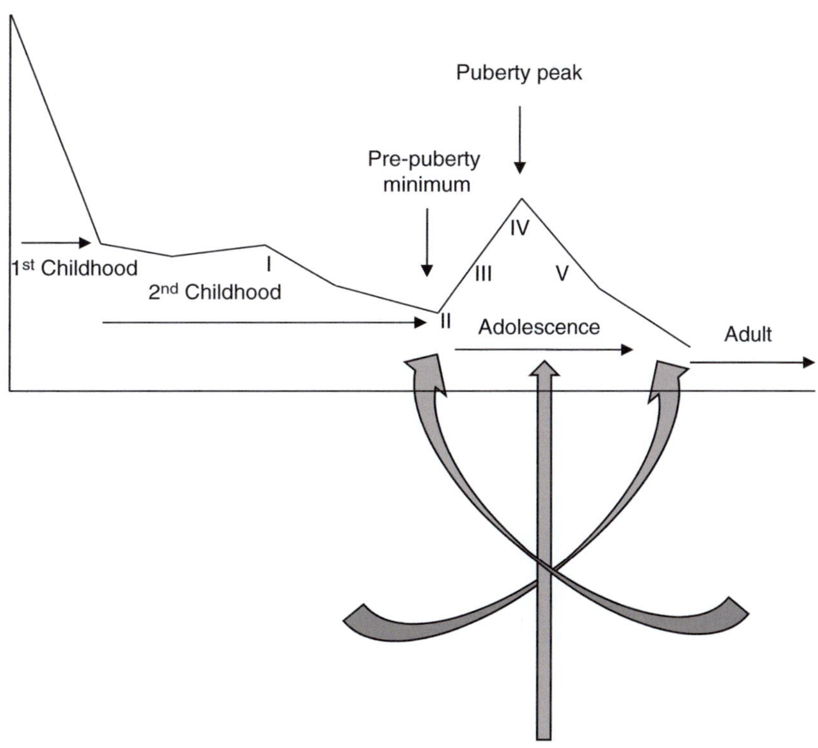

Fig. 5.1 Life stage of important physical and maturational changes

The biological age assessment model most used by sports coaches and specialists is that proposed by Marshall and Tanner for boys [11] and girls [12]. This model uses secondary sexual characteristics, such as the stage of development of pubic hair, breasts, and genitals, as standards. The most appropriate procedure involves an experienced pediatrician or pediatric endocrinologist performing the assessment; however, clinical evaluation of secondary sexual characteristics requires invading the adolescent's privacy at a time when young people are learning to cope with important physiological changes. Therefore, monitoring these characteristics requires the utmost care and sensitivity for the young person undergoing the evaluation [13].

Accordingly, other options are used to evaluate puberty in boys and girls, such as the self-assessment of pubertal stages proposed by Marshall and Tanner. However, the literature still shows controversial results on the use of self-evaluation; for example, Jaruratanasirikul et al. [14] evaluated the reliability of self-assessment and concluded that the method is reliable for assessing pubic maturation in boys and girls and less reliable for assessing breast maturation in girls. Conversely, Rasmussen et al. [15] examined the reliability of assessment by parents, boys, and girls and found that younger children tend to underestimate, whereas older children tended to overestimate development. Furthermore, girls and their parents tended to underestimate their pubertal stage, whereas boys tended to overestimate theirs. Therefore, the authors concluded that pubertal assessments performed by children or their parents are not a reliable measure of pubertal stage and that these assessments should be performed by physicians. However, for large epidemiological studies, self-assessment may be considered sufficiently precise for making a simple distinction between prepuberty and puberty.

These results show that self-assessment is a flawed procedure for evaluating the pubertal stage of children and adolescents. Furthermore, the assessment proposed by Marshall and Tanner reveals the degree of maturity of an individual according to stages, such as prepubertal, pubertal, and postpubertal, without identifying how long the individual remains in the same stage (beginning, middle, and end of the stage), complicating the design of training programs because each stage has a different length (the prepubertal stage lasts approximately 10 years, puberty lasts 2–4 years, and postpuberty is indefinite).

Thus, in order to solve the problems associated with pubertal stage assessments, noninvasive, simple methods have been suggested for the assessment of biological maturity, such as PHV prediction using sex-specific regression equations found in the literature.

Mirwald et al. [9] proposed a noninvasive and practical method of assessing maturity based on measurements that predict years from peak height velocity (a maturity compensation value) and maturity offset (MO) (Eqs. 5.1 and 5.2), wherein (decimal) age is determined by calculating the decimal fraction [16]. To define age groups, after determining the decimal age, the intervals of each age are determined for subjects ranging from −0.50 to 0.49 of the integer of each age. For example, the age of 10 years includes all individuals with a decimal age ranging from 9.50 to 10.49 years.

The age at PHV is also estimated from measures required by the model presented above. Because this model returns continuous values and maturity is categorized into integer values, for descriptive purposes, these values are rounded to the nearest integers. Because Yi is the level of maturity of the i-th individual, the classification is defined into eight levels (−4 to 3 years), with a negative sign indicating time before PHV and a positive sign indicating time after PHV. This categorization makes it possible to identify the maturity stage with the shortest interval from the model by Marshall and Tanner and, therefore, the most precise interval for designing training programs for young athletes.

Sex-specific multiple regression equations are derived, and the coefficient of determination (R^2) can be calculated for models for boys and girls. These models are described below:

Predictive equation for boys:

$$\textbf{Maturity offset} = -9.236 + 0.0002708 \times (\text{leg length and sitting height interaction}) - 0.001663 \times (\text{age and leg length interaction}) + 0.007216 \times (\text{age and sitting height interaction}) + 0.02292 \times (\text{weight by height ratio}) \quad (5.1)$$

Wherein, $R = 0.94$, $R^2 = 0.891$, and SEE = 0.592.

Predictive equation for girls:

$$\textbf{Maturity offset} = -9.376 + 0.0001882 \times (\text{leg length and sitting height interaction}) + 0.0022 \times (\text{age and leg length interaction}) + 0.005841 \times (\text{age and sitting height interaction}) - 0.002658 \times (\text{age and weight interaction}) + 0.07693 \times (\text{weight by height ratio}) \quad (5.2)$$

Wherein, $R^2 = 0.890$ and SEE = 0.569.

However, the results from three longitudinal studies [11, 12, 17] published in the last decade highlight the possible limitations of these equations. In their study, Moore et al. [18] identified and addressed issues relating to the correlation between subjects and an over-fit of the original study by Mirwald et al. [9]. Considering these issues, specific regression equations (Eqs. 5.3–5.5) have been reconstructed for each sex and may more adequately predict MO and PHV in growing children.

Predictive equation for boys:

$$\textbf{Maturity offset} = -8.128741 + (0.0070346 \times (\text{age} \times \text{sitting height})) \quad (5.3)$$

Wherein, $R^2 = 0.906$ and SEE = 0.514.

$$\textbf{Maturity offset} = -7.999994 + (0.0036124 \times (\text{age} \times \text{height})) \quad (5.4)$$

Wherein, $R^2 = 0.896$ and SEE = 0.542.

Predictive equation for girls:

$$\textbf{Maturity offset} = -7.709133 + (0.0042232 \times (\text{age} \times \text{height})) \quad (5.5)$$

Wherein, $R^2 = 0.898$ and SEE = 0.528.

In another study, Campos et al. [19] also adjusted the equations (Eqs. 5.6 and 5.7) proposed by Mirwald et al. [9] and derived the following equations:

Predictive equation for boys:

$$\textbf{Maturity offset} = -12.8 + (0.444 \times \text{age}) + (0.0746 \times \text{body mass}) + (0.084 \times \text{height}) - (0.103 \times \text{length of lower limbs}) - (11.6 \times (\text{body mass / height}) \quad (5.6)$$

Wherein, $R^2 = 0.99$ and SEE = 0.090.

Predictive equation for girls:

$$\textbf{Maturity offset} = -12.5 + (0.732 \times \text{age}) + (0.168 \times \text{body mass}) + (0.0442 \times \text{height}) - 0.052 \times \text{length of lower limbs}) - (20.6 \times (\text{body mass / height})) \quad (5.7)$$

Wherein, $R^2 = 0.99$ and SEE = 0.130.

Some studies related to sports [20, 21] have employed equations to assess the maturity status of athletes, to identify talent, or to assess functional or performance changes after activity-related interventions. However, developing a classification model for young people for sports participation [22] and competition remains challenging. Prediction errors likely remain slightly higher in children with early or late maturation, and, unsurprisingly, prediction errors also increase with the distance from the expected PHV [18].

In addition to these means of evaluating or predicting the biological age of children and young people, some authors have used the allometric scale function (Eq. 5.8) to mathematically demonstrate how much a physiological, anatomical, or temporal variable is related to body size (usually body mass) [1].

The allometric analysis or classification is described by the following equation:

$$Y = \alpha \cdot X^b \quad (5.8)$$

Wherein Y is the dependent variable, X is the independent variable, α is the regression intercept in the Y axis, and b is the slope used to model the relationship between Y and X. The values of α

and b are derived from linear regressions by logarithmic transformation (Eq. 5.9) [23]:

$$\log Y = \log \alpha + b \cdot \log X \quad (5.9)$$

The exponent b can be found by transforming the equation of the allometric scale into a linear logarithmic model to fit the chosen independent variable. An example is the estimate by MacAn and Adams [24] of the resting metabolic rate in children (6–12 years), which was the exponent of 0.67 and determined to be more appropriate (mL $kg^{-0.67}$ min^{-1}) [23].

In the context of sports, some authors have used the allometric scale to better understand the relationship between physical fitness variables and the size of individuals in sports such as soccer [25, 26], long-distance running [27], and basketball [24], to name a few examples.

It should be noted that using these equations is more useful in similar populations, and models should also be externally validated using data acquired from children with early or late maturity, such as athletes, clinical populations, or ethnic groups.

Furthermore, regarding sports, tools that are easy to use and understand must be developed to enable their application to various contexts of sports training in young athletes.

Despite all the limitations mentioned herein, assessing the maturity stage of young athletes is still of paramount importance for adjusting the planned training loads and abilities and/or skills that will be developed throughout the season.

Finally, the models should be used carefully, making the necessary adjustments to obtain more reliable parameters.

5.3 Tailoring Training to the Growth Phases of Young Athletes

Discourses and studies on the training of young athletes remain somewhat controversial because the approach is complex considering the various growth stages: prepuberty, puberty, and adolescence. The introduction of a competitive level of performance for younger age groups has been increasing worldwide, which may affect the development of children. This aspect may lead to mistakes in the development of young athletes because trainers who focus on competition show a markedly increased use of training volumes and intensities inappropriate for children and adolescents.

The methodological techniques used (short-term development) cause competitive specialization, leading to training specialization and, consequently, early specialization. Thus, these treatments, both by sports bodies and teachers and/or coaches, should be reviewed given the importance of risk factors for the development of young athletes. Furthermore, the norms proposed by the organization should also be reviewed according to the development of the sport in the case of competitions at early ages (under-12 and under-13) because these ages are inappropriate for unilateral training or for participation in competitions in their current form.

Regardless of how careful the training protocol is or whether alternative programs and diet are chosen, many factors may positively or negatively affect the training of young athletes because the physical and psychological skills required for success change and evolve with age. In addition, assuming what skills are required for success early is risky because with the shift from an early to an advanced stage, extensive practice, and experience, the pattern of key support skills required for successful performance gradually changes.

Most professionals managing children and adolescents under pressure to show results sometimes fail to respect the biological individuality of the children and to provide sufficient preparation time. This may cause physical and mental fatigue and may adversely affect both training and school performance, hindering certain developmental areas. If this becomes routine in a child's lives, the child could drop out of school (more commonly) or stop participating in the sport.

Trudeau and Shephard [28] found that the available literature suggests that academic performance is more likely to benefit from sporting activities when they are offered at school and not in other contexts, given the close proximity to educational resources and the school environment. Thus, because the high-intensity training of young athletes occurs in its own setting (i.e., outside the school) and requires maximum effort, this training should not occur after school activities with a high intellectual demand and vice versa.

Corroborating Trudeau and Shephard's findings [28] regarding the possibilities of individuals being subjected to technical/physical training mistakes, Carazzato [29] classified these areas of development as physical-motor, mental, and technical development. Each area has specific characteristics of development. For example, in the area of physical motor development, 40% of development occurs up to 7 years of age and 50% from 8 to 20 years of age. In the area of mental development, 35% of development occurs up to 7 years and 40% from 8 to 17 years of age. Conversely, in the area of technical development, 15% of development occurs up to 7 years of age and 70% from 8 to 20 years. The remainder of all areas of development occurs until 25 years of age, as shown in Fig. 5.2.

The analysis of the training of young athletes in team sports (Fig. 5.2) shows a similar pattern of development in the physical and mental development curves; therefore, it is a mistake to select young athletes only based on physical skills. Accordingly, training programs should integrate physical and mental/cognitive activities, whereas technical development in the first training stage should focus on motor coordination activities because the neurological system has already reached 90% of its development at this stage, thereby enabling the training of coordination skills.

However, early specialization is a major pitfall due to its possible cascade effect. Bringing forward the process of physical-motor development directly compromises the motor apparatus, resulting in a loss of approximately 20% of its maximum potential. At the same time, mental development is impaired because early "professionalization" impairs school performance, preventing the athlete from reaching their mental and intellectual peak and, indirectly, from gaining a full understanding of sports tactics. Technical development is further impaired because early specialization before completing the myelination process compromises the athlete's full development.

It should be noted that these skills may or may not be affected by external factors, namely, the

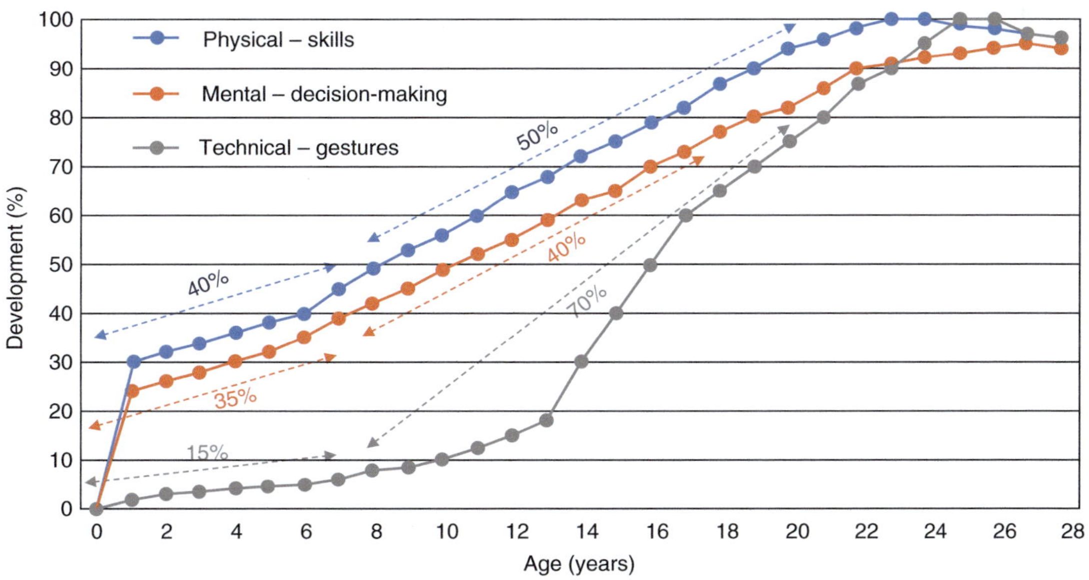

Fig. 5.2 Classification of physical, motor, mental, and technical development according to age (adapted from Carazzato, 1999)

work environment offered to these people. Thus, each coach should adjust the maturity stage and the physical, technical, and tactical stimuli and their development rhythms to the specificity of the sport, ensuring the proportional development of these training variables.

In the case of team sports, the training process should enable the children/young people to perform their technical, tactical, and affective skills and to develop their biological potential. Accordingly, numerous authors advocate that the training process should be divided into stages. Among these authors, Bompa and Haff [30] indicated the need for three stages of development in training young athletes. The first stage encompasses general training subdivided into initiation (6–10 years of age) and athletic training (11–14 years of age); the second stage comprises specialized training (15–18 years of age), and the third stage is characterized by high-performance training. Thus, the biological and psychological changes common to these stages of life are preserved.

Greco and Benda [31] suggest a model consisting of nine phases covering all developmental stages and age groups. In this chapter, universal sports initiation, or the approach from the universal stage, is highlighted. The universal phase (6–12 years of age) is the broadest and richest within the sports training process, during which the aim is to generally develop all conditioning and coordination skills through fun and games (often using popular culture games), thus creating a wide and varied base of movements emphasizing playfulness. The orientation phase (from 11–12 to 13–14 years of age) is the most indicated for initiating and developing technical sports skills because, by this age, the athletes' ability to perceive other stimuli is already well developed, which simultaneously enables the automatization of most movements. The direction phase (from 13–14 to 15–16 years of age) is marked by improvement and technical specialization in one sport. The specialization phase (from 15–16 to 17–18 years of age) is the peak of the development process, when technical and tactical potential should be optimized toward enhancing high-level tactical performance and stabilizing psychological skills. The approach phase (18–21 years) may be considered the most important period in the young athlete's transition to a possible high-performance and professional sports career. Therefore, in addition to perfecting technical, tactical, and physical skills, the optimization of psychological and social skills should be prioritized. The high-level phase is characterized by the stabilization, improvement, and mastery of technical-tactical performance and physical and psychological skills attained in the previous phases. This phase, which usually starts at 21 years, has no predicted length because it will depend on many variables affecting sports performance (Fig. 5.3).

Another compromising factor that should be considered is the training system used to develop the young athlete because the training plan should be designed to avoid physical or mental overload.

Most athlete development models are coupled to the long-term training process, which partly ensures their success. However, some difficulties and limitations must not be overlooked, including the cultural characteristics of the society, socioeconomic level, poor analysis of the results, lack of statistical models, and lack of specific tests. These difficulties are further highlighted when the process is accompanied by prediction mistakes, particularly when using a single variable as a predictor of talent and the same model for both team and individual sports.

This process does not guarantee permanent success because the stability of physical skills or even of a single variable in an individual may remain in a relative position within a group over time. Therefore, the efficiency of the training model of young athletes should be linked to the monitoring of the growth, development, and maturation process.

5.4 Physical Skills and Sensitive Phases in the Training of Young Athletes

Age periods when specific training effects on the human body trigger a strong reaction response, which ensures the considerable growth rates of the trained function, are termed sensitive (or critical) periods. If, in the athlete's process of

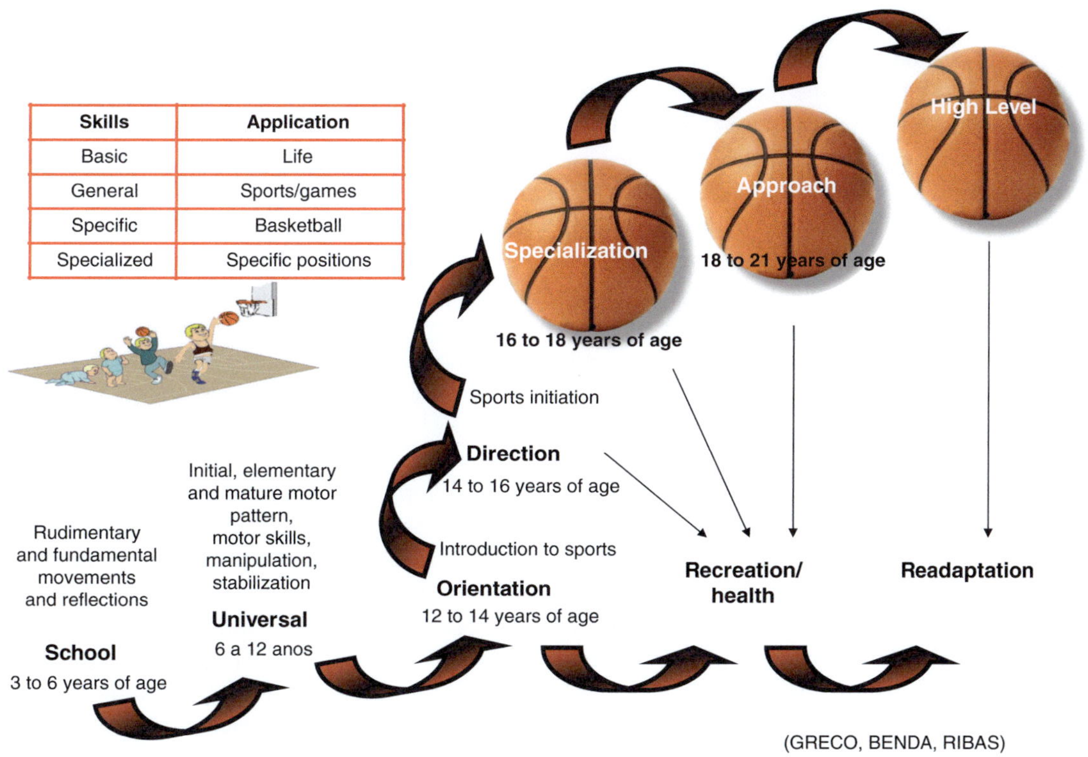

Fig. 5.3 Timeline, from initiation to high performance (adapted from Brenda and Greco)

> *preparation, for many years, favorable periods are not used to improve motor skills, it is often impossible to recover what was lost. (Zacharov & Gomes, 1992)* [32]

The process of using organizational means, methods, and forms of monitoring the development of young athletes ensures the focus on training redirection toward avoiding the negative consequences of training effects and introducing the necessary content correction in the training process at all phases of the long-term preparation by respecting the biological growth of young athletes. This monitoring may be performed using different protocols addressed in Sect. 5.2 of this chapter.

Conversely, motor skills and abilities must be assessed as young athletes develop their potential through tests and assessment criteria for specific indices of high-performance athletes in the same age group. Through this process, coaches should seek to proportionally develop the main physical abilities in each training phase, ensuring an optimal correlation with the development of young athletes.

The proportional development of these skills is crucial for the preparation process. However, this process should be combined with the technical/tactical improvement process. Accordingly, Gallahue [33] describes the stages of development of motor skills in terms of levels, from the development of fundamental motor skills through specialized motor skills to the development of special skills characterized by the enhancement of sports skills. Training should predominate only after completing the motor development stage. Training cannot precede teaching!

In the early stages of motor development, movement should be used to positively affect both cognitive and affective development.

> *[...] skills relevant to affectivity, cognition, and movement not only interact but also have the potential to modify and be modified by each other when fighting for motor control and motor competence. (Gallahue, 2012)*

Similarly, no human behavioral skill will be superior to or more important than any other, and all of them will have to be related/connected to and communicate/cooperate with each other. Thus, no single dimension will be more necessary, superior to, or more important than any other, and all of them will have to be compatible. Similarly, all of them will have to communicate and cooperate with each other.

Using team sports as an analogy, training a muscle in isolation from others (e.g., through exercise performed outside the context of a sport) neither encompasses the contemporary perspective of sports training nor the training process of young athletes.

According to Choshi [34], researchers excessively focus on energy aspects when seeking to understand human movement. The author uses the term "horse" to represent energy and "rider" to represent the information guiding and controlling the horse. In an organism, the horse corresponds to the muscle system and the rider to the central nervous system. However, this way of conceiving movement overlooks a key aspect: energy only becomes effective (capable of producing effective work) when it is controlled, and what controls it is information.

Accordingly, Hollmann et al. [35] indicated that performance capacity is, in turn, a somatic value consisting of isolated strengths, such as physical skills, specific intelligence, technical and tactical skills, and specific experience.

Thus, when addressing motor development studies, although the focus is on motor skills, this does not mean that the other skills are disregarded. On the contrary, all skills are strongly related, and the focus on one in particular is merely an issue of predominance. Conversely, the principle of specificity suggests that although all skills may be involved in a behavior, each skill must be analyzed specifically to account for the predominance of some over others. The contributions of studies and analyses of each specific skill, albeit without forgetting their interactions with others, presumably makes it possible to understand and examine overall human behavior [33].

These considerations lead to the important conclusion that training young athletes involves finding optimal values for critical system variables, which are more sensitive to appropriate interventions, thus favoring positive development approaches more than the same intervention performed earlier or later. In the training phase of young athletes, attempting to maximize rather than optimize any variable alone will invariably lead to the destruction of the system as a whole.

Considering the different training stages, the main objective of training young athletes is special technical preparation toward learning and improving the technique of competitive exercises.

The effectiveness of sports improvement for athletes depends on the optimal balance between physical preparation and technical learning. Therefore, the technique should be analyzed in close relationship with the level of development of the physical skills of young athletes.

The models traditionally used (Fig. 5.4) to classify motor skills aim to gather data from two clearly defined segments: (a) the group of coordination skills and (b) the group of conditioning skills.

The first group (a), coordination skills, is based on collecting, preparing, and processing information and on controlling the execution of movements through tactile, visual, acoustic, static-dynamic, and kinesthetic analyzers. The second group (b) consists of the set of motor skills whose main factors are muscle activity characteristics, biological energy availability, and, therefore, organic conditions of the motor control of the young athlete that are responsible for organizing and forming movements. Thus, conditioning skills are identified as traits associated with endurance, strength, speed, and combinations of these phenomena [36].

Thus, the potential of the athletes' sports results depends on their level of development of physical skills and on their rate of biological growth and development (Fig. 5.5 and Box 5.1). Furthermore, mental and technical development should be respected (Fig. 5.2).

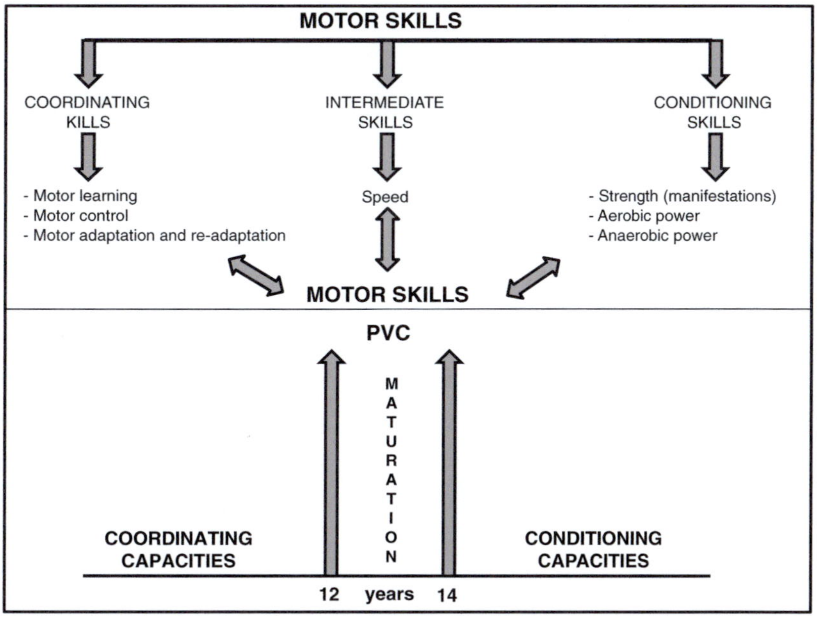

Fig. 5.4 Classification model of motor skills

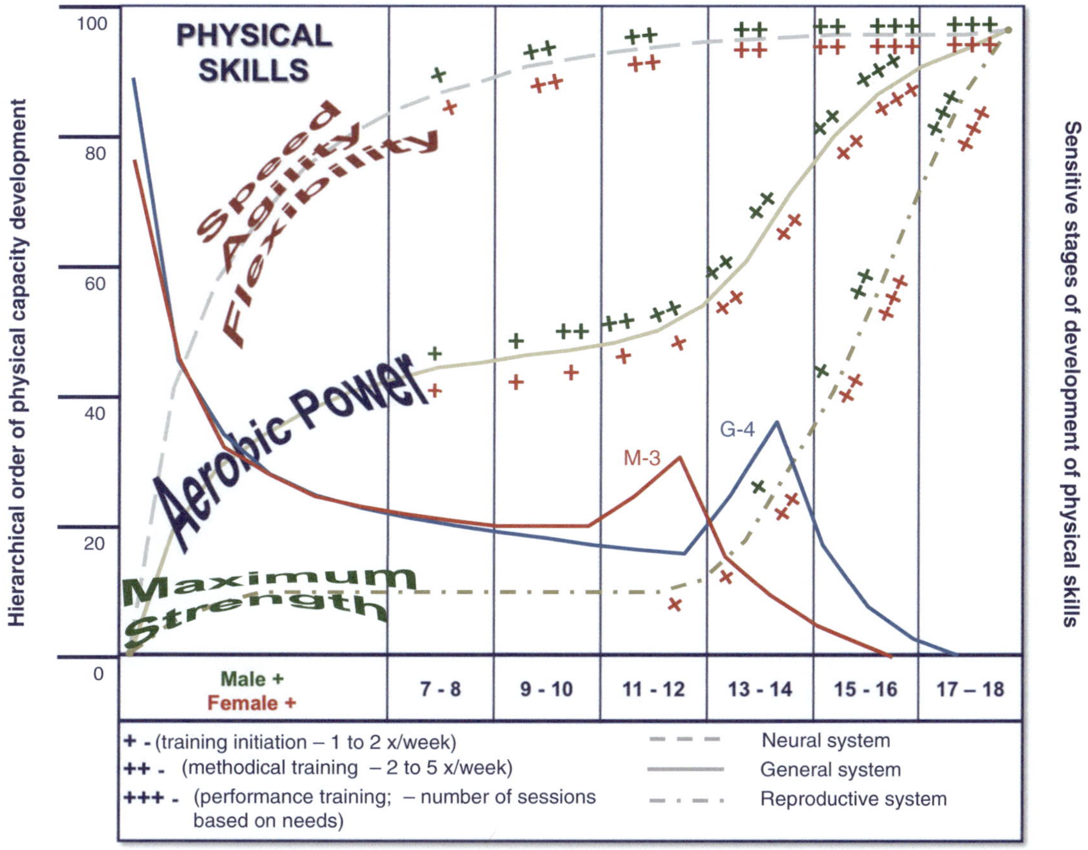

Fig. 5.5 Favorable conditions for training toward developing physical skills

Box 5.1 Sensitive Phases of Training in Young Athletes

PHYSICAL QUALITIES	AGE IN YEARS										
	6	7	8	9	10	11	12	13	14	15	16
Maximum strength									+ ++	+ ++	++ +++
Speed strength					 +	 +	+ ++	+ ++	++ +++	++ +++	+++ +++
Endurance strength							 +	 +	+ ++	+ ++	++ +++
Aerobic power	+	+ +	+ +	+ +	++ +	++ +	++ +	++ +	++ ++	++ ++	+++ +++
Anaerobic power							 +	 +	+ ++	+ ++	++ +++
Reaction time		+ +	+ +	++ ++	++ ++	++ ++	++ ++	++ ++	++ ++	++ ++	+++ +++
Gestural speed		+ +	+ +	++ ++	++ ++	++ ++	++ ++	++ ++	++ ++	++ ++	+++ +++
Travel speed		+ +	+ +	++ ++	++ ++	++ ++	++ ++	++ ++	++ ++	++ ++	+++ +++
Flexibility	++ ++	++ ++	++ ++	++ ++	++ ++	+++ +++	+++ +++	+++ +++	+++ +++	+++ +++	+++ +++
Male + **Female +**	+ (training initiation – 1 to 2 ×/week) ++ (methodical training – 2 to 5 ×/week) +++ (performance training; number of sessions based on needs)										

The analysis of Fig. 5.5 and Box 5.1 clearly shows that in the initial stage (from 6 to 12 years of age), the training of young athletes must focus on coordination skills because the neurodevelopmental curve responsible for the motor coordination process reaches 90% of maximum development at 6 years of age before considerably decreasing in the following ages. In this period, reaction speed and agility during work and jumps should be incorporated into coordination training because coordination skills are based on collecting, preparing, and processing information and on controlling the execution of movements through tactile, visual, acoustic, static-dynamic, and kinesthetic analyzers. Coaches should focus on the rapid development of this system because, as previously described, an intervention applied outside the sensitive period does not have the same effect as an intervention performed during this period.

In the 12–14 years age group, during which adolescents experience a growth spurt, the focus should shift to conditioning speed, mobility, flexibility, and aerobic power skills because these skills require methodical and flexibility training for performance due to early maturity.

Sometimes, speed-related attributes are considered intermediate motor skills (Fig. 5.4) and not necessarily conditioning skills because, when required, there may be no predominance of limiting energy factors other than a close relationship and effect of regulatory and therefore coordinative mechanisms. Flexibility-derived attributes should not be characterized solely by conditioning or coordination factors but by the involvement of both types of factors.

Assuming that motor performance is characterized by the high specificity of each motor skill and replacing the notion of general motor performance by the concept that each young athlete shows a specific performance of each motor skill, another proposal has emerged more recently.

Adolescents older than 14 years have already experienced their growth spurt, and, after this time, they should undergo performance training to maximize conditioning skills, including aerobic and lactic anaerobic endurance and muscle strength. Performance training should start 1 year after PHV.

Long-term preparation aims to enhance the potential development of children and adolescents at different stages of biological development while favoring the final selection process because the ideal type of children with the morphological, functional, and psychological qualities crucial for further specialization cannot be identified.

This system enables children and adolescents to reveal their potential for physical, technical, and tactical accomplishments at the appropriate time [37].

Hence, in addition to biological aspects, professionals must assess the effects of integrating variables classified as compensation, potentiation, and suppression phenomena, particularly in team sports and especially in younger age groups. The integration of these phenomena is related to the fact that performance in a specific sport involves several combinations of biopsychosocial phenomena, enabling young athletes, regardless of the maturity stage, to reach the optimal level, namely, physiological development that is considered not ideal for the time and/or sport but that may be offset by motor, cognitive, and/or socio-affective development. Therefore, individual diagnosis must be conducted at all training stages.

5.5 Final Considerations

Professionals working with children and young people should receive good technical, pedagogical, and ethical training and some discernment to plan and develop appropriate training because numerous transformations occur during the growth and development of children that directly affect their sports performance.

Considering the differences between individual and team sports, specific conditions must be created to improve analysis during the training process of young athletes.

Another key factor in the development of young athletes is knowing how to understand the performance of physical skills according to their phases of growth and development and how to estimate the growth curve according to the individual level of maturity and the future level based on the potential of each skill (sensitive phases) according to information present and its relationship with sports-specific criteria and/or tactical function. Therefore, this is a continuous and cyclical process.

Thus, all training stages, particularly for physical skills, must be designed not based on chronological age but on biological age, especially in the prepubertal and pubertal phases.

Therefore, training prescription is crucial for promoting development before specialization, making it possible to prescribe training programs according to the biological evolution of each variable while prioritizing variables that mature earlier to avoiding overloading physical variables that have not yet reached maturity.

It should be noted that at this phase, a training program will succeed only if the training system observes the stages of development of young athletes, avoiding the physical and mental overloads that explain many cases of early dropout.

Therefore, physical training based on these criteria should be prescribed considering not only the absolute value, which provides a temporary diagnosis, but also the variable maturation curve, which provides a dynamic and prognostic perspective.

Thus, we believe that the training of young athletes should be periodically reconsidered, restructured, and redesigned according to the needs of the child in each growth stage. Accordingly, professionals responsible for training athletes in this age group must base their decision-making process on research, considering new sports training methods and approaches.

References

1. Rowland TW. Children's exercise physiology. 2nd ed. Champaign: Human Kinetics; 2005.
2. Malina RM, Bouchard C, Bar-Or O. Growth, maturation, and physical activity. 2nd ed. Champaign: Human Kinetics; 2004.

3. Armstrong N, Van Mechelen W. Paediatric exercise science and medicine. 2nd ed. New York: Oxford University Press; 2008.
4. Silva L, Barros A, Matta M, Teoldo I. The relative age effect during the editions of FIFA world cup™ and the possible cultural differences in between the national teams. Rev Bras Futeb. 2014;7:13–31.
5. Parent AS, Teilmann G, Juul A, Skakkebaek NE, Toppari J, Bourguignon JP. The timing of normal puberty and the age limits of sexual precocity: variations around the world, secular trends, and changes after migration. Endocr Rev. 2003;24:668–93.
6. Bertelloni S, Ruggeri S, Baroncelli GI. Effects of sports training in adolescence on growth, puberty and bone health. Gynecol Endocrinol. 2006;22:605–12.
7. Myer GD, Lloyd RS, Brent JL, Faigenbaum AD. How young is too young to start training? ACSMs Health Fit J. 2013;17:14–23.
8. Brown KA, Patel DR, Darmawan D. Participation in sports in relation to adolescent growth and development. Transl Pediatr. 2017;6:150–9.
9. Mirwald RL, Baxter-Jones ADG, Bailey DA, Beunen GP. An assessment of maturity from anthropometric measurements. Med Sci Sports Exerc. 2002;34:689–94.
10. Beunen GP, Rogol AD, Malina RM. Indicators of biological maturation and secular changes in biological maturation. Food Nutr Bull. 2006;27:244–56.
11. Malina RM, Koziel SM. Validation of maturity offset in a longitudinal sample of Polish boys. J Sports Sci. 2014;414:1–9.
12. Malina RM, Kozieł SM. Validation of maturity offset in a longitudinal sample of Polish girls. J Sports Sci. 2014;32:1374–82.
13. Baxter-Jones ADG. Growth and maturation in elite young female athletes. Sports Med Arthrosc. 2002;10:42–9.
14. Jaruratanasirikul S, Kreetapirom P, Tassanakijpanich N, Sriplung H. Reliability of pubertal maturation self-assessment in a school-based survey. J Pediatr Endocrinol Metab. 2015;28:367–74.
15. Rasmussen AR, Wohlfahrt-Veje C, Tefre de Renzy-Martin K, Hagen CP, Tinggaard J, Mouritsen A, et al. Validity of self-assessment of pubertal maturation. Pediatrics. 2015;135:86–93.
16. Eveleth PH, Tanner J. Worldwide variation in human growth. Cambridge: Cambridge University Press; 1976.
17. Malina RM, Claessens AL, Van Aken K, Thomis M, Lefevre J, Philippaerts R, et al. Maturity offset in gymnasts: application of a prediction equation. Med Sci Sports Exerc. 2006;38:1342–7.
18. Moore SA, McKay HA, Macdonald H, Nettlefold L, Baxter-Jones ADG, Cameron N, et al. Enhancing a somatic maturity prediction model. Med Sci Sports Exerc. 2015;47:1755–64.
19. Campos RG, Hespanhol JE, Portella D, Vargas Vitoria R, De Arruda M, Cossio-Bolaños MA. Predicting somatic maturation from anthropometric variables: validation and proposed equations to school in Brazil. Nutr Clín Dietética Hosp. 2012;32:7.
20. Sherar LB, Cumming SP, Eisenmann JC, Baxter-Jones ADG, Malina RM. Adolescent biological maturity and physical activity: biology meets behavior. Pediatr Exerc Sci. 2010;22:332–49.
21. Matthys SPJ, Fransen J, Vaeyens R, Lenoir M, Philippaerts R. Differences in biological maturation, anthropometry and physical performance between playing positions in youth team handball. J Sports Sci. 2013;31:1344–52.
22. Baxter-Jones ADG, Eisenmann JC, Sherar LB. Controlling for maturation in pediatric exercise science. Pediatr Exerc Sci. 2005;17:18–30.
23. Carvalho HM, Coelho-E-Silva MJ, Gonçalves CE, Philippaerts RM, Castagna C, Malina RM. Age-related variation of anaerobic power after controlling for size and maturation in adolescent basketball players. Ann Hum Biol. 2011;38:721–7.
24. McCann DJ, Adams WC. A theory for normalizing resting. VO(2) for differences in body size. Med Sci Sports Exerc. 2002;34:1382–90.
25. Chamari K, Moussa-Chamari I, Boussaïdi L, Hachana Y, Kaouech F, Wisløff U. Appropriate interpretation of aerobic capacity: allometric scaling in adult and young soccer players. Br J Sports Med. 2005;39:97–101.
26. Valente-Dos-Santos J, Coelho-E-Silva MJ, Tavares ÓM, Brito J, Seabra A, Rebelo A, et al. Allometric modelling of peak oxygen uptake in male soccer players of 8-18 years of age. Ann Hum Biol. 2015;42:125–33.
27. Eisenmann JC, Pivarnik JM, Malina RM. Scaling peak VO2 to body mass in young male and female distance runners. J Appl Physiol. 2001;90:2172–80.
28. Trudeau F, Shephard RJ. Physical education, school physical activity, school sports and academic performance. Int J Behav Nutr Phys Act. 2008;5:10.
29. Carazzato JG. Atividade física na criança e no adolescente. In: Ghorayeb N, Barros T, editors. O exercício. Rio de Janeiro: Atheneu; 1999. p. 498.
30. Bompa TO, Haff G. Periodization: theory and methodology of training. 5th ed. Champaign: Human Kinetics; 2009.
31. Greco PJ, Novellino Benda R. Iniciaçao esportiva universal. Ed. Belo Horizonte: UFMG; 1998.
32. Zakharov A, Gomes AC. Ciência do treinamento desportivo. 2nd ed. São Paulo: Grupo Palestra; 2003.
33. Gallahue DL, Ozmun JC, Goodway J. Understanding motor development: infants, children, adolescents, adults. 7th ed. New York: McGraw-Hill Education; 2012.
34. Choski K. The concept of system and the human perceptual-motor behavior. In: Hagiwara H, Chosi K, editors. Human perceptual-motor behavior. Tokyo: Fumaido; 1975.
35. Hollmann W, Hettinger T, Strüder HK, Guarany R, Barbanti VJ, Gonçalves JP. Medicina do esporte: fundamentos anatômico-fisiológicos para a prática esportiva. 4th ed. São Paulo: Manole; 2013.
36. Guedes DP. Growth and development applied to physical education and sport. Rev Bras Educ Fís Esporte, São Paulo, 25 N. esp. 2011. p. 127–40.
37. Matveev LP. Teoría general del entrenamiento deportivo. Badalona: Editorial Paidotribo; 2001.

Physical Activity at Adulthood and Old Age

6

Sérgio Rocha Piedade, Mauro Mitsuo Inada, Gerson Muraro Laurito, Diego Navarro e Paiva, Gustavo Pereira Fraga, Rodrigo Goncalves Pagnano, Andre luis Lugnani de Andrade, and Tulio Pereira Cardoso

6.1 Introduction

Biological growth and development guide our lifetime via dynamic process of changes in the human body, clearly manisfeted by the musculoskeletal system development. Despite being extremely powerful during childhood and adolescence, this biological process is continuous and follows a hierarchical sequence of tissue maturity, natural weakness and deterioration, and death [1–3]. Musculoskeletal and neurological systems have their process of maturity starting with the fine motor development, which is followed by improvement in human skills to perform physical and sports activities as well as daily tasks [4, 5].

Adulthood and old age play a distinct part of our biological development, as they prsent the final phases of biological maturity. However, the exact period that involves early and late adulthood and also old age has been changing over decades as life expectancy has increased. Nowadays, it is accepted that early adulthood starts in the 20s, while the apex of human maturity arrives around 30s, when late adulthood starts, ending around 50s, reinforcing the premisse that human biological development is a dynamic process. At this stage, huge biomechanical changes will occur in the human body because a natural biological deterioration takes place slowly and progressively during the following years of our lifetime [6, 7]. Regarding the life-span, Fig. 6.1 shows the bone mass density according to age and gender.

In the past, it was believed that most of the biological growth and development occurred during infancy and adolescence, and, consequently, sports practice was not a common activity in adulthood and old age. Sun et al. [8] published a systematic literature revision of 53 papers since 2000, searching the involvement of adults over 60 years old in physical activities. They found a great variation related to sex, different age groups, and regularity of practising exercises and concluded that further studies are necessary to validate any conclusion.

S. R. Piedade (✉) · M. M. Inada · G. M. Laurito
R. G. Pagnano · A. l. L. de Andrade
Department of Orthopedics and Traumatology, State University of Campinas—UNICAMP, Exercise and Sports Medicine, Campinas, SP, Brazil
e-mail: piedade@fcm.unicamp.br; rpagnano@fcm.unicamp.br

D. Navarro e Paiva
Department of Radiology, State University of Campinas—UNICAMP, Exercise and Sports Medicine, Campinas, SP, Brazil

G. P. Fraga
State University of Campinas—UNICAMP, Campinas, SP, Brazil

T. P. Cardoso
Pontifícia Universidade Católica—PUC, Soracaba, SP, Brazil

S. Rocha Piedade et al. (eds.), *The Sports Medicine Physician*,
https://doi.org/10.1007/978-3-030-10433-7_6

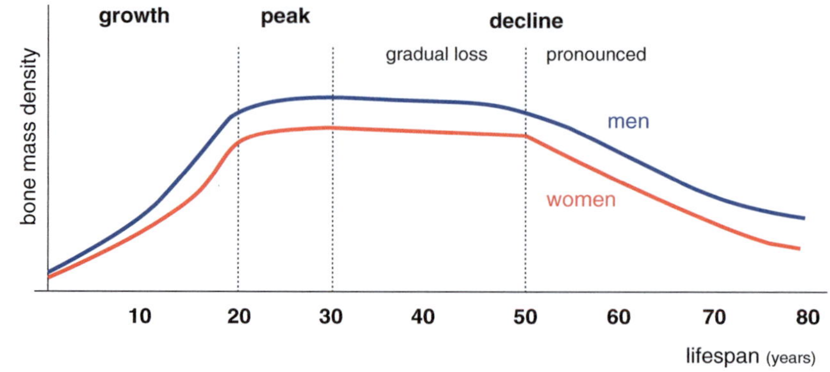

Fig. 6.1 Bone mass density growth, peak, and loss during male and female life-span

Considering that life expectancy has increased every decade, people should be aware of that. Ageing is defined as a time-dependent functional decline of the human body, where the elderly's capacity to remain independent is reduced and fall risks are higher; therefore, staying inactive could be risky for the elderly population as it increases neuromuscular impairment [9, 10].

The quality of life is directly related to how prepared we are to live longer because a price should be paid for it. Nevertheless, the speed of this process could vary from person to person, according to their genetics, nutrition, social behavior (sedentarism, smoking, alcohol), and comorbidities such as hypertension, diabetes, cardiopathy, as well as psychological impairment, reflecting on the person's behavior [11, 12]. It is well-known that sedentarism could impact people's lives negatively, and changing human behavior remains a huge challenge for the government, medical institutions, and physicians [13]. Moreover, osteoporosis, overweight, and obesity is an epidemic behavior worldwide. The literature has emphasized that sports practice presents one of the key healthy behaviors to improve human health and quality of life [14, 15].

Fighting against these health problems and human health behavior, it has been emphasized that sports practice and regular physical activities critically contribute to human health, especially in adult life and old age [16]. Physical activity could be defined as any voluntary movement that causes energy expenditure, while exercising comprises of planning, regularity, load, speed, and intensity, aiming for the improvement of fitness and physical capacity. Moreover, sports practice and regular physical activity could impact on the prevention, onset, and control of the main chronic diseases of ageing which are directly related to the high mortality rate worldwide [17].

This chapter aims to discuss the effects of aging, physical performance, sarcopenia, senescence of the metabolic axis, and related clinical conditions such as osteoporosis and osteoarthritis as well as the importance of sports practice and regular physical activity in adults and elderly population. Moreover, the chapter will discuss the best strategy to design a customized plan for sports practice and/or physical activity according to the individual needs of this age group.

6.2 Ageing, Physical Performance, and Sarcopenia

The increasing worldwide aging has stimulated the need to understand aging consequences, and how to manage the modifiable factors to promote quality of life, and consequently minimizing the impact of chronic diseases. Among the modifiable factors, physical activity and sports practice are well-recognized as a powerful modifier on aging effects [18, 19].

Ageing is a biological process that impacts different aspects of physical performance such as power, strength, and endurance [20, 21]. After 50s, the ability to perform daily tasks progressively weakens, falls happen due to muscle imbalance with all its negative impacts such as fractures, and restriction mobility occurs more frequent [22].

The progressive loss of the maximum capacity of an individual's strength is clinically observed after 50s, being more pronounced at 60s. The last factor, involving the senescence of muscle cells, is muscle endurance, defined as "failure of muscles to maintain a required or determined force, characterizing the inability to withstand exertion before muscle fatigue [23, 24]".

6.3 The Pathophysiology of Sarcopenia

Sarcopenia is defined as a progressive and global loss of skeletal muscle mass that involves endocrine, metabolic and nutritional factors, and cytological aspects of the senescence of muscle cells. In the endocrinological viewpoint, the progressive reduction of the secretion and sensitivity to anabolic hormones (growth hormone, testosterone, and insulin-like growth factor) affects the maintenance of muscle mass. Due to a lower degradation of proinflammatory cytokines (particularly, interleukin 6), the catabolic action enhances, consequently increasing muscle loss [25–27].

Imbalance progressively grows owing to lower muscle function and decrease of the anabolic hormone production. Besides that, a remarkable progressive loss of the absorption capacity and protein synthesis in muscle cells occurs in the elderly [22]. The protein metabolism falls because of the low response to hyperaminoacidemia, causing an enhancement of adipose deposition, and, consequently, a lower muscle mass per body mass takes place. This process potentializes the deleterious effects of obesity in the population named "sarcopenic obesity [28, 29]."

in the 60s, lower muscle stimulation as well as direct denervation cause a progressive loss of motor neurons in the spinal cord, loss of peripheral neurons, and degeneration of the neuromuscular units, and consequently, sarcopenia takes place at the cellular level [30]. Some studies have shown up to 25% of motor functioning unit loss in senility that is a useful marker in the differentiation between other causes of muscle function loss [31, 32].

6.4 The Senescence of the Metabolic Axis and Sarcopenia

A remarkable decline of the anabolic hormone production is expected in advanced ages and a stressed fall of total testosterone level, particularly their metabolic active portion (free portion), in elderly men [33, 34]. Although this mechanism has not been fully understood, it seems to have a cross-reaction with exercise practice and the level of this hormone, as observed by its increased response to sports and physical activity, suggesting that the sarcopenia cycle, activity, and muscle function loss can be directly related to sports and physical activity practice.

The decline of the hypothalamic-pituitary-gonadal axis as well as insulin-like growth factor 1 (IGF-1), both linked to loss of muscle mass in elderly, is more pronounced in women, given its relevance to an anabolic hormone in this group [35–37]. Moreover, the skeletal muscle shows an increase of insulin resistance and a closer relationship to the loss of muscle function and development of diabetes type II, especially among people with sarcopenic obesity [38]. It results in muscle contraction and increased glucose uptake into the muscle cell, a process that involves adenosine 5′-monophosphate-activated protein kinase (AMPK), and also relates to increased insulin secretion, activation of adipose metabolism, cholesterol, and triglycerides [39].

Although multiple attempts at supplementation of these hormones to treat sarcopenia were tested, the isolated approach did not have a satisfactory response [40], possibly due to other mechanisms involved in the perpetuation of the sarcopenic cycle.

6.5 The Relationship Between Diabetes Type II, Aging, and Physical Activity

Metabolic changes take place in the aging process, where the loss of muscle function and neuroendocrine system regulate the predisposition to develop diabetes type II. Nevertheless, physical activity and sports practice are an important and modifiable factor in this cascade of events, as it potentializes muscle mass gain and generates direct and indirect valuable effects on the neuroendocrine axis [18].

Randomized studies have found that physical activity and weight loss correlate with diet, reducing glucose intolerance progression to diabetes by up to 58%, and reinforce the benefits of physical activity on controlling patients' glycemia and decreasing cardiovascular risk and mortality rate in general. Therefore, there is a formal recommendation for sports and physical exercise practice [41, 42].

A Korean study [43] has demonstrated a clear connection between diabetes and sarcopenia, with a threefold risk of developing this condition in this group of patients. This correlation makes us think about how much physical activity can impact on the treatment of these patients. Also, it can be a double benefit when a physical activity causes muscle mass improvement and glycemic control, with a possible feedback mechanism between these two factors with cumulative benefits.

6.6 Osteopenia and Osteoporosis

Bones are living tissues that have the ability to adapt to biomechanical stress and to remodel. The bone mass density (BMD) increases until 20s and 30s, stabilizes during maturity, and becomes negative after 40s, presenting 1% of BMD loss each year (primary osteoporosis). Osteopenia is defined as a decrease of BMD that precedes osteoporosis, a systematic and metabolic disease which causes bone weakness and a higher risk of fracture because of BMD decrease and deterioration of bone tissue microarchitecture [44, 45]. Due to its clinical and biological behavior, it is manifested insidiously and silently. A bone fracture occurs when there is 30–40% of BMD loss, especially on the trabecular bone, and the vertebrae, distal third of the radius, humerus, proximal femur, and metatarsal bones are commonly affected [46–48].

In athletes, osteopenia and osteoporosis could be caused by higher intensity and volume of training, nutrition, psychological disorders (stress), and chronological age [49]. Besides that, sex (women), age, familial history (genetics), the bone (small bones), and ethnic features (white, oriental descendants) have implications for osteoporosis onset. Also, it is essential to evoke that hyperparathyroidism, diabetes, sedentarism, and even metastasis (bone or others) could be present as co-existing causes in adulthood and old age. Therefore, regarding all of these aspects, the sports physician should carefully investigate and rule out other causes of osteopenia and osteoporosis when dealing with reduced BMD.

The diagnosis is based on clinical history, laboratory exams, and BMD quantification through dual-energy X-ray absorptiometry (DXA), comparing the obtained values to the normal range for each age and gender. Osteoporosis is confirmed when the levels are below 2.5 SD (*T*-score of −2.5), while osteopenia is between −1 and −2.5 SD [50].

Risk factors that involve osteoporosis are didactically classified as non-modifiable and modifiable [51]. Sex, age, family history, bone size, and ethnicity are non-modifiable factors because they comprise of biological conditions inherent to each of them. Women are more affected because they are submitted to the effects of menopause and have lighter and thinner bones compared to men.

Although not all older adults present the clinical picture of osteoporosis, longevity implies a more significant risk. It is estimated that 15% of women aged 50 years have osteoporosis while 50% at 80 years of age. Some studies have reported the genetic potential for osteoporosis-specific genes [52]. Individuals with white and eastern ethnicity are more likely to develop osteoporosis and twice to have fractures when compared to African descendants.

Certain diseases such as hyperthyroidism, hyperparathyroidism, diabetes, and other chronic diseases, ingestion of some medications such as anticonvulsants, aluminum-based antacids, and others may affect bone metabolism. Bone metabolism monitoring is done by measuring hormone levels of estrogens (women) and testosterone (men), as they play an important role in guiding drug prescription.

Therefore, the treatment approach of osteoporosis includes a proper diet, adding supplements (calcium, sodium, vitamin D, estrogens, alendronate, risedronate, and other drugs), reducing ingestion of alcohol and coffee, and smoking, and agents such as anabolics and parathyroid hormones. Even though, new drugs have been introduced on the market, sports activity remains as one of the most important modifiable factors in osteopenia and clinical osteoporosis onset. Physical exercises promote an essential mechanical stimulus to bone formation due to muscle actions and weight-bearing [53, 54].

Although new drugs have been developed for the treatment of osteoporosis, the importance of regular physical activity and sports practice in controlling BMD loss in old age is well-known. In this context, high-impact exercises like jumping, aerobics, and running, as well as low-impact workouts such as walking, and weightlifting training, resistance load training and repeated exercises, such as plyometrics training (rapid and muscle blast exercises in eccentric and concentric contraction sequences), and weight lifting, showed positive effects on bones of all ages [55].

The efficacy of moderate to vigorous physical activities in maintaining bone health has been demonstrated [56, 57]. Exercises such as walking are part of the initial approach as it helps to restore body balance, reducing the risk of falls in sedentary and old age population. Cycling, yoga, and swimming comprise of activities commonly prescribed to older adults to improve their physical fitness condition. They are considered low impact activity and, like walking, have low osteogenic potential. On the other hand, weightlifting training and aerobic training are high impact exercises that contribute to the prevention of senile bone loss as it increases hip and spine BMD. Specific training programs and multicomponent strength training, aerobic, high-impact and/or weight-bearing exercises, as well as whole-body vibration (IVC), exercises alone or in combination with exercises, can help increase or at least prevent the decline of bone mass with aging, especially in postmenopausal women [54, 57, 58].

6.7 Osteoarthritis

Physical exercises can have antagonistic facets as they may contribute to the development of osteoarthritis as well as they may act as adjuvants in the treatment and prevention of osteoarthritis. Whereas physical activity causes joint overload, excessive immobility also impairs joint functioning, contributing to weakness, muscle retraction, joint stiffness, loss of bone mass, and consequent early joint "wear and tear". Thus, all these have to be taken into consideration when trying to reach an appropriate balance of joint functioning. It reinforces that the best exercise program should be customized, and, therefore, it should take into account the athlete's age, his prior level of sports practice (if sedentary or not), and mainly his physical status [59–61].

There is a considerable gap between medical recommendations on the benefits of regular physical exercise and how people are involved in performing exercises in their daily practice. Different causes could be responsible for that, such as lack of time, motivation, difficulty in moving, and resources to perform exercises in health clubs and centers of sports practice. Moreover, there seems to be a lack of information on the benefits of sports or regular physical exercises in improving the symptoms of osteoarthritis and quality of life [62].

Although joints can tolerate prolonged and even strenuous exercise without causing injury or symptomatology, a biological threshold exists and should be respected. When it is overtaken, an imbalance between injury and cartilage repair and regeneration occurs, and joint degeneration takes place. In some work and sports activities, joints are submitted to important and constant overload that can cause injury, and high-yielding athletes are more likely to develop early joint degeneration as they are commonly exposed to this condition.

The body's physical performance could be expanded and improved by guided training; moreover, physical exercises and sports practice play an essential role in muscle balance, improving joint functioning and the nutrition of articular cartilage. As for the elderly, physical activity is recommended for patients with rheumatic diseases like spondyloarthritis, rheumatoid arthritis, and hip and knee arthritis. The EULAR—European League Against Rheumatism—organized in 2018, developed a physical activity recommendation applicable for inflammatory and degenerative arthritis patients. It suggests that physical activity is beneficial for people suffering from spondyloarthritis, rheumatoid arthritis, and hip and knee arthritis [60].

Physical exercises have been used both in the treatment and in the prevention of osteoarthritis since they lead to an improvement in pain, joint function, and quality of life [59, 60]. In Denmark, after 3 years of initiation of the neuromuscular exercise program supervised by physiotherapists for the prevention and treatment of osteoarthritis, patients showed an improvement in symptoms and joint function, with less need of analgesic and less abscence from work, improvinge lifestyle, general health, and reduced health costs. Rehabilitation with physiotherapy for analgesia, and later for joint mobility, strength and proprioception. Physical exercises, and reduction of mechanical overload on the affected joint can provide an improvement in pain and maintenance of joint function, reflecting positively on the patients' quality of life [59].

Exercise prescription should be individualized, based on the patient's clinical and cardiovascular conditions, pain intensity, and joint impairment (limitation) phases, according to the degree of joint wear, physical capacity, biological threshold, and individual physical tolerance, oriented by physiotherapists and physical educators. Regarding exercise intensity, more studies are needed to determine the minimum intensity to obtain a clinical improvement as well as to assess the level of tolerance of patients for high-intensity exercises [63, 64].

Osteoarthritis can affect shoulders, elbows, hands, hips, knees, ankles, feet, and cervical spine causing pain, weakness, joint stiffness, and functional limitation for daily activities. The benefits of exercise in the clinical improvement of patients with hip and knee osteoarthritis are well established in the literature as well as improvement of pain relief and joint mobility [7–9]. However, the effects of exercises on the treatment of osteoarthritis of shoulders, elbows, hands, ankles, feet, and cervical spine need further studies [65, 66].

Among the exercise modalities for the treatment of hip and knee osteoarthritis, there are reports of aquatic exercises, stretching and muscular training, walking, isometric exercises, and isotonic and isokinetic exercises, with benefits in improving clinical symptoms and joint function [64, 67, 68]. Hanada et al. 2018 [69] reported functional improvement in patients who underwent quadriceps muscle strengthening exercises while maintaining the tibia in the internal rotation when compared to groups of patients maintaining neutral rotation of the tibia in patients with medial knee arthrosis. However, c onservative treatment for lumbar osteoarthritis is inconsistent. Most studies show improvement of chronic low back pain with exercise therapy and improvement in cases of lumbar osteoarthritis [70].

The lack of randomized studies, range of varieties in the types of physical exercise modalities, associated comorbidities, unicompartmental or polyarticular joint degeneration, and no uniformity of study methodology makes it difficult to have a consensus on the type, intensity, duration, and modality of exercises to osteoarthritis treatment [63–67]. Therefore, the exercise prescription should be individualized, based on individuals' clinical and cardiovascular conditions, intensity of pain, and joint impairment (limitation) according to the stage of joint degeneration. In addition to the physical capacity, individual's physical tolerance should be considered by physiotherapists and physical educators [62, 68].

6.8 Physical Activity and Sports Practice

There is no doubt that physical activity is very important to maintain healthy body and mind shape (*Mens sana in corpore sano*), and it is critical in preventing diseases, keeping independence and quality of life in adulthood and definetely in old age. Over the years, life-span has become longer, changing people's behavior and increasing the number of adults and older adults that are starting or even maintaining regular sports activity. Physical activity could be defined as any voluntary movement that causes energy expenditure, while exercising and sports practice comprise planning, regularity, load, speed, and intensity, aiming the improvement of fitness and physical capacity. Physical activities done in later life can bring health benefits reducing disabilities and increasing years of independent life, presenting one of the most promising non-pharmacological, noninvasive, and cost-effective methods of health promotion, and even a modest increase in physical activity can have a significant impact on health and quality of life. Older populations adopting physical activities will diminish the health and social care burden due to healthy aging [71–73].

A Chinese prospective cohort study published in 2011 found that for every 15 min of daily physical activity, up to 100 min per day decreases 4% of any mortality cause [74]. von Berens et al. [75] observed community-dwelling older adults, 71–86 years old, with minor mobility limitations, reporting the negative health effects of sedentary lifestyle and how to begin to change it. Although, the patients' main objective was to lose weight, while the authors' aim was to prevent *sarcopenia*, and a combination of regular exercise with nutritional support proved to be effective in controlling loss of muscle mass and strength.

The British *NHS Guidelines for older adults aged 65 and over* consider different age ranges, fitness condition, and health state to determine the recommended physical activity (duration, intensity, modality) [76]. It is advisable for people who have a sedentary lifestyle or do not practise regular physical activity for a long time, to start with exercises targeting balance and coordination, like yoga, tai chi, and light dancing. Two types of physical activity should be done every week: aerobic and strength exercises. It is also important to improve flexibility.

Sports practice and regular physical activity are well-known as a key healthy behavior that could impact on the prevention and onset of main chronic diseases of aging which are directly related to high mortality rate worldwide. In the musculoskeletal system, it improves muscle and bone mass, minimizing the risk of falls and also controlling weight gain. Besides that, it has a positive effect on depression and dementia as it may improve sleep and control anxiety [77, 78]. As a rule, 1 minute of vigorous activity provides the same health benefits as 2 minutes of moderate activity. Therefore, performing 75 minutes of vigorous activity can give similar health benefits to 150 minutes of moderate activity.

Sedentary behavior is considered an independent risk factor for ill health, no matter how much exercise you do. It is recommended to break long periods of sitting with light activities such as little shopping, cooking, or light housework. Peak muscle mass is reached in the third decade of life, with a progressive decline in muscle power, starting in the fifth decade of life, but becoming more prominent in the sixth decade.

Ageing is directly linked to progressive loss of muscle mass and muscle strength, which is called sarcopenia.The literature has pointed out that after 50s, the human body will present a muscle mass reduction of 40–50%, presenting a deficit in muscle control, worsening musculoskeletal balance [18, 21, 24].

Moreover, ageing could be associated with loss of quality of life due to different factors, and not only by musculoskeletal imbalance. The process of ageing has a clsoe link to chronic diseases responsible for great morbidity and increase in health costs, such as osteoporosis , type II diabetes mellitus, coronary disease, primary hypertension, osteoarthritis, and obesity [18, 42, 43, 46, 47].

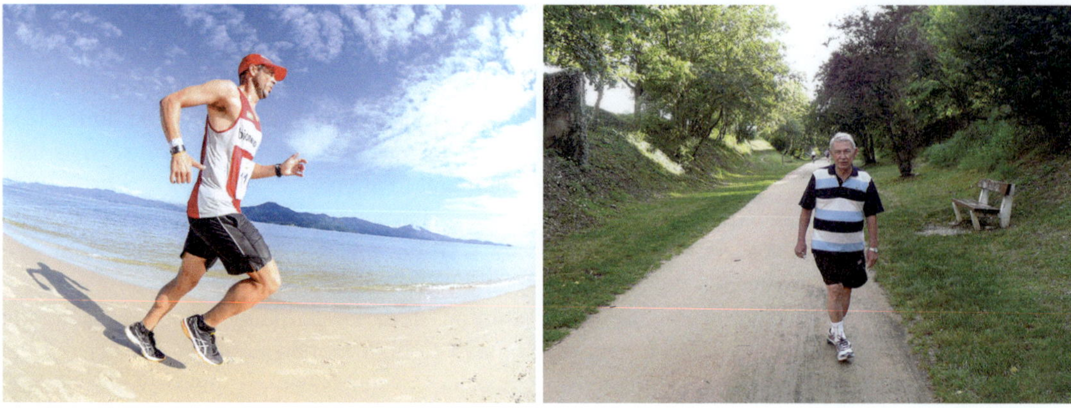

Fig. 6.2 Physical activity: vigorous aerobic activity of a 45-year-old runner and moderate activity of a 72-year-old man walking

In this context, sports practice and regular physical activities improve muscle and bone mass, minimizing the risk of falls and also controlling weight gain. As general recommendations for prescribing physical activity for adults and the elderly population, the sports physician as well the physical educator should focus on the individual's cardiorespiratory fitness, muscle strength, flexibility, neuromotor performance, comorbidities, individual's reported preferences of sports, and physical activity to define a customized approach. Physical activity can be classified as ***moderate aerobic activity***: walking, water aerobics, dancing, riding a bike on level ground, double tennis, pushing a lawn mower, canoeing, and volleyball. ***Vigorous aerobic activity*** includes jogging or running, gym aerobics, fast swimming, fast biking or on hills, single tennis, football, martial arts, hiking uphill, and energetic dancing. Figure 6.2 presents two examples of different levels of physical activity.

Activities to strengthen muscles are necessary for all daily movement, building and maintaining strong bones, regulating blood sugar and blood pressure, and maintaining a healthy weight. Examples of muscle-strengthening activities include carrying or moving heavy loads, such as groceries; activities that involve stepping and jumping, such as dancing; heavy gardening, such as digging or shoveling; and exercises that use your body weight for resistance, such as push-ups or sit-ups, yoga, and, of course, lifting weights. Remember that muscle-strengthening exercises are not an aerobic activity; therefore, they should be added to the exercise program. Some vigorous activities like circuit training, running, football, basketball, rugby, hockey, netball, and aerobics count as both an aerobic activity and a muscle-strengthening activity.

Take-Home Messages

- Ageing involves a series of metabolic, endocrine and muscular system dysfunctions that impacts negatively on one's quality of life, and is also related to chronic diseases.
- Regular physical activity contributes in reducing the overall risk of mortality and morbidity, and also acting in the treatment of many chronic diseases in adulthood and the elderly;
- Customized physical activity is the safer strategy in adulthood and the elderly population, because its focus is on the patient's profile of cardiorespiratory fitness, muscle strength, flexibility, neuromotor performance, co-morbidities, and preferences of sports and physical activity.

References

1. Hirvensalo M, Lintunen T. Life-course perspective for physical activity and sports participation. Eur Rev Aging Phys Act. 2011;8:13–22.
2. Diloreto R, Murphy CT. The cell biology of aging. Mol Biol Cell. 2015;26(25):4524–31.
3. López-Otín C, Blasco MA, Partridge L, Serrano M, Kroemer G. The hallmarks of aging. Cell. 2013;153(6):1194–217.
4. de Rezende Pinto WB, de Souza PV, Oliveira AS. Normal muscle structure, growth, development, and regeneration. Curr Rev Musculoskelet Med. 2015;8(2):176–81.
5. Liu CJ, Shiroy DM, Jones LY, Clark DO. Systematic review of functional training on muscle strength, physical functioning, and activities of daily living in older adults. Eur Rev Aging Phys Act. 2014;11:95–106.
6. Papadakis M, Sapkas G, Papadopoulos EC, Katonis P. Pathophysiology and biomechanics of the aging spine. Open Orthop J. 2011;5:335–42.
7. John EB, Liu W, Gregory RW. Biomechanics of muscular effort: age-related changes. Med Sci Sports Exerc. 2009;41(2):418–25.
8. Sun F, Norman IJ, While AE. Physical activity in older people: a systematic review. BMC Public Health. 2013;13:449. https://doi.org/10.1186/1471-2458-13-449.
9. Colón-Emeric CS, Whitson HE, Pavon J, Hoenig H. Functional decline in older adults. Am Fam Physician. 2013;88(6):388–94.
10. Lockhart TE, Smith JL, Woldstad JC. Effects of aging on the biomechanics of slips and falls. Hum Factors. 2005;47(4):708–29.
11. Iulian-Doru T, Maria T. Leisure sports activities impact on adults personal development and quality of life. Procedia Soc Behav Sci. 2013;84(9):1090–4.
12. Booth FW, Roberts CK, Laye MJ. Lack of exercise is a major cause of chronic diseases. Compr Physiol. 2012;2(2):1143–211.
13. Jaul E, Barron J. Age-related diseases and clinical and public health implications for the 85 years old and over population. Front Public Health. 2017;5:335.
14. Baker J, Fraser-Thomas J, Dionigi RA, Horton S. Sport participation and positive development in older persons. Eur Rev Aging Phys Act. 2010;7:3.
15. Wannamethee SG, Shaper AG. Physical activity and cardiovascular disease. Semin Vasc Med. 2002;2:257–66.
16. Ross R, Janssen I. Physical activity, total and regional obesity: dose–response considerations. Med Sci Sports Exerc. 2001;33:S521–7.
17. Caspersen CJ, Powell KE, Christenson GM. Physical activity, exercise, and physical fitness: definitions and distinctions for health-related research. Public Health Rep. 1985;100:126–31.
18. Steffl M, Bohannon RW, Sontakova L, Tufano JJ, Shiells K, Holmerova I. Relationship between sarcopenia and physical activity in older people: a systematic review and meta-analysis. Clin Interv Aging. 2017;12:835–45.
19. Krampe RT, Smolders C, Doumas M. Leisure sports and postural control: can a black belt protect your balance from aging? Psychol Aging. 2014;29(1):95–102.
20. Deschenes MR. Effects of aging on muscle fiber type and size. Sports Med. 2004;34(12):809–24.
21. Lexell L, Taylor CC, Sjostrom M. What is the cause of ageing atrophy? Total number, size and proportion of different fiber types studied in whole vastus lateralis muscle from 15- to 83-year-old-men. J Neurol Sci. 1988;84:275–94.
22. Skelton DA, Kennedy J, Rutherford OM. Explosive power and asymmetry in leg muscle function in frequent fallers and non-fallers aged over 65. Age Ageing. 2002;31(2):119–25.
23. Cruz-Jentoft AJ, Baeyens JP, Bauer JM, Boirie Y, Cederholm T, Landi F, Martin FC, Michel JP, Rolland Y, Schneider SM, Topinková E, Vandewoude M, Zamboni M. European Working Group on sarcopenia in older people. Age Ageing. 2010;39(4):412–23.
24. Macaluso A, De vito G. Muscle strength, power and adaptations to resistance training in older people. Eur J Appl Physiol. 2004;91(94):450–72.
25. Vermeulen A. Ageing, hormones, body composition, metabolic effects. World J Urol. 2002;20:23–7.
26. Ferrucci L, Penninx BW, Volpato S, Harris TB, Bandeen-Roche K, Balfour J, Leveille SG, Fried LP, Md JM. Change in muscle strength explains accelerated decline of physical function in older women with high interleukin-6 serum levels. J Am Geriatr Soc. 2002;50(12):1947–54.
27. Zoico E, Roubenoff R. The role of cytokines in regulating protein metabolism and muscle function. Nutr Rev. 2002;60(2):39–51.
28. Polyzos SA, Margioris AN. Sarcopenic obesity. Hormones (Athens). 2018;17(3):321–31. https://doi.org/10.1007/s42000-018-0049-x.
29. Barazzoni R, Bischoff S, Boirie Y, Busetto L, Cederholm T, Dicker D, Toplak H, Van Gossum A, Yumuk V, Vettor R. Sarcopenic obesity: time to meet the challenge. Obes Facts. 2018;11(4):294–305.
30. Rowan SL, Rygiel K, Purves-Smith FM, Solbak NM, Turnbull DM, Hepple RT. Denervation causes fiber atrophy and myosin heavy chain co-expression in senescent skeletal muscle. PLoS One. 2012;7:e29082.
31. Edström E, Altun M, Bergman E, Johnson H, Kullberg S, Ramírez-León V, Ulfhake B. Factors contributing to neuromuscular impairment and sarcopenia during aging. Physiol Behav. 2007;92(1–2):129–35.
32. Faulkner JA, Larkin LM, Claflin DR, Brooks SV. Age-related changes in the structure and function of skeletal muscles. Clin Exp Pharmacol Physiol. 2007;34(11):1091–6.

33. Stanworth RD, Jones TH. Testosterone for the aging male; current evidence and recommended practice. Clin Interv Aging. 2008;3(1):25–44.
34. Craig BW, Brown R, Everhart J. Effects of progressive resistance training on growth hormone and testosterone levels in young and elderly subjects. Mech Ageing Dev. 1989;49(2):159–69.
35. Veldhuis JD. Aging and hormones of the hypothalamo-pituitary axis: gonadotropic axis in men and somatotropic axes in men and women. Ageing Res Rev. 2008;7(3):189–208.
36. Kraemer WJ, Gordon SE, Fleck SJ, et al. Endogenous anabolic hormonal and growth factor responses to heavy resistance exercise in males and females. Int J Sports Med. 1991;12:228–35.
37. Rudman D. Growth hormone, body composition, and aging. J Am Geriatr Soc. 1985;33(11):800–7.
38. Cleasby ME, Jamieson PM, Atherton PJ. Insulin resistance and sarcopenia: mechanistic links between common co-morbidities. J Endocrinol. 2016;229(2):R67–81.
39. Ryan AS. Insulin resistance with aging: effects of diet and exercise. Sports Med. 2000;30(5):327–46.
40. Copras E, Harman SM, Blackman MR. Human growth hormone and human aging. Endocr Rev. 1993;14(1):20–39.
41. Boulé NG, Haddad E, Kenny GP, Wells GA, Sigal RJ. Effects of exercise on glycemic control and body mass in type 2 diabetes mellitus: a meta-analysis of controlled clinical trials. JAMA. 2001;286:1218–27.
42. Wei M, Gibbons LW, Kampert JB, Nichaman MZ, Blair SN. Low cardiorespiratory fitness and physical inactivity as predictors of mortality in men with type 2 diabetes. Ann Intern Med. 2000;132(8):605–11.
43. Kim TN, Park MS, Yang SJ, Yoo HJ, Kang HJ, Song W, Seo JA, Kim SG, Kim NH, Baik SH, Choi DS, Choi KM. Prevalence and determinant factors of sarcopenia in patients with type 2 diabetes: the Korean Sarcopenic Obesity Study (KSOS). Diabetes Care. 2010;33:1497–9.
44. Weaver CM, Gordon CM, Janz KF, Kalkwarf HJ, Lappe JM, Lewis R, O'Karma M, Wallace TC, Zemel BS. The national osteoporosis foundation's position statement on peak bone mass development and lifestyle factors: a systematic review and implementation recommendations. Osteoporos Int. 2016;27(4):1281–386.
45. Heaney RP, Abrahams S, Dawson-Hughes B, Looker A, Marcus R, Matkovic V, Weaver C. Peak bone mass. Osteoporos Int. 2000;11(12):985–1009.
46. Tsuda T. Epidemiology of fragility fractures and fall prevention in the elderly: a systematic review of the literature. Curr Orthop Pract. 2017;28(6):580–5.
47. WHO Scientific Group. Prevention and management of osteoporosis. WHO Technical Report Series. World Health Organ Tech Rep Ser. 2003;921:1–164.
48. Kanis JA. Assessment of fracture risk and its application to screening for postmenopausal osteoporosis: synopsis of a WHO report. WHO Study Group. Osteoporos Int. 1994;4:368–81.
49. MacKnight JM. Osteopenia and osteoporosis in female athletes. Clin Sports Med. 2017;36(4):687–702.
50. NIH Consensus Development Panel on Osteoporosis Prevention, Diagnosis, and Therapy. Osteoporosis prevention, diagnosis, and therapy. JAMA. 2001;285(6):785–95.
51. Snelling AM, Crespo CJ, Schaeffer M, Smith S Walbourn L. Modifiable and nonmodifiable factors associated with osteoporosis in postmenopausal women: results from the third national health and nutrition examination survey, 1988-1994. J Womens Health Gend Based Med. 2001;10(1):5765.
52. Xia B, Li Y, Zhou J, Tian B, Feng L. Identification of potential pathogenic genes associated with osteoporosis. Bone Joint Res. 2017;6(12):640–8.
53. Maïmoun L, Sultan C. Effects of physical activity on bone remodeling. Metabolism. 2011;60(3):378–88.
54. Russo CR. The effects of exercise on bone. Basic concepts and implications for the prevention of fractures. Clin Cases Miner Bone Metab. 2009;6(3):223–8.
55. Troy KL, Mancuso ME, Butler TA, Johnson JE. Exercise early and often: effects of physical activity and exercise on women's bone health. Int J Environ Res Public Health. 2018;15(5). pii: E878. https://doi.org/10.3390/ijerph15050878.
56. Gomes-Cabello A, Ara I, Gonzales-Aguero A, Casajus JÁ, Vicente-Rodrigues G. Effects of training on bone mass in older adults. Sports Med. 2012;42(4):301–25.
57. Carrasco Poyatos M, Navarro Sanches MD, Martinez-Moro I, Reche Orenes D. Daily physical activity impact in old women bone density and grip strength. Nutr Hosp. 2016;33(6):1305–11.
58. Layne JE, Nelson ME. The effects of progressive resistance training on bone density: a review. Med Sci Sports Exerc. 1999;31(1):25–30.
59. Skou ST, Roos EM. Good life with osteoarthritis in Denmark (GLAS:D™): evidence-based education and supervised neuromuscular exercise delivered by certified physiotherapists nationwide. BMC Musculoskelet Disord. 2017;18(1):72. https://doi.org/10.1186/s12891-017-1439-y.
60. Waugh E, King L, Gakhal N, Hawker G, Webster F, White D. Physical activity intervention in primary care and rheumatology for the management of knee osteoarthritis: a review. Arthritis Care Res (Hoboken). 2019;71(2):189–97.
61. Duarte VS, Santos ML, Rodrigues KA, Ramires JB, Areas GPT, Borges GF. Exercícios físicos e osteoartrose: uma revisão sistemática. Fisioter Mov. 2013;26(1):193–202.
62. Bennell KL, Dobson F, Hinman RS. Exercise in osteoarthritis: moving from prescription to adherence. Best Pract Res Clin Rheumatol. 2014;28(1):93–117.
63. Fransen M, McConnell S, Harmer AR, Van der Esch M, Simic M, Bennell KL. Exercise for osteoarthritis of the knee. Cochrane Database Syst Rev. 2015;1:CD004376. https://doi.org/10.1002/14651858.CD004376.pub3.
64. Fransen M, McConnell S, Hernandez-Molina G, Reichenbach S. Exercise for osteoarthritis of the hip.

Cochrane Database Syst Rev. 2014;(4):CD007912. https://doi.org/10.1002/14651858.CD007912.pub2.
65. Østerås N, Kjeken I, Smedslund G, Moe RH, Slatkowsky-Christensen B, Uhlig T, Hagen KB. Exercise for hand osteoarthritis. Cochrane Database Syst Rev. 2017;1:CD010388. https://doi.org/10.1002/14651858.CD010388.pub2.
66. Rao S, Riskowski JL, Hannan MT. Musculoskeletal conditions of the foot and ankle: assessments and treatment options. Best Pract Res Clin Rheumatol. 2012;26(3):345–68.
67. Bossen D, Veenhof C, Van Beek KE, Spreeuwenberg PM, Dekker J, De Bakker DH. Effectiveness of a web-based physical activity intervention in patients with knee and/or hip osteoarthritis: randomized controlled trial. J Med Internet Res. 2013;15(11):e257.
68. Bartels EM, Juhl CB, Christensen R, Hagen KB, Danneskiold-Samsøe B, Dagfinrud H, Lund H. Aquatic exercise for the treatment of knee and hip osteoarthritis. Cochrane Database Syst Rev. 2016;3:CD005523.
69. Hanada K, Hara M, Hirakawa Y, Hoshi K, Ito K, Gamada K. Immediate effects of leg-press exercises with tibial internal rotation on individuals with medial knee osteoarthritis. Physioher Res Int. 2018;2:e1725. https://doi.org/10.1002/pri.1725.
70. Goode AP, Carey TS, Jordan JM. Low back pain and lumbar spine osteoarthritis: how are they related? Curr Rheumatol Rep. 2013;15(2):305. https://doi.org/10.1007/s11926-012-0305-z.
71. Lachman ME, Lipsitz L, Lubben J, Castaneda-Sceppa C, Jette AM. When adults don't exercise: behavior strategies to increase physical activity in sedentary middle-aged and older adults. Innov Aging. 2018;2(1):igy007. https://doi.org/10.1093/geroni/igy007. Epub 2018 Apr 5.
72. Chase JA. Interventions to increase physical activity among older adults: a meta-analysis. Gerontologist. 2015;55(4):706–18.
73. Davis MG, Fox KR. Physical activity patterns assessed by accelerometry in older people. Eur J Appl Physiol. 2007;100(5):581–9.
74. Wen CP, Wai JP, Tsai MK, Yang YC, Cheng TY, Lee MC, Chan HT, Tsao CK, Tsai SP, Wu X. Minimum amount of physical activity for reduced mortality and extended life expectancy: a prospective cohort study. Lancet. 2011;378(9798):1244–53.
75. von Berens Å, Koochek A, Nydahl M, Fielding RA, Gustafsson T, Kirn DR, Cederholm T, Södergren M. "Feeling more self-confident, cheerful and safe". Experiences from a health-promoting intervention in community dwelling older adults—a qualitative study. J Nutr Health Aging. 2018;22(4):541–8.
76. NHS Guidelines for older adults aged 65 and over. https://www.nhs.uk/live-well/exercise/physical-activity-guidelines-older-adults/#guidelines-for-older-adults-aged-65-and-over.
77. Warburton DE, Nicol CW, Bredin SS. Health benefits of physical activity: the evidence. CMAJ. 2006;174(6):801–9.
78. Guure CB, Ibrahim NA, Adam MB, Said SM. Impact of physical activity on cognitive decline, dementia, and its subtypes: meta-analysis of prospective studies. BioMed Res Int. 2017;2017:9016924.

Oriented Warm-Up

7

Karina Mayumi Hatano

7.1 Introduction

Participation in sports has experienced huge growth in the last decade. People are practicing sports for different reasons, such as promoting health or improving performance, and the American College of Sports Medicine (ACSM) has recommended regular moderate and intensive exercises for optimal health [1]. However, for any physically active individual, there is the possibility of sustaining an injury. While some injuries are difficult to prevent, such as an ankle sprain or fracture, many other injuries are indeed preventable. In this article, I will discuss techniques that can be used by anyone to minimize common preventable sports-related injuries.

One of the major concerns facing today's athletes, both recreational and professional, is skeletal muscle injury. Indeed, damage to skeletal muscle is estimated to comprise over 30% of the injuries seen in sports medicine clinics [2]. It has been shown that mechanical joint loading during various sports has the potential to exceed the tensile capacities of connecting tissue surrounding musculature [3]. Even recreational activities such as stand-up paddle boarding can lead to injury, most commonly to muscles/tendons (50.4%) and to joints/ligaments (22.6%) [4]. The risk of musculoskeletal injury increases dramatically for professional athletes, as observed in such high-speed contact sports as football [5]. It is impressive that noncontact sports also have a high prevalence of this type of injury, as muscle injuries were the most prevalent type to be sustained among both male and female tennis players during the Australian Open Grand Slam event [6].

As a result of muscle concern injuries, it is imperative to utilize the most effective means to aid in deterring these injuries [2]. By following a few simple guidelines, injuries including muscle strains, tendonitis, and overuse injuries can be reduced. Warm-up prior to the start of physical activities is one of the most common methods recommended by health professionals, coaches, and athletes [7]. The beneficial effects of warm-up are seen in the overall improvement in sports performance and reduction in sports injuries due to physiological factors [8]. However, there are conflicting opinions regarding different methods of reducing muscular injury through warm-up and stretching techniques [2].

- Thirty percent of the injuries seen in sports medicine are skeletal muscle injury.
- Warm-up may prevent muscle/tendon and joint/ligament injuries.

K. M. Hatano (✉)
Instituto Cohen Ortop, Sao Paulo, Brazil

S. Rocha Piedade et al. (eds.), *The Sports Medicine Physician*,
https://doi.org/10.1007/978-3-030-10433-7_7

7.2 Definition

Warm-up can be defined in different ways:

- Any activity that increases the body temperature by a few degrees Celsius [9]
- A protocol or session specifically undertaken prior to and in preparation for the onset of subsequent physical activity [7]
- Simply as an activity that "prepares the body for exercise" [10]

7.3 Types of Warm-Up

Warm-up can be either passive or active. Active warm-up can further be classified as either a general warm-up or a specific warm-up [11]. A passive warm-up is one in which muscle temperature or core body temperature is increased by external means, without depleting energy substrate stores, as occurs during the physical activity associated with active warm-up [11]. Passive warm-up can include, for example, hot showers, saunas, or heating pads. The general active warm-up involves some type of physical activity featuring non-specific body movements such as jogging, cycling, or calisthenics. In contrast, the specific warm-up utilizes activities and stretches that are specific to the sports for which one is preparing [2].

The preferred mode is active warm-up in professional athletes, but the cumulative effects of passive or active warm-up on muscle performance and dynamic stability seem to be equally effective in recreational sports players [8]. The most effective of the warm-up techniques appears to be the specific warm-up, likely due to the fact that it mimics the activity to be performed [2]. However, the choice of best warm-up program must consider the age, sex, physical condition, type of sport to be practiced, and level of competition [12]. A typical warm-up protocol of a physical education lesson consists of low-intensity aerobic activity followed by a variety of stretching methods [13].

7.4 Physiological Effects of Warm-Up

The human body can adjust to almost anything. But one thing it cannot do is adjust immediately from rest to exercise. Instead, we need to gradually shift from rest to almost any level of physical work. Going from rest to very hard work without a warm-up is hard on the heart and skeletal muscle system. When a proper warm-up is applied, the subsequent exercise is more comfortable, and the risk of injury is reduced [14]. Warm-up is intended to perform the following two major functions: improve a muscle's dynamics so that it is less inclined to injury, and prepare the athlete for the demands of exercise [15]. Thus, the purpose of warm-up is to prepare the body to transition from rest to the maximally active state of the body. The warm-up should produce a mild sweat without fatiguing the individual [2]. Both passive and active warm-ups can evoke temperature and metabolic, neural, and psychological effects, including increased anaerobic metabolism, elevated oxygen uptake kinetics, and postactivation potentiation [11]. Active warm-up induces greater metabolic changes, leading to increased preparedness for a subsequent exercise task.

Physiologically, warm-up raises body and muscle temperature, and subsequent power output is increased by accelerating metabolic reactions [16]. As a result, exercise performance is proposed to be improved via decreased muscle and joint viscous resistance, greater unloading of oxygen from hemoglobin and myoglobin, speeding of oxygen kinetics, increased anaerobic metabolism, and increased nerve conduction rates [17]. Moreover, warm-up elevates muscle enzyme activity while dilating blood vessels that provide blood flow for better muscle oxidation during work [18]. The elevation of body temperature also augments the release of oxygen from hemoglobin in active muscles, so that the time to exhaustion at maximal endurance exercise is extended. These physiological changes induced by warm-up may enhance performance in not only maximal and supramaximal exercise but also submaximal endurance exercises [16].

Warming up gently raises the work demands on the cardiovascular system, and at the same time, the body is diverting blood flow away from areas not directly involved in exercise (e.g., the gastrointestinal system) to areas with higher blood requirements (e.g., working muscles and skin). The extra energy expended raises temperature, and warmer blood gives up oxygen to the working muscles faster than resting body temperature blood. Muscle is actually not as dense as people think, so when body temperature rises, muscle becomes suppler and more compliant which helps with circulation and flexibility. The added blood flow and elevated temperature also help increase the elasticity of tendons and ligaments, which gives more benefits with respect to flexibility [14]. An active warm-up has also been proposed to impart non-temperature-related benefits on subsequent exercise performance, such as increased blood flow and oxygen delivery to the working muscles, elevation of baseline oxygen consumption, and postactivation potentiation [17].

The aforementioned physiological mechanisms facilitate greater muscle force and power production which are important in team sports requiring acceleration, deceleration, or change of direction [13, 18]. Combine all those mechanisms together, and it should be apparent that a well-thought-out warm-up regimen has effects all over the body [14]. Consequently, acute effects of warm-up protocols may improve change-of-direction speed, reaction time, and movement time in sport [13].

Warm-Up Physiological Effects

- Elevate body and muscle temperature
- Increase muscle oxygenation
- Increase nerve conductions
- Elevate muscle enzyme activity
- Increase the elasticity of tendon and ligaments

7.5 Warm-Up Prevents Injuries and Improves Performance?

As discussed above, the effectiveness of warm-up in different types of sports has been demonstrated for all ages and types of athletes. Most professional and recreational athletes perform preconditioning warm-up exercises to prepare for a competitive task or routine exercises. The main objective of warming-up is to induce both temperature- and non-temperature-related responses to optimize performance. These responses include increasing muscle temperature, initiating metabolic and circulatory adjustments, and preparing psychologically for the upcoming task [19]. Also important for sports is having an appropriate level of range of movement and flexibility at specific joints and soft tissues in order to perform, as enhanced flexibility and musculoskeletal compliance have been associated with protection from injury [3].

However, the exact mechanisms and outcomes of various warm-up modes are still not fully clear [7]. Even though warm-up is a well-accepted practice and considered to be essential by many athletes for optimum performance, there is conflicting evidence in the scientific literature about the effectiveness of various methods to prevent muscle injuries and enhance performance [15]. Although there is no agreement on which is the best heating protocol, it is accepted that the protocol should be as sport-specific as possible [20].

Based on players' perceptions on injury prevention, 91.5% of athletes perform stretching to prevent injuries, and 54% do neuromuscular warm-up exercises. The perception of risk factors and performed preventive strategies is inconsistent with scientific evidence. Generally, current approaches regarding injury prevention focus on the transfer of evidence into daily practice, but future transfer strategies should incorporate the players' beliefs and attitudes [21].

The research into injury prevention programs has been of keen interest over the past 10–15 years, and a number of programs have been shown to reduce overall injuries by approximately one-third, with much more dramatic reductions for specific injuries [14]. In particular for soccer, this pre-workout focuses on (a) spatial orientation, anticipation, and attention, particularly while dual-tasking (to avoid unintended contact with other players or objects); (b) body stability and movement coordination (more general than specific neuromuscular or proprioceptive training); and (c) learning appropriate fall techniques (to minimize the consequences of unavoidable falls) [22].

Warm-Up Routine

- Well-accepted by athletes and coaches.
- 91.5% of athletes perform stretching to prevent injuries.
- Fifty-four percent do neuromuscular warm-up exercises.

Some protocols have been shown to be effective in preventing injuries for soccer. Implementation of a specific warm-up protocol improved physical performance compared with traditional warm-up routines in youth soccer players [22]. Additionally, this protocol reduced all injuries by 32%, training injuries by 32%, match injuries by 28%, severe injuries by 45%, and overuse injuries by 53%. Further evidence that generalized warm-up effectively reduces injuries comes from a Canadian program tested on girls' and boys' soccer that resulted in a 38% reduction in all injuries, 43% reduction in acute injuries, 50% reduction in ankle injuries, and 62% fewer knee injuries [14].

Similar programs have been reported to reduce injury in a wide variety of sports such as basketball, netball, team handball, and Australian rules football [14]. Another study confirmed the effectiveness of cycling warm-up as a preparatory activity for sprint bicycle exercises [23]. Additionally, a specific warm-up program led to a low prevalence of musculoskeletal injuries in recreational volleyball and was positively assessed by volleyball players and coaches with respect to its relevancy, suitability, and usability [24].

Furthermore, warm-up has a positive effect on swimmer's performance, especially for distances greater than 200 m, demonstrating that warm-up can prevent the early onset of fatigue. It is recommended that swimmers warm up for a relatively moderate distance (between 1000 and 1500 m) with a proper intensity (a brief approach to race-pace velocity), as well as sufficient recovery time to prevent the early onset of fatigue and allow restoration of energy reserves (8–20 min) [25].

As injuries can often lead to extended time lost to training and competition, as well as substantial healthcare expenses, everyone involved should welcome injury reductions like those highlighted above. One critical factor that is an underlying requirement to any program's effectiveness is compliance. The programs are only effective if players perform the warm-up before at least 75% of the training sessions. When there is poor compliance with the programs, little difference in injury rates is reported [14].

7.6 Science and Practice

Warm-up strategies have continued to develop largely on a trial-and-error basis, utilizing coach and athlete experiences rather than scientific evidence. However, over the past decade, new research has emerged, providing greater insight into how and why warm-up influences subsequent performance [11]. Warming up prior to exercise is vital for the attainment of optimum performance. The aim of warm-up is not overload of the musculoskeletal system but to do slow movements activating all the muscles and joints involved in the sport [11]. The most important reason for doing a warm-up is to prevent injury during exercise, as keeping the muscles warm will prevent acute injuries such as hamstring strains and will stave off overuse injuries by allowing the body to prepare steadily and safely.

In more static sports, such as cricket, it is a good idea to stretch throughout the game as this activity will keep the muscles warm and allow them to function effectively; substitutes should also continue to run and stretch while they are waiting to join a game. This strategy is commonly seen in football matches where the substitutes jog, jump, and stretch along the sidelines [14]. Recent studies suggest that aerobic warm-up and dynamic stretching are beneficial for sprint, jump, and agility tasks. On the other hand, static stretching schemes with intensity at or above a point of discomfort or used with duration not longer than 45 s are discouraged in performance settings for delivering detrimental effects; in contrast, a cyclic static stretch may reduce the debilitative effects of static stretching [18].

Some coaches use complex training in warm-up sessions. Complex training involves a set of strength training exercise (isometric or dynamic) followed by a biomechanically similar plyometric exercise. This concept is based on a phenomenon called postactivation potentiation and has presented positive results for muscle performance, especially in terms of twitch contractions, rate of force development, and explosive movements [26].

For some sports, studies have suggested the use of maximum or near-maximum loaded isometric warm-up schemes. Using a protocol based on prolonged intermittent low-intensity isometric exercises in warm-up settings in soccer players, a low-intensity intermittent isometric exercise as a preconditioning stimulus in warm-up would positively influence the jump, sprint, and agility performance [18].

Sprint performance may show greatest improvement without stretching and through the use of a walking generalized warm-up on a treadmill. According to Wallmann et al., these findings have clinically meaningful implications for recreational and competitive runners who include iliopsoas muscle stretching as a component of the warm-up [27].

Sports Aspects That May Be Improved by Warm-Up

- Endurance
- Strength
- Flexibility
- Agility
- Motor control
- Balance

Lastly, the use of equipment can increase performance effectiveness during warm-up. A dynamic warm-up performed with a vest weighted with 2% of body mass may be the most effective warm-up protocol for enhancing jumping performance in high school female athletes [28].

7.7 Warm-Up Intensity

The warm-up effect on performance is determined by the intensity, duration, and recovery interval between warm-up and exercise [29]. The purpose of warm-up is to prepare the athlete's body for sports, without requiring great energetic demand. The warm-up should produce a mild sweat without fatiguing the individual [2]. The warm-up should be structured in such a way that the individual experiences an increase in muscle temperature but does not experience a significant decrease in high-energy phosphate availability. The intensity of the warm-up should be tailored to meet the needs and abilities of each individual. For example, a poorly conditioned athlete will not require the same intensity or duration of warm-up as the well-conditioned athlete to achieve the same elevation in muscle temperature [15].

Many studies have used percent maximal oxygen uptake (VO_2 max) as a guide for warm-up intensity [17]. Maximal oxygen consumption (VO_2), is defined by the Fick equation $VO_2 = CO * a\text{-}VO_2diff$, where a-$VO_2$ difference is the arteriovenous oxygen difference [30]. Usually, it is suggested that moderate volume and that an intensity of 40–60% of a person's VO_2 max should be utilized to increase muscle temperature while also limiting high-energy phosphate depletion [15].

The heart rate and lactate concentrations could be used to control the intensity of warm-up. However, it must be considered that it has previously been shown that heart rate and blood lactate concentrations differed between participants of varying fitness levels when exercise was performed at a percent of VO_2 max but were similar during exercise performed at a percentage of the anaerobic threshold depicted as a rapid rise in blood lactate concentrations during incremental tests [17].

There are many sports medicine tools to estimate the intensity of warm-up exercises: field tests (e.g., Cooper test) and ergospirometry [31]. The Borg scale is a classic and easy tool to orientate the recreational and competitive athlete to achieve the proposed protocol [32]. However, in the absence of appropriate measurement instruments, it appears to be the general consensus that under normal conditions, light to mild sweating, without fatigue, is a reliable indicator of an adequate increase in muscle temperature [15].

7.8 Warm-Up Duration

There are more aspects to consider besides the intensity of the warm-up program. Physically active people, competitive athletes, and coaches must take into account the duration of warm-up and the subsequent recovery interval when practicing or assessing activities requiring powerful lower limb muscle contractions [29].

Warm-up enhances anaerobic performance through increasing muscle temperature and concomitantly enhancing muscular power [29]. There is no consensus on the effects of short (specific) or long (general+ specific) warm-up, and it must be specifically tailored for the athlete and sport to optimize its benefits [33]. Most warm-up sessions last between 20 min and half an hour; this gives the body plenty of time to gradually get ready for physical activity and gives the player time to prepare themselves mentally [14].

A short warm-up is as effective as a long warm-up for intermediate performance. Therefore, athletes can choose for themselves if they want to include a general part in their warm-up routines, even though it would not enhance their performance more compared with only using a short, specific warm-up. However, to increase efficiency of time for training or competition, these short, specific warm-ups should be performed instead of long warm-ups [33].

Another important aspect is the recovery interval between the warm-up activities. According to Frikha et al., a 5-min aerobic warm-up is a sufficient duration for the improvement of muscular power, essentially when the anaerobic exercise performance is applied immediately after the warm-up. However, the 15-min warm-up duration is better when followed by a 5-min rest interval. This recovery interval did not cause a drop in core temperature or in anaerobic performance [29].

Duration and Intensity

- Intensity and duration should be enough to activate the body muscles, without causing exhaustion.
- Generally the intensity of exercises is 40–60% VO_2 max or light to moderate level.
- Generally duration is about 20–30 min.
- Recovery interval should be considered between the exercises.

7.9 Types of Warm-Up Programs

An effective warm-up protocol provides the athlete increased flexibility, balance, agility, motor control, endurance, strength, and power output specific for the sport played. A smooth transition from the warm-up to a specific activity is an optimal way to prevent injuries. For example, a soccer player could pass, dribble, and shoot a ball; a weightlifter could lift light weights before moving onto greater resistance [34]. Sprint drills or jumps gently increase the level of intensity and prepare the body for sudden movements in the game [14].

7.9.1 Passive Heat and Cooling

Passive warm-up includes heating and/or cooling strategies. This method has limited use as a warm-up mode and is indicated more for light to moderate physically active people. Passive heating or cooling warm-ups do not affect endurance outcomes but might benefit strength training for improving muscle mass [35] and positively affect flexibility [7]. This type of pre-workout warm-up that passively heats muscles before a fatiguing eccentric exercise is likely to significantly minimize losses in flexibility for up to 8 days following the fatiguing exercise [7].

Historically, heat has been used in various clinical and sports rehabilitation settings to treat soft tissue injuries. More recently, interest has emerged in using heat to precondition muscle against injury. Heating muscle may also enhance the benefits of strength training for improving muscle mass in humans. Further research is needed to identify the most effective forms of heat therapy and to investigate the benefits of heat therapy for restricting muscle wasting in the elderly and those individuals recovering from serious injury or illness [35].

7.9.2 Stretching

The warm-up should gently prepare the body for exercises by gradually increasing the heart rate and circulation; this will loosen the joints and increase blood flow to the muscles. Stretching helps prepare your body for your workout and aids in your body's recovery process after your workout preventing injuries [36]. ACSM recommends that flexibility exercises should be a part of an overall fitness program, sufficient to develop and maintain range of motion. These exercises should stretch the major muscle groups and be performed a minimum of 2 to 3 days a week [9, 34, 37].

Flexibility is an important part of physical fitness and thereby can allow people to more easily do activities that require greater range of motion. Although flexibility may not impact health indicators as shown with aerobic or muscular fitness, stretching exercises should be considered as a valuable component of a complete exercise program [9, 34, 37].

There are several distinct types of stretches. Static stretching involves slowly moving a muscle to the end of its range of motion and then holding the position for a period of time. Some examples of static stretching include calf stretch, sitting hamstring stretch, and shoulder stretch. In contrast, dynamic stretching consists of controlled movement (arm or leg swings) through the active range of motion for a joint [13].

Proprioceptive neuromuscular facilitation is a different type of stretching. The PNF protocol used a "contract-relax-agonist-contraction" method (contract-release-contract) to minimize the intrusion of autogenic inhibition, myostatic reflexes, and neural activity in the involved musculature [3]. That PNF was also equally effective in flexibility conditioning would suggest that this mode of flexibility training should be used over passive to help preserve dynamic joint stability capabilities at this extended and vulnerable joint position [3]. Also, PNF stretching causes significant decrements in the bilateral and unilateral flexibility limitations on the body [38].

In moderately active individuals, short durations of stretching seem to temporarily improve flexibility without the detrimental strength losses [39]. Lobel et al. demonstrated that static, dynamic, and PNF stretching increases flexibility in *dancers* [40]. Some authors and athletes agree that if stretching is to *be performed* as part of a warm-up, dynamic stretching should *be favored* over static stretching [41], especially for upper extremity sports [42]. Flexibility programs (including static, dynamic, and PNF methods) should be *designed specifically* to meet the needs and demands of the individual's lifestyle. For most adults, flexibility training will help to improve balance and postural stability. Figure 7.1 shows examples of static stretching, while Figs. 7.2, 7.3, and 7.4 present examples of dynamic stretching.

7.9.3 Foam Rolling

Foam rolling has been proposed to improve muscle function, performance, and joint range of motion in order to improve flexibility and muscle strength. According to Su et al., comparing the acute effects of foam rolling with static stretching and dynamic stretching, foam rolling is more effective in acutely increasing flexibility and may be recommended as part of a warm-up program [43].

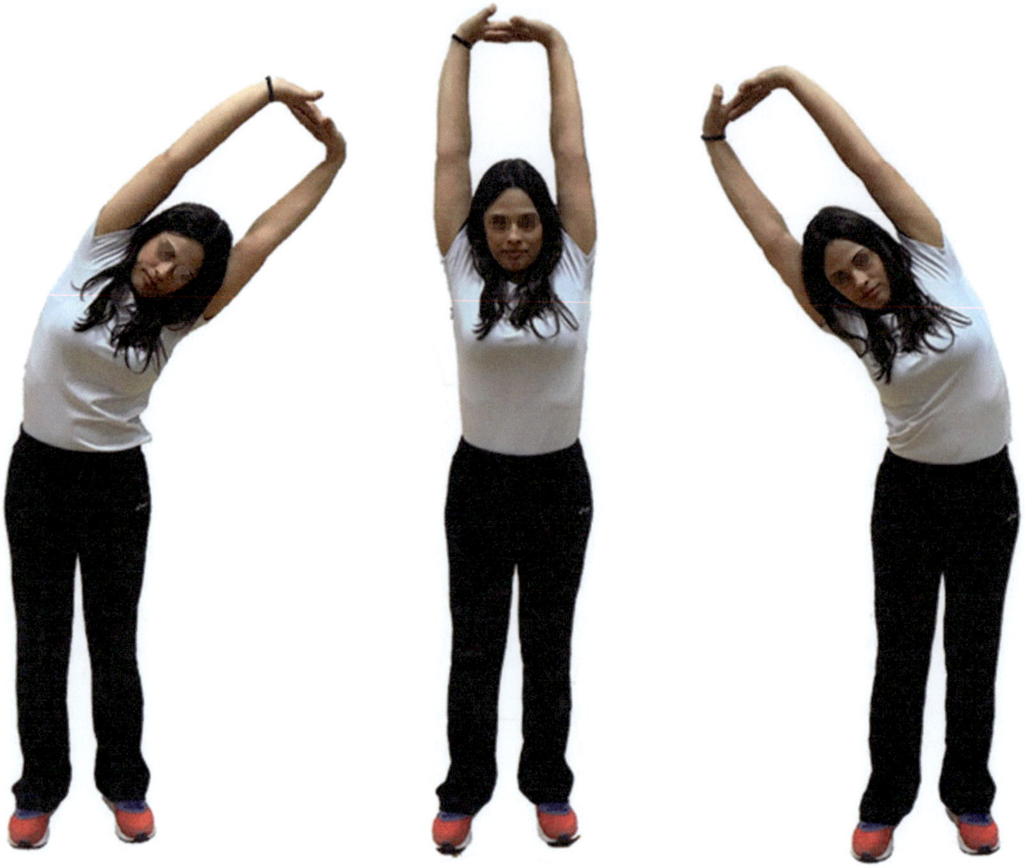

Fig. 7.1 Static stretching of upper body

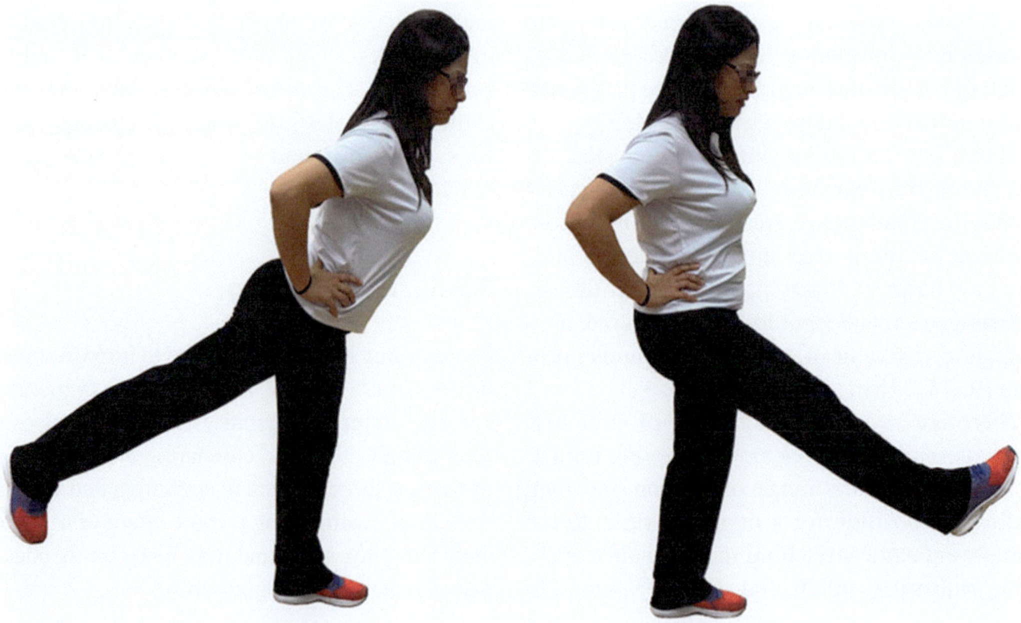

Fig. 7.2 Dynamic stretching, balance, and body control

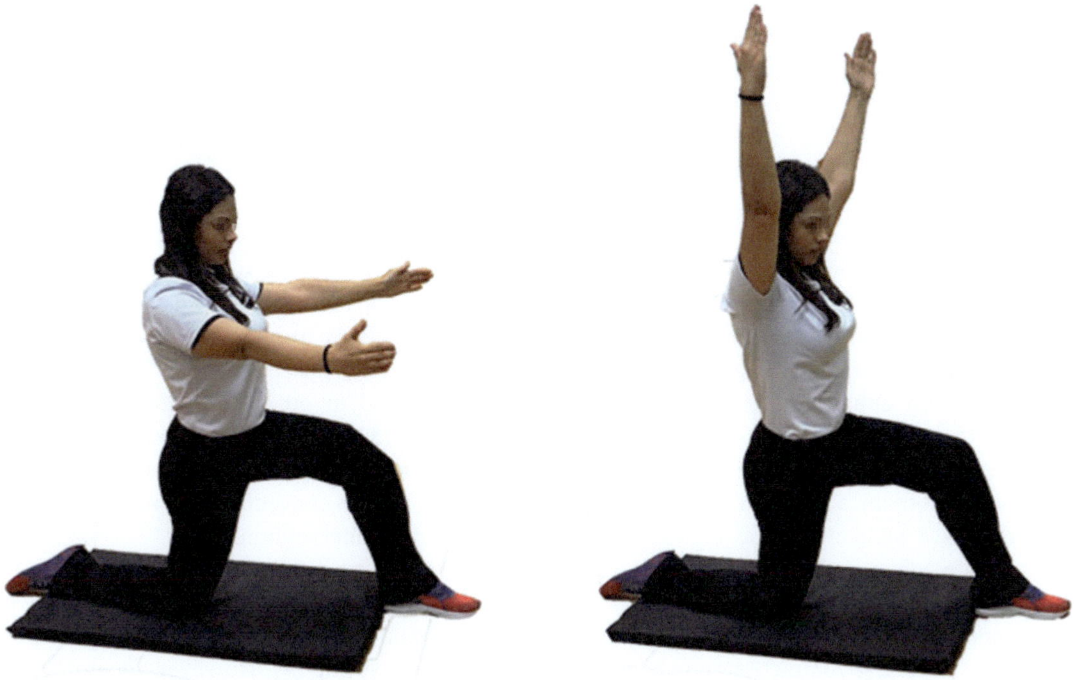

Fig. 7.3 Dynamic stretching using the whole body

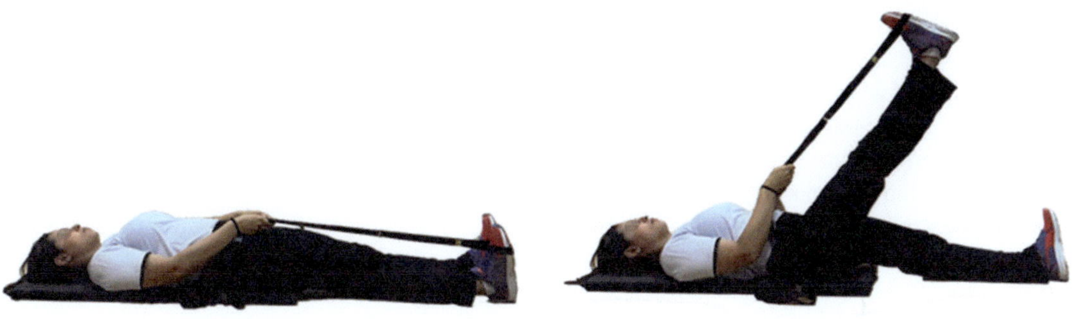

Fig. 7.4 Dynamic stretching using hip and leg accessories

7.9.4 Isometric Exercises

A low-intensity intermittent isometric exercise with maximum or near-maximum isometric load, as a preconditioning stimulus in warm-up, would positively influence the jump, sprint, and agility performance [18].

7.9.5 Postactivation Potentiation Theory (PAP)

Postactivation potentiation theory is a phenomenon in which muscular force is acutely enhanced as a result of prior contractile activity [44]. PAP is defined as the acute enhancement of muscular power output produced by performing a preload stimulus before an actual activity. It is known that any previous muscle activity can trigger both PAP and fatigue mechanisms. Contractile history of a muscle is said to have a positive effect on muscle performance, especially in terms of twitch contractions, the rate of force development, and explosive movements. This improved muscular performance can be attributed to increased phosphorylation of myosin light chains and increased motor neuron excitability [26].

After maximal muscular contraction, the muscles are in both a potentiated and fatigued state. However, fatigue dissipates faster than potentiation, creating a window of opportunity for possible performance enhancement [45]. PAP was shown to enhance vertical and horizontal jump performance, shot put performance, and sprint performance among collegiate male and female athletes [45], and PAP may improve sprint performance [46], suggesting that strength and conditioning practitioners should potentially alter their warm-up programs to include PAP protocols to enhance performance of power athletes [45].

Moreover, PAP substantially enhances 100 m freestyle performance in collegiate swimmers and presents a valid technique for competitive performance enhancement [45]. Some sports as judo and baseball can result in improved performance and peak power using PAP [7, 47]. Sport-specific conditioning contractions can be used to enhance performance [44] and association with other warm-up methods, as whole-body vibration has been suggested as a potential way to acutely improve sprint performance in cycling [48].

Hammami et al. studied the efficacy and characteristics of warm-up in soccer players and showed that static stretching reduced subsequent acute performance, while warm-up activities that include dynamic stretching and PAP-based exercises can elicit positive effects in soccer players [49].

7.9.6 Plyometric Exercises

Plyometric training is used to increase movement speed and power. This is a type of physical conditioning that emphasizes the stretch-shortening cycle and typically involves both open and closed kinetic chain exercises, such as jumping or medicine ball throws [50]. PAP in the form of a plyometric during warm-ups has been shown to improve performance in some speed/power events. Including a plyometric exercise during warm-ups can improve sprint performance in collegiate-aged male sprinters during short sprints [51]. Plyometric training on young soccer players revealed significant increases in performance when compared with regular soccer training [52].

7.9.7 Vibration

Vibration exercise is a safe modality with the capability to be included or used as a stand-alone warm-up modality to increase the intramuscular temperature at a faster rate with low metabolic cost compared to other conventional warm-up modalities [53]. However, vibration exercise does not provide any additional neurogenic benefits compared to conventional dynamic and passive warm-up interventions [53].

Body vibration alone showed some positive effects on flexibility [53] but no evidence to improve endurance, strength, power, and performance in sports [7]. However, the combination with other warm-up modalities could improve performance, as a study revealed that body-loaded squats with whole-body vibration could be incorporated into preparations for specific sprint training to improve the quality of the sprint training and also in order to improve sprint performance in relevant competitions [54].

7.9.8 Training Accessories

For improved practice assistance, some accessories can be helpful to improve the warm-up program. It is important to use proper equipment that fits correctly and meets safety standards. Too often, old, faulty, or improperly fitted equipment (such as footwear, mouth guards, helmets, goggles, or shin pads) can cause injuries.

A practical warm-up using relatively inexpensive and portable equipment such as elastic resistance bands were just as effective as a warm-up protocol that requires more substantial and less transportable equipment such as a squat rack and associated free weights [55].

Types of Warm-Up Programs
- Passive heat and cooling
- Stretching (static, dynamic, PNF)
- Foam rolling
- Isometric exercises
- Postactivation potentiation exercises
- Plyometric exercises
- Vibration

7.10 Weather Conditions

7.10.1 Warm-Up in Cold Weather

Passive and active warm-up, alone or in combination, should be practiced in cold weather [7]. Endurance performance does not seem to be affected by cold weather, but the benefit of warm-up during cold days is almost self-evident, as the blood flow increases body temperature and activates muscles for exercise [56].

7.10.2 Warm-Up in High Temperature and Humidity

Athletes generally perform active warm-up to prepare for an upcoming event, which is proposed to induce beneficial physiological responses. However, warm-up also elevates the core temperature; as a result, this effect may precipitate neuromuscular and cardiovascular impairments limiting endurance capacity [19], resulting in fatigue and reduced endurance performance in the heat [57].

Preparations for competing in the heat should include an acclimatization regimen and manipulation of the warm-up to suit the demands of competition in hot environments, along with other strategies to avoid heating up [19]. Athletes should also consider cooling interventions to curtail heat gain during the warm-up and minimize dehydration. Indeed, although it forms an essential part of the pre-competition preparation in all environmental conditions, the rise in whole-body temperature should be limited in hot environments [19].

Combining precooling (ice slurry and ice vest) and warm-up prior to endurance exercise in the heat may exploit the benefits of both strategies while avoiding the potential negative consequences of each on performance [58].

7.11 Warm-Up Plan Program

Typically, an optimized warm-up will consist of light cardiovascular exercises combined with stretches. The warm-up can be important not just for metabolic responses but also will involve cardiovascular exercises, stretching, and strength drills, to work agility, coordination, and balance. The combination of these can be worked in uni- and multilateral directions [14].

- Choose a general warm-up (jogging, cycling) and/or warm-up modalities: stretching, vibration, PAP, plyometric exercises, isometric, foam rolling, and other passive and active techniques.
  For recreational physical activities, the warm-up plan can include jumping jacks, walking knee hugs, arm circles, side shuffles, back pedaling, lungs, squats, leg swings, inchworms, and karaoke.
  For competitive or professional athletes, it is recommended to include activities involving the movements and muscles used in the sport.
- Equipment use.
  Choose equipment in proper maintenance and suitable for the athlete and the sporting activity.
- Always prepare your body for an upcoming event
  It is important to warm up in hot weather because even though the environment temperature is elevated, the athlete's muscle and articulations are not ready to start exercising.
- Wear comfortable clothes.
- Start easy and slow.

Start slowly with a general cardiovascular exercise such as walking, jogging, or biking for at least 5 min.

- Warm-ups can also be used to practice skills and team drills.
  Include light running exercises, dynamic flexibility, some agility work, motor control activities, some static and dynamic balance, and plyometrics.
- Smooth transition from the warm-up to a specific activity.
  The warm-up should focus on muscles and movements more specific to the exercise activity planned and work up to the harder work that precedes training or competition. For example, a soccer player could pass, dribble, and shoot a ball; a weightlifter could lift light weights before moving onto greater resistance.
- Slowly increase the amount of time of each workout, the intensity of the workout, and the resistance of the weights. ACSM recommends a 5% increase is a safe progression as the exercise becomes too easy
- Stretch the major and minor muscles.
  It is essential to activate all the muscles involved in the sports activity, especially areas known to be a problem.
  Perform static stretching after working out or alone on its own, and avoid bouncing while stretching, as this can cause injuries.
  For dynamic stretching, it is best to hold the stretch in one position and slowly move it through its range of motion.

7.12 ACSM Flexibility Exercise Recommendations

Variable	Evidence-based recommendation
Frequency	≥2–3 days/week of stretching the major muscle groups; greater gains will be attained if done daily
Intensity	Stretch to the point of slight discomfort or feeling of tightness in muscle
Time	10–30 s of static stretching holds for older persons; 30–60 s of static stretching holds for most adults
PNF stretches	3–6 s of a muscle contraction at 20–75% of maximum intensity followed by 10–30 s of an assisted stretch
Pattern	Two to four repetitions of each stretch is recommended
Volume	Provide a total of 60 s of stretching time per target muscle group for any stretching method utilized

- Multidirectional.
  Do exercises in 360°, in order to activate muscles and work equilibrium and coordination
- Stay hydrated.
  Hydration is very important, particularly for children and the elderly, since they are more susceptible to dehydration. Be sure to drink fluids frequently before, during, and after exercise [39].
  - Drink 16–20 fluid ounces of water or sports beverage at least 4 h before exercise.
  - Drink 8–12 fluid ounces of water 10–15 min before exercise.
  - During exercise, drink 3–8 fluid ounces of water every 15–20 min when exercising for less than 60 min.
  - Drink 3–8 fluid ounces of a sports beverage (5–8% carbohydrate with electrolytes) every 15–20 min when exercising greater than 60 min. Do not drink more than one quart/hour during exercise.
  - Enhancing palatability of fluid will help to encourage fluid consumption. This can be done with proper flavoring, proper salt (sodium) content, and drinking a cold beverage (15–21 °C)
- Body signs.
  The muscle should be heated and stretched enough to feel light to moderate discomfort, but not to feel pain.
- The warm-up is also a good opportunity for an individual to prepare themselves mentally for the game ahead and for a team to work together before starting of the game.

Oriented Warm-Up

- Plan a specific program for the sport/physical activity.
- Choose warm-up modalities (general and specific),
- Start easy and slow (walking, jogging, or biking).

- Soothe transition to a specific activity (jumping, lifting weights, throwing a ball).
- Slowly increase the intensity.
- Multidirectional.
- Stretch.
- Stay hydrated.
- Listen to body signs.
- Choose proper training equipments.
- Use it as a mental work.

Take-Home Message

The warm-up is a well-accepted strategy for athletes and coaches. Although the literature differs in what type of scheme is the best to use, there is general agreement that it is essential to prepare your muscles for the activity. Proper progression is the key to preventing injuries. An effective warm-up program prepares the muscles, tendons, and joints for work by allowing them to move freely through a full active range of motion. The more prepared the body is, the less likely it is to get injured, and better sports performance will be achieved.

References

1. American College of Sports Medicine. Health Fitness J. 2017;21(6):10–19.
2. Woods K, Bishop P, Jones E. Warm-up and stretching in the prevention of muscular injury. Sports Med. 2007;37(12):1089–99.
3. Minshull C, et al. The differential effects of PNF versus passive stretch conditioning on neuromuscular performance. Eur J Sport Sci. 2014;14(3):233–41.
4. Furness J, et al. Epidemiology of injuries in stand-up paddle boarding. Orthop J Sports Med. 2017;5(6):2325967117710759.
5. Arliani GG, et al. Orthopaedics injuries in male professional football players in Brazil: a prospective comparison between two divisions. Muscles Ligaments Tendons J. 2017;7(3):524–31.
6. Gescheit DT, et al. Injury epidemiology of tennis players at the 2011-2016 Australian Open Grand Slam. Br J Sports Med. 2017;51(17):1289–94.
7. McCrary JM, Ackermann BJ, Halaki M. A systematic review of the effects of upper body warm-up on performance and injury. Br J Sports Med. 2015;49(14):935–42.
8. Gogte K, Srivastav P, Miyaru GB. Effect of passive, active and combined warm up on lower limb muscle performance and dynamic stability in recreational sports players. J Clin Diagn Res. 2017;11(3):YC05–8.
9. Andrade DC, et al. Effects of general, specific and combined warm-up on explosive muscular performance. Biol Sport. 2015;32(2):123–8.
10. Landry M. Brukner & Khan's clinical sports medicine. Physiother Can. 2014;66(1):109–10.
11. McGowan CJ, et al. Warm-up strategies for sport and exercise: mechanisms and applications. Sports Med. 2015;45(11):1523–46.
12. Slauterbeck JR, et al. Characterization of prepractice injury prevention exercises of high school athletic teams. Sports Health. 2017;9(6):511–7.
13. Chatzopoulos DE, et al. Warm-up protocols for high school students. Percept Mot Skills. 2015;121(1):1–13.
14. Donald K. Warm-up & injury prevention in football. Aspetar Sports Med J. 2012;1(2):128–35.
15. Bishop D. Warm up II: performance changes following active warm up and how to structure the warm up. Sports Med. 2003;33(7):483–98.
16. Takizawa K, Yamaguchi T, Shibata K. Warm-up exercises may not be so important for enhancing submaximal running performance. J Strength Cond Res. 2017.
17. Anderson P, Landers G, Wallman K. Effect of warm-up on intermittent sprint performance. Rev Sports Med. 2014;22(1):88–99.
18. Pojskic H, et al. Acute effects of prolonged intermittent low-intensity isometric warm-up schemes on jump, sprint, and agility performance in collegiate soccer players. Biol Sport. 2015;32(2):129–34.
19. Racinais S, Cocking S, Periard JD. Sports and environmental temperature: from warming-up to heating-up. Temperature (Austin). 2017;4(3):227–57.
20. Ghareeb DM, et al. Effects of two warm-up programs on balance and isokinetic strength in male high school soccer players. J Strength Cond Res. 2017;31(2):372–9.
21. Zech A, Wellmann K. Perceptions of football players regarding injury risk factors and prevention strategies. PLoS One. 2017;12(5):e0176829.
22. Pomares-Noguera C, et al. Training effects of the FIFA 11+ kids on physical performance in youth football players: a randomized control trial. Front Pediatr. 2018;6:40.
23. Teles MC, et al. Comparison between whole-body vibration, light-emitting diode, and cycling warm-up on high-intensity physical performance during sprint bicycle exercise. J Strength Cond Res. 2015;29(6):1542–50.
24. Gouttebarge V, et al. The prevention of musculoskeletal injuries in volleyball: the systematic development of an intervention and its feasibility. Inj Epidemiol. 2017;4(1):25.
25. Neiva HP, et al. Warm-up and performance in competitive swimming. Sports Med. 2014;44(3):319–30.
26. Scott DJ, Ditroilo M, Marshall P. Complex training: the effect of exercise selection and training status on post-activation potentiation in rugby league players. J Strength Cond Res. 2017;31:3694–703.
27. Wallmann HW, et al. The acute effects of various types of stretching static, dynamic, ballistic, and no stretch of the iliopsoas on 40-yard sprint times in recreational runners. Int J Sports Phys Ther. 2012;7(5):540–7.
28. Faigenbaum AD, et al. Dynamic warm-up protocols, with and without a weighted vest, and fitness

performance in high school female athletes. J Athl Train. 2006;41(4):357–63.
29. Frikha M, et al. Influence of warm-up duration and recovery interval prior to exercise on anaerobic performance. Biol Sport. 2016;33(4):361–6.
30. Lavie CJ, et al. Exercise and the cardiovascular system: clinical science and cardiovascular outcomes. Circ Res. 2015;117(2):207–19.
31. Batista MB, et al. Validity of field tests to estimate cardiorespiratory fitness in children and adolescents: a systematic review. Rev Paul Pediatr. 2017;35(2):222–33.
32. Borg GA. Psychophysical bases of perceived exertion. Med Sci Sports Exerc. 1982;14(5):377–81.
33. van den Tillaar R, Vatten T, von Heimburg E. Effects of short or long warm-up on intermediate running performance. J Strength Cond Res. 2017;31(1):37–44.
34. ACSM's Health Fitness J. 2016;20.
35. McGorm H, et al. Turning up the heat: an evaluation of the evidence for heating to promote exercise recovery, muscle rehabilitation and adaptation. Sports Med. 2018;48(6):1311–28.
36. Wilkins LW. American College of Sports Medicine. 40:1529–7.
37. Blazevich AJ, et al. No effect of muscle stretching within a full, dynamic warm-up on athletic performance. Med Sci Sports Exerc. 2018;50(6):1258–66. https://doi.org/10.1249/MSS.0000000000001539.
38. Cengiz A. EMG and peak force responses to PNF stretching and the relationship between stretching-induced force deficits and bilateral deficits. J Phys Ther Sci. 2015;27(3):631–4.
39. ACSM's guidelines for exercise testing and prescription. 10 ed. 2017.
40. Lobel EE. The influence of two stretching techniques on standing hip range of motion. J Dance Med Sci. 2016;20(1):38–43. https://doi.org/10.12678/1089-313X.20.1.38.
41. Walsh GS. Effect of static and dynamic muscle stretching as part of warm up procedures on knee joint proprioception and strength. Hum Mov Sci. 2017;55:189–95.
42. Chatzopoulos D, et al. Acute effects of static and dynamic stretching on balance, agility, reaction time and movement time. J Sports Sci Med. 2014;13(2):403–9.
43. Su H, et al. Acute effects of foam rolling, static stretching, and dynamic stretching during warm-ups on muscular flexibility and strength in young adults. J Sport Rehabil. 2017;26(6):469–77.
44. Simpson CL, et al. Increase in post activation potentiation in females following a cycling warmup. Hum Mov Sci. 2018;57:171–7.
45. Hancock AP, Sparks KE, Kullman EL. Postactivation potentiation enhances swim performance in collegiate swimmers. J Strength Cond Res. 2015;29(4):912–7.
46. Ronnestad BR, Slettalokken G, Ellefsen S. Adding whole body vibration to preconditioning exercise increases subsequent on-ice sprint performance in ice-hockey players. J Strength Cond Res. 2016;30(4):1021–6.
47. Lum D. Effects of various warm up protocol on special judo fitness test performance. J Strength Cond Res. 2017. https://doi.org/10.1519/JSC.0000000000001862.
48. Ronnestad BR, Falch GS, Ellefsen S. The effect of whole-body vibration on subsequent sprint performance in well-trained cyclists. Int J Sports Physiol Perform. 2017;12(7):964–8.
49. Hammami A, et al. The efficacy and characteristics of warm-up and re-warm-up practices in soccer players: a systematic review. J Sports Med Phys Fitness. 2018;58(1-2):135–49.
50. Egan-Shuttler JD, et al. The effect of concurrent plyometric training versus submaximal aerobic cycling on rowing economy, peak power, and performance in male high school rowers. Sports Med Open. 2017;3:7.
51. Creekmur CC, et al. Effects of plyometrics performed during warm-up on 20 and 40 m sprint performance. J Sports Med Phys Fitness. 2017;57(5):550–5.
52. Ramirez-Campillo R, et al. Sequencing effects of plyometric training applied before or after regular soccer training on measures of physical fitness in young players. J Strength Cond Res. 2018.
53. Cochrane D. The sports performance application of vibration exercise for warm-up, flexibility and sprint speed. Eur J Sport Sci. 2013;13(3):256–71. https://doi.org/10.1080/17461391.2011.606837.
54. Duc S, Ronnestad BR, Bertucci W. Adding whole body vibration to preconditioning squat exercise increases cycling sprint performance. J Strength Cond Res. 2017. https://doi.org/10.1519/JSC.0000000000002236.
55. Buttifant D, Hrysomallis C. Effect of various practical warm-up protocols on acute lower-body power. J Strength Cond Res. 2015;29(3):656–60.
56. Renberg J, et al. Effect of ambient temperature on female endurance performance. J Therm Biol. 2014;45:9–14.
57. Levels K, et al. Effect of warm-up and precooling on pacing during a 15-km cycling time trial in the heat. Int J Sports Physiol Perform. 2013;8(3):307–11.
58. Al-Horani RA, et al. Precooling and warm-up effects on time trial cycling during heat stress. Aerosp Med Hum Perform. 2018;89(2):87–93.

8 Nutrition and Hydration

Daniéla Oliveira Magro

8.1 Introduction

The purpose of this chapter is to provide evidence-based information regarding nutrition and hydration for physical sports and their benefits as well as recommendation to prevent nutrition deficits, low performance during the sports exercises and recovery, and health risks.

To support and promote optimal performance, various aspects related to nutrition can cause fatigue and deterioration in the outputs of performance (e.g., power strength, agility, skill, and concentration) throughout or toward the end of the sporting event. These factors include dehydration, electrolyte imbalances, glycogen depletion, hypoglycemia, gastrointestinal discomfort, and disturbances to acid-base balance.

The amount of food intake throughout the day must provide to athlete's adequate proportion of macro- and micronutrients according to the timing and exercise type.

Macronutrients are carbohydrates, protein, and fat which are important for athletes' nutrition to keep performance up, avoid fatigue and associated injuries, maintain immune function, prevent overtraining, and achieve goals. Vitamins and mineral are micronutrients that are essential for the metabolism and athletes' performance.

D. O. Magro (✉)
Department of Surgery, Faculty of Medical Sciences, State University of Campinas (Unicamp), Campinas, SP, Brazil

This chapter will be divided mainly into the following topics: (a) energy needs, (b) carbohydrate in exercise (before, during, after), (c) protein in exercise, (d) fat in exercise, (e) hydration in exercise (before, during, after), and (f) vitamins and minerals and strategic of exercise length accordingly.

The aspects related to nutrition and hydration in sports will be discussed for the main categories of sports: endurance and resistance training.

8.2 Energy Needs During Exercise

According to the International Olympic Committee (IOC), an athlete's energy requirements consist of several components: baseline metabolic needs (such as the energy required to support cellular maintenance, temperature regulation, and immune health) and growth and physical activity [1].

Energy balance occurs when total energy intake (EI) equals total energy expenditure (TEE), which then consists of the summation of basal metabolic rate (BMR), the thermic effect of food (TEF), and the thermic effect of activity (TEA = planned exercise expenditure, more spontaneous physical activity, more no-exercise activity thermogenesis) [2].

$$\mathbf{TEE = BMR + TEF + TEA}$$

S. Rocha Piedade et al. (eds.), *The Sports Medicine Physician*,
https://doi.org/10.1007/978-3-030-10433-7_8

BMR can be obtained by using Cunningham [3] or Harris-Benedict [4] equations, as an appropriate activity factor to estimate TEE. The first component to optimize training and performance through nutrition is to ensure the athlete is consuming enough calories to offset energy expenditure [5].

Athlete's energy requirements depend on the periodized training and competition cycle and will vary from day to day according to volume and intensity. Factors that increase energy needs above normal baseline levels include exposure to cold or heat, fear, stress, high altitude, and others [2]. Athletes are vulnerable to changes in energy availability and fast weight loss programs, or those who are afraid of eating proper fuel are associated with health and performance decrements, including impairment of hormone, immune, and metabolic function and irreversible loss of bone mass [1].

According to the International Society for Sports Nutrition (ISSN), people who participate in a general fitness program (e.g., exercising 30–40 min per day, three times per week) need to follow a normal diet (e.g., 1800–2400 kcal/day or about 25–35 kcal/day for a 50–80 kg individual) because their caloric demands to exercise are not too great (e.g., 200–400 kcal/session). Athletes involved in moderate levels of intense training (e.g., 2–3 h/day, 5–6 times a week) need 50–80 kcal/kg/day (2500–8000 kcal/day for a 50–100 kg athlete). For elite athletes, energy expenditure during heavy training or competition may be huge (e.g., 100–150 kcal/kg/day for a 60–80 kg athlete may range between 6000 and 12,000 kcal/day) depending on the volume and intensity of different training phases [5, 6].

8.3 Carbohydrate in Exercise

Carbohydrates are the main energy source during high-intensity activity [6] for the central nervous system as well as muscle fuel [2, 6]. The inadequate endogenous carbohydrate availability is associated with an impaired team sports performance [7], fatigue in the form of reduced work rates, impaired skill and concentration, and increased perception of effort [2].

From a historical perspective, the nutrient timing was first conceptualized in the 1970s and 1980s with the initial work that examined the effects of increased carbohydrate feedings on glycogen status and exercise performance [8]. A variety of carbohydrate sources from both food and fluids are effective in restoring glycogen stores, the choices being determined by athlete preference (taste), practicality, and availability [7]. Ivy and collaborators were one of the first groups to demonstrate that carbohydrate timing could influence postexercise rates of glycogen resynthesis [9]. Moderate to high glycemic index carbohydrate choices are adequate because glycogen storage will, in part, be regulated by rapid glucose supply and insulin response [7] and the intake of carbohydrates is suboptimal; the addition of protein (0.3–4 g/kg/h) may help maximize glycogen resynthesis during recovery [10].

There are differences in the quantity of carbohydrate requirement that vary according to athletes' needs, based on training intensity, type of workout, and timing during the session. Higher intakes of carbohydrate are associated with better performance.

In general, athletes will need to consume 3–5 g per kilogram body weight (BW) daily for low activity [1–3] and 8–12 g per kg BW per day for high intense training (≥70% VO_2 max) of 12 h per week [2, 6, 8]. The carbohydrate intake level has been shown to maximize glycogen storage and to avoid muscle damage. The dietary reference intake (DRI) for carbohydrate (60–70% of total daily caloric intake) has fallen out due to inability to appropriately prescribe required carbohydrate amounts in athletes eating high amounts of food or in those who may be following a restricted energy intake [8] (Table 8.1).

Carbohydrate intake should be consumed throughout the day, as well as before or during the session or recovery period.

Before session, the carbohydrate choice may be poor fat, protein, fiber, and residues and easily consumed and to meet goals, gut comfort and "racing weight" [2]. Athletes' individual preferences and experiences should be respected. Carbohydrate-rich food and drink may help to achieve target and consumption during the

Table 8.1 Summary of carbohydrate intake guideline: daily needs for fuel and recovery

Sports activity level/organization	The timing of carbohydrate intake	g/kg body weight per day
Low		
ISSN	Physical activities in general, 30–60 min/day, 3–4 times a week	3–5
IOC		3–5
Moderate		
ISSN	2–3 h/day, 5–6 times a week	5–8
IOC	Exercise program—1 h/day	5–7
High		
ISSN	3–6 h/day, 1–2 sessions, 5–6 times a week	8–10
IOC	Endurance program—1–3 h/day	6–10
Very high		
IOC	Extreme commitment >4–5 h/day	8–12
Strength-trained athletes		
IOC	Undetermined period	4–7
Acute fueling strategies (high carbohydrate to promote optimal performance)		
General fueling up	Preparation for events <90 min	7–12 g/kg/24 h as for daily fuel needs
Carbohydrate loading	Preparation for events >90 min of sustained/intermittent exercise	10–12 g/kg/24 h (by 36–48 h)
Speedy refueling	<8 h recovery between two fuel-demanding sessions	1–1.2 g/kg/h for first 4 h and then resume daily fuel needs
Pre-event fueling	Before exercise >60 min	1–4 g/kg consumed, 1–4 h before exercise
Fueling strategies during exercise		
During brief exercise	<45 min	Not needed
During sustained high-intensity exercise	45–75 min	Small amount including mouth rinse
During endurance exercise, including "stop-and-start" sports	1–2.5 h	30–60 g/h
During ultra-endurance exercise	≥2.5–3 h	Up to 90 g/h

ISSN International Society for Sports Nutrition, *IOC* International Olympic Committee [1]
Table adapted by Thomas et al. [2] and Jeffrey R. Bytomski, DO [6]

sessions according to rules and nature of each sport. Sports products (sports drinks, gels, and bars) with multiple transportable carbohydrates (glucose, fructose mixtures) achieve high rates of oxidation of carbohydrate consumed during exercise [2]. Consumption of 1.5–2 cups fluid with 6–8% carbohydrate solution per 100 mL sustains blood glucose levels and maximizes performance [8].

According to the IOC, several everyday food and drink such as fruit, juices, and soft drinks may also be suitable. The athlete should practice in training to develop a race or event fueling plan. This plan will need to take into account the opportunities provided in the athlete's event to consume drink or food [1].

8.4 Protein in Exercise

Proteins are at the macronutrients' level. They are comprised of two types of amino acids, essential (phenylalanine, valine, threonine, tryptophan, methionine, leucine, isoleucine, lysine, and histidine) and nonessential (alanine, arginine, aspartic acid, cysteine, glutamic acid, glutamine, glycine, proline, serine, tyrosine, asparagine, selenocysteine, pyrrolysine), with the former only being fully obtained through nutrition because our bodies cannot produce them [6], and the latter is synthesized by our organism.

There are many questions on how much protein is needed for athletes. DRI [11] for protein is 0.8 g per kilogram body weight for sedentary individuals [6, 11, 12]. Many studies showed that athletes have higher daily protein requirements [13, 14]. Proteins are important for several metabolic processes. They are responsible for building blocks of the muscle and tendons and essential for building enzymes, hormones, and neurotransmitters for several bodily functions which include facilitating muscle repair, muscle and immune function remodeling, and injury recovery [6, 7, 8, 15]. Protein provides only a small source of fuel for the exercising muscle but has a substantial anabolic effect on protein synthesis when combined with exercise [1].

The key component of the muscle remodeling is muscle protein synthesis (MPS), the synthesis of amino acids into functional contractile myofibrillar proteins and end-energy-producing mitochondrial proteins [7]. Multiple factors, including the source, per meal dose, daytime pattern, and timing (about exercise) of ingested protein, as well as co-ingestion of other nutrients, all modulate the response of MPS to protein intake [7, 15, 16].

The American College of Sports Medicine (ACSM), International Society for Sports Nutrition (ISSN), and International Olympic Committee (IOC) provide a consensus which stated that the daily protein requirements of athletes range between 1.2 and 2.0 per kilogram body weight per day. IOC recommends 1.8–2.7 g per kilogram BW per day when the athlete is trying to lose fat while gaining lean mass in a slight caloric deficit and proper training program [1, 6, 15]. It should be taken into consideration whether the athlete has a normal kidney function because some authors discussed the deleterious effects of high-protein diets including kidney failure and osteoporosis [6]. Recommended sources of protein for athletes include lean meats (chicken, pork, beef) and fish, cottage cheese, eggs, milk, Greek yogurts, and protein shakes. Protein sources for vegetarian athletes may include beans, lentils, quinoa, black beans, peas, chickpeas, almonds, and vegetarian protein shakes. The protein supplements are used when needed.

Leucine supplement, essential amino acid, such as whey protein is rapidly digested. Both have been shown to elicit a greater stimulation of MPS during recovery compared with a slowly digested protein of lower leucine composition, such as soy, micellar casein, and wheat [7, 15]. Endurance exercise increases leucine oxidation [14].

It is known that resistance training is very different from endurance training, and the result is that the muscle requires more of the specific proteins needed to reach a higher level of performance. A recent updated published by ISSN, in 2017 [14], included new information on the most important dietary protein for exercise performance, categorized in endurance and resistance exercise performance (increases in maximal strength). The main information is described in Table 8.2.

There is consensus from ACSM, ISSN, and IOC on the beneficial effect of the ingestion of ~20 g protein with carbohydrates within 30 min postexercise because it might support an enhanced performance, to facilitate muscle protein synthesis; however, no plausible mechanism for this effect is readily available until now [1, 2, 9]. Protein serves both as a substrate and a trigger for adaptation after both resistance and aerobic exercises. Protein intake that exceeds this recommended amount does not promote MPS but can result in protein oxidation. This recovery strategy can be achieved through dietary sources. Additional supplementation is not essential [1].

ISSN recommends and IOC recognizes that the addition of creatine monohydrate as a supplement after exercise can increase skeletal muscle hypertrophy after resistance training. The practical application of this is questionable [2, 13]. Creatine is a nonessential nutrient that is produced endogenously in the liver, pancreas, and kidneys and is also consumed through the diet [7]. It is normally found in meat and fish, but the doses that are commonly used (20 g per day for 4–5 days to load and then 2–3 g per day for maintenance) are more than those found in normal food. Supplementation of creatine after exercise is not necessary and can even be harmful to health [1]. The same results can be achieved with the ingestion of sufficient carbohydrate and high biological value protein after exercise [2]. Creatine supplementation might be important for vegan

Table 8.2 Summary of protein intake guideline

	Endurance exercise performance	Resistance exercise performance
Protein recommendation	• Adequate carbohydrate is delivered; adding protein to carbohydrate does not appear to improve endurance performance over the course of a few days or weeks • Protein doses should contain 700–3000 mg of leucine and a higher relative leucine content, in addition to a balanced array of the essential amino acids (EAAs). These protein doses should ideally be evenly distributed, every 3–4 h, across the day. Rapidly digested proteins that contain high proportions of EAAs and adequate leucine are most effective in stimulating MPS	• Hyperenergetic diet, a heavy resistance training program, and protein supplementation may promote increases in skeletal muscle cross-sectional area and lean body mass • An elevated daily intake of protein (2–3 × the RDA) can promote greater losses of fat mass and greater overall improvements in body composition • Resistance exercise and protein ingestion both stimulate synthesis MPS and are synergistic when protein consumption occurs before or after resistance exercise. There is novel evidence that suggests higher protein intakes (>3.0 g/kg/day) may have positive effects on body composition • Recommendations regarding the optimal protein intake per serving for athletes to maximize MPS are mixed and are dependent upon age and recent resistance exercise stimuli
Protein before exercise	• Endurance athletes should focus on achieving adequate carbohydrate intake to promote optimal performance; the addition of protein may help to offset muscle damage and promote recovery	• Pre-event meal resistance exercise can be achieved by including 0.15–0.25 g/kg BW protein with the recommended 1–2 g/kg BW carbohydrates, 3–4 h before training or competition
Protein during exercise	• Adding protein during an intensive endurance exercise may suppress the rise in plasma proteins linked to myofibrillar damage and reduce feelings of muscle soreness 12–24 h post-exercise. • It is recommended for endurance athletes to ingest approximately 0.25 g of protein/kg body weight per hour of endurance exercise (in addition to the athlete's regular carbohydrate intake) • The addition of protein to carbohydrates (carbohydrates to protein ratio of 3–4:1) during exercise has shown promise • Ingestion of carbohydrate + protein or amino acids (EAAs) during endurance exercise can help to maintain a favorable anabolic hormone profile, promote increases in muscle cross-sectional area, and increase the time to exhaustion during prolonged training	Not needed
Post-exercise	• Administration of protein when combined with suboptimal intake of carbohydrates (<1.2/kg/day) can increase muscle glycogen recovery and may help mitigate changes in muscle damage • Adding protein after an intensive endurance exercise may damage and reduce feelings of muscle soreness 12–24 h post-exercise. The recommendation for recovery is a carbohydrate to protein ratio of 3–4:1 or 0.2–0.5 g/kg BW protein • ISSN also recommends that ingestion of essential amino acid (EAA) stimulates by adding 6–20 g EAA to at least 30–40 g high glycemic carbohydrates which should be ingested immediately or within 3 h post-exercise	• General recommendations are 0.25 g of a high-quality protein per kg of body weight, or an absolute dose of 20–40 g (10–12 g of EAAs, 1–3 g of leucine) stimulates MPS, which can help to promote a positive nitrogen balance • Skeletal muscle is sensitized to the effects of protein and amino acids (EAAs) for up to 24 h after completion of a bout of resistance exercise

athletes to consider and compensate for reduced muscle creatine stores experienced as a result of their lifestyle choices [17].

8.5 Fat in Exercise

Fat requirements for athletes are similar to those for nonathletes (20–35% total daily calories) [12]. IOC does not recommend consuming less than 15–20% of total calories from fat, because it is essential for many metabolic processes, including cell membrane structure, absorption of fat-soluble vitamins, hormone regulation, brain health, and energy for muscle metabolism [2, 13].

There are two essential fatty acids, alpha-linolenic acid (omega-3 fatty acid—fish, nuts, chia) and linoleic acid (omega-6 fatty acid—vegetable oils, margarine, grains, fast and processed food), that our organism cannot synthesize them and must be supplied by food [2]. The main symptoms of essential fatty acid deficiencies are skin lesions, infertility, and increased susceptibility to infections.

Athletes should focus on good sources of fat which are high in unsaturated fats and essential fatty acids (requirement: 2% total calories omega-6; at least 1.3% total calories omega-3). The proportion of energy from saturated fats should be limited to less than 10% and trans fat ingestion avoided [2, 6]. Healthy sources of fat include salmon, nuts and nut butters, and avocado, as well as olive oil. Athletes may also consider taking omega-3 (PUFA) supplements (3 g/day, of 1.3 g of EPA and 0.3 g of DHA), as they can also counteract inflammatory (increased interleukin (IL)-2 production and the cytotoxic activity of natural killer cells during 3 h of exercise recovery) and free radical formation sustained from training. Recently studies showed that omega-3 promoted muscle remodeling, muscle repair, and immune surveillance and also exhibit immunomodulatory properties [7, 13].

Fat in the form of plasma-free fatty acids, intramuscular triglycerides, and adipose tissue provides a fuel substrate that is both relatively plentiful and increased in availability to the muscle as a result of endurance exercise (>90 min). Athletes consuming less than 10% of their calories from carbohydrates can oxidize fat between 1.2 and 1.5 g/min during a progressive-intensity exercise near 65% VO_2 max. A fat-burning adapted ironman triathlete can use the fat stored in his/her body to fuel the race effectively at that oxidation rate for the entire race compared with a carbohydrate-burning athlete who needed to consume another 90–105 g per hour to maintain performance [2, 6, 7].

During resistance training, such as weight lifting, creatine phosphate (CP) and carbohydrate are predominant as an energy source, being proportionally lower to the contribution of lipids to energy synthesis [18].

8.6 Hydration in Sports

Athletes usually need to hydrate before, during, and after exercise. The main goals of hydration are optimization of the performance, prevention of metabolic strain, and thermoregulation during exercise. Most authorities warn that athletes losing >2% body weight during activity (e.g., 1.0 kg for 50 kg person, 1.5 kg for a 75 kg person, and 2 kg for a 100 kg person) may show decrease in cognitive function and performance [1, 2, 6, 19, 20]. Thirst is often not a good indicator of dehydration. An athlete can lose until 1.5 L before thirst is perceived [6]. Athletes may lose from 0.3 to 2.4 L per hour of sweat, and rates vary based on environment, sex, body size, and type and length of activity [1]. Sweat comprises water, sodium, potassium, calcium, magnesium, and chloride, so athletes should replace both fluids and electrolytes with their recovery strategy [6]. Dehydration refers to the process of losing body water and leads to hypohydration [2].

8.6.1 Is There Any Need to Hydrate If Training Session Lasts Less Than an Hour?

It is not necessary to drink during exercise that lasts less than about 40 min unless the athlete starts the session dehydrated. When it is not possible to drink during "heavy-sweating"-type exercise lasting longer than 30 min, an alternative is to hydrate 15 min before starting the session (e.g., 300–800 mL) [1].

8.6.2 Hot Days/Cold Days: Is There Any Difference Regarding How to Hydrate?

Hot environments (when the ambient temperature exceeds body temperature heat) and exercise reinforce a higher risk of impaired performance and heat illness. A more feasible alternative is to try to minimize dehydration. In some situations, athletes overhydrate during exercise if they are drinking more than their sweat losses. The problems can occur when the fluid intake is rapid and excessive leading to hyponatremia (dilution of blood sodium concentration) [1, 2].

Strategies to reduce high skin temperatures and large sweat (fluid and electrolyte) in hot environments should include acclimatization, individualized hydration plans, regular monitoring of hydration status, beginning exercise hydrated, consuming cold fluids during exercise, and the inclusion of electrolyte [2] (Fig. 8.1).

In cold environments, the primary strategy is the maintenance of euhydration and body temperature with appropriate clothing. Several factors can increase the risk of hypohydration, such as cold-induced diuresis, impaired thirst sensation, reduced desire to drink, limited access to fluids, self-restricted fluid intake to minimize urination, sweat losses from overdressing, and increased respiration with high-altitude exposure. Fluid intakes should be regularly assessed and changes in BW and hydration status when exercising in both hot and cold environments [2].

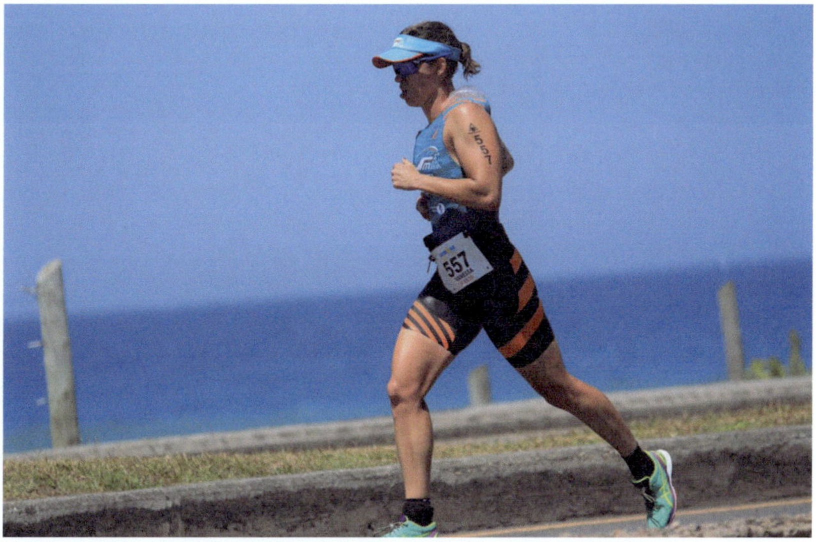

Fig. 8.1 Athlete with *ice bag* in her back

Table 8.3 How to estimate sweat losses and sweat rates[a]

1. Measure body mass before and after at least 1 h of exercise under conditions similar to competition or a hard practice
2. Take these body mass measurements wearing minimal clothing and while bare footed. Towel dry after exercise, and obtain body mass as soon as is practical after exercise (e.g., less than 10 min and before eating, drinking, or going to the toilet)
Example: Pre-exercise weight = 74.5 kg. Post-exercise weight = 72.8 kg. Fluid deficit = 1.7 kg
3. Estimate the weight of any fluid or food you have consumed during the workout
Example: 800 mL of fluid = 800 g or 0.8 kg
4. Sweat loss (liters) = body mass before exercise (in kg) – body mass after exercise (kg) + weight of fluids/foods consumed (kg)
Example: 74.5 kg – 72.8 kg = 1.7 kg deficit + 0.80 kg (800 mL fluid) = sweat loss of 2.5 kg or 2500 mL
To convert to a sweat rate per hour, divide by the exercise time in minutes, and multiply by 60
5. Weight deficit at the end of the session provides a guide to hydrate during the session and how much is needed to rehydrate afterward. To convert kg to % body mass, divide the weight deficit by starting body mass, and multiply by 100:
Example: 1.7 kg/74.5 × 100 = 2.3%
Note: 2.2 pounds equals 1.0 kg and converts to a volume of 1000 mL or 1 L

[a]**Source: Nutrition for athletes—A practical guide to eating for health and performance IOC** [1]

Before exercise. Athletes should intake a fluid volume equivalent to 5–10 mL/kg BW (~2–4 mL/lb) for 2–4 h pre-session to achieve pale yellow urine color allowing enough time to empty excess fluid. Sodium consumed in pre-exercise fluids and food may help with fluid retention. Glycerol and other plasma expanders for this purpose are prohibited by the World Anti-Doping Agency (WADA) [2, 21].

During exercise. An hour exercise duration can lead to fatigue, so athletes are advised to consume some liquid carbohydrate source that is rapidly converted to blood glucose [1]. Routine measurement of body weight pre- and post-exercise, in addition to urinary losses and drink volume, can help athletes estimate sweat losses during sporting activities and customize their fluid replacement strategies (Table 8.3). Fluid plan that suits most athletes and athletic events will typically achieve an intake of 0.4–0.8 L/h, although it is needed to customize the athlete's tolerance and experience, their opportunities for drinking fluids, and the benefits of consuming other nutrients (e.g., carbohydrate) in drink form (Figs. 8.2 and 8.3).

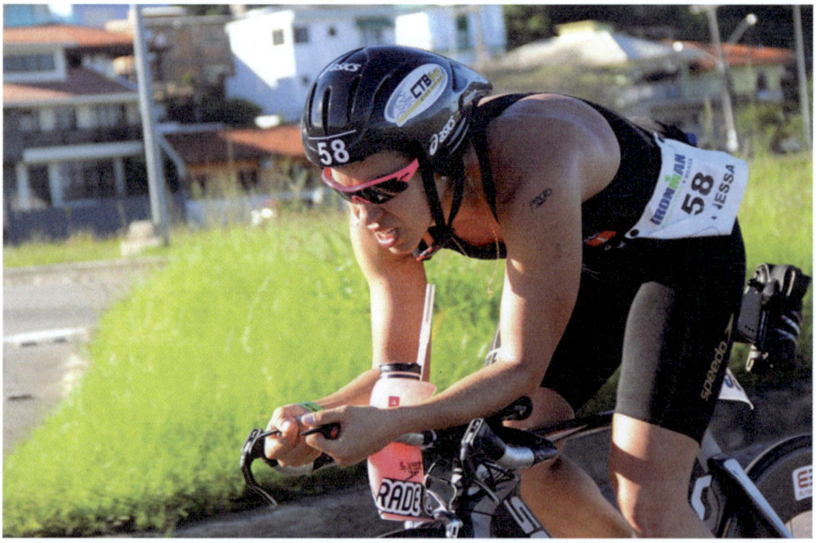

Fig. 8.2 An athlete having fluid drinks during Ironman Brazil, on a sunny day

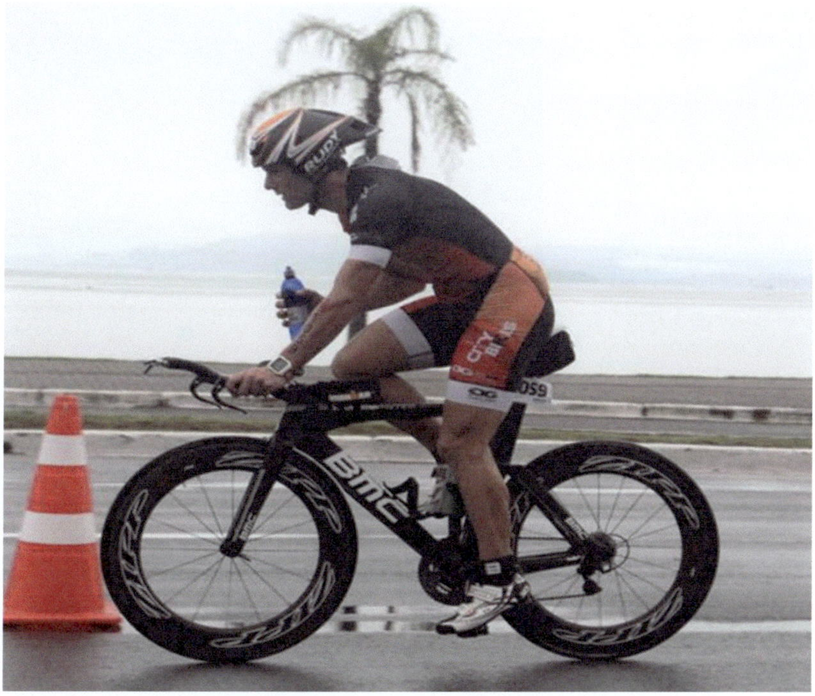

Fig. 8.3 An athlete having fluid drinks during Ironman Brazil, on a cloudy day

8.6.3 Overhydration or Hypohydration: What Might Happen?

Overdrinking fluids and sweat and urinary losses in excess might be the primary cause of hyponatremia (plasma sodium <135 mmol/L), also known as water intoxication, although this can be exacerbated in cases where there are excessive losses of sodium in sweat and fluid replacement involving low sodium beverages. Symptoms of hyponatremia include bloating, puffiness, weight gain, nausea, vomiting, headache, confusion, delirium, seizures, respiratory distress, loss of consciousness, and possibly death if untreated [2].

Sodium should be ingested during exercise when large sweat sodium losses (>1.2 L/h), salty sweat, or prolonged exercise exceeding 1–2 h in duration (e.g., 3–4 g of sodium, in hot and humid climate) occurs [1, 2].

Skeletal muscle cramps are typically caused by muscle fatigue and may be associated with hypohydration and electrolyte imbalances. Sports drinks with sodium (e.g., 300–500 mg sodium per 500 mL liquid) may help reduce the risk of cramps [1].

After exercise. Most athletes need to restore euhydration during recovery period consumption of water and sodium at a modest rate that minimizes diuresis and urinary losses. The increase in plasma sodium concentration and osmolality with sodium ingestion stimulates renal water reabsorption (e.g., decreases diuresis) and promotes plasma volume restoration [7]. Sodium replacement can be achieved via sodium-containing fluids such as sports drinks and pharmacy oral rehydration solutions. However, a meal (e.g., bread, cheese, and breakfast cereal), snack (e.g., peanuts, crackers), or use of table salt added on food can supply the sodium necessity. Effective rehydration requires volume of fluid intake (e.g., 125–150%) greater than the final fluid deficit (e.g., 1.25–1.5 L fluid for every 1 kg BW lost) to restore fluid losses and optimize glycogen resynthesis when the length of time separating one bout of exercise from another is 8 h [2, 16]. Excessive intake of alcohol in the recovery period is discouraged due to its diuretic effects [2] (Fig. 8.4).

An important and easy hydration indicator can be urine color post training. The darker is the color (copper brown until ruby brown), the more

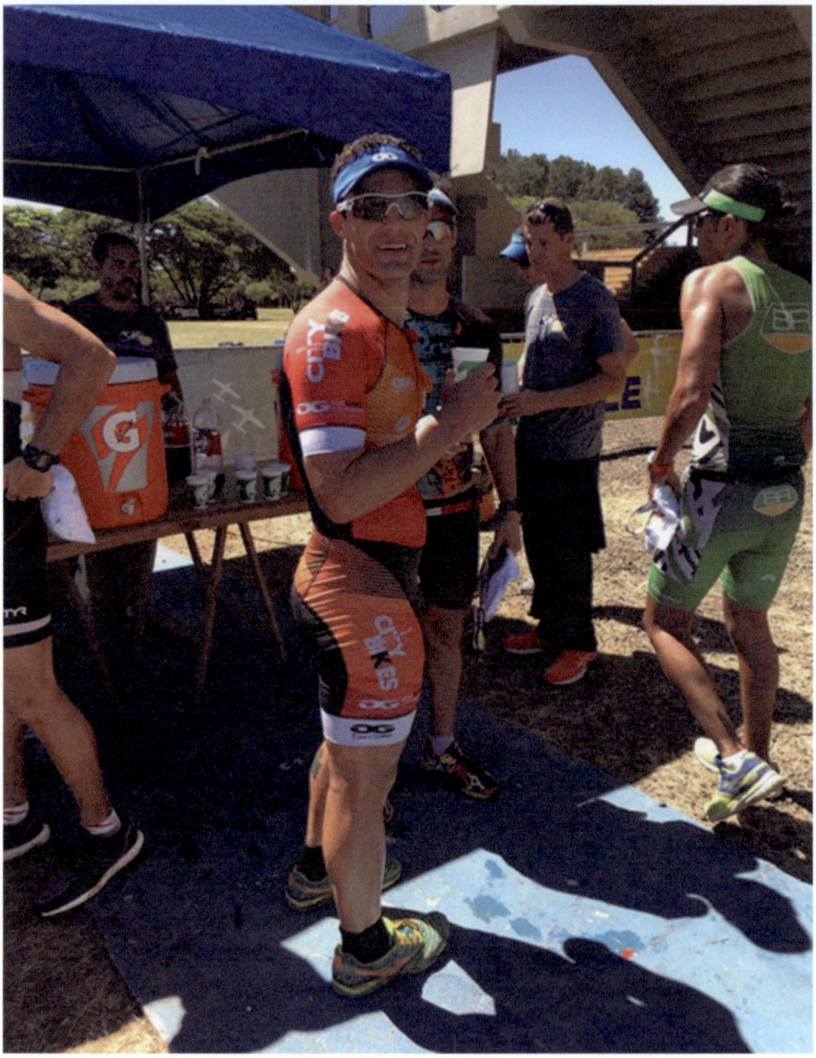

Fig. 8.4 Post-race Hydration, ironman Brazil

is dehydration, requiring larger quantities of liquids for recovery. Recovery after exercise is part of the preparation for the next exercise session, and rehydration should be considered as an important part of the strategy.

IOC presents a very interesting guide to assess the level of post-training dehydration (Table 8.3) [1].

8.7 Micronutrients in Exercise

Micronutrients are comprised of vitamins and minerals which help the body to function, acting as cofactors in metabolism. Vitamins' and minerals' requirements may be increased during athletes training. Most athletes should obtain sufficient micronutrients through a balanced diet, but athletes who practice extreme dietary or weight loss patterns or eliminate whole food groups such as vegetarians may be a risk for certain deficiencies and need micronutrient supplementation, as well as in special conditions with illness, injury, and recovery [1, 2, 6].

Some vitamin and mineral deficiency may decrease performance. The most common deficiencies are iron, vitamin D, calcium, and some antioxidants such as vitamins E and C, vitamin B12, and zinc, mainly for vegetarian athletes [2, 6, 17]. Monitoring blood levels of these

Table 8.4 Deficiencies, requirement, and supplementation of the micronutrients in sports

Micronutrients	Function	Deficiencies	Requirement and supplementation	Toxicity and adverse effects
Iron	A key component in oxygen transport via hemoglobin (blood) and myoglobin (muscle) in energy pathways in the body [1, 6]	Most common in female athletes. Causes include heavy menstruation, inadequate dietary intake (vegan diet), gastrointestinal losses, and training losses both intravascularly and via sweat Athletes can be iron deficient without anemia Serum ferritin is the best indicator of the iron store; levels between <35 and <10 ng/mL and hemoglobin of <12 g/dL have been used to describe deficiency with or without anemia [2, 6]	**DRI**—18 mg for women and 8 mg for men/day [11] Female athletes may have increased requirement of 70% which is more than the average [6] **Vegan athletes:** 33 mg for women and 14 mg for men/day [17] Treatment includes dietary intake (with heme iron (from meats)), oral supplementation (with vitamin C), and intramuscular injections Routine use of iron supplements is not recommended [1] Dosages are controversies but 20 mg of elemental iron 6–8 weeks is recommended [6] Intramuscular and/or intravenous injections should be used only in severe deficiency or those who do not respond to dietary and oral supplementation [6]	Effects of supplementation include gastrointestinal discomfort, constipation, and nausea [2, 6]
Vitamin D (25OHD)	It is essential for calcium absorption. Helps regulate many metabolic pathways in bone health, inflammation, immune function, and muscle function [6, 17, 22] Vitamin D status (blood 25OHD) 30–50 ng/L [7] The major source of vitamin D is provided through the interaction of the skin with UVB light, and its production is affected by age, season, geographic location, and skin pigmentation [1, 22]	Low exposure to ultraviolet B (UVB), stress fracture (overtraining), muscle pain, or weakness. Insufficiency is defined as <30 ng/mL and deficiency as <20 ng/mL [2, 6, 17]	**DRI** recommends 600 IU/day [11], and the UK Department of Health recommends 400 IU/day [17]. Sources of dietary include fish, dairy, and eggs **Supplementation:** **Daily** (2–4000 IU) or weekly (25–50,000 IU) or 4–500 IU/day for vegan athletes [6, 17]. Testing 8 weeks to avoid toxicity [6] 5–30 min of direct sun exposure (arms and legs) several times per week between 10:00 and 14:00 hrs is recommended [13]	Blood 25 OHD values >150 ng/mL (plus hypercalcemia); include nausea, vomiting, poor appetite, weight loss, constipation, weakness, mental confusion, irregularities in cardiac rhythm, and calcification of soft tissues [6, 17]

(continued)

Table 8.4 (continued)

Micronutrients	Function	Deficiencies	Requirement and supplementation	Toxicity and adverse effects
Calcium	It is important for metabolic processes, including bone health (with vitamin D) and muscle contraction, nerve conduction, and clotting functions [6]	Low dietary calcium is associated with disordered eating and low energy availability, especially in adolescents and in female athletes [1] Stress fractures are increased, and low bone mineral density may occur [6] Vegan athletes have a higher risk of fracture due to lower calcium intake [17]	**DRI** for calcium (1000 mg/day) [11] **IOC** recommends 1500 mg per day of calcium, with 1500–2000 IU vitamin D [1, 2, 6]	Intake of calcium through diet is preferable, considering the increased risk of adverse effects, which are kidney stones and cardiovascular events
Antioxidants (vitamins C and E)	Antioxidants have important roles in protecting cell membranes from oxidative damage. Vitamin C promotes collagen synthesis, facilitates glycogen storage, and may prevent exercise-induced oxidative changes Vitamin E blocks the propagation of free radical formation [6]	Increase oxidative stress [6] Greatest risks for poor antioxidant intakes are those who restrict energy intake, follow a chronic low-fat diet, or limit dietary intake of fruits, vegetables, and whole grains [2]	Increase food that is higher in antioxidants such as vitamins C and E (fruits, vegetables, and whole grains) There is little evidence that antioxidant supplementation enhances athletic performance but may be beneficial in athletes recovering from injury [1]	High doses of vitamins C and E can be prooxidant, and large doses of vitamin E can also impede vitamin K metabolism and platelet function [6]
Vitamin B12	Vitamin B12 (cobalamin) is essential for normal nervous system function, homocysteine metabolism, and DNA synthesis [17]	Lead to morphological chances to the blood cells, megaloblastic anemia, and neuropathy [17]	**DRI—**2.4 μg day, both sexes [11] Vegan athletes—6.0 μg day Monitoring B12 status carefully might be necessary for vegan athletes [17]	The body appears to have a limited capacity to absorb vitamin B12 supplements orally which is limited by the presence of intrinsic factor, a glycoprotein secreted by the stomach's parietal cells that combine with B12 before absorption in the distal ileum via receptor-mediated endocytosis [17]
Zinc	It is an essential trace element with numerous biological functions, including immunity, energy metabolism, and antioxidative processes [23]	Impaired immunity and growth retardation [23]	**DRI**— 11 mg for men and 8 mg/day for women [11] Vegan athletes: 16.5 mg for men and 12 mg/day for women [17] Source of dietary include meat, beans, nuts, seeds, oats, wheat germ, egg, and dairy	

micronutrients should be mandatory; whenever they are deficient, supplementation is needed, as well as periodical evaluations. There are no general micronutrient guidelines for athletes. Public health guidelines such as the DRIs provide micronutrient intake recommendations for sports dietitians to help athletes avoid both deficiency and safety concerns associated with excessive intake [2, 11].

Below, Table 8.4 describes the main deficiencies, requirement, and supplementation of micronutrients for athletes.

8.8 Final Considerations

Appropriate nutritional recommendations for macronutrients, micronutrients, and fluids constitute the pinnacle to promote optimal performance and recovery after training and competition. Sports nutrition practice should help athletes and teams work toward their performance-related goals, avoid fatigue and deterioration in skill, or concentrate over the course of the event. All athletes should adopt specific nutritional strategies before, during, and after training and competition. These aspects may depend on the sports categories as well as the timing and intensity of the session.

Athletes are different, and diet and their needs cannot be generalized. Nutritional recommendations need to be individualized for each athlete; they also need to change across the season and training goals.

Essential nutrients can be obtained in adequate amounts from normal foods. A varied and wholesome nutrient-rich diet that encompasses vegetables, fruits, beans, legumes, grains, lean animal meats, fish, oil, and carbohydrates should ensure an adequate intake of all essential vitamins and

Fact Box 1
- Exercise produces catabolic conditions in skeletal muscle, and these effects depend on the intensity and duration.
- The inadequate intake of carbohydrates leads to damage to muscle contraction process, while its availability is inversely related to the rate of protein catabolism during the exercise.
- General recommendation post-exercise is 0.25 g of a high-quality protein per kg of body weight, or an absolute dose of 20–40 g (10–12 g of EAAs, 1–3 g of leucine) stimulates MPS.
- Protein intake that exceeds this recommended amount does not promote MPS, but it can result in protein oxidation.

Fact Box 2
- Hydration aims to optimize the performance, prevention of metabolic strain, and thermoregulation during exercise.
- Athletes losing <2% body weight during activity may show a decrease in cognitive function and performance.
- Sodium should be ingested during exercise when large sweat sodium losses occur.
- Appropriate fluid intake before, during, and after is important for health and performance.
- Overdrinking fluids and sweat and urinary losses in excess might be the primary causes of hyponatremia.
- Vitamin D, iron, and omega-3 polyunsaturated fatty acids are potentially beneficial micronutrients and supplements to help support performance and recovery, when necessary.
- A well-balanced diet with the inclusion of fruits and vegetables to obtain a variety of antioxidants may be more appropriate supplementation.
- Monitoring micronutrients status carefully might be necessary for vegan athletes.

minerals. Supplementation recommendations should always be individualized, granting that targeted supplementation may be warranted to treat or prevent deficiency.

Evidence-based guidelines on the amount, composition, and timing of food intake have been defined to help athletes perform and train more effectively, with less risk of illness and injury.

Athletes should be careful about the indiscriminate use of dietary supplements. The use of a small and lawful number of supplements and sports food may benefit some athletes.

References

1. Nutrition for athletes—a practical guide to eating for health and performance [Internet]. Lausanne: International Olympic Committee; 2016. 37 p. www.olympic.org.
2. Thomas DT, Erdman KA, Burke LM. Position of the Academy of Nutrition and Dietetics, Dietitians of Canada, and the American College of Sports Medicine: nutrition and athletic performance. J Acad Nutr Diet. 2016;116(3):501–28.
3. Cunningham J. A reanalysis of the factors influencing basal metabolic rate in normal adults. Am J Clin Nutr. 1980;33(11):2372–4.
4. Roza A, Shizgal H. The Harris Benedict equation reevaluated: resting energy requirements and the body cell mass. Am J Clin Nutr. 1984;40(1):168–82.
5. Kreider RB, Wilborn CD, Taylor L, Campbell B, Almada AL, Collins R, et al. ISSN exercise & sport nutrition review: research & recommendations. J Int Soc Sports Nutr. 2010;7(1):7.
6. Bytomski JR. Fueling for performance. Sports Health Multidiscip Approach. 2018;10(1):47–53.
7. Heaton LE, Davis JK, Rawson ES, Nuccio RP, Witard OC, Stein KW, et al. Selected in-season nutritional strategies to enhance recovery for team sport athletes: a practical overview. Sports Med. 2017;47(11):2201–18.
8. Kerksick CM, Arent S, Schoenfeld BJ, Stout JR, Campbell B, Wilborn CD, et al. International Society of Sports Nutrition Position Stand: nutrient timing. J Int Soc Sports Nutr [Internet]. 2017 Dec [cited 2017 Dec 27];14(1). Available from: http://jissn.biomedcentral.com/articles/10.1186/s12970-017-0189-4.
9. Ivy JL, Katz AL, Cutler CL, Sherman WM, Coyle EF. Muscle glycogen synthesis after exercise: effect of time of carbohydrate ingestion. J Appl Physiol. 1988;64(4):1480–5.
10. Howarth KR, Moreau NA, Phillips SM, Gibala MJ. Coingestion of protein with carbohydrate during recovery from endurance exercise stimulates skeletal muscle protein synthesis in humans. J Appl Physiol. 2009;106(4):1394–402.
11. Institute of Medicine, Food and Nutrition Board. Dietary reference intakes for energy, carbohydrate, fiber, fat, fatty acids, cholesterol, protein, and amino acids. Washington, DC: The National Academies; 2005.
12. US Department of Health and Human Services and US Department of Agriculture. 2015–2020 dietary guidelines for Americans [Internet]. 8th ed. 2015 [cited 2018 Jan 18]. Available from: http://health.gov/dietaryguidelines/2015/guidelines.
13. Potgieter S. Sport nutrition: a review of the latest guidelines for exercise and sport nutrition from the American College of Sport Nutrition, the International Olympic Committee and the International Society for Sports Nutrition. Afr J Clin Nutr. 2013;26(1):6–16.
14. Jäger R, Kerksick CM, Campbell BI, Cribb PJ, Wells SD, Skwiat TM, et al. International Society of Sports Nutrition Position Stand: protein and exercise. J Int Soc Sports Nutr [Internet]. 2017 Dec [cited 2018 Jan 2];14(1). Available from: http://jissn.biomedcentral.com/articles/10.1186/s12970-017-0177-8.
15. Phillips SM, Van Loon LJC. Dietary protein for athletes: from requirements to optimum adaptation. J Sports Sci. 2011;29(Suppl 1):S29–38.
16. McCartney D, Desbrow B, Irwin C. Post-exercise Ingestion of carbohydrate, protein and water: a systematic review and meta-analysis for effects on subsequent athletic performance. Sports Med [Internet]. 2017 Nov 2 [cited 2018 Jan 6]. Available from: http://link.springer.com/10.1007/s40279-017-0800-5.
17. Rogerson D. Vegan diets: practical advice for athletes and exercisers. J Int Soc Sports Nutr [Internet]. 2017 Dec [cited 2018 Jan 18];14(1). Available from: http://jissn.biomedcentral.com/articles/10.1186/s12970-017-0192-9.
18. Chidnok W, Fulford J, Bailey SJ, DiMenna FJ, Skiba PF, Vanhatalo A, et al. Muscle metabolic determinants of exercise tolerance following exhaustion: relationship to the "critical power". J Appl Physiol. 2013;115(2):243–50.
19. Akerman AP, Tipton M, Minson CT, Cotter JD. Heat stress and dehydration in adapting for performance: good, bad, both, or neither? Temperature. 2016;3(3):412–36.
20. Jeukendrup AE. Periodized nutrition for athletes. Sports Med. 2017;47(S1):51–63.
21. Martínez-Sanz J, Sospedra I, Ortiz C, Baladía E, Gil-Izquierdo A, Ortiz-Moncada R. Intended or unintended doping? A review of the presence of doping substances in dietary supplements used in sports. Nutrients. 2017;9(10):1093.
22. Goolsby MA, Boniquit N. Bone health in athletes: the role of exercise, nutrition, and hormones. Sports Health Multidiscip Approach. 2017;9(2):108–17.
23. Chu A, Holdaway C, Varma T, Petocz P, Samman S. Lower serum zinc concentration despite higher dietary zinc intake in athletes: a systematic review and meta-analysis. Sports Med. 2018;48(2):327–36.

Sports Rehabilitation

9

Knut Beitzel, Daniel Berthold, and Manuel Klose

9.1 Introduction

Sports injuries, such as damage to the muscles, ligaments or bone, often require surgery as well as a developed rehabilitation protocol. The rehabilitation process should be focused on the initial diagnosis of the injured athlete and include a wide number of therapeutic approaches. The primary aim is a return to sports at a preinjury physical and emotional level and, with injury, prevention as key point. However, tissue healing after injury as the natural healing process should be considered while developing a rehabilitation programme.

Focuses on sports rehabilitation are physiotherapy, performed by an experienced therapist, medical training therapy and sports-specific training. Further therapies such as ergotherapy, massage, electrotherapy, hydrotherapy, kinesiology and osteopathy should be considered individually in each rehabilitation protocol. Modern rehabilitation protocols require teamwork and proper rehabilitation planning, with sports physiotherapist and sports physician in leading positions. The team should be completed by an experienced athletic (strength and conditioning) coach and, in some cases, a sports psychologist and a dietitian.

Close coordination with trainers and coaches and the understanding of injury and subsequent problems by athlete and coaches are key in each rehabilitation protocol. Injury prevention during the reconditioning phase is crucial and requires data maintenance by teams and trainers.

Rehabilitation protocols should be focused on early passive mobilization considering the initial diagnosis of the patient. An experienced physiotherapist should guide the patient through the different phases of rehabilitation. Understanding the sports, biomechanical and physiological demands are crucial.

Rehabilitation includes immediate immobilization up to early, passive postoperative and early active exercises such as shoulder pendulum exercise or slight knee extensions/flexions. Meta-analyses of randomized clinical comparative studies showed no significant differences between early and delayed passive exercise in terms of clinical outcome and re-rupture rate regarding shoulder injuries. The full range of motion (ROM) can be achieved more quickly after early passive exercise. However, early aggressive active exercise can affect the healing and should not be performed in the first weeks after injury or surgery. Athlete and therapist should take into account the change of biomechanical properties of the injured part of the body in the first weeks and months. The length of immobilization varies

K. Beitzel (✉) · D. Berthold · M. Klose
Abteilung für Sportorthopädie, Klinikum rechts der Isar, München, München, Germany
e-mail: beitzel.knut@mri.tum.de; beitzelknut@tum.de; daniel.berthold@mri.tum.de; manuel.klose@mri.tum.de

S. Rocha Piedade et al. (eds.), *The Sports Medicine Physician*,
https://doi.org/10.1007/978-3-030-10433-7_9

between 4 and 8 weeks. The orthosis can be used to avoid aggressive active exercise or inappropriate movements, especially in patients with reduced compliance. Regarding shoulder injuries such as rotator cuff lesions, studies showed increased blood circulation in the repaired tendon and significantly reduced stress on tendon-suture construct in patients with abduction (15–45°) orthosis. Therefore, immobilization in slight abduction should be considered.

Recent studies investigated different rehabilitation approaches, especially in patients suffering from ACL injuries. Criterion-based protocols seem to be significantly superior in athletes after undergoing ACL surgery than time-based protocols. Time-based protocols are standardized rehabilitation protocols with fixed time tables and deadlines. Patients undergoing a time-based protocol seem to undergo less physiotherapy and shorter rehabilitation time which leads to a quicker return to sports. Risks and complications such as ACL elongations, re-rupture or injuries can be the causes. Patients undergoing criterion-based programmes need to achieve fixed goals in order to proceed in their rehabilitation. For example, running can only be allowed after finishing strength or coordination training. This leads to a more individualized rehabilitation protocol, taking into account the different characteristics of the athlete as well as the initial diagnosis, in order to decrease potential injury risks.

9.2 Physiotherapy

The first principle of the rehabilitation should take into account the different diagnoses and surgeries of the injured athlete. Physician or surgeon should define a postoperative protocol for the upcoming weeks which takes into account the different stages of wound healing, as well as the biomechanical aspects of the sport, injury and/or surgery.

The second principle pays careful attention to signs or indications of progressive overload, overtraining or stress. First hints of overloading can be signs of inflammation such as dolour, rubor, calor, tumour or functio laesa. This also includes general symptoms of exhaustion and fatigue (tiredness, fatigue, lack of motivation), caused by too much training or too intense rehabilitation.

The third principle of a rehabilitation protocol is seen as the "cause-effect chain". In other words, rehabilitation should take into account the complex reactions and compensation strategies of the body after injuries or surgeries.

As injured athletes tend to be impatient after long injuries or absences from sports activities, secondary dysfunctions seen as the "cause-effect chain" can cause problems during rehabilitation. The body and the related diagnosis or surgery should be seen as a whole complex unit. Injured parts of the body are linked to physical dysfunction in a chain of effects. An experienced therapist has to take care of dysfunctions and include them in training.

Core stability is seen as the fourth principle in physiotherapist protocols. A well-trained core is essential to optimal force flow in the kinetic chain (Figs. 9.1 and 9.2), as all the force couples are generated from our core. Injured athletes should be aware of the importance of core stability and

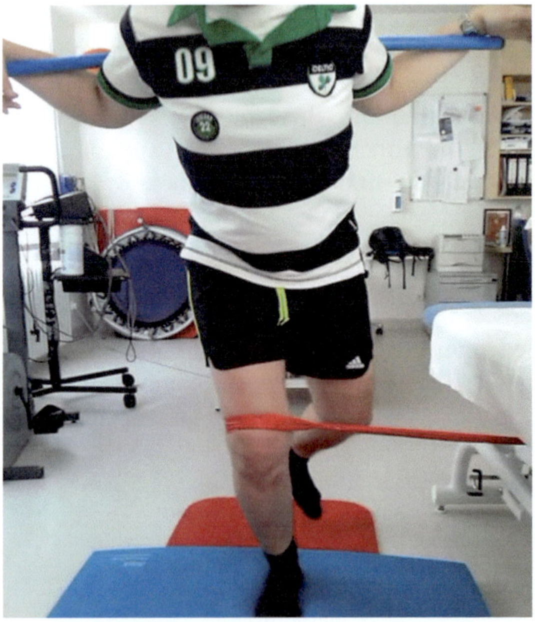

Fig. 9.1 Training of the leg axis with combined training of core strength

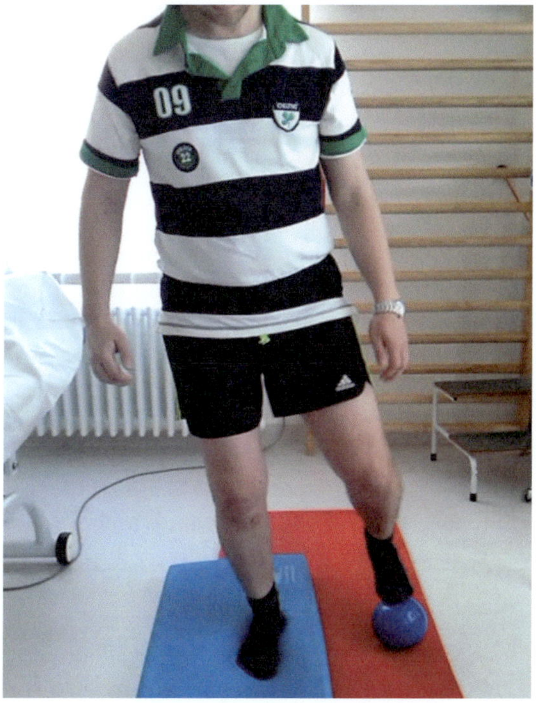

Fig. 9.2 Proprioceptive training of the lower extremity

include coordination, core strength and functional training in their rehabilitation protocol.

The fifth principle includes continuous communication between the patient and the whole rehabilitation team such as physiotherapist, physician or coaches.

The athlete should be informed in detail about his injury, the biomechanical aspects of his injury/surgery or the planed therapies. The more the patient brings understanding about the details, the higher should be the compliance, especially in activity restriction or absence from sports.

As those five principles are the spine of each rehabilitation protocol, physiotherapist should be aware of compliance, subjective feeling and pain of the athlete. Furthermore, each rehab can be classified into four phases. Immediately after injury or surgery, the first phase is defined as the post-injury or acute postoperative phase. During this time, the importance should be set on rest and reducing inflammatories such as swelling with ice and cold therapy and compression. Medication can also be taken into account. Recent studies also showed the importance of clean and healthy eating and adequate water supply during this time. This can help to eliminate metabolites much faster and increase recovery time.

Soon after completing the first phase, the inflammatory phase in injured athletes starts. Anti-inflammatory measures can also be applied.

The proliferation phase is seen as the third phase in physiotherapy. While starting with mobilization, the therapist should start with light endurance activities in order to increase the oxygen input.

Functional training and return to sports-related activities or movements are seen as the remodelling phase.

In summary, therapist and athlete should work on individual rehabilitation protocols with the main focus on personal aspects of the injured patient. All the activities should be performed without greater pain (VAS 1–3). Communications between all people included can prevent overtraining, dysfunction or reduced compliance.

Key Facts
- Criterion-based protocols are superior than time-based protocols.
- The five principles of physiotherapy are diagnosis, indications of overload, cause-effect chain, core strength and communication between athlete and rehabilitation team.

9.3 Manual Therapy

While completing the different stages of physiotherapy, the rehabilitation process is enhanced by manual therapy. Manual therapy involves examining, detecting, assessing and treating reversible disorders of the locomotor system. This means that the therapist must be familiar with the mutual influence of arthrogenous, muscular and neurogenic structures, filter out the primary symptomatic structure, consider possible contraindications and recognize the sensitivity of the structure to be treated, in order to be able to draw up an individual treatment plan. Medical training therapy is an equipment-supported form of training for

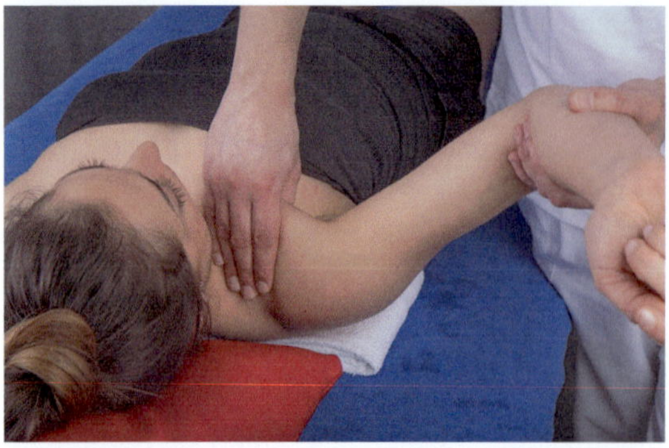

Fig. 9.3 Technique of manual therapy to detonize the pectoralis group

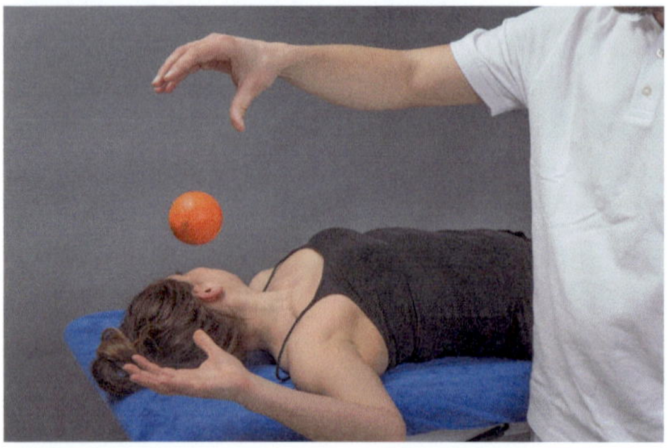

Fig. 9.4 Proprioceptive training and strengthening of the shoulder muscles

strength, endurance, coordination and movement under medical supervision. The objective of medical training therapy (MTT) is to regain and stabilize a person's physical capabilities.

The main focus should be set on optimizing the quality of the movement. As soon as an optimal quality of the movement, rhythm and extent is achieved, the load can be increased. The physiotherapist and the athlete should work on coordination, proprioception (Figs. 9.3 and 9.4) as well as the interaction between different muscles and core. In addition to passive and active exercises, fitness equipment can be a useful asset in manual therapy. It allows working step by step on strength, power and endurance. An experienced athlete can even perform their training after an appropriate introduction and under constant control.

9.4 Core Strength

Core training is vital for each rehabilitation protocol. It provides stability and increases efficiency in force production as well as movement patterns. The literature showed that strong extremities in combination with weak core strength result in less force production and muscular dysfunction. It helps reducing pain in the lower back, sacroiliac joint, hamstring, shoulders and groin. Elite athletes require much higher levels of core stability, in order to maintain and maximize sports performances and promote efficient biomechanics. Core stabilization exercises should be integrated in rehabilitation programmes, as it shows decreased injury rates, especially for the lower extremity.

Core musculature can be divided into local and global categories. Muscles attached to the lumbar vertebrae are defined as local muscles. They can influence intersegmental motion and improve the coordination and proprioception. Global muscles attach to the hips and pelvis and increase the mobility of the spine. If there is a dysfunction in one of the local muscles, this can cause a significant imbalance between all the muscles involved. This leads to inefficient movements and increases the risk of injuries, with a high number of musculoskeletal injuries. The abdominal muscles such as rectus abdominis, transversus abdominis and internal or external obliques are the key muscles in positioning spine and pelvis correctly. Up to this, intra-abdominal pressure, as well as stabilization of the spine, is guaranteed by the transversus abdominis and the thoracolumbar fascia. The thoracolumbar fascia is seen as the connection of the upper and lower extremities. It maintains the kinetic chain and guarantees an optimal force couple for the extremities involved. Trapezius, latissimus dorsi, deltoid and pectoralis major can be seen as axial-appendicular attachments, which transfer force and momentum between extremities and core.

Even the diaphragm plays its own role in core strength and stabilization by contracting and increasing intra-abdominal pressure and generating a co-contraction of the pelvic floor muscles

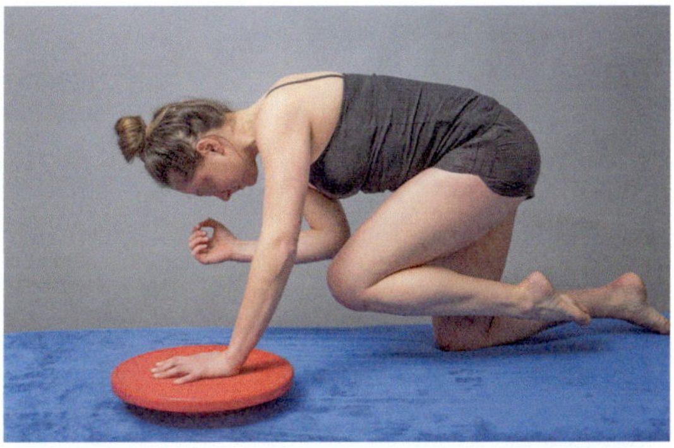

Fig. 9.5 Training of core strength combined with proprioceptive training

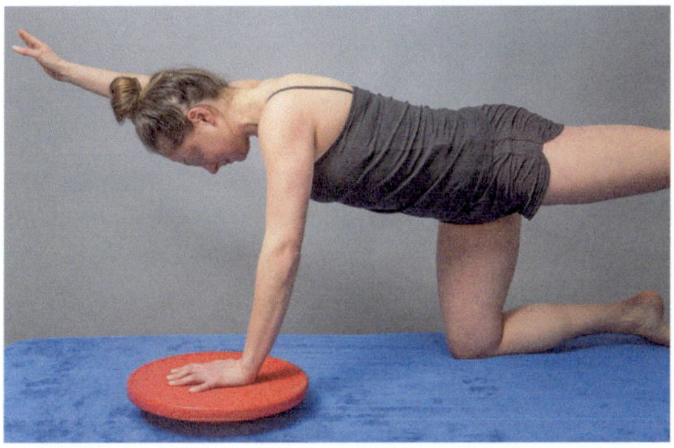

Fig. 9.6 Training of core strength combined with proprioceptive training

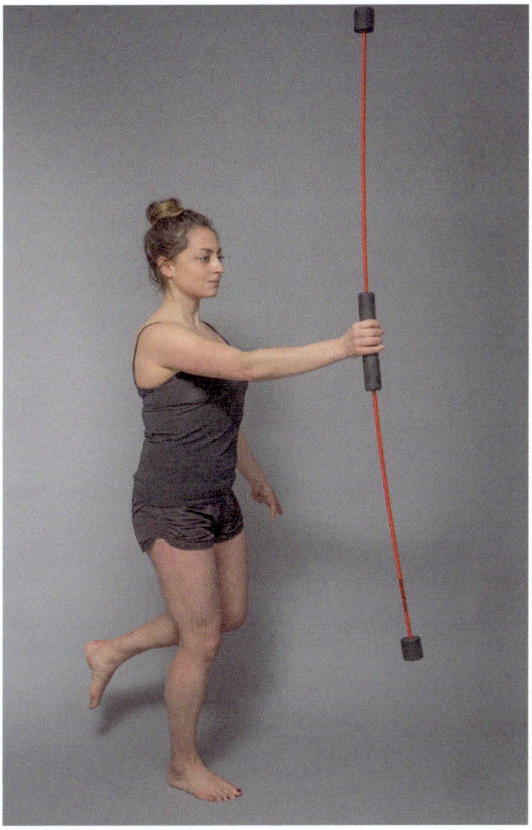

Fig. 9.7 Training of core strength combined with proprioceptive training

prior to limb movement. Diaphragmatic breathing exercises can improve core stability, as it serves as the superior boundary of the abdominal cavity.

The lumbopelvic hip complex, like the gluteal muscles, pelvic floor and hip girdle, provides a corset-lie stabilization on the trunk and spine. Gluteus maximus and medius, hip adductors, rectus femoris and iliopsoas are seen as the core stabilization muscles.

The focus on core stability lays on keeping a neutral spinal alignment, optimal trunk position and the transfer of loads along the kinetic chain.

Core stability needs be trained in a progressive way (Figs. 9.5, 9.6 and 9.7) beginning with recruitment of local muscle, moving it to core stabilization and total body dynamic movements. Overall deficiencies in core stabilization and load transfer muscles are be related to lower extremity function and injury.

9.5 Mobility

Stretching and continuous increase of flexibility and mobility should be part of each rehabilitation protocol, as it increases muscles length and full range of motion.

Reduced joint flexibility or range of motion can be caused by many reasons or factors such as muscles or capsuloligamentous structures surrounding the joint.

The anatomy of a muscle provides both passive and active tension. The passive tension is dependent on the surrounding fascia as well as the anatomic properties of the muscle. Active tension is given by dynamic muscle contraction and results from neuroreflexive properties as peripheral motor neuron innervation and reflexive activation.

Athletes often describe a stiff muscle as muscle "tightness". In fact, muscles can become significantly shorter due to contraction or spasm. Overall, this can prevent optimal healing during rehabilitation or cause muscle or joint damage and lead to absence from sports.

In sports rehabilitation, three muscle stretching techniques are applied and described in the literature: static, dynamic and pre-contraction. Static stretching can be either performed actively by the subject or passively by a partner and is the most common type of stretching. A specific position is held with the muscle on tension to the point of a stretching feeling and can be repeated from seconds up to few minutes.

Dynamic stretching is described as active or ballistic stretching. While active stretching is performed in order to restore the full range of motion of a limb while moving it through its full range of motion to the end range, ballistic stretching includes rapid or alternating movements at end range of motion. Studies showed an increased risk of injury for ballistic stretching which is no longer recommended in sports rehabilitation.

The third form of stretching is described as pre-contraction stretching. While stretching, the muscle should be contracted up to 75–100% of maximal contraction. One of the most described techniques is proprioceptive neuromuscular facilitation (PNF) stretching.

In terms of orthopaedic and sport orthopaedic injuries, stretching should be seen as effective physiotherapeutic tool. In patients with hamstring strains, one of the most common injuries in soccer players, static stretching is seen as more effective as dynamic stretching. In addition, intensive stretching was shown as more effective than by less intensive stretching. Overall, studies showed that 6–8 weeks of static stretching is sufficient to increase hamstring length.

9.6 Nutrition

During sports rehabilitation, nutrition is seen as one of the most important factors in the overall healing and post-injury performance. Injuries, which limit limb or body mobility, will lead after few weeks to a significant lower metabolic turnover. Athletes can suffer from an increase of muscle strength or neuromuscular control by losing proteins or carbohydrates. Deficiencies of energy, protein and other nutrients should be avoided, as it can lead to a longer absence from sports. The right diet, in combination with the right rehabilitation protocol, should see the athlete back to his performance faster than expected.

During injury, immobilization or reduced physical activity can be divided in two main stages. The first stage is seen as the healing and recovery phase with inflammation, proliferation and remodelling. The second stage is the return to activity with increased activity and rehabilitation. Both stages can be influenced by nutrition or a right diet.

In severe injuries, the metabolic outcome can decrease up to 20%. In order to prevent muscle loss, a small weight gain can be beneficial. If there is a loss in energy, muscle growth can be limited, and the overall loss can be greater. During the rehabilitation, protein (2–2.5 g/kg/day), carbohydrate and fat intake (esp. omega-3) as well as vitamins (esp. vitamins A and C) and minerals should be part of each diet. Sports beverages, gels, sodas, concentrated sweets and alcohol should be avoided.

Key Facts

- Manual therapy treats reversible structures in the locomotor system.
- It is important to restore the perfect interaction between core stability and mobility in order to achieve the best possible result of the rehab.
- Unfortunately, often neglected, a balanced diet supports sports rehab in all areas.

Take-Home Message

Rehabilitation protocols require teamwork, steady communication between athlete, medical team and coaches as well as a detailed understanding of injury or surgery. Vital to each rehabilitation are physiotherapy and manual therapy. Signs of overtraining, stress, inflammation or pain should be considered carefully. Core strength, mobility and nutrition should be seen as the key facts in order to prevent from injury through dysfunction. Criteria-based protocols should be favoured in injured athletes, as time-based protocols do not take individual characteristics of patients into account and increase risks of failure or injury.

The Role of a Strength and Conditioning Coach

10

Telmo Sousa

10.1 Introduction

Working in elite level teams requires that professionals from interrelated fields have expertise and knowledge to reach the collective goal—achieving sports success. Establishing optimal communication between diverse professionals is crucial to upgrade your system and benefit your athletes.

With the advances in sports science, monitoring software and technology, the amount of data we have available is huge, but the key is not the amount of data we collect. The winning formula is to select and monitor important data, to share information with all collaborators, and to understand a common strategy of intervention in order to optimize performance.

It seems easy, but it isn't. With the level of specialization required by high-performance training, we usually have more staff members than athletes. Throughout this chapter, my examples are mostly related to football, as it is my daily sport. An elite football team can have around 25–30 players but a greater number of staff, including technical, medical, strength and conditioning (S&C), and sports science staff.

Whether integrated into the technical or medical department, or as an independent department, a S&C coach should be a part of an integrated system. The main actions of a coach include communicating, motivating, and relating with various people. Technical qualities, acquired mainly by the permanent search for updated scientific evidence, are the basis for high-quality work, but besides that, as in any other profession, soft skills are a very important part of the work: motivation, commitment, creativity, problem solving, flexibility, and teamwork are keys for implementing proper strategies and achieving success.

The closest analogy for an elite athlete is to compare him with a Formula 1 car. When this special car has a "screw" that is not properly attached, it can work with minor problems for a short period of time, but later, this minor issue will become bigger and affect performance. We also have to remind ourselves that we are not the only person working with players. Injury prevention and athletic performance directly depend on the sum of a player's multidisciplinary interventions. In his daily routine, a player will work with a masseur, physio, nutritionist, and S&C coach, among others, and will also have team training, so it's crucial to understand the dynamic and the influence of all these workers in a highly complex global system. Also, the relation between accumulating fatigue and recovering effectively during a competitive week cycle determines what we usually call training load (Fig. 10.1).

Elite athletes, particularly football players, are often exposed to year-long training with congested

T. Sousa (✉)
Futebol Clube do Porto, Porto, Portugal
e-mail: telmo.sousa@fcporto.pt

S. Rocha Piedade et al. (eds.), *The Sports Medicine Physician*,
https://doi.org/10.1007/978-3-030-10433-7_10

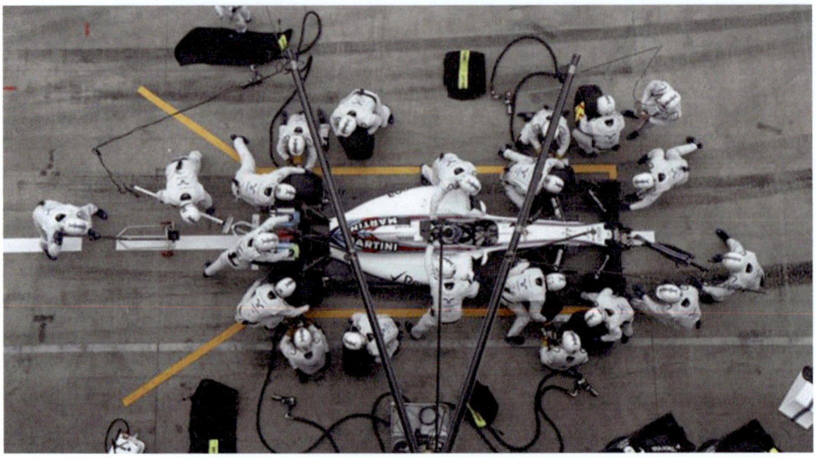

Fig. 10.1 Example of a Formula 1 pit crew

fixtures competition, play consecutive matches, and are frequently limited to 3 days of recovery [1]. Therefore, a minor problem can easily result in a major problem. In this case, a major problem is an injury that stops an athlete from training and competition. Also, it will automatically decrease his performance and athletic capacities. We need to individualize and adapt programs, as their responses to training and competition depend on several factors and vary from day to day and week to week. We always have to interpret, make decisions, and adapt strategies in a permanent search to improve performance. This means that we want to have athletes always in their best condition for training and competition. They should be able to tolerate high training loads and therefore maximize exposure to technical and tactical coaching. We have to prepare them for thousands of hours of training and competition.

In my opinion, the most important of all is to have a club vision of developing athleticism through the physical aspects of high performance. The head coach and coaching staff should valorize and share this philosophy of work, understand the importance of complementary work, and define global strategies with S&C coaches and medical staff in order to have a common strategy and implementation. Above all, players should feel that this is a global strategy and that we all must have mental resilience to create a culture of success through hard work in order to achieve our main goal: excellence in a long-term season.

As long as the coaches are not involved in the strategies of complementary work, the system of injury prevention and performance simply will not work.

Collective strategies should be made according to a global model while respecting individual needs.

In my perspective, instead of talking about injury prevention, we should talk about training. We should speak about making players robust enough to withstand technical and tactical training without getting injured.

10.2 Characterizing the Game/Physical Parameters

Different sports require different approaches to physical training programs. To improve physical conditioning, and thereby enhance sports performance, at both the individual and collective levels, it is extremely important to have deep knowledge regarding the physiological demands of the game. It is likewise essential to have a baseline testing battery, early in the preparatory phase, to realize where we stand and to define a plan for where we want to go.

In a football match, according to several studies [2, 3], the total distance covered in the 1950s was between 4000 and 5000 m, which increased to 10,000 m in the 1990s.

Today, the mean total distance covered is reported to be between 10,000 and 11,000 m, with some players covering up to 14,000 m, and almost one-fourth of this distance is covered in high-intensity running (>14.4 km/h) [4].

Clearly, the total distances covered in the modern elite-standard English League are much higher than 40 years ago [5]. Also, the amount of high-intensity running is similar to that in the Italian *Serie A* and the *Spanish La Liga* [6].

Thus, in terms of physical demands, team sports are becoming more and more intense.

Barnes et al. studied more than 1000 individual players across 7 seasons (between 2006/2007 and 2012/2013 in the English Premier League) and concluded [7]:

- The total distance covered during a match was 2% lower, which means that there were no significant changes between those 7 seasons.
- The mean total of high-intensity running distance (19.8–25.1 km/h) increased by 30%, with an associated increase of 50% in the number of high-intensity running actions.
- High-intensity running (with ball possession) was lower in 2006/2007 (373 ± 238 m) compared with other seasons, apart from 2008/2009 (389 ± 242 m), peaking in 2012/2013 (478 ± 260 m).
- High-intensity running (without ball possession) was lower in 2006/2007 (451 ± 162 m) compared to other seasons, peaking in 2012/2013 (589 ± 198 m), as well as increasing in mean by 22%.
- Total sprint distance increased by 50% density, as estimated by the number of sprints against the percentage of explosive sprints over the 7 premiership seasons.
- The number of sprints increased by 80%, and an increased proportion of these sprints were explosive in nature (38%).
- Maximal running speed attained increased 5%.
- Mean sprint distance was shorter by −15%, but the proportion of explosive sprints increased by 35%.

In conclusion, everything that is considered an intense action during the game, actions that are decisive in the creation of imbalances and that can decide a game, have become more frequent and intense.

Over the years, from the physical point of view, football has become increasingly demanding. Players are fitter, faster, and stronger than ever before. Therefore, we must create strategies to develop our athletes in terms of physical capacities if we want to reach and stay at the top.

Football is characterized as a high-intensity, intermittent game with both aerobic and anaerobic elements.

Based on several studies [6, 8, 9], Solé J. cited the distribution of effort time and the intensity at which it is performed [10]:

- 49–54′—The player is standing or walking.
- 30–35′—Efforts of intensity less than 15 km/h (70–80% VO2 max).
- 3–5′—Effort at intensities 15–25 km/h (90–115% VO2 max).
- 2–3′—Effort at intensities greater than 25 km/h (alactic-lactic).

Most of the investigations agree that the match HR average intensity is close to the anaerobic threshold (80–90% of maximal heart rate) [11, 12].

Match average oxygen consumption is 3.5 L/m, which is equivalent to 76% of VO2 max. Different percentages of VO2 max are presented, depending on the position occupied: 69% defenses, 66% midfielders, and 43.3% forwards. The approximate energy expenditure is 1530 kcal in 90 min [13].

Therefore, athletes should be prepared to perform with relative ease these physical demands, without showing symptoms of excessive fatigue.

Fatigue following a soccer match is multifactorial and related to dehydration, glycogen depletion, muscle damage, and mental fatigue [14].

The level of dehydration depends upon climatic and atmospheric conditions (weather, wind, temperature, humidity, and altitude). Moderate fluid deficits corresponding to ~2% of body mass are common even in football matches played in neutral conditions [15].

Scientific research helps to recognize the evolution of sports' physical parameters, particularly in football. This knowledge should be useful in talent identification and also when designing and monitoring training processes. Therefore, clubs should invest in the individual development of young players if they want to increase the possibility of achieving first team and higher competition levels.

10.3 Monitoring Training Load

Load is determined by the interaction of exercise duration, intensity, and frequency and can be quantified by external and/or internal parameters [16].

Load monitoring is a common practice in professional sports, with 40 of 41 surveyed professional soccer teams reporting that they collect load data for every player during every field training session [17].

Enhancing performance requires a scientific approach to load monitoring, managing risks associated with possible inappropriate designs of training programs.

Appropriate monitoring of training load can provide important information to coaches, athletes, and support staff. Monitoring systems should be intuitive and provide efficient data that can be easy-to-interpret in order to have proper feedback and understand individual and group responses to training stimuli.

In elite sports, optimizing performance requires exposing athletes to high training loads, at their limits, so the associated probability of injury is high. At this level, that often means training stimuli are on the borderline between optimal outcomes and injury risk.

To achieve the best physical condition requires optimal adaptation. For example, in team sports, postsession and accumulative fatigue must occur during a match-to-match microcycle in order to create proper adaptations and recovery and have athletes be fresh and better prepared for the weekend competition.

With an increased number of technologies available, coaches should adopt scientifically valid tools to monitor internal and external loads and to understand the training load impact and its effect on each athlete and the entire group.

Today, it is recognized that external and internal loads are relevant components of load quantification for an effective monitoring system [18]. However, there is frequently dissociation between external and internal load units. So, to monitor an athlete's state of fatigue, individualization cannot be over emphasized. External and internal measurements must be taken in account to make individual adjustments and design programs.

But how can we monitor internal and external loads in our team sports teams?

There is no absolute truth about the type of monitoring tools that coaches should adopt [17]. They should consider what is really important to evaluate and select effective tools for this purpose.

10.3.1 Internal Load

Recent evidence suggests the importance of individual load monitoring for detecting possible negative outcomes and reducing the risk of overtraining, illness, and injury. Also, the relationship between internal load (in the form of athlete self-reported wellness and subjective measurements) and external load (objective measurements) on match performance should be considered.

In this way, coaches and support staff are increasingly seeking a more current and scientific approach for the monitoring process.

Rating of perceived exertion (RPE) is probably the most common means of assessing internal load. Foster developed the session-RPE method, and evidence shows it to be a simple, free, valid, and reliable tool of quantifying training load [19]. Workload is quantified by multiplying the athlete's RPE (on a 1–10 scale) by the duration of the session (in min).

Although moderate to strong correlations exist between s-RPE- and HR-based measures of internal load, none of these methods are considered preferential or superior than the other. If possible, they should be used together because they give complementary information.

The mean of the overall daily wellness scores can include athlete self-report questionnaire and also can be used to quantify weekly wellness. Coaches can use pre-training self-reported wellness to make adjustments to training if warranted.

Results in Australian football confirm the value of quantifying load and determining training status using self-reported measures and highlight the importance of a mixed-method approach to comprehensively assess athlete status [20].

Monitoring internal loads will give coaches feedbacks of athletes at risk of overtraining and others failing to reach a sufficient training stimulus.

Furthermore, the positive association between field-based loads and objective match performance suggests higher loads improved performance, particularly when combined with reduced wellness scores.

10.3.1.1 Heart Rate Monitoring

Heart rate monitors have become commonly used in all sports. In the last years, heart rate variability (HRV) has become more popular. HRV can be measured during ultrashort recordings (1–3 min) with the athlete in standing, seated, or supine positions. HRV reflects the variation in time between each heartbeat and appears to correlate with recovery status.

Research has focused on identifying its association with athletic performance and recovery and illness. Furthermore, HRV has been investigated as a diagnostic marker of overreaching and overtraining [21]. It can also be used to identify when the athlete may be more or less adaptive to training (aiding training prescription) and potentially predict when an athlete may perform better or worse on a particular day [22]. It is agreed that athletes with higher scores in HRV will be more able to perform in endurance activities and athletes with higher markers of stress will be less available for strength training. Scientific insights derived from HR and HRV data suggest the need for individualized training and recovery guidance.

Also, real-time HR monitors permit knowing and adjusting the time spent in HR zones.

However, measures of heart rate cannot provide data on all aspects of wellness, fatigue, and performance, so they are still not widely implemented to monitor athletes' responses to training load, probably because of apparent contradictory findings in the literature [23].

Therefore, it is important to cross-check all information combining internal and external loads to take a more holistic approach to monitoring training status.

10.3.1.2 Self-Reported Wellness/s-RPE/A/C RPE Workload

Internal training load represents the psychobiological response to a given external load and can be measured via numerous objective and subjective parameters.

Daily and/or weekly questionnaires and the rate of perceived exertion are commonly used in field-based sports. However, like any subjective parameter, consideration should be given to playing experience, position, and time-trial performance when interpreting athletes' internal load.

Research suggests that monitoring pre-training perceived wellness may provide coaches with information about the intensity of output that can be expected from individual players during a training session [24]. Daily questionnaires commonly include rating of fatigue, sleep quality, general muscle soreness, stress levels, and mood.

The acute/chronic workload ratio (A/C) has received growing interest in recent years for monitoring injury risk in a variety of team sports.

$$\text{Workload ratio acute / chronic} = (\text{accumulated last 7 days}) / (\text{accumulated last 21 or 28 days})$$

According to Malone S. and colleagues [25], players who were exposed to large and rapid increases in high-speed distance (HSR) and sprint distance (SR) had increased odds of injury. Conversely, better intermittent aerobic fitness and higher chronic training loads (weekly sums ≥2584 AU) counterbalance by decreasing the lower limb injury risk associated with these running distances. An A/C workload at 1:3 weeks between 1.00 and 1.25 is considered to be protective for professional soccer players [25].

A/C workload ratios at 1:3 and 1:4 weeks were associated with noncontact injury. Recently, in a study of elite football, a greater risk of injury was found for players with A/C workloads at 1:4 weeks of 0.97–1.38 and >1.38, compared with players whose A/C workloads were 0.60–0.97. An A/C workload at 1:3 weeks of >1.42 compared with 0.59–0.97 displayed 1.94 times higher risk of injury. In conclusion, internal A/C workload ratio (measured using s-RPE) is considered to be predictive of risk factors for noncontact injuries in elite European footballers; however, it should be complemented by other methods [26].

This A/C workload ratio can be used for internal load (session-rate of perceive exertion (session-RPE) × duration) and external load (often tracking variables such as total distance or high-speed running distance).

10.3.2 External Load

For external load monitoring, elite sports teams usually adopt Global Positioning System (GPS), time motion analyses, and power output measuring devices, such as strength training machines with the possibility to test, monitor, and analyze performance.

10.3.2.1 GPS Analysis Software

Athlete performance tracking systems are used by elite teams all over the world in training and competition. This type of monitoring can have different approaches, such as by installing cameras around the facility (e.g., stadium or training ground) or, most commonly, having athletes wear vests with small devices that can be tracked by satellite. Then, at the end of a training session, data will be downloaded to software for further analysis. This software must be easy-to-use and intuitive and give coaches information on total distance covered, high-speed distance, maximal speed, number of accelerations and decelerations, player load, and acute/chronic workload ratio, as well as many other parameters that can be chosen.

In addition, this software allows coaches to select the type of parameters they wish to analyze and also perform cuts to each exercise to understand and analyze the behavior of each athlete in each exercise. Essentially, it gives coaches the possibility to interpret and make better decisions when planning training sessions and to adapt according to individual needs when necessary. Also, in terms of the rehabilitation process after injury, it is an excellent tool that allows comparing players' individual values before being injured, as well as comparing with team demands during each training day and cumulative training load for a week microcycle before the match. Thus, GPS allows for progressive and controlled integration in the training process, thereby reducing the risk of reinjury and allowing a secure and successful return to play.

10.3.2.2 Neuromuscular Function and Assessment

For S&C coaches, neuromuscular function is of crucial importance. Therefore, special emphasis is given to monitoring devices that can evaluate different movements/actions. Jump tests; isokinetic, isoinertial flywheel equipment for eccentric training (also known as Yoyos such as squat, hamstrings, and VersaPulley™); forces platforms; linear and rotational encoders; electromyography sensors; and dynamometers are often utilized in the team sport environment (Figs. 10.2 and 10.3).

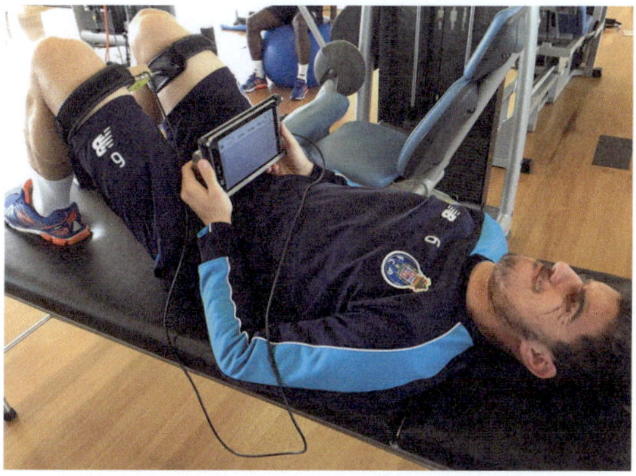

Fig. 10.2 Dynamometer testing adductor strength

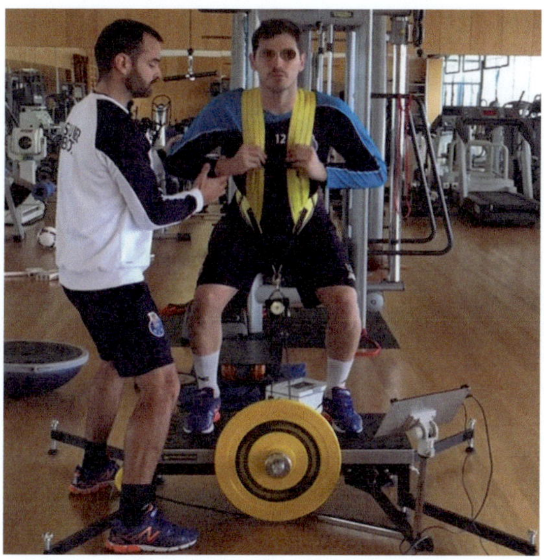

Fig. 10.3 Flywheel Yoyo squat

10.4 Principles for Developing Athletic Performance

About 20 years ago, a group of professionals with diverse experiences but linked to team sports emerged in Barcelona under the leadership of Paco Seirul-lo. A new training paradigm was emerging for team sports, and Julio Tous was responsible for developing and specializing the theme of *Strength* (Fig. 10.4).

I have been positively influenced by Julio Tous' guiding principles and methodology, along with other decisive factors such as my ongoing reflective practice, experience, training, and the expertise of many professionals that I have had the privilege of working with over the years. These crucial factors have both inspired and molded my work in this field and lay the foundation for what I believe to be the decisive premises for a "*Strength Training*" approach at a professional level for team athletes.

10.4.1 Robustness as Primary Prevention

Strength is surely the best prevention tool in elite sports, and every S&C should always be alert to injuries. Above, I discussed monitoring tools, assessments/measurements, and different types of tests. Testing is very important to achieve individual enhancement, but there is another determining factor—*training*!

Fig. 10.4 Adapted by: Fajardo T. J. "Strength as a fundamental physical capacity. El entrenamiento en los deportes de equipo" (2017) (RPA repeated power ability: ROM range of motion)

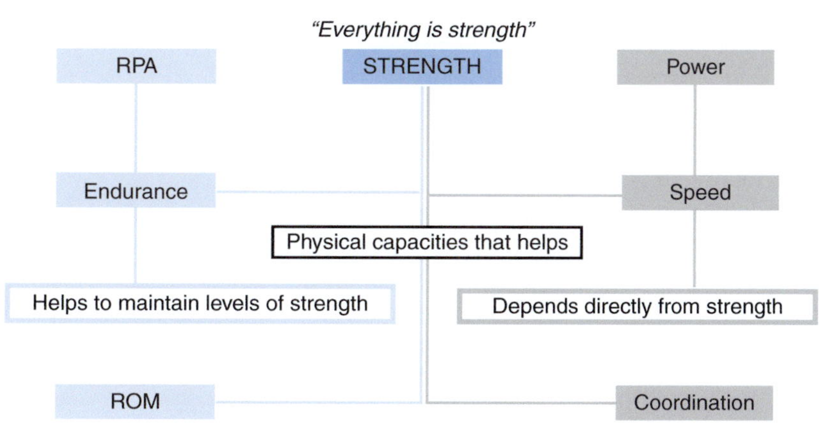

The road to success is to study extensively, regularly apply science-based evidence, and be assertive in the implementation of training programs. That makes the difference in terms of injury reduction (because injuries will always happen) and keeping athletes performing on the field. Some trainers spend a lot of time testing and little time investing in what is really important—*training*!

In my opinion, in team sports, the application of individual programs to improve performance makes perfect sense as a complementary strategy. That is, in the preseason, detailed evaluation (energy systems, strength, power, speed, flexibility, and detecting postural imbalances) should be made of all players that compose the team, and a collective strategy should be defined. Then, based on the individual responses that are daily evaluated with the available monitoring systems, individual adjustments should be made in order to enhance performance and reduce the risk of injury for each player.

Thus, individual strategies must be as the name implies complementary work. They cannot overlap collective strategies. Usually when this happens, it means that either there are no collective strategies or they are inadequate.

In professional football, muscle injuries are the most common injury type [27].

Hamstring strains are the most prevalent muscle injuries reported in sport [28] and also have a high recurrence rate [29, 30], with lost training and playing time in running-based sports [31].

Hamstring injuries are estimated to cost elite soccer clubs as much as €280,000 per injury [32].

Top-level professional football teams regularly play within a 72-h interval (representing one-third of matches), which increases neuromuscular fatigue and the risk of injury [4].

According to Bengtsson [33], in a 14-year prospective study with more than 130,000 match observations, there were no match congestion-related differences in total match injury rates, but muscle injury rates during matches were lower when players were given at least 6 days between their match exposures. Furthermore, statistically significant more hip/groin muscle injuries were observed when matches were separated by ≤3 days compared with ≥6 days since the last match exposure, for male professional football players [33]. Therefore, in order to decrease the odds for injury, coaching staff must consider player rotation, even when time between matches is up to 5 days.

Hamstring strain injury is the most common injury in football, and there is scientific evidence for large-scale interventions employing the Nordic hamstring. This exercise has reported 50–70% reductions in hamstring injuries in football when athletes are compliant [34–36].

In addition, hamstring rehabilitation protocols applying long length exercises are significantly more effective in accelerating time to return to play from injury than conventional exercises [37].

Besides these observations, hamstring injury prevention using Nordic hamstring protocols and evidence-based injury prevention has not been adopted by the majority of Champions League football teams [38] (Fig. 10.5).

As cited by Bourne M. et al. [39], scientific research has established that eccentric knee flexor strength reduces the risk of hamstring strain injury when compliance is adequate and also partly mediated by increases in biceps femoris long head fascicle length and, possibly, a rightward shift in the angle of peak knee flexor torque, as well as other adaptations that can also occur. The authors also claim that acute responses and chronic adaptations to training with different hamstring exercises are heterogeneous. Muscle activation may be an important determinant of training-induced hypertrophy; however, contraction mode appears to be the largest driver of architectural changes within the hamstring [39].

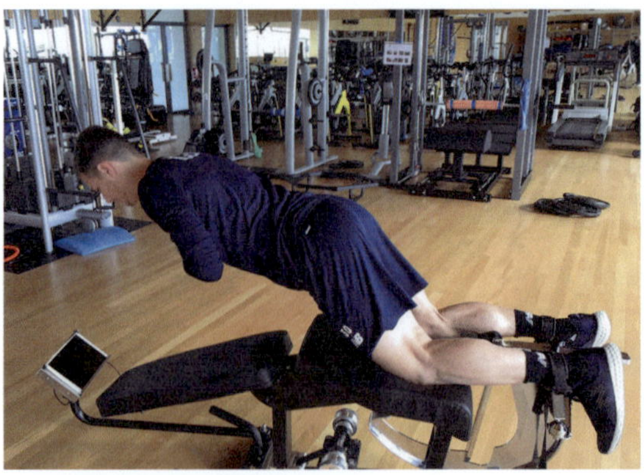

Fig. 10.5 Nordic hamstring exercise

Strength training appears to be the most effective way of reducing hamstring injury rates, although acute responses and chronic adaptations to training with different exercises are not uniform. Furthermore, S&C coaches may design training interventions based on scientific evidence, sensitivity, and expertise. It's also very important to take into account players' experiences and histories of practice because different players can have different responses to the same stimulus. The nature of the exercise stimulus (i.e., the intensity, duration, and number of series performed, as well as the duration and activity patterns during recovery) and timing of applying these exercises should depend on the best day, according to a match-to-match microcycle. In addition, players' levels of experience and individual responses, team periodization, and accumulative fatigue should be considered when carrying out these programs before (having fresh athletes) or after training (consider training under fatigue). For example, when planning an in-season 7-day microcycle (if matches always fall on a Sunday) and including one gym session to maintain strength levels, the best day would probably be Wednesday (+72 h after the match day —MD + 3) or Thursday (−72 h before the match, MD − 3). In this case, taking advantage of the midweek means having athletes be fresh and recovered from the game and still having time for the athletes to recover fully from the strength stimulus before the next game.

In my personal opinion, the most effective way to reduce hamstring injury rates is to define global strategies (in agreement with technical and medical staff) and then make adjustments for individual needs. It's important to involve everyone in the process, especially the athletes.

10.4.2 Developing Single-Leg Strength

Over the years, team sports have adapted strength methods, characterized by classical bilateral movements and which predominantly occur in the vertical plane, from weightlifting. In team sports, movements are mostly unilateral, and lower body strength must be used to improve agility (commonly called COD ability).

These whole-body movements involve decelerating, changing direction, and accelerating while also maintaining balance during these maneuvers. Figure 10.6 shows an example of a VersaPulley exercise based on horizontal forces to improve COD ability, thus ensuring best transfer from the weight room to the playing field.

Taking another example, now in a vertical exercise, a squat in a unilateral pattern (single-leg squat) will be substantially more demanding from a neuromuscular point of view. Doing this obtains a greater activity of action of the hamstrings, gluteus medius, and trunk stabilizers. The one-leg box squat is the most "famous" of the single-leg exercises. It requires stability from the opposite leg and pelvic stabilizers must function as stabilizers. This stabilization is needed for acceleration and sprinting actions. Therefore, this exercise is closer to game actions in team sports.

S&C should create efficient and effective workouts based on:

- Working with body weight
- Improving core stability and strength
- Adding functionality to your program
- Enhancing/optimizing movement efficiency
- Building strength in key movement patterns
- Looking for "movement quality" instead of repetitions/series

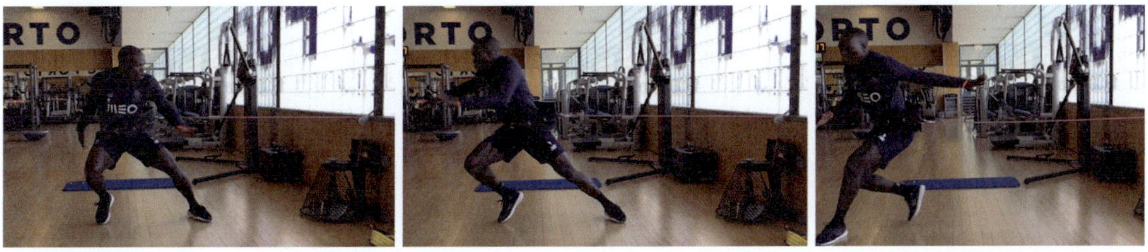

Fig. 10.6 VersaPulley crossed COD

10.4.3 Taking Advantages of Eccentric Training

The benefits of eccentric overload training are well accepted and well-known by professionals in the field of injury prevention and sports training.

Maximal decelerations are key movements in team sports, and deceleration (eccentric action) reduces the great moment of horizontal force, thereby facilitating a more efficient support in the moment to apply a greater propulsive force (acceleration—concentric action).

Eccentric contractions force muscles to lengthen and concentric contractions force muscles to shorten. Depending on periodized training, the athlete's level and historical of practice, after eccentric exercise muscle pain can occur, the so-called delayed onset muscle soreness (DOMS). Periodizing your training session carefully is crucial in order to achieve the best results. Thus, when planning workouts, coaches must be conscious of athletes that are unaccustomed to eccentric training and thus increase the intensity and duration of the proposed exercises in a progressive way.

The available evidence indicates that eccentric overload exercises are more effective in strength gains and hypertrophy, and there is scientific evidence showing positive effects after the damage caused by lengthened muscle contractions. As a consequence, this causes an adaptation process with an increase in sarcomere numbers in muscle fibers.

Following the damage created by eccentric exercises, muscles rapidly adapt to the optimum length for active tension, thereby decreasing the injury risk by protecting muscles against more major injuries.

While concentric contractions initiate movements, eccentric contractions slow or stop them. The figure below shows an example of a crossed change of direction (COD) in VersaPulley. This exercise simulates the deceleration-acceleration that happens in the field when a player changes direction (eccentric overload monitored with Smartcoach analysis software) (Fig. 10.7). In this way, it allows us to have real-time feedback of the intensity of each repetition (and the type of contraction—concentric or eccentric), as well as to record and compare different moments and follow its progression.

10.4.4 Power Sessions/Explosive Performance

Examining the great players of modern-day team sports shows that they all share common characteristics—speed and power. Thus, all coaches try to enhance these characteristics in their players so that they can put them into practice in the field.

What a few years ago would be unthinkable, such as doing power sessions on the day before an important game, is now a regular practice in many teams.

There is increasing scientific evidence that shows the benefits of these low volume sessions, with long and full recovery rests, which include exercises with low/moderate loads executed at maximal speed. Tsoukos and colleagues [40] concluded that five sets of four repetitions of jump squats with 3 min of rest improved neuromuscular performance in the lower limbs 24 as well as 48 h after a resistance

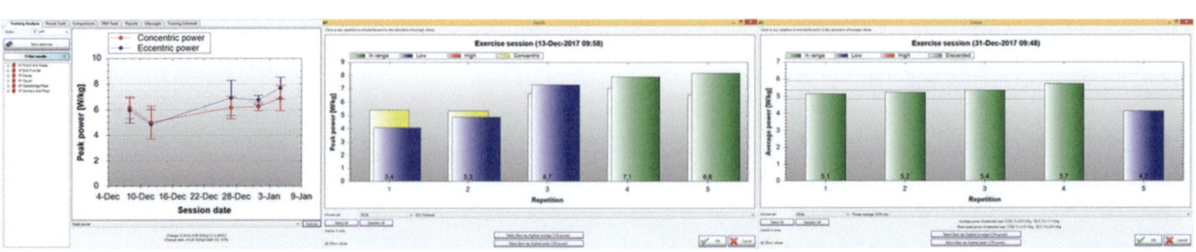

Fig. 10.7 Examples of Smartcoach overviews

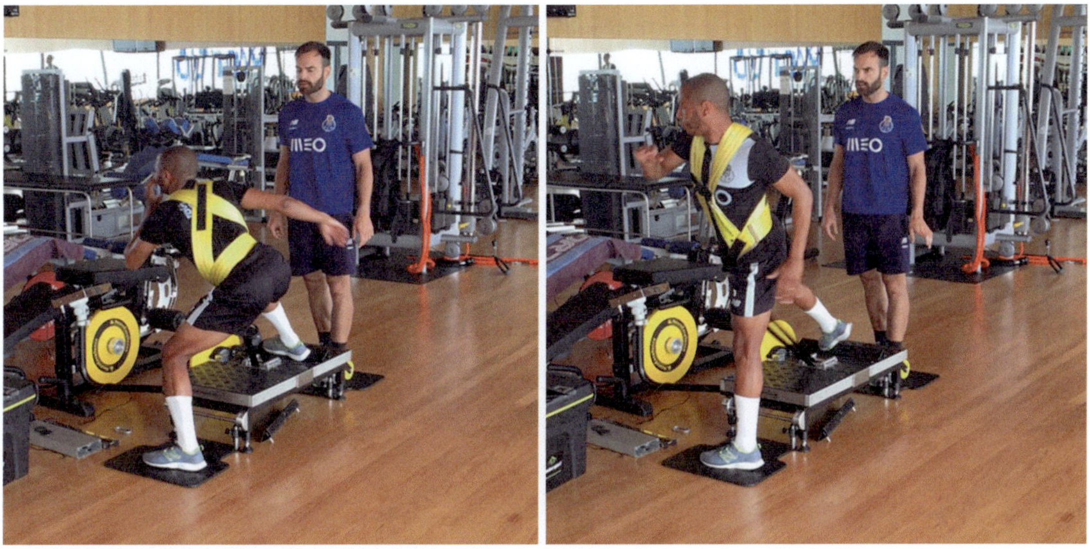

Fig. 10.8 Lateral eccentric squat (COD)

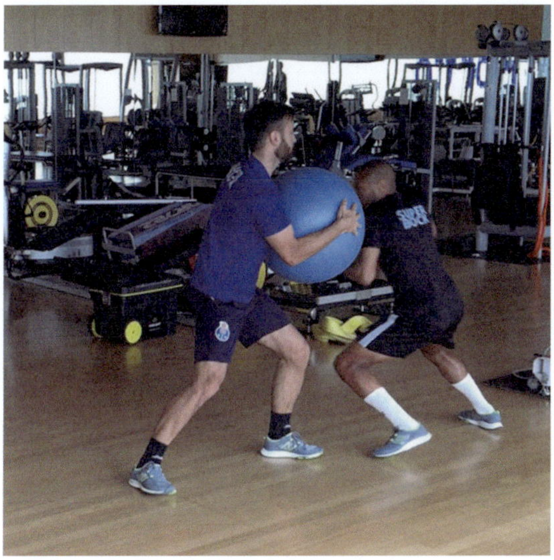

Fig. 10.9 Example of COD exercise transfer

training session, with greater enhancement observed after 24 h. Therefore, low volume resistance training and a high-quality training session 1 day before an important competition improve athletes' performance in all power-based sports [40].

The images below show an example of combining a sequence of two exercises with a COD transfer (with a low number of repetitions, full rest, and low load and based on speed execution) (Figs. 10.8 and 10.9).

Take-Home Messages

- Build robust players to reduce the odds of injury.
- Develop athleticism to support technical skills.
- Don't forget that athletes should perform on the pitch, as many times as possible, in training and competition.
- Design workout programs based on "high-quality movements," speed, power, and agility.
- Develop unilateral (single arm/leg), multidirectional, and velocity-based workouts.
- Individual approaches should focus on an athlete's weaknesses.
- Athletes benefit from eccentric overload, either for enhancing their performance or helping them recover from injuries. Even so, it may induce DOMS, especially in the case of an unusual exercise.

The success of a "strength program" depends on everyone involved in the training process: coaches, medical staff, and athletes.

References

1. Nédélec M, Halson S, Abaidia AE, Ahmaidi S, Dupont G. Stress, sleep and recovery in elite soccer: a critical review of the literature. Sports Med. 2015;45(10):1387–400.
2. Moreno M. Consideraciones a las tendencias del fútbol actual. El Entrenador Español. 1993;57:24–8.
3. Dufour W. Las técnicas de observación del comportamiento motor. Fútbol. Rev Entren Deport. 1990;4(4):16–24.
4. Bengtsson H, Ekstrand J, Hägglund M. Muscle injury rates in professional football increase with fixture congestion: an 11-year follow-up of the UEFA champions league injury study. Br J Sports Med. 2013;47:743–7.
5. Reilly T, Thomas V. A motion analysis of work-rate in different positional roles in in professional football match-play. J Hum Mov Stud. 1976;2:87–9.
6. Di Salvo V, Baron R, Tschan H, Calderon Montero FJ, Bachl N, Pigozzi F. Performance characteristics according to playing position in elite soccer. Int J Sports Med. 2007;28:222–7.
7. Barnes C, et al. The evolution of physical and technical performance parameters in the English premier league. Int J Sports Med. 2014;35:1095–100.
8. Gorrostiaga E. Bases científicas del fútbol: aplicación al entrenamiento I y II parte. El Entrenador Español. 1993:56–7.
9. Di Salvo V, Gregson W, Atkinson G, Tordoff P, Drust B. Analysis of high intensity activity in premier league soccer. Int J Sports Med. 2009;30:205–12.
10. Solé J. Entrenamiento de la resistencia en los deportes de equipo. Apuntes del Master de alto rendimiento en deportes de equipo 2002, vol. 80. Barcelona: Byomedic System; 2002. p. 81.
11. Bangsbo J, Mohr M, Krustrup P. Physical and metabolic demands of training and match-play in the elite football player. J Sports Sci. 2006;24(7):665–74.
12. Stolen T, Chamari K, Castagna C, Wisloff U. Physiology off soccer. An update. Sports Med. 2005;35:501–36.
13. Rodriguez FA, Iglesias X, Tapiolas J. Gasto energético y valoración metabólica en el fútbol. Train fútbol. 1996;9:25–33.
14. Nédélec M, McCall A, Carling C, Legall F, Berthoin S, Dupont G. Recovery in soccer: part I—post-match fatigue and time course of recovery. Sports Med (Auckland, NZ). 2012;42:997–1015. https://doi.org/10.2165/11635270-000000000-00000.
15. Edwards AM, Noakes TD. Dehydration: cause of fatigue or sign of pacing in elite soccer? Sports Med. 2009;39(1):1–13. https://doi.org/10.2165/00007256-200939010-00001.
16. Halson SL. Monitoring training load to understand fatigue in athletes. Sports Med (Auckland, NZ). 2014;44(Suppl 2):139–47. https://doi.org/10.1007/s40279-014-0253-z.
17. Akenhead R, Nassis GP. Training load and player monitoring in high-level football: current practice and perceptions. Int J Sports Physiol Perform. 2016;11(5):587–93. https://doi.org/10.1123/ijspp.2015-0331.
18. Akubat I, Barrett S, Abt G. Integrating the internal and external training loads in soccer. Int J Sports Physiol Perform. 2014;9(3):457–62. https://doi.org/10.1123/IJSPP.2012-0347.
19. Foster C, Florhaug JA, Franklin J, Gottschall L, Hrovatin LA, Parker S, et al. A new approach to monitoring exercise training. J Proc Natl Acad Sci USA. 2001;15:109–15. https://doi.org/10.1519/00124278-200102000-00019.
20. Gallo TF. Monitoring athlete preparedness in professional Australian football: load, self-report measures and performance (doctoral thesis, Australian Catholic University). 2016.
21. Hottenrott K, Hoos O, Esperer HD. Heart rate variability and physical exercise. Current status. Herz. 2006;31(6):544–52.. Review. German.
22. Flatt A. HRVtraining. Heart rate variability explained: part 1|HRVtraining. 2016. https://hrvtraining.com/2012/01/16/heart-rate-variability-explained-part-1/. Accessed 1 June 2016.
23. Buchheit M. Monitoring training status with HR measures: do all roads lead to Rome? Front Physiol. 2014;5:73.
24. Gallo TF. Pre-training perceived wellness impacts training output in Australian football players. J Sports Sci. 2016;34(15):1445–51. https://doi.org/10.1080/02640414.2015.1119295.. Epub 2015 Dec 4
25. Malone S, Owen A, Mendes B, Hughes B, Collins K, Gabbett TJ. High-speed running and sprinting as an injury risk factor in soccer: can well-developed physical qualities reduce the risk? J Sci Med Sport. 2018;21(3):257–62.
26. McHall A, Dupont G, Ekstrand J. Internal workload and non-contact injury: a one-season study of five teams from the UEFA Elite Club Injury Study. Br J Sports Med. 2018;52(23):1517–22. https://doi.org/10.1136/bjsports-2017-098473.
27. Ekstrand J, Hägglund M, Kristenson K, Magnusson H, Waldén M. Fewer ligament injuries but no preventive effect on muscle injuries and severe injuries: an 11-year follow-up of the UEFA champions. Br J Sports Med. 2013;47(12):732–7. https://doi.org/10.1136/bjsports-2013-092394.. Epub 2013 Jun 29.
28. Goode AP, Reiman MP, Harris L, et al. Eccentric training for prevention of hamstring injuries may depend on intervention compliance: a systematic review and meta-analysis. Br J Sports Med. 2015;49:349–56.
29. Orchard J, Best TM. The management of muscle strain injuries: an early return versus the risk of recurrence. Clin J Sport Med. 2002;12:3–5.
30. De Vos RJ, Reurink G, Goudswaard GJ, et al. Clinical findings just after return to play predict hamstring

re-injury, but baseline MRI findings do not. Br J Sports Med. 2014;48:1377–84.
31. Opar DA, Williams MD, Shield AJ. Hamstring strain injuries: factors that lead to injury and re-injury. Sports Med. 2012;42(3):209–26.
32. Ekstrand J. Keeping your top players on the pitch: the key to football medicine at a professional level. Br J Sports Med. 2013;47:723–4.
33. Bengtsson H, Ekstrand J, Waldén M, Hägglund M. Muscle injury rate in professional football is higher in matches played within 5 days since the previous match: a 14-year prospective study with more than 130 000 match observations. Br J Sports Med. 2018;52(17):1116–22. https://doi.org/10.1136/bjsports-2016-097399.
34. Arnason A, Andersen TE, Holme I, et al. Prevention of hamstring strains in elite soccer: an intervention study. Scand J Med Sci Sports. 2008;18(1):40–8.
35. Petersen J, Thorborg K, Nielsen MB, et al. Preventive effect of eccentric training on acute hamstring injuries in men's soccer: a cluster-randomized controlled trial. Am J Sports Med. 2011;39(11):2296–303.
36. Van der Horst N, Smits DW, Petersen J, et al. The preventive effect of the Nordic hamstring exercise on hamstring injuries in amateur soccer players: a randomized controlled trial. Am J Sports Med. 2015;43(6):1316–23.
37. Askling CM, Tengvar M, Tarassova O, et al. Acute hamstring injuries in Swedish elite sprinters and jumpers: a prospective randomised controlled clinical trial comparing two rehabilitation protocols. Br J Sports Med. 2014;48(7):532–9.
38. Bahr R, Thorborg K, Ekstrand J. Evidence-based hamstring injury prevention is not adopted by the majority of champions league or Norwegian premier league football teams: the Nordic hamstring survey. Br J Sports Med. 2015;49(22):1466–71.
39. Bourne MN, et al. An evidence-based framework for strengthening exercises to prevent hamstring injury. New York: Springer; 2017.
40. Tsoukos A, et al. Delayed effects of a low volume, power-type resistance exercise session on explosive performance. J Strength Cond Res. 2018;32(3):643–50.

Sport Injury Primary and Secondary Prevention

11

Rogério Pereira, Renato Andrade, Alexandre Rebelo-Marques, and João Espregueira-Mendes

11.1 Background

In the former three decades, there is a growing body of evidence concerning the efficacy of preventive measures of sports injuries [1–3] and reinjuries (defined as an injury of the same type and at the same site as an index injury in the preceding year) [4, 5]. This comes handy as the number of participants in organized youth sports is on the rise, with increasing number of games, and more competitive sporting modalities seem to be demanding more from human development domains (and these are not discrete, i.e., they constantly interact). Athletes and other sports agents are always in a hurry to return to play after injury, and more people in general are being enrolled on large-scale actions striving for physically active life styles' promotion as it is the case of the World Health Organization (WHO) Global action plan on physical activity and health 2018–2030: "More active people for a healthier world." Hence, sports injury preventive evidence-based measures should be strongly stimulated, continuously developed, and widely and systematically implemented in broad ecological settings to reduce injuries, narrow gaps between research

R. Pereira (✉)
Clínica do Dragão, Espregueira-Mendes Sports Centre—FIFA Medical Centre of Excellence, Porto, Portugal

Dom Henrique Research Centre, Porto, Portugal

Faculty of Sports, University of Porto, Porto, Portugal

University Fernando Pessoa, Porto, Portugal
e-mail: rp@espregueira.com

R. Andrade
Clínica do Dragão, Espregueira-Mendes Sports Centre—FIFA Medical Centre of Excellence, Porto, Portugal

Dom Henrique Research Centre, Porto, Portugal

Faculty of Sports, University of Porto, Porto, Portugal
e-mail: randrade@espregueira.com

A. Rebelo-Marques
Clínica do Dragão, Espregueira-Mendes Sports Centre—FIFA Medical Centre of Excellence, Porto, Portugal

Dom Henrique Research Centre, Porto, Portugal

Faculty of Medicine, University of Coimbra, Coimbra, Portugal

Coimbra Institute for Clinical and Biomedical Research (iCBR), Coimbra, Portugal

J. Espregueira-Mendes
Clínica do Dragão, Espregueira-Mendes Sports Centre—FIFA Medical Centre of Excellence, Porto, Portugal

Dom Henrique Research Centre, Porto, Portugal

Medicine School of Minho University, Braga, Portugal

ICVS/3B's–PT Government Associate Laboratory, Braga/Guimarães, Portugal
e-mail: espregueira@dhresearchcentre.com

S. Rocha Piedade et al. (eds.), *The Sports Medicine Physician*,
https://doi.org/10.1007/978-3-030-10433-7_11

and athletic community uptake, decrease the asymmetries in access, and aim for comprehensive public health strategies. Risk management strategies may lead the way to reduce the sport activity-related injuries and increase the outcome of benefit-risk ratio in all participation levels. These strategies comprehend injury surveillance, pre- and in-season meetings to refine strategies with technical staff, accounting with their planning, overlooked and/or unpredictable facts, regular screening of athletes, and implementation of prevention programs. All stakeholders should work together to provide regular participation in sports or physical activity, ensuring a safe and effective exposure to reach the most from health-related benefits and performance goals. This must be accomplished as part of health professionals' governance and will impact positively in sports and health achievements and, at the same time, reduce the societal and economic burden from injuries. In the European Union, there is a cost higher than two billion euros only with direct medical costs associated with sports injuries treatment [6].

There is strong scientific evidence reporting efficacy and effectiveness particularly of exercise-based interventions in reducing most common sports injuries within adult semi- and professional levels [2, 7–9]. Beneficial effects of injury-specific and multimodal exercise-based prevention programs have also been reported in youth athletes with high efficiency in reducing sports injuries (injury reduction superior to 40%) [6, 10]. For purposes of intelligibility of this chapter, the authors consider primary prevention as all actions aiming to avoid a first-time injury, which may imply a functional or structural impairment, and secondary prevention as incidence of a reinjury of early recurrence (within 2 months after full return to participation from the index injury), late recurrence (after more than 2 months), or delayed recurrence (after more than 12 months).

Despite the need to acknowledge and work on its complexity—if we are to truly address the dynamic web of causation—to enable and facilitate fundamentals acquisition, some simplified pedagogic exercises will be presented as fast and significant facts to lever all stakeholders embracing injury prevention mandatory cause. If up to today prediction is not possible [11, 12], effective and cost-effective preventive interventions associated with sports-related injuries are not utopic [13]. Compliance and maintenance of evidence-based injury prevention programs and broad community adoption is what is lacking the most [14]. A more comprehensive knowledge of the risk factors and injury mechanisms, with their complex interplay, and to what extent they could work in a synergistic manner to influence the outcome is also lagging. This will certainly allow improved interventions aiming for prevention within an ever-changing context, in which a sports-related injury may occur or prevail.

This chapter will address in a step-by-step (with chronological sequences of knowledge development and with incidence on research translation into practice) and critical approach the sports injuries challenge. This, fortunately will engage readers by providing key rationales and facts to keep athletes healthy while continuous and simultaneously developing their athletic skills and teams' sporting and financial performance [15].

11.2 Predisposing Risk Factors and Injury Mechanisms

Several risk factors have been identified that may predispose the athlete to risk of injury including anatomical, biomechanical, neuromuscular, environmental, developmental, hormonal, and genetical [16–18]. These can be divided into intrinsic (within the body) and extrinsic (outside the body) and to modifiable and non-modifiable risk factors. Both the intrinsic and the extrinsic risk factors may interact making the athlete susceptible to injury [19, 20]. Intrinsic risk factors often include occurrence of previous injury, increased body mass index, gender, age, individual genetic predisposition, neuromuscular and strength impairments, anatomical malalignments, anthropometric variations, abnormal kinematics, and genetic predisposition. In turn, extrinsic risk factors comprise environmental conditions, training and match surfaces, high total exposures hours, inappropriate training (volume, magnitude, speed of loading, frequency, inclination, fatigue, wrong sportive gesture, abrupt or acute modifications in amount or type of load), player position, and poor equipment utilization (e.g., wrong footwear). Still, these risk factors will not directly cause an injury, but rather predispose the athlete to a certain level of risk, before an injury-inciting event takes place [19]. Inciting events can appear at any time (training or match situations) and comprise several factors, such as playing situation, player and/or opponent behavior, individual gross (whole body), and specific biomechanical characteristics [20, 21]. Thus, a precise and comprehensive description of the inciting event, by extending the traditional biomechanical model, is key to better understand the multifactorial nature of injuries and better match prevention strategies that can either address intrinsic and extrinsic risk factors, proxies, and their interplay. This interplay can be illustrated by picturing a player with an increased risk of sustaining an anterior cruciate ligament (ACL) tear, which is a female (intrinsic and non-modifiable risk factor for ACL), associated with artificial floors [22] when playing handball (extrinsic and modifiable factor and proxy that seems to predispose to an injury mechanism), which may be augmented by unanticipated perturbation of the trunk [23] and/or gender differences in proximal control of the knee joint [24]. Thus, knowing facts, it becomes evident that preventive strategies must address several dimensions of the player and the game including athletes' physical and motor preparation, floor type, rules of the game, and others identified either as risk factors or injury-inciting event components, particularly, if these are prone to modification or manageable in nature. The main focus of preventive measures is on those risk factors that are modifiable, but all those players and individuals that are at higher risk of injury (either modifiable or non-modifiable) should take part in prevention programs.

The intrinsic risk factors are directly related to the individual characteristics, and its modifiability is not always possible. Nevertheless, knowledge regarding both modifiable and non-modifiable intrinsic risk factors may be used to target intervention strategies of those at risk of sustaining injury. These are often related with biomechanical, neuromuscular, and structural deficits which can be addressed in order to reduce the predisposition to the specific injury. On the other hand, although most of extrinsic risk factors can be modifiable, these depend upon on a myriad of external factors, which may be due to random circumstances (e.g., environmental conditions of the training or match or a player-to-player interaction).

As female athletic participation has been fast growing worldwide—in Europe there are 6 countries with more than 100,000 football players and 30 million at worldwide level [25]—it is of upmost importance to understand the gender-specific risk factors, such as developmental differences; anatomical, biomechanical, and neuromuscular differences; hormonal-specific characteristics; sexual maturation; and anthropometric specifications [26–28]. Moreover, female athletes have different sport-specific biomechanical and skills performance [29–33], and there is a need to adapt the training loads and intensities to their physical demands and capacities [26].

In the last few decades, a considerable amount of research has been conducted to explain the aetiology of sports injuries and to propose implementation models for sports injury prevention (Table 11.1). Initially, there was a trend to linear causal-effect models, i.e., identify a specific predisposing risk factor and implement a preventive strategy on this specific risk factor [34]. Then, it was understood that there was no linear casual-effect relationship between a single risk factor, but an interaction of a complex web of several different factors which led to the development of several multifactorial risk of injury models [35, 36].

More recently, the exposure to training and workload-injury relationships has gained increasing interest as one of the main risk factors for athletic injury and reinjury. Within this line, Gabbett has disseminated the training-injury prevention paradox based on a ratio of the athlete loading exposure—the acute-chronic workload ratio (last week load, divided by the last 4 weeks load) [46]. The workloads may be internal (e.g., individual perceived effort) or external (e.g., exposure measured as training and match

Table 11.1 Relevant scientific references on aetiology of sports injuries and models for injury prevention

Year	Model	First author	Reference	Citations
1983	First randomized controlled trial on sports injury prevention [37]	J. Ekstrand	Ekstrand et al. (1983). Int J Sports Med. 4:124–28	438
1992	Stage sequence of prevention [34]	W. van Mechelen	van Mechelen et al. (1992) Sports Med. 14:82–99	1341
1994	Dynamic, multifactorial model of sports injury aetiology [38]	W. Meeuwisse	Meeuwisse (1994). Clin J Sport Med. 4:171–5	417
2003	Adapted Meeuwisse model [14]	R. Bahr	Bahr et al. (2003). Br J Sports Med. 37:384–92	636
2005	Injury risk model [39]	A. McIntosh	McIntosh (2005). Br J Sports Med. 39:2–3	95
2005	Understanding injury mechanisms [21]	R. Bahr	Bahr et al. Br J Sports Med. 39:324–9	817
2006	TRIPP framework [40]	C. Finch	Finch (2006). J Sci Med Sport. 9:3–9	508
2007	A dynamic, recursive model of aetiology in sports injury [19]	W. Meeuwisse	Meeuwisse et al. (2007). Clin J Sport Med. 17:215–9	330
2010	Behavior factor for sports injury prevention [41]	E. Verhagen	Verhagen et al. (2010). Sports Med. 40:899–906	91
2010	RE-AIM framework expanded [42]	C. Finch	Finch et al. (2010). Br J Sport Med. 44:973–8	163
2011	"No long lost in translation"—Implementation science notes [43]	C. Finch	Finch (2011). Br J Sports Med. 45:1253–7	92
2014	Seven steps for developing and implementing a prevention model [44]	D. Padua	Padua et al. (2014) Clin Sport Med. 33:615–32	25
2015	Complementary and alternative conceptual approach for prevention of sports injury [36]	A. Hulme	Hulme et al. (2015). Inj Epidemiol. 2:31	22
2016	Complex model for sports injuries [35]	N. Bittencourt	Bittencourt et al. (2016). Br J Sports Med. 50:1309–14	66
2018	Revisiting the first step of the "sequence of prevention" [45]	C. Bolling	Bolling et al. (2018). Sports Med. (Epub)	NA

hours). The concept suggests that inadequate planning of periodization of team may raise the probability of players sustaining an injury. Thus, it is important to both consider the acute and chronic workloads and, through a detailed and programed training schedule, find the so-called sweet spot for the individual athlete and, considering the athlete's profile, manage the acceptable level of injury risk if beyond. This will vary for each individual or team and depends on the current athlete characteristics (development stage, recovery of an injury, specific physical demands) and the sport-specific and extrinsic factors (type of sports, season timing, proximity of an important game). Nevertheless, this should not lead to the misconception that the acute-chronic workload ratio is capable of predicting injuries and should be rather used to make informed decisions when the athlete's injury risk may be increased or decreased [47]. Despite the athlete's cumulative training workloads, load spikes should be avoided especially in undertrained athletes, as they may lead to fatigue and increase the injury risk [46, 48–50]. Rather, a consistent training may provide resilience and result in protection from injuries [49]. This concept is not exclusive to the individual athlete and may be used planning the periodization of a team [47]. Guidelines for interpreting and applying training monitoring data have been published [51, 52]. Recently, the acute-chronic workload ratio has been reported considering different sports, including football [53, 54], rugby [55–57], gaelic football [58], and others.

One of the cornerstones of injury prevention programs is correctly identify and describe the extent of sports injury, i.e., the injury incidence and severity. While it is only possible to treat or prevent what is known, the extent of injury is also determinant to achieve risk matrix calculations, i.e., to support risk assessment by considering the category of probability or likelihood against the category of consequence severity. This qualitative risk analysis is a simple mechanism to increase visibility of risks and assist stakeholders to effectively manage it within a sporting setting. Along with the promotion of sport and physical activity and acknowledgment of all the related benefits, there is a risk to sustain injuries. In turn, this correlates to dropouts of youth participation in sport and physical activity which can hamper long-term health and well-being. Thus, evidence-based injury prevention programs and their translation to community-based scenarios—with a strong focus on adherence and its evaluation—are a priority to make the most from countermeasures. This implies a previous assessment of causation by a multifactorial point of view, weighing how potential interactions between intrinsic and extrinsic risk factors predispose an individual to injury.

The inciting event (e.g., pitch with greater grip, slippery surface, contact with an opponent) is the final and proximal link in the web causation which enables an injury mechanism lead to injury [38]. A comprehensive and multidimensional characterization of the inciting event is important to underpin the different domains, including the athlete's (physical fitness, skill level) and sports' (rules, turf type) related factors and others which may be addressed to prevent injuries [21]. Even though injury mechanisms—especially under a classical and isolated biomechanical point of view—often received the focus from the health professionals actuating within sports medicine, prevention practices have been evolving. Fortunately, the neuromuscular and biomechanical screening and load management strategies that are being applied more frequently nowadays are good examples that more attention is being directed to risk factors that, even being distant to the outcome and/or injury, need to be managed to reduce likelihood and/or severity of sports injuries. These may be referred to as prospective risk factors (e.g., strength deficits and/or bilateral or unilateral asymmetries, motor control impairments, previous injury) which reveal an association with a specific type of injury and may be manageable by effective evidence-based preventive interventions. While some of these are modifiable (e.g., strength and neuromuscular deficits), others are not (e.g., previous injury). Thus, the dynamic nature of some risk factors and recursive nature of athletes' participation endorse periodic surveillance in order to update and manage risk profile. A more comprehensive understanding of causality supports the development and implementation of more effective preventive strategies and suitable countermeasures. Ditto, this will reduce the number of athletes that will experience potential injury mechanisms if the number needed to treat is observed according to the absolute risk reduction. Despite that effective sports injury prevention to some extent is an option and taken just by a few, those with delayed onset of call of duty are in opposition to another reality where some athletes could be spared from injury.

11.3 Exposure

A comprehensive and precise registration of athlete exposure is crucial as denominator for accurate data collection procedures. This, especially within prospective cohort studies, allows to seek for relationships between the number of new injuries during a specified time period and the variables or risk factors within a population of athletes. Beyond attendance and duration (in minutes) in training and matches, other descriptive information for each individual may be explored. This may include weather conditions [59, 60], floor or turf type [22, 61], training and match load [53, 54], pitch count [62, 63], and compliance with use of protective equipment [64, 65], just to mention a few. These variables may be sorted according to study-related specific purposes [66]. The incidence of injuries should preferably be reported as the number of injuries per 1000 player-hours, rather than athlete-exposures (being an exposure a training session or match), as the duration of exposure units will vary. Naturally, it is also interesting to have incidence rates in relation to training or match exposures or type of floor (wooden or artificial) exposures, and these can and should also be recorded. When reporting injuries or reinjuries—irrespective of type of exposure—it is also essential to adopt the same definition of injury [66] (i.e., "all," "medical-attention," or "time-loss" injuries) as it is well known that the injury definition can often underestimate the extent of overuse injuries. The modified version of the overuse injury questionnaire (mOIQ) which was developed and validated by the Oslo Sports Trauma Research Center (OSTRC) [67] provided a superior insight of the magnitude and burden of knee injuries in volleyball players. Using the time-loss definition—an injury that results in a player being unable to take full part in future training or match—20% of participants reported that they had knee injuries, but, in opposition, when using the mOIQ, 85% reported a knee problem and 67% sustained a substantial knee problem [68]. Therefore, along with surveillance methodology, it is determinant to be aware of the injury definition used in order to provide consistency in injury occurrence and burden reporting and interstudy comparison [66, 68].

11.4 Models for Research on Sports Injuries Prevention and Translation of Evidence into Practice

The "sequence of prevention" of sports injuries of van Mechelen et al. [34] has been revisited for more than 25 years. First, Finch [40] added two steps to the "sequence of prevention," advancing a new sports injury prevention research framework—the Translating Research into Injury Prevention Practice (TRIPP) framework. This was intended to overcome the real-world implementation limitations of the former model by describing and assessing the intervention implementation context and the effectiveness of injury prevention programs. The two steps added include:

1. The need for understanding the implementation context (personal, environmental, societal, and sports delivery factors).
2. The evaluation of implementation process of preventive measures.

TRIPP model builds on the unquestionable fact that only research that can and will be adopted by sports main stakeholders (such as participants and their coaches or health providers) will prevent injuries. This is critical, since it is known that even having identified effective interventions, the process frequently falters at the dissemination, implementation, and maintenance phases. Moreover, feasibility assessment and potential for broad uptake of preventive interventions should precede large investments in trial-based evaluation as there is little to be gained from proving efficacy of an intervention that, for whatever the reasons may be, will never be accepted by sports main stakeholders [69]. The TRIPP framework was considered to provide a practical and meaningful approach to research within sports injury prevention, and therefore its adoption was recommended to all researchers in the field [69].

Later, Padua and colleagues [44] reported that the TRIPP framework did not provide specific guidance on the steps required to develop (TRIPP stage 3) and implement injury prevention programs (TRIPP stage 5) that have been proven to be effective. The seven steps are indexed to the stages 3 and 5 of the TRIPP framework (Fig. 11.1), being highlighted that key stakeholder's involvement and the development of an interdisciplinary implementation team facilitates the identification of barriers and solutions for the development of an evidence-based and context-specific exercise-based injury prevention program. This increases odds of buy-in, high-level implementation compliance and maintenance of the program, and related implementation strategies, i.e., these seven new steps optimize the translation into practice of evidence-based prevention programs within real-world settings. Nonetheless, it has to be acknowledged that Finch and Donaldson [42] had previously recognized that despite the availability of evidence-based interventions, there was a

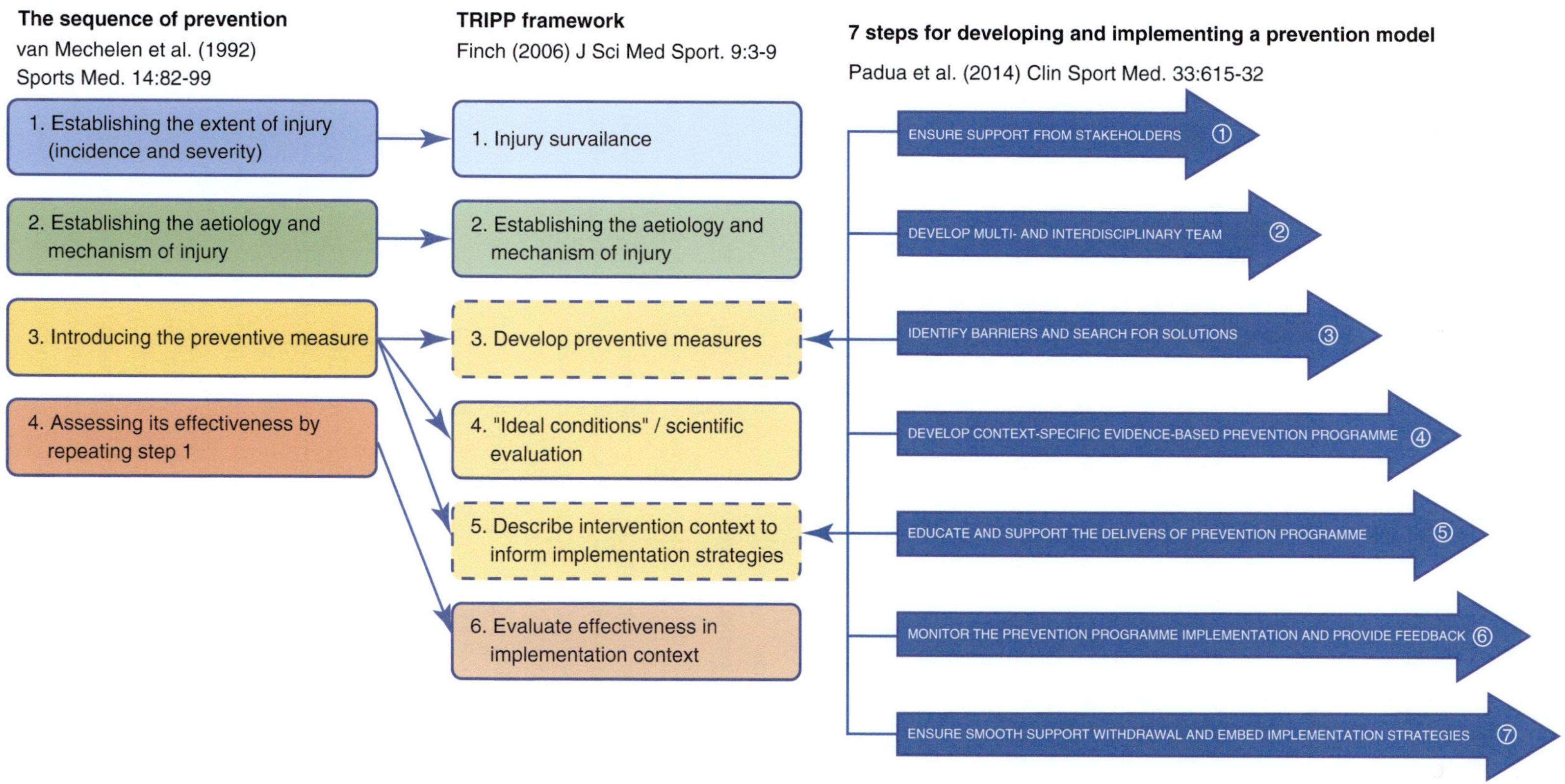

Fig. 11.1 Adaptation of the seven-step model for effective injury prevention program design and implementation from Padua et al. [44], incorporating the "sequence of prevention" [34] and TRIPP [40] models

major gap in injury prevention implementation and, therefore, provided a novel extension to the RE-AIM framework (Reach, perceived Effectiveness, Adoption, Implementation, and Maintenance)—the RE-AIM Sports Setting Matrix—as a way to embrace the delivery-setting complexity and optimize intervention delivery and evaluation. Additionally, Finch [43] previously discussed that the way interventions were developed and delivered was the reason why implementation of preventive strategies often fail and that scientific literature of injury intervention implementation studies was lagging. Thus, supported on the six steps of the Intervention Mapping protocol, an iterative path from problem identification to problem-solving or mitigation developed a scaffold within which empirical evidence, relevant theoretical constructs, contextual knowledge, and context-specific experience come together to inform the development, implementation, and evaluation of injury prevention programs—https://interventionmapping.com/. Finch [43] also gave insight on social theories such as diffusion of innovations theory which relies on communication of new ideas within multilevel ecological structures, with the purpose of achieving some form of behavioral or social change, outlining an agenda for sports injury intervention implementation research. In a subsequent publication [70] extends the discussion on the need to use concepts from *Implementation Science* as requirements for successful intervention implementation. In fact, to make a point on the relevance of implementation drivers, Finch and colleagues [71] show how they could be applied to facilitate the widespread and adherence of an evidence-based coach-delivered lower limb injury prevention program in a community-level Australian football clubs [71]. Also in this line, Bolling et al. [45] recently revisited the first step of the "sequence of prevention" and acknowledged the complexity of sports injuries and their prevention and, particularly, the need to establish the extent of the injury problem considering the athlete in the center of a socioecological model. Interestingly, a work done by Klügl et al. [13] found that only 1% of all English language publications related to sports injury prevention research (up to March 2010) investigated implementation and effectiveness. This fact reflects part of why implementation and maintenance of preventive measures often fail and the existing gaps that separate the complementary different kinds of content, process, and context experts [14]. Particularly, stepwise approaches for implementation and evaluation of evidence- and exercise-based injury prevention programs are still lagging. Thus, studies such as the one above referred by Finch et al. facilitating the widespread and adherence of an evidence-based injury prevention program [71], the one of Bizzini et al. [72] developed to implement the FIFA 11+ in national member football associations, that on awareness and use of the 11+ injury prevention program among coaches of adolescent female football teams in Football Federation Victoria [73], and the above referred of Padua et al. [44] are crucial for an effective reduction of sports injuries and optimization of the benefit-risk ratio.

11.4.1 Gap into Practice

Even when a specific prevention program proves its efficacy under controlled study conditions, this rarely translates into practice. Thus, it is crucial to advance with implementation research, providing detailed information about context-specific implementation strategies. These must be supported by a strong theoretical basis and should cover questions such as why and how the injury prevention program or specific exercises were selected and delivered and to what extent these were effective in reaching and changing the behavior of targeted audience [70]. Thus, the health belief model [74] and RE-AIM framework [42] can help to systematize outcomes of the interventions and knowledge about drivers for engagement [75]. Despite that underpinning concepts of *Implementation Science* such as engaging intervention end users in the planning and operationalizing of implementation activities were already adopted into sports injury prevention implementation, it seems that implementation drivers such as competency, organizational, and leadership need to be considered with a profound understanding of their purpose and application within an ecological setting of a sports injury prevention evidence-based program [70].

The wide variety of effective prevention strategies reported in the literature did not close the gap between injury prevention research and player safety behavior and practices [14]. In fact, looking at sports-related injury prevention interventions, the involvement from context and process experts is scarce. Therefore, if multiple interrelated contextual factors are not addressed, a big gap between efficacy and effectiveness will persist. Moreover, it must be kept in mind that internal validity does not assure external validity.

The transition from stage 3 (scientific development and testing of interventions) to stage 4 (dissemination and widespread adoption) of the public health model [14] is the greater challenge. However, even within the third step of the public health model, there are several challenges that need to be overcome. Compliance (often used interchangeably as implementation fidelity [76]) is used to indicate if the athlete is correctly following prescribed instructions of a sports injury prevention program, for example, dosage, timing, and frequency. In an intention-to-treat approach, compliance to the injury prevention program is crucial to better judge the efficacy of a preventive strategy. In large RCTs on injury prevention, controlling and influencing the individuals may become an almost impossible task as this is dependent on their own motivation levels and others stakeholders' interference [77]. Thus, prevention strategies should be designed considering the end-user context [78]. Higher compliance to injury prevention programs has shown to significantly decrease the overall injury rate [79–83]. In turn, adherence involves behavioral changes which may be influenced by the environment, social and personal contexts, motivations, skills, and resources [84, 85]. However, the often-long follow-up periods required in injury prevention studies for behavior changes can take place can lead to a significant loss to follow-up [86–88]. Even at the elite European football clubs (UEFA Elite Club Injury Study), the number of players that adhere to injury prevention programs is still insufficient [89]. Responsibility and governance have to be called into action with particular incidence in children and adolescent in sport. Hence, the sports medicine professionals supported on evidence-based preventable measures and their positive outcomes at different levels (health-related, competitive, and financial) must play a major role bringing together a responsibility hierarchy based on potential influence [90]. Injury prevention measures have to merge as core value and culture signature of every sports organization and ruling bodies.

11.5 Injury Primary Prevention

Ekstrand et al. [30] published in 1983 the first randomized controlled trial (RCT) reporting the results of the implementation of an injury prevention program in 180 amateur male football players achieving 75% of reduction of the injury rates. Since this major landmark study, injury prevention programs have been evolving, and there is a growing body of evidence of their substantial injury-preventing effect.

11.5.1 Multimodal Injury Prevention Programs

Multimodal injury prevention programs often include general and specific muscle strengthening and conditioning activities as running drills (recently with special focus on running technique), motor learning and motor control exercises, strengthening, plyometrics, proper technique during landing, agility, specific anatomical regions mobility, and kinetic chain improvement [91]. All these exercise categories are intended to improve general health, prevent sports injuries, and scale up general sports and skills performance, either gender- or sports- or position-specific skills, or even related to environmental conditions. These hardly take more than 20 minutes and often replace the traditional warm-up. This is in favor of overruling barriers such as adding additional time to training sessions which is definitely going to boost player compliance.

This is often an issue along with lack of awareness [73, 79]. More importantly, exercise-based programs have been found efficacious in reducing lower and upper limbs injury incidence, prevalence, and burden [1–3, 92, 93]. This is accomplished due to the fact that the exercise categories are intended to manage the already known risk factors and reduce the probability and/or severity of injury. Due to their easy accessibility and efficacy, exercise-based injury prevention programs became frequent within the context of RCTs applied to different sports. Their dissemination and potential for broad uptake at the sporting community level may yield significant societal and economic positive impact. There is convincing evidence that multimodal injury prevention programs can reduce the overall injury rate by 40% in child and adolescent, both those aiming all or specific injuries [94]. These programs improve several neuromuscular performance measures as balance/stability and leg power (small effects), reaching medium effect for isokinetic leg strength at low speeds and large effects for sprint abilities and sport-specific tests [95].

The ideal combination of training components within multimodal programs remains unclear [91]. Thus, injury prevention programs (such as FIFA 11+, PEP, IPEP, OSTRC shoulder injury prevention program) can be enhanced in open source way, i.e., these may benefit from the addition of one or more evidence-based exercises or components. For example, low adductor strength has been shown to represent a risk factor for groin injury in soccer [96]. Therefore, Harøy et al. [97] suggested the inclusion of the Adductor Strengthening Programme into the FIFA 11+ multimodal exercise-based program, to match the specificity principle of exercise, as there is an improvement of eccentric force of the adductors and, more importantly, a reduction in 41% of the risk of reporting groin problems in football players, through the Copenhagen Adduction exercise [98]. Naturally, the implementation of the exercise is not program-dependent.

A good example of efficacious and collaborative program is the FIFA 11+ Neuromuscular Training Programme developed by the Medical Assessment and Research Center of FIFA (F-MARC) in collaboration with the OSTRC and the Santa Monica Sports Medicine Foundation (SMSMF). It includes 15 structured exercises including core stabilization, eccentric thigh muscle training, proprioceptive training, dynamic stabilization, and plyometric exercises, all performed focusing postural alignment. This program has proven to reduce 39% of football injuries in female, male adolescent, and senior football players [2].

In the particular case of children, the injury prevention program for children's football ("11+ Kids") reduced the overall injury risk by 48% and the risk for severe injuries by 74% [94]. The "icing in the cake" is that after a cost-effectiveness analysis, comparing the "11+ Kids" with a usual warm-up, it was reported that a countrywide implementation (in Switzerland) would be dominant, i.e., lower injuries and 1.48 million Swiss Francs in healthcare costs could be avoided in just one season [99]. This adds strength to its widespread implementation and makes room for political actions.

In the year 2000, the SMSMF presented the Prevent Injury and Enhance Performance (PEP) program. The PEP program focused on proper landing, cutting, and decelerating techniques. It takes 20 minutes and can replace a traditional warm-up. In a cohort study involving competitive female youth football players, there was an 88% overall reduction in ACL injury in the first year of study and 74% in the second [100]. In turn, the OSTRC performed a cluster RCT in female adolescent handball (16-year and 17-year division), reporting that acute knee or ankle injuries can be reduced by 50% and severe injuries even more [10]. The intervention consisted in a structured warm-up program to improve running, cutting, and landing technique as well as neuromuscular control, balance, and strength.

In Sweden, the Knee Control Injury Prevention Exercise Programme (IPEP) is a project initiated in 2008 by the Swedish Football Association and the insurance company Folksam, aiming to reduce the burden of severe knee injuries. The IPEP contains six different principal exercises focusing on neuromuscular control, landing and cutting technique, core and lower limb strength, and lower limb alignment. All exercises have four levels of progression, and the entire program takes about 15 minutes to perform. It was reported to be the largest RCT on sports injury prevention (230 clubs, 4564 players). The IPEP resulted in a 64% lower rate of ACL injury in the intervention group, 82% reduction in the rates of severe knee injury and 47% reduction in any acute knee injury. Compliance with the program was decisive [3].

Due to the lacking evidence on implementation of preventive measures of overuse shoulder injuries, which are common within several overhead and throwing sports, research on overuse shoulder injury prevention was mandatory [1]. For elite handball players, the average prevalence of shoulder problems throughout the season was reported to be 28% (95% confidence interval 25–31%) and 12% (95% CI 11–13%) for substantial shoulder problems (leading to moderate or severe reductions in handball participation or performance). Among others, reduced glenohumeral rotation, external rotators weakness, and scapular dyskinesis were identified as risk factors for elite shoulder injuries in male handball players [101]. Thus, Stig and collaborators [1] recently performed the first RCT in overuse shoulder-specific injury prevention to implement the OSTRC Shoulder Injury Prevention Programme based on identified risk factors. It includes five exercises that were prescribed to increase the glenohumeral internal range of motion, external rotation strength, and scapular muscle strength, as well to improve the kinetic chain and thoracic mobility. Despite that compliance was challenging (1.6 times per week of the recommended three weekly sessions), it did not influence the risk of shoulder problems. Moreover, a 28% lower risk of shoulder problems (odds ratio of 0.72, 95% confidence interval 0.52–0.98, $p = 0.038$) and 22% lower risk of substantial shoulder problems (odds ratio of 0.78, 95% confidence interval 0.53–1.16, $p = 0.23$) were observed in the intervention group. Thus, the OSTRC Shoulder Injury Prevention Programme, which takes only 10 min to perform, can have an important role in preventing shoulder overuse injuries with plausible application in other overhead and/or throwing sports.

11.5.2 Injury-Specific Prevention: Fast Facts

This subsection will cover some of the best evidence available of four injury-specific prevention measures and their respective implementation outcomes (fast facts). The classical four-step model is still part of the foundations for research on sports injury prevention, even acknowledging to be supported in a linear framework. However, the "sequence of prevention" allows a first approach to fundamental literacy within sports-related injuries knowledge and competencies. Thus, examples of pedagogic exercises will be presented covering all the four below-discussed injuries as a path to match facts and build a first and determinant layer of knowledge for intervention purposes. Naturally, these steps should all be fed by evidence-based data, context-driven as discussed before, and public health models and Implementation Science are mandatory if success is an option.

11.5.2.1 ACL Injury Prevention: Fast Facts

ACL ruptures are severe injuries with high negative impact in individual and team performance, substantial economic burden (total healthcare utilization cost is $13,403 to $38,121 for each patient undergoing arthroscopic ACL reconstruction [102, 103]), and potential negative impact in long-term health and well-being [104, 105]. According a recent systematic review with meta-analysis [106], the incidence rate of ACL injury in sports is 0.9 per 10,000 athlete-exposures in male players and 1.5 per 10,000 exposures in female players. Irrespective of the participation level, the incidence rate among women was 1.5 times higher than in men.

While evidence regarding neuromuscular and biomechanical risk factor for ACL injury in male athletes is lagging [18], risk factors for ACL injuries female athletes seem to be well established [16, 23, 107]. Increased dynamic knee valgus, high knee abduction loads, dynamic trunk instability, and gender-specific asymmetries after puberty—females exhibit measurable quadriceps dominance, ligament dominance, leg dominance, and trunk dominance [108–111]. The multimodal injury prevention programs may play a major role in injury prevention in female adolescent since they may induce the neuromuscular spurt, tackling several of the referred risk factors.

A video analysis of 39 ACL injury cases reported that 85% of the ACL injuries in male professional football players resulted either from non-contact or indirect contact mechanisms, being the three predominant mechanisms: pressing situations, regaining balance after kicking, and landing after heading. While knee valgus was frequent, dynamic valgus collapse was not [112]. It was reported that 77% of ACL ruptures occur while defending which is consistent with a previous work—73% [113]. Video analysis of ACL injuries on other sports has been published, including American football [100], rugby [114], netball [115], alpine skiing [116], basketball, and handball [117, 118]. An overview of several video analysis studies suggested that ACL injury prevention programs should focus on enhancing cutting and landing technique that avoids knee valgus and internal rotation during knee flexion, as well as proper hip flexion to absorb energy from ground reaction force and avoid excessive hip internal rotation [119].

More recently, a systematic review and meta-analysis of overlapping meta-analyses on ACL injury prevention programs reported conclusive evidence that they reduce the risk of all ACL injuries in 50% in all athletes and non-contact ACL injuries in 67% in female athletes [120]. A total of 108 (95% confidence interval, 86–150) and 120 (95% confidence interval, 74–316) individuals would need to be trained to prevent one non-contact or one overall ACL injury over the course of one competitive season, respectively [121]. In female athletes, lower body strengthening, proximal control exercises (specific focus on landing stabilization), and multi-exercise genres increase the efficacy of ACL neuromuscular interventions [122, 123], while age, dosage, exercise variations, and utilization of verbal feedback are predictors for optimization of prophylactic effects in ACL neuromuscular training [124]. These exercises have the potential to enhance cutting and landing biomechanics by improving neuromuscular deficits linked to ACL rupture, especially when emphasizing the individualized biomechanical technique correction [125, 126]. Recently, clinical practice guidelines on exercise-based knee and ACL injury prevention report useful recommendations that may be used by clinicians, coaches, parents, and athletes [127].

A pedagogic example of the four-step injury prevention model applied to ACL injury is presented in Fig. 11.2.

11.5.2.2 Ankle Injury Prevention: Fast Facts

The incidence rates of lateral ankle sprains are high, vary significantly according to sports, and are one of the most common musculoskeletal injuries. The direct costs of ankle sprain management range from \$292 to \$2268 per patient, depending on the injury severity and treatment strategy [128]. Pooled cumulative incidence of ankle sprains is 7 per 1000 exposures (95% confidence interval 6.8–7.2) for court sports, 3.7 per 1000 exposures (95% CI 3.3–4.17) for ice/water sports, 1.0 per 1000 exposures (95% CI 0.95–1.05) for field sports, and 0.88 per 1000 exposures (95% CI 0.73–1.02) for outdoor sports. Additionally, females are at a higher risk of sustaining an ankle sprain compared with males, as well as children compared with adolescents and adults [129].

Considering best-evidence recommendations from a recent evidence-based clinical guideline, the intrinsic modifiable risk factors included limited dorsiflexion range of motion, reduced proprioception and (preseason) deficiencies in single-leg postural balance test, which substantially increase the risk of sustaining a lateral ankle sprain (level 1). In turn, considering extrinsic modifiable risk factors, irrespective of its likelihood of modification, included type of sport (e.g., basketball, indoor volleyball; level 2), male participation, landing after a jump in volleyball, playing soccer in natural grass, and being defender (level 3) [130]. In volleyball lateral ankle sprains were found to be the most frequent injury (54% of all injuries, with 89% of this occurring at the net), being 68% result of landing in the foot of an opponent and 19% in a

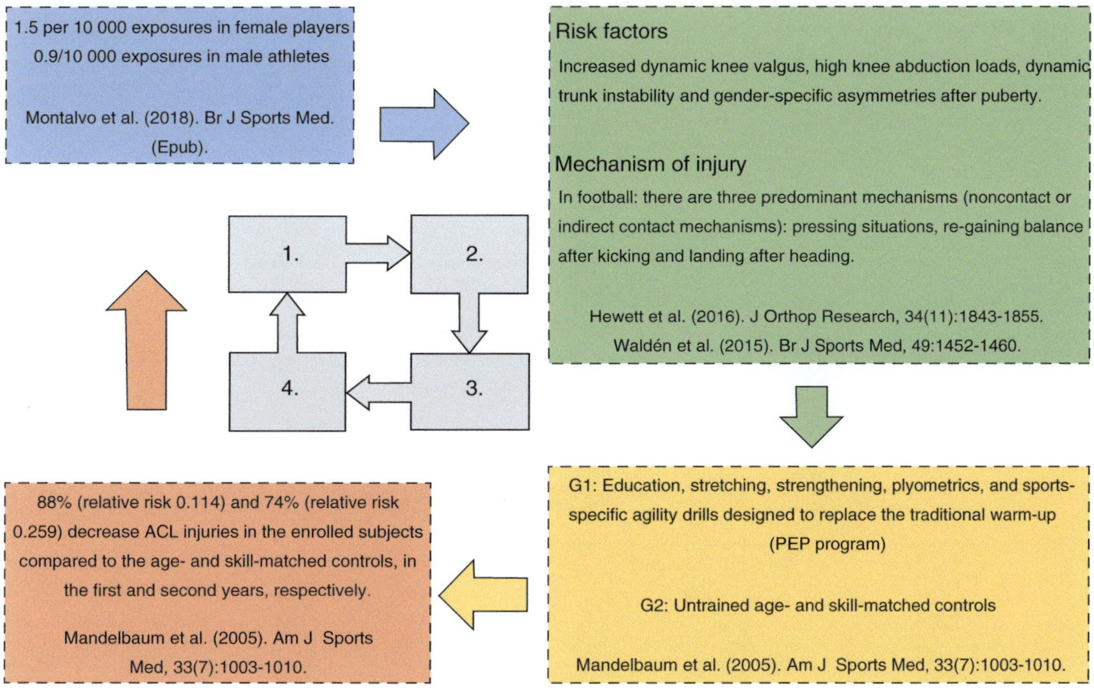

Fig. 11.2 Pedagogic example of the four-step injury prevention model applied to ACL injury: (*1*) establishing the extent of the sports injury problem [106]; (*2*) establishing aetiology [23] and mechanism of injury [112]; (*3*) introducing preventive measure [93]; (*4*) assessing its effectiveness by repeating step 1 [93]

teammate's foot [131]. Recent evidence supports this finding reporting that majority of injuries occur while blocking, often landing on an opponent with rapid inversion with no plantarflexion, rather than previously thought that these occurred in plantarflexion [132]. This playing situation related to inversion injury mechanisms is also common in basketball [133]. In turn, in football the injury mechanism usually comprises player-to-player contact with impact by an opponent on the medial aspect of the leg just before or at foot strike, resulting in a laterally directed force causing the player to land with the ankle in a vulnerable, inverted position or a forced plantar flexion where the injured player hit the opponent's foot when attempting to shoot or clear the ball [134].

In a Cochrane review, it was reported that using an external ankle support, there is significant reduction in the number of ankle sprains (relative risk 0.53, 95% CI 0.40–0.69) [135]. More recently, it was reported that the use of ankle braces or tape can reduce the risk of first-time lateral ankle sprains (relative risk of 0.30, 95% confidence interval 0.21–0.43) [130]. For recurrence of ankle sprains, the use of ankle bracing is more effective (relative risk 0.69, 95% confidence interval 0.49–0.96) [130]. When comparing ankle bracing to neuromuscular training, the relative risk is 0.53 (95% confidence interval 0.29–0.97). An unsupervised proprioceptive training program to reduce the recurrence of lateral ankle sprains can reduce a mean of €81 (standard deviation, €134) per athlete and €114 (€325) per injured athlete [136].

A pedagogic example of the four-step injury prevention model applied to lateral ankle sprains is presented in Fig. 11.3.

11.5.2.3 Muscle Injuries Prevention: Fast Facts

Muscle injuries represent more than one third of all time-loss injuries (elite European professional football clubs) [140]. A recurrence rate of 17% has been reported in elite football players [141]. The hamstring, quadriceps (mainly the rectus femoris), the adductor, and the calf muscles are

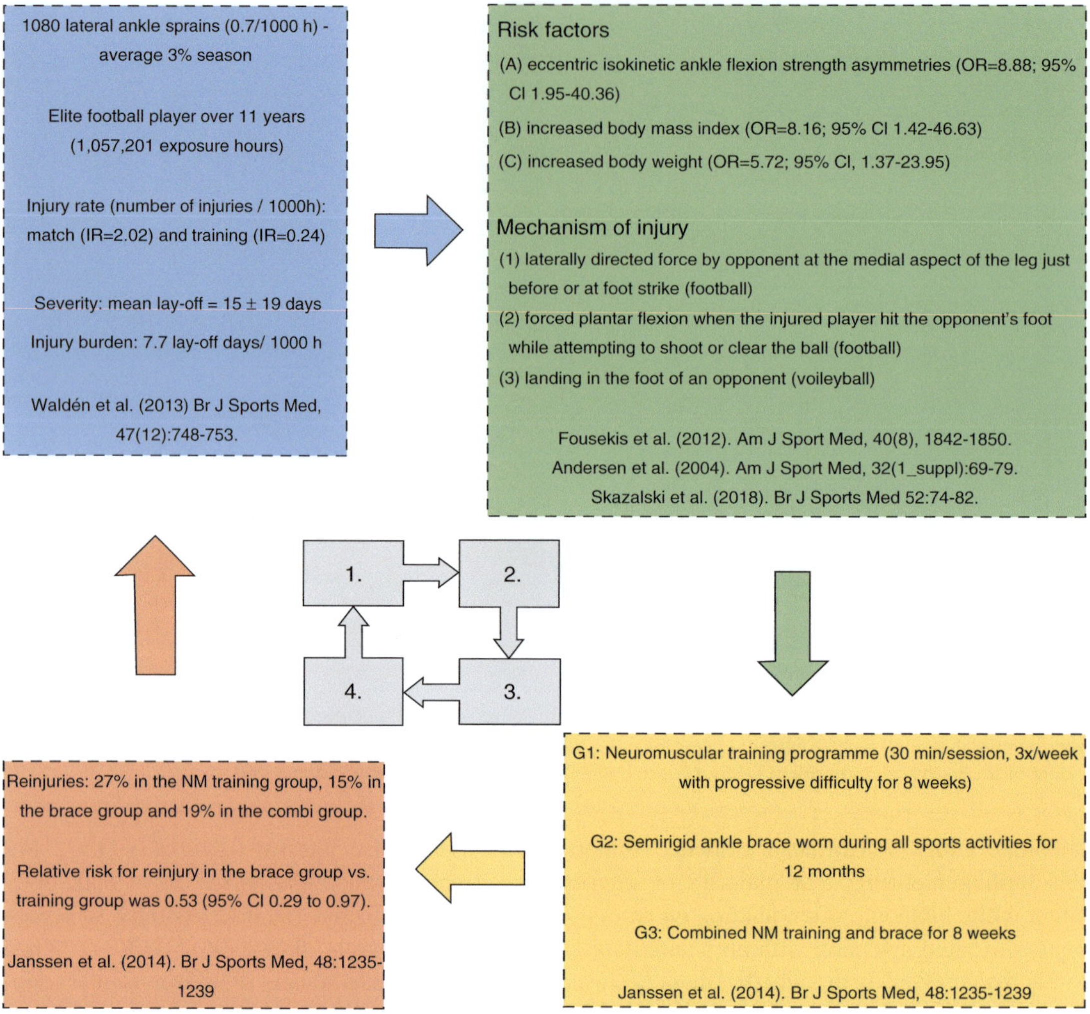

Fig. 11.3 Pedagogic example of the four-step injury prevention model applied to lateral ankle sprains: (*1*) establishing the extent of the sports injury problem [137]; (*2*) establishing aetiology [138] and mechanism of injury [132, 134]; (*3*) introducing preventive measure [139]; (*4*) assessing its effectiveness by repeating step 1 [139]

the most affected accounting for 92% of all muscle injuries, being the hamstring the most common subtype, representing 12% of all injuries [140]. This means that, within a team with 25 players, around 5–6 hamstring injuries will occur each season [140]. In addition, the average injury burden is 19.7 days/1000 h [142]. This has a very high financial impact as the average cost for a first team player being injured for 1 month is around 500,000 € [143]. According to more recent reports, the training-related hamstring injury rate and injury burden is on the raise since 2001 (2.3% increase in the injury rate and 4.1% increase in the total hamstring injury burden) [142]. Hamstring reinjuries most commonly occur in biceps femoris injuries than semitendinosus and semimembranosus [144].

There is evidence on the association of older age, increased quadriceps peak torque, past history of hamstring injury, and kicking leg with increased risk of hamstring muscle strain-type injuries in sport [145, 146]. For recurrent hamstring injuries, there is limited evidence that athletes with a larger volume size of initial trauma, a Grade 1 hamstring injury, and a previous ipsilateral ACL reconstruction are at increased risk [147]. Direct muscle injuries are caused by an external force (contusion or laceration) and by

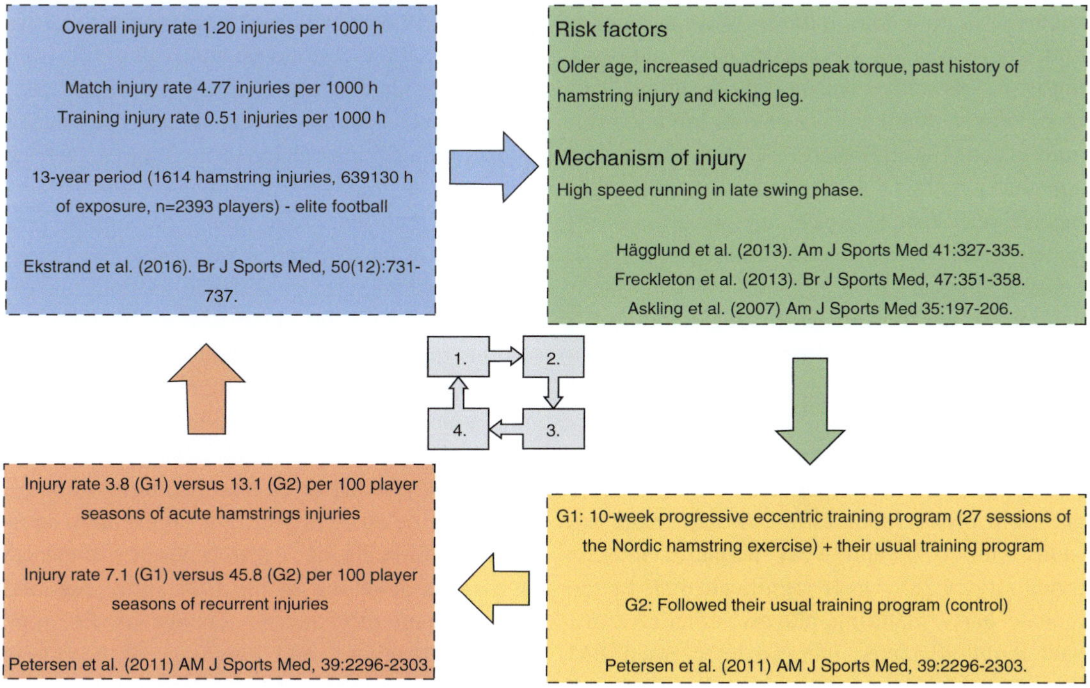

Fig. 11.4 Pedagogic example of the four-step injury prevention model applied to hamstring injuries: (*1*) establishing the extent of the sports injury problem [142]; (*2*) establishing aetiology [145, 146] and mechanism of injury [149]; (*3*) introducing preventive measure [152]; (*4*) assessing its effectiveness by repeating step 1 [152]

their nature cannot be prevented. In turn, indirect muscle injuries occur without an external trauma and are classified as either functional (nonstructural)—without evidence of a tear—or structural [148]. Acute hamstring injuries often occur at high-speed running in late swing phase [149] and are often considered as either a sprinting or stretching type [149, 150]. Stretching injuries affect more often the proximal semimembranosus at the muscle or tendon level [149, 151].

Despite that there is evidence-based hamstring injury prevention available to reduce the risk of new acute hamstring injuries in football up to 59% [152, 153], the adoption and implementation of the Nordic hamstring exercise at the highest level of football in Europe is low [154]. At amateur football level, the Nordic hamstring exercise also significantly reduces hamstring injury incidence with an excellent compliance level (91%) [155]. Nevertheless, when translating the evidence into practice, the Nordic hamstring exercise does not act directly to the main injury mechanism of hamstring injury which is, as previously described, high sprint running [156]. Thus, this exercise could be complemented with other potential preventive measures, such as the core stability training reducing hamstring stiffness [157] and pelvic stability, as hip flexor tightness leads to reciprocal inhibition of gluteus maximus and synergistic dominance of the hamstrings [158]. Moreover, when managing players with very high volumes of high sprint running—in which the risk of hamstring injury is higher—ensuring an adequate acute-chronic workload ratio (as described previously), controlling fatigue (often due to insufficient recovery), and avoiding acute load peaks has a key role in preventing hamstring injuries [159, 160].

A pedagogic example of the four-step injury prevention model applied to hamstring injuries is presented in Fig. 11.4.

11.5.2.4 Groin Pain Prevention: Fast Facts

At the European professional football (UEFA elite study), hip and groin injuries account for 12–16% of all time-loss injuries per season. However, in the last years, it was reported a slight decrease in time-loss injuries rates but not in injury burden [161]. In another report, comprising two consecutive seasons of the entire Qatar Stars League, the incidence rate of hip and groin injuries was 1.0 injuries/1000 h (time-loss injury approach), being 68% of all time-loss groin injuries adductor-related [162]. Hip and groin injury is the most common non-time-loss injury in female amateur football, and around three-quarters of the players with long-standing hip and groin injuries within the previous season show residual problems at the start of the following season [163].

Most relevant risk factors for hip and groin injuries in field-based sports are a previous groin/hip injury (odds ratio 2.6–7.3), older age (odds ratio 0.9), and weak adductor muscles (odds ratio 4.28). Other significant risk factors include early maturing players, smaller dominant femur diameter, increased/decreased BM, decreased hip abduction and total hip rotation range of motion, abduction and adduction-with-rotation peak torque, strength ratio of hip muscle groups, and bilateral difference in extension peak torque [164]. More recently, a systematic review concluded that there is strong evidence that total bilateral hip rotation (<85°) measured at the preseason screening is a risk factor for groin pain development and that internal rotation, abduction, and extension are not associated with the risk or presence of groin pain [165]. A recent video analysis study [166] identified that 71% of acute adductor longus injuries in male football players resulted from non-contact mechanisms, both in closed and open chain mechanisms. Four distinct predominant mechanisms were reported: change of direction (35%), kicking (29%), reaching (24%), and jumping (12%). The adductor longus injury accounts for 90% of the two-thirds of hip adductor-related acute groin injuries and a rapid muscle activation, while the muscle that is rapidly lengthened was admitted to be its fundamental injury mechanism.

Evidence on the prevention of hip and groin injuries is still evolving. A meta-analysis of RCTs showed a 19% reduction of groin injuries (relative risk 0.81; 95% confidence intervals 0.60–1.09) following specific groin injury prevention programs but without a statistically significant reduction in sports-related groin injuries. Despite the lack of statistical significance, the authors reported that the groin injury prevention programs may be of clinical relevance and potentially worthwhile to consider in football players [167]. Based on the video analysis of adductor longus injuries, it is suggested a focus on triplanar exercises leading to an increased capacity of the adductor longus/muscle-tendon unit withstand a rapid activation at a lengthened state (which may be achieved with eccentric training). This may be an effective injury prevention strategy. Additionally, it is also advised a focus on synergists actuating in the four above reported predominant mechanisms (change of direction, kicking, reaching, and jumping), as a way to reducing load on the adductor longus which may decrease injury risk [166]. Considering exercise selection and progression, particularly, for targeting the adductor longus, evidence exists for the Copenhagen Adduction exercise on both muscle activation patterns [168] and strength gains [97, 128, 169]. In a cluster RCT, the Copenhagen Adduction exercise reduced the prevalence and risk of groin problems in male football players by 41%. Considering all physical complaints, the average weekly prevalence of all groin problems during the competitive season was 13.5% in the intervention group and 21.3% in the control group [98]. Moreover, if strong evidence exists based on a single-exercise approach, a more comprehensive and now informed preventive strategy may even lead to superior outcomes. The authors point out that similarities related to structural adaptations from eccentric strengthening and its preventive effect on hamstrings and mechanisms in open chain category [170–172] may raise similar benefits in relation to adductor longus injuries.

A pedagogic example of the four-step injury prevention model applied to groin injuries is presented in Fig. 11.5.

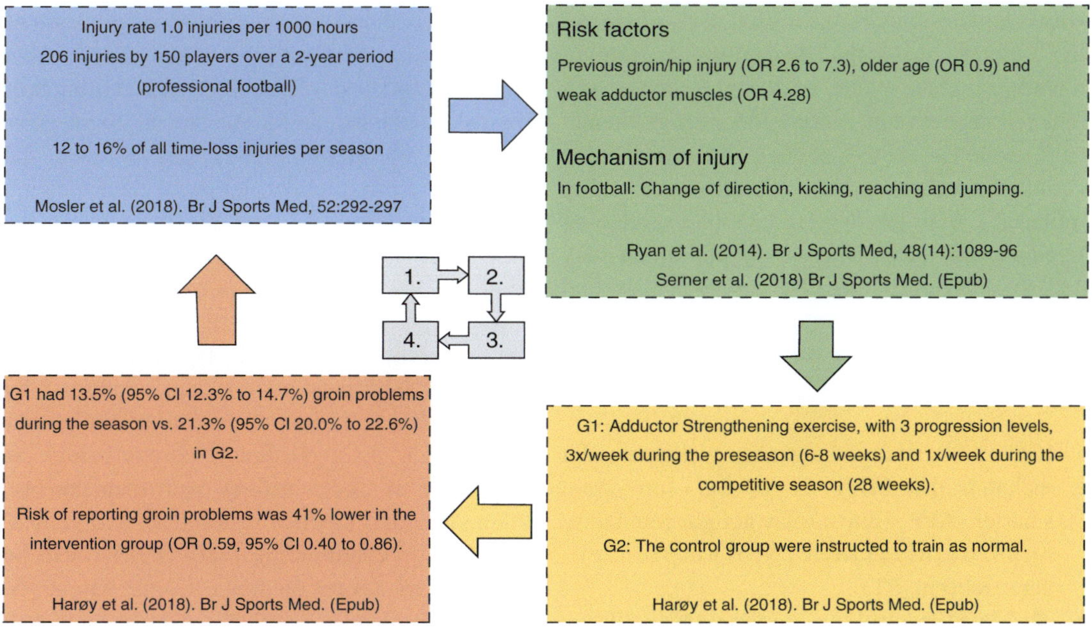

Fig. 11.5 Pedagogic example of the four-step injury prevention model applied to groin injuries: (*1*) establishing the extent of the sports injury problem [162]; (*2*) establishing aetiology [164] and mechanism of injury [166]; (*3*) introducing preventive measure [98]; (*4*) assessing its effectiveness by repeating step 1 [98]

11.5.3 Improving Reach of Proven Exercise-Based Prevention Programs Through mHealth

Despite large-scale RCTs proving that exercise-based programs substantially decrease injuries and are cost-effective [136, 139], broad uptake by sports teams and community is lagging [154], i.e., even the most effective programs will fail if you do not actually do it. Moreover, recent reports on elite football pointed out a raise in injuries as it is the case of hamstring injuries [142]—the number 1 lesion in elite professional football. Among other reasons, this paradox may be explained by lack of reach and/or awareness of the injury prevention programs by different stakeholders as coaches and players; lack of fidelity when implementing them (which may affect effectiveness); coaches and/or players may opt not to use it; and poor compliance (only compliant athletes will benefit from the preventive effect) or maintenance. Although a prevention program delivered either through a mobile App or a booklet has led to similar results in compliance rates, mobile health (mHealth), as a branch of information and communications technology (ICT), may help at fostering widespread adoption of those programs. In particular, using a mobile App ("Strengthen your ankle") in comparison to a printed booklet produced an incremental cost-effectiveness of 361.5€ [173] and a higher level of satisfaction [174], which can lead to potential changes in practice guidelines for general practitioners [175]. Given the continuous growing uptake of smartphones and consume of mobile Apps, this may be a smart way to channel opportunities. What digital tools bring may be supported by the implicit buy-in from policy makers. In fact, this is implicit to the eHealth Action Plan 2012–2020—Innovative healthcare for the twenty-first century from the European Union—which also includes a special focus on mHealth. Familiarity and high penetration of smartphones among general population and in particular within athletes may frame digital tools as part of the solution to stimulate injury prevention measures uptake while enabling feedback and interaction between stakeholders (e.g., health staff, technical team, athletes). Therefore, while gamification techniques [176] and virtual reality (clinical trials.gov/NCT02933008) ongoing research may yield positive results which may add to prevention interventions, we may find free-downloadable injury prevention mobile phone applications via App Store and Google Play such as:

- IOC's APP (so far 7 languages available and it includes the FIFA 11+): Get set—Train smarter APP (https://play.google.com/store/apps/details?id=org.olympic.app.getset&hl=pt_PT).
- The knee control programme (available in german): KnieKontrolle (https://play.google.com/store/apps/details?id=de.inventivo.kniekontrolle).
- "Strengthen Your Ankle" by VeiligheidNL (available in dutch): Versterk je enkel (https://play.google.com/store/apps/details?id=nl.veiligheid.versterkjeenkel).

11.6 Secondary Prevention

The likelihood of sustaining a reinjury is often higher compared with uninjured athletes. Compared with uninjured adolescents, a young athlete who returns to sport after ACL reconstruction may be at a 30–40 times greater risk of ACL injury [177]. Reinjuries are often more severe [178]. In football, previous injury is probably the most reported and prominent risk factor for injury. Reinjuries overall rate is about 17%, which is low if compared with amateur football teams (35%). Early recurrences (within 2 months) stand for 77% of those [179].

Primary prevention and evidence-based management of rehabilitation, return to play, and secondary prevention should be major priorities concerning health and well-being, with performance and financial implications. When facing an injury, there is an evolutive process of rehabilitation to accomplish. There are possible and/or established validated criteria (chronobiological, functional, and psychosocial) to progress within rehabilitation phases and to clear the player to return to play (please see the following chapter on return to play). For instance, in the case of ACL reconstruction, if the established return to play criteria are not matched, there is a fourfold greater risk of re-rupture [180]. Thus, the rehabilitation should be stepwise with criterion-based progressions and supported by the available and most up-to-date scientific evidence [181, 182]. Different domains such as timeframe of tissue healing, pain management, kinematics and kinetics restoration, and general and specific conditioning [180–183] have to be mastered by sports medicine teams. Moreover, when an athlete is reintegrated to training and competition, extrinsic factors (along with eventual unmatched rehabilitation goals and criteria categories to return to play) such as load and match congestion may particularly predispose an athlete to reinjury [184]. Along with this line, prospective surveillance of predisposing risk factors and potentially identified deficits is important to prevent the occurrence of a reinjury.

Athletes younger than 25 years old who return to play have a secondary ACL injury rate of 23%. This means that almost one in four young players that return to play after an ACL reconstruction will have a retear [177]. Also, poor self-confidence, poor performance on the triple hop for distance, hip and knee altered neuromuscular control during a dynamic landing task, and postural stability deficits after ACL reconstruction may be managed in a subgroup of individuals that may require extended rehabilitation to decrease the risk of reinjury [185, 186]. An approximation to neurosciences for improving rehabilitation techniques, skills, and efficacy may yield good results in motor control development, restoration, or enhancement, suppressing, for instance, deficits in motor control that were reported to persist even after 2 years of ACL reconstruction [187]. In this sense, novel video feedback, virtual reality, and verbally directed optimization techniques have emerged to enhance the ACL injury prevention programs [188–193]. Fortunately, it appears that following simple decision rules (meeting the return to play criteria) can reduce the reinjury risk by 84% [183]. But, are we followers of available good practices while pursuing new evidence?

Hamstring reinjuries are very frequent in professional football, and most of all recurrent hamstring injuries occur within the first month after returning to competition [22, 178, 194, 195]. Additionally, an increased susceptibility for reinjury seems to be present for several months after the initial injury [22, 195–199]. This high recurrence rate may be related to the fact that these players may have been exposed inappropriately to high training and competition loads or inappropriate rehabilitation (e.g., returned to play too soon without meeting the clearance criteria). Thus, a judicious and stepwise rehabilitation and return to play to minimize the risk of recurrence is key [178]. In fact, although accumulating higher training loads during rehabilitation delays the return to play after muscle injuries, accumulating moderate to high sprint running loads has protective effects against reinjury [200]. Thus, it is very interesting to recall the cluster RCT on the preventive effect of eccentric training on acute hamstring injuries in men's football, to point out the fact the recurrent injuries were reduced in almost 85% [152]. Additionally, performing agility and stabilization exercises rather than strengthening and stretching exercises during rehabilitation led to a lower risk for reinjury (7.7% vs. 70%) [147].

Concerning secondary preventable measures of ankle sprains recurrence, exercise interventions (odds ratio 0.59, 95% confidence interval 0.51–0.68) and external support interventions (odds ratio 0.38, 95% confidence interval 0.30–0.47) significantly decrease the risk of sustaining a recurrent ankle sprain, and thus, both interventions are supported in the prevention of chronic ankle instability [201]. However, evidence indicates that bracing dominates over both neuromuscular training and a combination of both regarding the potential savings and preventive effect [139].

Take-Home Message

Prevention of sports-related injury is an exercise of professionalism and governance. Knowledge and its translation into practice require hard work and bringing together the competencies of many professionals from different areas. There is a responsibility hierarchy that needs to be definitely and entirely called into action. However, every sports medicine health professional entails part of a mission that could and should be accomplished. No doubts could subsist that *Prevention is the best remedy* (Portuguese saying) for the health and well-being, societal and economic partial achievable goals of the whole sports family.

References

1. Andersson SH, Bahr R, Clarsen B, Myklebust G. Preventing overuse shoulder injuries among throwing athletes: a cluster-randomised controlled trial in 660 elite handball players. Br J Sports Med. 2017;51:1073.
2. Thorborg K, Krommes KK, Esteve E, Clausen MB, Bartels EM, Rathleff MS. Effect of specific exercise-based football injury prevention programmes on the overall injury rate in football: a systematic review and meta-analysis of the FIFA 11 and 11+ programmes. Br J Sports Med. 2017;51:562–71.
3. Waldén M, Atroshi I, Magnusson H, Wagner P, Hägglund M. Prevention of acute knee injuries in adolescent female football players: cluster randomised controlled trial. BMJ. 2012;344:e3042.
4. Hägglund M, Waldén M, Bengtsson H, Ekstrand J. Re-injuries in professional football: the UEFA Elite Club Injury Study. In: Return to play in football. Berlin: Springer; 2018. p. 953–62.
5. Fuller CW, Ekstrand J, Junge A, Andersen TE, Bahr R, Dvorak J, Hägglund M, McCrory P, Meeuwisse WH. Consensus statement on injury definitions and data collection procedures in studies of football (soccer) injuries. Scand J Med Sci Sports. 2006;16:83–92.
6. Bauer R, Kisser R, Macey S, Thayer D. Injuries in the European Union: statistics summary 2008–2010. European Association for Injury Prevention and Safety Promotion (EuroSafe). 2013.
7. Sewry N, Verhagen E, Lambert M, van Mechelen W, Viljoen W, Readhead C, Brown J. Exercise-based interventions for injury prevention in tackle collision ball sports: a systematic review. Sports Med. 2017;47:1847–57.
8. van der Horst NN, van de Port II, Backx FF. How effective are exercise-based injury prevention

programmes for soccer players? A systematic review. Sports Med. 2017;43:257.
9. Silva PV, Kamper SJ, LDCM C. Exercise-based intervention for prevention of sports injuries (PEDro synthesis). Br J Sports Med. 2017;52(6):408–9.
10. Olsen O-E, Myklebust G, Engebretsen L, Holme I, Bahr R. Exercises to prevent lower limb injuries in youth sports: cluster randomised controlled trial. BMJ. 2005;330:449.
11. Bahr R. Why screening tests to predict injury do not work—and probably never will…: a critical review. Br J Sports Med. 2016;50:776.
12. van Dyk N, Clarsen B. Prevention forecast: cloudy with a chance of injury. London: BMJ Publishing Group Ltd and British Association of Sport and Exercise Medicine; 2017.
13. Klügl M, Shrier I, McBain K, Shultz R, Meeuwisse WH, Garza D, Matheson GO. The prevention of sport injury: an analysis of 12 000 published manuscripts. Clin J Sport Med. 2010;20:407–12.
14. Hanson DW, Finch CF, Allegrante JP, Sleet D. Closing the gap between injury prevention research and community safety promotion practice: revisiting the public health model. Public Health Rep. 2012;127:147–55.
15. Rohde M, Breuer C. Europe's elite football: financial growth, sporting success, transfer investment, and private majority investors. Int J Financial Stud. 2016;4:12.
16. Posthumus M, Collins M, September AV, Schwellnus MP. The intrinsic risk factors for ACL ruptures: an evidence-based review. Phys Sportsmed. 2011;39:62–73.
17. Andrade R, Vasta S, Sevivas N, Pereira R, Leal A, Papalia R, Pereira H, Espregueira-Mendes J. Notch morphology is a risk factor for ACL injury: a systematic review and meta-analysis. J ISAKOS. 2016;1:70–81.
18. Alentorn-Geli E, Mendiguchia J, Samuelsson K, Musahl V, Karlsson J, Cugat R, Myer GD. Prevention of anterior cruciate ligament injuries in sports. Part I: systematic review of risk factors in male athletes. Knee Surg Sports Traumatol Arthrosc. 2014;22:3–15.
19. Meeuwisse WH, Tyreman H, Hagel B, Emery C. A dynamic model of etiology in sport injury: the recursive nature of risk and causation. Clin J Sport Med. 2007;17:215–9.
20. Bahr R, Holme I. Risk factors for sports injuries—a methodological approach. Br J Sports Med. 2003;37:384–92.
21. Bahr R, Krosshaug T. Understanding injury mechanisms: a key component of preventing injuries in sport. Br J Sports Med. 2005;39:324–9.
22. Olsen O, Myklebust G, Engebretsen L, Holme I, Bahr R. Relationship between floor type and risk of ACL injury in team handball. Scand J Med Sci Sports. 2003;13:299–304.
23. Hewett TE, Myer GD, Ford KR, Paterno MV, Quatman CE. Mechanisms, prediction, and prevention of ACL injuries: cut risk with three sharpened and validated tools. J Orthop Res. 2016;34:1843–55.
24. Mendiguchia J, Ford KR, Quatman CE, Alentorn-Geli E, Hewett TE. Sex differences in proximal control of the knee joint. Sports Med. 2011;41:541–57.
25. UEFA UEFA report. https://www.uefa.com/insideuefa/football-development/womens-football/news/newsid=2516070.html.
26. Martinez-Lagunas V, Niessen M, Hartmann U. Women's football: player characteristics and demands of the game. J Sport Health Sci. 2014;3:258–72.
27. Hewett TE, Myer GD, Ford KR. Decrease in neuromuscular control about the knee with maturation in female athletes. J Bone Joint Surg Am. 2004;86-a:1601–8.
28. Schilaty ND, Bates NA, Nagelli CV, Krych AJ, Hewett TE. Sex-based differences of medial collateral ligament and anterior cruciate ligament strains with cadaveric impact simulations. Orthop J Sports Med. 2018;6:2325967118765215.
29. Sigward SM, Powers CM. Loading characteristics of females exhibiting excessive valgus moments during cutting. Clin Biomech. 2007;22:827–33.
30. Sakamoto K, Sasaki R, Hong S, Matsukura K, Asai T. Comparison of kicking speed between female and male soccer players. Procedia Eng. 2014;72:50–5.
31. Sakamoto K, Hong S, Tabei Y, Asai T. Comparative study of female and male soccer players in kicking motion. Procedia Eng. 2012;34:206–11.
32. Ball K. Loading and performance of the support leg in kicking. J Sci Med Sport. 2013;16:455–9.
33. Jones PA, Herrington LC, Graham-Smith P. Technique determinants of knee joint loads during cutting in female soccer players. Hum Mov Sci. 2015;42:203–11.
34. Van Mechelen W, Hlobil H, Kemper HC. Incidence, severity, aetiology and prevention of sports injuries. Sports Med. 1992;14:82–99.
35. Bittencourt N, Meeuwisse W, Mendonça L, Nettel-Aguirre A, Ocarino J, Fonseca S. Complex systems approach for sports injuries: moving from risk factor identification to injury pattern recognition—narrative review and new concept. Br J Sports Med. 2016;50(21):1309–14.
36. Hulme A, Finch CF. From monocausality to systems thinking: a complementary and alternative conceptual approach for better understanding the development and prevention of sports injury. Injury Epidemiol. 2015;2:31.
37. Ekstrand J, Gillquist J. The avoidability of soccer injuries. Int J Sports Med. 1983;4:124–8.
38. Meeuwisse WH. Assessing causation in sport injury: a multifactorial model. Clin J Sport Med. 1994;4:166–70.
39. McIntosh AS. Risk compensation, motivation, injuries, and biomechanics in competitive sport. Br J Sports Med. 2005;39:2–3.
40. Finch C. A new framework for research leading to sports injury prevention. J Sci Med Sport. 2006;9:3–9. discussion 10.

41. Verhagen EA, van Stralen MM, van Mechelen W. Behaviour, the key factor for sports injury prevention. Sports Med. 2010;40:899–906.
42. Finch CF, Donaldson A. A sports setting matrix for understanding the implementation context for community sport. Br J Sports Med. 2010;44:973–8.
43. Finch CF. No longer lost in translation: the art and science of sports injury prevention implementation research. Br J Sports Med. 2011;45:1253–7.
44. Padua DA, Frank B, Donaldson A, de la Motte S, Cameron KL, Beutler AI, DiStefano LJ, Marshall SW. Seven steps for developing and implementing a preventive training program: lessons learned from JUMP-ACL and beyond. Clin Sports Med. 2014;33:615–32.
45. Bolling C, van Mechelen W, Pasman HR, Verhagen E. Context matters: revisiting the first step of the 'Sequence of Prevention' of sports injuries. Sports Med. 2018;48(10):2227–34.
46. Gabbett TJ. The training—injury prevention paradox: should athletes be training smarter <em>and</em> harder? Br J Sports Med. 2016;50:273–80.
47. Hulin BT, Gabbett TJ. Indeed association does not equal prediction: the never-ending search for the perfect acute:chronic workload ratio. Br J Sports Med. 2018.
48. Windt J, Zumbo BD, Sporer B, MacDonald K, Gabbett TJ. Why do workload spikes cause injuries, and which athletes are at higher risk? Mediators and moderators in workload–injury investigations. Br J Sports Med. 2017;51:993–4.
49. Gabbett TJ, Hulin BT, Blanch P, Whiteley R. High training workloads alone do not cause sports injuries: how you get there is the real issue. Br J Sports Med. 2016;50:444–5.
50. Hulin BT, Gabbett TJ, Blanch P, Chapman P, Bailey D, Orchard JW. Spikes in acute workload are associated with increased injury risk in elite cricket fast bowlers. Br J Sports Med. 2014;48:708–12.
51. Gabbett TJ, Nassis GP, Oetter E, et al. The athlete monitoring cycle: a practical guide to interpreting and applying training monitoring data. Br J Sports Med. 2017;51:1451–2.
52. Gabbett TJ, Kearney S, Bisson LJ, Collins J, Sikka R, Winder N, Sedgwick C, Hollis E, Bettle JM. Seven tips for developing and maintaining a high performance sports medicine team. Br J Sports Med. 2018;52:626–7.
53. McCall A, Dupont G, Ekstrand J. Internal workload and non-contact injury: a one-season study of five teams from the UEFA Elite Club Injury Study. Br J Sports Med. 2018;52(23):1517–22.
54. Fanchini M, Rampinini E, Riggio M, Coutts AJ, Pecci C, McCall A. Despite association, the acute:chronic work load ratio does not predict noncontact injury in elite footballers. Sci Med Football. 2018;2:108–14.
55. Hulin BT, Gabbett TJ, Caputi P, Lawson DW, Sampson JA. Low chronic workload and the acute:chronic workload ratio are more predictive of injury than between-match recovery time: a two-season prospective cohort study in elite rugby league players. Br J Sports Med. 2016;50:1008–12.
56. Windt J, Gabbett TJ, Ferris D, Khan KM. Training load--injury paradox: is greater preseason participation associated with lower in-season injury risk in elite rugby league players? Br J Sports Med. 2017;51:645–50.
57. Quarrie KL, Raftery M, Blackie J, et al. Managing player load in professional rugby union: a review of current knowledge and practices. Br J Sports Med. 2017;51:421–7.
58. Malone S, Roe M, Doran DA, Gabbett TJ, Collins K. High chronic training loads and exposure to bouts of maximal velocity running reduce injury risk in elite Gaelic football. J Sci Med Sport. 2017;20:250–4.
59. Cappaert TA, Stone JA, Castellani JW, Krause BA, Smith D, Stephens BA. National Athletic Trainers' Association position statement: environmental cold injuries. J Athl Train. 2008;43:640–58.
60. Castellani JW, Young AJ, Ducharme MB, Giesbrecht GG, Glickman E, Sallis RE. Prevention of cold injuries during exercise. Natick, MA: Army Research Institute of Environmental Medicine, Thermal and Mountain Medicine Division; 2006.
61. Orchard JW, Chivers I, Aldous D, Bennell K, Seward H. Rye grass is associated with fewer non-contact anterior cruciate ligament injuries than Bermuda grass. Br J Sports Med. 2005;39:704.
62. Kerut EK, Kerut DG, Fleisig GS, Andrews JR. Prevention of arm injury in youth baseball pitchers. J La State Med Soc. 2008;160:95–8.
63. Zaremski JL, Krabak BJ. Shoulder injuries in the skeletally immature baseball pitcher and recommendations for the prevention of injury. PM R. 2012;4:509–16.
64. Marshall SW, Loomis DP, Waller AE, Chalmers DJ, Bird YN, Quarrie KL, Feehan M. Evaluation of protective equipment for prevention of injuries in rugby union. Int J Epidemiol. 2004;34:113–8.
65. Benson BW, Hamilton GM, Meeuwisse WH, McCrory P, Dvorak J. Is protective equipment useful in preventing concussion? A systematic review of the literature. Br J Sports Med. 2009;43:i56–67.
66. Hägglund M, Waldén M, Bahr R, Ekstrand J. Methods for epidemiological study of injuries to professional football players: developing the UEFA model. Br J Sports Med. 2005;39:340–6.
67. Clarsen B, Myklebust G, Bahr R. Development and validation of a new method for the registration of overuse injuries in sports injury epidemiology: the Oslo Sports Trauma Research Centre (OSTRC) overuse injury questionnaire. Br J Sports Med. 2012;47(8):495–502.
68. MacDonald KJ, Palacios-Derflingher LM, Emery CA, Meeuwisse WH. The effect of injury definition and surveillance methodology on measures of injury occurrence and burden in elite volleyball. Int J Sports Med. 2018;39(11):860–6.

69. Gabbe BJ. Re: a new framework for research leading to sports injury prevention. J Sci Med Sport. 2006;9:10.
70. Donaldson A, Finch CF. Applying implementation science to sports injury prevention. London: BMJ Publishing Group Ltd and British Association of Sport and Exercise Medicine; 2013.
71. Finch CF, Gabbe BJ, Lloyd DG, Cook J, Young W, Nicholson M, Seward H, Donaldson A, Doyle TL. Towards a national sports safety strategy: addressing facilitators and barriers towards safety guideline uptake. Inj Prev. 2011;17:e4.
72. Bizzini M, Junge A, Dvorak J. Implementation of the FIFA 11+ football warm up program: how to approach and convince the football associations to invest in prevention. Br J Sports Med. 2013;47:803–6.
73. Donaldson A, Callaghan A, Bizzini M, Jowett A, Keyzer P, Nicholson M. Awareness and use of the 11+ injury prevention program among coaches of adolescent female football teams. Int J Sports Sci Coach. 2018.
74. Skinner CS, Tiro J, Champion VL. The health belief model. Health behavior: theory, research, and practice. 5th ed. San Francisco: Jossey-Bass; 2015. p. 75–94.
75. Finch CF, White P, Twomey D, Ullah S. Implementing an exercise-training programme to prevent lower-limb injuries: considerations for the development of a randomised controlled trial intervention delivery plan. Br J Sports Med. 2011;45:791–6.
76. Breitenstein SM, Gross D, Garvey C, Hill C, Fogg L, Resnick B. Implementation Fidelity in community-based interventions. Res Nurs Health. 2010;33:164–73.
77. Verhagen EA, Hupperets MD, Finch CF, van Mechelen W. The impact of adherence on sports injury prevention effect estimates in randomised controlled trials: looking beyond the CONSORT statement. J Sci Med Sport. 2011;14:287–92.
78. McKay CD, Verhagen E. 'Compliance' versus 'adherence' in sport injury prevention: why definition matters. Br J Sports Med. 2016;50:382–3.
79. Silvers-Granelli HJ, Bizzini M, Arundale A, Mandelbaum BR, Snyder-Mackler L. Higher compliance to a neuromuscular injury prevention program improves overall injury rate in male football players. Knee Surg Sports Traumatol Arthrosc. 2018;26:1975–83.
80. van Reijen M, Vriend I, van Mechelen W, Finch CF, Verhagen EA. Compliance with sport injury prevention interventions in randomised controlled trials: a systematic review. Sports Med. 2016;46:1125–39.
81. Soligard T, Nilstad A, Steffen K, Myklebust G, Holme I, Dvorak J, Bahr R, Andersen TE. Compliance with a comprehensive warm-up programme to prevent injuries in youth football. Br J Sports Med. 2010;44:787.
82. Hupperets MDW, Verhagen EALM, Mechelen WV. Effect of unsupervised home based proprioceptive training on recurrences of ankle sprain: randomised controlled trial. BMJ. 2009:339.
83. Hägglund M, Atroshi I, Wagner P, Waldén M. Superior compliance with a neuromuscular training programme is associated with fewer ACL injuries and fewer acute knee injuries in female adolescent football players: secondary analysis of an RCT. Br J Sports Med. 2013;47:974–9.
84. Luftey K, Wishner W. Beyond "compliance" is adherence. Diabetes Care. 1999;22:635–9.
85. Vrijens B, De Geest S, Hughes DA, et al. A new taxonomy for describing and defining adherence to medications. Br J Clin Pharmacol. 2012;73:691–705.
86. Verhagen E, van der Beek A, Twisk J, Bouter L, Bahr R, van Mechelen W. The effect of a proprioceptive balance board training program for the prevention of ankle sprains: a prospective controlled trial. Am J Sports Med. 2004;32:1385–93.
87. Lun V, Meeuwisse WH, Stergiou P, Stefanyshyn D. Relation between running injury and static lower limb alignment in recreational runners. Br J Sports Med. 2004;38:576–80.
88. Stevenson MR, Hamer P, Finch CF, Elliot B, Kresnow M. Sport, age, and sex specific incidence of sports injuries in Western Australia. Br J Sports Med. 2000;34:188–94.
89. McCall A, Dupont G, Ekstrand J. Injury prevention strategies, coach compliance and player adherence of 33 of the UEFA Elite Club Injury Study teams: a survey of teams' head medical officers. Br J Sports Med. 2016;50:725–30.
90. Emery CA, Hagel B, Morrongiello BA. Injury prevention in child and adolescent sport: whose responsibility is it? Clin J Sport Med. 2006;16:514–21.
91. Taylor JB, Waxman JP, Richter SJ, Shultz SJ. Evaluation of the effectiveness of anterior cruciate ligament injury prevention programme training components: a systematic review and meta-analysis. Br J Sports Med. 2015;49:79.
92. Soligard T, Myklebust G, Steffen K, et al. Comprehensive warm-up programme to prevent injuries in young female footballers: cluster randomised controlled trial. BMJ. 2008;337:a2469.
93. Mandelbaum BR, Silvers HJ, Watanabe DS, Knarr JF, Thomas SD, Griffin LY, Kirkendall DT, Garrett W Jr. Effectiveness of a neuromuscular and proprioceptive training program in preventing anterior cruciate ligament injuries in female athletes: 2-year follow-up. Am J Sports Med. 2005;33:1003–10.
94. Rossler R, Donath L, Verhagen E, Junge A, Schweizer T, Faude O. Exercise-based injury prevention in child and adolescent sport: a systematic review and meta-analysis. Sports Med. 2014;44:1733–48.
95. Faude O, Rössler R, Petushek EJ, Roth R, Zahner L, Donath L. Neuromuscular adaptations to multimodal injury prevention programs in youth sports: a systematic review with meta-analysis of randomized controlled trials. Front Physiol. 2017;8:791.

96. Whittaker JL, Small C, Maffey L, Emery CA. Risk factors for groin injury in sport: an updated systematic review. Br J Sports Med. 2015;49(12):803–9.
97. Haroy J, Thorborg K, Serner A, Bjorkheim A, Rolstad LE, Holmich P, Bahr R, Andersen TE. Including the Copenhagen adduction exercise in the FIFA 11+ provides missing eccentric hip adduction strength effect in male soccer players: a randomized controlled trial. Am J Sports Med. 2017;45:3052–9.
98. Haroy J, Clarsen B, Wiger EG, Oyen MG, Serner A, Thorborg K, Holmich P, Andersen TE, Bahr R. The adductor strengthening programme prevents groin problems among male football players: a cluster-randomised controlled trial. Br J Sports Med. 2018.
99. Rössler R, Verhagen E, Rommers N, Dvorak J, Junge A, Lichtenstein E, Donath L, Faude O. Comparison of the '11+ Kids' injury prevention programme and a regular warmup in children's football (soccer): a cost effectiveness analysis. Br J Sports Med. 2018.
100. Johnston JT, Mandelbaum BR, Schub D, et al. Video analysis of anterior cruciate ligament tears in professional American football athletes. Am J Sports Med. 2018;46:862–8.
101. Clarsen B, Bahr R, Andersson SH, Munk R, Myklebust G. Reduced glenohumeral rotation, external rotation weakness and scapular dyskinesis are risk factors for shoulder injuries among elite male handball players: a prospective cohort study. Br J Sports Med. 2014;48:1327–33.
102. Herzog MM, Marshall SW, Lund JL, Pate V, Spang JT. Cost of outpatient arthroscopic anterior cruciate ligament reconstruction among commercially insured patients in the United States, 2005-2013. Orthop J Sports Med. 2017;5:2325967116684776.
103. Mather RC III, Koenig L, Kocher MS, Dall TM, Gallo P, Scott DJ, Bach BR Jr, Spindler KP, Group MK. Societal and economic impact of anterior cruciate ligament tears. J Bone Joint Surg Am. 2013;95:1751.
104. Lohmander LS, Englund PM, Dahl LL, Roos EM. The long-term consequence of anterior cruciate ligament and meniscus injuries: osteoarthritis. Am J Sports Med. 2007;35:1756–69.
105. Filbay S, Culvenor A, Ackerman I, Russell T, Crossley K. Quality of life in anterior cruciate ligament-deficient individuals: a systematic review and meta-analysis. Br J Sports Med. 2015;49:1033–41.
106. Montalvo AM, Schneider DK, Yut L, Webster KE, Beynnon B, Kocher MS, Myer GD. "What's my risk of sustaining an ACL injury while playing sports?" A systematic review with meta-analysis. Br J Sports Med. 2018.
107. Anderson MJ, Browning WM III, Urband CE, Kluczynski MA, Bisson LJ. A systematic summary of systematic reviews on the topic of the anterior cruciate ligament. Orthop J Sports Med. 2016;4:2325967116634074.
108. Ford KR, Myer GD, Hewett TE. Valgus knee motion during landing in high school female and male basketball players. Med Sci Sports Exerc. 2003;35:1745–50.
109. Hewett TE, Stroupe AL, Nance TA, Noyes FR. Plyometric training in female athletes: decreased impact forces and increased hamstring torques. Am J Sports Med. 1996;24:765–73.
110. Hewett TE, Ford KR, Hoogenboom BJ, Myer GD. Understanding and preventing acl injuries: current biomechanical and epidemiologic considerations-update 2010. N Am J Sports Phys Ther. 2010;5:234.
111. Myer GD, Brent JL, Ford KR, Hewett TE. Real-time assessment and neuromuscular training feedback techniques to prevent ACL injury in female athletes. Streng Cond J. 2011;33:21.
112. Walden M, Krosshaug T, Bjorneboe J, Andersen TE, Faul O, Hagglund M. Three distinct mechanisms predominate in non-contact anterior cruciate ligament injuries in male professional football players: a systematic video analysis of 39 cases. Br J Sports Med. 2015;49:1452–60.
113. Brophy RH, Stepan JG, Silvers HJ, Mandelbaum BR. Defending puts the anterior cruciate ligament at risk during soccer: a gender-based analysis. Sports Health. 2015;7:244–9.
114. Montgomery C, Blackburn J, Withers D, Tierney G, Moran C, Simms C. Mechanisms of ACL injury in professional rugby union: a systematic video analysis of 36 cases. Br J Sports Med. 2016;52(15):994–1001.
115. Stuelcken MC, Mellifont DB, Gorman AD, Sayers MG. Mechanisms of anterior cruciate ligament injuries in elite women's netball: a systematic video analysis. J Sports Sci. 2016;34:1516–22.
116. Bere T, Flørenes TW, Krosshaug T, et al. Mechanisms of anterior cruciate ligament injury in World Cup alpine skiing: a systematic video analysis of 20 cases. Am J Sports Med. 2011;39:1421–9.
117. Koga H, Nakamae A, Shima Y, Iwasa J, Myklebust G, Engebretsen L, Bahr R, Krosshaug T. Mechanisms for noncontact anterior cruciate ligament injuries: knee joint kinematics in 10 injury situations from female team handball and basketball. Am J Sports Med. 2010;38:2218–25.
118. Olsen O-E, Myklebust G, Engebretsen L, Bahr R. Injury mechanisms for anterior cruciate ligament injuries in team handball: a systematic video analysis. Am J Sports Med. 2004;32:1002–12.
119. Koga H, Muneta T, Bahr R, Engebretsen L, Krosshaug T. ACL injury mechanisms: lessons learned from video analysis. In: Rotatory knee instability. Berlin: Springer; 2017. p. 27–36.
120. Webster KE, Hewett TE. Meta-analysis of meta-analyses of anterior cruciate ligament injury reduction training programs. J Orthop Res. 2018;36(10):2696–708.
121. Sugimoto D, Myer GD, McKeon JM, Hewett TE. Evaluation of the effectiveness of neuromuscular training to reduce anterior cruciate ligament injury in female athletes: a critical review of relative

risk reduction and numbers-needed-to-treat analyses. Br J Sports Med. 2012;46(14):979–88.
122. Sugimoto D, Myer GD, Barber Foss KD, Hewett TE. Specific exercise effects of preventive neuromuscular training intervention on anterior cruciate ligament injury risk reduction in young females: meta-analysis and subgroup analysis. Br J Sports Med. 2015;49:282.
123. Petushek EJ, Sugimoto D, Stoolmiller M, Smith G, Myer GD. Evidence-based best-practice guidelines for preventing anterior cruciate ligament injuries in Young female athletes: a systematic review and meta-analysis. Am J Sports Med. 2018:0363546518782460.
124. Sugimoto D, Myer GD, Barber Foss KD, Pepin MJ, Micheli LJ, Hewett TE. Critical components of neuromuscular training to reduce ACL injury risk in female athletes: meta-regression analysis. Br J Sports Med. 2016;50:1259.
125. Pappas E, Nightingale EJ, Simic M, Ford KR, Hewett TE, Myer GD. Do exercises used in injury prevention programmes modify cutting task biomechanics? A systematic review with meta-analysis. Br J Sports Med. 2015;49:673.
126. Lopes TJA, Simic M, Myer GD, Ford KR, Hewett TE, Pappas E. The effects of injury prevention programs on the biomechanics of landing tasks: a systematic review with meta-analysis. Am J Sports Med. 2017;46:1492–9.
127. Arundale AJ, Bizzini M, Giordano A, et al. Exercise-based knee and anterior cruciate ligament injury prevention: clinical practice guidelines linked to the international classification of functioning, disability and health from the academy of orthopaedic physical therapy and the American Academy of sports physical therapy. J Orthop Sports Phys Ther. 2018;48:A1–A42.
128. Bielska IA, Wang X, Lee R, Johnson AP. The health economics of ankle and foot sprains and fractures: a systematic review of English-language published papers. Part 2: the direct and indirect costs of injury. Foot (Edinburgh, Scotland). 2017.
129. Doherty C, Delahunt E, Caulfield B, Hertel J, Ryan J, Bleakley C. The incidence and prevalence of ankle sprain injury: a systematic review and meta-analysis of prospective epidemiological studies. Sports Med. 2014;44:123–40.
130. Vuurberg G, Hoorntje A, Wink LM, et al. Diagnosis, treatment and prevention of ankle sprains: update of an evidence-based clinical guideline. Br J Sports Med. 2018;52:956.
131. Bahr R, Bahr IA. Incidence of acute volleyball injuries: a prospective cohort study of injury mechanisms and risk factors. Scand J Med Sci Sports. 1997;7:166–71.
132. Skazalski C, Kruczynski J, Bahr MA, Bere T, Whiteley R, Bahr R. Landing-related ankle injuries do not occur in plantarflexion as once thought: a systematic video analysis of ankle injuries in world-class volleyball. Br J Sports Med. 2018;52:74–82.
133. Panagiotakis E, Mok KM, Fong DT, Bull AMJ. Biomechanical analysis of ankle ligamentous sprain injury cases from televised basketball games: understanding when, how and why ligament failure occurs. J Sci Med Sport. 2017;20:1057–61.
134. Andersen TE, Floerenes TW, Arnason A, Bahr R. Video analysis of the mechanisms for ankle injuries in football. Am J Sports Med. 2004;32:69–79.
135. Handoll HH, Rowe BH, Quinn KM, de Bie R. Interventions for preventing ankle ligament injuries. Cochrane Database Syst Rev. 2001:CD000018.
136. Hupperets MD, Verhagen EA, Heymans MW, Bosmans JE, van Tulder MW, van Mechelen W. Potential savings of a program to prevent ankle sprain recurrence: economic evaluation of a randomized controlled trial. Am J Sports Med. 2010;38:2194–200.
137. Walden M, Hagglund M, Ekstrand J. Time-trends and circumstances surrounding ankle injuries in men's professional football: an 11-year follow-up of the UEFA Champions League injury study. Br J Sports Med. 2013;47:748–53.
138. Fousekis K, Tsepis E, Vagenas G. Intrinsic risk factors of noncontact ankle sprains in soccer: a prospective study on 100 professional players. Am J Sports Med. 2012;40:1842–50.
139. Janssen KW, van Mechelen W, Verhagen EALM. Bracing superior to neuromuscular training for the prevention of self-reported recurrent ankle sprains: a three-arm randomised controlled trial. Br J Sports Med. 2014;48:1235–9.
140. Ekstrand J, Hägglund M, Waldén M. Epidemiology of muscle injuries in professional football (soccer). Am J Sports Med. 2011;39:1226–32.
141. Petersen J, Thorborg K, Nielsen MB, Hølmich P. Acute hamstring injuries in Danish elite football: a 12-month prospective registration study among 374 players. Scand J Med Sci Sports. 2010;20:588–92.
142. Ekstrand J, Waldén M, Hägglund M. Hamstring injuries have increased by 4% annually in men's professional football, since 2001: a 13-year longitudinal analysis of the UEFA Elite Club injury study. Br J Sports Med. 2016;50:731–7.
143. Ekstrand J. Keeping your top players on the pitch: the key to football medicine at a professional level. London: BMJ Publishing Group Ltd and British Association of Sport and Exercise Medicine; 2013.
144. Hallén A, Ekstrand J. Return to play following muscle injuries in professional footballers. J Sports Sci. 2014;32:1229–36.
145. Freckleton G, Pizzari T. Risk factors for hamstring muscle strain injury in sport: a systematic review and meta-analysis. Br J Sports Med. 2013;47:351.
146. Hägglund M, Waldén M, Ekstrand J. Risk factors for lower extremity muscle injury in professional soccer: the UEFA Injury Study. Am J Sports Med. 2013;41:327–35.
147. de Visser HM, Reijman M, Heijboer MP, Bos PK. Risk factors of recurrent hamstring injuries: a systematic review. Br J Sports Med. 2012;46:124–30.

148. Mueller-Wohlfahrt H-W, Haensel L, Mithoefer K, et al. Terminology and classification of muscle injuries in sport: a consensus statement. Br J Sports Med. 2013;47(6):342–50.
149. Askling CM, Tengvar M, Saartok T, Thorstensson A. Acute first-time hamstring strains during high-speed running: a longitudinal study including clinical and magnetic resonance imaging findings. Am J Sports Med. 2007;35:197–206.
150. Askling CM, Malliaropoulos N, Karlsson J. High-speed running type or stretching-type of hamstring injuries makes a difference to treatment and prognosis. London: BMJ Publishing Group Ltd and British Association of Sport and Exercise Medicine; 2012.
151. Askling CM, Tengvar M, Saartok T, Thorstensson A. Proximal hamstring strains of stretching type in different sports: injury situations, clinical and magnetic resonance imaging characteristics, and return to sport. Am J Sports Med. 2008;36:1799–804.
152. Petersen J, Thorborg K, Nielsen MB, Budtz-Jørgensen E, Hölmich P. Preventive effect of eccentric training on acute hamstring injuries in men's soccer: a cluster-randomized controlled trial. Am J Sports Med. 2011;39:2296–303.
153. Arnason A, Andersen T, Holme I, Engebretsen L, Bahr R. Prevention of hamstring strains in elite soccer: an intervention study. Scand J Med Sci Sports. 2008;18:40–8.
154. Bahr R, Thorborg K, Ekstrand J. Evidence-based hamstring injury prevention is not adopted by the majority of Champions League or Norwegian Premier League football teams: the Nordic Hamstring Survey. Br J Sports Med. 2015;49:1466–71.
155. van der Horst N, Smits DW, Petersen J, Goedhart EA, Backx FJ. The preventive effect of the nordic hamstring exercise on hamstring injuries in amateur soccer players: a randomized controlled trial. Am J Sports Med. 2015;43:1316–23.
156. Buckthorpe M, Gimpel M, Wright S, Sturdy T, Stride M. Hamstring muscle injuries in elite football: translating research into practice. Br J Sports Med. 2018;52:628–9.
157. Kuszewski M, Gnat R, Saulicz E. Stability training of the lumbo-pelvo-hip complex influence stiffness of the hamstrings: a preliminary study. Scand J Med Sci Sports. 2009;19:260–6.
158. Mills M, Frank B, Goto S, Blackburn T, Cates S, Clark M, Aguilar A, Fava N, Padua D. Effect of restricted hip flexor muscle length on hip extensor muscle activity and lower extremity biomechanics in college-aged female soccer players. Int J Sports Phys Ther. 2015;10:946.
159. Duhig S, Shield AJ, Opar D, Gabbett TJ, Ferguson C, Williams M. Effect of high-speed running on hamstring strain injury risk. Br J Sports Med. 2016;50(24):1536–40.
160. Bowen L, Gross AS, Gimpel M, Li F-X. Accumulated workloads and the acute: chronic workload ratio relate to injury risk in elite youth football players. Br J Sports Med. 2017;51(5):452–9.
161. Werner J, Hägglund M, Waldén M, Ekstrand J. UEFA injury study: a prospective study of hip and groin injuries in professional football over seven consecutive seasons. Br J Sports Med. 2009;43:1036–40.
162. Mosler AB, Weir A, Eirale C, Farooq A, Thorborg K, Whiteley RJ, Hlmich P, Crossley KM. Epidemiology of time loss groin injuries in a men's professional football league: a 2-year prospective study of 17 clubs and 606 players. Br J Sports Med. 2018;52:292–7.
163. Langhout R, Weir A, Litjes W, Gozeling M, Stubbe JH, Kerkhoffs G, Tak I. Hip and groin injury is the most common non-time-loss injury in female amateur football. Knee Surg Sports Traumatol Arthrosc. 2018.
164. Ryan J, DeBurca N, Mc Creesh K. Risk factors for groin/hip injuries in field-based sports: a systematic review. Br J Sports Med. 2014;48:1089–96.
165. Tak I, Engelaar L, Gouttebarge V, Barendrecht M, Van den Heuvel S, Kerkhoffs G, Langhout R, Stubbe J, Weir A. Is lower hip range of motion a risk factor for groin pain in athletes? A systematic review with clinical applications. Br J Sports Med. 2017;51:1611–21.
166. Serner A, Mosler AB, Tol JL, Bahr R, Weir A. Mechanisms of acute adductor longus injuries in male football players: a systematic visual video analysis. Br J Sports Med. 2018.
167. Esteve E, Rathleff MS, Bagur-Calafat C, Urrutia G, Thorborg K. Prevention of groin injuries in sports: a systematic review with meta-analysis of randomised controlled trials. Br J Sports Med. 2015;49:785–91.
168. Serner A, Jakobsen MD, Andersen LL, Holmich P, Sundstrup E, Thorborg K. EMG evaluation of hip adduction exercises for soccer players: implications for exercise selection in prevention and treatment of groin injuries. Br J Sports Med. 2014;48:1108–14.
169. Ishøi L, Sørensen C, Kaae N, Jørgensen L, Hölmich P, Serner A. Large eccentric strength increase using the Copenhagen Adduction exercise in football: a randomized controlled trial. Scand J Med Sci Sports. 2016;26:1334–42.
170. Goode AP, Reiman MP, Harris L, DeLisa L, Kauffman A, Beltramo D, Poole C, Ledbetter L, Taylor AB. Eccentric training for prevention of hamstring injuries may depend on intervention compliance: a systematic review and meta-analysis. Br J Sports Med. 2014;49(6):349–56.
171. Heiderscheit BC, Hoerth DM, Chumanov ES, Swanson SC, Thelen BJ, Thelen DG. Identifying the time of occurrence of a hamstring strain injury during treadmill running: a case study. Clin Biomech. 2005;20:1072–8.
172. Chumanov ES, Schache AG, Heiderscheit BC, Thelen DG. Hamstrings are most susceptible to injury during the late swing phase of sprinting. London: BMJ Publishing Group Ltd and British Association of Sport and Exercise Medicine; 2012.
173. Van Reijen M, Vriend I, van Mechelen W, Verhagen EA. Preventing recurrent ankle sprains: is the use of an App more cost-effective than a printed

booklet? Results of a RCT. Scand J Med Sci Sports. 2018;28:641–8.
174. van Reijen M, Asscheman M, Vriend I, van Mechelen W, Verhagen E. Users' perspectives, opportunities, and barriers of the strengthen your ankle app for evidence-based ankle sprain prevention: mixed-methods process evaluation for a randomized controlled trial. JMIR. 2018;5:e13.
175. Mailuhu AK, Verhagen EA, van Ochten JM, Bindels PJ, Bierma-Zeinstra SM, van Middelkoop M. The trAPP-study: cost-effectiveness of an unsupervised e-health supported neuromuscular training program for the treatment of acute ankle sprains in general practice: design of a randomized controlled trial. BMC Musculoskelet Disord. 2015;16:78.
176. Burgess JD, Cameron CM, Watt K, Kimble RM. Cool Runnings—an app-based intervention for reducing hot drink scalds: study protocol for a randomised controlled trial. Trials. 2016;17:388.
177. Wiggins AJ, Grandhi RK, Schneider DK, Stanfield D, Webster KE, Myer GD. Risk of secondary injury in younger athletes after anterior cruciate ligament reconstruction: a systematic review and meta-analysis. Am J Sports Med. 2016;44:1861–76.
178. Wangensteen A, Tol JL, Witvrouw E, Van Linschoten R, Almusa E, Hamilton B, Bahr R. Hamstring reinjuries occur at the same location and early after return to sport: a descriptive study of MRI-confirmed reinjuries. Am J Sports Med. 2016;44:2112–21.
179. Hagglund M, Walden M, Ekstrand J. Injury recurrence is lower at the highest professional football level than at national and amateur levels: does sports medicine and sports physiotherapy deliver? Br J Sports Med. 2016;50:751–8.
180. Kyritsis P, Bahr R, Landreau P, Miladi R, Witvrouw E. Likelihood of ACL graft rupture: not meeting six clinical discharge criteria before return to sport is associated with a four times greater risk of rupture. Br J Sports Med. 2016;50:946–51.
181. Adams D, Logerstedt DS, Hunter-Giordano A, Axe MJ, Snyder-Mackler L. Current concepts for anterior cruciate ligament reconstruction: a criterion-based rehabilitation progression. J Orthop Sports Phys Ther. 2012;42:601–14.
182. Andrade R, Pereira R, Bastos R, Pereira H, Oliveira JM, Reis RL, Espregueira-Mendes J. Return to play following cartilage injuries. In: Musahl V, Karlsson J, Krutsch W, Mandelbaum B, Espregueira-Mendes J, d'Hooghe P, editors. Return to play in football. Berlin: Springer; 2018. p. 593–610.
183. Grindem H, Snyder-Mackler L, Moksnes H, Engebretsen L, Risberg MA. Simple decision rules can reduce reinjury risk by 84% after ACL reconstruction: the Delaware-Oslo ACL cohort study. Br J Sports Med. 2016;50:804–8.
184. Carling C, McCall A, Le Gall F, Dupont G. The impact of short periods of match congestion on injury risk and patterns in an elite football club. Br J Sports Med. 2016;50:764.
185. Paterno MV, Huang B, Thomas S, Hewett TE, Schmitt LC. Clinical factors that predict a second ACL injury after ACL reconstruction and return to sport: preliminary development of a clinical decision algorithm. Orthop J Sports Med. 2017;5:2325967117745279.
186. Paterno MV, Schmitt LC, Ford KR, Rauh MJ, Myer GD, Huang B, Hewett TE. Biomechanical measures during landing and postural stability predict second anterior cruciate ligament injury after anterior cruciate ligament reconstruction and return to sport. Am J Sports Med. 2010;38:1968–78.
187. Paterno MV, Ford KR, Myer GD, Heyl R, Hewett TE. Limb asymmetries in landing and jumping 2 years following anterior cruciate ligament reconstruction. Clin J Sport Med. 2007;17:258–62.
188. Benjaminse A, Welling W, Otten B, Gokeler A. Novel methods of instruction in ACL injury prevention programs, a systematic review. Phys Ther Sport. 2015;16:176–86.
189. Benjaminse A, Gokeler A, Dowling AV, Faigenbaum A, Ford KR, Hewett TE, Onate JA, Otten B, Myer GD. Optimization of the anterior cruciate ligament injury prevention paradigm: novel feedback techniques to enhance motor learning and reduce injury risk. J Orthop Sports Phys Ther. 2015;45:170–82.
190. Welling W, Benjaminse A, Gokeler A, Otten B. Retention of movement technique: implications for primary prevention of acl injuries. Int J Sports Phys Ther. 2017;12:908–20.
191. Gokeler A, Benjaminse A, Seil R, Kerkhoffs G, Verhagen E. Using principles of motor learning to enhance ACL injury prevention programs. Sports Orthopaed Traumatol. 2018;34:23–30.
192. Benjaminse A, Welling W, Otten B, Gokeler A. Transfer of improved movement technique after receiving verbal external focus and video instruction. Knee Surg Sports Traumatol Arthrosc. 2018;26:955–62.
193. Gokeler A, Seil R, Kerkhoffs G, Verhagen E. A novel approach to enhance ACL injury prevention programs. J Exp Orthopaed. 2018;5:22.
194. Brooks JH, Fuller CW, Kemp SP, Reddin DB. Incidence, risk, and prevention of hamstring muscle injuries in professional rugby union. Am J Sports Med. 2006;34:1297–306.
195. Orchard J, Best TM. The management of muscle strain injuries: an early return versus the risk of recurrence. Clin J Sport Med. 2002;12:3–5.
196. De Vos R-J, Reurink G, Goudswaard G-J, Moen MH, Weir A, Tol JL. Clinical findings just after return to play predict hamstring re-injury, but baseline MRI findings do not. Br J Sports Med. 2014;48(18):1377–84.
197. Gibbs N, Cross T, Cameron M, Houang M. The accuracy of MRI in predicting recovery and recur-

rence of acute grade one hamstring muscle strains within the same season in Australian Rules football players. J Sci Med Sport. 2004;7:248–58.
198. Malliaropoulos N, Isinkaye T, Tsitas K, Maffulli N. Reinjury after acute posterior thigh muscle injuries in elite track and field athletes. Am J Sports Med. 2011;39:304–10.
199. Verrall GM, Slavotinek JP, Barnes PG, Fon GT, Esterman A. Assessment of physical examination and magnetic resonance imaging findings of hamstring injury as predictors for recurrent injury. J Orthop Sports Phys Ther. 2006;36:215–24.
200. Stares J, Dawson B, Peeling P, Drew M, Heasman J, Rogalski B, Colby M. How much is enough in rehabilitation? High running workloads following lower limb muscle injury delay return to play but protect against subsequent injury. J Sci Med Sport. 2018;21(10):1019–24.
201. Doherty C, Bleakley C, Delahunt E, Holden S. Treatment and prevention of acute and recurrent ankle sprain: an overview of systematic reviews with meta-analysis. Br J Sports Med. 2017;51(2):113–25.

Return to Play (RTP) 12

Alexandre Rebelo-Marques, Renato Andrade, Rogério Pereira, and João Espregueira-Mendes

12.1 Background

The popularity of sports in all of its forms continues to steadily increase. We live in an age where sport became a business. Winning or losing has a tremendous impact; it is more than just pride but also an important financial and social aspect. Thus, there are a wide number of different circumstances that play a role in the decision-making process that determine when an athlete should return to competition [1]. Return-to-play (RTP) decisions are often difficult and complex [2]. These circumstances involve an array of individuals that are involved in this decision, including the medial department with the sports physicians and physiotherapists, the athlete, parents or guardians, coaches, the athletic trainer, and many others. The appropriate synergy of these views and inputs, along with the athlete's own feelings and self-efficacy, makes a significant contribution and is the key to a successful outcome.

A. Rebelo-Marques (✉)
Clínica do Dragão, Espregueira-Mendes Sports Centre—FIFA Medical Centre of Excellence, Porto, Portugal

Dom Henrique Research Centre, Porto, Portugal

Faculty of Medicine, University of Coimbra, Coimbra, Portugal

Coimbra Institute for Clinical and Biomedical Research (iCBR), Coimbra, Portugal

R. Andrade
Clínica do Dragão, Espregueira-Mendes Sports Centre—FIFA Medical Centre of Excellence, Porto, Portugal

Dom Henrique Research Centre, Porto, Portugal

Faculty of Sports, University of Porto, Porto, Portugal
e-mail: randrade@espregueira.com

R. Pereira
Clínica do Dragão, Espregueira-Mendes Sports Centre—FIFA Medical Centre of Excellence, Porto, Portugal

Dom Henrique Research Centre, Porto, Portugal

Faculty of Sports, University of Porto, Porto, Portugal

University Fernando Pessoa, Porto, Portugal
e-mail: rp@espregueira.com

J. Espregueira-Mendes
Clínica do Dragão, Espregueira-Mendes Sports Centre—FIFA Medical Centre of Excellence, Porto, Portugal

Dom Henrique Research Centre, Porto, Portugal

Medicine School of Minho University, Braga, Portugal

ICVS/3B's–PT Government Associate Laboratory, Braga/Guimarães, Portugal
e-mail: espregueira@dhresearchcentre.com

S. Rocha Piedade et al. (eds.), *The Sports Medicine Physician*,
https://doi.org/10.1007/978-3-030-10433-7_12

The RTP decision will be better understood and accepted if all stakeholders are properly informed and considered. However, determining prognosis could be tricky, and including the inputs of such a wide range of specialist staff in a fully integrated way is very complex, often leading to disagreements regarding the RTP [3]. The clinician is expected to provide an opinion based on a large number of factors including the history of the injury, physical examination, type of injury, rehabilitation, type of activity psychological state, competitive level, and ability to protect the injury [4]. Yet, sociocultural and clinical differences and perspectives between the stakeholders involved may lead to a number of negative scenarios, such as (1) miscommunication, (2) loss of trust, (3) potential litigation, (4) decrease in sport participation rates as sometimes the player cannot "get back in the game," and (5) potentially coming back with serious medical complications after unsuccessful RTP or return while still at unacceptable levels of risk for subsequent sport-related injury [5–7].

Returning to competition can be a confusing scenario when all the possible circumstances that might be involved are considered. Thus, it is important to consider the expectations of the athlete when they return to training and competition, such as [1]:

(a) Pain-free, normal range of motion (ROM) (if applicable), and reestablishment of sport-specific movements.
(b) Restored power and strength to approximately the preinjury levels.
(c) Metabolic and neuromuscular fatigue resistance to high-intensity sporting performance.
(d) Self-confidence and competitiveness in the technical performance of sporting skills.

Moreover, it is also essential to minimize the risk of potential conflicts in the process, and this is only achieved through two important factors:

(a) A well-defined process outlining how the RTP decision should be made.
(b) A formal process to guide the individuals' interactions between those contributing to the RTP process.

Regarding the cultural context, we know we can find different approaches of dealing the RTP process: (1) the athlete could be capable of an autonomous decision, and (2) the decision could be left to the medical staff or (3) is expected that the clinician determine the course of action. Anyway, the clinician is usually legally responsible for any consequences of the decision. Besides that, a transparent framework for arriving RTP decision is indispensable to downplay potential conflicts.

12.2 Reconditioning and Performance Enhancement

Sports are complex and present a considerable number of factors affecting performance. Injuries are one of the athlete's major fears and that is why the reliable understanding of injury mechanisms and etiology are crucial steps in any effective injury prevention. For a successful return to performance, athletes need to be healthy (proper nutrition [8] and sleep [9], as well as, adequate psychological status and well-being), since injury load is correlated to team performance [10, 11].

A successful rehabilitation is of utmost importance to return the player as fast and as safe as possible to sports competition within the preinjury level and prevent reinjury and long-term sequelae. Within this line, a stepwise and individualized rehabilitation program with criteria-based progression should be followed to ensure safe progression through the different phases based on objective criteria and allow the RTP with lower risk of reinjuries. Many progression objective criteria can be applied through different phases of the rehabilitation and may involve effusion grading [12], muscle soreness [13], running progression [14], sport-specific agility progression [15, 16], and functional testing [17].

Reconditioning is a crucial component of the stepwise rehabilitation program (Fig. 12.1) and has a major role on making sure the injured ath-

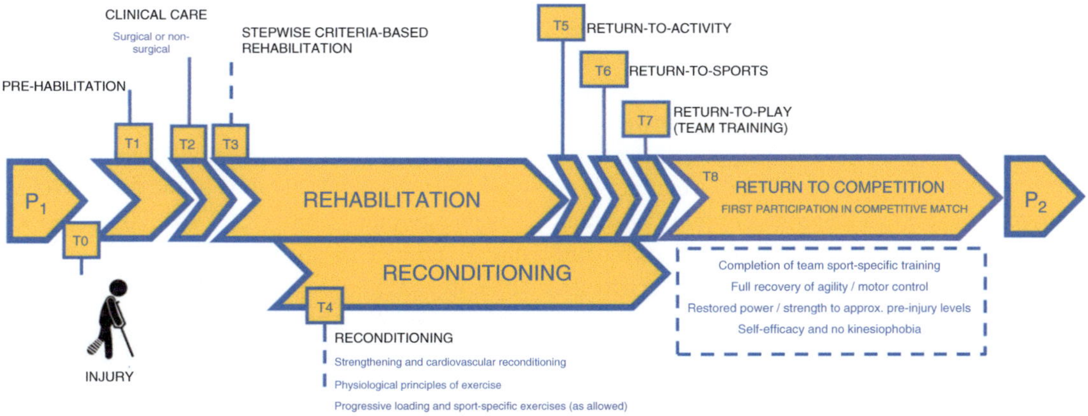

Fig. 12.1 Progressive stepwise criteria-based diagram, from injury to RTP and competition (P1 primary prevention, T0 injury occurrence, T1 pre-habilitation before treatment, T2 treatment (surgical or nonsurgical care), T3 beginning of rehabilitation, T4 beginning of physical reconditioning, T5 criteria to return to activity, T6 criteria to return to sports, T7 criteria to RTP, T8 criteria to return to competition, P2 secondary prevention). Adapted from [18]

lete is ready to perform at 100 percent when he or she returns to competition. For the injured athlete return to training, it is important to demonstrate the physical and technical qualities required by their particular sport of participation. Regardless of the affected area (excluding some cases that require complete rest, such as concussion or a severe cardiac condition), the reconditioning should start as soon as possible and can be introduced into the rehabilitation process in many ways. For instance, if a lower limb injury is involved (e.g., an anterior cruciate ligament injury), cardiovascular and respiratory systems may be challenged with upper limb cycle ergometer and upper body muscle strengthening. Moreover, when involving athletes, including sport-specific exercises will increase their adherence and compliance to the rehabilitation. Thus, in case of the previous example, the athlete may perform a single-leg stance on an unstable board with the uninvolved lower limb (maintaining/increasing balance skills and strengthening the uninjured lower limb and core muscles) while performing non-weight-bearing sport-specific exercises with the injured limb (Fig. 12.2).

It is extremely important to develop the athlete up to preinjury fitness levels in order to promote the best and safest return. In order to achieve this, we must prepare the athlete in terms of (1) power, (2) speed, (3) strength, (4) endurance, and (5) metabolic/cardiovascular capacity.

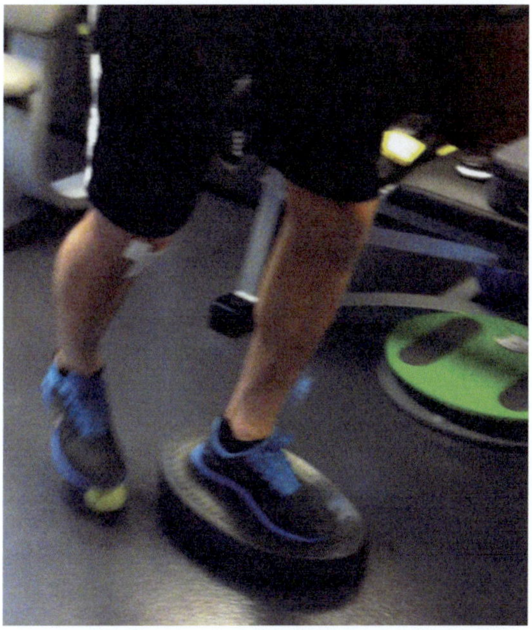

Fig. 12.2 Example of a non-weight-bearing sport-specific exercise of the injured lower limb

Strength is an essential component of all rehabilitation and performance enhancement programs. It is the ability of the muscle to exert force or torque at a specified velocity [19]. Because all muscles function concentrically, isometrically, and eccentrically in the frontal, sagittal, and transverse planes, an integrated training program should use a wide training approach using the entire muscle and velocity contraction spectrum [20, 21]. Eccentric training produces more force than concentric training [22–24].

Training programs for power demand both high-force and high-quality movements. Power is characterized by work per unit of time (force × distance/time) or force × velocity (distance × time). Rate of force development is the rate at which strength increases [25], and it is the most important neural adaptation for the majority of athletes [26]. Complex training could be used to improve power in the athlete by alternating biomechanically similar high-load weight training with plyometric exercises in the same workout [27].

Speed production have two components: stride frequency and stride length [28]. Stride length can be developed by bounding drills, running uphill, or power skips [28, 29]. Stride frequency can be upgraded with fast leg drills, resisted sprints, or assisted sprints [29]. When training for speed, intensity and training volume must be monitored. In addition, volume should increase gradually, as proper technique is required to prevent compensations or altered movement patterns. With fatigue, sprinting form is potentially sacrificed, thereby overcoming the positive effects of speed training. Therefore, to maximize speed production, speed practice drills should be performed at the beginning of training sessions, before the player getting fatigued. Rest periods are necessary and should allow full recovery between sets.

Increasing aerobic sources of energy can enhance endurance, by delaying the onset of blood lactate accumulation [25], which is dependent on maximal oxygen consumption and the intramuscular adaptations that facilitate prolonged work [25]. To improve endurance, muscles must oxidize lactate during work and decrease dependence on glycolysis to supply energy. Endurance training eliminates the disparity between the anaerobic and aerobic abilities of muscles and lactate accumulation [25]. Nowadays we can differentiate two types of endurance: general endurance, the base level of cardiorespiratory ability, and special endurance that is related to specific activities (metabolic capacity) [25].

In addition, plyometric, agility and sport-specific activities to the patient's home exercise program can be added, as long as the patient has no contraindications (e.g., loading restrictions or increased effusion) and exhibits pain-free and full-ROM performance of loading activities. Before adding these higher-level activities to a home program, it is important that the athlete show proper technique under supervision. Agility drills can assist the athlete in most of sport-specific activities, such as changing directions, accelerating, and decelerating [30]. Plyometrics can improve neuromuscular control in athletes, which can become a learned skill that transfers to return to competitive play [31].

With all this, it is well accepted that loading can change and develop fitness, and it's known that different fitness areas involved at the same time modulate sports performance. In addition, other areas of extreme importance cannot be ignored: sleep, rest, and nutrition. Like Pickett and Morris [32] said, "next to the air we breathe, food and sleep are the most crucial physical essentials for maintaining a sound and healthful state of living." The foods and liquids ingested will provide energy during physical activity and help the body recover from strenuous activity [33]. Sleep is recognized as a critical factor in athlete's performance. Sleep is thought to affect both physiological and cognitive function, which can affect sports performance. Athletes have lower quality of sleep as well as lower quantity of sleep, compared with the nonathlete, particularly during periods of intensified training [34–36].

Hence, a manifold of loading features and fitness areas are involved in the players' reconditioning, and an attempt to simplify this giant and complex relationship is displayed on Fig. 12.3.

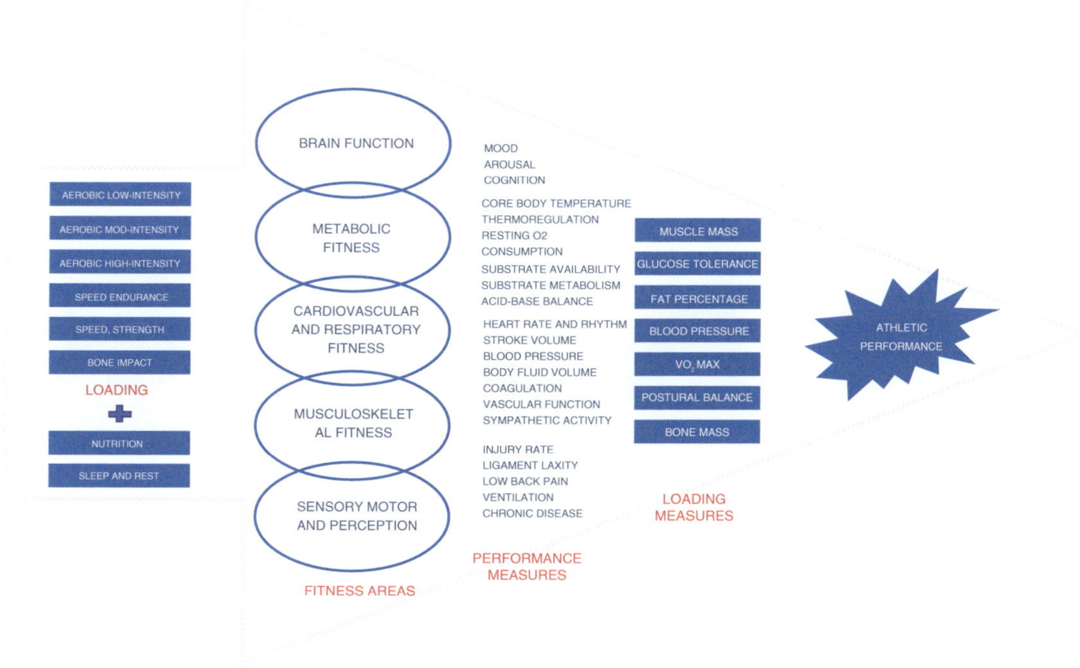

Fig. 12.3 Overview of the impact of different types of physical loading on various fitness capacities and its influence on the different components of physical performance. Adapted from [37–39]

Nowadays, there is a dogma that higher training load has been linked to higher injury rates [40]. Gabbett and his team introduce in this fitness area the training-injury prevention paradox, where there is a relationship between high training loads and injury, but the problem is not with training per se but more likely the inappropriate training that is being prescribed [40]. So, they consider that both acute (previous week) and chronic (previous 4 weeks) training loads have a better way to model the training and to minimize injury risk. Training loads have also a major role during the reconditioning and RTP phases. Recording and monitoring the individual player loads allow to follow the player's rehabilitation and reconditioning progress and maintain within safer load ranges and avoid load spikes [41, 42]. Several biofeedback wearable devices have been developed that can be used to monitor the player's loading progression [43–46].

At a high level, sports imply massive social media coverage and tremendous financial impact encompassing great pressure from the club stakeholders. With all this, it is natural that there is also great pressure from all the related stakeholders on health professionals responsible for health and recovery of athletes. Therefore, considering relevant factors including level of competition, season time, age, and career status is crucial to take part of the injury clinical reasoning [18]. When involved in team sports, it is important to also consider the individual response to the stimulus. Performance of a sports team is multifactorial and depends on several factors such as team spirit, technique, tactics, team organization, fan support, and other private circumstances. Legal, religious, cultural, linguistic, and family norms play also a role. Hence, it is important to understand the theoretical model on the influence of the load on the different systems (fitness), how this variation is perceived, and how it can be assessed. Independent from the league or the degree of professionalism, team sports lead to considerable physiological and psychological challenges. It is important for the team physician to recognize all pathological states, which may require treatment or rest. Nowadays, it is known that certain subgroups of players like females or veterans need additional attention to phenomena which are specific for them.

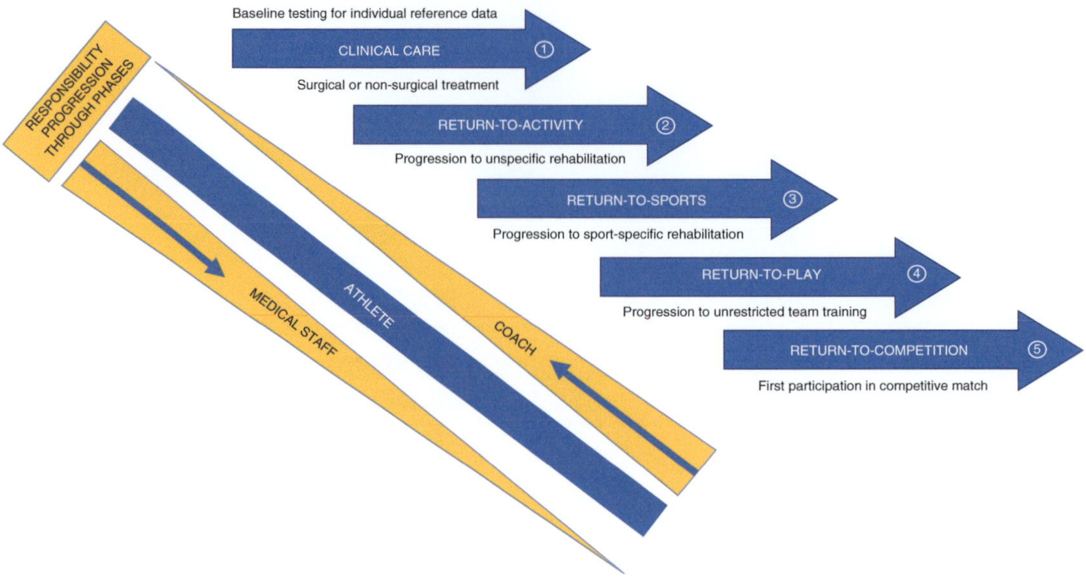

Fig. 12.4 Milestones of the RTP process and the compilation of responsibilities from the medical staff, coaches, and the athlete. Adapted from [48, 50]

12.3 Return-To-Play (RTP) Milestone

Establishing and setting up RTP guidelines are essential for a safe and effective RTP. RTP criteria are always dependent on the type and severity of injury, demands of the specific sport, the affected body region, and potential associated lesions [47]. These should be shared with the coaches, athletes, parents, and all other stakeholders. Confusing or absent criteria and policies can lead to challenges for all. Thus, the RTP milestone is crucial and has a particular importance for clubs, insurance institutions, and the injured athlete, as it marks the athlete's end of short-term disability and herewith associated remuneration payments [48]. Nevertheless, there is no single formula that can serve as an RTP guideline for all conditions. Still, a panel of experts agreed on five distinctive milestones in which the injured athletes will go through during an ideal rehabilitation process [48]. Milestones are passages from one rehabilitation phase to the next, which are mostly associated to significant gains in performance and progress in specific skills and based on objective verifiable criteria. These findings allow the involved professionals to control, monitor, and adjust the rehabilitation process in order to ensure a safe progression. The prioritized balance of all factors will depend upon the type and severity of the initial injury and a coordinated and truly integrated team effort, which involves respecting each other's professionals' abilities [49]. These milestones include several progressions of rehabilitation and RTP process, and the involvement and responsibility of the coach and medical staff change as the rehabilitation and RTP progress overtime (Fig. 12.4).

12.3.1 Preinjury Screening and Clinical Care (PRE-CC)

Sports participation has always an inherent risk of injury. Before the clinical approach to the injury, it is crucial to have a preseason or baseline screening (preinjury screening), which is no more than a prospective data collection that provides the rehabilitation staff with important reference values for the injured athlete that can be used in the event of an injury. Besides that, the preinjury screening offers the opportunity to identify any underlying performance deficits and abnormalities. This is helpful to modulate the training process and derive targeted individual primary prevention measures before an injury occurs. Deficits in regarding proprioception, muscular strength, and neuromuscular control (i.e., activation patterns) are extremely common.

It is very important to establish a treatment plan with achievable goals. Moreover, this can be started through conservative or surgical treatment or even a combination of both.

12.3.2 Return to Activity (RTA): Progression to Unspecific Rehabilitation

Return to activity is the progression to unspecific rehabilitation—a transition from the clinical care (phase I) to general rehabilitation training (phase II)—and describes the first posttraumatic milestone that the injured athlete can achieve. The clinician should perform a clinical examination and decide whether the athlete can start the general rehabilitation training, which is often focused on symptomatic control, regaining pain-free range of motion, stability, and movement control during basic movement patterns. The biologic rebuilding mechanisms are part of the rehabilitation process, so when establishing the treatment plan, examining the athlete is essential to recognize the biological healing process timeframes so as not to advance steps faster than it should.

12.3.3 Return to Sport (RTS): Progression to Sport-Specific Rehabilitation

Return to sport is a crucial phase since it marks the starting point of including the athlete in the sport-specific rehabilitation training and individualized competition training (phase III). At this milestone, the athlete should already meet basic clinical and functional requirements as a result from the previous rehabilitation phase.

12.3.4 Return to Play (RTP): Progression to Unrestricted Team Training

RTP is the progression to unrestricted team training, i.e., from the individualized and restricted team training to unrestricted participation in team and pre-competition training. This is an extremely sensitive progression for all involved, as in one hand for the athlete who wants to return as soon as possible and, in the other hand, for the medical department who wants to prevent further injuries. Following a comprehensive test battery, it is important to have a multidisciplinary decision-making team. After consensus, it should be the team physician responsible to make the RTP decision and, in a manner, promote unrestricted participation in competitive training.

12.3.5 Return to Competition (RTC): First Participation in Competitive Match

The return to competition milestone corresponds to the first participation in competition, which is the ultimate athlete's main goal. This phase is the culmination of the whole process of treatment and rehabilitation, comprising the entire reintegration process from the time of the injury to the first competition play.

The agreement between medical department, technical team, and the athlete is recommended for a safe and effective integration into competition. However, the time span from the positive RTP decision and the athlete's first selection is mainly the responsibility of the head coach.

12.4 Strategic Assessment of Risk and Risk Tolerance (StARRT)

In 2010, a group of researchers [51] adapted a three-step decision-based theoretic model for RTP. The medical factors and sport risk modifiers assess the risk, and the third step evaluates the effect of decision modifiers. However, categorizing biological and physiological causes into sociological constructs may lead to significant challenges and confusion, so they realized that they need to improve their first work.

In 2015 Shrier and colleagues [52] proposed a modified model, the Strategic Assessment of Risk and Risk Tolerance (StARRT) framework for RTP decisions. This framework addresses the limitations of the original three-step model and can be applied to any injury or RTP definition. This framework organizes the available information into different factors that determine the risk of participation and risk tolerance.

The StARRT framework (Fig. 12.5) simply uses the risk assessment of the outcome. If the risk assessment is greater than the risk tolerance, the decision should indicate to not allow to RTP. Injury or reinjury may occur whenever the stress applied to the tissue is greater than the stress the tissue can absorb. The next sections expand on these principles and show how the new terminology provides a more consistent framework.

12.4.1 Medical Factors: Step 1, The Tissue Health

The first step is to assess the amount of stress that the tissue can absorb before becoming damaged—tissue function health. Usually, tissue damage is assessed through the presence or absence of symptoms and signs, such as pain or

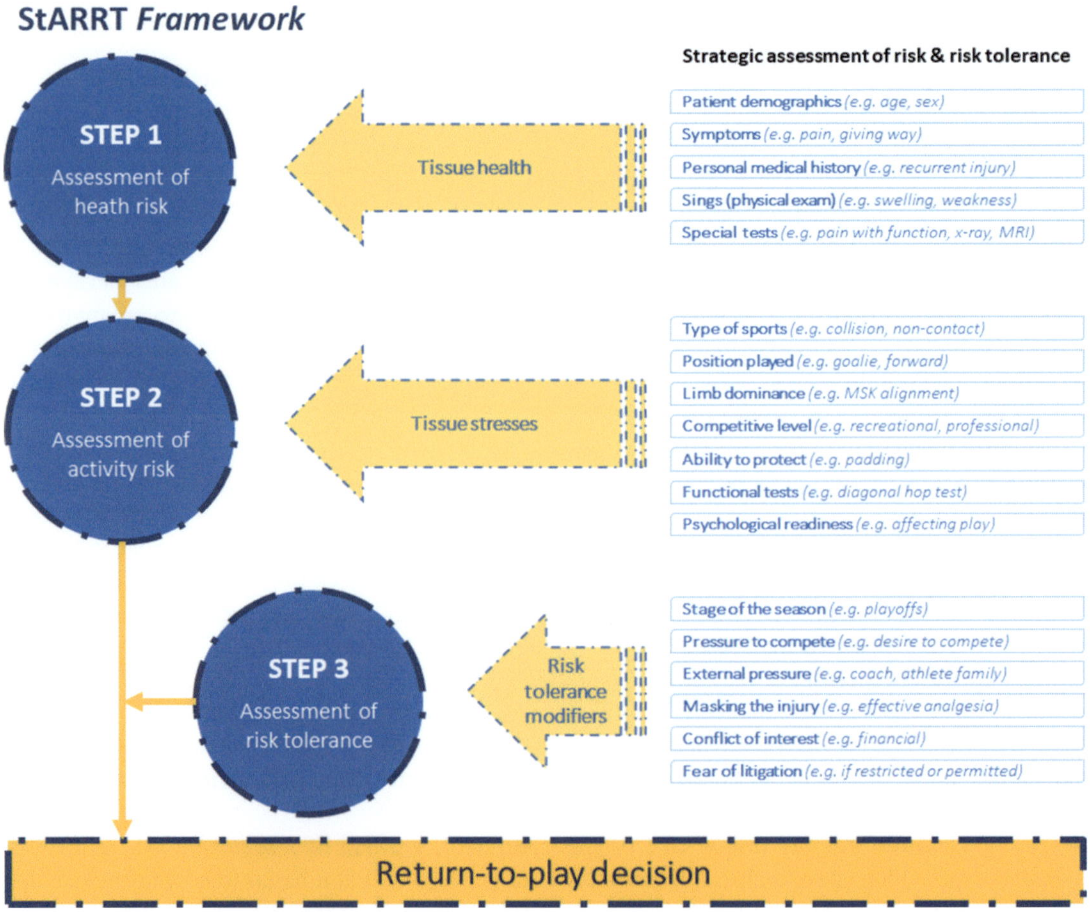

Fig. 12.5 The Strategic Assessment of Risk and Risk Tolerance (StARRT) framework. Adapted from [52]

swelling, or through diagnostic tests. For the same level of activity, the risk of reinjury increases with increasing damage to the tissue. This information comes from the health professional, so these factors were considered “medical.”

12.4.2 Sport Risk Modifiers: Step 2, The Tissue Stresses

The second step is to assess the stress that will be applied to the tissue. If an unhealthy tissue is exposed to only minimal stress, it continues the healing process. But, if the stress exceeds the capacity of the tissue, a new injury or reinjury will occur. Nowadays, there are many different ways to categorize activity. It is possible to use the “FITT” training principle and modify activity through the frequency (F), intensity (I), time (T), or type (T), for instance, 4 days per week, vigorous intensity, 45 min per session, and playing football. Within this line, tissue stress is directly related to the planned activity. Within this biological framework, it is best to think of “type” in relation to the biological stresses that increase with the specific activity and might cause injury rather than in general terms such as running or swimming. This is important because the biomechanics requirement is different between positions (football or handball), styles (swimming), and others and may impose different tissue stress (e.g., in football a wing player will have more sprint and deceleration situations than a center back player). The medical staff should focus on activities that increase stress in the musculoskeletal system. By changing or reducing stress (e.g., switching players positions or style), the injury risk will decrease.

Psychological readiness (in the original framework was in step 1) measures of functional capacity, and it’s here in step 2, because we know they can affect risk of reinjury via the way the athlete approaches and plays the game and therefore the potential stresses applied to the body. You can read more about this subject later in this chapter.

12.4.3 Decision Modifiers: Step 3, The Risk Tolerance Modifiers

The third step is clearly designed to express the clinician’s threshold for an acceptable risk (risk tolerance), which factors affect this risk, and why two athletes with same risk assessment may lead to different RTP decisions. The risk of new injury or reinjury represents one of the several outcomes that affect the athlete’s overall health or well-being. For instance, if the athlete is a 15-year-old male track and field high school athlete, the clinician’s risk tolerance is different when compared to an athlete on the way to an Olympic competition.

Regardless who is responsible for the RTP decision, it should be considered if there is any context where changing the factor would shift the threshold of an acceptable risk [4]. So, this relates the risk tolerance to the patient’s well-being and is consistent with societal values.

12.4.4 The Integrated Model: Beyond Injury Risk

The purpose of the StARRT framework is to reach at a decision based on whether the risk assessment exceeds the risk tolerance. It is important to understand that in clinical terms, the RTP may be referred to “full return without restrictions,” “partial return,” “allowed to practice,” and so forth. The StARRT framework can be applied to any decision-making process and will work uniformly with any definition of RTP. Any decision-maker can follow this process, whether it is a clinician, an athlete, a judge, or a shared decision-making process. In summary, this framework organizes the available information into different factors that determine the risk of participation and risk tolerance. Thus, the risk of participation depends on the interaction between the tissue health and tissue stresses (steps 1 and 2). These decisions are inappropriate when the risk assessment is poor or when (1) risk tolerance depends on factors unrelated to the patient’s well-being or (2) personal values conflict with societal values.

12.5 Injury-Psychological Readiness to Return to Sports

Sport psychology is the discipline that uses psychological knowledge and skills to give optimal performance and well-being of athletes and developmental and social aspects of sports participation [53]. Since the psychological part is related with injuries, this area becomes a topic of considerable investigation. When athletes get injured, the experiences are not only physical loss but also psychological loss [54–56], that is why this must be a priority for clinicians.

Sport psychology researchers have examined athletes' emotional, cognitive, and behavioral responses to injury. Because cognitive and emotional responses may affect physiological healing processes, the understanding of this responses is important for facilitating adaptive forms of coping, enhancing key rehabilitation behaviors such as adherence and compliance [57]. Advances in treatment and rehabilitation interventions have helped advance recovery processes. Unfortunately, the athletes' physical recovery is not always matched with athletes' perceptions of psychological readiness to return to competitive sport [58–60].

Neurocognitive, behavioral, and psychophysiological changes can be behind the increase of the risk of acute or overuse injuries (or increased risk of injury and/or increased injury time-loss) through the individual psychosocial characteristics [61]. Appropriate use of psychological interventions can modify each of these potential mechanisms [62, 63].

To optimize the RTP, it is very important that clinicians should be empowered to consider confidently all the psychological aspects. There are several intervention techniques with potential injury reduction benefits [61–65], such as:

1. Progressive muscular relaxation that potentially decreases muscle tension and increases rate of recovery.
2. Mindfulness-acceptance and commitment that can reduce attention disruption and distractions by paying attention to the present moment can improve attentional processes.
3. Cognitive behavioral stress management that through imagery and cognitive restructuring, the control of diaphragmatic breathing and incorporating relaxation can help deal with stressful situations and with emotions, thus impact behavioral compliance.
4. Combined imagery and positive self-talk, which help athletes cope with the pressure, increasing confidence and coping with adversity, thus improving concentration on appropriate environmental conditions.

12.5.1 Psychological Readiness to Return to Sport Assessment

Addressing the multitude of challenges faced by returning athletes, a number of investigators have examined constructs associated with psychological readiness to return to sport. The athlete's psychological readiness to return to sports assessment is of upmost importance for the RTP decision [66, 67]. Although multifactorial, psychological readiness is majorly influenced by an athlete's emotions and self-confidence [68]. The Injury-Psychological Readiness to Return to Sport (I-PRRS) scale [58] and the Reinjury Anxiety Inventory [60] have been developed to assess athletes' psychological mind-set during the reentry period. In addition to the I-PPRS scale, injury-specific scales have been developed, such as in the case of anterior cruciate ligament (ACL) injuries and anterior cruciate ligament-return to sport after injury (ACL-RSI) [69]. These scales represent an important advance in terms of objective measurement and assessment of the athlete's psychological readiness to return to sports.

Kinesiophobia, fear of reinjury, and lack of self-efficacy are often barriers that inhibit the athlete's readiness to return to sport and may also affect the quality of their performance. The capacity to believe in being successful in a given situation, it is called self-efficacy. As the athlete recovers from the injury, there is a significant improvement of this. In addition, higher levels of self-efficacy are associated with patient satisfaction and better outcomes [70]. Self-efficacy following knee injuries may be assessed by the knee self-efficacy scale [71], and, in the case of ACL reconstruction, it was reported that higher levels of self-efficacy are positively correlated with higher levels of postoperative activity [72]. Kinesiophobia and/or fear of reinjury has been reported as one of the main reasons for not returning to the previous level of activity [73] and can be assessed through the Tampa Scale of Kinesiophobia [74]. Yet, the exact constitution of what is fear of reinjury is unclear. It might be the fear implications for time off work and the related loss of income, fear of not being able to return to the previous level, fear of the pain of injury itself, or any combination of these [70]. Fear of reinjury is often referred as main reason to not returning to sports, and there are studies that fear of reinjury precludes RTP in nearly half of the ACL-reconstructed patients [75]. Moreover, athletes who had successfully returned to their preinjury sport generally participated without fear of reinjury [76].

Returning injured athletes to sport before they are psychologically ready can lead to anxiety, fear, reinjury, depression, injury to different body parts, and a decrease in performance [77] and potentially to greater risk of secondary injury [67, 78]. In turn, positive psychological responses including motivation, confidence, and low fear are associated with a higher likelihood of returning to the preinjury level of sports participation and returning faster [79]. Glazer [58] established the six-item I-PRRS scale (Table 12.1) to assess athletes' psychological readiness to RTP after an injury, which was validated through the Delphi method with numerous experts and achieved good reliability and validity. Scoring of each item of the scale ranges from 0 to 100 with intervals of 10. A score of 0 implies that the athlete has little to no confidence, a score of 50 indicates moderate confidence, and a score of 100 implies that the athlete had utmost confidence for that item. Then, the final scores of the 6 items are summed and divided by 10, with a final score up to 60 points. A score of 60 implies that an athlete is confident to return to sport at that time; 40, the athlete has only moderate confidence; and 20, the athlete had low overall confidence. A scale like this is necessary to determine when the athlete is ready for RTP since this preparation is personal and each injured athlete regain their confidence at different times during their own rehabilitation [80].

Table 12.1 Example of Injury-Psychological Readiness to Return to Sport (I-PRRS) scale

Item	Scoring (rate the current level of confidence, 0 = no confidence to 100 = complete confidence)
1. Overall confidence to play	0–100
2. Confidence to play without pain	0–100
3. Confidence to give 100% effort	0–100
4. Confidence in the injured body part to handle the demands of the situation	0–100
5. Confidence in skill level/ability	0–100
6. Confidence to not concentrate on the injury	0–100
Total score =	Sum of items 1 to 6 divided by 10

This scale is simple, can be easily used throughout the rehabilitation process, and can be applied by health professionals or coaches for monitoring athletes' psychological readiness to return to sport participation. Besides that, professionals involved (health or training) can determine with greater accuracy a more appropriate time for injured athletes return to competition [58]. Therefore, this scale should be applied to every RTP progression and can help identify those athletes that are not ready to return to competition and provide the health professional any eventual psychological readiness deficits that may require intervention before the athlete return to competition.

12.6 Decision-Maker Process: Who's Responsibility?

RTP decisions can be complex, multifactorial, and many times specific to the athlete and type of sport and often influenced by "decision modification" factors (e.g., pressure to return for a major event)

[51]. There are implications for the injured athlete, organizations, and technical department, and even the medical personnel can be impacted. On the other hand, these decisions are often made in team environments comprised by individuals with vast experience and knowledge surrounding athletic injuries [81]. Yet, the goal would be to achieve a unanimous decision concerning RTP of a given athlete for optimal congruency and management [52]. But this is not always easy to conquer.

Power relationships are widely studied in medical sociology, but this has not occurred within the RTP context [4]. Shrier et al. [82] conducted a survey questionnaire of Canadian sports medical department to determine which profession is best perceived to evaluate an athlete's RTP. It was concluded that medical doctors, physiotherapists, and athletic therapists were considered best able to assess factors related to risk of injury and associated complications.

Informed decisions require information from several sources. Besides that, it is important to eliminate all potential sources of bias, for example, any professional (from the medical doctor to the athlete) that is worried about losing his/her status or position, can make unconscious decision, and put all his work at risk. A shared decision-making process is the best way to achieve an effective result. However, each professional has duties in the process. There are three key steps in this decision: (1) choice, athlete and coach should be aware of the options; (2) option, different options must be detailed; and (3) decision, guiding the athlete and coach to consider and decide what is best [83, 84].

When several healthcare professionals are involved, a straight line of communication and authority must be clearly defined [2]. This professional group is the most appropriated to assess the health status of the athlete and provide advice on management options and possible clinical outcomes following RTP (usually a sports physician and/or physiotherapist). When taking care of the athlete, it is important to consider the external pressure always present in sports environment (social and financial factors) and minimize the influence of own values and beliefs [2, 81].

In elite sports, the RTP advice is usually informed. Short- and long-term consequences must be evaluated. When fully competent, the athlete will decide based in professional and personal circumstances and experience. Nevertheless, at the highest-level sports, there are a wide range of implications in individual events and team performance. Therefore, this is not an isolated decision, but the athlete's input is a prerequisite [83].

The primary role of the coach is to maximize athletic performance. They see their role as managing the unrealistic athlete expectations about the RTP process [4]. The main contribution from the coach to the RTP process is related with the sport-specific context. In elite sports, the coach is the only one that can take the "ability-to-perform" decision, by evaluating the athlete knowledge and missing training, functional progression, and the information provided by the healthcare professional.

Friends, family, agent, and corporate or institutional managers have interests in the RTP decision; however, their interactions can be misleading. Since the decision should always be in the best interest of the athlete, their role should be to support and comfort.

The involvement of different professions in the RTP process calls for a multilateral implementation strategy to enable a widespread distribution within the target group of elite and semi-elite football clubs (i.e., players, coaches, athletic coaches, physiotherapists, team physicians, club decision-makers) is essential. The healthcare professional's role or objective is to inform the athlete and coach about healthcare status and risk [83]. Clear, effective, and consistent communication is vital to achieve trust among the key people involved and to a good RTP decision.

12.7 Injury-Focused Examples of Return to Play

RTP is multifactorial and is dependent of a myriad of intrinsic and extrinsic factors. These may affect the rate of RTP at the preinjury level and the time to RTP. Intrinsic factors may include the damaged tissue healing timeframes, reestablishment of muscle strength and joint ROM, regaining of proper motor control and proprioception, psychological readiness, recovery of functional ability (e.g., hop test for lower limb injuries or Y balance test for upper limb injuries), and sport-specific skills, among others. Extrinsic factors often include the time into the season, career or contract status, proximity of an important competition, and pressure from related stakeholders (e.g., the coach or the club directors). The next subsections of this chapter explore the RTP rates and respective time to RTP of some common sports injuries.

12.7.1 ACL Reconstruction

A systematic review of the scientific literature [85] reported that following ACL reconstruction, a pooled rate of 83% of athletes return to sports within 6–13 months. Despite the athletic performance was decreased overtime from the preinjury levels, when comparing to the uninjured control group, no significant deterioration of the athletic performance was found. However, around 5% of those who RTP reported re-rupture.

The return to sports timing after ACL reconstruction is multifactorial and may depend on several factors including the level of participation and sports type. Thus, mean ranges of time to return to sports vary considerably according to the sports type: football from 6.0 to 10.2 months [86–89], basketball from 10.7 to 11.8 months [90–92], American football from 7.8 to 12.8 months [93–97], ice hockey from 9.8 to 13 months [98, 99], and rugby under or equal to 6 months [100].

When focusing adolescent and children with ACL reconstruction, the pooled rates were 92% of return to any sport participation, 79% return to preinjury level of sport, and 81% to competitive level of sport. A total of 13% ($n = 93$ of the 717 athletes) reported graft ruptures, and 14% ($n = 91$ of 652 patients) reported contralateral ACL injuries [101].

12.7.2 Knee Cartilage Injuries

Several systematic reviews have been published reporting the RTP rates and timing after knee cartilage surgery. Although RTP rates are similar across the surgical techniques employed, the time to RTP varies considerably and should be considered when the surgical decision is made (may depend level of competition, time into the season, and career status). Hence, the return to sports at any level, at the preinjury level, and time to return to sports are reported below according to the surgical technique employed [102–104]:

- Osteochondral autologous transplantation: RTP is 89–93% at any level, 70% at the preinjury level, and 5.2–7.1 months for return to sports.
- Osteochondral allograft transplantation: RTP is 88% at any level, 79% at the preinjury level, and 9.2–9.6 months for return to sports.
- Microfracture: RTP is 58–75% at any level, 68–69% at the preinjury level, and 7.0–9.1 months for return to sports.
- Autologous chondrocyte implantation: RTP is 67–84% at any level, 71–76% at the preinjury level, and 11.8–18.0 months for return to sports.

Similarly, when focusing football players [105], the return to sports rates were similar, with the osteochondral autologous transplantation providing a faster return (4.5 months), followed by microfractures (8 months) and autologous chondrocyte implantation (13.1 months).

12.7.3 Meniscal Surgery

Just as previously seen for knee cartilage injuries, the timing to RTP in meniscal injuries may vary considerably according to the approach employed. The indications of each surgical technique may often reflect the surgeon's preference but mostly depend on the pattern of the tear, the presence of associated injuries, the age and goals of the patient, and the level of competition [106]. In competing athletes, the surgical options mostly include partial meniscectomy, meniscal allograft transplantation, and meniscal repair:

- Partial meniscectomy: 61% of RTP at the preinjury level ($n = 47$ of 77 lateral partial meniscectomies in American football players) within an average of 8.5 months [107]. If considering football players (n = 90, n = 42 lateral, and n = 48 medial partial meniscectomy), the median time to RTP was longer in the lateral partial meniscectomies (7 weeks, range 5–18 weeks) than the medial group (5 weeks, range 3–6 weeks). However, the cumulative probability of returning to play was six times greater for players with a partial medial meniscectomy when comparing to partial lateral meniscectomy [108].

- Meniscal allograft transplantation: Reports of RTP following meniscal allograft transplantation are scarce, and only a few case series have been reported [109–111]. The return to preinjury levels of competition mean rates range from 77 to 96% (pooled sample size of 39 athletes, n = 26 football, and n = 13 multiple sports) within an average of 7.6–16.5 months.
- Meniscal repair: A pooled 89% of RTP at the preinjury level was reported (86% in professional athletes) within a mean time to return to sports of 4.3–6.5 months. Failure rate was lower in professional athletes (9%) when comparing to samples comprising different levels of competition (22%) [112].

12.7.4 Muscle Injuries

Muscle injuries account for 35% of all injuries in professional football and cause 25% of total absence. Within this line, a male elite football team of 25 players can expect 15 muscle injuries each season. Overall, muscle injuries affect mostly four muscle groups (the hamstring, the quadriceps (mainly rectus femoris), the adductor, and the calf muscles) accounting for 92% of all muscle injuries [113]. Return to training in elite professional men's football players is significantly faster in groin muscle injuries (median, 9 days) than hamstring (median, 13 days), quadriceps (median, 12 days), and calf muscle (median, 13 days) injuries [114].

The UEFA elite study (years 2001–2013) reported a total of 2287 thigh muscle injuries (25% of all injuries), of these 11.5% were direct injuries (contusion) and 88.5% indirect injuries (strain). Mean absence (time to full training) of all thigh muscle injuries was 17.2 ± 18.9 (range, 0–247) days. After indirect injury, the absence time was significantly longer 18.5 ± 19.5 (range, 1–247) days compared to direct injuries 7.0 ± 9.1 (range, 0–93) days [115]. In the case of hamstring injuries (UEFA study, years 2007–2014), the magnetic resonance parameters, more specifically the radiological grade and size of the edema, correlate with time to RTP for both grade 1 and 2 injuries. However, no correlations were found between time to RTP and the location and type of injury [116]. Reinjuries are most common in biceps femoris injuries but rare in semitendinosus and semimembranosus injuries [114].

Hip and groin injuries constitute a considerable part of all time-loss injuries in men's professional football. In the elite UEFA study (years 2001–2016) [117], hip and groin injuries accounted for 14% of all injuries (n = 1812, 11% were reinjuries), with adductor-related injury as the most common of hip and groin injuries (n = 1139, 63%; incidence rate 0.6/1000 h). The mean layoff for all hip and groin pain was 16 ± 23 days and 15 ± 20 for adductor-related injuries.

12.7.5 Shoulder Surgery

RTP after rotator cuff tears is challenging and few guidelines have been published. According to the type of lesion, its symptoms, and the player role, the treatment of rotator cuff tears can be surgical (tendon repair) or conservative (shoulder immobilization, pain control, and restoring full range of motion with physiotherapy) [118]. A systematic review [119] accounting 635 athletes (n = 286 professional and n = 349 recreational) and different sports (baseball, n = 224; tennis, n = 104; and golf, n = 54) reported an overall rate of return to any level of sports of 85 and 66% to the preinjury level of sports, after 4–17 months. Focusing the professional athletes, half of them returned to the preinjury level of sports.

Anterior shoulder dislocation and subsequent chronic instability are common in young athletes.

Athletes managed nonoperatively often show unacceptably high rates of recurrent instability and are less likely to successfully RTP [120]. Hence, athletes with recurrent instability that are unable to perform the sport-specific drills are indicated for surgical stabilization. Within this line, arthroscopic approaches have become popular with high rates of success [121]. In a comparative study [122], 90% of athletes who underwent arthroscopic stabilization returned to sports in the subsequent season without recurrent instability and were 5.8 times more likely return to competition without recurrent instability in the subsequent season compared to athletes who underwent nonoperative management. In a systematic review, 1036 patients that underwent surgical management of shoulder stabilization reported higher RTP rates at the preinjury level following arthroscopic Bankart repair (71%) or the Latarjet procedure (73%) than open stabilization (66%).

12.7.6 Ankle Lateral Ligamentous Injury

After a lateral ligamentous injury, it is difficult to determine when a football player can RTP. The non-elite or recreational player will undergo a conservative three-phase rehabilitation program for 3 months and in case of continued instability will follow for stabilization surgery [123]. In the case of elite athletes, the acute repair is most often considered [124].

In the elite UEFA study, within a timeframe of 11 years, a total of 729 ankle sprains were recorded (68% of all ankle injuries and an incidence rate of 0.7/1000 h), accounting with 10% of those classified as reinjuries. The mean layoff time (time to training) was 15 days. The average layoff days was not significantly different between recurrent sprains and other sprains [125].

Following lateral ligament surgery, a systematic review reported a return to sports rate of 85% within an average of 4.7 months (range, 2.4–6.8 months) [126]. When considering professional players, a case series of 42 athletes reported a median RTP of 77 days (range, 56–127 days) for isolated lateral ligamentous injuries and 105 days (range, 82–178 days) for those with concomitant injuries [127].

12.7.7 Patellar Dislocation

Acute lateral patellar dislocations are common in the active young population. Around 50–60% of initial first-time lateral patellar dislocations will occur secondary to a sports-related injury [128]. Depending on the underlying individual risk factors for dislocation recurrence, conservative or surgical management may be applied efficiently.

Nonoperative management still remains the standard of care for first-time patellar dislocations [129]. A retrospective review of patients with primary lateral patellar dislocations treated conservatively showed that 73% of patients reported no further dislocation events. Of these, 86% of the patients returned to their most important physical activity, but only 26% were able to return without limitations [130]. In another report, although 69% of patients RTP within 6 months without recurrence episodes, 58% reported limitations upon intense activity [131]. Surgical stabilization surgery most often includes medial patellofemoral ligament reconstruction, tibial tubercle osteotomy, or trochleoplasty, which is performed in isolate or in combination. The RTP rate varies from 84 to 100%, with 33–77% of return to the preinjury level. The time to RTP is highly variable, ranging from 3 to 12 months [132].

12.8 Summary

A successful RTP program returns the athlete as fast and as safe to preinjury levels of competition, without fear or increase risk of reinjury and without long-term comorbidities. This process should be progressive in terms of loading and movement complexity and should drive by "what" the athlete is able to do rather than "when." The final decision to return an athlete to competition should be given when all the stakeholders—from the medical team and coaches to the athlete as well—have the evidence each needs to confirm the athlete is recovered close to the preinjury levels and as the minimum risk of reinjury.

Fact Box
1. A successful rehabilitation is of utmost importance to return the player as fast and as safe as possible to sports competition within the preinjury level and prevent reinjury and long-term sequelae.
2. RTP guidelines are essential, and the criteria are always dependent on the type and severity of injury, demands of the specific sport, the affected body region, and potential associated lesions.
3. Psychological readiness and proper reconditioning are crucial and present throughout all the RTP spectrum.
4. The final decision to return an athlete to competition should be given when all the stakeholders have the evidence each needs to confirm the athlete is recovered close to the preinjury levels and as the minimum risk of reinjury.

References

1. Joyce D, Lewindon D. Sports injury prevention and rehabilitation: integrating medicine and science for performance solutions. New York: Routledge; 2015.
2. Ardern CL, Glasgow P, Schneiders A, et al. 2016 Consensus statement on return to sport from the first world congress in sports physical therapy, Bern. Br J Sports Med. 2016;50:853–64.
3. Wiese-bjornstal DM, Smith AM, Shaffer SM, Morrey MA. An integrated model of response to sport injury: psychological and sociological dynamics. J Appl Sport Psychol. 1998;10:46–69.
4. Brukner P, Khan K. Brukner & Khan's clinical sports medicine. 5th ed. New York: McGraw-Hill Education; 2017.
5. Roderick M. The work of professional football. London: Routledge; 2006.
6. Safai P. Negotiating with risk: exploring the role of the sports medicine clinician. In: Young K, editor. Sporting bodies, damaged selves: sociological studies of sports-related injury (research in the sociology of sport); 2004. p. 269–86.
7. Safai P. Sports medicine, health, and the politics of risk. In: Andrews DL, Carrington B, editors. A companion to sport. Malden, MA: Blackwell; 2013. p. 112–28.
8. Manikandan S, Selvam D. Nutrition and sports performance. Br J Sports Med. 2010;44.
9. Watson AM. Sleep and athletic performance. Curr Sports Med Rep. 2017;16:413–8.
10. Eirale C, Tol JL, Farooq A, Smiley F, Chalabi H. Low injury rate strongly correlates with team success in Qatari professional football. Br J Sports Med. 2012;47:807–8.
11. Hägglund M, Waldén M, Magnusson H, Kristenson K, Bengtsson H, Ekstrand J. Injuries affect team performance negatively in professional football: an 11-year follow-up of the UEFA Champions League injury study. Br J Sports Med. 2013;47:738–42.
12. Sturgill LP, Snyder-Mackler L, Manal TJ, Axe MJ. Interrater reliability of a clinical scale to assess knee joint effusion. J Orthop Sports Phys Ther. 2009;39:845–9.
13. Fees M, Decker T, Snyder-Mackler L, Axe MJ. Upper extremity weight-training modifications for the injured athlete. A clinical perspective. Am J Sports Med. 1998;26:732–42.
14. Rambaud AJM, Ardern CL, Thoreux P, Regnaux J-P, Edouard P. Criteria for return to running after anterior cruciate ligament reconstruction: a scoping review. Br J Sports Med. 2018;52(22):1437–44. https://doi.org/10.1136/bjsports-2017-098602.
15. Adams D, Logerstedt DS, Hunter-Giordano A, Axe MJ, Snyder-Mackler L. Current concepts for anterior cruciate ligament reconstruction: a criterion-based rehabilitation progression. J Orthop Sports Phys Ther. 2012;42:601–14.
16. Fitzgerald GK, Axe MJ, Snyder-Mackler L. Proposed practice guidelines for nonoperative anterior cruciate ligament rehabilitation of physically active individuals. J Orthop Sports Phys Ther. 2000;30:194–203.
17. Abrams GD, Harris JD, Gupta AK, McCormick FM, Bush-Joseph CA, Verma NN, Cole BJ, Bach BRJ. Functional performance testing after anterior cruciate ligament reconstruction: a systematic review. Orthop J Sports Med. 2014;2(1):2325967113518305. https://doi.org/10.1177/2325967113518305.
18. Andrade R, Pereira R, Bastos R, Pereira H, Oliveira JM, Reis RL, Espregueira-Mendes J. Return to play following cartilage injuries. In: Return to play footb. Berlin: Springer; 2018. p. 593–610.
19. Lorenz DS, Reiman MP, Walker JC. Periodization: current review and suggested implementation for athletic rehabilitation. Sports Health. 2010;2:509–18.
20. Bompa T. Theory and methodology of training: the key to athletic performance. 3rd ed. Dubuque, IA: Kendall Hunt; 1994.

21. Fleck SJ, Kraemer WJ. Designing resistance training programs. 3rd ed. Champaign, IL: Human Kinetics; 2004.
22. Knuttgen HG, Kraemer WJ. Terminology and measurement in exercise performance. J Appl Sport Sci. 1987;1–10.
23. Maganaris CN, Narici MV, Almekinders LC, Maffulli N. Biomechanics and pathophysiology of overuse tendon injuries: ideas on insertional tendinopathy. Sports Med. 2004;34:1005–17.
24. Leadbetter WB. Cell-matrix response in tendon injury. Clin Sports Med. 1992;11:533–78.
25. Siff MC. Supertraining. 4th ed. Denver, CO: Supertraining Institute; 2003.
26. Clark M. Integrated training for the new millennium. Thousand Oaks, CA: National Academy of Sports Medicine; 2001.
27. Maio Alves JMV, Rebelo AN, Abrantes C, Sampaio J. Short-term effects of complex and contrast training in soccer Players' vertical jump, Sprint, and agility abilities. J Strength Cond Res. 2010;24:936–41.
28. Cissik JM. Means and methods of speed training, part I. Streng Cond J. 2004;26:24–9.
29. Cissik JM. Means and methods of speed training: part II. Streng Cond J. 2005;27.
30. Risberg MA, Ekeland A. Assessment of functional tests after anterior cruciate ligament surgery. J Orthop Sports Phys Ther. 1994;19:212–7.
31. Myer GD, Schmitt LC, Brent JL, Ford KR, Barber Foss KD, Scherer BJ, Heidt RSJ, Divine JG, Hewett TE. Utilization of modified NFL combine testing to identify functional deficits in athletes following ACL reconstruction. J Orthop Sports Phys Ther. 2011;41:377–87.
32. Pickett GF, Morris AF. Effects of acute sleep and food deprivation on total body response time and cardiovascular performance. J Sports Med Phys Fitness. 1975;15:49–56.
33. Beck KL, Thomson JS, Swift RJ, von Hurst PR. Role of nutrition in performance enhancement and postexercise recovery. Open Access J Sports Med. 2015;6:259–67.
34. Killer SC, Svendsen IS, Jeukendrup AE, Gleeson M. Evidence of disturbed sleep and mood state in well-trained athletes during short-term intensified training with and without a high carbohydrate nutritional intervention. J Sports Sci. 2017;35:1402–10.
35. Halson SL, Bridge MW, Meeusen R, Busschaert B, Gleeson M, Jones DA, Jeukendrup AE. Time course of performance changes and fatigue markers during intensified training in trained cyclists. J Appl Physiol. 2002;93:947–56.
36. Halson SL, Lancaster GI, Achten J, Gleeson M, Jeukendrup AE. Effects of carbohydrate supplementation on performance and carbohydrate oxidation after intensified cycling training. J Appl Physiol. 2004;97:1245–53.
37. Meyer T, Julian R, Thompson C. Exercise physiology of football: factors related to performance and health. In: Musahl V, Karlsson J, Krutsch W, Mandelbaum BR, Espregueira-Mendes J, D'Hooghe P, editors. Return to play football. An evidence-based approach. Berlin: Springer; 2018. p. 85–95.
38. Lebrun CM, Joyce SM, Constantini NW. Effects of female reproductive hormones on sports performance. In: Constantini N, Hackney AC, editors. Endocrinology of physical activity and sport. 2nd ed. Totowa, NJ: Humana Press; 2013. p. 281–322.
39. Krustrup P, Aagaard P, Nybo L, Petersen J, Mohr M, Bangsbo J. Recreational football as a health promoting activity: a topical review. Scand J Med Sci Sports. 2010;20(Suppl 1):1–13.
40. Gabbett TJ. The training—injury prevention paradox: should athletes be training smarter and harder? Br J Sports Med. 2016;50:273–80.
41. Bourdon PC, Cardinale M, Murray A, et al. Monitoring athlete training loads: consensus statement. Int J Sports Physiol Perform. 2017;12:S2161–70. https://doi.org/10.1123/IJSPP.2017-0208.
42. Hulin BT, Gabbett TJ, Blanch P, Chapman P, Bailey D, Orchard JW. Spikes in acute workload are associated with increased injury risk in elite cricket fast bowlers. Br J Sports Med. 2014;48:708–12.
43. Cardinale M, Varley MC. Wearable training-monitoring technology: applications, challenges, and opportunities. Int J Sports Physiol Perform. 2017;12:255–62.
44. Akenhead R, Nassis GP. Training load and player monitoring in high-level football: current practice and perceptions. Int J Sports Physiol Perform. 2016;11:587–93.
45. Vanrenterghem J, Nedergaard NJ, Robinson MA, Drust B. Training load monitoring in team sports: a novel framework separating physiological and biomechanical load-adaptation pathways. Sports Med. 2017;47:2135–42.
46. Peake JM, Kerr G, Sullivan JP. A critical review of consumer wearables, mobile applications, and equipment for providing biofeedback, monitoring stress, and sleep in physically active populations. Front Physiol. 2018;9:743.
47. Ardern CL, Bizzini M, Bahr R. It is time for consensus on return to play after injury: five key questions. Br J Sports Med. 2016;50:506–8.
48. Bloch H, Klein C, Luig P, Riepenhof H. Development and implementation of a modular return-to-play test battery after ACL reconstruction. In: Return to play football. Berlin: Springer; 2018. p. 217–36.
49. Ardern CL. Anterior cruciate ligament reconstruction-not exactly a one-way ticket Back to the preinjury level: a review of contextual factors affecting return to sport after surgery. Sports Health. 2015;7:224–30.
50. Krutsch W, Wormuth F, Schweinsteiger T. Expectations and responsibilities of players and team coaches in the return-to-play process. In: Musahl V, Karlsson J, Krutsch W, Mandelbaum BR, Espregueira-Mendes J, D'Hooghe P, editors. Return to play football. An evidence-based approach. Berlin: Springer; 2018. p. 793–809.

51. Creighton DW, Shrier I, Shultz R, Meeuwisse WH, Matheson GO. Return-to-play in sport: a decision-based model. Clin J Sport Med. 2010;20:379–85.
52. Shrier I. Strategic assessment of risk and risk tolerance (StARRT) framework for return-to-play decision-making. Br J Sports Med. 2015;49:1311–5.
53. Podlog L. Sports injury. In: Schinke RJ, McGannon KR, Smith B, editors. The Routledge International handbook of sport psychology. New York: Routledge; 2016. p. 167–75.
54. Andersen MB, Williams JM. A model of stress and athletic injury: prediction and prevention. J Sport Exerc Psychol. 1988;10:294–306.
55. Wiese-bjornstal DM, Smith AM, LaMott EE. A model of psychologic response to athletic injury and rehabilitation. Athl Train Sports Health Care Perspect. 1995;1:17–30.
56. Williams JM, Andersen MB. Psychosocial antecedents of sport injury: review and critique of the stress and injury model. J Appl Sport Psychol. 1998;10:5–25.
57. Brewer BW. Psychology of sport injury rehabilitation. In: Handbook of sport psychology. Hoboken, NJ: Wiley; 2012. p. 404–24.
58. Glazer DD. Development and preliminary validation of the injury-psychological readiness to return to sport (I-PRRS) scale. J Athl Train. 2009;44:185–9.
59. Podlog L, Eklund RC. A longitudinal investigation of competitive athletes' return to sport following serious injury. J Appl Sport Psychol. 2006;18:44–68.
60. Walker N, Thatcher J, Lavallee D. A preliminary development of the re-injury anxiety inventory (RIAI). Phys Ther Sport. 2010;11:23–9.
61. Gledhill A, Forsdyke D. An ounce of prevention is better than a pound of cure: shouldn't we be doing EVERYTHING to reduce sports injury incidence and burden?. Br J Sports Med. 2018;52.
62. Ivarsson A, Johnson U, Andersen MB, Tranaeus U, Stenling A, Lindwall M. Psychosocial factors and sport injuries: meta-analyses for prediction and prevention. Sports Med. 2017;47:353–65.
63. Gledhill A, Forsdyke D, Murray E. Psychological interventions used to reduce sports injuries: a systematic review of real-world effectiveness. Br J Sports Med. 2018;52:967–71.
64. Perna FM, Antoni MH, Baum A, Gordon P, Schneiderman N. Cognitive behavioral stress management effects on injury and illness among competitive athletes: a randomized clinical trial. Ann Behav Med. 2003;25:66–73.
65. Ivarsson A, Johnson U, Andersen MB, Fallby J, Altemyr M. It pays to pay attention: a mindfulness-based program for injury prevention with soccer players. J Appl Sport Psychol. 2015;27:319–34.
66. Ardern CL, Taylor NF, Feller JA, Whitehead TS, Webster KE. Psychological responses matter in returning to preinjury level of sport after anterior cruciate ligament reconstruction surgery. Am J Sports Med. 2013;41:1549–58.
67. Ardern CL, Osterberg A, Tagesson S, Gauffin H, Webster KE, Kvist J. The impact of psychological readiness to return to sport and recreational activities after anterior cruciate ligament reconstruction. Br J Sports Med. 2014;48:1613–9.
68. Ardern CL, Kvist J, Webster KE. Psychological aspects of anterior cruciate ligament injuries. Oper Tech Sports Med. 2016;24:77–83.
69. Webster KE, Feller JA, Lambros C. Development and preliminary validation of a scale to measure the psychological impact of returning to sport following anterior cruciate ligament reconstruction surgery. Phys Ther Sport. 2008;9:9–15.
70. Webster KE, Feller JA. Psychological factors influencing return to sport after anterior cruciate ligament reconstruction. In: Musahl V, Karlsson J, Krutsch W, Mandelbaum BR, Espregueira-Mendes J, D'Hooghe P, editors. Return to play football. An evidence-based approach. Berlin: Springer; 2018. p. 73–83.
71. Thomee P, Wahrborg P, Borjesson M, Thomee R, Eriksson BI, Karlsson J. A new instrument for measuring self-efficacy in patients with an anterior cruciate ligament injury. Scand J Med Sci Sports. 2006;16:181–7.
72. Thomee P, Wahrborg P, Borjesson M, Thomee R, Eriksson BI, Karlsson J. Determinants of self-efficacy in the rehabilitation of patients with anterior cruciate ligament injury. J Rehabil Med. 2007;39:486–92.
73. Kvist J, Ek A, Sporrstedt K, Good L. Fear of re-injury: a hindrance for returning to sports after anterior cruciate ligament reconstruction. Knee Surg Sports Traumatol Arthrosc. 2005;13:393–7.
74. French DJ, France CR, Vigneau F, French JA, Evans RT. Fear of movement/(re)injury in chronic pain: a psychometric assessment of the original English version of the Tampa scale for kinesiophobia (TSK). Pain. 2007;127:42–51.
75. Flanigan DC, Everhart JS, Pedroza A, Smith T, Kaeding CC. Fear of reinjury (kinesiophobia) and persistent knee symptoms are common factors for lack of return to sport after anterior cruciate ligament reconstruction. Arthroscopy. 2013;29: 1322–9.
76. Ardern CL, Taylor NF, Feller JA, Webster KE. Fear of re-injury in people who have returned to sport following anterior cruciate ligament reconstruction surgery. J Sci Med Sport. 2012;15:488–95.
77. Wiese DM, Weiss MR. Psychological rehabilitation and physical injury: implications for the sportsmedicine team. Sport Psychol. 1987;1:318–30.
78. Podlog L, Banham SM, Wadey R, Hannon JC. Psychological readiness to return to competitive sport following injury: a qualitative study. Sport Psychol. 2015;29:1–14.
79. Ardern CL, Taylor NF, Feller JA, Webster KE. A systematic review of the psychological factors associated with returning to sport following injury. Br J Sports Med. 2013;47:1120 LP–1126.

80. Quinn AM, Fallon BJ. The changes in psychological characteristics and reactions of elite athletes from injury onset until full recovery. J Appl Sport Psychol. 1999;11:210–29.
81. Safai P. Healing the body in the "culture of risk": examining the negotiation of treatment between sport medicine clinicians and injured athletes in Canadian intercollegiate sport. Sociol Sport J. 2003;20:127–46.
82. Shrier I, Safai P, Charland L. Return to play following injury: whose decision should it be? Br J Sports Med. 2014;48:394.
83. Dijkstra HP, Pollock N, Chakraverty R, Ardern CL. Return to play in elite sport: a shared decision-making process. Br J Sports Med. 2017;51:419–20.
84. Elwyn G, Frosch D, Thomson R, et al. Shared decision making: a model for clinical practice. J Gen Intern Med. 2012;27:1361–7.
85. Lai CCH, Ardern CL, Feller JA, Webster KE. Eighty-three per cent of elite athletes return to preinjury sport after anterior cruciate ligament reconstruction: a systematic review with meta-analysis of return to sport rates, graft rupture rates and performance outcomes. Br J Sports Med. 2018;52:128 LP–138.
86. Howard JS, Lembach ML, Metzler AV, Johnson DL. Rates and determinants of return to play after anterior cruciate ligament reconstruction in National Collegiate Athletic Association Division I Soccer Athletes: a study of the Southeastern Conference. Am J Sports Med. 2016;44:433–9.
87. Zaffagnini S, Grassi A, Marcheggiani Muccioli GM, Tsapralis K, Ricci M, Bragonzoni L, Della Villa S, Marcacci M. Return to sport after anterior cruciate ligament reconstruction in professional soccer players. Knee. 2014;21:731–5.
88. Walden M, Hagglund M, Magnusson H, Ekstrand J. Anterior cruciate ligament injury in elite football: a prospective three-cohort study. Knee Surg Sports Traumatol Arthrosc. 2011;19:11–9.
89. Erickson BJ, Harris JD, Cvetanovich GL, Bach BR, Bush-Joseph CA, Abrams GD, Gupta AK, McCormick FM, Cole BJ. Performance and return to sport after anterior cruciate ligament reconstruction in male Major League Soccer players. Orthop J Sports Med. 2013;1(2):2325967113497189. https://doi.org/10.1177/2325967113497189.
90. Namdari S, Scott K, Milby A, Baldwin K, Lee G-C. Athletic performance after ACL reconstruction in the Women's National Basketball Association. Phys Sportsmed. 2011;39:36–41.
91. Harris JD, Erickson BJ, Bach BRJ, Abrams GD, Cvetanovich GL, Forsythe B, McCormick FM, Gupta AK, Cole BJ. Return-to-sport and performance after anterior cruciate ligament reconstruction in National Basketball Association Players. Sports Health. 2013;5:562–8.
92. Busfield BT, Kharrazi FD, Starkey C, Lombardo SJ, Seegmiller J. Performance outcomes of anterior cruciate ligament reconstruction in the National Basketball Association. Arthroscopy. 2009;25:825–30.
93. Erickson BJ, Harris JD, Heninger JR, Frank R, Bush-Joseph CA, Verma NN, Cole BJ, Bach BR. Performance and return-to-sport after ACL reconstruction in NFL quarterbacks. Orthopedics. 2014;37:728–34.
94. Shah VM, Andrews JR, Fleisig GS, McMichael CS, Lemak LJ. Return to play after anterior cruciate ligament reconstruction in National Football League athletes. Am J Sports Med. 2010;38:2233–9.
95. Erickson BJ, Harris JD, Fillingham YA, Cvetanovich GL, Bhatia S, Bach BR, Bush-Joseph CA, Cole BJ. Performance and return to sport after anterior cruciate ligament reconstruction in X-games skiers and snowboarders. Orthop J Sports Med. 2013;1(6):2325967113511196. https://doi.org/10.1177/2325967113511196.
96. Daruwalla JH, Greis PE, Hancock R, Xerogeanes JW. Rates and determinants of return to play after anterior cruciate ligament reconstruction in NCAA division 1 college football athletes: a study of the ACC, SEC, and PAC-12 conferences. Orthop J Sports Med. 2014;2(8):2325967114543901. https://doi.org/10.1177/2325967114543901.
97. Carey JL, Huffman GR, Parekh SG, Sennett BJ. Outcomes of anterior cruciate ligament injuries to running backs and wide receivers in the National Football League. Am J Sports Med. 2006;34:1911–7.
98. Sikka R, Kurtenbach C, Steubs JT, Boyd JL, Nelson BJ. Anterior cruciate ligament injuries in professional hockey players. Am J Sports Med. 2016;44:378–83.
99. Erickson BJ, Harris JD, Cole BJ, Frank RM, Fillingham YA, Ellman MB, Verma NN, Bach BR. Performance and return to sport after anterior cruciate ligament reconstruction in National Hockey League Players. Orthop J Sports Med. 2014;2(9):2325967114548831. https://doi.org/10.1177/2325967114548831.
100. Fabbriciani C, Milano G, Mulas PD, Ziranu F, Severini G. Anterior cruciate ligament reconstruction with doubled semitendinosus and gracilis tendon graft in rugby players. Knee Surg Sports Traumatol Arthrosc. 2005;13:2–7.
101. Kay J, Memon M, Marx RG, Peterson D, Simunovic N, Ayeni OR. Over 90% of children and adolescents return to sport after anterior cruciate ligament reconstruction: a systematic review and meta-analysis. Knee Surg Sport Traumatol Arthrosc. 2018;26:1019–36.
102. Mithoefer K, Hambly K, Della Villa S, Silvers H, Mandelbaum BR. Return to sports participation after articular cartilage repair in the knee: scientific evidence. Am J Sports Med. 2009;37(Suppl 1):167S–76S.
103. Campbell AB, Pineda M, Harris JD, Flanigan DC. Return to sport after articular cartilage repair in athletes' knees: a systematic review. Arthroscopy. 2016;32:651–68.e1.

104. Krych AJ, Pareek A, King AH, Johnson NR, Stuart MJ, Williams RJ 3rd. Return to sport after the surgical management of articular cartilage lesions in the knee: a meta-analysis. Knee Surg Sports Traumatol Arthrosc. 2017;25:3186–96.
105. Andrade R, Vasta S, Papalia R, Pereira H, Oliveira JM, Reis RL, Espregueira-Mendes J. Prevalence of articular cartilage lesions and surgical clinical outcomes in football (soccer) players' knees: a systematic review. Arthroscopy. 2016;32:1466–77.
106. Batailler C, Servien E, Magnussen R, Lustig S, Neyret P. Return to play following meniscal injuries. In: Musahl V, Karlsson J, Krutsch W, Mandelbaum BR, Espregueira-Mendes J, D'Hooghe P, editors. Return to play football. An evidence-based approach. Berlin: Springer; 2018. p. 583–92.
107. Aune KT, Andrews JR, Dugas JR, Cain EL. Return to play after partial lateral meniscectomy in National Football League Athletes. Am J Sports Med. 2014;42:1865–72.
108. Nawabi DH, Cro S, Hamid IP, Williams A. Return to play after lateral meniscectomy compared with medial meniscectomy in elite professional soccer players. Am J Sports Med. 2014;42:2193–8.
109. Marcacci M, Marcheggiani Muccioli GM, Grassi A, Ricci M, Tsapralis K, Nanni G, Bonanzinga T, Zaffagnini S. Arthroscopic meniscus allograft transplantation in male professional soccer players: a 36-month follow-up study. Am J Sports Med. 2013;42:382–8.
110. Chalmers PN, Karas V, Sherman SL, Cole BJ. Return to high-level sport after meniscal allograft transplantation. Arthroscopy. 2013;29:539–44.
111. Alentorn-Geli E, Vazquez RS, Diaz PA, Cusco X, Cugat R. Arthroscopic meniscal transplants in soccer players: outcomes at 2- to 5-year follow-up. Clin J Sport Med. 2010;20:340–3.
112. Eberbach H, Zwingmann J, Hohloch L, Bode G, Maier D, Niemeyer P, Südkamp NP, Feucht MJ. Sport-specific outcomes after isolated meniscal repair: a systematic review. Knee Surg Sport Traumatol Arthrosc. 2018;26:762–71.
113. Ueblacker P, Mueller-Wohlfahrt H-W. Return to play in muscle injuries. In: Musahl V, Karlsson J, Krutsch W, Mandelbaum BR, Espregueira-Mendes J, D'Hooghe P, editors. Return to play football. An evidence-based approach. Berlin: Springer; 2018. p. 441–52.
114. Hallén A, Ekstrand J. Return to play following muscle injuries in professional footballers. J Sports Sci. 2014;32:1229–36.
115. Ueblacker P, Müller-Wohlfahrt H-W, Ekstrand J. Epidemiological and clinical outcome comparison of indirect ('strain') versus direct ('contusion') anterior and posterior thigh muscle injuries in male elite football players: UEFA Elite League study of 2287 thigh injuries (2001–2013). Br J Sports Med. 2015;49:1461–5.
116. Ekstrand J, Lee JC, Healy JC. MRI findings and return to play in football: a prospective analysis of 255 hamstring injuries in the UEFA Elite Club Injury Study. Br J Sports Med. 2016;50:738–43.
117. Werner J, Hägglund M, Ekstrand J, Waldén M. Hip and groin time-loss injuries decreased slightly but injury burden remained constant in men's professional football: the 15-year prospective UEFA Elite Club Injury Study. Br J Sports Med. 2018.
118. Pulici L, Zanini B, Carrai L, Menon A, Compagnoni R, Randelli P. Return to play after rotator cuff surgery. In: Musahl V, Karlsson J, Krutsch W, Mandelbaum BR, Espregueira-Mendes J, D'Hooghe P, editors. Return to play football. An evidence-based approach. Berlin: Springer; 2018. p. 313–20.
119. Klouche S, Lefevre N, Herman S, Gerometta A, Bohu Y. Return to sport after rotator cuff tear repair: a systematic review and meta-analysis. Am J Sports Med. 2016;44:1877–87.
120. Elsenbeck MJ, Dickens JF. Return to sports after shoulder stabilization surgery for anterior shoulder instability. Curr Rev Musculoskelet Med. 2017;10:491–8.
121. Horner NS, Ekhtiari S, Chan AA, Choudur HN, Ayeni OR. Joint specific return to play recommendations: "return to play in non-operative hip/groin pain". In: Musahl V, Karlsson J, Krutsch W, Mandelbaum BR, Espregueira-Mendes J, D'Hooghe P, editors. Return to play football. An evidence-based approach. Berlin: Springer; 2018. p. 331–46.
122. Dickens JF, Rue J-P, Cameron KL, Tokish JM, Peck KY, Allred CD, Svoboda SJ, Sullivan R, Kilcoyne KG, Owens BD. Successful return to sport after arthroscopic shoulder stabilization versus nonoperative management in contact athletes with anterior shoulder instability: a prospective multicenter study. Am J Sports Med. 2017;45:2540–6.
123. Loeffen FGJ, Shimozono Y, Kerkhoffs GMMJ, Kennedy JG. Return to play after ankle injuries. In: Musahl V, Karlsson J, Krutsch W, Mandelbaum BR, Espregueira-Mendes J, D'Hooghe P, editors. Return to play football. An evidence-based approach. Berlin: Springer; 2018. p. 365–86.
124. van den Bekerom MPJ, Kerkhoffs GMMJ, McCollum GA, Calder JDF, van Dijk CN. Management of acute lateral ankle ligament injury in the athlete. Knee Surg Sports Traumatol Arthrosc. 2013;21:1390–5.
125. Waldén M, Hägglund M, Ekstrand J. Time-trends and circumstances surrounding ankle injuries in men's professional football: an 11-year follow-up of the UEFA Champions League injury study. Br J Sports Med. 2013;47:748 LP–753.
126. Hunt KJ, Fuld RS, Sutphin BS, Pereira H, D'Hooghe P. Return to sport following lateral ankle ligament repair is under-reported: a systematic review. J ISAKOS Jt Disord Orthop Sport Med. 2017;2:234–40.

127. Pearce CJ, Tourne Y, Zellers J, Terrier R, Toschi P, Silbernagel KG. Rehabilitation after anatomical ankle ligament repair or reconstruction. Knee Surg Sports Traumatol Arthrosc. 2016;24:1130–9.
128. Laidlaw M, Diduch D. Current concepts in the management of patellar instability. Indian J Orthop. 2017;51:493–504.
129. Magnussen RA, Schmitt LC, Arendt EA. Return to soccer following acute patellar dislocation. In: Musahl V, Karlsson J, Krutsch W, Mandelbaum BR, Espregueira-Mendes J, D'Hooghe P, editors. Return to play football. An evidence-based approach. Berlin: Springer; 2018. p. 649–60.
130. Magnussen RA, Verlage M, Stock E, Zurek L, Flanigan DC, Tompkins M, Agel J, Arendt EA. Primary patellar dislocations without surgical stabilization or recurrence: how well are these patients really doing? Knee Surg Sport Traumatol Arthrosc. 2017;25:2352–6.
131. Atkin DM, Fithian DC, Marangi KS, Stone ML, Dobson BE, Mendelsohn C. Characteristics of patients with primary acute lateral patellar dislocation and their recovery within the first 6 months of injury. Am J Sports Med. 2000;28:472–9.
132. Sherman SL, Deasis DP, Garrone AJ, Voss EE, Oliver HA. Return to play after patellar stabilization. Curr Rev Musculoskelet Med. 2018;11:280–4.

Part II

Overtraining Injuries

Treatment of Achilles Tendinopathies

13

Jon Karlsson, Annelie Brorsson, Unnur Jónsdóttir,
and Karin Grävare Silbernagel

13.1 Achilles Tendinopathy

The ***overuse type*** of injury to the Achilles tendon is a painful type of injury that occurs when the body's reparative capability is exceeded by repetitive microtrauma [1, 2]. The injury can be in an acute or chronic phase. The exact time criteria that are used to classify the injury as acute or chronic are arbitrary. In the literature, definitions for the injury to be chronic range from 4 weeks to 3 months or pain on and off for more than 6 months [3–6]. The injury can be divided into distal Achilles tendinopathy and midportion Achilles tendinopathy depending on the location of the pain (Fig. 13.1).

Achilles tendinopathy is particularly common in recreational athletes, and the annual incidence in runners is between 7 and 9% [7, 8]. However, Achilles tendinopathy may also occur in individuals that are not physically active [9]. Risk factors may be intrinsic or extrinsic. Examples of intrinsic risk factors are abnormal tendon structure, high BMI,

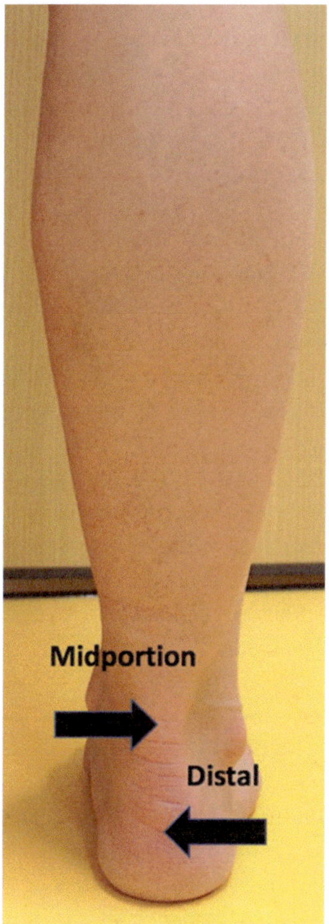

Fig. 13.1 Location of the pain for midportion and distal Achilles tendinopathy

J. Karlsson (✉) · A. Brorsson · U. Jónsdóttir
Department of Orthopaedics, Institute of Clinical Sciences at Sahlgrenska Academy, Gothenburg University, Gothenburg, Sweden
e-mail: jon.karlsson@telia.com

K. G. Silbernagel
Department of Physical Therapy, University of Delaware, Newark, DE, USA

S. Rocha Piedade et al. (eds.), *The Sports Medicine Physician*,
https://doi.org/10.1007/978-3-030-10433-7_13

decreased ankle plantar flexion strength, or increased foot pronation, while repetitive overuse injuries and inappropriate equipment are extrinsic risk factors [10–12]. In 163 patients with Achilles tendinopathy, surgical and histopathological findings showed that 90% had degenerative changes, the so-called tendinosis [13]. On the other hand, degenerative changes were also found in 20% of non-symptomatic tendons. Another finding showed that 19% of the patients had partial ruptures that always occurred in the tendinosis area. There was also a lack of inflammatory cells and poor healing response in the biopsies.

The degenerative changes in the tendon can be divided into several subcategories such as hypoxic, mucoid, hyaline, lipoid, fibrinoid, calcific, or a combination of these [14, 15]. The degenerative changes can be the result of a variety of causes such as aging, microtrauma, vascular compromise, or other reasons, and they may vary from tendon to tendon [14]. The histopathological findings of tendinosis are collagen disorientation, disorganization, and fiber separation. Tendinosis might also occur together with the involvement of the paratenon. This can present itself as crepitation due to adhesions between the tendon and the paratenon. In addition to degenerative changes in the tendon, it has recently been suggested that sensitization of the central nervous system may play a part in the pain presented in patients with Achilles tendinopathy [16, 17].

13.2 Diagnosis

Achilles tendinopathy is a clinical diagnosis for the clinical syndrome, characterized by a combination of pain, swelling (diffuse or localized), and impaired performance of the Achilles tendon. Pain on palpation of the tendon (sensitivity 84%) and the subjective reporting of pain 2–6 cm above the insertion into the calcaneus (sensitivity 78%) has also been found to be reliable and valid tests for diagnosing Achilles tendinopathy in the midportion of the tendon when compared to ultrasound scanning [18]. Clinically, a distinction between midportion (2–6 cm proximal to tendon insertion) and distal (insertion to the calcaneus) Achilles tendinopathy can be made on the basis of the location of the pain. The typical symptoms of Achilles tendinopathy are pain during and after physical activity, tenderness on palpation, and morning stiffness [19–21]. With increased severity, patients may also have pain during daily functional activities [20, 21].

13.2.1 Midportion Achilles Tendinopathy

Midportion Achilles tendinopathy is reported to account for 55–65% of all the Achilles tendon injuries [22–25]. Patients usually describe a gradual onset of pain. Many patients have had pain for many months or on and off for many years. Initially, the symptoms occur after heavy physical activity, but as the injury progresses, some patients develop pain during physical activity. Patients may also have pain with daily activities, such as walking. Morning stiffness and/or stiffness after sitting for longer periods of time are also common. Correlation between pain level, morning stiffness, and severity of disease is reported in the literature [20, 21, 26, 27]. Clinically, the patients report pain on palpation in the middle part of the tendon (2–6 cm proximal to the tendon insertion), and sometimes there is a palpable thickening in the same area, usually in the more chronic stages. With these findings together with the arc sign [28] and Royal London Hospital [28] test (Fig. 13.2), it is possible to diagnose midportion Achilles tendinopathy [29]. Noticeable crepitation can be indicative of adhesions of the paratenon and paratendinopathy in more acute stages. A thorough physical examination is important in order to rule out any other causes of the pain. Examples of differential diagnosis are involvement of the plantaris tendon [30], acute Achilles tendon rupture or partial tear of the Achilles tendon [31, 32], os trigonum syndrome [33], accessory soleus muscle [34], and irritation or neuroma of the sural nerve [31].

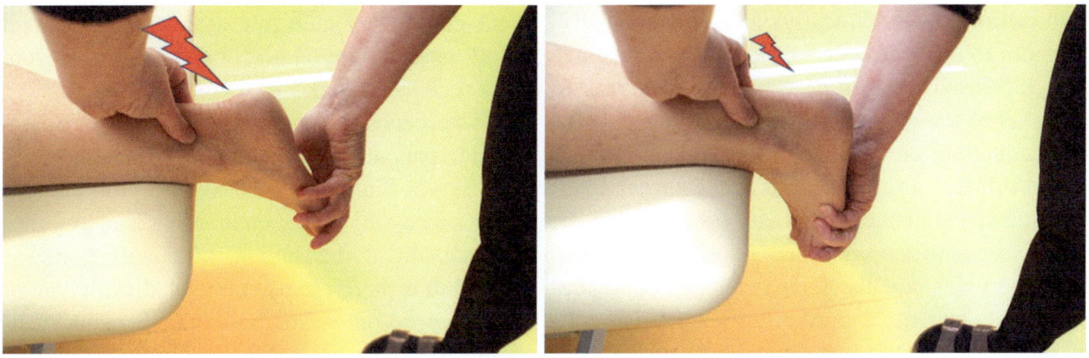

Fig. 13.2 Royal London Hospital test

13.2.2 Distal Achilles Tendinopathy

Approximately 20–25% of all Achilles tendon injuries are reported to be distal. This condition is also called insertional Achilles tendinopathy [35]. In a study of patients with Achilles tendon injury during the years 1976–1986, 23% had pain distally, and, of these, 61% were diagnosed with insertion tendinitis, 21% with retrocalcaneal bursitis, and 18% with both [25]. These patients report the same complaints as in midportion injury and/or pain related to the type of shoe/athletic wear. In this case the pain can occur due to external compression on the tendon insertion. Swelling around the Achilles tendon insertion to the calcaneus, with redness and warmth, could also be present and might be related to active bursitis. The patients sometimes also report pain after having run uphill, standing on a ladder, or walking barefoot on sand. Clinically, there is pain when the tendon insertion is palpated. This type of injury can also be caused by compression injury of the tendon and the bursa onto the calcaneus, the so-called posterior impingement. A prominent superior projection of the calcaneus, i.e., Haglund's deformity, can be the cause of the posterior impingement. Magnetic resonance imaging (MRI) as well as ultrasound imaging can be used for examination both of soft tissue and bony changes [36] even if 0–19% of the patients with symptomatic Achilles tendinopathy present normal appearance when examined with MRI or ultrasound imaging [37].

13.3 Treatment

In the literature various types of treatments such as ultrasound, deep friction massage, anti-inflammatory medication, surgery, injection therapies, extracorporeal shock wave therapy, photobiomodulation (laser) therapy, and exercise are described to be used as treatments for Achilles tendinopathy [29]. Systematic reviews indicate that exercise, especially eccentric exercise, has the most evidence of effectiveness but has been less successful in the patients with insertional Achilles tendinopathy compared to those with midportion injury [38, 39]. Today the consensus is that Achilles tendinopathy should initially be treated with exercise for at least 3–6 months. Even with other types of treatments, some type of exercise is recommended.

13.3.1 Therapeutic Exercise

The basis of exercise as treatment for Achilles tendinopathy is to address possible impairments and deficiencies in strength, range of motion, balance, proprioception, and function and to promote healing of the tendon. Since the tendon is subjected to the highest loads eccentrically, eccentric training has always been an important part of the prescribed exercise. However, it has been questioned if there is a need for an eccentric-only exercise protocol since it can be difficult to isolate eccentric contractions from concentric and there is little evidence that isolated eccentric contractions are clinically and mechanically superior to concentric-eccentric contractions [40, 41]. Increased speed of movement also increases the load of the tendon during the eccentric muscle activation, and, to increase the load on the tendon during exercise, both the external load and the speed of movement can be increased. It has also been found that heavy-load slow-speed exercise gives equally good results as eccentric training in patients with Achilles tendinopathy. It is important to note that for patients with distal Achilles tendinopathy, it is recommended to perform the heel-rises on a plain surface and avoid excessive dorsiflexion during exercise [42].

13.3.1.1 Current Rehabilitation Protocols

There are currently three exercise programs that have been used in various studies evaluating treatment in patients with Achilles tendinopathy. One of the protocols, the so-called eccentric-only protocol [43], uses eccentric loading only, whereas another protocol, the so-called comprehensive treatment protocol [44], includes both concentric and eccentric strengthening. These two protocols have been shown to have good short-term results in patients with midportion tendinopathy. When evaluating the long-term outcome of the protocols, it was found that with the eccentric-only protocol, 38% of the patients were completely pain-free at 5 years and, with the comprehensive treatment protocol, 80% were fully recovered after 5 years [45, 46].

The eccentric-only protocol has also been evaluated in patients with distal Achilles tendinopathy [42]. It was found that this exercise program was more successful in patients with distal Achilles tendinopathy if the amount of dorsiflexion was limited. It is therefore recommended, with both of the eccentric-only and the comprehensive treatment protocols, that patients with distal Achilles tendinopathy should be standing flat on the ground instead of standing at the edge of a step.

The third exercise protocol is the heavy slow resistance protocol [47]. This protocol showed superior patient satisfaction after 3 months compared to the eccentric-only protocol [43] but equally good results after 1 year.

13.3.1.2 Eccentric-Only Exercise Protocol

Alfredson et al. [43] published in 1998 a nonrandomized study using a protocol with only eccentric heel-rises with both the knee straight and the knee bent. The patients are instructed to use the uninjured side to get up on the toes and then place the weight on the injured side and then lower the heel all the way down (Fig. 13.3). The patient performs 3 sets of 15 repetitions of the 2 exercises, twice a day for a total of 12 weeks.

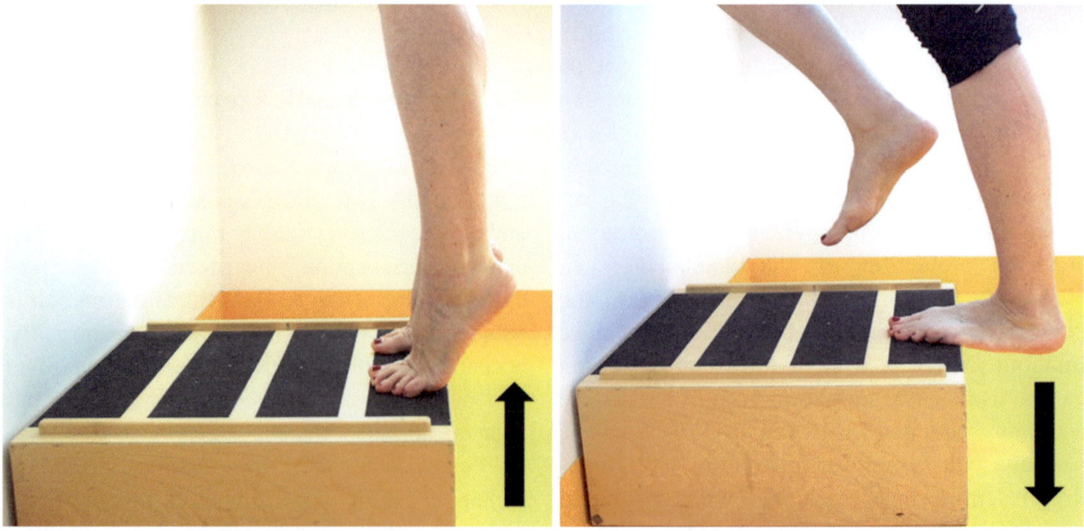

Fig. 13.3 Eccentric heel-rise

The treatment program is also supposed to be painful, and if the exercises could be performed without experiencing any minor pain or discomfort, the patients were instructed to increase the load by wearing a backpack with added weights.

13.3.1.3 A Comprehensive Treatment Protocol

This protocol includes both concentric and eccentric exercises of the calf muscles together with a pain-monitoring model and a training log [44]. The reason for this is that both concentric and eccentric activations are included in all physical activities and it has been shown that patients with Achilles tendinopathy have both concentric and eccentric strength deficits [48]. The program consists of single- (Fig. 13.4) and double-legged standing heel-rises (Fig. 13.5), seated heel-rises, eccentric heel-rises, and quick rebounding heel-rises.

There are four different phases of the program with gradually increasing strength

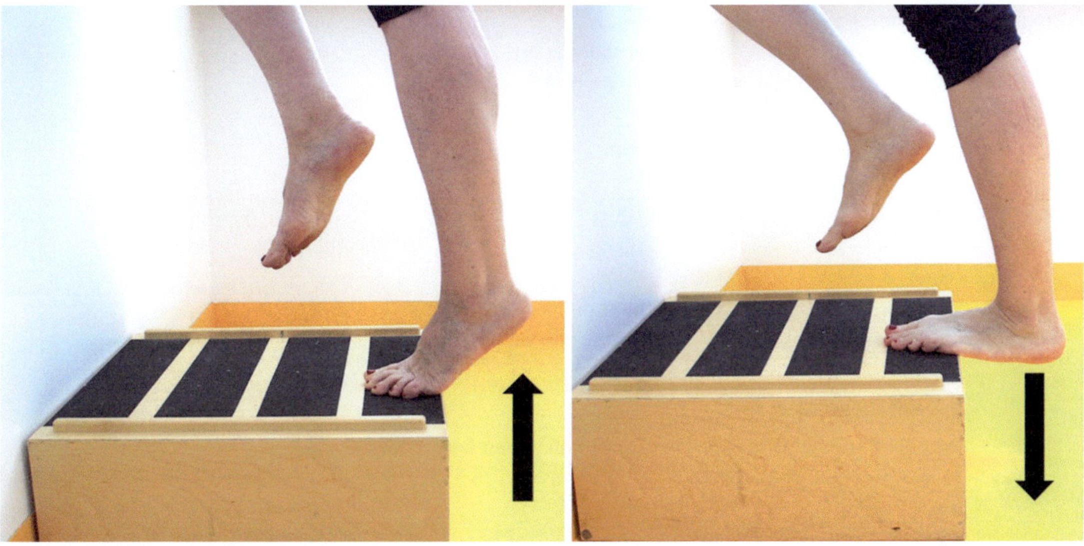

Fig. 13.4 Single-legged standing heel-rise

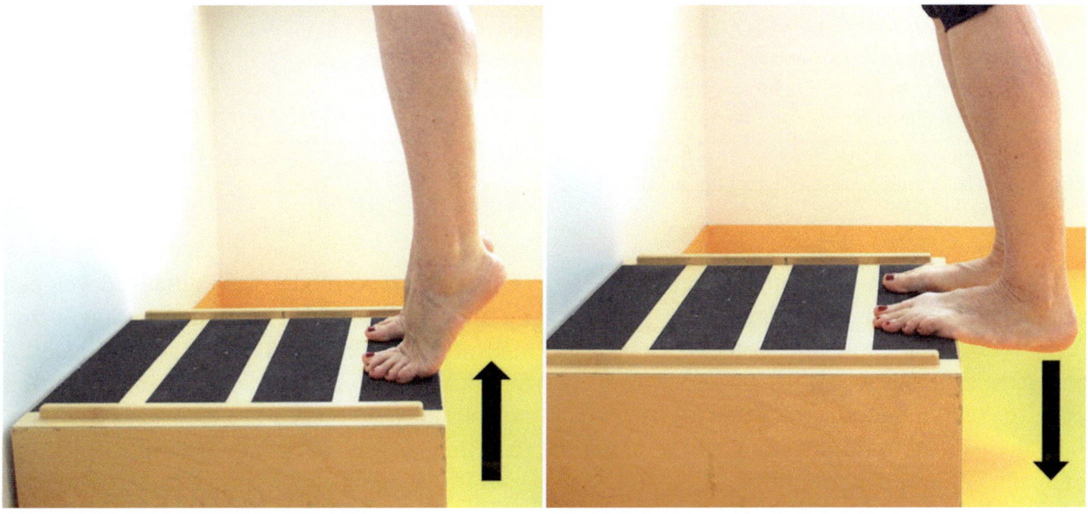

Fig. 13.5 Double-legged standing heel-rise

Phase 1: Week 1-2

Patient status: Pain and difficulty with all activities, difficulty performing 10 single-leg heel-rises

Goal: Start to exercise, understanding nature of their injury and of ***pain monitoring model***

Treatment program: Perform exercises every day

- Pain monitoring model information and advice on exercise activity
- Circulation exercises (foot up/down)
- Double-leg heel-rises standing on the floor (3x10-15)
- Single-leg heel-rises standing on the floor (3x10)
- Sitting heel-rises (3x10)
- Eccentric heel-rises standing on the floor (3x10)

Phase 2: Week 2-5 *(If pain distally continue standing on the floor)*

Patient status: Pain with exercise, morning stiffness, pain when performing heel-rises

Goal: Start strengthening

Treatment program: Perform exercises every day

- Double-leg heel-rises standing on edge of stair (3x15)
- Single-leg heel-rises standing on edge of stair (3x15)
- Sitting heel-rises (3x15)
- Eccentric heel-rises standing on edge of stair (3x15)
- Quick rebounding heel-rises 3x20

Phase 3: Week 3-12 (or longer if needed) *(If pain distally continue standing on the floor)*

Patient status: Handle the phase 2 exercise program, no pain distally in tendon insertion, possibly decreased or increased morning stiffness

Goal: Heavier strength training, increase or start running and/or jumping activity

Treatment program: Perform exercises every day and with heavier load 2-3 times per week

- Single-leg heel-rises standing on edge of stair with added weight (3x15)
- Sitting heel-rises (3x15)
- Eccentric heel-rises standing on edge of stair with added weight (3x15)
- Quick rebounding heel-rises (3x20)
- Plyometrics training

Phase 4: *3-6 months (or longer if needed)* *(If pain distally continue standing on the floor)*

Patient status: Minimal symptoms, not morning stiffness every day, can participate in sports without difficulty

Goal: Maintenance exercise, No symptoms

Treatment program: Perform exercises 2-3 times per week

- Single-leg heel-rises standing on edge of stair with added weight (3x15)
- Eccentric heel-rises standing on edge of stair with added weight (3x15)
- Quick rebounding heel-rises (3x20)

Fig. 13.6 The comprehensive treatment protocol

demands, and what phase the patient is in is dependent on their symptoms and function (Fig. 13.6). This treatment protocol allows the patient to experience pain during and after exercise. The pain-monitoring model is used to facilitate the patients' understanding of the amount of pain allowed during and after exercise (Fig. 13.7). The model was initially developed by Thomeé [49] and presented in a randomized controlled trial in 1997 for patients with patellofemoral pain syndrome. The pain-monitoring model and training log are tools that also help the clinician and patient to determine how the exercise program should progress and also how much is the optimal amount of exercise overall. The exercise program, complemented with the pain-monitoring model, has been evaluated in two randomized controlled trials and led to significant improvements in patients with midportion Achilles tendinopathy [44, 50].

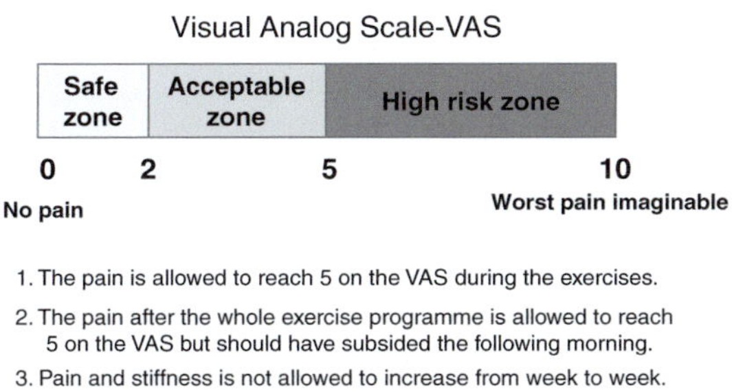

Fig. 13.7 The pain-monitoring model

13.3.1.4 Heavy Slow Resistance Protocol

Beyer et al. [47] presented in 2015 a heavy-load slow-speed protocol for patients with midportion Achilles tendinopathy. The program consists of three bilateral heel-rises in full range of motion: (1) seated with the knees in 90° in a calf muscle weight-training machine, (2) standing with extended knees with a barbell on shoulders, and (3) a leg press machine with extended knees (Fig. 13.8). Every repetition was performed at a speed of 6 s. The program went on for 12 weeks, and during this time the weight was progressively

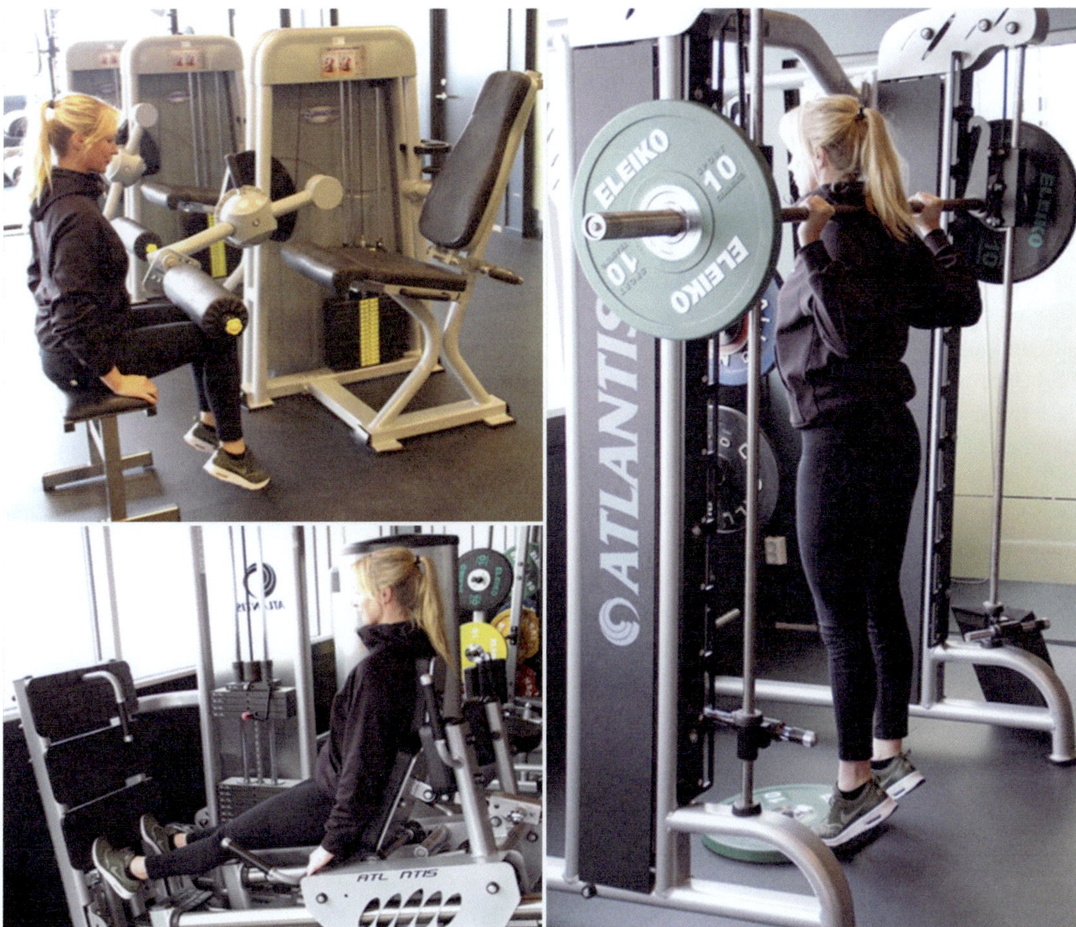

Fig. 13.8 The heavy slow resistance protocol

increased, while the numbers of repetitions successively decreased. This study was a prospective randomized single-blind controlled trial, and the patients were randomized to either the heavy slow resistance protocol or the eccentric-only exercise protocol. The heavy slow resistance protocol showed superior patient satisfaction after 3 months compared to the eccentric-only protocol but equally good results after 1 year [47].

13.3.1.5 Stretching

Stretching of the ankle plantar flexors may be used to reduce pain in patients with midportion Achilles tendinopathy if the patient experience limited ankle dorsiflexion [51]. The stretching can be performed both with the knee extended and flexed.

13.3.1.6 Neuromuscular Reeducation

It has been found that runners with Achilles tendinopathy present decreased muscle activity in the lower extremity compared to a control group [52]. Chang and Kulig [53] have also presented evidence for if tendinotic changes are present within the Achilles tendon, this may lead to adaptations in motor control within the central nervous system. However, it can be discussed if decreased muscle activation is a cause or a result in patients with midportion Achilles tendinopathy. Clinicians can be recommended to use neuromuscular exercises for lower leg with the aim to avoid an atypical biomechanical movement pattern.

13.3.1.7 Manual Therapy

There is some evidence that soft tissue mobilization can be used to improve mobility and function [54], but no studies have investigated soft tissue mobilization particularly for patients with Achilles tendinopathy.

13.3.2 Orthotics

It has been suggested that biomechanical malalignments are risk factors for Achilles tendinopathy. Corrective orthotics is therefore often prescribed for patients with Achilles tendinopathy. No difference has been found between patients who had customized orthosis compared to sham orthoses [55], and systematic reviews have not been able to prove that orthotics for patients with Achilles tendinopathy is beneficial [39, 56]. Clinically, some patients report no effects with orthotics, whereas others report significant improvements with its use. Until there is research showing that corrective orthotics is effective in relieving symptoms, its use should be based on clinical judgment.

13.3.3 Taping

There is limited evidence that taping can reduce pain, but rigid taping can be used to alter foot posture or reduce strain on the Achilles tendon [56, 57].

13.3.4 Nonsteroidal Anti-Inflammatory Drugs (NSAIDs)

Since Achilles tendinopathy is mainly a non-inflammatory condition, apart from a possible short initial inflammatory phase, the use of NSAIDs will have no major therapeutic effect [13, 58, 59]. NSAIDs might, however, have an analgesic effect for the patient. Åström and Westlin [60] found no beneficial effect from NSAIDs in patients with Achilles tendinopathy. In a review of the literature, the investigators report insufficient evidence for determining the efficacy of NSAIDs in chronic tendon injury [61].

13.3.5 Injections

A systematic review investigating platelet-rich plasma (PRP) injections, autologous blood injections, sclerosing polidocanol injections, and corticosteroid injections could not find any evidence that injections of any kind alone could be favorable for patients with Achilles tendinopathy even if there could be some benefits used together with physical therapy [62]. Total and partial ruptures in the Achilles tendon have been reported as a complication after injections with corticosteroids and polidocanol [63, 64].

13.3.5.1 Platelet-Rich Plasma Injection

The use of platelet-rich plasma injections has mainly been investigated in midportion Achilles tendinopathy. There are some evidences that this type of injection may have benefits together with eccentric training [65] even if recent meta-analyses have not been able to confirm these findings [66, 67].

13.3.5.2 High-Volume Image-Guided Injection

High-volume image-guided injection (HVIGI) is a technique where ultrasound image is used to guide the needle with the aim to reach the area between the anterior aspect of the Achilles tendon and Kager's fat pad. It is believed that this area has the maximal neovascularization around the Achilles tendon. The injection consists of saline and local anesthetic with or without added corticosteroids [68].

In a randomized double-blinded prospective study, Boesen et al. [65] found that high-volume injection together with eccentric training had superior effect on chronic midportion Achilles tendinopathy than eccentric training alone. The effect has been confirmed in other studies [68–70], but there is, at this time point, a lack of high-level evidence in this field.

13.3.5.3 Sclerotherapy

Sclerotherapy means injections with the substance polidocanol in the neovascularization zone in a pathological Achilles tendon. Early studies showed excellent results [71], but more recent studies and systematic reviews have not been able to confirm these results [64, 72].

13.3.5.4 Corticosteroids

Corticosteriods are commonly used for their anti-inflammatory effect. In a review of the use of corticosteroids in chronic tendon injuries, it was found that they might provide some initial pain relief but that their beneficial effect on the outcome remained uncertain [61]. One systematic review reported that corticosteriod injections for tendinopathy may show positive short-term results, but this treatment was found to be worse than other options in the intermediate and long terms [73]. A recent study has shown more positive results [74]. The effects might also vary depending on the site for tendinopathy, and due to the heavy load on the Achilles tendon and the potential increased risk for Achilles tendon rupture, it is not recommended as an option.

13.3.6 Extracorporeal Shock Wave Therapy

Extracorporeal shock wave therapy (ESWT) is used for pain relief and to promote tendon healing; however, the underlying mechanism is not clear (Fig. 13.9). The published trials for the use of ESWT in tendinopathy also vary in intensity, frequency, and duration [75–79]. A systematic review including 11 trails concluded that for patients with distal Achilles tendinopathy, ESWT was superior to eccentric loading in the short term, while for patients with midportion Achilles tendinopathy, a combination with ESWT and eccentric loading was the best choice [80]. The general recommendation is that it might be beneficial to use ESWT in conjunction with optimal therapeutic exercise and patients with distal Achilles tendinopathy might benefit more than patients with midportion injury. However, the optimal dosage is still unclear [29].

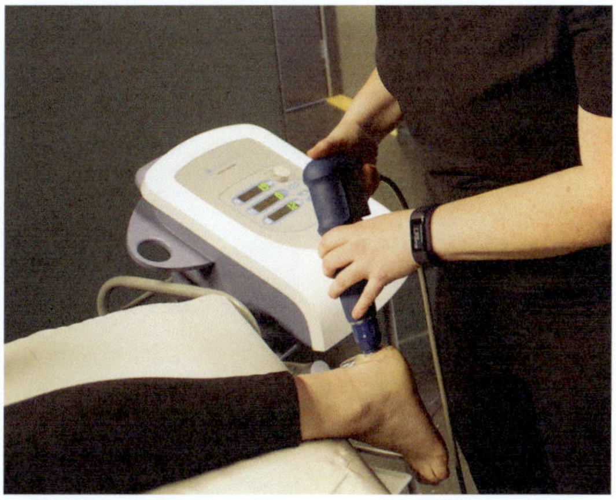

Fig. 13.9 Treatment with extracorporeal shock wave therapy (ESWT)

13.3.7 Laser

The photobiostimulation that occurs when treating the tissue with laser has been reported to reduce inflammation [81] and have positive effects on angiogenesis [82] and collagen synthesis [83]. Controversy exists over dosage recommendations, and consensus does not exist of the most efficacious dose [84]. A systematic review evaluating the effect of low-level laser therapy (LLLT) on tendinopathy indicated favorable outcome with this treatment, but the results vary between different studies [84]. However, none of the studies has evaluated the effect of LLLT on patients with the distal-type injury. More recent studies have showed conflicting results; Hutchison et al. [85] found no difference between LLLT and placebo laser, while Tumilty et al. [86] concluded that LLLT together with exercise could be as beneficial compared to exercise together with placebo laser. Because of this conflicting results, a recent published guideline cannot recommend LLLT for patients with Achilles tendinopathy [29].

13.3.8 Therapeutic Ultrasound

In animal studies therapeutic ultrasound has been found to enhance tendon healing [87], but few clinical studies show positive results. For Achilles tendinopathy therapeutic ultrasound has been shown to be inferior to eccentric exercise [88]. Systematic reviews and meta-analyses have failed to show that active ultrasound is more effective than placebo [89].

13.3.9 Surgery

There appears to be consensus in the literature that surgery should only be performed after patients have been treated unsuccessfully with a treatment protocol involving exercise for a minimum of 6 months [20, 21, 58, 90]. The surgical techniques vary but usually include removing abnormal tendon tissue and releasing adhesion and scarring [20, 21, 90]. In patients with distal Achilles tendinopathy, the surgical methods often include removal of the calcaneal prominence, the retrocalcaneal bursa, and, if present, calcifications together with pathological parts of the Achilles tendon [37] (Fig. 13.10). It is not clear why surgery sometimes helps and the postoperative rehabilitation may be as important as the actual surgery [58]. The success rates for surgery vary between 70 and 90% in different studies [21, 91, 92], and the mean success rate (according to Coleman et al. [93]) for surgery performed in

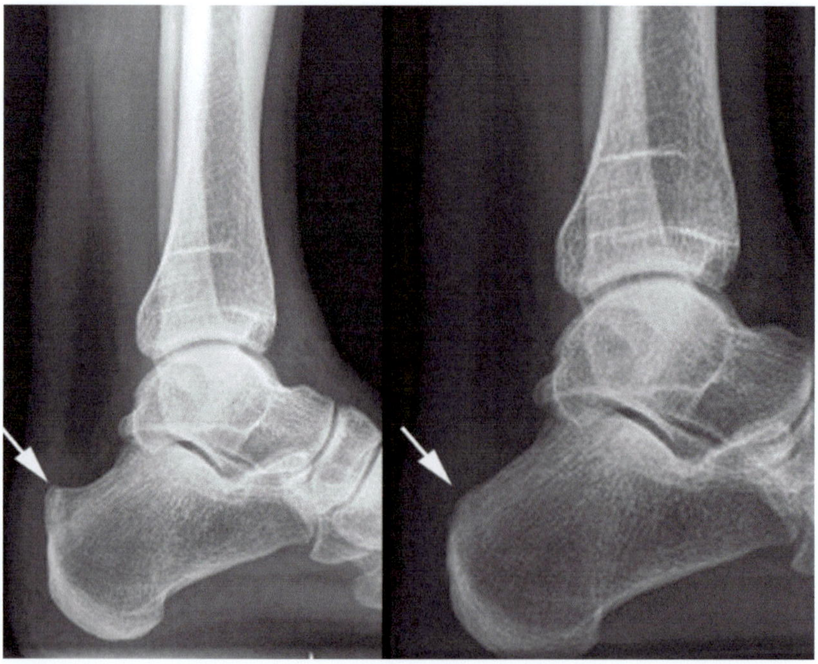

Fig. 13.10 Before and after removal of the calcaneal prominence

midportion Achilles tendinopathy is recently reported to be 83.4% [91]. Complications after surgery also need to be considered, and, in a systematic review included 20 studies with 714 patients and 801 tendons altogether, the complication rate was reported to be 6.3% [91]. With improvements in nonsurgical treatment, there will, however, be fewer requests for surgery.

13.3.10 Nitric Oxide

Nitric oxide (NO) is a small free radical generated by a family of enzymes, the nitric oxide synthase (NOSs). In the animal model, tendon healing was found to be enhanced when additional NO was added [94]. Clinical trials have reported that treatment with NO delivered via a transdermal patch enhances the subjective and objective recovery in patients with tendinopathy [95, 96]. It is important to note however that the results have not been found to be superior to exercise and side effects such as severe headaches are reported with this treatment.

13.3.11 Wait-And-See

It has been shown that a 4-month wait-and-see strategy was ineffective compare to eccentric training and low-energy shock wave therapy (SWT) when treating patients with midportion Achilles tendinopathy [75].

13.4 Conclusion

The treatment with the highest level of evidence is rehabilitation exercises. To experience a favorable outcome from the exercise program, the exercises need to be individualized and are allowed to cause pain. The use of a pain-monitoring model together with a training log helps the patient and the clinician to balance between overload and loading enough to achieve a positive response to the exercises. The exercise program needs to continue for at least 12 weeks, but more often it needs to be continued for up to a year. It might also be beneficial to combine the exercise treatment with other treatments, such as shock wave therapy, laser therapy, and the use of orthotics. Surgery is to be considered as the last option, and when performed, there is a need for the patient to complete an individualized rehabilitation program designed for gradually loading. Patients with insertional Achilles tendinopathy are more likely to need surgery compared to patients with midportion Achilles tendinopathy.

References

1. Leadbetter WB. Cell-matrix response in tendon injury. Clin Sports Med. 1992;11:533–78.
2. Magnan B, Bondi M, Pierantoni S, Samaila E. The pathogenesis of Achilles tendinopathy: a systematic review. Foot Ankle Surg. 2014;20:154–9.
3. el Hawary R, Stanish WD, Curwin SL. Rehabilitation of tendon injuries in sport. Sports Med. 1997;24:347–58.
4. Angermann P, Hovgaard D. Chronic Achilles tendinopathy in athletic individuals: results of nonsurgical treatment. Foot Ankle Int. 1999;20:304–6.
5. Mafi N, Lorentzon R, Alfredson H. Superior short-term results with eccentric calf muscle training compared to concentric training in a randomized prospective multicenter study on patients with chronic Achilles tendinosis. Knee Surg Sports Traumatol Arthrosc. 2001;9:42–7.
6. Roos EM, Engström M, Lagerquist A, Söderberg B. Clinical improvement after 6 weeks of eccentric exercise in patients with mid-portion Achilles tendinopathy—a randomized trial with 1-year follow-up. Scand J Med Sci Sports. 2004;14:286–95.
7. Kujala UM, Sarna S, Kaprio J. Cumulative incidence of Achilles tendon rupture and tendinopathy in male former elite athletes. Clin J Sport Med. 2005;15:133–5.
8. Nielsen RO, Ronnow L, Rasmussen S, Lind M. A prospective study on time to recovery in 254 injured novice runners. PLoS One. 2014;9:e99877.
9. Holmes GB, Lin J. Etiologic factors associated with symptomatic Achilles tendinopathy. Foot Ankle Int. 2006;27:952–9.
10. Dowling GJ, Murley GS, Munteanu SE, et al. Dynamic foot function as a risk factor for lower limb overuse injury: a systematic review. J Foot Ankle Res. 2014;7:53.
11. Jhingan S, Perry M, O'Driscoll G, et al. Thicker Achilles tendons are a risk factor to develop Achilles tendinopathy in elite professional soccer players. Musc Ligam Tendons J. 2011;1:51–6.
12. Klein EE, Weil L Jr, Weil LS Sr, Fleischer AE. Body mass index and Achilles tendonitis: a 10-year retrospective analysis. Foot Ankle Spec. 2013;6:276–82.
13. Astrom M, Rausing A. Chronic Achilles tendinopathy. A survey of surgical and histopathologic findings. Clin Orthop Relat Res. 1995:151–64.

14. Józsa L, Kannus P. Human tendons. Anatomy, physiology and pathology. Champaign, IL: Human Kinetics; 1997. p. ix, 574 p.
15. Maffulli N, Wong J, Almekinders LC. Types and epidemiology of tendinopathy. Clin Sports Med. 2003;22:675–92.
16. Heales LJ, Lim EC, Hodges PW, Vicenzino B. Sensory and motor deficits exist on the non-injured side of patients with unilateral tendon pain and disability—implications for central nervous system involvement: a systematic review with meta-analysis. Br J Sports Med. 2014;48:1400–6.
17. Tompra N, van Dieen JH, Coppieters MW. Central pain processing is altered in people with Achilles tendinopathy. Br J Sports Med. 2016;50:1004–7.
18. Hutchison AM, Evans R, Bodger O, et al. What is the best clinical test for Achilles tendinopathy? Foot Ankle Surg. 2013;19:112–7.
19. Alfredson H. Chronic midportion Achilles tendinopathy: an update on research and treatment. Clin Sports Med. 2003;22:727–41.
20. Kader D, Saxena A, Movin T, Maffulli N. Achilles tendinopathy: some aspects of basic science and clinical management. Br J Sports Med. 2002;36:239–49.
21. Paavola M, Kannus P, Järvinen TA, Khan K, Jozsa L, Järvinen M. Achilles tendinopathy. J Bone Joint Surg Am. 2002;84-A:2062–76.
22. Järvinen M. Epidemiology of tendon injuries in sports. Clin Sports Med. 1992;11:493–504.
23. Jarvinen TA, Kannus P, Maffulli N, Khan KM. Achilles tendon disorders: etiology and epidemiology. Foot Ankle Clin. 2005;10:255–66.
24. Kvist M. Achilles tendon injuries in athletes. Sports Med. 1994;18:173–201.
25. Kvist M. Achilles tendon injuries in athletes. Ann Chir Gynaecol. 1991;80:188–201.
26. Vora AM, Myerson MS, Oliva F, Maffulli N. Tendinopathy of the main body of the Achilles tendon. Foot Ankle Clin. 2005;10:293–308.
27. Sandmeier R, Renström PA. Diagnosis and treatment of chronic tendon disorders in sports. Scand J Med Sci Sports. 1997;7:96–106.
28. Maffulli N, Kenward MG, Testa V, Capasso G, Regine R, King JB. Clinical diagnosis of Achilles tendinopathy with tendinosis. Clin J Sport Med. 2003;13:11–5.
29. Pain A. Stiffness, and muscle power deficits: midportion Achilles tendinopathy revision 2018: using the evidence to guide physical therapist practice. J Orthop Sports Phys Ther. 2018;48:425–6.
30. Pollock N, Dijkstra P, Calder J, Chakraverty R. Plantaris injuries in elite UK track and field athletes over a 4-year period: a retrospective cohort study. Knee Surg Sports Traumatol Arthrosc. 2016;24:2287–92.
31. Alfredson H, Cook J. A treatment algorithm for managing Achilles tendinopathy: new treatment options. Br J Sports Med. 2007;41:211–6.
32. Chan O, Morton S, Pritchard M, et al. Intratendinous tears of the Achilles tendon—a new pathology? Analysis of a large 4-year cohort. Musc Ligam Tendons J. 2017;7:53–61.
33. Tu P, Bytomski JR. Diagnosis of heel pain. Am Fam Physician. 2011;84:909–16.
34. Luck MD, Gordon AG, Blebea JS, Dalinka MK. High association between accessory soleus muscle and Achilles tendonopathy. Skeletal Radiol. 2008;37:1129–33.
35. van Dijk CN, van Sterkenburg MN, Wiegerinck JI, Karlsson J, Maffulli N. Terminology for Achilles tendon related disorders. Knee Surg Sports Traumatol Arthrosc. 2011;19:835–41.
36. Chimenti RL, Chimenti PC, Buckley MR, Houck JR, Flemister AS. Utility of ultrasound for imaging osteophytes in patients with insertional Achilles tendinopathy. Arch Phys Med Rehabil. 2016;97:1206–9.
37. Chimenti RL, Cychosz CC, Hall MM, Phisitkul P. Current concepts review update: insertional Achilles tendinopathy. Foot Ankle Int. 2017;38:1160–9.
38. Sussmilch-Leitch SP, Collins NJ, Bialocerkowski AE, Warden SJ, Crossley KM. Physical therapies for Achilles tendinopathy: systematic review and meta-analysis. J Foot Ankle Res. 2012;5:15.
39. Magnussen RA, Dunn WR, Thomson AB. Nonoperative treatment of midportion Achilles tendinopathy: a systematic review. Clin J Sport Med. 2009;19:54–64.
40. Couppe C, Svensson RB, Silbernagel KG, Langberg H, Magnusson SP. Eccentric or concentric exercises for the treatment of tendinopathies? J Orthop Sports Phys Ther. 2015;45:853–63.
41. Malliaras P, Barton CJ, Reeves ND, Langberg H. Achilles and patellar tendinopathy loading programmes : a systematic review comparing clinical outcomes and identifying potential mechanisms for effectiveness. Sports Med. 2013;43:267–86.
42. Jonsson P, Alfredson H, Sunding K, Fahlstrom M, Cook J. New regimen for eccentric calf-muscle training in patients with chronic insertional Achilles tendinopathy: results of a pilot study. Br J Sports Med. 2008;42:746–9.
43. Alfredson H, Pietila T, Jonsson P, Lorentzon R. Heavy-load eccentric calf muscle training for the treatment of chronic Achilles tendinosis. Am J Sports Med. 1998;26:360–6.
44. Silbernagel KG, Thomee R, Eriksson BI, Karlsson J. Continued sports activity, using a pain-monitoring model, during rehabilitation in patients with Achilles tendinopathy: a randomized controlled study. Am J Sports Med. 2007;35:897–906.
45. van der Plas A, de Jonge S, de Vos RJ, et al. A 5-year follow-up study of Alfredson's heel-drop exercise programme in chronic midportion Achilles tendinopathy. Br J Sports Med. 2012;46:214–8.
46. Silbernagel KG, Brorsson A, Lundberg M. The majority of patients with Achilles tendinopathy recover fully when treated with exercise alone: a 5-year follow-up. Am J Sports Med. 2011;39:607–13.
47. Beyer R, Kongsgaard M, Hougs Kjaer B, Ohlenschlaeger T, Kjaer M, Magnusson SP. Heavy

slow resistance versus eccentric training as treatment for Achilles tendinopathy: a randomized controlled trial. Am J Sports Med. 2015;43:1704–11.
48. Silbernagel KG, Gustavsson A, Thomee R, Karlsson J. Evaluation of lower leg function in patients with Achilles tendinopathy. Knee Surg Sports Traumatol Arthrosc. 2006;14:1207–17.
49. Thomee R. A comprehensive treatment approach for patellofemoral pain syndrome in young women. Phys Ther. 1997;77:1690–703.
50. Silbernagel KG, Thomee R, Thomee P, Karlsson J. Eccentric overload training for patients with chronic Achilles tendon pain—a randomised controlled study with reliability testing of the evaluation methods. Scand J Med Sci Sports. 2001;11:197–206.
51. Verrall G, Schofield S, Brustad T. Chronic Achilles tendinopathy treated with eccentric stretching program. Foot Ankle Int. 2011;32:843–9.
52. Franettovich Smith MM, Honeywill C, Wyndow N, Crossley KM, Creaby MW. Neuromotor control of gluteal muscles in runners with Achilles tendinopathy. Med Sci Sports Exerc. 2014;46:594–9.
53. Chang YJ, Kulig K. The neuromechanical adaptations to Achilles tendinosis. J Physiol. 2015;593: 3373–87.
54. Cheatham SW, Lee M, Cain M, Baker R. The efficacy of instrument assisted soft tissue mobilization: a systematic review. J Can Chiropr Assoc. 2016;60:200–11.
55. Munteanu SE, Scott LA, Bonanno DR, et al. Effectiveness of customised foot orthoses for Achilles tendinopathy: a randomised controlled trial. Br J Sports Med. 2015;49:989–94.
56. Rowe V, Hemmings S, Barton C, Malliaras P, Maffulli N, Morrissey D. Conservative management of midportion Achilles tendinopathy: a mixed methods study, integrating systematic review and clinical reasoning. Sports Med. 2012;42:941–67.
57. Firth BL, Dingley P, Davies ER, Lewis JS, Alexander CM. The effect of kinesiotape on function, pain, and motoneuronal excitability in healthy people and people with Achilles tendinopathy. Clin J Sport Med. 2010;20:416–21.
58. Khan KM, Cook JL, Bonar F, Harcourt P, Åstrom M. Histopathology of common tendinopathies. Update and implications for clinical management. Sports Med. 1999;27:393–408.
59. Alfredson H, Thorsen K, Lorentzon R. In situ microdialysis in tendon tissue: high levels of glutamate, but not prostaglandin E2 in chronic Achilles tendon pain. Knee Surg Sports Traumatol Arthrosc. 1999;7:378–81.
60. Åström M, Westlin N. No effect of piroxicam on achilles tendinopathy. A randomized study of 70 patients. Acta Orthop Scand. 1992;63:631–4.
61. Almekinders LC, Temple JD. Etiology, diagnosis, and treatment of tendonitis: an analysis of the literature. Med Sci Sports Exerc. 1998;30:1183–90.
62. Maffulli N, Papalia R, D'Adamio S, Diaz Balzani L, Denaro V. Pharmacological interventions for the treatment of Achilles tendinopathy: a systematic review of randomized controlled trials. Br Med Bull. 2015;113:101–15.
63. Alfredson H. Conservative management of Achilles tendinopathy: new ideas. Foot Ankle Clin. 2005;10:321–9.
64. Kearney RS, Parsons N, Metcalfe D, Costa ML. Injection therapies for Achilles tendinopathy. Cochrane Database Syst Rev. 2015:CD010960.
65. Boesen AP, Hansen R, Boesen MI, Malliaras P, Langberg H. Effect of high-volume injection, platelet-rich plasma, and sham treatment in chronic midportion Achilles tendinopathy: a randomized double-blinded prospective study. Am J Sports Med. 2017;45:2034–43.
66. Lin MT, Chiang CF, Wu CH, Hsu HH, Tu YK. Meta-analysis comparing autologous blood-derived products (including platelet-rich plasma) injection versus placebo in patients with Achilles tendinopathy. Arthroscopy. 2018;34:1966–75.e5.
67. Zhang YJ, Xu SZ, Gu PC, et al. Is platelet-rich plasma injection effective for chronic Achilles tendinopathy? A meta-analysis. Clin Orthop Relat Res. 2018;476:1633–41.
68. Maffulli N, Spiezia F, Longo UG, Denaro V, Maffulli GD. High volume image guided injections for the management of chronic tendinopathy of the main body of the Achilles tendon. Phys Ther Sport. 2013;14:163–7.
69. Wheeler PC, Tattersall C. Novel interventions for recalcitrant Achilles tendinopathy: benefits seen following high-volume image-guided injection or extracorporeal shockwave therapy—a prospective cohort study. Clin J Sport Med. 2018.
70. Chaudhry FA. Effectiveness of dry needling and high-volume image-guided injection in the management of chronic mid-portion Achilles tendinopathy in adult population: a literature review. Eur J Orthop Surg Traumatol. 2017;27:441–8.
71. Alfredson H, Ohberg L. Sclerosing injections to areas of neo-vascularisation reduce pain in chronic Achilles tendinopathy: a double-blind randomised controlled trial. Knee Surg Sports Traumatol Arthrosc. 2005;13:338–44.
72. Ebbesen BH, Molgaard CM, Olesen JL, Gregersen HE, Simonsen O. No beneficial effect of Polidocanol treatment in Achilles tendinopathy: a randomised controlled trial. Knee Surg Sports Traumatol Arthrosc. 2018;26:2038–44.
73. Coombes BK, Bisset L, Vicenzino B. Efficacy and safety of corticosteroid injections and other injections for management of tendinopathy: a systematic review of randomised controlled trials. Lancet. 2010;376:1751–67.
74. Wetke E, Johannsen F, Langberg H. Achilles tendinopathy: a prospective study on the effect of active rehabilitation and steroid injections in a clinical setting. Scand J Med Sci Sports. 2015;25:e392–9.
75. Rompe JD, Nafe B, Furia JP, Maffulli N. Eccentric loading, shock-wave treatment, or a wait-and-see policy for tendinopathy of the main body of tendo

Achillis: a randomized controlled trial. Am J Sports Med. 2007;35:374–83.
76. Rompe JD, Furia J, Maffulli N. Eccentric loading versus eccentric loading plus shock-wave treatment for midportion Achilles tendinopathy: a randomized controlled trial. Am J Sports Med. 2009;37:463–70.
77. Furia JP, Rompe JD, Cacchio A, Del Buono A, Maffulli N. A single application of low-energy radial extracorporeal shock wave therapy is effective for the management of chronic patellar tendinopathy. Knee Surg Sports Traumatol Arthrosc. 2013;21:346–50.
78. Haake M, Konig IR, Decker T, Riedel C, Buch M, Muller HH. Extracorporeal shock wave therapy in the treatment of lateral epicondylitis: a randomized multicenter trial. J Bone Joint Surg Am. 2002;84-A:1982–91.
79. Furia JP. High-energy extracorporeal shock wave therapy as a treatment for insertional Achilles tendinopathy. Am J Sports Med. 2006;34:733–40.
80. Mani-Babu S, Morrissey D, Waugh C, Screen H, Barton C. The effectiveness of extracorporeal shock wave therapy in lower limb tendinopathy: a systematic review. Am J Sports Med. 2015;43:752–61.
81. Bjordal JM, Lopes-Martins RA, Iversen VV. A randomised, placebo controlled trial of low level laser therapy for activated Achilles tendinitis with microdialysis measurement of peritendinous prostaglandin E2 concentrations. Br J Sports Med. 2006;40:76–80.. discussion 76-80.
82. Salate AC, Barbosa G, Gaspar P, et al. Effect of In-Ga-Al-P diode laser irradiation on angiogenesis in partial ruptures of Achilles tendon in rats. Photomed Laser Surg. 2005;23:470–5.
83. Reddy GK, Stehno-Bittel L, Enwemeka CS. Laser photostimulation of collagen production in healing rabbit Achilles tendons. Lasers Surg Med. 1998;22:281–7.
84. Tumilty S, Munn J, McDonough S, Hurley DA, Basford JR, Baxter GD. Low level laser treatment of tendinopathy: a systematic review with meta-analysis. Photomed Laser Surg. 2010;28:3–16.
85. Hutchison AM, Pallister I, Evans RM, et al. Intense pulsed light treatment of chronic mid-body Achilles tendinopathy: a double blind randomised placebo-controlled trial. Bone Joint J. 2013;95-b:504–9.
86. Tumilty S, Mani R, Baxter GD. Photobiomodulation and eccentric exercise for Achilles tendinopathy: a randomized controlled trial. Lasers Med Sci. 2016;31:127–35.
87. Enwemeka CS. The effects of therapeutic ultrasound on tendon healing. A biomechanical study. Am J Phys Med Rehabil. 1989;68:283–7.
88. Chester R, Costa ML, Shepstone L, Cooper A, Donell ST. Eccentric calf muscle training compared with therapeutic ultrasound for chronic Achilles tendon pain—a pilot study. Man Ther. 2008;13:484–91.
89. Robertson VJ, Baker KG. A review of therapeutic ultrasound: effectiveness studies. Phys Ther. 2001;81:1339–50.
90. Wilson JJ, Best TM. Common overuse tendon problems: a review and recommendations for treatment. Am Fam Physician. 2005;72:811–8.
91. Lohrer H, David S, Nauck T. Surgical treatment for achilles tendinopathy—a systematic review. BMC Musculoskelet Disord. 2016;17:207.
92. Tallon C, Coleman BD, Khan KM, Maffulli N. Outcome of surgery for chronic Achilles tendinopathy. A critical review. Am J Sports Med. 2001;29:315–20.
93. Coleman BD, Khan KM, Maffulli N, Cook JL, Wark JD. Studies of surgical outcome after patellar tendinopathy: clinical significance of methodological deficiencies and guidelines for future studies. Victorian Institute of Sport Tendon Study Group. Scand J Med Sci Sports. 2000;10:2–11.
94. Yuan J, Murrell GA, Wei AQ, Appleyard RC, Del Soldato P, Wang MX. Addition of nitric oxide via nitroflurbiprofen enhances the material properties of early healing of young rat Achilles tendons. Inflamm Res. 2003;52:230–7.
95. Paoloni JA, Appleyard RC, Nelson J, Murrell GA. Topical glyceryl trinitrate treatment of chronic noninsertional achilles tendinopathy. A randomized, double-blind, placebo-controlled trial. J Bone Joint Surg Am. 2004;86-A:916–22.
96. Paoloni JA, Murrell GA. Three-year followup study of topical glyceryl trinitrate treatment of chronic noninsertional Achilles tendinopathy. Foot Ankle Int. 2007;28:1064–8.

Muscle Injuries

14

Gian Luigi Canata, Valentina Casale, Marco Davico, and Simone Lapi

14.1 Overreaching and Overtraining

Musculoskeletal overuse injuries are of important concern in athletics, especially in endurance sports where the balance between workload and rest is often ignored for obtaining maximal performance results [1–3].

In fact, overloading is often deliberately programmed as part of the endurance in the athlete's training process, stimulating physiological and psychological adaptations and improving physical performance. To do that, the training stimuli must be high enough to cause disturbance of homeostasis: this way the body is forced to adaptation [4]. Unfortunately, excessive and repetitive overloading followed by inadequate recovery may lead to overreaching and overtraining syndrome, characterized by acute feelings of fatigue and decreases in performance [3, 5]. Hooper et al. suggest that volume of training rather than intensity may be the primary cause of development of the overtraining syndrome [6].

The spectrum of underperformance conditions includes:

- Functional overreaching (FOR): A short-term reduction of performance (days to few weeks) followed by a *supercompensation* after recovery, with a consequent improvement of performance
- Nonfunctional recovery (FNOR): A short-term decrease in performance (weeks to months, longer than FOR) followed by a full recovery, but the previous performance abilities may not always be reestablished
- Overtraining syndrome (OTS): After a long-term recovery (usually several months), combines decrease of performance abilities and psychological symptoms

While an overreaching condition frequently affects athletes with an incidence between 5 and 60% [7–9], the OTS is much less prevalent [3, 10]. The OTS may be described as a condition caused by training too hard for too long, leading to a general breakdown in physiological functions [4].

It is difficult to draw a clear distinction among these three conditions [5]. The clinical signs and symptoms caused by the imbalance between training and recovery may be confused with illness, stress, sleep disorders, or inadequate nutrition [3]. Several synonyms around overreaching conditions do exist: training stress syndrome, under-recovery, failure adaptation, burnout, muscle failure syndrome, and excessive exercise [11]. However, as cited before, the ultimate result consists in dysfunctions of immune, inflammatory,

G. L. Canata (✉) · V. Casale · M. Davico · S. Lapi
Centre of Sports Traumatology, Koelliker Hospital, Torino, Italy
e-mail: studio@ortosport.it

S. Rocha Piedade et al. (eds.), *The Sports Medicine Physician*, https://doi.org/10.1007/978-3-030-10433-7_14

neurological, hormonal, and metabolic system, causing the inability to manage chronic exposure to intensive metabolic and tissue stresses [5].

Establishing the optimal training regimen is difficult, because the volume of training and the best rest period to improve performance are not easily determined: the suitable scheme for some athletes may cause undertraining or overtraining in others [12]. Furthermore, if the interval between workouts is too long, the overcompensation may impair the original function conditions, and progressive improvement will not occur; conversely, too frequent training stimulus may reduce the recovery ability, and adaptation will not be possible [13].

Overreaching and overtraining negatively affect muscle strength, power, and velocity [14–16]. Unlike overreaching subjects, the reduction in maximal force production persists in overtrained athletes, even after several weeks of recovery [14].

14.2 Overtraining Syndrome Pathophysiology

Overtraining pathophysiology hypothesis
1. Glycogen hypothesis
2. Central fatigue hypothesis
3. Glutamine hypothesis
4. Oxidative stress hypothesis
5. Autonomic nervous system hypothesis
6. Cytokine hypothesis

Numerous hypotheses which should consider the complexity and variability of symptoms have been suggested to explain the development of the overtraining fatigue [17, 18].

The "glycogen hypothesis" indicates the low muscle glycogen levels as the cause of increased oxidation and decreased branched chain amino acids, leading to an altered synthesis of central neurotransmitters involved in fatigue [19]. Although these concepts are not strictly connected to the overtraining syndrome onset, they explain how the exercise-induced fatigue develops [11].

The "central fatigue hypothesis" describes the connection between increased levels of serotonin and a reduction of performance [10, 20, 21]. Well-trained athletes show a low sensitivity to serotonin [22]; in fact, marathon runners receiving branched chain amino acids supplementation feel energized and mentally clear, showing lower levels of serotonin synthesis [21]. Conversely, overtrained athletes have an increased neurologic sensitivity to serotonin, even though few studies have analyzed serotonin activity in overtrained athletes so far [21].

The "glutamine hypothesis" is related to the immune cell functions. Low glutamine levels after exercise may cause upper respiratory tract infections in overtrained athletes [23–25]. The low levels of glutamine after activity are related to an overutilization and/or a reduced production by overworked muscles [26]. Although the glutamine amount in immune cells does not necessarily change after its reduction caused by exercise [26], the glutamine supplementation has been proved to decrease early rates of infection [27]. It is important to remind that the connection between low levels of glutamine and upper respiratory tract infections is not clear, even because glutamine amount is influenced by nutritional state, trauma, or infections [26].

The "oxidative stress hypothesis" focuses on the role of reactive oxygen species (ROS) released from damaged muscles (i.e., superoxide, hydrogen peroxide, and hydroxyl radical) [17]. Initially, these species regulate cellular repair [28], with positive effects for muscular homeostasis; nevertheless, when oxidative stress becomes pathologic, the reactive oxygen species may cause inflammation, muscle fatigue, and soreness, leading to reduced performance [29]. Overtrained athletes show high resting markers of oxidative stress, which raise during exercise [29, 30]. Among damages to proteins and lipids in the contracting myocytes, it has been reported that oxidants regulate several cell signaling pathways and influence the expression of numerous genes [31], resulting in changes at transcriptional, mRNA stability, and signal transduction levels [31]. What is more, ROS may promote an inflammatory response during repair of the damaged overtrained muscles, leading to neutrophil and macrophage infiltration of muscles [28, 32] and a consequent leukocytosis which lasts several days [33].

The "autonomic nervous system hypothesis" explains a reduced sympathetic activation and a parasympathetic dominance typically present in overtrained athletes, responsible for muscle fatigue, bradycardia, and performance inhibition [20, 34]. The balance between sympathetic and parasympathetic systems is restored after a week of rest [35].

The "hypothalamic hypothesis" explores the alterations among the hypothalamic-pituitary-adrenal and hypothalamic-pituitary-gonadal axes: the results are variations in cortisol, adrenocorticotropic hormone (ACTH), testosterone, and other hormone levels [20, 34, 36–38]. Nevertheless, several other stimuli influence these hormonal axes; thus the correlation with the overtraining condition is not such clear [17].

The "cytokine hypothesis" analyzes the inflammatory cascade induced by repetitive microtrauma on tissues. Tissue healing and strengthening derives from the recruitment of cytokines (i.e., interleukin 1 beta or IL-1ß, IL-6, and the tumor necrosis factor α or TNF-α) as a physiological reaction to exercise, although amplification and pathological response may occur if the required resting phase is not respected [24, 34, 39]. Although this theory may explain "why" the overtraining injuries develop, the exact correlation between cytokines and overtraining remains unclear [34].

A further reference deals with the predisposing factors to overuse injuries. For example, the structure of coordinative variability may reduce or increase the injury rates [40]. Nevertheless, it is still unclear if a low coordinative variability is a cause or an effect of overuse injuries, as well as a too high variability sometimes may be associated to higher lesions rates [40].

As for running overuse injuries, van der Worp et al. reported the risk factors associated with running and training, such as the surface and running distance, the shoe used, the running participation rates, and the athlete experience [41].

14.2.1 Overtraining Effects on Skeletal Muscle Metabolism and Homeostasis

Overtrained athletes show an altered hormonal response to stress, such as lower heart rate, blood lactate, and plasma cortisol reduction by downregulation, as a consequence of repetitive large stress responses [42]. Gleeson summarized the most commonly reported physiological and psychological changes as:

- Underperformance
- Muscle weakness
- Chronic fatigue and muscles soreness
- Increased perceived stress during activity
- Reduced motivation
- Sleep disturbance
- Increased early morning or sleeping heart rate
- Altered mood state
- Loss of appetite
- Gastrointestinal disturbance
- Recurrent infection

As for the musculoskeletal metabolic changes, the three major adaptations to exercise determine an increase in density of mitochondria, a modification of muscle types, and an orientation of the use of energy substrates [43]. The resulting conditions consist in a capillary proliferation around muscles, higher intramuscular glycogen and triglyceride reserves, and an increase in maximal oxygen uptake [44]. The higher volume of mitochondria per muscle unit promotes a preferential use of lipids, which is further simplified by an increase in intramuscular lipid content [45]. Furthermore, since moderate- to high-intensity exercises use carbohydrates as the primary source of energy, overtraining has been demonstrated to reduce levels of muscle glycogen despite the dietary intake remains unchanged [46]. Muscle glycogen resynthesis delays and performance levels decrease [47]. Along with a reduced energy storage, low muscle glycogen levels may also cause a dropping of the branched amino acids due to oxidation of glucose, thus developing a central fatigue [48]. The reflection of overtraining on the ultrastructural level of skeletal muscle highlights that the negative effect depends on the muscle fiber type [49]. It has been well reported that endurance training produces a change from glycolytic-type fibers (type II) to slower oxidative-type fibers (type I) [43] and from type IIb glycolytic fast fibers to type IIa oxidative fast fibers [50]. This entails a decrease of the muscle fatigue due to a better diffusion of oxygen toward the mitochondria, but a concurrent reduction of the force capacity per motor unites [43]. During overtraining, changes in the skeletal muscle myofibrillar apparatus may develop, especially the destruction of contractile proteins [13], with a final development of an *exercise myopathy* [49]. Furthermore, it has been reported a diminished synthesis of muscle proteins, especially myofibrillar proteins, as well as an increased protein degradation in skeletal muscles [4]. Overtraining affects neuromuscular junctions too. The nerve-muscle transfer is gradually disrupted in overtrained muscles, cell regeneration slows down, and muscle fiber atrophy develops. An initial clinical sign may be the delayed onset muscle soreness (DOMS). It usually begins 12–24 h after an excessive workload. Tenderness and stiffness develop, soreness reaches the climax 48 h later, and then symptoms resolve within 10 days [51]. As the severity of this condition depends on the intensity and volume of training, persisting in hard workload during the DOMS symptomatic period may compromise shock wave absorption ability, strength output, force steadiness, and coordination [52], finally resulting in overtraining muscle lesions.

14.3 Diagnosis of Overtrained Muscle Injuries

As several reviews discuss, there is no definitive biomarker able to differentiate functional overreaching, nonfunctional overreaching, and overtraining syndromes [11]. Therefore, it is essential to rule out the more common medical diseases, such as anemia, asthma, cardiovascular affections (especially in masters athletes), mood disorder, and infections [11, 18].

Nevertheless, some markers may be helpful if evaluated once an athlete reports clinical signs of overtraining muscle fatigue [3, 17, 38].

Since several metabolic and psychologic diseases may cause underperformance and symptoms of overtraining syndrome, a thorough clinical history must always be collected [3, 10, 17, 18]. Furthermore, the patient usually reports a persisting, reduced performance despite weeks or months of rest, as well as disorders of mood, without clear signs of other possible causes of underperformance [3].

Significant organic diseases must be excluded, as well as infection diseases, endocrinological disorders, autoimmune diseases, deficiencies of carbohydrate/protein intake, iron, vitamin D, and magnesium [3, 9, 17, 21, 30]. In particular, monitoring heart rate and blood lactate seems to be effective to classify a high percentage of athletes who may be entering overtraining fatigue [53, 54]. Part of the clinical diagnosis of overtraining fatigue takes into account mood changes. The Profile of Mood States questionnaire (POMS) is widely used for diagnosing alterations of the mood among athletes [55].

Among the triggers for a correct diagnosis of overtraining injuries, there are training errors which imply an imbalance between load and recovery, the monotony of training, too many competitions, and psychological issues [3]. However, the diagnosis of overtraining syndrome is still possible only after the exclusion of all the other possible causes of underperformance [3, 11].

In case a DOMS is suspected, magnetic resonance (MR) imaging may be helpful [56], while ultrasound (US) is considered not sensitive enough to detect the changes secondary to this condition [57] (Fig. 14.1a, b). In particular, muscle edema may be found as a high-intensity signal at the muscle belly on MRI, and perifascial fluid may be present in the early injury stage [56] (Fig. 14.2a, b). Usually, no fiber disruption or tears are associated with DOMS

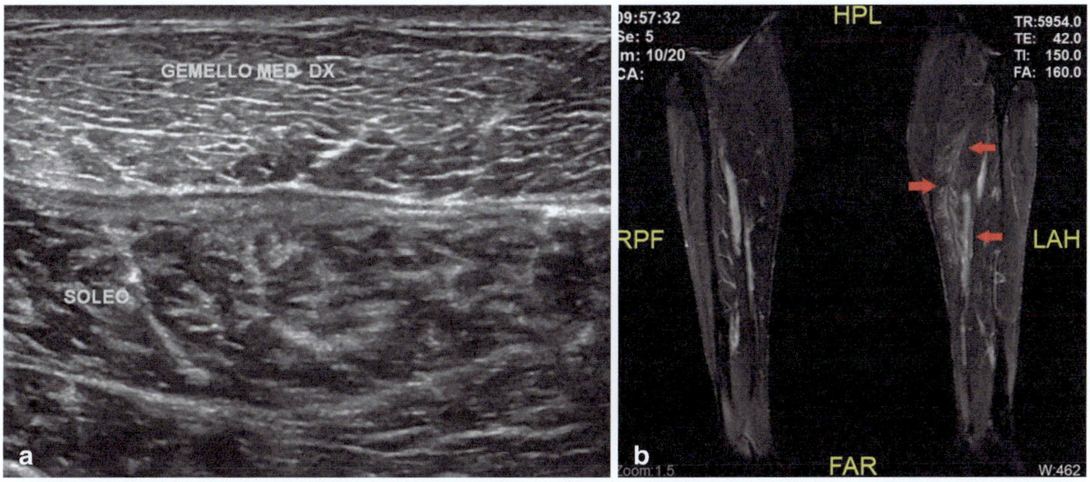

Fig. 14.1 The absence of any muscular alteration on US (**a**). MRI shows a perivascular myofascial edema with high signal intensity of the perivascular venous spaces (**b**)

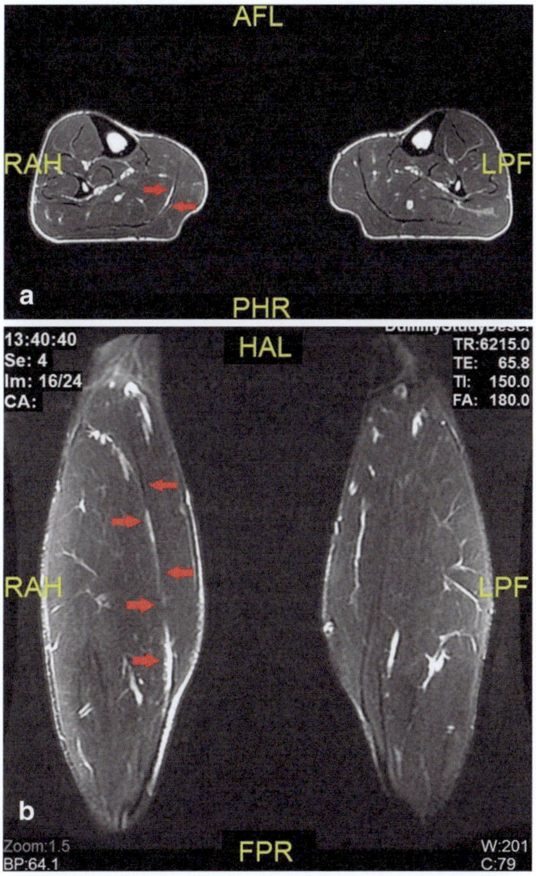

Fig. 14.2 Axial (**a**) and coronal (**b**) MR images show interfascial edema, with hyperemia and thickening of the fascia between soleus and the medial head of gastrocnemius. No alterations of muscular trophism are detectable

(Fig. 14.3a, b). It is important to remember that though symptoms have been completely solved, usually within 10–12 days, the MR images may take even 80 days to detect no abnormal signal intensity [58]. To assess the muscle healing response, US can be used to look for persistent focal abnormality, although MRI is highly sensitive and more specific for detecting small residual areas of injury that US cannot be visualized [59].

14.4 How to Manage Overtraining Muscle Injuries

As Kreher and Schwartz underline, when the cause of OTS is an organic disease, an appropriate treatment is strongly recommended [17]. In case of functional overreaching condition, the most effective management is balancing overload training with appropriate rest [10]. If nonfunctional or overtraining syndrome is present, the only effective treatment is rest [17]. Rest may be absolute or relative; in any case it is important to introduce physical activity gradually, for example, starting from 5 to 10 min daily until 1 h if the athlete tolerates it [60]. If stress, depression, or anxiety does not reduce or even increase during full rest, relative rest is advisable [10].

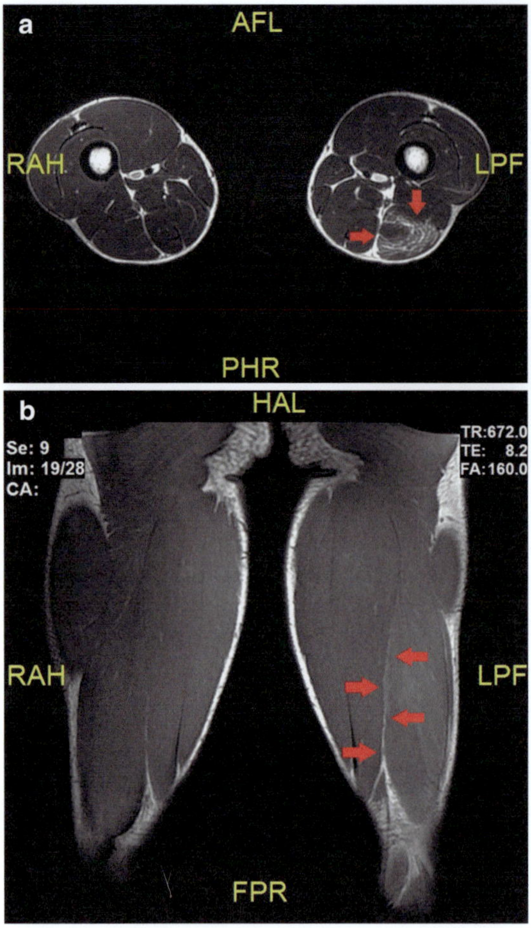

Fig. 14.3 The high-definition axial (**a**) and coronal (**b**) MR images are enable to diagnose a typical DOMS condition. An edema of the contractile fibrils is evident, without discontinuity of myofascial bands

14.5 Prevention of Overtrained Muscle Injuries

How to Prevent Overtraining Syndrome
1. To monitor athlete's daily training loads
2. To consider psychological aspects
3. To work on modifiable risk factors (i.e., high training frequency, running distance)
4. To adopt a standardized performance test to be done periodically
5. To remember that every athlete has different tipping points for overtraining fatigue
6. To educate athletes, coaches, and sports medicine professionals to recognize first signals and to communicate with each other

Prevention of the overtraining syndrome is widely approved as fundamental [3]. Since the main cause of overtraining injuries is the imbalance in the training recovery ratio, an effective prevention injury program is to monitor the athlete daily training loads [61, 62]. The most used methods are training diaries, retrospective questionnaires, physiological screenings, and direct observation [63]. The psychological aspects also need to be considered, as well as the rate of perceived exertion (RPE) [3, 11] and the periodization and individualization of the athlete's nutritional requirements [64]. Among the several biochemical processes as causes of overtraining injuries, much of the prevention may be simply the education to risk factors and the ways to avoid excessive stress without adequate rest [11].

Working on modifiable risk factors can be a further effective prevention strategy. For example, it is well known that high training frequency and running distance are more susceptible to overuse injuries [65], but even one run a week prevents the musculoskeletal system adapting to that type of exercise [66, 67]. In fact, it has been reported that training may play a protective role and undertraining may increase injury risks [68]. Pluim and Drew proposed six load management tips to optimize this concept related to tennis overload injuries [69]:

1. Establish a basic fitness level
2. Minimize the week-to-week changes
3. Try to avoid peaks in load
4. Make sure you maintain a correct work-rest balance
5. Maintain a minimum training load
6. Do not overdo it!

It is also suggested to adopt a standardized workout routine or to do a performance test periodically, for relating any possible variation in the results to the athlete's condition [17, 18, 38].

Nevertheless, every athlete has to be considered as an individual with different tipping points for overtraining fatigue and different stress capacities [19]. The main purpose should be identifying overreaching episodes to allow the athlete recognize them and to prevent by further damages [11]. In fact, an important warning sign an athlete should recognize is a minor performance despite increased efforts [3, 17]. It is fundamental having a proper education among athletes, coaches, and sports medicine providers, showing how to ensure an adequate recovery, for example, measuring physiologic marker such as weight, morning heart rate, and maximal heart rate [11]. Communication between the athlete and his/her coach is equally paramount: if present, every subjective feeling of fatigue and increased RPE should be promptly reported. The first hypothesis will trace back to a medical cause, but it is important to remember that, while medical diseases are usually present at the onset of the exercises, the overtraining fatigue appears during activity, and the athlete feels incapable of completing the workload [17, 60]. Last but not the least, athletes, coaches, and sports medicine professionals must remember that the psychological aspects of endurance training are often associated with the development of fatigue [11]. They should consider depressed and anxious moods as symptoms of excessive exercise, talking about that and not classifying them as mood disorders [11].

Take-Home Message
Overloading and subsequent recovery are part of athlete's training. A constant balance of training charges is advisable, but a careful individual planning is needed to maximize performance without risking muscle overuse injuries. Several physiologic and psychologic diagnostic signals must be checked on a regular basis to effectively manage an optimal sequence of overload training and moderate rest avoiding an undesired functional impairment. MR is the most reliable imaging tool to detect excessive muscle overload. Prevention is of paramount importance with a constant training load monitoring based on a constant communication between athletes, coaches, and sports medicine professionals. Rest is the best treatment, being aware that full recovery from overload injuries may take several weeks.

References

1. Tonoli DC, Cumps E, Aerts I, et al. Incidence, risk factors and prevention of running related injuries in long-distance running: a systematic review. Geneeskd Sport. 2010;43(5):12–8.
2. Clarsen B, Ronsen O, Myklebust G, et al. The Oslo Sports Trauma Research Center questionnaire on health problems: a new approach to prospective monitoring of illness and injury in elite athletes. Br J Sports Med. 2014;48(9):754–60.
3. Meeusen R, Duclos M, Foster C, et al. Prevention, diagnosis, and treatment of the overtraining syndrome: joint consensus statement of the European College of Sport Science and the American College of Sports Medicine. Med Sci Sports Exerc. 2013;45(1):186–205.
4. Seene T, Umnova M, Kaasik P, et al. Overtraining injuries in athletic population. In: Tiidus PM, editor. Skeletal muscle damage and repair. Champaign: Human Kinetics; 2008. p. 173–84.
5. Cadegiani FA, Kater CE. Hormonal aspects of overtraining syndrome: a systematic review. BMC Sports Sci Med Rehabil. 2017;9:14.
6. Hooper S, Mackinnon L, Howard A, et al. Markers for monitoring overtraining and recovery. Med Sci Sports Exerc. 1995;27:106–12.
7. Hooper S, MacKinnon LT, Hanrahan S. Mood states as an indication of staleness and recovery. Int J Sport Psychol. 1997;28:1–12.
8. Koutedakis Y, Sharp NC. Seasonal variations of injury and overtraining in elite athletes. Clin J Sport Med. 1998;8(1):18–21.
9. Matos NF, Winsley RJ, Williams CA. Prevalence of nonfunctional overreaching/overtraining in young English athletes. Med Sci Sports Exerc. 2011;43(7):1287–94.
10. Meeusen R, Duclos M, Gleeson M, et al. Prevention, diagnosis and treatment of the overtraining syndrome: ECSS Position Statement "Task Force". Eur J Sport Sci. 2006;6(1):1–14.
11. Kreher JB. Diagnosis and prevention of overtraining syndrome: an opinion on education strategies. Open Access J Sports Med. 2016;7:115–22.
12. O'Toole ML. Overreaching and overtraining in endurance athletes. In: Kreider RB, Fry AC, O'Toole ML, editors. Overtraining in sport. Champaign: Human Kinetics; 1998. p. 3–17.
13. Seene T, Kaasik P, Alev K, et al. Composition and turnover of contractile proteins in volume-overtrained skeletal muscle. Int J Sports Med. 2004;25(6):438–45.
14. Fry AC, Kraemer WJ, van Borselen F, et al. Performance decrements with high intensity resistance exercise overtraining. Med Sci Sports Exerc. 1994;26:1165–73.
15. Ratamess NA, Kraemer WJ, Volek JS, et al. The effects of amino acid supplementation on muscular performance during resistance training overreaching. J Strength Cond Res. 2003;17(2):250–8.

16. Wilson JM, Joy JM, Lowery RP, et al. Effects of oral adenosine-5′-triphosphate supplementation on athletic performance, skeletal muscle hypertrophy and recovery in resistance-trained men. Nutr Metab. 2013;10(1):57.
17. Kreher JB, Schwartz JB. Overtraining syndrome: a practical guide. Sports Health. 2012;4(2):128–38.
18. Carfagno DG, Hendrix JC 3rd. Overtraining syndrome in the athlete: current clinical practice. Curr Sports Med Rep. 2014;13(1):45–51.
19. Costill DL, Flynn MG, Kirwan JP, et al. Effects of repeated days of intensified training on muscle glycogen and swimming performance. Med Sci Sports Exerc. 1988;20(3):249–54.
20. Lehmann M, Foster C, Keul J. Overtraining in endurance athletes: a brief review. Med Sci Sports Exerc. 1993;25(7):854–62.
21. Budgett R, Newsholme E, Lehmann M, et al. Redefining the overtraining syndrome as the unexplained underperformance syndrome. Br J Sports Med. 2000;34(1):67–8.
22. Budgett R, Hiscock N, Arida E, et al. The effects of the 5-HT2C agonist m-chlorophenylpiperazine on elite athletes with unexplained underperformance syndrome (overtraining). Br J Sports Med. 2010;44(4):280–3.
23. Mackinnon LT, Hooper SL. Plasma glutamine and upper respiratory tract infection during intensified training in swimmers. Med Sci Sports Exerc. 1996;28(3):285–90.
24. Smith LL. Overtraining, excessive exercise, and altered immunity: is this a T helper-1 versus T helper-2 lymphocyte response? Sports Med. 2003;33(5):347–64.
25. Walsh NP, Blannin AK, Robson PJ, et al. Glutamine, exercise and immune function. Links and possible mechanisms. Sports Med. 1998;26(3):177–91.
26. Hiscock N, Pedersen BK. Exercise-induced immunodepression—plasma glutamine is not the link. J Appl Physiol. 2002;93(3):813–22.
27. Castell LM, Poortmans JR, Leclercq R, et al. Some aspects of the acute phase response after a marathon race, and the effects of glutamine supplementation. Eur J Appl Physiol. 1997;75:47–53.
28. Tiidus PM. Radical species in inflammation and overtraining. Can J Physiol Pharmacol. 1998;76(5):533–8.
29. Tanskanen M, Atalay M, Uusitalo A. Altered oxidative stress in overtrained athletes. J Sports Sci. 2010;28(3):309–17.
30. Margonis K, Fatouros IG, Jamurtas AZ, et al. Oxidative stress biomarkers responses to physical overtraining: implications for diagnosis. Free Radic Biol Med. 2007;43(6):901–10.
31. Powers SK, Ji LL, Kavazis AN, et al. Reactive oxygen species: impact on skeletal muscle. Compr Physiol. 2011;1(2):941–69.
32. Evans WJ, Cannon JG. Metabolic effects of exercise-induced muscle damage. Exerc Sport Sci Rev. 1991;19:99–125.
33. Fielding RA, Manfredi TJ, Ding W, et al. Acute phase response to exercise. III. Neutrophil and IL-1 beta accumulation in skeletal muscle. Am J Phys. 1993;265(1 Pt 2):R166–72.
34. Smith LL. Cytokine hypothesis of overtraining: a physiological adaptation to excessive stress? Med Sci Sports Exerc. 2000;32(2):317–31.
35. Pichot V, Roche F, Gaspoz JM, et al. Relation between heart rate variability and training load in middle-distance runners. Med Sci Sports Exerc. 2000;32(10):1729–36.
36. Angeli A, Minetto M, Dovio A, et al. The overtraining syndrome in athletes: a stress-related disorder. J Endocrinol Investig. 2004;27(6):603–12.
37. Halson SL, Jeukendrup AE. Does overtraining exist? An analysis of overreaching and overtraining research. Sports Med. 2004;34(14):967–81.
38. Urhausen A, Kindermann W. Diagnosis of overtraining: what tools do we have? Sports Med. 2002;32(2):95–102.
39. Robson P. Elucidating the unexplained underperformance syndrome in endurance athletes: the interleukin-6 hypothesis. Sports Med. 2003;33(10):771–81.
40. Hamill J, Palmer C, van Emmerik RE. Coordinative variability and overuse injury. Sports Med Arthrosc Rehabil Ther Technol. 2012;4(1):45.
41. van der Worp MP, ten Haaf DS, van Cingel R, et al. Injuries in runners; a systematic review on risk factors and sex differences. PLoS One. 2015;10(2):e0114937.
42. Gleeson M. Biomechanical and immunological markers of over-training. J Sports Sci Med. 2002;1(2):31–41.
43. Guezennec CY, Krentowski R. Muscle physiology in athletes. In: Roger B, Guermazi A, Skaf A, editors. Muscle injuries in sport athletes. Sports and traumatology. 1st ed. Berlin: Springer; 2017. p. 3–18.
44. Hoppeler H, Howald H, Conley K, et al. Endurance training in humans: aerobic capacity and structure of skeletal muscle. J Appl Physiol. 1985;59(2):320–7.
45. Jeppesen J, Jordy AB, Sjøberg KA, et al. Enhanced fatty acid oxidation and FATP4 protein expression after endurance exercise training in human skeletal muscle. PLoS One. 2012;7(1):29–39.
46. Costill DL, Bowers R, Branam G, et al. Muscle glycogen utilization during prolonged exercise on successive days. J Appl Physiol. 1971;31(6):834–8.
47. Karlsson J, Saltin B. Diet, muscle glycogen and endurance performance. J Appl Physiol. 1971;31(2):203–6.
48. Newsholme EA, Parry-Billings M, McAndrew N, et al. A biochemical mechanism to explain some characteristics of overtraining. In: Brouns F, Saris WHM, Newsholme EA, editors. Advances in nutrition and top sport. 32nd ed. Basel: Karger; 1991. p. 79–93.
49. Seene T, Umnova M, Kaasik P. The exercise myopathy. In: Lehmann M, Foster C, Gastmann U, et al., editors. Overload, performance incompetence, and regeneration in sport. 1st ed. Berlin: Springer; 2007. p. 119–30.
50. Seene T, Kaasik P, Umnova M. Structural rearrangements in contractile apparatus and resulting skeletal muscle remodeling: effect of exercise training. J Sports Med Phys Fitness. 2009;49(4):410–23.

51. Nelson N. Delayed onset muscle soreness: is massage effective? J Bodyw Mov Ther. 2013;17(4):475–82.
52. Vila-Chã C, Hassanlouei H, Farina D, et al. Eccentric exercise and delayed onset muscle soreness of the quadriceps induce adjustments in agonist-antagonist activity, which are dependent on the motor task. Exp Brain Res. 2012;216(3):385–95.
53. Le Meur Y, Hausswirth C, Natta F, et al. A multidisciplinary approach to overreaching detection in endurance trained athlete. J Appl Physiol. 2012;114(3):411–20.
54. Bosquet L, Léger L, Legros P. Blood lactate response to overtraining in male endurance athletes. Eur J Appl Physiol. 2001;84(1–2):107–14.
55. Biehl B, Landauer A. Das profile of mood states (POMS). Mannheim: Universität; 1975.
56. Guermazi A, Roemer FW, Robinson P, et al. Imaging of muscle injuries in sports medicine: sports imaging series. Radiology. 2017;282(3):646–63.
57. Dierking JK, Bemben MG, Bemben DA, et al. Validity of diagnostic ultrasound as a measure of delayed onset muscle soreness. J Orthop Sports Phys Ther. 2000;30(3):116–22.
58. Shellock FG, Fukunaga T, Mink JH, et al. Exertional muscle injury: evaluation of concentric versus eccentric actions with serial MR imaging. Radiology. 1991;179(3):659–64.
59. Woodhouse JB, McNally EG. Ultrasound of skeletal muscle injury: an update. Semin Ultrasound CT MR. 2011;32(2):91–100.
60. Budgett R. Fatigue and underperformance in athletes: the overtraining syndrome. Br J Sports Med. 1998;32(2):107–10.
61. Foster C. Monitoring training in athletes with reference to overtraining syndrome. Med Sci Sports Exerc. 1998;30(7):164–8.
62. Foster C, Daines E, Hector L, et al. Athletic performance in relation to training load. Wis Med J. 1996;95:370–4.
63. Hopkins W. Quantification of training in competitive sports. Methods and applications. Sports Med. 1991;12:161–83.
64. Lewis NA, Collins D, Pedlar CR, et al. Can clinicians and scientists explain and prevent unexplained underperformance syndrome in elite athletes: an interdisciplinary perspective and 2016 update. BMJ Open Sport Exerc Med. 2015;1(1):e000063.
65. van Gent RN, Siem D, van Middelkoop M, et al. Incidence and determinants of lower extremity running injuries in long distance runners: a systematic review. Br J Sports Med. 2007;41(8):469–80.
66. Hreljac A. Impact and overuse injuries in runners. Med Sci Sports Exerc. 2004;36(5):845–9.
67. Taunton JE, Ryan MB, Clement DB, et al. A prospective study of running injuries: the Vancouver sun run "in training" clinics. Br J Sports Med. 2003;37(3):329–44.
68. Drew MK, Finch CF. The relationship between training load and injury, illness and soreness: a systematic and literature review. Sports Med. 2016;46(6):861–83.
69. Pluim BM, Drew MK. It's not the destination, it's the "road to load" that matters: a tennis injury prevention perspective. Br J Sports Med. 2016;50(11):641–2.

Stress Fractures

15

Timothy L. Miller and Christopher C. Kaeding

Stress fractures of bone, also known as fatigue fractures or march fractures, are common and troublesome injuries in athletes in military personnel. A multitude of biological and mechanical factors influence the body's ability to remodel bone and impact an individual's risk for developing a bony stress injury. These factors include sex, age, race, hormonal status, nutrition, neuromuscular function, and genetic factors. Other predisposing factors to consider include abnormal bony alignment, improper technique/biomechanics, poor running form, inadequate blood supply to specific bones, improper or worn-out footwear, and hard training surfaces. Understanding the classification and grade of stress fractures and their implications is the key to providing optimal care to all patients with stress fractures, especially those with an injury at a high-risk site.

15.1 The Holistic Approach to Stress Fractures

Stress fractures are the result of the loss of the normal balance between the creation and repair of microcracks in bone. Treatment principles include taking a holistic and systemic approach to individuals presenting with this injury. In order to decrease the creation of microcracks, one must evaluate the patient's training regimen, biomechanics, and equipment. Maximizing the patient's biologic capacity to repair microcracks requires an assessment of the athlete's general health. This includes nutritional status, hormonal status, emotional status, and medication use.

Stress fractures are not a single consistent entity. They occur along a continuum of severity which can impact treatment and prognosis [1–4]. Not only does the extent of these injuries vary, but the clinical behavior of these injuries varies by location and causative activity [5, 6]. It should be borne in mind that no two stress fractures behave exactly alike. Treatment protocols should be individualized to the patient, the causative activity, the anatomical site, and the severity of the fracture. The key principles for

T. L. Miller (✉)
Orthopaedic Surgery and Sports Medicine, The Ohio State University Wexner Medical Center, Jameson Crane Sports Medicine Institute, Columbus, OH, USA

Ohio State University Athletics, The Ohio State University Wexner Medical Center Endurance Medicine Team, Columbus, OH, USA
e-mail: timothy.miller@osumc.edu

C. C. Kaeding
Department of Orthopaedics, The Ohio State University Wexner Medical Center Sports Medicine, Jameson Crane Sports Medicine Institute, Columbus, OH, USA

Department of Athletics, The Ohio State University, Columbus, OH, USA
e-mail: Christopher.Kaeding@osumc.edu

S. Rocha Piedade et al. (eds.), *The Sports Medicine Physician*,
https://doi.org/10.1007/978-3-030-10433-7_15

treating stress fractures in athletes are summarized in Table 15.1, and a treatment algorithm that has been successfully employed by the authors is shown in Fig. 15.1.

Table 15.1 Key treatment principles for a holistic approach to bony stress injuries

• Biomechanical and technique modification
• Alternative training including training surfaces
• Nutritional optimization
• Hormonal balance
• Mental and emotional fitness and coping skills
• Surgical stabilization

The goal of treating bony injuries is to decrease the repetitive stress at the fracture site enough to allow the body to restore the dynamic balance between damage and repair. This may include decreasing volume and intensity of activity, equipment changes, technique changes, or cross-training. One benefit to such a strategy is that the individual typically does not endure a substantial loss of conditioning while still allowing his or her body to repair the bony damage. If pain intensifies and activity modification alone is inadequate for healing, treatment should be intensified to include complete rest, immobilization, or surgical intervention.

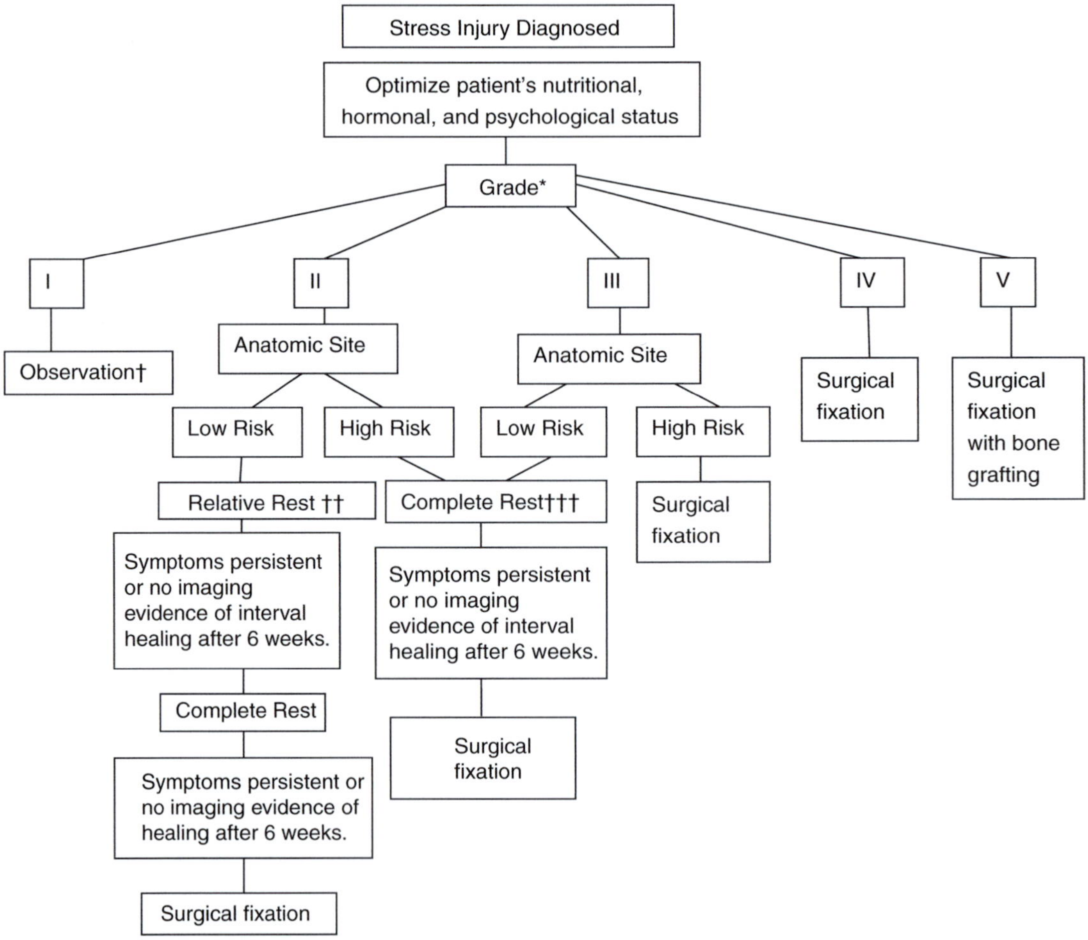

Fig. 15.1 Recommended treatment algorithm for stress injuries of bone (Reproduced from Rockwood and Wilkins, *Fractures in Adults*, 9th Edition). *Grading based on the Kaeding-Miller classification system presented in Table 15.2 [1]. †**Observation** = Return to activity with close follow-up. Consider relative rest and cross-training. ††**Relative Rest** = Decrease frequency or intensity of inciting activity. May cross-train. Gradual return to full pain-free activity. †††**Complete Rest** = Discontinuation of any activity that places stress at fracture site. May include immobilization

15.2 Athletes at Risk for Stress Fractures

15.2.1 Vitamin D Insufficiency

It is recommended that most athletes receive at least 800–1000 IU (or perhaps as much as 5000 IU) of vitamin D_3 daily. This level of supplementation is safe and has a high therapeutic index. Serum 25(OH)D_3 level is the study of choice for identifying Vitamin D deficiency [7]. In those individuals with low vitamin D or low bone mineral density, the therapeutic goal for supplementation should range from at least 50 nmol/L (20 ng/mL) to as high as 90–100 nmol/L (36–40 ng/mL) based on the Food and Nutrition Board recommendations [7]. In general a serum level the ideal level for the athlete is 40–50 ng/mL. To achieve this goal as much 50,000 IU per may be prescribed for individuals with severe hypovitaminosis D. Although higher dietary intake of Vitamin D_3 may provide some protective effect against fractures, the exact role of Vitamin D in fracture prevention is still up for debate.

Recent studies have evaluated the potential association between serum Vitamin D_3 levels and stress fractures. A prospective study of Finnish military recruits found that the average serum vitamin D_3 concentration was significantly lower in the group that had sustained a stress fracture [8]. Another randomized, double-blind, placebo-controlled study examined whether calcium and Vitamin D_3 intervention could reduce the incidence of stress fractures in female recruits during basic training [8]. This level 1 study suggested that calcium and Vitamin D_3 supplementation may have prevented a significant percentage of their recruits from sustaining a stress fracture and led to a significant decrease in morbidity and financial burden [8].

15.2.2 The Female Athlete Triad and Caloric Insufficiency

Inadequate caloric intake may play a role in amenorrhea, which has been linked to an increased incidence of stress fractures [9, 10]. Dietary intake and disordered eating patterns have been linked to amenorrhea in a number of studies. A concept that has been developed supporting the link between dietary intake and amenorrhea is the so-called energy drain hypothesis. If caloric intake is too low, production of hormones such as estrogen and progesterone is moved lower on the body's list of priorities. These hormones may not be produced in amounts high enough to allow menstruation to occur [11]. Oligomenorrheic or amenorrheic female athletes are at increased risk secondary to decreased estrogen levels and increased osteoclastic activity [12].

Endocrine and malabsorption conditions can impair the delicate balance between bone formation and resorption, thus predisposing athletes to bony stress injuries. Stress fractures are associated with lower fat intake, lower calorie intake, eating disorders, and body weight of less than 75% of ideal body weight. The female athlete triad (menstrual irregularity, inadequate caloric intake, and decreased bone mineral density) has been associated with increased susceptibility to stress fractures. This increased risk is most commonly seen among female distance runners and military recruits and is increased compared with males performing the same activities [13]. High-intensity training may suppress menses, which may exacerbate these risk factors [10].

Muscle fatigue may be a collaborative culprit in the development of stress fractures in overtrained athletes. Since the late twentieth century, it has been widely accepted that neuromuscular conditioning plays a significant role in enhancing the shock-absorbing and energy-dissipating function of muscles to the ground reaction forces occurring during impact loading. This neuromuscular tone is able to decrease the amount of energy being directly absorbed by the bones and joints [14]. Thus, as muscles fatigue, they are less apt to dissipate the applied external forces, allowing for more rapid accumulation of microtrauma to the bone [3]. A recent study of female track-and-field/cross-country runners indicated an increased risk of developing stress fractures if body mass index (BMI) was less than 19. The authors of this case series found that female athletes with BMI of 19 or lower took significantly longer to return to unrestricted training and competition than those with a BMI above 19 [15, 16]. The authors further suggested that decreased muscle mass is a risk factor for stress injuries and poor healing [15, 16].

15.2.3 The Male Endurance Athlete Tetrad

Recent literature suggests that male runners may also be predisposed to decreased bone mineral density [10]. This has been shown to be most notable in the lumbar spine and radius. The cause of this decreased density is most likely multifactorial. Inadequate caloric intake, decreased testosterone levels, and a genetic predilection are suspected to be the main culprits. Decreased energy availability may be the key factor for low bone mineral density, and decreased testosterone levels have been shown to be present in males who participate in prolonged endurance events. To prevent severe or irreversible effects of low bone mineral density, it is necessary to assess the nutritional behaviors of male endurance athletes as well as their female counterparts.

15.3 Pathophysiology

Healthy bone is constantly in balanced homeostasis between microcrack creation and repair. The key modifiable risk factors in the development of overuse injuries of bone relate to the preparticipation condition of the bone and the frequency, duration, and intensity of the causative activity [17]. Without preconditioning and acclimation to a particular activity, athletes are at significantly increased risk for the development of overuse and fatigue-related injuries of bone [18, 19]. Repeated episodes of bone strain can result in the accumulation of enough microdamage to become a clinically symptomatic stress reaction or stress fracture [2–4]. Fatigue failure of bone has three stages: crack initiation, crack propagation, and complete fracture.

Crack initiation typically occurs at sites of stress concentration during bone loading [3]. Stress concentration occurs at sites of differential bone consistency such as the lacunae or canuliculi [3]. Initiation of the microcrack alone is not sufficient to cause a symptomatic fracture. It is the first step in bone remodeling and may serve to increase bone density and strength. Crack propagation occurs if loading continues at a frequency or intensity above the level at which new bone can be laid down and microcracks repaired. Propagation, or extension of a microcrack, typically occurs along the cement lines of the bone and is considered pathologic. Continued loading and crack propagation allows for the coalescence of multiple cracks to the point of becoming a clinically symptomatic stress fracture [3]. If the loading episodes are not modified or the reparative response is not increased, crack propagation can continue until a complete fracture occurs [3, 20].

15.4 Clinical Presentation

Pain that is initially present only during activity is common in patients presenting with a stress fracture. Symptom onset is usually insidious, and typically patients cannot recall a specific injury or trauma to the affected area. If activity level is not decreased or modified, symptoms persist or worsen. Those who continue to train without modification of their activities may develop pain with normal daily activity and potentially sustain a complete fracture [4].

Physical examination reveals reproducible point tenderness with direct palpation of the affected bone site. There may or may not be swelling or a palpable soft tissue or bone reaction. Physical examination tests commonly used for assessing for stress fractures include the fulcrum test for long bones (Fig. 15.2a, b) where a

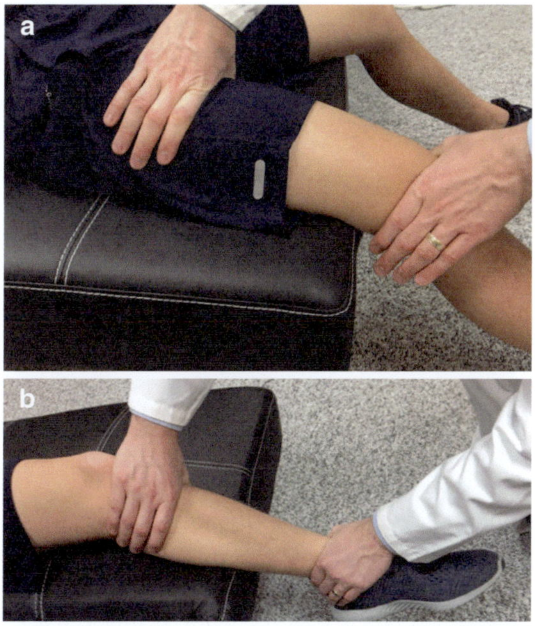

Fig. 15.2 Fulcrum test of the long bones. (**a**) Femoral shaft fulcrum test. (**b**) Tibial shaft fulcrum test

3-point bending moment is applied to a long bone and the single leg stance and hop tests (Fig. 15.3) for evaluating pelvic and lower extremity stress injuries [7, 21]. The tuning fork test for identifying sites of bone stress fractures has not been shown to be adequately sensitive or specific and should not be relied upon routinely [7, 22].

15.5 Radiologic Evaluation

15.5.1 Radiographs

Radiographs are most often negative early in the course of a stress fracture, especially in the first 2–3 weeks [23, 24]. As healing progresses, radiographic findings may be subtle and easily overlooked if the images are not thoroughly evaluated. Two-thirds of radiographs are initially normal, but about half ultimately provide evidence of a bony stress injury as healing progresses

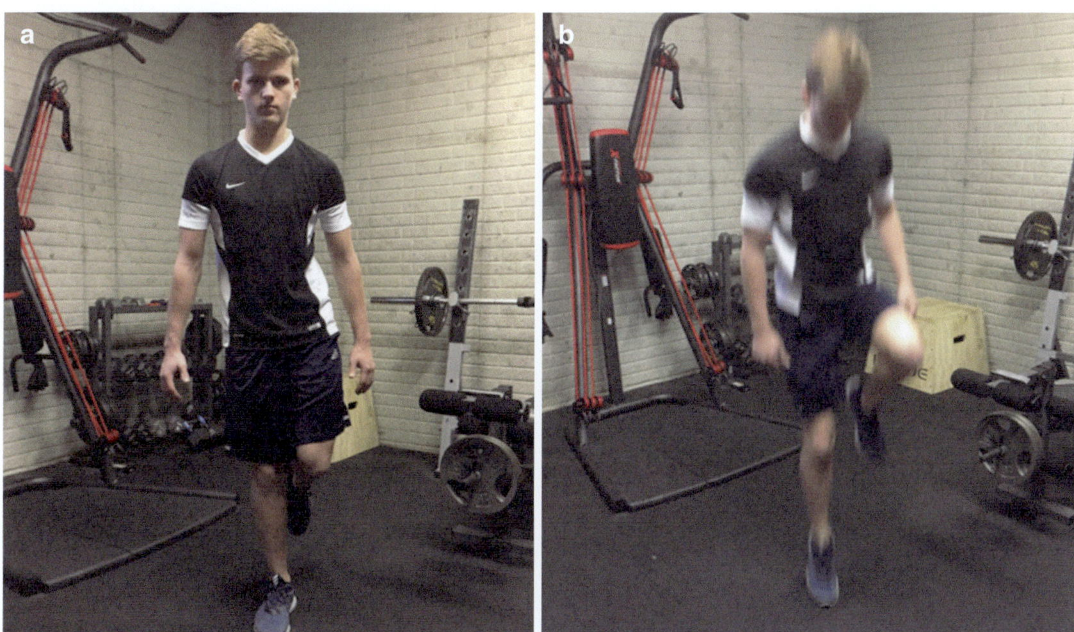

Figs. 15.3 (**a–c**) Soccer goalie demonstrates single leg stance and hop tests

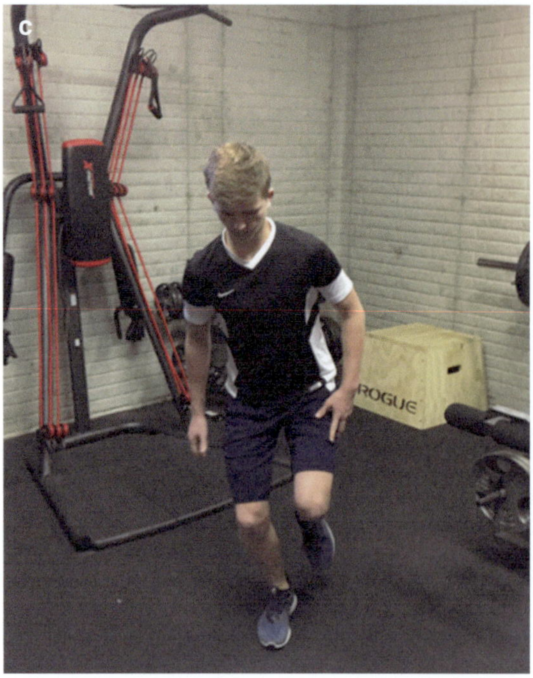

Fig.15.3 (continued)

(Fig. 15.4a) [25]. This makes plain radiographs specific but not sensitive for identifying and categorizing stress fractures.

15.5.2 Bone Scintigraphy

Bone scintigraphy has been shown to be nearly 100% sensitive for bony stress injuries, although it has a lower specificity than MRI [26]. It is especially useful for identifying rib, pelvic, femoral, pelvic, tibial, and tarsal stress fractures. Bone scans are typically positive in all phases of a triple-phase technetium scan (angiogram, blood pool, delayed). This allows for easier differentiation of stress fractures from periostitis, or medial tibial stress syndrome (shin splints), as periostitis is often negative in the angiogram and blood pool phases and positive in the delayed image phase. Medial tibial stress syndrome has also been shown to have a more diffuse distribution along the medial border of the tibia as opposed to a

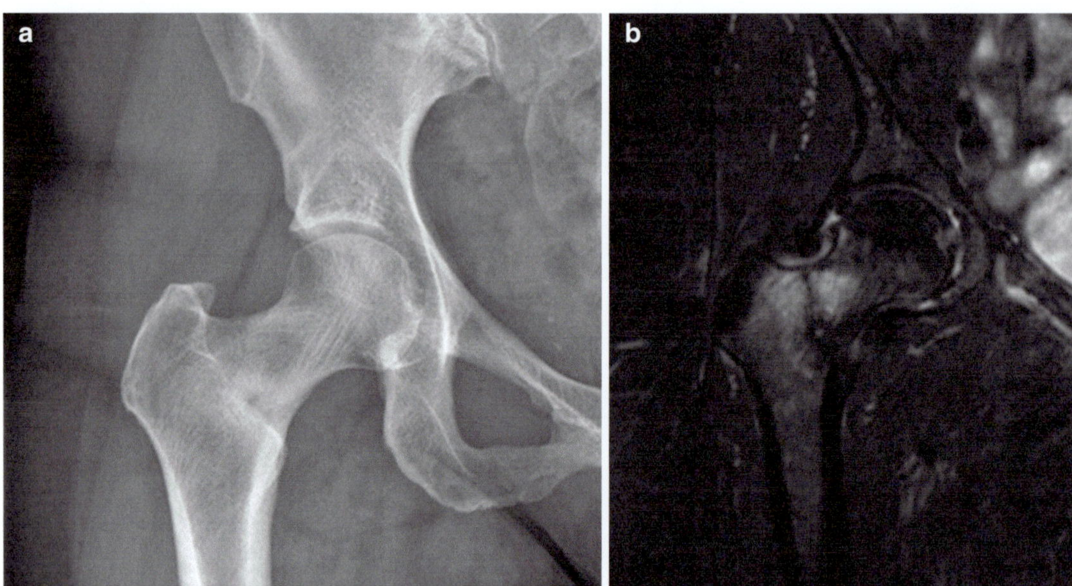

Fig. 15.4 (**a**) Anteroposterior radiograph of the hip in a 47-year-old female marathon runner with tension side femoral neck stress fracture with early callus formation. (**b**) T2 coronal MRI demonstrating nondisplaced transcervical femoral neck stress fracture in a 47-year-old female marathon runner

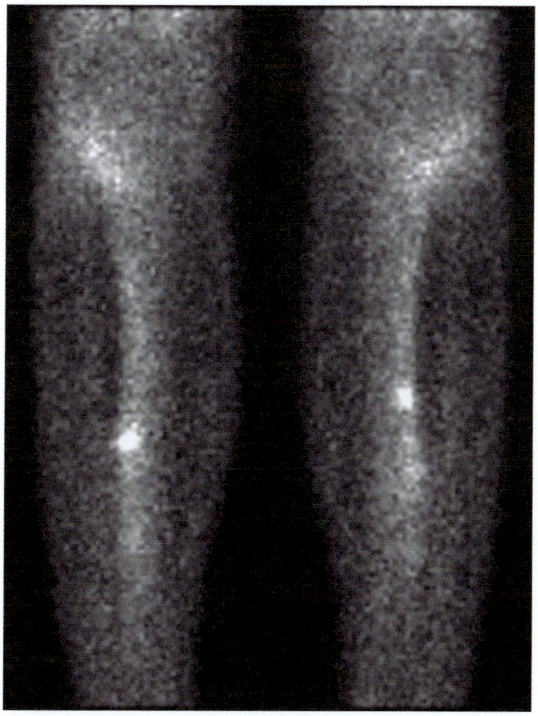

Fig. 15.5 Bone scan of bilateral tibias of a 19-year-old female college basketball player with multiple stress fractures of the bilateral anterior tibial diaphyses

focal "hotspot" indicating a stress fracture [27]. The greatest value of bone scintigraphy is its ability to diagnose multiple stress injuries. Bone scans will often demonstrate increased uptake in the affected bone 1–2 weeks before radiographic changes occur (Fig. 15.5). However, given that uptake on bone scan requires 12–18 months to normalize, bone scintigraphy is less helpful for guiding return to sports participation [26].

15.5.3 Computed Tomography (CT Scan)

In the setting of a chronic stress fracture, computed tomography scan is beneficial for demonstrating evidence of healing by clearly showing the presence or absence of a nonunion [28, 29]. CT scan delineates bone well and is of high utility for

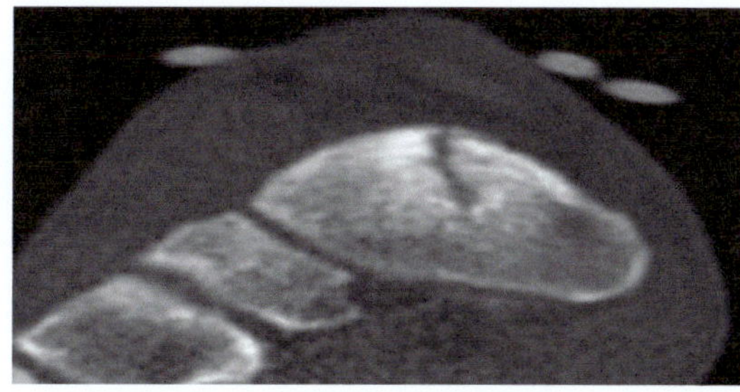

Fig. 15.6 Coronal CT scan demonstrating sagittal dorsal navicular stress fracture

determining if the fracture is complete or incomplete [29]. It is of particular use in the case of tarsal navicular stress fractures (Fig. 15.6) and for stress injuries of the pars interarticularis [30].

15.5.4 Magnetic Resonance Imaging (MRI)

In 2018, magnetic resonance imaging is the gold standard for diagnosing and classifying bony stress injuries. It has demonstrated superior sensitivity and specificity to bone scan and CT for associated soft tissue abnormalities and may delineate injury earlier than bone scan [26]. Typical MRI findings on T2 sequences include a band of low signal corresponding to the fracture line, surrounded by diffuse high signal intensity representing marrow edema (Fig. 15.4b) [31]. Its sensitivity is similar to that of a bone scan, and it is much more precise in delineating the anatomic location, acuity, and extent of a bony injury [26]. It has additionally shown prognostic ability regarding time to healing a stress fracture and time to return to sports [15, 16].

15.5.5 Classification/Grading

Stress fractures are classified in a variety of ways [32]. They are most commonly categorized by the size of the fracture line, the anatomic site of injury, the biologic healing potential of the injury

Table 15.2 Kaeding-Miller stress fracture classification system—shown is a combined clinical and radiographic classification system for stress fractures that has shown high intra- and inter-observer reliability and prognostic ability for healing

Grade	Pain	Radiographic findings (CT, MRI, bone scan or X-ray)
I	–	Imaging evidence of stress FX *No* fracture line
II	+	Imaging evidence of stress FX *No* fracture line
III	+	Nondisplaced fracture line
IV	+	Displaced fracture (>2 mm)
V	+	Nonunion

Table 15.3 Anatomic sites for high-risk stress fractures [6]

• Femoral neck (tension side)
• Patella (tension side)
• Anterior tibial cortex
• Medial malleolus
• Talar neck
• Dorsal tarsal navicular cortex
• 5th metatarsal proximal metaphysis
• Sesamoids of great toe

location, the natural history of the particular fracture, or a combination of these features [1–7, 31]. Multiple authors have advocated classifying stress fractures as either "high-risk" or "low-risk." [3–6] High-risk sites have at least one of the following characteristics: relative avascularity with or without retrograde blood supply and high tensile forces [7, 32]. These characteristics increase the risk of delayed or nonunion, refracture, and significant long-term consequences if a complete fracture occurs including avascular necrosis.

In addition to determining the risk level of a stress fracture, the extent of the fatigue failure or "grade" of the injury is necessary to describe and treat it [1, 4, 31]. A combined clinical and radiographic classification system developed by the authors of this chapter is shown in Table 15.2. This system has shown high inter- and intra-observer reliability among sports medicine and orthopedic clinicians [1]. Additionally, this system has been shown to have high prognostic ability for time to healing and return to sports participation [3, 4, 15, 16]. The recommended treatment algorithm included in this chapter is based on the Kaeding-Miller classification system for stress fractures.

15.6 Risk Assessment

15.6.1 High-Risk, Intermediate-Risk, and Low-Risk Stress Fractures

Low-risk stress fractures include the distal femur, the medial tibia, the ribs, the ulnar shaft, and the first through fourth metatarsals, all of which have a consistent blood supply and favorable natural history. These sites tend to be on the compressive side of the bone and respond well to activity modification. Low-risk stress fractures are less likely to recur, develop nonunion, or have a significant complication should they progress to complete fracture [5].

Intermediate-risk stress fractures are those that occur near a high-risk site but have a favorable healing potential and biomechanical forces acting on them. Anatomic sites included in this group are the inferior surface of the femoral neck, the proximal femoral shaft, the inferior pubic ramus, and the pars intra-articularis. Rarely do these sites require surgical stabilization to allow healing, but given their biomechanical features and proximity to high-risk sites, they have an increased potential to extend into a high-risk site if the fracture propagates.

Table 15.3 presents a list of anatomic locations considered high risk for stress fracture propagation along with their recommended treatment strategies. A delay in treatment for a high-risk site may prolong the patient's period of complete rest and potentially alter the treatment strategy to include surgical fixation with or without bone grafting. Due to their location on the tension side of their respective bones, these fractures possess biomechanical properties that predispose them to propagation of the fracture line. In comparison to low-risk stress fractures, high-risk injuries are not likely to heal without complete rest and surgical stabilization. With less aggressive treatment, high-risk stress fractures tend to progress to nonunion or complete fracture, require operative management, and recur in the same location [3, 4, 6].

15.6.2 Management of High-Risk Stress Fractures

Treatment decision-making for high-risk stress fractures should be based on radiographic findings with less consideration given to symptom severity. The immediate goal of treatment of a high-risk stress fracture is to avoid propagation of the fracture. Typically this requires either limited resistance, protected weight-bearing, or surgical stabilization. Ideally while the fracture is healing, a balance is maintained between the athlete maintaining fitness and minimizing the risk of fracture progression. While overtreatment of a low-risk stress fracture may result in unnecessary deconditioning and loss of playing time, undertreatment of a high-risk injury puts the athlete at risk of significant long-term complications.

The presence of a visible fracture line on a plain radiograph in a high-risk stress fracture should prompt serious consideration for surgical stabilization. Depending on injury severity, patients with stress injuries in high-risk locations may require immediate immobilization and/or restriction from weight-bearing activities with close monitoring. If an incomplete fracture is present on plain radiographs with evidence of fracture on MRI or CT in a high-risk location, immobilization and strict non-weight-bearing is indicated. Worsening symptoms or radiographic evidence of fracture progression despite non-operative treatment is an indication for operative treatment. All complete fractures at high-risk sites should receive serious consideration for surgical treatment. In general, a low threshold for surgical fixation should be maintained for high-risk stress fractures for several reasons. These include expediting healing, allowing earlier return to activity, and minimizing the risk of delayed union and refracture. In the case of a tension-sided femoral neck stress fracture (Fig. 15.4a, b), urgent surgical intervention may be necessary to prevent a catastrophic fracture (Fig. 15.7) [6, 7, 21].

15.6.3 Management of Low-Risk Stress Fractures

Low-risk stress fractures may be treated most often with relative rest and activity modification.

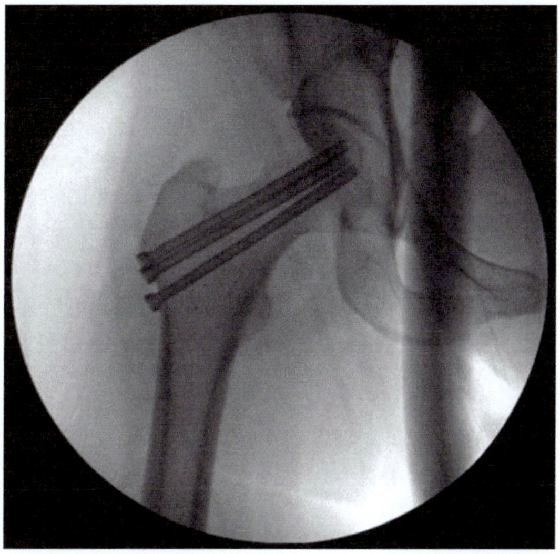

Fig. 15.7 Fluoroscopic radiographic image of the right hip following closed reduction and percutaneous screw fixation of a femoral neck stress fracture

Decision-making should be based in part on symptom severity. Those who experience enough pain to limit function should be treated with relative, if not complete, rest. The decision to continue activity despite the presence of a low-risk stress fracture and titrate the volume of activity to a low but functional pain level can be made after a discussion with the athlete. A key point in this discussion is the possibility of progression to a complete fracture with this approach. If the goal is not to continue activity but to completely heal the fracture, then rest to a pain-free level is required before return to athletic participation. Unless otherwise contraindicated, a patient may be permitted to maintain fitness by cross-training during this time with low-impact alternatives such as cycling, swimming, elliptical, antigravity treadmill, or aquatic running.

15.7 Insufficiency Fractures

A distinction should be made between stress fractures and insufficiency fractures although they are not mutually exclusive. Both are the result of the loss of balance between the creation and repair of microdamage in bone. A stress fracture is the result of high loads placed on relatively normal bone, whereas an insufficiency fracture is the result of normal loads placed on bone with decreased osseous density or impaired healing capacity [33]. Insufficiency fractures occur most commonly in elderly females but may occur in athletes with malabsorption conditions of the gastrointestinal tract. An example of a subchondral insufficiency fracture of the medial femoral condyle is shown along with an intraoperative fluoroscopic image posttreatment with intraosseous bioplasty procedure (Fig. 15.8a, b).

15.8 Return to Sports Participation

For most athletes, return to sports should only be allowed after proper treatment and complete healing of a stress fracture. Given the heterogeneity of these injuries, however, the time to return is difficult to predict. The Kaeding-Miller classification system presented in Table 15.2 has shown the ability to predict the expected time to return to athletic activity with the average to time to return to competitive running being 11–14 weeks with female athletes requiring greater time to return to sports [15, 16, 18].

The majority of early stress reactions at high-risk sites heal with non-operative management [6]. The key difference between a low-grade stress fracture at a high-risk location and a low-risk location is that with the low-risk site, the athlete may be allowed to continue to train, whereas the high-risk injury requires complete healing prior to return to unrestricted activity. Regardless of the grade and location, the risk of continued participation should be discussed with each athlete, and the management of each fracture should be individualized. Cross-training while resting from the inciting activity allows maintenance of cardiovascular fitness while decreasing tensile, bending, and rotational forces at the healing fracture site [3, 7, 21, 34]. Return to participation should be a joint decision between the physician, athletic trainer, coach, and athlete.

15.9 Prevention of Stress Injuries to Bone

Prevention is the ideal treatment of stress injuries of bone and most other overuse injuries. An assessment of the athlete's risk should be made at pre-participation evaluations, especially in those with a history of previous stress fractures women with light or absent menses [2, 12, 21]. Correction of amenorrhea in females and calcium and Vitamin D_3 supplementation is recommended in addition to general nutritional optimization. If biomechanical abnormalities are encountered, the use of appropriately designed orthotic devices should be considered as an initial corrective measure. However, running gait analysis (Fig. 15.9) and appropriate running form or technique changes may be necessary to prevent future injuries. Unfit or unconditioned athletes including military recruits, particularly female athletes with menstrual irregularities, are at peak risk for stress injuries to bone and increased utilization of healthcare resources [18].

15.10 Biologic Healing Enhancement

15.10.1 Electrical Osseous Stimulation

Recent technological developments have given rise to the use of biologic treatment modalities for stress injuries to bone. These include the use of electronic bone stimulators, pulsed parathyroid hormone (teriparatide), subchondroplasty, and concentrated bone marrow aspirate. Pulsed electromagnetic fields (PEMF) and low-intensity pulsed ultrasound (LIPU) are FDA-approved, noninvasive tools which increase the production of regulatory mediators required for physiological bone healing [35]. PEMF creates a magnetic field and a secondary electric impulse activating a series of enzyme reactions that upregulate growth factors such as bone morphogenetic proteins, transforming growth factor-β, and calmodulin

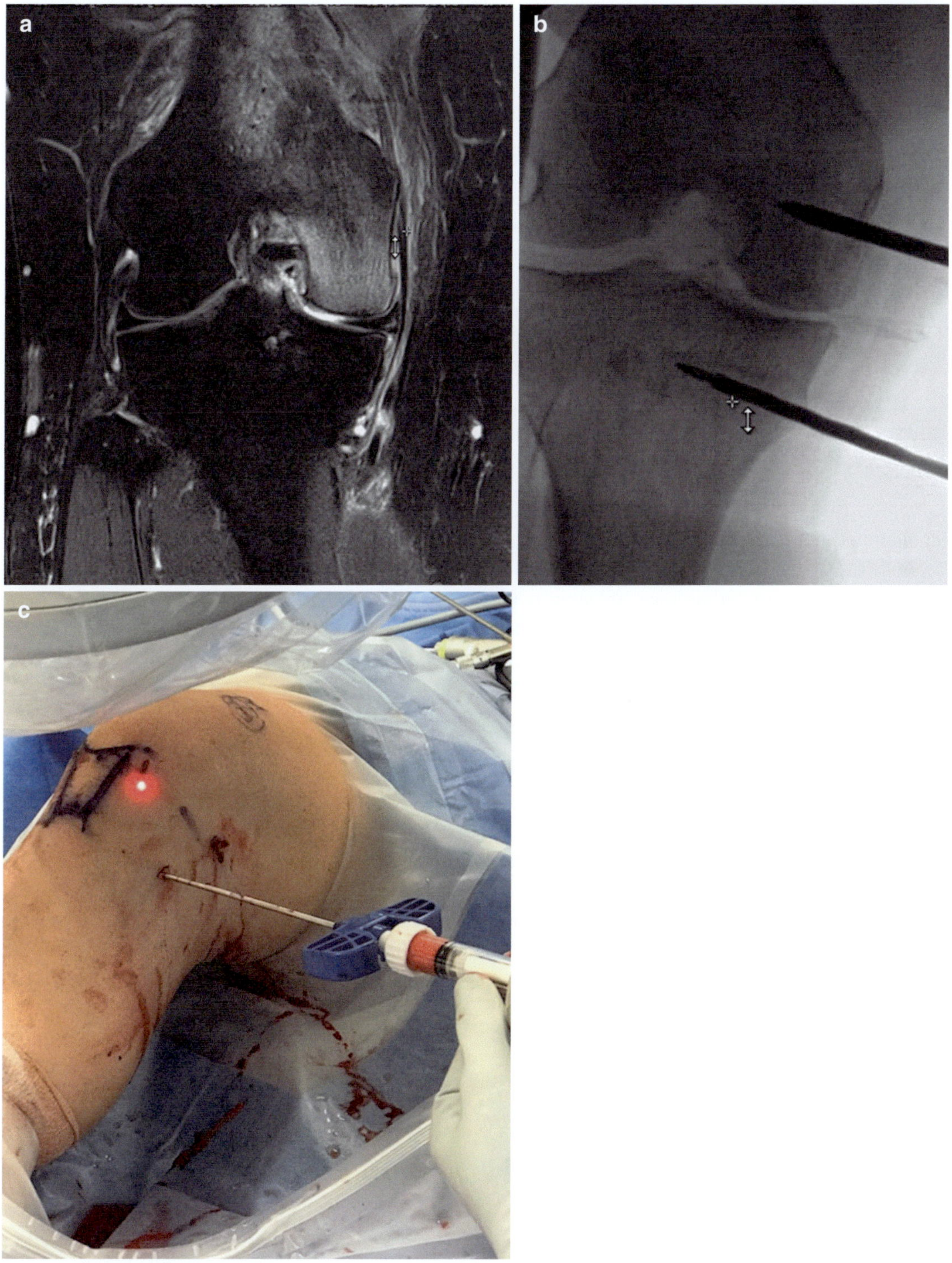

Fig. 15.8 (**a**) T2 coronal MRI demonstrating subchondral insufficiency fracture of the medial femoral condyle. (**b**) Intraoperative fluoroscopic radiograph during intraosseous bioplasty of the medial femoral condyle and medial tibial plateau. (**c**) Intraosseous bioplasty performed at the medial proximal tibia. Mixture of demineralized bone matrix and concentrated bone marrow aspirate is injected after core decompression has been completed

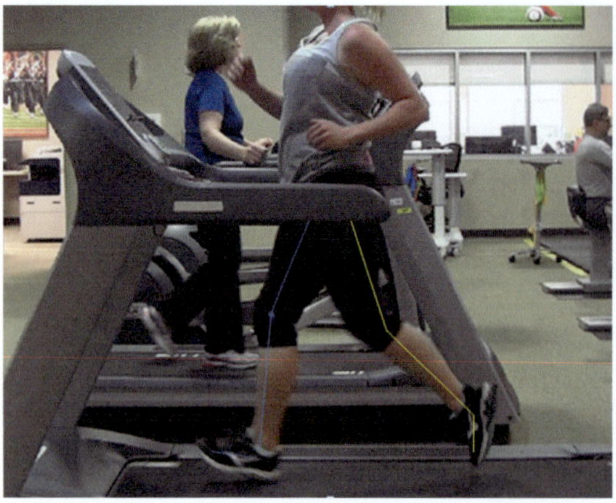

Fig. 15.9 Video running gait analysis performed on a 29-year-old female runner with recurrent tibial stress fractures

leading to bone cell proliferation and fracture healing. LIPU appears to have a direct effect on ion channels for stimulating bone cell activity via mechanoreceptors [36]. Bone stimulators have been shown to be the most effective for delayed unions of the tibial shaft and fifth metatarsal shaft.

15.10.2 Parathyroid Hormone Stimulation

The effect of teriparatide on fracture healing has been evaluated with mixed results. However, teriparatide has been shown to achieve the primary endpoint of accelerated healing with improved early fracture callus formation compared to placebo [37]. Preclinical studies on rat models have shown that supraphysiologic doses of parathyroid hormone have demonstrated increased fracture site strength and callus quantity, with greater mineralization at the fracture site [37, 38].

15.10.3 Subchondroplasty and Intraosseous Bioplasty

Subchondroplasty is a recently developed procedure for increasing the density and structural integrity of subchondral bone. This surgical technique is performed by drilling into subchondral bone with a cannulated guide pin. Under fluoroscopy engineered calcium phosphate paste is injected into subchondral bony defects forming a macroporous scaffold for bone. Its application includes the treatment of subchondral insufficiency fractures most commonly of the distal femur and proximal tibia (Fig. 15.8b) [39]. Initial short-term results of the procedure have shown that it provides significant improvement in the parameters of pain and functional capacity over the first 24 weeks following surgery [40]. Intraosseous bioplasty involves percutaneously performing a core decompression of the affected metaphyseal bone site and injecting a mixture of bone marrow concentrate, calcium chloride clot, and demineralized bone matrix (Fig. 15.8c). Long-term results of these treatment options are currently being investigated.

15.10.4 Bone Marrow Aspirate Concentrate (BMAC)

Bone marrow aspirate concentrate is a biologic treatment employing an individual's own stem cells to stimulate bony healing. Osteoblastic progenitor cells are available in the bone marrow aspirate of the iliac crest, proximal aspect of the tibia, and calcaneus. The iliac crest provides the highest yield of osteoblastic progenitor cells though it can be extracted locally from other sites including the proximal tibial metaphysis (Fig. 15.10) [41]. Percutaneous screw fixation of proximal fifth metatarsal fractures augmented with bone marrow aspirate concentrate has been shown to provide predictable healing results while permitting athletes a return to sports at their previous levels of competition with few complications [42]. Autologous BMAC combined with PRP injection has been shown to improve bone healing in distraction osteogenesis of the tibia [43]. The local application of BMAC in the treatment of delayed healing is a promising alternative to autogenous bone grafting and may help to reduce donor site morbidity [44].

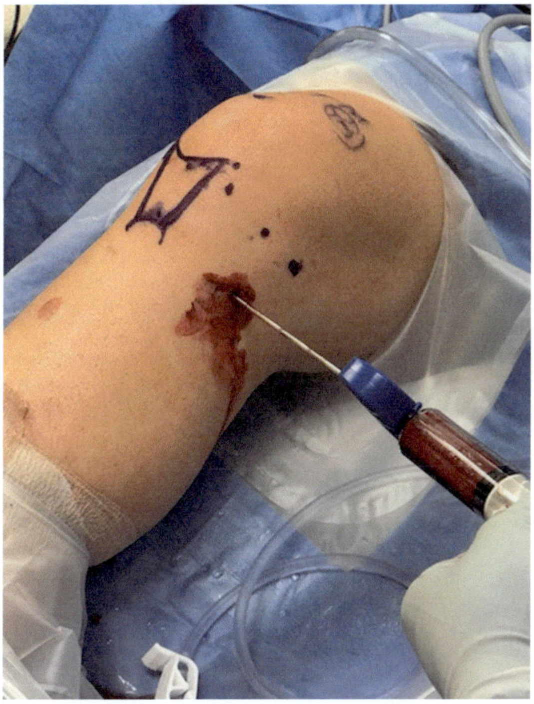

Fig. 15.10 Aspiration of bone marrow concentrate from the medial proximal tibial metaphysis

15.11 Summary

Stress fractures are common injuries particularly in endurance athletes and military recruits. The diagnosis can be made if a high index of suspicion is maintained and the proper imaging studies are obtained. The Kaeding-Miller classification system for stress fractures characterizes these injuries based on the patient's symptoms as well as their position on a radiologic continuum of severity. A holistic approach to treatment that takes into account the importance of nutritional, hormonal, psychologic, and biomechanical factors is necessary for treatment success. Stress fracture management should be individualized to the patient or athlete by taking into consideration injury site (low versus high risk), grade (extent of microdamage accumulation), the individual's activity level, competitive situation, and risk tolerance. High-risk stress fractures are primarily loaded in tension, have a poor natural history, and commonly require surgical intervention. Low-risk fractures are most often those loaded in compression, have a better prognosis, and are unlikely to progress to complete fracture. The recommended treatment algorithm stratifies these injuries based upon injury severity and the biomechanical environment in which they are located. In addition to the traditional treatment strategies of rest, immobilization, and surgical stabilization, recent modalities for enhancing healing potential have been utilized with some success from further research being required to fully confirm their efficacy.

References

1. Kaeding CC, Miller TL. The comprehensive description of stress fractures: a new classification system. J Bone Joint Surg. 2013;95(13):1214–20.
2. Kaeding CC, Yu JR, Wright R, et al. Management and return to play of stress fractures. Clin J Sport Med. 2005;15(6):442–7.
3. Kaeding CC, Spindler KP, Amendola A. Management of troublesome stress fractures. Am Acad Orthop Surg Instr Course Lect. 2004;53:455–69.
4. Kaeding CC, Najarian R. Stress fractures—classification and management. Phys SportsMED. 2010;38(3):45–54.
5. Boden BP, Osbahr DC, Jimenez C. Low-risk stress fractures. Am J Sports Med. 2001;29(1):100–11.
6. Boden BP. High-risk stress fractures: evaluation and treatment. J Am Acad Orthop Surg. 2000;8:344–53.
7. McInnis KC, Ramey LN. High-risk stress fractures: diagnosis and management. PMR. 2016;8(3 Suppl):S113–24.
8. Lappe J, Cullen D, Haynatzki G, Recker R, Ahlf R, Thompson K. Calcium and vitamin D supplementation decreases incidence of stress fractures in female navy recruits. J Bone Miner Res. 2008;23(5):741–9.
9. Pouilles JM, Bernard J, Tremollières F, Louvet JP, Ribot C. Femoral bone density in young male adults with stress fractures. J Bone. 1989;10:105–8.
10. Rettig AC, Shelbourne KD, McCarroll JR, Bisesi M, Watts J. The natural history and treatment of delayed union stress fractures of the anterior cortex of the tibia. Am J Sports Med. 1988;16(3):250–5.
11. Brukner P, Bennell K, Matheson G. Stress fractures of the trunk. In: Brukner P, editor. Stress fractures. Victoria: Blackwell Science; 1999. p. 119–38.
12. Tenforde AS, Carlson JL, Chang A, Sainani KL, Shultz R, Kim JH, Cutti P, Golden NH, Fredericson M. Association of the female athlete triad risk assessment stratification to the development of bone stress injuries in collegiate athletes. Am J Sports Med. 2017;45(2):302–10.

13. Eller DJ, Katz DS, Bergman AG, et al. Sacral stress fractures in long-distance runners. Clin J Sport Med. 1997;7:222–5.
14. Jones BH, Harris JM, Vinh TN, Rubin C. Exercise-induced stress fractures and stress reactions of bone: epidemiology, etiology, and classification. Exerc Sport Sci Rev. 1989;17:379–422.
15. Jamieson M, Everson S, Siegel C, Miller TL. Expected time to return to athletic participation following stress fracture in division I collegiate athletes. Sport Health. 2018;10(4):340–4.
16. Jamieson M, Schroeder A, Day J, et al. Time to return to running after tibial stress fracture in female division I collegiate track and field. Currt Orthop Pract. 2017;31(4):393–7.
17. Hosey RG, Fernandez MM, Johnson DL. Evaluation and management of stress fractures of the pelvis and sacrum. Orthopedics. 2008;31(4):383–5.
18. Krauss MR, Garvin NU, Boivin MR, Cowan DN. Excess stress fractures, musculoskeletal injuries, and health care utilization among unfit and overweight female army trainees. Am J Sports Med. 2017;45(2):311–6.
19. Miller TL, Harris JD, Kaeding CC. Stress fractures of the ribs and upper extremities: causation, evaluation, and management. Sports Med. 2013;43(8):665–74.
20. Bennell K, Brukner P. Epidemiology and site specificity of stress fractures. Clin Sports Med. 1997;16:179–96.
21. Miller TL, Best TM. Taking a holistic approach to managing difficult stress fractures. J Orthop Surg Res. 2016;11(1):98.
22. Toney CM, Games KE, Winkelmann ZK, Eberman LE. Using tuning-fork tests in diagnosing fractures. J Athl Train. 2016;51(6):498–9.
23. Coughlin MJ, Grimes JS, Traughber PD, Jones CP. Comparison of radiographs and CT scans in the prospective evaluation of the fusion of hindfoot arthrodesis. Foot Ankle Int. 2006;27(10):780–7.
24. Wall J, Feller JF. Imaging of stress fractures in runners. Clin Sports Med. 2006;25(4):781–802.
25. Brukner P, Bradshaw C, Khan KM, White S, Crossley K. Stress fractures: a review of 180 cases. Clin J Sport Med. 1996;6(2):85–9.
26. Dobrindt O, Hoffmeyer B, Ruf J, Seidensticker M, Steffen IG, Zarva A, Fischbach F, Wieners G, Furth C, Lohmann CH, et al. MRI versus bone scintigraphy. Evaluation for diagnosis and grading of stress injuries. Nuklearmedizin. 2012;51(3):88–94.
27. Dutton J. Clinical value of grading the scintigraphic appearances of tibial stress fractures in military recruits. Clin Nucl Med. 2002;27(1):18–21.
28. Gaeta M, Minutoli F, Vinci S, Salamone I, D'Andrea L, Bitto L, Magaudda L, Blandino A. High-resolution CT grading of tibial stress reactions in distance runners. Am J Roentgenol. 2006;187:789–93.
29. Bradshaw C, Khan K, Brukner P. Stress fracture of the body of the talus in athletes demonstrated with computer tomography. Clin J Sport Med. 1996;6:48–51.
30. Standaert CJ. Spondylolysis in the adolescent athlete. Clin J Sport Med. 2002;12(2):119–22.
31. Arendt EA, Griffiths HJ. The use of MR imaging in the assessment and clinical management of stress reactions of bone in high-performance athletes. Clin Sports Med. 1997;16:291–306.
32. Miller T, Kaeding CC, Flanigan D. The classification systems of stress fractures: a systematic review. Phys Sportsmed. 2011;39(1):93–100.
33. Cabarrus MC, Ambekar A, Lu Y, Link TM. MRI and CT of insufficiency fractures of the pelvis and the proximal femur. AJR Am J Roentgenol. 2008;191(4):995–1001.
34. Jensen J. Stress fracture in the world class athlete: a case study. Med Sci Sports Exerc. 1998;30: 783–7.
35. Longhino V, Bonora C, Sansone V. The management of sacral stress fractures: current concepts. Clin Cases Miner Bone Metab. 2011;8(3):19–23.
36. Massar L, Caruso G, Sollazzo V, Setti S. Pulsed electromagnetic fields and low intensity pulsed ultrasound in bone tissue. Clin Cases Miner Bone Metab. 2009;6(2):149–54.
37. Aspenberg P, Johansson T. Teriparatide improves early callus formation in distal radial fractures. Acta Orthop. 2010;81(2):234–6.
38. O'Loughlin PF, Cunningham ME, Bukata SV, et al. Parathyroid hormone (1-34) augments spinal fusion, fusion mass volume, and fusion mass quality in a rabbit spinal fusion model. Spine. 2009;34(2): 121–30.
39. Cohen SB, Sharkey PF. Subchondroplasty for the treating bone marrow lesions. J Knee Surg. 2016;29(7):555–63.
40. Bonadio MB, Giglio PN, Helito CP, et al. Subchondroplasty for treating bone marrow lesions in the knee—initial experience. Rev Bras Ortop. 2017;52(3):325–30.
41. Hyer CF, Berlet GC, Bussewitz BW, Hankins T, Ziegler HL, Philbin TM. Quantitative assessment of the yield of osteoblastic connective tissue progenitors in bone marrow aspirate from the iliac crest, tibia, and calcaneus. J Bone Joint Surg Am. 2013;95(14):1312–6.
42. Murawski CD, Kennedy JG. Percutaneous internal fixation of proximal fifth metatarsal jones fractures (zones II and III) with Charlotte Carolina screw and bone marrow aspirate concentrate: an outcome study in athletes. Am J Sports Med. 2011;39(6): 1295–301.
43. Lee DH, Ryu KJ, Kim JW, Kang KC, Choi YR. Bone marrow aspirate concentrate and platelet-rich plasma enhanced bone healing in distraction osteogenesis of the tibia. Clin Orthop Relat Res. 2014;472(12):3789–97.
44. Jäger M, Jelinek EM, Wess KM, Scharfstädt A, Jacobson M, Kevy SV, Krauspe R. Bone marrow concentrate: a novel strategy for bone defect treatment. Curr Stem Cell Res Ther. 2009;4(1):34–43.

Shin Pain

16

Sérgio Rocha Piedade, Luis António Mendes,
Leonardo Manoel Carvalho,
Ramon Medeiros Fagundes dos Santos,
Luis Carlos Marques, and Daniel Miranda Ferreira

16.1 Introduction

Anatomically, the leg is described as the segment of the lower limb localized between the knee and ankle joint. It provides part of the bone structure of both joints and has muscles arranged in four compartments, each one of them bound by fascia, anterior, lateral, and posterior (superficial and deep) compartments [1, 2] (Fig. 16.1). Due to its anatomical location and the presence of biarticular muscles, the leg plays an essential role in daily-activity physical tasks.

In sports, the physical demands are greater compared to daily activity home, as they comprise of running, jumping/landing, changing direction, and acceleration/deceleration and impose to axial, shearing, and rotational loads to the lower limbs. Despite that, the legs are structurally highly prepared to bear the load and intensity of regular sports training as well as to provide body support, balance, and propulsion [3–6].

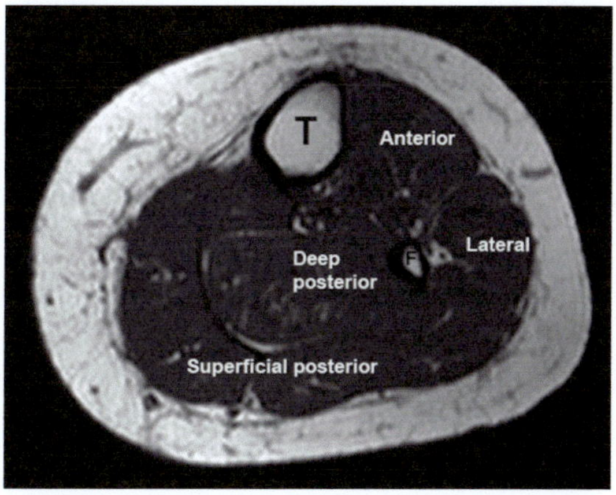

Fig. 16.1 Axial view of T1-weighted magnetic resonance image of four muscle compartments of the lower leg (*T* tibia, *F* fibula)

However, the ability of the lower limb to absorb stress can be reduced, and also impaired, by different clinical settings such as strenuous training, insufficient time of rest, inadequate sports material (shoes), axis and postural deformities **of** the knee and/or foot, as well as poor athlete's physical status. Therefore, it is easy to understand why leg pain is a common clinical complaint **in sports practice** [7, 8].

"Shin" (leg) pain, "shin splints," and medial tibial stress syndrome, are general terms used to describe pain and discomfort localized on the front outside **or** medial side of the lower leg, a

S. R. Piedade (✉) · R. M. F. dos Santos
L. C. Marques
Department of Orthopedics and Traumatology, State University of Campinas—UNICAMP, Exercise and Sports Medicine, Campinas, SP, Brazil
e-mail: piedade@fcm.unicamp.br

L. A. Mendes · L. M. Carvalho
State University of Campinas—UNICAMP, Exercise and Sports Medicine, Campinas, SP, Brazil
e-mail: luiz.mendes@hc.fm.usp.br

D. M. Ferreira
Department of Radiology, State University of Campinas—UNICAMP, Exercise and Sports Medicine, Campinas, SP, Brazil

S. Rocha Piedade et al. (eds.), *The Sports Medicine Physician*,
https://doi.org/10.1007/978-3-030-10433-7_16

clinical entity that affects recreational and professional athletes, indiscriminately. A close relationship has been reported with distance runners, athletes of endurance sports, dancers, and the military, confirming the huge the influence of the physical demands (amount and intensity of load) present in these physical activities [9, 10].

Regarding risk factors, the literature has shown no influence of anthropometric characteristics and body composition on the genesis of shin pain, but extrinsic factors such as the amount of training, training surface (field), sports material (shoes), as well as intrinsic factors (athlete's phenotype and anatomy) play an essential role in shin pain development and progression [11, 12].

Although shin pain has been described as an exercise-related problem, i.e., overuse injury, it has a broad differential diagnosis, as different pathologies and structures can be implicated in clinical presentation. In this context, soft tissue inflammation (tendons, muscle, and fascia), exertional compartment syndrome, vascular deficiency, medial tibial stress syndrome, and stress fracture can be a possible diagnosis [13–16].

The aim of this chapter is to discuss athletes' complaints, intensity and load of sports training, physical and radiological assessment of different clinical problems related to shin pain symptoms (leg tendinopathies, vascular deficiency, stress fracture, and exertional compartment syndrome), and treatment approach.

16.2 Physical Assessment

Considering that shin pain could involve several conditions, the sports medicine physician should closely observe the athlete's response to the intensity and load of training as well as the periodicity of competition events, especially when he/she starts complaining about leg pain.

Like any medical problem, anamnesis plays a vital role. The previous history of MTSS, running inexperience, inappropriate sports material (shoes), high body mass index, smoking, and increased external rotation of the hip in males should be investigated as they are related to greater risk of developing MTSS [17, 18].

Therefore, the athletes' complaint and also the training program should be carefully explored during anamnesis, and the athlete should answer the following questions:

- How long have you been feeling pain and discomfort in your legs?
- Is it the first time?
- Can you pinpoint when it started?
- Are you in a regular training program?
- Do you have close supervision from a coach?
- Have you changed your training program?
- What do you think of your intensity of training?
- What are your training shoes like?
- What is the training surface like?
- How do you feel during your training?

All these questions are an important part of the strategy used to formulate the diagnosis and treatment approach.

16.3 Symptoms and Complaints

In general, shin pain primary clinical symptoms are pain and discomfort. Usually, the athlete complains about tenderness, pain, or discomfort along the inner edge of the shinbone, mainly the two-thirds below the knee joint (Fig. 16.2). Generally, the pain increases with sports activity and relieves with rest. Sometimes, shin pain comprises of redness and swelling [19, 20].

Regarding pain, it could have some particularities inherent to each clinical condition. In the exertional compartment syndrome, the pain starts 10 min after sports, followed by sensory and motor loss, and relieves with 30 min of rest. In the medial tibial stress, the pain is described as vague and diffuse, while in the tendinopathies, it is related to tendon and its movement, where the Achilles tendon, tibialis posterior, and fibular tendons are the commonly affected structures [20].

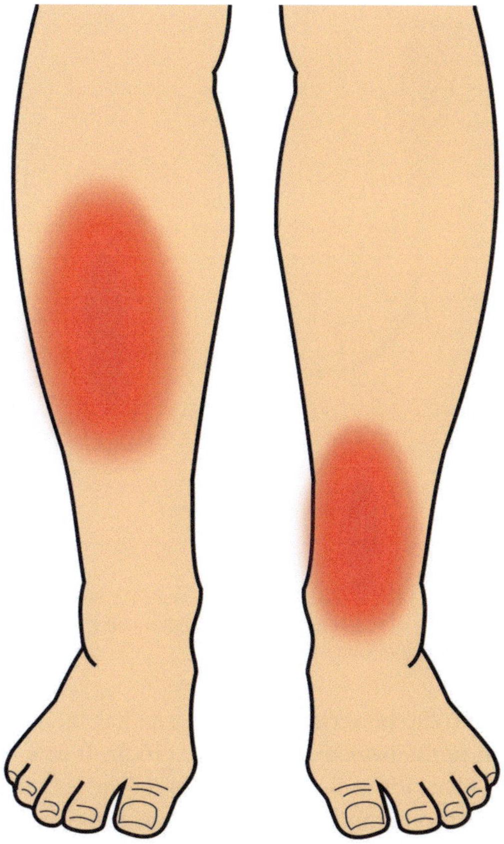

Fig. 16.2 Common shin pain sites

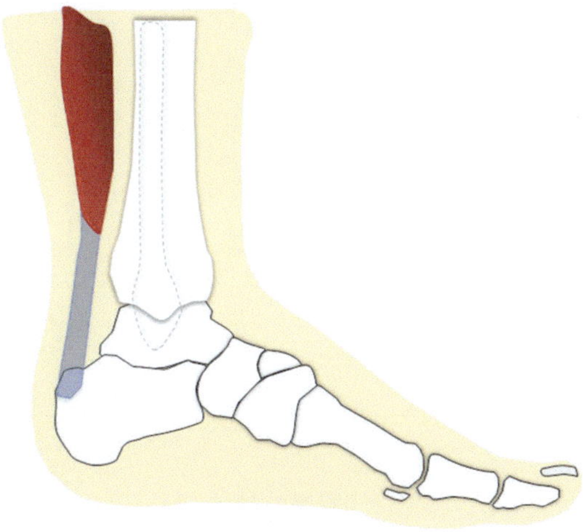

Fig. 16.3 Topography of Achilles tendon and its insertion in the calcaneus bone

16.4 Differential Diagnosis

As pointed out above, shin pain is a clinical symptom that could express different pathologies, and, therefore, it is essential to investigate carefully differential diagnoses such as tendinitis, stress fracture, tendonosis, chronic exertional compartment syndrome, and popliteal artery entrapment syndrome [9, 12, 14, 15, 19, 20].

16.4.1 Lower Leg Tendinopathy

Firstly, it should be emphasized that tendinopathy includes pathological conditions such as tendinosis and peritendinitis and is commonly associated with overuse injuries. Clinically, it can be manifested by pain, discomfort, diffuse, or localized swelling, impairing the athlete's sports performance.

Undoubtedly, Achilles tendinopathy is more prevalent than the other one, but it can also affect the anterior tibial, posterior tibial, and peroneal tendons. All of them will cause lower leg pain and discomfort according to the tendinopathy, tendon anatomy, topography, and sports dynamic performed.

16.4.2 Achilles Tendon

The Achilles tendon starts at the middle of the calf and attaches the calf (gastrocnemius and plantaris) and soleus muscles to the calcaneus bone. It is the strongest and thickest tendon but also the most often ruptured in the human body [21].

The configuration of its insertion on the calcaneus bone helps to dissipate tendon-bone stress (Fig. 16.3). The Achilles tendinitis is commonly described as a sport-related injury, touching recreational and professional athletes in more than two-thirds of cases.

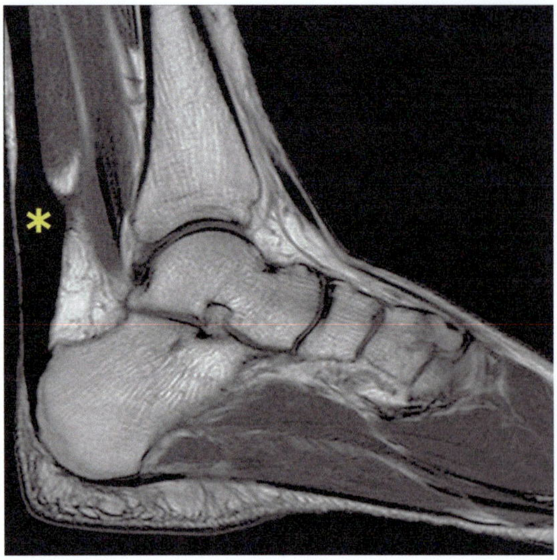

Fig. 16.4 Sagittal view of T1-weighted magnetic resonance image (MRI) of the ankle showing fusiform thickening of the Achilles tendon (tendinosis)*

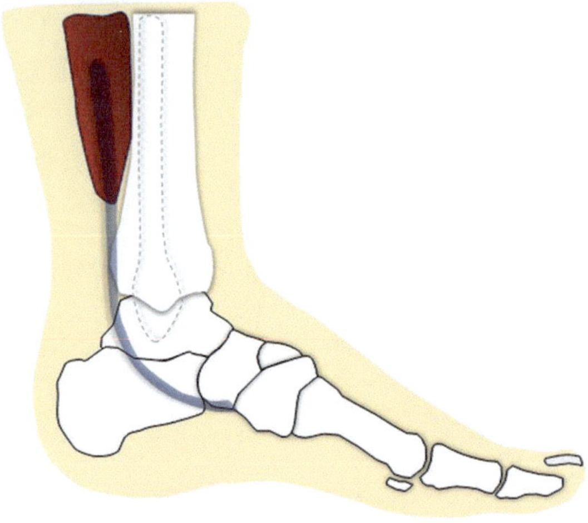

Fig. 16.5 Medial side of the ankle and foot, showing the topography of the posterior tibial tendon and its insertion in the navicular bone

Generally, athletes complain about pain and tenderness on the medial and posteriormedial aspect of the distal third of the lower leg. This pain could increase with sports practice, and during a clinical exam, it may be observed when the athlete performs plantar flexion against resistance. In chronic cases, edema, hyperemia, and decreased loss of function are gradually established. This clinical symptom is a prevalent problem in runners due to sports dynamic and effort.

The main etiological risk factors related to Achilles tendon are overuse, lower limb malalignment (genu valgum, genu varum, pes cavus, pes planovalgus), problems related to uneven and unstable training surfaces, and previous injury [22–24].

Ultrasound and MRI (Fig. 16.4) are commonly used exams in these cases as they allow, more appropriately, the visualization of soft tissues, while X-rays can be used to rule out associated injuries.

16.4.3 Posterior Tibial Tendon

The posterior tendon muscle is located on the posterior medial side of the calf, rising from the posterior rear of the tibia and fibula, and runs behind the posterior malleolus and has its insertion in the navicular bone (Fig. 16.5). It acts on the inversion and plantar flexion of the foot and plays a vital role in the maintenance of the medial arch of the foot.

The onset of tendon dysfunction is gradual and worse if the volume and intensity of sports activity remain or increase, especially in running and jumping activities [25]. In general, athletes complain about pain along the posterior tibial tendon topography until its insertion in the medial side of the foot.

In more advanced stages, the medial longitudinal arch of the foot is attenuated progressively and can disappear causing the acquired adult flatfoot, presented by a clinical sign called "too many toes". Other clinical signs are, a decreased in the movements of foot supination and eversion (Fig. 16.6).

Radiological evaluation can show a medial talar displacement and also a decrease of the medial longitudinal arch of the foot, clinical signs related to more advanced stages of tendon dysfunction. However, MRI is the best exam to evaluate the initial stages of posterior tendon tendinopathy [25–27].

In the early stages, conservative treatment offers satisfactory outcomes for most of the

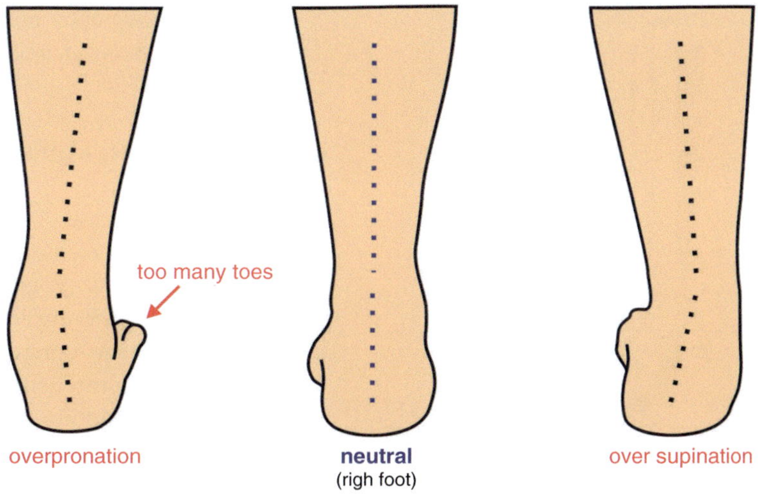

Fig. 16.6 Posterior view of the foot, showing the foot in a neutral (middle), **overpronated** (left), and over supinated (right) position

athletes. Relief of the symptoms, physiotherapy, shoe modifications, orthosis and exercise programs are part of the treatment approach. The use of orthosis aims to provide hindfoot eversion and longitudinal medial arch support and may include a heel lift if there is a gastrocnemius contracture [26–28]. Surgery is commonly performed in advanced stages of tendon dysfunction.

16.4.4 Anterior Tibial Tendon

The anterior tibial muscle starts in the two-thirds of the lateral side of the tibia and runs along to be inserted in the first cuneiform and the first metatarsal. It is responsible for foot dorsiflexion and inversion. Its tendinopathy impairs these muscle functions, and consequently, the athletes' sports performance for running, kicking, and many other sport movements decreases.

Clinically, the athlete complains of pain and discomfort as well as swelling on the medial side of the leg, following the anterior tibial tendon topography (Fig. 16.7) and can be exacerbated by active foot dorsiflexion and inversion performed against resistance.

Foot overpronation, overtraining, excessive tendon stretching, and footwear are common causes of anterior tibial tendinopathy.

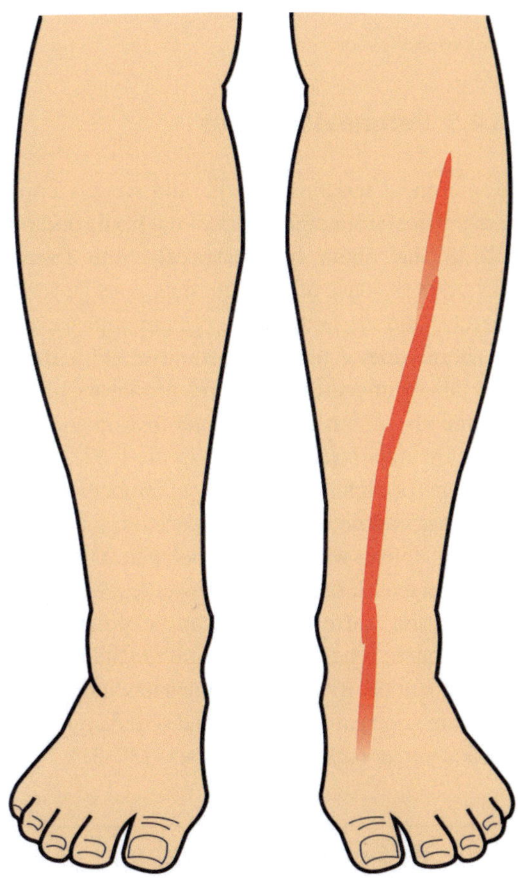

Fig. 16.7 Topography of pain and discomfort related to anterior tibial tendon tendinopathy

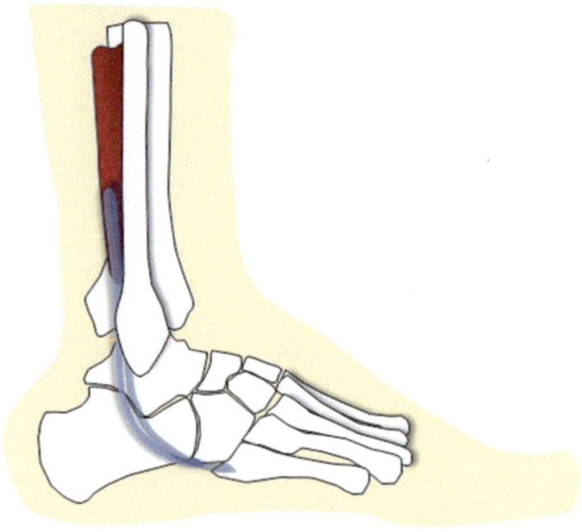

Fig. 16.8 Topography of the peroneal tendons and their insertions in the foot

16.4.5 Peroneal Tendons

The peroneal tendons, brevis, and longus come from the posterolateral aspect of the fibula and run over to the fibula tip posteriorly: the former inserted in the base of the fifth metatarsal (inferior tubercle) and the latter in the plantar superface of the lateral side of the first metatarsal (Fig. 16.8). They are primary evertors and pronators of the foot and also contribute to plantar flexion and foot and ankle stabilization against sprain [29].

The peroneal tendon injury is commonly seen in sports that impose repetitive ankle motion and also affecting athletes with a higher foot arch. The pain is located on the lateral site of the lower leg. Moreover, swelling and warm to touch can be present. The most frequent types of injuries are tendinitis, tears, and subluxation. In case of peroneal tendon instability, subluxation can be elicited and observed by foot eversion and dorsiflexion maneuvers [30, 31].

16.5 Radiological Evaluation in Tendinitis of the Lower Leg

In a complementary investigation, X-rays do not usually add more accurate information but may be useful for ruling out other diagnostic suspicions. Ultrasonography and magnetic resonance imaging are more accurate diagnostic strategies [31].

16.5.1 Treatment

As in any case of tendinopathies, with an initial phase of decreased load, followed by eccentric training with progressive loads. The use of ice and analgesic medications may be necessary for symptomatic control at the start of treatment. Sports biomechanics management and ankle alignment during gait and run should be considered because of the possibility of biomechanical errors increasing the overload on these tendons. Injection of corticosteroids is not classically indicated because of tendon rupture risk. In cases of tendon instability, surgical treatment is usually necessary [29, 30].

16.5.2 Chronic Exertional Compartment Syndrome

Chronic exertional compartment syndrome (CECS) is a relatively common condition that could touch recreational and professional athletes indistinctly. The prevalence is uncertain, and most of the athletes affected are younger than 30 years old [32]. Although several sports can be involved, running is the main sports activity related to this syndrome [1, 32]. It is defined as a recurrent and exercise-induced leg pain characterized by pain, tightness, cramp, and weakness [1, 2, 32, 33].

Many theories have been proposed for CECS pathophysiology. One of them is transient ischemia that would be caused by a greater intercompartment pressure of the lower leg induced by sports activity, impairing neuromuscular blood flow.

Although muscle volume could increase by 20% during physical activity, the compliance of muscle compartment is vital to keep ICP control. Other described theories involve muscle hypertrophy, decreased venous return, muscular microtrauma, and myopathies [1]. Moreover, Edmundsson and colleagues showed that lower capillarity related to muscle fiber could be involved in CECS's pathophysiology [34]. However, further investigation is needed to reach a consensus; the hypotheses match the patient's symptoms.

Usually, patients/athletes do not present symptoms at rest, but clinical complaints arise sometimes after physical activity and are described as full, achy cramping or pressure in the lower leg according to the compartment involved, but the pain and discomfort stop when the activity is interrupted [1, 2, 32]. The incidence is equal in both genres.

16.5.3 Physical Assessment

Physical examination and anamnesis are fundamental tools for CECS diagnosis. Although athletes could not present symptoms at rest, recurring and exercise-induced pain are clinical signs that require further assessment [32].

On the other hand, CECS could be manisfested by indirect signs even at rest such as muscle hardness and muscle hernias [2, 35]. Paresthesia, post-effort muscle weakness, and postexercise hypertrophy may also be reported. Moreover, the absence of pain during palpation at rest has been described as a signal associated with CECS.

16.5.4 Imaging Evaluation

Therapeutic approach requires imaging exams such as radiographs, bone scintigraphy, and MRI. If neurological symptoms are persistent, an electroneuromyography should be performed. Moreover, when the clinical exam is compatible, and images exclude other causes for pain, the postexercise needle manometry features could help to confirm CECS.

The measurement of ICP implies an exercise before the procedure. The exercise ought to be enough for surging symptoms. The measurement is taken in all of the leg compartments even in the absence of pain. Pedowitz and colleagues [36] have described objective diagnostic criteria for CECS:

- A preexercise pressure greater than or equal to 15 mmHg
- A 1-min postexercise pressure of greater than or equal to 30 mmHg
- A 5-min postexercise pressure of greater than or equal to 20 mmHg

If at-rest measurement or 1-min postexercise measurement is confirmatory, further measuring shall not be necessary.

16.5.5 Therapeutic Approach

Conservative management is usually chosen as the treatment in the first moment. First, the treatment plan could be with the cessation or reduction of causative activity. In fact, most athletes are unwilling to avoid sport practice as CECS management [1, 33]. Furthermore, the non-operative treatment has included anti-inflammatory medication, stretching, and an alternative exercise program. This apart, there has been a physical rehabilitation program involving massage, gait changes, foot orthotics, botulinum toxin, and USG percutaneous needle fascial fenestration [2]. Adopting a forefoot strike while running was shown to be an effective conservative treatment strategy in a runner. Usually, the side effect of botulinum toxin A was a loss of strength [1, 35]. If the non-operative management has not worked as well, then the operative treatment becomes a good option to be considered.

Currently, the open fasciotomy has been considered the gold standard treatment for CECS because of the positive outcomes related to relieving pain and return to sport in most cases [1, 37, 38]. Endoscopic techniques have also shown favorable outcomes in athletes. In spite of that, there are no studies comparing non-operative and operative treatments. The complications reported after surgery could include wound infection, peripheral nerve injury, hematoma, and deep vein thrombosis. The failure of surgical treatment is linked more to localized constrictions from postsurgical fibrosis than the involvement of the entire compartment [37]. It may be related to incomplete fascial release.

16.5.6 Popliteal Artery Entrapment Syndrome

Popliteal artery entrapment syndrome (PAES) is a symptomatic compression or occlusion of the popliteal artery, typically manifested with claudication symptoms due to a developmentally abnor-

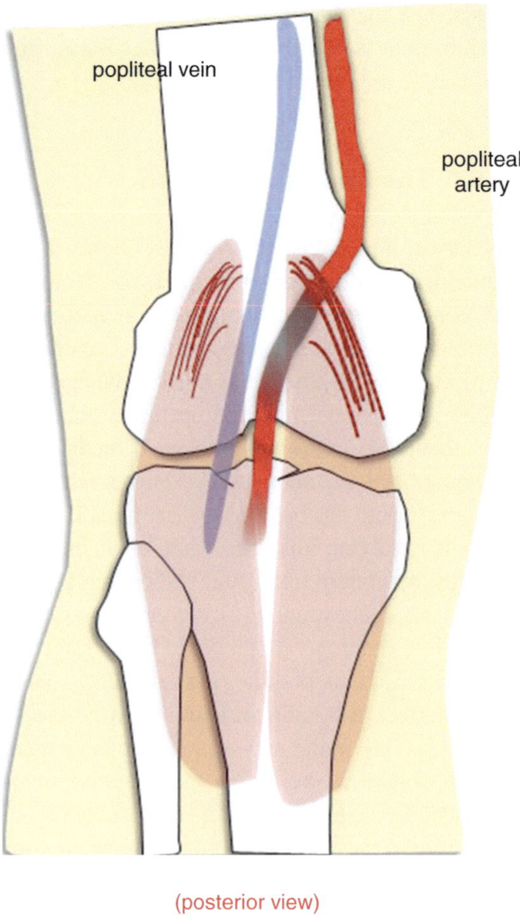

Fig. 16.9 Popliteal artery entrapment

mal anatomic positioning of the popliteal artery (PA) in relation to its surrounding structures [39, 40]. Figure 16.9 shows the close relationship of PA to the medial head of the gastrocnemius (MHG). According to the different anatomical features involving PA, five types of entrapment are described (classification of PAES) [41].

Type 1—PA (popliteal artery) has an aberrant medial course around the medial head of gastrocnemius (MHG) which has a normal insertion above the femoral condyle.

Type 2—MHG is inserted more laterally in the distal femur but PA not displaced.

Type 3—An aberrant accessory slip of MHG slings around and surrounds PA.

Type 4—PA is located deep in the popliteal fossa and entrapped by the popliteus muscle or fibrous bands.

Type 5—Any form of entrapment that involves both PA and popliteal vein (PV).

16.5.7 Medial Tibial Stress Syndrome

Similarly to shin pain, stress fracture can also result from repetitive stress, an overuse injury. The clinical complaints and site of pain can be similar, but the physical examination performing palpation and passive and active tibial rotation and valgus and varus stress can clarify the diagnosis. An example of an elicit maneuver is the "one-leg hop test" that can be used to distinguish MTSS from stress fracture. An athlete with MTSS can hop at least ten times on the affected leg, while in the case of stress fracture, the attempt of hopping is followed by severe pain, preventing the athlete from continuing the test [7, 8, 42, 43].

Regarding MTSS, running/jumping activities, elevated BMI, overtraining and inadequate rest, training on hard and irregular surfaces, and the female sex are reported as risk factors in developing MTSS.

The radiological evaluation should be done to confirm the diagnosis, and guide the therapeutic approach, even though, in most cases, the X-ray examination can show no abnormality (no injury). Although CT scan is not a sensitive exam for this pathology, it can show mild osteopenia related to the early stage of cortical bone damage in tibial diaphysis [44–46]. Bone scintigraphy can also be useful to establish the diagnosis, but MRI is the most sensitive radiological exam to confirm the diagnosis.

An MRI classification for tibial stress injuries was developed by Fredericson et al. [47] based on radiological findings such as periosteal edema, bone marrow edema, and intracortical signal abnormality. This classification defines grade 1 as isolated periosteal edema; grade 2 is outlined by T2-weighted images of visible bone marrow edema. Grade 3 shows bone marrow

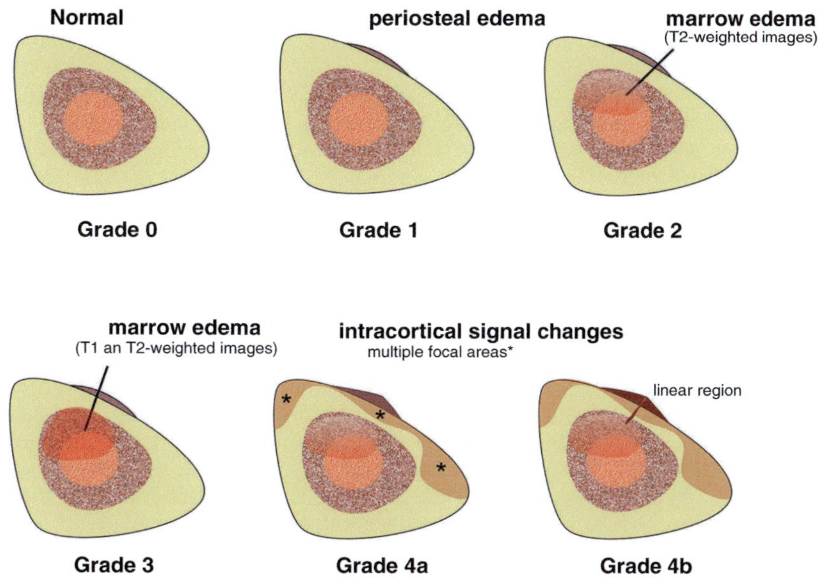

Fig. 16.10 Fredericson's classification

edema on both T1-weighted and T2-weighted images, while grade 4 presents an intracortical abnormality (4A) or linear area(s) of intracortical signal changes correlated to stress fracture (4B).

This classification was validated by Kijowski et al. [48] who noted that grades 2, 3, and 4A stress injuries had similar degrees of periosteal and bone marrow edema and are also related to similar returns to sports activity, suggesting that these three grades can be combined into a single category in an abbreviated Fredericson's classification (Fig. 16.10).

Take-Home Messages

- Shin pain is a common clinical complaint that touches recreational and professional athletes.
- Distance runners, athletes of endurance sports, dancers, and the military are commonly affected.
- Shin pain is a clinical symptom referred by different pathologies.
- Changes in the intensity and load of training as well as the periodicity of competition should be carefully investigated.
- Footwear, training on hard and irregular surfaces, elevated BMI, and gender can also be also a trigger for MTSS.

References

1. Vajapey S, Miller T. Evaluation, diagnosis, and treatment of chronic exertional compartment syndrome: a review of current literature. Phys SportsMed. 2017;45:391–8.
2. Flick D, Flick R. Chronic exertional compartment syndrome testing. Curr Sports Med Rep. 2015;14:380–5.
3. Bloomfield J, Polman R, O'Donoghue P. Physical demands of different positions in premier league soccer. J Sports Sci Med. 2007;1:63–70.
4. Heiderscheit BC, Chumanov ES, Michalski MP, Wille CM, Ryan MB. Effects of step rate manipulation on joint mechanics during running. Med Sci Sports Exerc. 2011;43(2):296–302.
5. Gabbett TJ. Quantifying the physical demands of collision sports: does microsensor technology measure what it claims to measure? J Strength Cond Res. 2013;27(8):2319–22.
6. Read D, Weaving D, Phibbs P, Darrall-Jones J, Roe G, Weakley J, Hendricks S, Till K, Jones B. Movement and physical demands of school and university rugby union match-play in England. BMJ Open Sport Exerc Med. 2017;2(1):e000147.
7. Brewer RB, Gregory AJ. Chronic lower leg pain in athletes: a guide for the differential diagnosis, evaluation, and treatment. Sports Health. 2012;4(2):121–7.
8. Burrus MT, Werner BC, Starman JS, Gwathmey FW, Carson EW, Wilder RP, Diduch DR. Chronic leg pain in athletes. Am J Sports Med. 2015;43(6):1538–47.
9. Franklyn M, Oakes B. Aetiology and mechanisms of injury in medial tibial stress syndrome: current and future developments. World J Orthop. 2015;6(8):577–89.

10. Craig DI. Current developments concerning medial tibial stress syndrome. Phys Sportsmed. 2009;37(4):39–44.
11. Becker J, Nakajima M, Wu WFW. Factors contributing to medial tibial stress syndrome in runners: a prospective study. Med Sci Sports Exerc. 2018;50(10):2092–100.
12. Warden SJ, Burr DB, Brukner PD. Stress fractures: pathophysiology, epidemiology, and risk factors. Curr Osteoporos Rep. 2006;4(3):103–9.
13. Paik RS, Pepples D, Hutchinson MR. Chronic exertional compartment syndrome. BMJ. 2013;346(7896):35–7.
14. Dunn JC, Waterman BR. Chronic exertional compartment syndrome of the leg in the military. Clin Sports Med. 2014;33(4):693–705.
15. Wilder RP, Sethi S. Overuse injuries: tendinopathies, stress fractures, compartment syndrome, and shin splints. Clin Sports Med. 2004;23(1):55–81, vi.
16. Ringhof S, Stein T. Biomechanical assessment of dynamic balance: specificity of different balance tests. Hum Mov Sci. 2018;58:140–7.
17. Thacker SB, Gilchrist J, Stroup DF, Kimsey CD. The prevention of shin splints in sports: a systematic review of literature. Med Sci Sports Exerc. 2002;34:32–40.
18. Lieberman DE, Venkadesan M, Werbel WA, et al. Foot strike patterns and collision forces in habitually barefoot versus shod runners. Nature. 2010;463:531–5.
19. Kortebein PM, Kaufman KR, Basford JR, Stuart MJ. Medial tibial stress syndrome. Med Sci Sports Exerc. 2000;32(3 Suppl):S27–33.
20. Edwards PH Jr, Wright ML, Hartman JF. A practical approach for the differential diagnosis of chronic leg pain in the athlete. Am J Sports Med. 2005;33(8):1241–9.
21. Doral MN, Alam M, Bozkurt M, Turhan E, Atay OA, Dönmez G, Maffulli N. Functional anatomy of the Achilles tendon. Knee Surg Sports Traumatol Arthrosc. 2010;18(5):638–43.
22. Longo UG, Ronga M, Maffulli N. Achilles tendinopathy. Sports Med Arthrosc Rev. 2018;26(1):16–30.
23. Magnan B, Bondi M, Pierantoni S, Samaila E. The pathogenesis of Achilles tendinopathy: a systematic review. Foot Ankle Surg. 2014;20(3):154–9.
24. Rompe JD, Furia J, Maffulli N. Eccentric loading versus eccentric loading plus shock-wave treatment for midportion Achilles tendinopathy: a randomized controlled trial. Am J Sports Med. 2009;37(3):463–70.
25. Espinosa N, Maurer MA. Stage I and II posterior tibial tendon dysfunction: return to running? Clin Sports Med. 2015;34(4):761–8.
26. Alvarez RG, Marini A, Schmitt C, et al. Stage I and II posterior tibial tendo dysfunction by a structured nonoperative management protocol: an orthosis and exercise program. Foot Ankle Int. 2006;27(1):2–8.
27. Kulig K, Burnfield JM, Reischl S, et al. Effect of foot orthoses on tibialis posterior activation in persons with pes planus. Med Sci Sports Exerc. 2005;37(1):24–9.
28. Steb HS, Marzano R. Conservative management of posterior tibial tendon dysfunction, subtalar joint complex, and pes planus deformity. Clin Podiatr Med Surg. 1999;16(3):439–51.
29. Roster B, Michelier P, Giza E. Peroneal tendon disorders. Clin Sports Med. 2015;34(4):625–41.
30. Espinosa N, Maurer MA. Peroneal tendon dislocation. Eur J Trauma Emerg Surg. 2015;41(6):631–7.
31. Taljanovic MS, Alcala JN, Gimber LH, Rieke JD, Chilvers MM, Latt LD. High-resolution US and MR imaging of peroneal tendon injuries. Radiographics. 2015;35(1):179–99.
32. George C, Hutchinson M. Chronic exertional compartment syndrome. Clin Sports Med. 2012;31:307–19.
33. Rajasekaran S, Hall M. Nonoperative management of chronic exertional compartment syndrome. Curr Sports Med Rep. 2016;15:191–8.
34. Edmundsson D, Toolanen G, Thornell LE, et al. Evidence for low muscle capillary supply as a pathogenic factor in chronic compartment syndrome. Scand J Med Sci Sports. 2010;20(6):805–13.
35. Winkes M, Scheltinga M. Chronic exertional compartment syndrome of the deep posterior lower leg. Br J Sports Med. 2018;52(19):1279–80.
36. Pedowitz RA, Hargens AR, Mubarak SJ, et al. Modified criteria for the objective diagnosis of chronic compartment syndrome of the leg. Am J Sports Med. 1990;18:35–40.
37. Schepsis AA, Fitzgerald M, Nicoletta R. Revision surgery for exertional anterior compartment syndrome of the lower leg: technique, findings, and results. Am J Sports Med. 2005;33:1040–7.
38. Fouasson-Chailloux A, Menu P, Allorent J, Dauty M. Determination of the predictive clinical parameters to diagnose chronic exertional compartment syndrome. Eur J Sport Sci. 2017;18:279–85.
39. Carneiro Júnior FCF, Carrijo ENDA, Araújo ST, Nakano LCU, de Amorim JE, Cacione DG. Popliteal artery entrapment syndrome: a case report and review of the literature. Am J Case Rep. 2018;19:29–34.. Review.
40. Gaunder C, McKinney B, Rivera J. Popliteal artery entrapment or chronic Exertional compartment syndrome? Case Rep Med. 2017;2017:1–5.
41. Elias DA, White LM, Rubenstein JD, Christakis M, Merchant N. Clinical evaluation and MR imaging features of popliteal artery entrapment and cystic adventitial disease. AJR Am J Roentgenol. 2003;180(3):627–32.
42. Newman P, Witchalls J, Waddington G, Adams R. Risk factors associated with medial tibial stress syndrome in runners: a systematic review and meta-analysis. Open Access J Sports Med. 2013;4: 229–41.
43. Moen MH, Tol JL, Weir A, Steunebrink M, De Winter TC. Medial tibial stress syndrome: a critical review. Sports Med. 2009;39(7):523–46.
44. Gaeta M, Minutoli F, Scribano E, Ascenti G, Vinci S, Bruschetta D, et al. CT and MR imaging findings in athletes with early tibial stress injuries: comparison with bone scintigraphy findings and emphasis on cortical abnormalities. Radiology. 2005;235(2):553.

45. Gaeta M, Minutoli F, Vinci S, Salamone I, D'Andrea L, Bitto L, et al. High-resolution CT grading of tibial stress reactions in distance runners. AJR Am J Roentgenol. 2006;187(3):789–93.
46. Anderson MW, Ugalde V, Batt M, Gacayan J. Shin splints: MR appearance in a preliminary study. Radiology. 1997;204(1):177–80.
47. Fredericson M, Bergman AG, Hoffman KL, Dillingham MS. Tibial stress reaction in runners. Correlation of clinical symptoms and scintigraphy with a new magnetic resonance imaging grading system. Am J Sports Med. 1995;23(4):472–81.
48. Kijowski R, Choi J, Shinki K, Del Rio AM, De Smet A. Validation of MRI classification system for tibial stress injuries. AJR Am J Roentgenol. 2012;198(4):878–84.

Groin Injuries

17

Per Hölmich, Lasse Ishøi, Andreas Serner, and Kristian Thorborg

17.1 Introduction

In recent years, there have been great advances in our understanding of groin pain in athletes. In 2015, the Doha Agreement on terminology and definitions on groin pain in athletes was published [46]. To keep the terminology more clear and support both clinical and scientific communication, the consensus group agreed on four clinical entities to describe long-standing groin pain, including adductor-related, iliopsoas-related, inguinal-related, and pubic-related groin pain [46]. Thus, terms, such as adductor and iliopsoas tendinitis or tendinopathy, athletic groin pain, athletic pubalgia, biomechanical groin overload, Gilmore's groin, groin disruption, Hockey-goalie syndrome, Hockey groin, osteitis pubis, sports groin, sportsman's groin, sports hernia, and sportsman's hernia, which have been used frequently should be avoided [46]. The authors of this chapter fully support this recommendation.

Groin injuries are a common cause of sporting disability, particularly in football codes [9, 42]. A recent study investigating groin problems in football players during the preseason period observed a weekly prevalence of 29% [9]. Similarly, a large cross-sectional cohort study including 695 football players found that 49% reported hip and/or groin pain in the previous season, and 31% of those had pain lasting more than 6 weeks [42]. Acute groin injuries are also frequent in multidirectional sports, and a 25-player football squad can expect 2–4 acute groin injuries each season [5, 23].

However, as groin pain is the cardinal symptom in many diagnoses, the clinician should also seek to rule out other potential causes of groin pain such as intra-articular hip pathology or pelvic disorders [8, 20, 26].

17.2 Adductor Injuries

17.2.1 Longstanding Adductor-Related Pain

Adductor-related groin pain is a common cause of long-standing groin pain in athletes [46]. Although the hip adductor complex comprises of five muscles (pectineus, gracilis, adductor brevis, adductor magnus, and adductor longus), the most frequent

P. Hölmich (✉) · L. Ishøi · K. Thorborg
Sports Orthopedic Research Center—Copenhagen (SORC-C), Department of Orthopedic Surgery, Copenhagen University Hospital, Amager-Hvidovre, Denmark
e-mail: per.hoelmich@regionh.dk; lasse.ishoei@regionh.dk; kristian.thorborg@regionh.dk

A. Serner
Department Sports Groin Pain Center, Aspetar Orthopaedic and Sports Medicine Hospital, Doha, Qatar
e-mail: andreas.serner@aspetar.com

S. Rocha Piedade et al. (eds.), *The Sports Medicine Physician*, https://doi.org/10.1007/978-3-030-10433-7_17

type of long-standing adductor-related pain involves the adductor longus muscle [11]. The pain is typically present during athletic activities, such as sprinting, change of direction, and kicking, and is located medially in the groin in the region around the origin of the adductor longus muscle at the pubic bone. During activities such as kicking, acceleration and deceleration, and change of direction, the hip adductors are exposed to large eccentric forces, typically in combination with an abduction, external rotation, and extension movement of the femur putting further stress on the adductor muscle-tendon unit [3]. Although the specific etiology of long-standing adductor-related groin pain is unknown, repetitive microtrauma of the hip adductor structures may lead to long-standing adductor-related pain [4].

17.2.1.1 Diagnosis

According to the *DOHA* Agreement, long-standing adductor-related groin pain is diagnosed as adductor tenderness *AND* pain on resisted hip adduction [46]. Furthermore, subjects with current and/or previous long-standing adductor-related groin pain typically present with reduced hip adduction strength and/or reduced range of motion in passive abduction and bent knee fallout [22].

With the patient lying supine with the hip flexed, abducted, and externally rotated, and the knee slightly flexed, the adductor longus tendon can be easily palpated. The examiner, using the right hand on the right leg, and the left hand on the left leg, palpates the adductor longus tendon with two fingers and follows the tendon to the insertion at the pubic bone. The insertion area, including the bone, is tested with firm pressure at a radius of about 1 cm. Pain on palpation suggests adductor-related groin pain [11].

Pain on resisted hip adduction is examined using a long-lever hip adduction squeeze test, as this has been shown to elicit the largest torque output, hence stressing the muscle-tendon unit of the adductors the most [21]. The examiner stands at the end of the examination table with the hands and lower arms between the feet placed just proximal to the medial malleolus. The feet of the subject are pointing straight up, and the subject squeeze the legs together with maximal force without lifting the legs or pelvis. The test is positive if it reproduces pain from the insertion site of the adductor longus where the patient also was tender at palpation [11, 12].

17.2.1.2 Treatment

Consistent evidence suggests that athletes with long-standing groin pain present with reduced hip adduction strength specifically when measured during eccentric contractions [22, 39]. Consequently, the treatment is based upon active exercise therapy aiming to restore optimal hip adductor muscle function and increase load capacity [16]. In line with this, rest alone or passive treatment modalities do not seem to resolve symptoms effectively [16, 42].

Only few high-quality studies on the treatment of long-standing adductor-related pain exist [30], with a randomized controlled trial showing exercise therapy to be highly effective in comparison with passive treatment modalities, such as massage or laser therapy [16]. It should be noted that bony morphologies related to femoroacetabular impingement syndrome do not seem to prevent a successful treatment outcome at long-term follow-up [15]. The treatment program used in this study consists of two modules, with the first module lasting approximately 2 weeks and aiming to teach the patient to reactivate the adductor muscles using isometric and low-load exercises. The second module includes more demanding exercises targeting both the adductor muscles specifically and the stability of lumbopelvic region. The patient and clinician should be aware that at least 8–12 weeks of focused exercise therapy are usually needed to resolve symptoms and allow return to previous sporting activities [16]. In addition to exercise therapy, manual therapies may be used as a supplement [47]. Additionally, a progressive running and change of direction protocol appears beneficial [47]. Following return to sport activities, maintenance of eccentric hip adductor strength is considered important. This can be secured by performing the Copenhagen Adduction exercise [17] or hip adduction with an elastic band [19]. In line with this, football players with past-season groin pain for more than 6 weeks seem to begin the new season with hip adduction weakness, potentially increasing the risk of a new injury/pain [7].

Besides focus on restoring hip adduction strength, the clinician should also pay attention to other hip muscles such as the hip flexors and extensors. In an extended hip position, the adductor muscles are considered important hip flexor synergists, whereas adductor magnus is an effective hip extensor [24]. Thus, any impairments in hip flexor and/or extensor muscles should be addressed as part of treatment for adductor-related groin pain, to minimize the risk of continuously overloading the adductor muscles [24].

17.2.2 Acute Adductor Injuries

The adductors account for the majority of acute groin injuries in athletes [29], and similar to the long-standing adductor-related groin pain, the adductor longus accounts for the majority of the injuries. About 90% of acute adductor injuries involve the adductor longus [32]. The adductor brevis and pectineus are injured in about a fourth of cases, often in combination with an adductor longus injury, whereas obturator externus, gracilis, and adductor magnus injuries are rarer causes of acute groin pain [32]. Acute adductor magnus is in our experience more likely to give pain more posteriorly on the thigh and may therefore be more common in athletes presenting with acute posterior thigh pain.

17.2.2.1 Diagnosis

The diagnosis of an acute adductor injury can be comfortably made through a clinical examination consisting of adductor palpation, adductor stretch, and adductor resistance tests, with similar methods as described for long-standing adductor-related groin pain [31]. These tests have a high accuracy, which means they can be highly trusted to diagnose an adductor injury through clinical examination only. Furthermore, they can individually provide about 80% certainty of an adductor injury on magnetic resonance imaging (MRI) [31].

Imaging will be able to provide more detailed information regarding the specific location and extent of injuries, with MRI being slightly more sensitive than ultrasound [29]. A detailed MRI study of acute adductor injuries has shown that there are three characteristic locations of adductor longus injuries: (1) the proximal insertion, (2) the musculotendinous junction (MTJ) of the proximal tendon, and (3) the MTJ of the distal tendon. In the MTJ injuries at both the proximal and distal insertion, there is rarely any injury to the tendon structure itself, whereas at the proximal insertion, most injuries are complete avulsions [32]. It is unknown whether there is a difference in prognosis between injuries in the different muscles and whether clinical or imaging findings can improve prognostic accuracy in individual cases.

17.2.2.2 Treatment

There is currently no evidence to suggest optimal treatment methods for acute adductor injuries. Therefore, the current treatment follows the general recommendation of the POLICE acronym (protection, optimal loading, ice, compression, elevation) [2], with a high focus on progressive loading as soon as possible. Studies from elite football suggest that the rehabilitation duration will be less than a month in 90% of acute adductor injuries.

Avulsion injuries will usually require a discussion of a surgical reattachment. Both surgical and conservative treatments for adductor avulsion injuries are usually successful. The duration of conservative treatment is however reported considerably shorter (3–15 weeks) [28, 44] compared to surgical treatment (10–32 weeks) [1, 28, 34].

It is important to note that for both acute groin injuries in general and acute adductor injuries, specifically, there is a high risk of reinjury, with 18–27% reported in football [5, 23].

17.3 Hip Flexor Injuries

17.3.1 Long-Standing Iliopsoas-Related Pain

Iliopsoas-related groin pain is considered the second most common source of groin pain in athletes, affecting between 8 and 35% presenting with groin pain [11, 48]. The pain is typically present during athletic activities, such as sprinting and change of direction, and is in the anterior aspect of the thigh, lateral to the adductor-related pain. Due to the location of pain most often being on the anterior thigh, iliopsoas-related pain is an important differential diagnosis in subjects with suspected intra-articular hip joint pathology. Iliopsoas-related pain is frequently observed in conjunction with adductor-related groin pain [14, 35] and in patients presenting with intra-articular hip joint pathology [18].

17.3.1.1 Diagnosis

According to the DOHA Agreement, long-standing iliopsoas-related pain is diagnosed as iliopsoas tenderness [46]. Furthermore, pain in the iliopsoas muscle may also arise on passive stretching of the muscle during the Thomas test or when tested isometrically with 90° of hip flexion although these are not diagnostic criteria for long-standing iliopsoas-related pain.

When palpating the iliopsoas muscle-tendon, the subject is lying supine. The iliopsoas can be palpated both (1) proximal to the inguinal ligament at the level of the Anterior Auperior Iliac Spine and (2) under the inguinal ligament, medial to the sartorius muscle and lateral to the femoral artery. Abdominal palpation is performed with both hands using soft gentle fingers. The fingers are gently pressed posteriorly while pushing the abdominal structures away to reach the iliopsoas muscle. The patient is then asked to elevate the leg 5 cm, and the psoas can be felt and palpated for any pain. As this test can sometimes be painful in non-injured people, it is important to ask the patient whether any pain is similar to their injury pain. The palpation of the distal iliopsoas tendon is most easily performed by first locating the proximal part of the sartorius muscle just distal to the inguinal ligament and then moving the fingers slightly medially. The patient is then asked to elevate the examined leg 5 cm, and the finger position is adjusted until the tendon is clearly felt under the fingers. Then, the patient relaxes and the tendon can be palpated again for any pain [11].

17.3.1.2 Treatment

There is no evidence-based treatment of long-standing iliopsoas-related groin pain; however, it is advised to adopt an active exercise program focusing on strengthening the iliopsoas muscle. This can be done using a systematic and gradual strengthening program with a simple hip flexion exercise using an elastic band as external resistance [37]. If pain hinders the ability to perform the exercise program, it is our experience that an ultrasound-guided injection along the distal iliopsoas tendon with cortisone sometimes can be helpful to settle pain allowing the patient to perform the exercises without pain. In a retrospective review of athletes with iliopsoas-related groin pain without information on treatment, the mean (SD) duration to return to sport was 20 (±14) weeks [43].

17.3.2 Acute Hip Flexor Injuries

In athletes, around one third of acute groin injuries affect the hip flexor muscles, with the iliopsoas muscles accounting for about half of these [29]. Acute iliopsoas injuries most frequently occur during change of direction and kicking [33].

17.3.2.1 Diagnosis

The clinical diagnosis of acute iliopsoas injuries can be difficult in the initial examination. There is often a widespread pain in the area potentially coming from a number of muscles, which leads to specific hip flexor tests (palpation, stretch, and resistance tests) often being positive without positive MRI findings in the iliopsoas [29]. This results in general poor accuracy of the clinical examination tests [31]. A delayed clinical examination or imaging may therefore be helpful.

When positive, an MRI can provide detailed information on the location and extent of the injury, which may be relevant as complete tears are possible, although rare [33]. A detailed MRI study has shown that the iliacus muscle is more frequently injured than the psoas major [33]; however, it is still unclear whether this differentiation is clinically relevant for diagnosis or prognosis.

17.3.2.2 Treatment

Like the long-standing iliopsoas-related groin pain, there is no evidence-based treatment of acute iliopsoas injuries. Treatment therefore follows the general guidelines for acute muscle injuries, with a main focus on early load progression. Although clinicians usually consider acute iliopsoas injuries as minor, there appears to be a large variation in the time to return to sports with a mean duration reported to be 8.6 ± 8.3 weeks [43].

17.4 Abdominal Injuries

17.4.1 Long-Standing Inguinal-Related Groin Pain

Inguinal-related groin pain is a relatively rare diagnosis in the groin region, only affecting 4–8% of all injuries to the hip and groin in male elite soccer players [23, 49]. The majority soccer players with inguinal-related groin pain is absent from soccer for more than 4 weeks [23].

Although, the exact pathophysiology remains unclear, it is thought that inguinal-related groin pain may develop as an overuse injury, due to the accumulation of the large shear forces acting across the pelvis, trunk, and leg during athletic movements. Additionally, restricted hip range of motion may result in altered rotational pattern of the symphysis leading to excessive stress on the inguinal region [4].

Patients with inguinal-related groin pain typically complain of pain over the inguinal canal and at the pubic tubercle that may radiate to the medial groin and the scrotum.

17.4.1.1 Diagnosis

According to the DOHA Agreement, long-standing inguinal-related groin pain is diagnosed as tenderness at the insertion of the conjoined tendon at the pubic tubercle and pain when palpating the inguinal canal through the scrotum with the patient standing [46].

Palpation of the conjoined tendon insertion at the pubic tubercle is performed with the subjects lying supine. The examiner locates the proximal part of the pubic tubercle and follows the rim until reaching just medial to the inguinal ligament [11]. The inguinal canal is approximately the size of a fingertip and can be palpated supine or with the patient standing by invaginating the skin of the scrotum. During this palpation, the patient can be asked to perform the Valsalva maneuver. A palpable bulge of the posterior abdominal wall may be present and/or increased pain, which should be similar to the patient's injury pain.

17.4.1.2 Treatment

There is no evidence-based treatment of long-standing inguinal-related groin pain using a conservative treatment approach [30]; however, it is recommended to adopt an active exercise program focusing on strengthening the abdominal muscles including the muscles around the hip joint. The exercise program used for adductor-related groin pain [16] can be used as a base and be supplemented with progressive abdominal exercises such as long-lever planks and sit-ups lying on a Swiss ball, focusing on the deep and oblique abdominal muscles. Like adductor-related groin pain, treatment of inguinal-related groin pain often lasts for at least 8–12 weeks. Aggravating activities stressing the inguinal area such as kicking and forceful rotational movements of the trunk should be minimized during the initial treatment period and gradually re-introduced as the treatment progresses.

In cases where exercise therapy fails, surgery, either open or laparoscopic hernia repair, should be considered as a viable option. In a systematic review published in 2015, 38 studies regarding surgical treatment of inguinal-related pain were identified; however, only one study was deemed high quality [30]. In that study, 60 patients were randomized to either surgery (laparoscopic totally extraperitoneal repair) or conservative treatment consisting of exercise therapy, corticosteroid injections, and oral anti-inflammatory analgesics [25]. Almost all athletes (97%) returned to sport at 12 months following surgery compared to 50% of athletes treated conservatively. While this study suggests that surgery is superior to conservative treatment for athletes with inguinal-related groin pain, approximately one in two athletes can expect to return to sport following conservative exercise therapy, and thus it is our opinion this should be considered the initial choice of treatment.

17.4.2 Acute Abdominal Muscle Injuries

Acute abdominal injury is a rare isolated cause of acute groin pain; however, in about 10–20% of acute groin injuries, athletes will report pain in the lower abdominal area during clinical examination. Positive tests are usually found in combination with a larger injury in a different muscle in the groin (such as adductor longus avulsions), and positive imaging findings in the abdominal muscles will only be present in 1–6% cases [29, 31]. There are currently no evidence-based treatment guidelines for acute abdominal injuries.

17.5 Pubic Symphysis Pain

17.5.1 Pubic-Related Groin Pain

Pubic-related groin pain is considered a rare condition that remains poorly explored in the literature. As such the epidemiological data related to this entity is scarce; however, a recent report evaluating 100 athletes presenting multidisciplinary sports groin pain clinic showed that four athletes (4%) had pubic-related groin pain, but it was only considered as the primary cause of pain in one athlete [35].

17.5.1.1 Diagnosis

According to the DOHA Agreement, long-standing pubic-related groin pain is diagnosed as tenderness with palpation of the pubic symphysis and the immediately adjacent bone [46].

Palpation of the pubic symphysis is performed with the subject lying supine. The examiner locates the upper part of the pubic bone by palpating with a gentle finger followed by palpation of the pubic symphysis distally. It is important to note that most athletes are tender at the top of the pubic bone, and proper palpation at the distal part is therefore important to decrease the risk of a false-positive test [12].

17.5.1.2 Treatment

There is no high-level evidence to suggest the most appropriate treatment strategy for long-standing pubic-related groin pain. However, evidence from a case series study including professional Australian football players have reported favorable outcomes using an approach consisting mainly of load management and pelvic stability exercises. During the initial 12 weeks following the diagnosis, the athlete should refrain from all weight-bearing running activities, whereas stationary cycling may be introduced at week 4 given that no pain is elicited by the activity. After 12 weeks, running activities should be gradually introduced [45].

17.5.2 Pubic Apophysitis

Pubic apophysitis is a newly described groin entity, and very limited data exist. It should be suspected as a potential source of pain in skeletally immature athletes (up to 21 years old) presenting with long-standing adductor-related groin pain. It has been hypothesized that the development of pubic apophysitis may be due to a combination of traction and compressive forces, leading to excessive apophyseal plate stress in young athletes with non-fusion of the secondary ossification center of the pubic symphysis [27].

17.5.2.1 Diagnosis

The diagnosis of pubic apophysitis is based on a history of increasing pain during and after even careful adductor exercises in adolescent athletes including tenderness of the adductor longus insertion on the pubis on palpation including radiographic confirmation, preferable using CT scan [27].

With the patient lying supine with the hip flexed, abducted, and externally rotated, and the knee slightly flexed, the adductor longus tendon can be easily palpated. The examiner, using the right hand on the right leg, and the left hand on the left leg, palpates the adductor longus tendon with two fingers and follows the tendon to the insertion at the pubic bone. The insertion area, including the bone, is tested with firm pressure to a radius of about 1 cm [11].

It has been suggested that CT scan allows for the best visualization of the pubic apophysis, with 1.5 T MRI adding no value to the diagnosis. However, 3.0 T MRI may be promising and thus should be considered due to no radiation [27].

17.5.2.2 Treatment

There is no high-level evidence to suggest the most appropriate treatment strategy for pubic apophysitis; however, a combination of load management and gradual strengthening of the hip adductors seems promising [27].

17.6 Monitoring of Groin Function and Pain During Treatment

Effective and simple monitoring of groin function and pain before, during, and after the treatment period is advised to guide progression of the treatment.

Objective measures of groin function can easily be performed using a hand-held dynamometer [36, 41]. Additionally, self-reported groin function can be obtained using the Copenhagen Hip and Groin Outcome Score (HAGOS), which is the only validated patient-reported outcome measure in patients presenting with groin pain arising from musculotendinous structures [40].

Another quick assessment of the hip and groin function can be performed with the Copenhagen five-second squeeze test [38]. The test is performed as a regular long-lever squeeze test with the athlete instructed to score the experienced pain in the groin region on a Numerical Rating Scale going from 0 to 10 after a maximum adductor squeeze for 5 s. Based on the experienced pain level, the athlete can be given a green (0–2 NRS), yellow (3–5 NRS), or red (6–10 NRS) light representing an approximation of readiness to progress load during treatment or participate in training or matches [38].

17.7 Prevention of Groin Injuries

A 2015 systematic review and meta-analysis on prevention of groin injuries noted a clinically relevant reduction in groin injuries of 19%; however, few studies were specifically designed to reduce the risk of groin injuries [6]. Promising effect for groin injury prevention exists for a prevention program focused on active adductor exercises, where a reduction of 31% has been observed [13]. Additionally, a recent study including an exercise program consisting of only one adductor exercise (performed at three different levels) during the football season showed a reduction in groin problems of 41% [10].

References

1. Bharam S, Feghhi DP, Porter DA, Bhagat PV. Proximal adductor avulsion injuries: outcomes of surgical reattachment in athletes. Orthop J Sports Med. 2018;6:2325967118784898.
2. Bleakley CM, Glasgow P, MaCauley DC. PRICE needs updating, should we call the POLICE? Br J Sports Med. 2012;46:220–1.
3. Charnock BL, Lewis CL, Garrett WE Jr, Queen RM. Adductor longus mechanics during the maximal effort soccer kick. Sports Biomech. 2009;8:223–34.
4. Dimitrakopoulou A, Schilders E. Current concepts of inguinal-related and adductor-related groin pain. Hip Int. 2016;26(Suppl 1):2–7.
5. Ekstrand J, Hagglund M, Walden M. Epidemiology of muscle injuries in professional football (soccer). Am J Sports Med. 2011;39:1226–32.
6. Esteve E, Rathleff MS, Bagur-Calafat C, Urrutia G, Thorborg K. Prevention of groin injuries in sports: a systematic review with meta-analysis of randomised controlled trials. Br J Sports Med. 2015;49:785–91.
7. Esteve E, Rathleff MS, Vicens-Bordas J, Clausen MB, Holmich P, Sala L, Thorborg K. Preseason adductor squeeze strength in 303 Spanish male soccer athletes: a cross-sectional study. Orthop J Sports Med. 2018;6:2325967117747275.
8. Griffin DR, Dickenson EJ, O'Donnell J, Agricola R, Awan T, Beck M, Clohisy JC, Dijkstra HP, Falvey E, Gimpel M, Hinman RS, Holmich P, Kassarjian A, Martin HD, Martin R, Mather RC, Philippon MJ, Reiman MP, Takla A, Thorborg K, Walker S, Weir A, Bennell KL. The Warwick agreement on femoroacetabular impingement syndrome (FAI syndrome): an international consensus statement. Br J Sports Med. 2016;50:1169–76.
9. Haroy J, Clarsen B, Thorborg K, Holmich P, Bahr R, Andersen TE. Groin problems in male soccer

players are more common than previously reported. Am J Sports Med. 2017;45:1304–8.
10. Haroy J, Clarsen B, Wiger EG, Oyen MG, Serner A, Thorborg K, et al. The Adductor Strengthening Programme prevents groin problems among male football players: a cluster-randomised controlled trial. Br J Sports Med. 2018. https://doi.org/10.1136/bjsports-2017-098937.
11. Holmich P. Long-standing groin pain in sportspeople falls into three primary patterns, a "clinical entity" approach: a prospective study of 207 patients. Br J Sports Med. 2007;41:247–52; discussion 252.
12. Holmich P, Holmich LR, Bjerg AM. Clinical examination of athletes with groin pain: an intraobserver and interobserver reliability study. Br J Sports Med. 2004;38:446–51.
13. Holmich P, Larsen K, Krogsgaard K, Gluud C. Exercise program for prevention of groin pain in football players: a cluster-randomized trial. Scand J Med Sci Sports. 2010;20:814–21.
14. Holmich P, Thorborg K, Dehlendorff C, Krogsgaard K, Gluud C. Incidence and clinical presentation of groin injuries in sub-elite male soccer. Br J Sports Med. 2014;48:1245–50.
15. Holmich P, Thorborg K, Nyvold P, Klit J, Nielsen MB, Troelsen A. Does bony hip morphology affect the outcome of treatment for patients with adductor-related groin pain? Outcome 10 years after baseline assessment. Br J Sports Med. 2014;48:1240–4.
16. Holmich P, Uhrskou P, Ulnits L, Kanstrup IL, Nielsen MB, Bjerg AM, Krogsgaard K. Effectiveness of active physical training as treatment for long-standing adductor-related groin pain in athletes: randomised trial. Lancet. 1999;353:439–43.
17. Ishoi L, Sorensen CN, Kaae NM, Jorgensen LB, Holmich P, Serner A. Large eccentric strength increase using the Copenhagen adduction exercise in football: a randomized controlled trial. Scand J Med Sci Sports. 2016;26:1334–42.
18. Jacobsen JS, Hölmich P, Thorborg K, Bolvig L, Jakobsen SS, Søballe K, Mechlenburg I. Muscle-tendon-related pain in 100 patients with hip dysplasia: prevalence and associations with self-reported hip disability and muscle strength. J Hip Preserv Surg. 2017;5:39–46.
19. Jensen J, Holmich P, Bandholm T, Zebis MK, Andersen LL, Thorborg K. Eccentric strengthening effect of hip-adductor training with elastic bands in soccer players: a randomised controlled trial. Br J Sports Med. 2014;48:332–8.
20. Laslett M, Aprill CN, McDonald B, Young SB. Diagnosis of sacroiliac joint pain: validity of individual provocation tests and composites of tests. Man Ther. 2005;10:207–18.
21. Light N, Thorborg K. The precision and torque production of common hip adductor squeeze tests used in elite football. J Sci Med Sport. 2016;19:888–92.
22. Mosler AB, Agricola R, Weir A, Holmich P, Crossley KM. Which factors differentiate athletes with hip/groin pain from those without? A systematic review with meta-analysis. Br J Sports Med. 2015;49:810.
23. Mosler AB, Weir A, Eirale C, Farooq A, Thorborg K, Whiteley RJ, Hlmich P, Crossley KM. Epidemiology of time loss groin injuries in a men's professional football league: a 2-year prospective study of 17 clubs and 606 players. Br J Sports Med. 2018;52:292–7.
24. Neumann DA. Kinesiology of the hip: a focus on muscular actions. J Orthop Sports Phys Ther. 2010;40:82–94.
25. Paajanen H, Brinck T, Hermunen H, Airo I. Laparoscopic surgery for chronic groin pain in athletes is more effective than nonoperative treatment: a randomized clinical trial with magnetic resonance imaging of 60 patients with sportsman's hernia (athletic pubalgia). Surgery. 2011;150:99–107.
26. Reiman MP, Thorborg K. Clinical examination and physical assessment of hip joint-related pain in athletes. Int J Sports Phys Ther. 2014;9:737–55.
27. Sailly M, Whiteley R, Read JW, Giuffre B, Johnson A, Holmich P. Pubic apophysitis: a previously undescribed clinical entity of groin pain in athletes. Br J Sports Med. 2015;49:828–34.
28. Schlegel TF, Bushnell BD, Godfrey J, Boublik M. Success of nonoperative management of adductor longus tendon ruptures in National Football League athletes. Am J Sports Med. 2009;37:1394–9.
29. Serner A, Tol JL, Jomaah N, Weir A, Whiteley R, Thorborg K, Robinson M, Holmich P. Diagnosis of acute groin injuries: a prospective study of 110 athletes. Am J Sports Med. 2015;43:1857–64.
30. Serner A, Van Eijck CH, Beumer BR, Holmich P, Weir A, de Vos RJ. Study quality on groin injury management remains low: a systematic review on treatment of groin pain in athletes. Br J Sports Med. 2015;49:813.
31. Serner A, Weir A, Tol JL, Thorborg K, Roemer F, Guermazi A, Holmich P. Can standardised clinical examination of athletes with acute groin injuries predict the presence and location of MRI findings? Br J Sports Med. 2016;50:1541–7.
32. Serner A, Weir A, Tol JL, Thorborg K, Roemer F, Guermazi A, Yamashiro E, Holmich P. Characteristics of acute groin injuries in the adductor muscles: a detailed MRI study in athletes. Scand J Med Sci Sports. 2018;28:667–76.
33. Serner A, Weir A, Tol JL, Thorborg K, Roemer F, Guermazi A, Yamashiro E, Holmich P. Characteristics of acute groin injuries in the hip flexor muscles—a detailed MRI study in athletes. Scand J Med Sci Sports. 2018;28:677–85.
34. Tansey RJ, Benjamin-Laing H, Jassim S, Liekens K, Shankar A, Haddad FS. Successful return to high-level sports following early surgical repair of combined adductor complex and rectus abdominis avulsion. Bone Joint J. 2015;97-B:1488–92.
35. Taylor R, Vuckovic Z, Mosler A, Agricola R, Otten R, Jacobsen P, Holmich P, Weir A. Multidisciplinary assessment of 100 athletes with groin pain using the Doha agreement: high prevalence of adductor-related

groin pain in conjunction with multiple causes. Clin J Sport Med. 2018;28:364–9.
36. Thorborg K, Bandholm T, Holmich P. Hip- and knee-strength assessments using a hand-held dynamometer with external belt-fixation are inter-tester reliable. Knee Surg Sports Traumatol Arthrosc. 2013;21:550–5.
37. Thorborg K, Bandholm T, Zebis M, Andersen LL, Jensen J, Holmich P. Large strengthening effect of a hip-flexor training programme: a randomized controlled trial. Knee Surg Sports Traumatol Arthrosc. 2016;24:2346–52.
38. Thorborg K, Branci S, Nielsen MP, Langelund MT, Holmich P. Copenhagen five-second squeeze: a valid indicator of sports-related hip and groin function. Br J Sports Med. 2017;51:594–9.
39. Thorborg K, Branci S, Nielsen MP, Tang L, Nielsen MB, Holmich P. Eccentric and isometric hip adduction strength in male soccer players with and without adductor-related groin pain: an assessor-blinded comparison. Orthop J Sports Med. 2014;2:2325967114521778.
40. Thorborg K, Holmich P, Christensen R, Petersen J, Roos EM. The Copenhagen Hip and Groin Outcome Score (HAGOS): development and validation according to the COSMIN checklist. Br J Sports Med. 2011;45:478–91.
41. Thorborg K, Petersen J, Magnusson SP, Holmich P. Clinical assessment of hip strength using a hand-held dynamometer is reliable. Scand J Med Sci Sports. 2010;20:493–501.
42. Thorborg K, Rathleff MS, Petersen P, Branci S, Holmich P. Prevalence and severity of hip and groin pain in sub-elite male football: a cross-sectional cohort study of 695 players. Scand J Med Sci Sports. 2017;27:107–14.
43. Tsukada S, Niga S, Imamura S, Saito M, Hatanaka J. Iliopsoas disorder in athletes with groin pain: prevalence in 638 consecutive patients assessed with MRI and clinical results in 134 patients with signal intensity changes in the Iliopsoas. JB JS Open Access. 2018;3:e0049.
44. Ueblacker P, English B, Mueller-Wohlfahrt HW. Nonoperative treatment and return to play after complete proximal adductor avulsion in high-performance athletes. Knee Surg Sports Traumatol Arthrosc. 2016;24:3927–33.
45. Verrall GM, Slavotinek JP, Fon GT, Barnes PG. Outcome of conservative management of athletic chronic groin injury diagnosed as pubic bone stress injury. Am J Sports Med. 2007;35:467–74.
46. Weir A, Brukner P, Delahunt E, Ekstrand J, Griffin D, Khan KM, Lovell G, Meyers WC, Muschaweck U, Orchard J, Paajanen H, Philippon M, Reboul G, Robinson P, Schache AG, Schilders E, Serner A, Silvers H, Thorborg K, Tyler T, Verrall G, de Vos RJ, Vuckovic Z, Holmich P. Doha agreement meeting on terminology and definitions in groin pain in athletes. Br J Sports Med. 2015;49:768–74.
47. Weir A, Jansen JA, Van de Port IG, Van de Sande HB, Tol JL, Backx FJ. Manual or exercise therapy for long-standing adductor-related groin pain: a randomised controlled clinical trial. Man Ther. 2011;16:148–54.
48. Werner J, Hagglund M, Ekstrand J, Walden M. Hip and groin time-loss injuries decreased slightly but injury burden remained constant in men's professional football: the 15-year prospective UEFA Elite Club Injury Study. Br J Sports Med. 2018. https://doi.org/10.1136/bjsports-2017-097796.
49. Werner J, Hagglund M, Walden M, Ekstrand J. UEFA injury study: a prospective study of hip and groin injuries in professional football over seven consecutive seasons. Br J Sports Med. 2009;43:1036–40.

Part III

Neurological Disorders

Epilepsy and Seizures

18

Jorge Roberto Pagura and Rudá Alessi

18.1 Introduction

Epilepsy is defined by the International League Against Epilepsy as a brain disorder characterized by an enduring predisposition to generate epileptic seizures and by the neurobiologic, cognitive, psychological, and social consequences associated [1]. An epileptic seizure is a transient occurrence of signs and/or symptoms due to abnormal excessive or synchronous neuronal activity in the brain [1]. Not every patient that presents an epileptic seizure has epilepsy and/or must be treated to such condition, and even repeated seizures due to an acute identified etiology (e.g., alcohol withdraw, hypoglycemia) are not considered epilepsy.

Epileptic seizures are only one manifestation of neurologic or metabolic diseases, having many possible causes, from genetic predisposition to brain tumors and head trauma. The diagnosis of epilepsy requires (1) at least two unprovoked seizures occurring >24 h apart; (2) one unprovoked seizure and a probability of further seizures like the general recurrence risk (at least 60%) after two unprovoked seizures, occurring over the next 10 years; or (3) the diagnosis of an epileptic syndrome [2].

As seizures are nonspecific manifestations of neurologic injury or even clinical disease, the prevalence of seizures is high, with lifetime likelihood of one seizure of 9%, and of receiving a diagnosis of epilepsy is almost 3% [3, 4]. There is a very high incidence in the first year of life and in early childhood, with a relative decrease in adolescence.

Incidence is at its lowest between the ages of 20 and 40 and steadily increases after age 50, with the greatest increase seen in those over age 80 [5].

18.2 Pathophysiology

Although the pathophysiology of epilepsy and seizures is diverse and still poorly understood, there is an element in common across epilepsies: an imbalance between excitatory (via glutamatergic signaling) and inhibitory (via GABAergic signaling) activity, leading to excessive neuronal

J. R. Pagura (✉)
Neurosurgery, ABC Medical School—FMABC, Santo André, Brazil

Brazilian Neurosurgical Society, Paraíso, Brazil

Medical and Antidoping control-Brazilian Soccer Confederation (CBF), Rio de Janeiro, Brazil
e-mail: jorge.pagura@cbf.com.br

R. Alessi
Neuroscience Department, ABC Medical School—FMABC, Santo André, Brazil

Laboratory of Clinical Neurophysiology, Institute and Department of Psychiatry, University of Sao Paulo—USP, São Paulo, Brazil

S. Rocha Piedade et al. (eds.), *The Sports Medicine Physician*,
https://doi.org/10.1007/978-3-030-10433-7_18

activity. In order for a brain to become "epileptic," there is an understanding that it must go through a process called epileptogenesis. This process suggests a time interval between the insult (e.g., a physical insult) and the resultant epileptic condition [6].

Considering post-traumatic epilepsy as a model for symptomatic epilepsy, everything begins with injury, and often death, of a significant of neurons. Hyperexcitability arises from this lesion from the release of potassium [7, 8] and glutamate [9] to the extracellular space, which may be a reason to acute symptomatic seizures. Later, the glutamate release leads to a rise in the influx of calcium, with subsequent dysfunction of mitochondrial activity and release of cytochrome c [10]. It has been known for some time now that traumatic insult leads later on to altered gene expression, with possible loss of inhibitory constraints and altering synaptic and network organization [11].

Table 18.1 Types of seizures

Focal onset seizures	Generalized onset	Unknown onset
Motor onset	Motor	Motor
Automatisms	Tonic-clonic	
Atonic	Clonic	Tonic-clonic
Clonic	Tonic	
Epileptic spasms	Myoclonic	Epileptic spasms
Hyperkinetic		
Myoclonic	Myoclonic-tonic-clonic	Nonmotor
Tonic		Behavior arrest
Nonmotor onset		
Autonomic	Myoclonic-atonic	
Behavior arrest		
Cognitive	Atonic	
Emotional	Epileptic spasms	
Sensory		
Aware/impaired awareness	Nonmotor (absence)	
Focal to bilateral tonic-clonic	Typical	
	Atypical	
	Myoclonic	
	Eyelid myoclonia	

Adapted from Fisher RS, Cross JH, French JA, et al. Operational classification of seizure types by the International League Against Epilepsy: Position paper of the ILAE Commission for Classification and Terminology. Epilepsia 2017

18.3 Classification of Seizures and Epilepsy

After the diagnosis of epilepsy is made (other than other paroxysmal events, like psychogenic events or syncope), the physician must identify the seizure type [12].

Seizure type is classified based on clinical manifestation and is divided in generalized, focal, or unknown (seizure onset is missed or obscured) (Table 18.1) [12–14].

Generalized seizures are further divided into motor and nonmotor (absence) seizures, while focal seizures are subdivided on motor and nonmotor and on level of awareness (perceptive or disperceptive) [12, 13].

Generalized Tonic-Clonic seizures are those that originate at some point within or rapidly engage bilaterally distributed networks, which do not necessarily include the entire cortex [12, 13].

Focal seizures are the ones that originate in networks limited to one single hemisphere [12, 13].

Once seizure is a clinical manifestation of neuronal hyperactivity, its semiological classification allows the physician to infer the anatomical site on the brain of the seizure generation.

Focal seizures may evolve to both sides of the brain and are called focal to bilateral tonic-clonic seizure.

18.4 Approach to a First Seizure

The main objective when approaching a patient's first seizure is to determine whether there is a treatable (and potentially lethal) condition, such as a systemic condition or an intrinsic injury of the nervous system.

An acute symptomatic seizure is a seizure that occurs at the time of a systemic insult or in close temporal association with a brain insult (up to 1 week, if traumatic brain injury) [14].

Some of these patients may develop epilepsy in the future, but most of these patients do not recur in seizures nor develop epilepsy.

The causes of acute symptomatic seizures are many and vary according to the setting of the seizure and the type of seizure. Medical conditions associated are listed on Table 18.2, and virtually

Table 18.2 Clinical causes of acute symptomatic seizure

Hyponatremia (<115 mg/dL)
Hypomagnesemia (<0.8 mg/dL)
Hypocalcemia (<5 mg/dL)
Hypo- (<36 mg/dL) or hyperglycemia (>450 mg/dL)

Adapted from Beleza P. Acute Symptomatic Seizures. The Neurologist 2012;18(3):109–19

any acute brain injury can cause a seizure (e.g., TBI, acute ischemic or hemorrhagic stroke, brain hematomas, brain abscesses, encephalitis).

The evaluation must begin with medical history and description of the event and include the postictal event, any focal deficits, history of prior events, medications and substance in use, and past and family history. Laboratory tests must include electrolytes, glucose, calcium, magnesium, complete blood count, renal function tests, liver function tests, urinalysis, and toxicology screens [15].

Electroencephalography (EEG) is an essential tool to study and classify epileptic seizures. In patients that presented their first seizure, EEG must be performed, and the presence of epileptiform abnormalities increases the odds of a new event, but a normal EEG does not rule out the possibility of further seizures [15, 16].

Neuroimaging must be performed in all patients with a first seizure and with urgency in those with a new focal deficit or persistent altered mental status, fever, persistent headache, history of TBI, malignancy, immunocompromised, alcoholism, anticoagulation, or bleeding diathesis [15, 17, 18].

18.5 Epilepsy and Sports

The benefits and risks of sports practice in patients with epilepsy remain controversial although most authors in the last decades have reported more benefits than risks depending on the type of sports being practiced.

The advocates of the benefits of sports practice in epileptic patients for the improvement of health and psychosocial benefits athletes cite evidence that suggests that physical exercise and active participation in sports may favorably affect seizure control in addition to producing social integration [19].

Some studies show the comparison between matched controls and patients called "epilepsy only" in childhood [20] suggest that the sports activity when practiced under control surely benefits the patient.

Despite this tendency, it is fundamental that the person with epilepsy should be accompanied by a clinician and neurologist to perform their activities safely.

Among many variables, the current neurological situation, adherence to treatment, and time of crises control should be considered.

Another problem is the impact of stigma on exercising in epileptic people [21]. The stigma, unfortunately, influences the group negatively in team sports.

It is possible to reduce it by educating others about the effects of sports on epileptic athletes. All the clarification on this brings positive aspects to both the epilepsy patient and the other participants.

People with epilepsy increased self-esteem, socialization, and health benefits in general although they are often discouraged due to the overprotection and lack of knowledge about the subject.

Social exclusions occur frequently in the first ages when they are physically more fragile.

In any case, the benefit of sports in an epileptic person is indisputable, not only for the social inclusion but due to improvement of the cognitive function with effects in the psychosocial development and integration.

The consensus paper prepared by the International League Against Epilepsy (ILAE) divided the sports into three categories according to the risk of death or serious injury if a seizure occurs during the practice of it [19]:

1. Sports with no significant additional risk, like collective sports on the ground, golf, and racquet sports
2. Sports with moderate risk to epileptic athletes but no risks to bystanders like cycling, gymnastics, and weightlifting
3. Sports with major risk, like motor sports, parachuting, rodeo, and scuba diving

There is no doubt that sports where the head can be reached routinely like boxing, karate, taekwondo, judo, and MMA have to be avoided.

One of the causes of seizures during the sports is cerebral concussion, which occurs with the displacement of the brain inside the skull by impact or external displacement forces.

American football, rugby, hockey, and soccer with well-defined protocols are not only for withdrawal in cases of occurrence of the but also for the return to play.

Most of these sports are classified in category 1 by the ILAE, and although they possibly present concussion, they do not present absolute contraindication for the practice by athletes with epilepsy.

If the seizure after a cerebral concussion occurs, the evaluation for the return to play should follow the specific protocols, in relation to a non-epileptic athlete mainly in relation to the imaging and electroencephalogram examinations, besides the evaluation of the levels of medications previously used.

These athletes should be managed on an individualized basis by a multidisciplinary team of specialists with clinical expertise in epilepsy [22].

The high-performance athletes can use safely the antiepileptic drugs because they are not included in the list of forbidden drugs by World Anti-Doping Agency (WADA).

Even in high-performance sports where energy demand is much higher, and the hyperventilation can directly exacerbate the seizures, or the exercise indirectly can alter the level of anticonvulsants, [23] there are no clear restrictions on sports practice because the exercise benefits individuals with epilepsy. However neurological monitoring and adherence to the prescribed treatment are very important.

18.6 Post-traumatic Epilepsy

Post-traumatic epilepsy is lifelong complications of traumatic brain injury.

After the head injury, the seizure can occur, immediately related to the trauma itself or even after 1 week when it is considered to be post-traumatic seizure (PTS).

Some authors considered PTS, seizures up to 4 weeks after the head injury [24].

Normally the post-traumatic epilepsy occurs close to 80% in the first 2 years after the head injury [25].

There is a correlation between the severity of the head trauma and the development of post-traumatic epilepsy. Thus, in patients with brain contusion, intracerebral hematoma is more likely to develop PTE, when compared with mild injuries such as cerebral concussion.

For the diagnosis of brain lesions, magnetic resonance imaging (MRI) is the most indicated neuroimaging method.

The utility of the electroencephalogram in differentiating which patients are at an increased risk of developing PTE remains unclear. However, the use of prophylactic antiepileptic drugs for a short time after severe head trauma is advocated by some authors to prevent the PTE [26].

The treatment of post-traumatic epilepsy follows the same orientation of epileptic patients.

18.7 Management of Seizures and Epilepsy

For most patients with epilepsy, treatment does not aim to cure the condition but to control seizures and improve quality of life, with the minimum of side effects possible. The choice of lifestyles according to the patient's abilities is also a big factor in managing epilepsy [27].

The first data taken into account when treating a patient with epilepsy is the type of epilepsy. Seizure types and seizure syndromes have important implications in the choice of antiseizure drugs. When well chosen, and in adequate dosage, approximately half of the patients with a new diagnosis of epilepsy will remain seizure-free with the first antiseizure drugs prescribed, [28, 29] with another 10–20% of patients having a successful control with a second drug trial [30, 31], with the remaining, nonseizure-free patients, being called refractory [32], with low chances of becoming seizure-free.

Table 18.3 Antiseizure drugs according to seizure type

Broad spectrum (used for focal and generalized onset seizures)	Narrow spectrum (used for focal onset seizures)	Narrow spectrum (absence)
Valproate Levetiracetam Topiramate Lamotrigine Brivaracetam Clobazam Perampanel	Carbamazepine Oxcarbazepine Eslicarbazepine Gabapentin Phenytoin Pregabalin Lacosamide	Ethosuximide

Table 18.4 Antiseizure drugs with the potential to worsen generalized seizures

Generalized onset tonic-clonic seizures	Carbamazepine and phenytoin
Absence seizures in children	Carbamazepine, oxcarbazepine, phenobarbital, phenytoin, tiagabine, and vigabatrin
Absence seizures, myoclonic seizures, and in some cases generalized-onset tonic-clonic seizures in patients with juvenile myoclonic epilepsy	Carbamazepine, gabapentin, lamotrigine, oxcarbazepine, phenytoin, tiagabine, and vigabatrin

Adapted from Glauser T, Ben-Menachem E, Bourgeois B, et al. Updated ILAE evidence review of antiepileptic drug efficacy and effectiveness as initial monotherapy for epileptic seizures and syndromes. Epilepsia 54:551–63; 2013

Tables 18.3 and 18.4 give a broad idea of medical treatment of epilepsy.

Refractory patients should always be referred to a tertiary epilepsy center, in order to investigate if there is an indication of surgical treatment. Video-EEG and MRI are particularly important in this follow-up [33].

References

1. Fisher RS, van Emde Boas W, Blume W, et al. Epileptic seizures and epilepsy: definitions proposed by the International League Against Epilepsy (ILAE) and the International Bureau for Epilepsy (IBE). Epilepsia. 2005;46(4):470–2.
2. Fisher RS, Acevedo C, Arzimanoglou A, et al. ILAE official report: a practical clinical definition of epilepsy. Epilepsia. 2014;55(4):475–82.
3. Luders H, Acharya J, Baumgartner C, et al. Semiological seizure classification. Epilepsia. 1998;39(9):1006–13.
4. Hauser WA, Annegers JF, Kurland LT. Incidence of epilepsy and unprovoked seizures in Rochester, Minnesota: 1935–1984. Epilepsia. 1993;34:453.
5. Everitt P, Sander JW. Incidence of epilepsy is now higher in elderly people than children. Br Med J. 1998;316:780.
6. Schwartzkroin PA. Mechanisms of epileptogenesis in symptomatic epilepsy. In: The causes of epilepsy. Cambridge: Cambridge University Press; 2011.
7. Reinert M, Khaldi A, Zauner A, et al. High level of extracellular potassium and its correlates after severe head injury. J Neurosurg. 2000;93:800–7.
8. Gorji A, Speckmann EJ. Spreading depression enhances the spontaneous epileptiform activity in human neocortical tissues. Eur J Neurosci. 2004;19:3371–4.
9. Benardo LS. Prevention of epilepsy after head trauma: do we need new drugs or a new approach? Epilepsia. 2003;44(10):27–33.
10. Nizuma K, Endo H, Chan PH. Oxidative stress and mitochondrial dysfunction as determinants of ischemic neuronal death and survival. J Neurochem. 2009;109(1):133–8.
11. Pitkanen A, Karatishvili I, Karhunen H. Epileptogenesis in experimental models. Epilepsia. 2007;49(5):19–25.
12. Scheffer IE, Berkovic S, Capovilla G, et al. LAE classification of the epilepsies: position paper of the ILAE Commission for Classification and Terminology. Epilepsia. 2017;58(4):512–8.
13. Fisher RS, Cross JH, French JA. Operational classification of seizure types by the International League Against Epilepsy: position paper of the ILAE Commission for Classification and Terminology. Epilepsia. 2017;58(4):522.
14. Beghi E, Carpio A, Forsgren L, et al. Recommendation for a definition of acute symptomatic seizure. Epilepsia. 2010;51(4):671.
15. Krumholz A, Wiebe S, Gronseth G, et al. Practice parameter: evaluating an apparent unprovoked first seizure in adults (an evidence-based review): report of the Quality Standards Subcommittee of the American Academy of Neurology and the American Epilepsy Society. Neurology. 2007;69(21):1996.
16. van Donselaar CA, Schimsheimer RJ, Geerts AT. Value of the electroencephalogram in adult patients with untreated idiopathic first seizures. Arch Neurol. 1992;49(3):231.
17. Fountain NB, Van Ness PC, Swain-Eng R, et al. Quality improvement in neurology: AAN epilepsy quality measures: report of the Quality Measurement and Reporting Subcommittee of the American Academy of Neurology. Neurology. 2011;76(1):94.
18. ACEP Clinical Policies Committee, Clinical Policies Subcommittee on Seizures. Critical issues in the evaluation and management of adult patients presenting to the emergency department with seizures. Ann Emerg Med. 2004;43(5):605–25.
19. Capovilla G, Kaufman KR, Perucca E, Moshé SL, Arida RM, et al. Epilepsy, seizures, physical exercise,

and sports: a report from the ILAE task force on sports and epilepsy. Epilepsia. 2016;57(1):6–12.
20. Jalava M, Sillanpaa M. Physical activity, health-related fitness, and health experience in adults with childhood-onset epilepsy: a controlled study. Epilepsia. 1997;38(4):424–9.
21. Collard SS, Ellis-Hill C. 'I'd rather you didn't come': the impact of stigma on exercising with epilepsy. J Health Psychol. 2017:1359105317729560.
22. Ellis MJ, Ritchie L, Essig M, Ng M, Tamayo A, Serletis D. Management and return to play considerations in an Elite hockey player with temporal lobe epilepsy. Curr Sports Med Rep. 2018;17(1):10–2. https://doi.org/10.1249/JSR.0000000000000439.
23. Sahoo SK, Fountain NB. Epilepsy in football players and other land-based contact or collision sport athletes: when can they participate, and is there an increased risk? Curr Sports Med Rep. 2004;3(5):284–8.
24. Frey LC. Epidemiology of posttraumatic epilepsy: a critical review. Epilepsia. 2003;44(Suppl 10):11–7.
25. Haltiner AM, Temkin NR, Dikmen SS. Risk of seizure recurrence after the first late posttraumatic seizure. Arch Phys Med Rehabil. 1997;78:835–40.
26. Chen JW, Ruff RL, Eavey R, Wasterlain CG. Posttraumatic epilepsy and treatment. J Rehabil Res Dev. 2009;46(6):685–96.
27. Schachter SC. Advances in the assessment of refractory epilepsy. Epilepsia. 1993;34(Suppl 5):S24.
28. Kwan P, Brodie MJ. Effectiveness of first antiepileptic drug. Epilepsia. 2001;42(10):1255.
29. Brodie MJ, Perucca E, Ryvlin P. Comparison of levetiracetam and controlled-release carbamazepine in newly diagnosed epilepsy. Neurology. 2007;68(6):402.
30. Kwan P, Brodie MJ. Early identification of refractory epilepsy. N Engl J Med. 2000;342(5):314.
31. Bonnett LJ, Tudur Smith C, Donegan S, et al. Treatment outcome after failure of a first antiepileptic drug. Neurology. 2014;83(6):552–60.
32. Kwan P, Arzimanoglou A, Berg AT, et al. Definition of drug resistant epilepsy: consensus proposal by the ad hoc Task Force of the ILAE Commission on Therapeutic Strategies. Epilepsia. 2010;51(6):1069.
33. Labiner DM, Bagic AI, Herman ST, et al. Essential services, personnel, and facilities in specialized epilepsy centers—revised 2010 guidelines. Epilepsia. 2010;51(11):2322.

Spine Injuries

19

Elcio Landim, Paulo Tadeu Maia Cavali,
Marcelo Italo Risso Neto,
and Mauricio Coelho Lima

19.1 Introduction

The head, the neck, and the spinal cord are the costliest and potentially morbid among sports injuries. Although the practice of sports usually results in well-being while it aggregates lots of health benefits, no sport is immune to the risk of a spine injury. The spine may be affected during professional and recreational sports practice, both in training and competitions [1].

The spine is very sensitive to asymmetric sports, which may contribute to the postural imbalance or increase of pre-existing asymmetries. For the same reason, athletes with posture deviations are more susceptible to these types of lesions. As an example, studies on the relationship between posture and sports injuries in footballers have shown that back injuries are associated with the poor symmetry of shoulders and back, as well as to scapulae abduction [1].

There are specific lesions that are more common in sports practices, and these can be divided into those due to direct trauma in a specific anatomical structure or those due to supraphysiological stress on the spine [2]. Stress lesions can take place both in the individual as in collective sports. Special attention must, therefore, be given during the training phase in order to avoid excessive workloads in terms of intensity and frequency. Appropriate timing must be observed taking into account the period needed for recovery and the adaptation of the muscle and tendon involved; this way, this type of lesion can be avoided, as well as the pain associated with inflammatory phenom-

E. Landim (✉) · M. C. Lima
Spine Surgery Group of the German Hospital "Oswaldo Cruz", São Paulo, SP, Brazil

Department of Scoliosis, AACD (Associação de Assistência à Criança Deficiente), São Paulo, SP, Brazil

Spine Surgery Division of Orthopedics and Traumatology Department, State University of Campinas—UNICAMP, Campinas, SP, Brazil

Brazilian Society of Orthopedics and Traumatology, and the Brazilian Spine Society, São Paulo, SP, Brazil
e-mail: elciolandim@uol.com.br

P. T. M. Cavali
Spine Surgery Group of the German Hospital "Oswaldo Cruz", São Paulo, SP, Brazil

Department of Scoliosis, AACD (Associação de Assistência à Criança Deficiente), São Paulo, SP, Brazil

Brazilian Society of Orthopedics and Traumatology, and the Brazilian Spine Society, São Paulo, SP, Brazil
e-mail: pt.cavali@uol.com.br

M. I. Risso Neto
Spine Surgery Group of the German Hospital "Oswaldo Cruz", São Paulo, SP, Brazil

Spine Surgery Division of Orthopedics and Traumatology Department, State University of Campinas—UNICAMP, Campinas, SP, Brazil

Brazilian Society of Orthopedics and Traumatology, and the Brazilian Spine Society, São Paulo, SP, Brazil
e-mail: mrisso@me.com

S. Rocha Piedade et al. (eds.), *The Sports Medicine Physician*,
https://doi.org/10.1007/978-3-030-10433-7_19

ena and anatomical injuries of spine structures [3]. Traumatic lesions usually occur in speed and contact sports, both individual and collective.

19.2 Anatomy of Spine Lesions (Table 19.1)

19.2.1 Bone Lesions

Many types of fractures occur in sports injuries. The most common and frequently reported vertebral bone lesion is spondylolysis, the vertebra area that connects the upper and lower zygapophyseal joints. These lesions are related to repeated extension movements which impact the isthmus on the superior facet joint of the inferior vertebra. The symptoms are back pain whether or not associated with radiculopathy [4]. Fractures of the vertebral body may occur due to compression forces in high-energy sports accidents [5].

19.2.2 Muscle Lesions

Muscular lesions are probably the most common ones related to sports. Direct contusions, stretches, and ruptures may be caused by diverse mechanisms. Reflex contractions of muscles are another cause of pain, and they are usually secondary to another skeletal lesion.

19.2.3 Ligament Lesions

This type of lesion on the spine is related to hyperextension or hyperflexion in repeated movements or a traumatic condition. Incomplete lesions occur due to stretches and are not associated with instability. On the other hand, complete lesions are unstable and commonly associated with neurological deficit [6].

Table 19.1 Anatomical lesions on the spine

Muscle	Contusion, stretch, total or partial rupture
Ligaments	Stretch, total or partial rupture
Disc	Disc rupture, protrusion, extrusion
Bone	Fractures (compression, traction, rotations, and avulsion)
Joints	Sprain and dislocation
Neurological	Nerve root and spinal cord (partial or complete)

19.2.4 Disc Lesions

This condition is related to sport intensity and its repeated movements, as well as to a previous degenerative disease that leads to its worsening and becoming more frequent. A disc herniation seldom occurs due to a traumatic event even though it has been reported [7]. Neurological deficits and pain may occur due to disc compression.

19.2.5 Joint Lesions

Low-energy traumas may cause a sprain, while high-energy traumas may cause joint dislocations. Chronic lesions with mild instability are associated with synovial cysts and possible radiculopathy.

19.2.6 Neurological Lesions

Neurological spine lesions are among the worst and most devastating lesions in sports. They affect the spinal cord and/or spinal nerve roots, with different presentations and levels of severity. Contact sports are among the riskiest for these lesions. Many publications report severe spine lesions in ice hockey, rugby, and football [8–12]. Degenerative disease and congenital stenosis reduce available space in the vertebral canal of the spinal cord; there are findings concerning the risk of developing neurological injury in the practice of sports.

> Contact sports present the highest rates of severe injuries.

19.3 Cervical Spine Lesions in Sport

Cervical spine injuries are common in sports. Most injuries result from low-energy trauma causing sprains, which, in turn, lead to complete rehabilitation without sequelae. Although rare, cervical spine injuries involving the spinal cord and nerve roots can lead to potentially serious sequelae such as tetraplegia. The severity and extent of the injury depend fundamentally on the kinetics of trauma and is related to the type of sport and the technical level of the athlete. Contact sports, especially rugby; high-speed sports, such as skiing; and motorized sports have a greater risk of developing serious injuries [8–11].

> In general, lumbar injuries are the most common, but the cervical spine is subject to the most severe lesions.

The presence of previous lesions, such as congenital or acquired spinal canal stenosis, increases the risk of neurological damage and should be considered and evaluated before sports practices that expose the cervical spine to risk. Trauma in hyperextension of the cervical spine can cause a medullary contusion with the possibility of transient or permanent symptoms.

Cervical neurological lesions in the athlete are classified in three categories [13]:

- Type I—Permanent spinal cord injury.
- Type II—Transient medullary or root neurological deficit, with regression in a few minutes or hours.
- Type III—Post-traumatic lesion with purely radiological findings, without clinical correspondence.

In addition to acute traumas, repetitive traumatic injuries can cause or accelerate degenerative processes leading to lesions that may have clinical presentations ranging from asymptomatic to chronic axial pain and neurological root or spinal deficits.

19.3.1 Cervical Peripheral Nerve Injuries

19.3.1.1 Burners

"Burners" (also known as "stingers") are temporary symptoms of burn, pain, or sensitive and/or motor loss that happens involving the upper limbs [14]. They usually occur after a trauma to the brachial plexus or the exiting nerve roots in the cervical spine [15]. They frequently happen in contact sports, such as football and rugby. A high number of football players, most commonly defensive players, present burner symptoms at least once during their careers [16].

Burners can be caused by compression, distraction, or direct blow mechanisms. If an asymmetrical axial trauma to the neck causes a compression in the neuroforamen, it can damage the peripheral nerve root. Also, if the player falls on the shoulder and his head is distracted from the upper limb, traction is applied to the nerve root and the brachial plexus. Finally, when the cervical spine receives a force in hyperextension, hyperflexion, or lateral flexion to the opposite side, the distance and the angle between the shoulder and neck are excessively increased, thus stretching the brachial plexus. Compression combined with extension is the most common mechanism [17].

Symptoms of burners are usually severe pain in the shoulder and arm, with a loss of the sense of touch and weakness of the arm. The deltoid (C5), biceps (C5,6), and spinatus muscles (C5,6) are most commonly involved, and the symptoms typically last only a few seconds or minutes. Shoulder abduction may cause less pain, and the doctor can ask the player to place a hand on the top of the head. The Spurling maneuver reproduces the mechanism of the injury, and burning or pain is reported by the player when this movement is performed [16, 18] The symptoms can be presented in different degrees of severity ranging from a transient nerve irritation without residual damage (most common) to a complete avulsion of the nerve root from the spinal cord with permanent deficit (very rare) [17].

To prevent burners the player needs to wear appropriate protection equipment and to learn the correct way to block and to tackle during the practice, using only the shoulder, and never the head while keeping the head down [17].

Initial treatment involves removing the player from the game and allowing him/her to rest; this is followed by strengthening exercises of the neck and restoration of the range of motion. These injuries are classified using the Seddon classification of neurapraxia. Athletes with more severe lesions may require a longer period for recovery lasting from a few hours to a few weeks when the athlete will be away from the game [19–26].

19.3.1.2 Cervical Stenosis

Congenital cervical stenosis is a risk factor for cervical spine injuries [27]. Burners are more common in players with spinal stenosis as defined by the Torg ratio, which is defined as the ratio of the spinal canal width to the width of the vertebral body at the same level; the narrowest is at C7. A Torg ratio of 0.7 to 0.8, or lower, is high risk. For players with cervical stenosis, the risk of burners and other neurological complications during sports practice is three times as high as players without stenosis, and this ratio is usually used as a screening for football and rugby players to prevent neurological complications in those sports [20–31].

19.3.1.3 Transient Spinal Cord Compression

Torg and colleagues [32] related the syndrome of transient quadriplegia, which represents a "neuropraxia of the cervical spinal cord." The syndrome is characterized by bilateral upper and lower limbs' neurological involvement without any fracture or dislocation associated; in most cases, the problem is solved in 36 hours. There is a strong association between transient quadriplegia and developmental spinal stenosis; according to the current literature, all patients who presented transient quadriparesis had a diagnosis of spinal stenosis. However, there is no evidence that the occurrence of transient quadriplegia predisposes to permanent neurological injury [17, 32].

19.4 Thoracolumbar Lesions in Sports

The thoracolumbar lesions are more frequent than the cervical ones, and they represent 10% of the injuries caused by sports. Likewise, there is a broad clinical presentation spectrum ranging from non-specific low back pain to paraplegia [33, 34].

The different types of sports and mechanisms of thoracolumbar injury are related to the clinical findings. The lesions that occur in extension expose the risk of fracture of the pars or facet joints, and gymnasts are among the most affected athletes [35]; torsional injuries affect discs and facets and occur more often in sports such as golf and tennis; compression/flexion lesions expose the intervertebral disc to greater risk of damage; injury by fall or secondary to an external agent can cause unexpected and potentially more serious damages depending on the intensity and energy of the trauma [36].

The way energy is applied to the trauma can lead to different lesions and in different tissues: for example, lesions occurring at high speed can affect the vertebrae and cause fractures by abrupt deceleration, while the application of progressive and repetitive energy favors disc and ligament degeneration.

19.4.1 Spondylolysis

Spondylolysis is a stress fracture of the pars interarticularis. It is generally considered to be a low-risk fracture that occurs most frequently at L5, followed by L4 and L3. The mean rate of spondylolysis is 5–6% in the general population, [37] and, in general, it is asymptomatic. Repetitive stress generally produces fatigue fracture. These fractures may consolidate but develop fibrous nonunion or heal in an elongated state [38].

The incidence of pars defects is greater in athletes than in the nonathletic population, and it is a clinical problem for these patients [39]. Sports that require hyperextension associated with rotational movements such as gymnastics, wrestling, and weightlifting are associated with a stress fracture of the pars interarticularis. Some specific sports, such as diving, weightlifting, wrestling, and gymnastics, have extraordinarily high rates of this injury [40]. Many studies suggest that a variety of sports, such as soccer, volleyball, and baseball, increase the risk of spondylolysis [41].

Spondylolysis is a bone injury that, in most cases, does not produce neurological symptoms. Any nerve root signs would suggest an alternative diagnostic [37].

19.4.2 Spondylolisthesis

Spondylolisthesis occurs when there is a bilateral lesion in the pars interarticularis, and the vertebral body slips forward over the lower vertebra. The incidence of spondylolisthesis in athletes is the same as in the general population [37].

In the current literature, there are no criteria available for predicting which cases of spondylolysis will progressively slip, resulting in spondylolisthesis. Most cases of spondylolisthesis are low grade and unlikely to progress. With mild spondylolisthesis, there is no reason to forbid the athlete from participating in sports [37].

Isthmic spondylolisthesis is the most common type found in young athletes. Bilateral stress fractures of the pars are the distinguishing pathology of spondylolisthesis. The main risk factor, other than a familial predisposition for this injury, is hyperextension mechanism [37].

Symptoms of spondylolisthesis are low back pain worsened during activity, especially those that involve hyperextension and rotation. Sports with rotation and extension under load repeated a lot of times during practice such as gymnastics, football, wrestling, hockey, pole vaulting, diving, and throwing sports are related as causal factors in many reports [42, 43]. Typically for mechanical-type pain, rest tends to alleviate the pain [37].

During the investigation, it was found that, if radiculopathy is present, the L5 root is most commonly involved [44, 45]. Cases with neurological symptoms must be differentiated from disc herniation.

The lateral X-ray of the lumbar spine confirms the diagnostic, and the degree of the slip is graded according to the Meyerding classification. There is a consensus that kyphosis is a more important sign of severity measure of the deformity than displacement [45].

19.4.3 Apophyseal Ring Fracture

This injury is characterized by bone fragments at the posterior vertebral endplate and is also known as limbus fracture or fracture of the vertebral rim, ring, or endplate [46]. This lesion is exclusive of adolescents [47] and was reported by Skobowytsh-Okolot in 1962 [48, 49]. There is an overall prevalence of only 0.07%; there is also an 85% predominance in males; 66% have an association with a traumatic event, such as weightlifting or sports injury [46–49]. This is, also, associated with Scheuermann disease [50] and lumbar disc herniations [51].

Both hyperextension of the lumbar spine [52] and acute flexion associated with axial compression to the lumbar spine, such as it occurs with weightlifting, are the proposed mechanisms of this injury [47, 48, 53]. Symptoms of an apophyseal ring fracture are similar to Disc Herniation - pain in the back and buttock which gets worse after coughing, sports and sitting [48]. Pain may radiate down one or both legs. The straight-leg-raise test is positive, and contralateral straight-leg raise is frequently positive. Paraspinal muscle spasm, lumbar tenderness, scoliosis, intermittent claudication, paraparesis, and cauda equina syndrome have been reported [47, 48].

19.4.4 Disc Herniation

Disc herniation or Herniated Nucleus Pulposus is an injury related to sports, and surgeries for these conditions in athletes are performed many times during a sports season. High-risk activities include weightlifting and collision sports, such as football [48], and also basketball, baseball, and wrestling [50]. The incidence is 95% of herniations occurring from L4 to S1 and is fairly evenly distributed between L4–L5 and L5–S1. The L3–L4 herniation is present in 5% of patients [54].

The symptoms of HNP are leg pain with or without neurological issues. Rehabilitation is demanded as soon as the symptoms appear, and the return to sports is related to the severity of them and the moment of disappearance of these symptoms.

MRI is the gold standard, and the conservative treatment is effective in most cases, while surgery is reserved for the cauda equina syndrome, progressive motor deficits, or failure of the conservative care [37].

19.5 Common Spine Injuries in Sports

19.5.1 Football

In the United States, football is a very popular sport and leads all other sports in the number of injuries [55]. The football lesion rates are figured from 600,000 to 1.2 million injuries of the entire body every year in the United States [56]. As the number of football players continues to increase around the globe, the analysis of prevalent lesions in professional football is necessary in order to help health professionals to understand the risks that the athletes are exposed to during their practice [57].

Using a National Football League (NFL) injury database, recorded from years 2000 to 2010, Mall et al. [56] have identified 2208 axial skeleton lesions, including spinal injuries. This study demonstrates that injuries to the spine accounted for 7% of the lesions in the National Football League (NFL). The number of spinal injuries varied between 152 and 256 per year, during this 10-year follow-up, while 987 (44.7%) of these lesions were cervical injuries which account for the most frequently injured location of the axial skeleton during football practice. The lumbar spine was affected in 30.9% of the cases, the thoracic spine and ribs in 3.9%, and the sacrum, coccyx, and pelvis in 10.1% and the spinal cord was responsible for 0.6% of the injuries.

There are a high number of severe injuries during football practice [4]; because of this, there are probably only a few studies that have demonstrated data on fewer incapacitating injuries in football [58]. These include back contusions, lumbar back pain, back cramp/spasm, back muscle strain, back degeneration, and intervertebral disc disorders [56]. Disc herniations have accounted for 13% of all injuries affecting the entire spine and, more specifically, represented 28% of lumbar spine injuries, 6% of cervical spine injuries, and 5% of thoracic spine injuries [59].

Spondylolysis occurs most frequently among adolescents, with high rates of incidence among athletes, especially football players [60]. Also, the incidence of degenerative disc disease and facet degeneration is higher among the football population than in the general population [61]. Having spondylolysis is a very important risk factor when analyzing football athletes with low back pain [62]. The higher incidence of spine issues in football players is caused by the excessive compressive, torsional, and shearing forces produced in the spine during practice.

The cervical spine is the most affected anatomic location of the spine during football, and it is also where the most severe lesions occur [2]. In order of incidence, the lesions in the cervical spine are presented as follows: nerve root or brachial plexus neurapraxia (burners), cervical strains (muscular injury), disc injury with neck pain only, cervical sprains (ligament injury), disc herniation with radicular symptoms, transient spinal cord compression secondary to stenosis, and cervical fractures [32, 63–65].

Analyzing average time missed after an injury during the football practice, cervical fractures are responsible for the highest mean number of days missed during a season, among all injuries sustained in the National Football League (NFL) [56]. Their accounting for 120 days per injury and disc degeneration/ herniation was responsible for a mean time loss of 85 days per injury, while spinal cord injury responded for 77 days per injury [66].

Tackling is the football movement most related to cervical spine lesions, while blocking produces most of the lumbar spine injuries.

This injury mechanism suggests the reason why defensive players present a higher rate of spine injuries than their offensive teammates. Recent data suggest that these lesions are found not only among professional athletes but also among non-professional players [57].

American football players present a high risk for severe trauma, including spinal cord injury [67]. The incidence of serious cervical spine injuries was highest in early times but declined during the 1970s with the banning of head-down “spear tackling” as shown by Torg et al. [32, 62, 68]. The National Football League (NFL) began its efforts to address SRC (sport-related concussion) with the establishment of the Mild Traumatic Brain Injury Committee in 1994 [63]. In 2010 the committee was reconstituted as the Head, Neck and Spine (HN&S) Committee [69], which defines protocols and guidelines for the management and prevention of these important lesions and also contributes for a safer practice of this sport around the world.

The education of the athletes, coaches, and referees was responsible for the decrease of the serious cervical injuries in contact sports, especially football and rugby.

19.5.2 Rugby

Rugby is one of the most popular sports around the world [70] and the most popular collision sport. Rugby is a physical contact sport that presents a high risk for traumatic injury and the use of little or no body padding. This risk has increased with the professionalization of the sport, which stimulated players to become larger and stronger [71]. Rugby presents one of the highest overall injury rates of all team sports [72].

Epidemiological studies demonstrated that the most common injuries to the spine during rugby practice are less severe lesions to the lumbar spine as back pain, back muscle strain, and lumbar disc disorders [10, 73, 74]. Iwamoto and colleagues [75, 76] noted structural abnormalities in 74% of the rugby players assessed in the study. Severe lesions are rare in the lumbar spine, and disc herniation is the condition that most needs an intervention such as surgery or steroid injections [77, 78].

Despite all the concerns about the cervical spine during the rugby practice, Hind et al. showed that rugby players also had a higher risk for thoracolumbar fractures, presenting greater rates of this kind of fracture than the previously reported prevalence rates for the general population [79].

Injuries to the cervical spine are the most serious injuries during rugby practice. From the 1970s to the middle of the 1980s, an increase was found in the rates of rugby-related spinal lesions in countries where rugby was commonly played all over the globe. Many injury prevention measures were implemented worldwide by the International Rugby Board (IRB) aiming the alterations of the rules of the game and educational measures of the players searching for safer techniques in the game. The scrum was the part of the game most associated with spinal lesions until 1990; after the rule changed, the rates of spinal lesions occurring during tackle became higher [80].

The most common cervical spine injuries in rugby were facet dislocations. The injury often affects C4/C5 and C5/C6 levels. Hyperflexion of the neck was hypothesized to be the primary mechanism for cervical spine injury in rugby [17, 81–85], but recent studies have identified tackle as the moment of highest occurrence of the cervical injuries and buckling as the main biomechanical mechanism of cervical spine injury during rugby practice [17].

19.5.3 Tennis

Tennis athletes experience few severe injuries on average. Tennis lesions are due to repetitive overload and related with the increasing years of training. Although ankle and knee lesions are more common in tennis practice, lumbar spine lesions are more recurrent than others [86].

There is a paucity of published data in relation to elite athletes, with considerable variability in the reported incidence of lesions, ranging from 0.04 to 3.0 injuries per 1000 playing hours, not related to gender. Lumbar lesions account for around 12–13% and head and neck around 3% of all musculoskeletal lesions [87]. Regarding male athletes, the lumbar region is the third anatomical site of injury, and to female athletes, it is the fifth. This finding is due to the repetitive trunk movements required in tennis practice, especially hyperextension and rapid rotation of the lumbar spine during training and playing a match; this supports the frequent findings of low back pain in tennis athletes and its correlation with radiological abnormalities in this population [88, 89]. As a reference, the lumbar region undergoes substantial loading during the kick and flat tennis serves, including lateral flexion forces approximately eight times those experienced during running.

A study that describes lumbar MRI findings in asymptomatic young elite tennis players concluded that any abnormalities occurred with 84.8% of these players almost exclusively on L4 L5 and L5S1 levels, with facet joint arthropathy, pars, and intervertebral disc injuries [89, 90].

19.5.4 Winter Sports

Sports requiring ice or snow as a playing surface are called winter sports. Most of these sports are associated with high speed, thus susceptible to spine traumas.

After the head and the chest, spine injuries are the most common among these sports. Due to the association with high speed and high energy, the majority of these lesions is caused because of falls and collision against natural objects [91].

The literature contains a wide range of statistics related to lesions due to snow sports, especially depending on the age group, location, and the specific sport. Injuries associated with neurological deficit accounts for 42%, and males are more frequently injured [92, 93]. The most frequent lesions from skiing and snowboard are thoracolumbar junction fractures. Ice hockey presents an equal number of cervical and thoracolumbar fractures since two thirds of them are associated with neurological deficit. These lesions usually occur between levels C5 and C7, caused by head impact against the boards, sustaining an axial compression on the cervical spine [93].

19.5.5 Volleyball

Volleyball and beach volleyball are intensive sports, associated with high impact and repetition of similar movements that may cause spine injuries.

Volleyball is associated with a predominant forward bending and extension posture, which may cause changes in lumbar lordosis and sagittal imbalance. Lumbar lordosis flattening is associated with pelvic retroversion due to increased use of abdominal and gluteal muscles. The finding of a decrease of lumbar lordosis is associated with the increase of thoracic kyphosis.

These changes in lumbar lordosis may be associated with the findings of a higher incidence of low back pain and with a higher prevalence of degenerative findings on MRI, including disc degeneration and spondylolisthesis [94]. In professional volleyball players, the prevalence of disc degeneration is up to three times as high when compared to the normal population. Considering MRI findings in professional beach volleyball players, the prevalence of disc degeneration is 79%, and spondylosis is 21%. Despite these data, MRI findings do not correlate with back pain symptoms [95].

Traumatic lesions may occur due to repetitive stress, as well as impact or sudden and severe contraction of the muscles. The literature on volleyball practice reports few cases such as stable fractures in lower cervical spinous processes, called Clay shoveler's fracture [96], myelopathy due to acute disc herniation, and vertebral artery dissection [97].

Case 1

A 34-year-old female professional volleyball athlete in the national league refers to sudden neck pain during training, associated with right arm pain and weakness. She came to specialized evaluation after 2 days of conservative treatment with analgesics and physiotherapy. She complained of neck pain irradiating to the right arm on the C6 and C7 dermatomes, weakness of wrist and elbow extension, hyperreflexia, and clonus on upper and lower limbs. MRI of cervical spine showed a disc herniation at C5C6 level with medullar compression and hypersignal in the sagittal and axial views (Fig. 19.1a, b). Ten days after this injury, the patient was submitted to decompression and arthrodesis on C5/C6 levels with autologous iliac graft (Fig. 19.2a, b). The complete weakness she experienced improved, and she returned to play 3 months after the surgery when fusion occurred and was confirmed with CT scan (Fig. 19.3).

19.5.6 Boxing

Boxing is an Olympic sport [98–100]; however, it is classified as a dangerous sport by presenting severe neurological complications of head lesions which have been discussed in several studies [101, 102].

Many studies show a small number of severe injuries, but this modality is related to dangerous injuries, especially head and brain lesions. Previous studies on boxing practice showed low injury rates with 0.69 injuries per boxer per year and 2.0 injuries per 1000 h of training [102, 103]. Boxing athletes most often present head, upper limbs, and overall injuries; these injuries resulted in an average of 10.5 lost days [104].

Cervical spine injuries represent around 10–20% of the injuries found in boxing athletes. In the cervical spine, severe injuries as fractures or spinal cord injuries are described as rare ones, but contusions and muscular lesions are the main cervical injuries related to this sport [104, 105].

The lumbar spine is less affected, and the number of injuries is around 8%, while the low back accounts for the highest number of lesions. Disc herniations can also occur, but the mean number of lesions is around 0.5%. Lumbar spine injuries during boxing are classified as less severe injuries and are related to a low rate of lost days of practice [104, 105].

19.5.7 Baseball

Spinal injuries are relatively rare in sports with less contact between the players such as in baseball; yet, there are a reasonable number of writings on the possibility of baseball players having spinal lesions in the entire extension of the

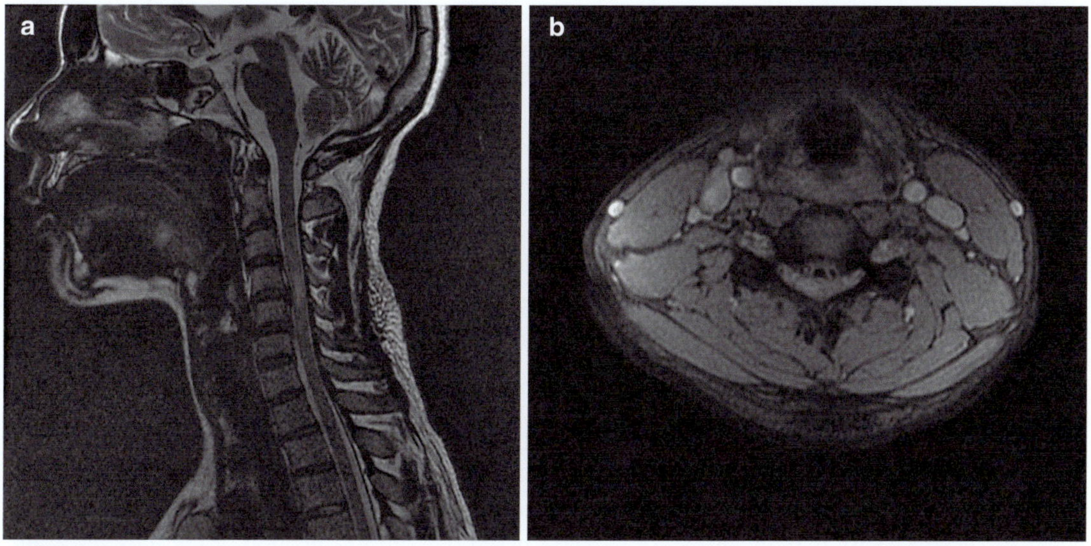

Fig. 19.1 (**a** and **b**) Cervical sagittal (**a**) and axial (**b**) MRI views of disc herniation at C5C6 level with medullar compression and hypersignal

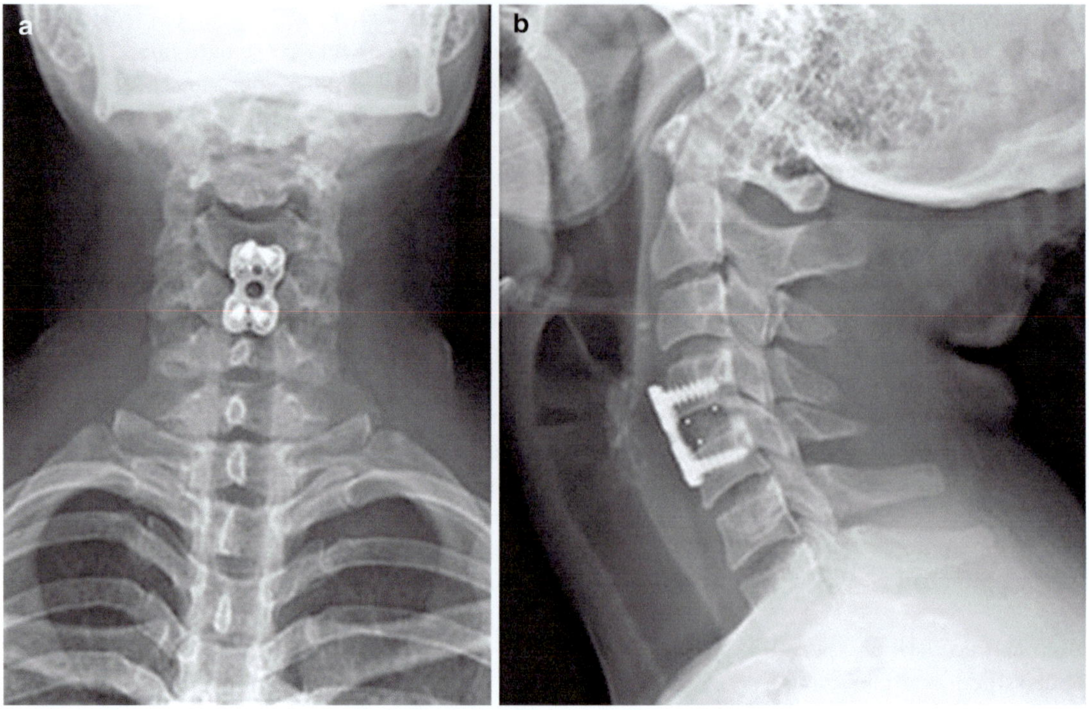

Fig. 19.2 (**a** and **b**) Decompression and arthrodesis on levels C5/C6 with autologous iliac graft 10 days after lesion, anteroposterior (**a**) and lateral (**b**) radiographic views

vertebral spine [106]. Spinal injuries during baseball practice are mostly found in the lumbar spine, and the correct diagnosis and treatment are necessary to allow the player to return to the sport as soon as possible [107].

Among baseball players, the injuries to the spine and core musculature respond with 11.7% of all sports injuries [108]. Lumbar disc herniation, spondylolysis, and spondylolisthesis are the most frequent injuries, while lumbar back pain is the main issue of the players [106, 107, 109–112].

19.5.7.1 Biomechanics of Baseball Injuries

Spinal stability depends on the structure of the bones and soft tissues and is achieved by the important role of the muscles that create dynamic and active support for the spine, allowing complex moves of torsion and extension of the trunk which are necessary for playing baseball.

The pitchers are the most commonly injured players. During a pitch, the torsion of the body begins in the lower limbs; then it raises to the pelvis, creating a hyperextension of the lumbar spine and a torsional movement of the thoracic spine, which produce the energy necessary for the upper limbs to perform the throw of the ball. This sequence of complex movements requires a higher strain on the facet joints [107, 110].

In spondylolysis and spondylolisthesis, the stress to the pars can lead to simple injuries as the local inflammatory response or to more severe lesions as fractures and dislocations. The pitchers present lumbar back pain in 15% of the cases during their careers, while around 9% of them present spondylolisthesis [109, 111, 112].

The treatment of the lumbar conditions in baseball players is widely discussed [113–116]. Low back pain has to be investigated, and other important diagnostics are excluded. The rehabilitation of low back pain without other lesions is based on core fortification of the muscles, training on stabilizers, and progressive stretching of lumbar and hamstrings [110].

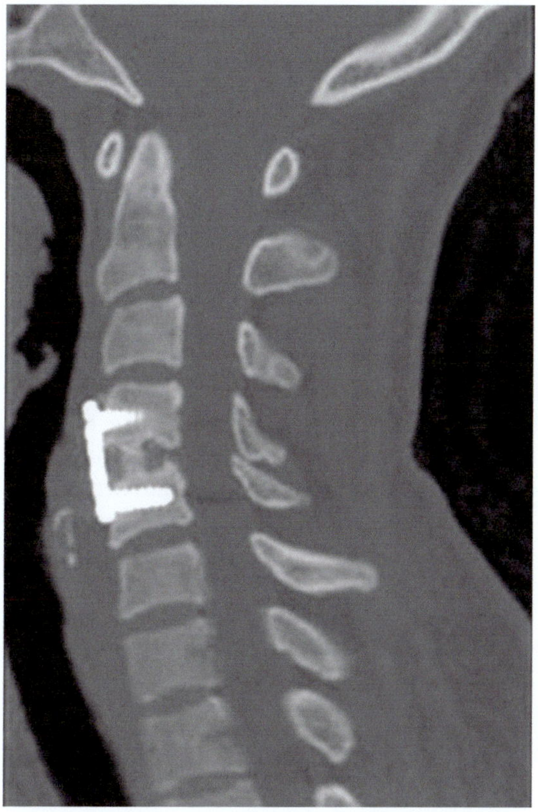

Fig. 19.3 Computed tomography showing evidence of bone marking and signs of consolidation at 3 months postoperative

Spondylolysis and spondylolisthesis treatment for baseball players follows the same principles of the guidelines of non-player patients. The choice between a surgical or conservative treatment is controversial, and most studies indicate surgery only after the failure of conservative treatment. Also, the average recovery time after surgery is longer (about 7 months) [114–116].

19.5.8 Soccer

Spinal injuries in soccer are not exclusive among elite or semiprofessional players; they have been reported in all ages and from amateurs to professional players [107]. Reducing injuries and improving the performance in soccer are directly related to neuromuscular control, which is defined as a dynamic process of maintaining balance during the practice [117]. In a physical contact sport, such as soccer, decreased core stability is associated with a higher incidence of low back pain.

Talib et al. collected prospective injury data for players of all 41 English professional soccer youth academies for 5 years, totalizing 12,306 academy players. These players presented 10,225 musculoskeletal injuries, resulting in 310 (4%) of lumbar spine injuries, and most of them was low back pain (49%), with strains being second (15%) and spondylolysis being third (4%). They also reported that there is an increased risk of lower back injury, according to the players' age and the contact mechanism, in the second part of the first half of competitive matches (a risk that was maintained throughout the second half), which was responsible for the majority of the lesions [118].

Back pain is the spinal symptom most frequently reported by the soccer players. The chronic lower back pain results in a time loss of 7–30 days of practice [119]. Longer training sessions, especially on artificial turf, are risk factors to develop back pain [120], and smoking and thigh muscle imbalance are reported with even worse symptoms [121, 122]. Early diagnosis allows appropriate management; the radiological investigation is indicated when this group of players presents back pain lasting longer than 3 weeks [119].

Rassi et al. (2005) [119] observed that 43% of the patients felt pain during the kicking movement, which is the most common moment to perceive pain. Sakai et al. (2010) [123] found that the incidence of spondylolysis was at 30% in the soccer-playing population. Most soccer players with spondylolysis had good or even excellent results after non-operative treatment. Cessation of sports for a period of 2–3 months can optimize the clinical outcome and is a strong predictor of a favorable return to sports. Similarly, Sys et al. (2001) [124] reported that early diagnosis of a fatigue fracture of the pars interarticularis is important because non-operative treatment of active spondylolysis leads to excellent results and sports resumption may be possible within 6 months for the majority of athletes.

19.6 Management of Sports Lesions

19.6.1 Lumbar Injuries

When pain is severe, rest may be necessary for a couple of days for initial pain management. A longer time of rest can start to cause muscular loss and is not recommended. The sooner the player starts some minor and tolerated activity, the quicker and more effective recovery is [125].

Anti-inflammatories and muscle relaxants are recommended for the maximum of 7–10 days, not more than that. Opioid administration can be used for a few days. Local anesthetic injections into the facet joints or into trigger points can be used and may help to establish a diagnostic while finding different causes for the symptoms [125].

Different modalities of physical therapy as ice, tens, massage, or heat can be used in initial treatment, but the player has to start active rehabilitation and strengthening as soon as possible; bracing should be avoided or minimized [125].

19.6.2 Cervical Injuries

During the sports practice, management of the injuries starting from the initial moment of the trauma may reduce long-term risk to the players and improve the return to playing [58]. If a cervical spine injury is suspected, the physician should investigate any spinal pain, search for the altered perception of touch, and interrogate numbness, weakness, or difficulty moving the extremities. Any player with these signs during an on-field examination should not participate in the game or training any longer, and cervical injuries need to be investigated [62].

When examining ambulatory athletes after a cervical trauma, the examiner should evaluate neck range of motion, and perform a motor and sensory examination of the extremities. Alterations observed during the exam mean that the athlete must be removed from competition and immobilized in a cervical collar. If the player is unconscious, it means that the physician should presume that a cervical spine injury exists, and the neck needs to be immobilized. A helmet should be placed and not removed, and the athlete must be immobilized before taken anywhere. Persistent or severe pain means that the player needs immediate radiologic evaluation. Returning to practice will occur when the symptoms have disappeared, and the image exams do not show any injury [125].

19.7 Return to Play

The return to the sport is very controversial, and there are many conflicting guidelines for each modality and injury. In general terms, for lumbar injuries, the athlete can return to play when there is no pain specifically related to the activity of the sport, and when the full range of motion is recovered. There is no definitive test to define when this point is reached. Gradual relief in pain and improvement in performance are predictive of a good prognosis.

The return to play after cervical spine trauma is based on guidelines which recommend waiting for the symptoms to disappear and for the player to have recovered the full range of motion and complete strength [125, 126]. Some studies recommend that the return to sport should be based on normal radiological exams as well [125, 127]. Less complex lesions, such as spinous process fractures, should have the treatment based on immobilization and return to activities only after healing. Patients with more than three burners in the same season should be clinically evaluated as well as with imaging, to make sure that there is no spinal stenosis or severe injury before returning to the sport. A single-level fusion, or one of two levels, may enable the return after healing. With three or more level fusions, the return to play is contraindicated [125, 128] (Table 19.2).

> Return to play is based on the type of injury, the relief of symptoms, and the recovery of the range of motion, but each case has to be analyzed for each sport and for each patient, also taking into account previous spine injuries, congenital stenosis, and surgeries for spinal conditions

Table 19.2 Traumatic and ligamentous injuries of the cervical spine: contraindication to return to play

No contraindications	Relative contraindications	Absolute contraindications
Neuropraxia or other neurological symptoms of spinal cord without radiological alterations and after complete resolution	Healed nondisplaced Jefferson fractures in patients who are also pain-free, have full range of cervical motion, and have no evidence of neurological injury	Injuries of C1-C2 that involve fracture or ligamentous laxity
	<3.5 mm of horizontal displacement of either vertebra in relation to the other and depending on the patient's level of performances, physical habits, and position played	>3.5 mm of horizontal displacement of either vertebra in relation to the other
	<11° of rotation of either adjacent vertebra and depending on the patient's level of performance, physical habits, and position played	>11° of rotation of either adjacent vertebra

Adapted from Torg JS. Cervical spine injuries and the return to football. Sports Health. 2009;1(5):376–83 [129]

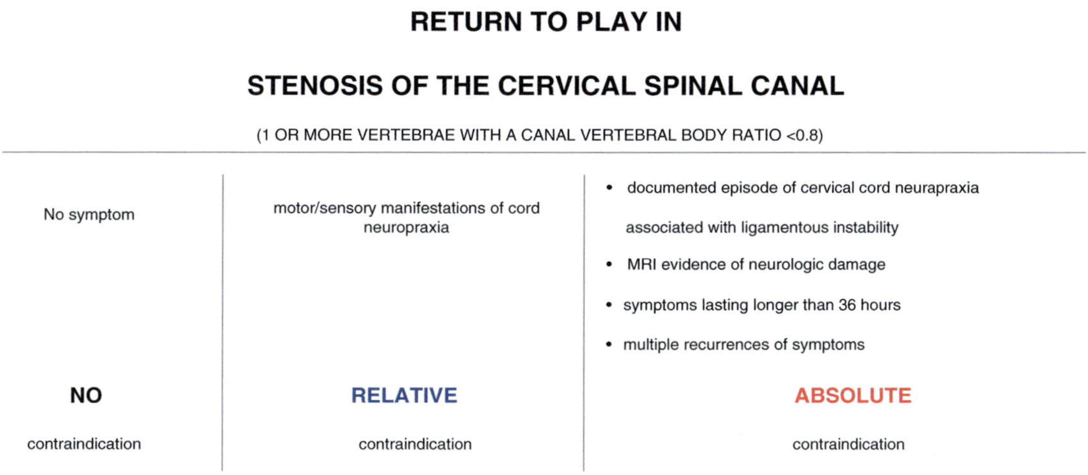

Fig. 19.4 Recommendations on return to play in stenosis of the cervical spinal canal

The suspicion, correct diagnosis, and treatment are the key to avoid permanent lesions and, in some cases, allow the athlete to return to amateur or professional sports practice. Prevention of lesions must be advised especially for those who are under risk due to pathological or congenital conditions, who are under risk for spine lesions and for the practice of sports that expose the spine to dangerous lesions.

The sports medicine physician must be aware of congenital stenosis, congenital intervertebral instability, congenital spondylolisthesis, disc herniation, spondylosis, degenerative stenosis, previous spine surgery, and antecedent spine lesion with temporary or definitive neurological sequel when conducting an initial or periodical evaluation regarding sports practice (Fig. 19.4).

Contact sports and those with the risk of collisions like rugby, football, hockey, and other snow sports expose the athlete to a higher risk of lesions. The association of a previous condition of the spine with the practice of a risk sport to spine lesion is what should be avoided, or, at least, the athlete should be warned about the potentiality of sequels.

Take-Home Messages

- Spine injuries are not only related to professional sports but also to recreational ones and can occur during competitions and training.
- The direct trauma and, also, supraphysiological stress on the spine are the most common mechanisms of spine injury in sports practice.

- Although most of these injuries are related to minor impairment to the athlete, such as lumbago, contusion, and paravertebral muscle contracture, the sports physician should keep in mind that devastating damage to spinal cord can occur in cases of high-energy trauma as well as contact sports.
- The knowledge of sports biomechanics helps the physician to suspect and identify traumas at higher risk to spinal cord injury and, therefore, define a more accurate approach to an athlete in the field.
- The sports physician on initial or periodical evaluation regarding sports practice must be aware of congenital stenosis, congenital intervertebral instability, congenital spondylolisthesis, disc herniation, spondylosis, degenerative stenosis, previous spine surgery, and antecedent spine lesion with a temporary or definitive neurological sequel and should rule them out before allowing the athlete's participation in contact sports such as martial arts, rugby, football, and ice hockey.

References

1. Tall RL, De Vault W. Spinal injury in sport: epidemiologic considerations. Clin Sports Med. 1993;12(3):441–8.
2. Powell JW, Barber-Foss KD. Injury patterns in selected high school sports: a review of the 1995-1997 seasons. J Athl Train. 1999;34(3):277–84.
3. Barile A, Limbucci N, Splendiani A, Gallucci M, Masciocchi C. Spinal injury in sport. Eur J Radiol. 2007;62(1):68–78.
4. Leone A, Cianfoni A, Cerase A, Magarelli N, Bonomo L. Lumbar spondylolysis: a review. Skeletal Radiol. 2011;40:683–700.
5. Katz DA, Scerpella TA. Anterior and middle column thoracolumbar spine injuries in young female gymnasts. Report of seven cases and review of the literature. Am J Sports Med. 2003;31:611–6.
6. De Palma MJ, Slipman CW, Siegelman E, Bayruns TJ, Bhargava A, Frey ME, Chin KR. Interspinous bursitis in an athlete. J Bone Joint Surg. 2004;86(7):1062–4.
7. Rouseau MA, Pascal-Moussellard H, Bellefqih S, Zeitoun D, Saillant G. Acute paralyzing sciatica due to traumatic lumbar disc herniation in grass hockey player. Eur J Trauma. 2005;6:590–2.
8. Bottini E, Poggi EJ, Luzuriaga F, Secin FP. Incidence and nature of the most common rugby injuries sustained in Argentina (1991-1997). Br J Sports Med. 2000;34:94–7.
9. McCoy GF, Piggot J, Macafee AL, AdairI V. Injuries of the cervical spine in schoolboy rugby football. J Bone Joint Surg. 1984;66:500–3.
10. Scher AT. Catastrophic rugby injuries of the spinal cord: changing patterns of injury. Br J Sports Med. 1991;25:57–60.
11. Sénégas J. Traumatisme grave du rachis cervical chez le rugbyman. Sports Med. 1997;92:36–9.
12. Wetzler MJ, Akpata T, Laughlin W, Levy AS. Occurrence of cervical spine injuries during the rugby scrum. Am J Sports Med. 1998;26:177–80.
13. Warren WL, Baisel JE. On the field evaluation of athletic neck injury. Clin Sports Med. 1998;17:99–110.
14. Ellis JL, Gottlieb JE. Return-to-play decisions after cervical spine injuries. Curr Sports Med Rep. 2007;6(1):56–61.
15. Concannon LG, Harrast MA, Herring SA. Radiating upper limb pain in the contact sport athlete: an update on transient quadriparesis and stingers. Curr Sports Med Rep. 2012;11(1):28–34.
16. Vaccaro AR, Klein GR, Ciccoti M, Pfaff WL, Moulton MJR, Hilibrand AJ, Watkins B. Return to play criteria for the athlete with cervical spine injuries resulting in stinger and transient quadriplegia/paresis. Spine. 2002;2(5):351–6.
17. Herkowitz HN, Garfin SR, Eismont FJ, Bell GR, Balderston RA. Rothman-Simeone the spine: expert consult. E-book, vol. 1. 6th ed. Philadelphia: Elsevier Health Sciences; 2017.
18. Meyer SA, Schulte KR, Callaghan JJ, et al. Cervical spinal stenosis and stingers in collegiate football players. Am J Sports Med. 1994;22:158–66.
19. Albright JP, McAuley E, Martin RK, Crowley ET, Foster DTY. Head and neck injuries in college football: an eight-year analysis. Am J Sports Med. 1985;13:147–52.
20. Albright JP, VanGilder J, El Khoury GY, et al. Head and neck injuries in sports. In: Scott WN, Nisonson B, Nicholas JA, editors. Principles of sports medicine. Baltimore: Williams & Wilkins; 1984. p. 40–86.
21. Bergfeld JA, Hershman E, Wilbourn A. Brachial plexus injury in sports: a five year follow-up. Orthop Trans. 1988;12:743–4.
22. Clancy WG Jr, Brand RL, Bergfield JA. Upper trunk brachial plexus injuries in contact sports. Am J Sports Med. 1977;5:209–16.
23. Funk FF, Wells RE. Injuries of the cervical spine in football. Clin Orthop Relat Res. 1975;109:50–8.
24. Rockett FX. Observations on the "burner": traumatic cervical radiculopathy. Clin Orthop Relat Res. 1982;164:18–9.
25. Speer KP, Bassett FH 3rd. The prolonged burner syndrome. Am J Sports Med. 1990;18:591–4.
26. Watkins RG. Neck injuries in football players. Clin Sports Med. 1986;5:215–46.
27. Eismont FJ, Clifford S, Goldberg M, Green B. Cervical sagittal spinal canal size in spine injury. Spine. 1984;9:663–6.

28. Quan D, Bird SJ. Nerve conduction studies and electromyography in the evaluation of peripheral nerve injuries. Univ PA Orthop J. 1999;12:45–51.
29. Seddon HJ. Three types of nerve injuries. Brain. 1943;66:237.
30. Sunderland SA. A classification of peripheral nerve injuries producing loss of function. Brain. 1951;74:491–516.
31. Castro FP Jr, Ricciardi J, Brunet ME, Busch MT, Whitecloud TS 3rd. Stingers, the Torg ratio, and the cervical spine. Am J Sports Med. 1997;25:603–8.
32. Torg JS, Pavlov H, Genuario SE, Sennett B, Wisneski RJ, Robie BH, Jahre C. Neurapraxia of the cervical spinal cord with transient quadriplegia. J Bone Joint Surg Am. 1986;68:1354–70.
33. Harvey J, Tanner S. Low back pain in young athletes. A practical approach. Sports Med. 1991;12:394–406.
34. Khan N, Husain S, Haak M. Thoracolumbar injuries in the athlete. Sports Med Arthrosc. 2008;16:16–25.
35. Ciullo JV, Jackson DW. Pars interarticularis stress reaction, spondylolysis, and spondylolisthesis in gymnasts. Clin Sports Med. 1985;4:95–110.
36. Gallo RA, Reitman RD, Altman DT, Altman GT, Jones CB, Chapman JR. Flexion-distraction injury of the thoracolumbar spine during squat exercise with the smith machine. Am J Sports Med. 2004;32:1962–7.
37. Herkowitz HN, Garfin SR, Eismont FJ, Bell GR, Balderston RA. Rothman-Simeone the spine: expert consult. E-book, vol. 1. 6th ed. Philadelphia: Elsevier Health Sciences; 2017.
38. Cyron BM, Hutton WC. The fatigue strength of the lumbar neural arch in spondylolysis. J Bone Joint Surg Br. 1978;60:234–8.
39. Herman MJ, Pizzutillo PD, Cavalier R. Spondylolysis and spondylolisthesis in the child and adolescent athlete. Orthop Clin North Am. 2003;34:461–7.
40. Jackson DW, Wiltse LL, Cirincoine RJ. Spondylolysis in the female gymnast. Clin Orthop Relat Res. 1976;117:68–73.
41. Soler T, Calderon C. The prevalence of spondylolysis in the Spanish elite athlete. Am J Sports Med. 2000;28:57–62.
42. Berk RH. Lumbar spine injuries in pediatric and adolescent athletes. Acta Orthop Traumatol Turc. 2004;38(suppl 1):S58–63.
43. Wimberly RL, Lauerman WC. Spondylolisthesis in the athlete. Clin Sports Med. 2002;21:133–45.
44. Teitz CC, Cook DM. Rehabilitation of neck and low back injuries. Clin Sports Med. 1985;4:455–76.
45. Burkus JK, Lonstein JE, Winter RB, Denis E. Long-term evaluation of adolescents treated operatively for spondylolisthesis: a comparison of in situ arthrodesis only with in situ arthrodesis and reduction followed by immobilization in a cast. J Bone Joint Surg Am. 1992;74:693–704.
46. Beggs I, Addison J. Posterior vertebral rim fractures. Br J Radiol. 1998;71:567–72.
47. Sassmannshausen G, Smith BG. Back pain in the young athlete. Clin Sports Med. 2002;21:121–32.
48. Martinez-Lage JF, Poza M, Arcas P. Avulsed lumbar vertebral rim plate in an adolescent: trauma or malformation? Childs Nerv Syst. 1998;14:131–4.
49. Skobowytsh-Okolot B. "Posterior apophysis" in L.IV—the cause of neuroradicular disturbance. Acta Orthop Scand. 1962;32:341–51.
50. Dietemann JL, Runge M, Badoz A, Dosch JC, Beaujeux R, Bonneville JF, Wackenheim A. Radiology of posterior lumbar apophyseal ring fractures: report of 13 cases. Neuroradiology. 1988;30:337–44.
51. Dang L, Liu Z. A review of current treatment for lumbar disc herniation in children and adolescents. Eur Spine J. 2010;19:205–24.
52. Keller RH. Traumatic displacement of the cartilaginous vertebral rim: a sign of intervertebral disc prolapse. Radiology. 1974;110:21–4.
53. Lippit A. Fracture of the vertebral body end plate and disk protrusion causing subarachnoid block in an adolescent. Clin Orthop Relat Res. 1974;11:112–5.
54. DeLuca PF, Mason DE, Weiand R, Howard R, Bassett GS. Excision of herniated nucleus pulposus in children and adolescents. J Pediatr Orthop. 1994;14:318–22.
55. Comstock RD, Knox C, Gilchrist J. Center for Disease Control and Prevention (CDC)Sports-related injuries among high school athletes—United States, 2005-06 school year. MMWR Morb Mortal Wkly Rep. 2006;55(38):1037–40.
56. Mall NA, Buchowski J, Zebala L, Brophy RH, Wright RW, Matava MJ. Spine and axial skeleton injuries in the National Football League. Am J Sports Med. 2012;40:1755–61.
57. Olson D, Sikka RS, Labounty A, Christensen T. Injuries in professional football. Curr Sports Med Rep. 2013;12(6):381–90.
58. Gray BL, Buchowski JM, Bumpass DB, Lehman RA Jr, Mall NA, Matava MJ. Disc herniations in the national football league. Spine. 2013;38(22):1934–8.
59. Proctor MR, Cantu RC. Head and neck injuries in young athletes. Clin Sports Med. 2000;19:693–715.
60. Iwamoto J, Abe H, Tsukimura Y, Wakano K. Relationship between radiographic abnormalities of lumbar spine and incidence of low back pain in high school and college football players: a prospective study. Am J Sports Med. 2004;32(3):781–6.
61. Ekstrom RA, Donatelli R, Carp K. Electromyographic analysis of core trunk, hip, and thigh muscles during 9 rehabilitation exercises. J Orthop Sports Phys Ther. 2007;37(12):754–62.
62. Torg JS, Vegso JJ, Sennett B, Das M. The National Football Head and neck injury registry. 14-year report on cervical quadriplegia, 1971 through 1984. JAMA. 1985;254:3439–43.
63. Tagliabue P. Tackling concussions in sports. Neurosurgery. 2003;53:796.
64. NFL Head, Neck & Spine Committee. Protocols regarding diagnosis and management of concussion. New York: National Football League; 2013.
65. Boden BP, Tacchetti RL, Cantu RC, Knowles SB, Mueller FO. Catastrophic cervical spine injuries

in high school and college football players. Am J Sports Med. 2006;34:1223–32.
66. Torg JS, Corcoran TA, Thibault LE, Pavlov H, Sennett BJ, Naranja RJ Jr, Priano S. Cervical cord neurapraxia: classification, pathomechanics, morbidity, and management guidelines. J Neurosurg. 1997;87:843–50.
67. Torg JS, Naranja RJ Jr, Pavlov H, Galinat BJ, Warren R, Stine RA. The relationship of developmental narrowing of the cervical spinal canal to reversible and irreversible injury of the cervical spinal cord in football players. J Bone Joint Surg Am. 1996;78:1308–14.
68. Torg JS, Guille JT, Jaffe S. Injuries to the cervical spine in American football players. J Bone Joint Surg Am. 2002;84-A:112–22.
69. Palmer-Green DS, Stokes KA, Fuller CW, England M, Kemp SP, Trewartha G. Match injuries in English youth academy and schools rugby union: an epidemiological study. Am J Sports Med. 2013;41: 749–55.
70. Kaplan KM, Goodwillie A, Strauss EJ, Rosen JE. Rugby injuries: a review of concepts and current literature. Bull NYU Hosp Joint Dis. 2008;66(2):86–93.
71. Patricios JS. Rugby contact and collisions—clinical challenges of a global game. Curr Sports Med Rep. 2014;13(5):326–33.
72. International Rugby Board. Available at www.irb.com. Accessed 27 Jul 2006.
73. Bishop PJ. Factors related to quadriplegia in football and the implications for intervention strategies. Am J Sports Med. 1996;24:235–9.
74. Iwamoto J, Abe H, Tsukimura Y, et al. Relationship between radiographic abnormalities of lumbar spine and incidence of low back pain in high school rugby players: a prospective study. Scand J Med Sci Sports. 2005;15:163–8.
75. Bennett DL, Nassar L, DeLano MC. Lumbar spine MRI in the elite-level female gymnast with low back pain. Skeletal Radiol. 2006;35:503–9.
76. Fuller CW, Brooks JHM, Kemp SPT. Spinal injuries in Professional Rugby Union: a prospective cohort study. Clin J Sport Med. 2007;17(1):10–6.
77. Hind K, Birrell F, Beck B. Prevalent morphometric vertebral fractures in professional male rugby players. PLoS One. 2014;9(5):e97427.
78. Quarrie KL, Cantu RC, Chalmers DJ. Rugby union injuries to the cervical spine and spinal cord. Sports Med. 2002;32(10):633–53.
79. Van Mechelen W, Hlobil H, Kemper HC. Incidence, severity, aetiology and prevention of sports injuries: a review of concepts. Sports Med. 1992;14(2):82–99.
80. Kew T, Noakes TD, Kettles AN, Goedeke RE, Newton DA, Scher AT. A retrospective study of spinal cord injuries in Cape Province rugby players, 1963- 1989: incidence, mechanisms and prevention. S Afr Med J. 1991;80(3):127–33.
81. Scher AT. Rugby injuries to the cervical spinal cord [letter]. S Afr Med J. 1980;57(2):37.
82. Taylor TK, Coolican MR. Spinal-cord injuries in Australian footballers, 1960-1985. Med J Aust. 1987;147(3):112–3, 116-8.
83. Jenner J, Scopes J, Yates D. Rugby injuries to the cervical cord [letter]. BMJ. 1979:193.
84. Kuster D, Gibson A, Abboud R, Drew T. Mechanisms of cervical spine injury in rugby union: a systematic review of the literature. Br J Sports Med. 2012;46(8):550–4.
85. Dunn RN, van der Spuy D. Rugby and cervical spine injuries–has anything changed? A 5-year review in the Western Cape. S Afr Med J. 2010;100(4):235–8.
86. McCurdie I, Smith S, Bell PH, Batt ME. Tennis injury data from The Championships, Wimbledon, from 2003 to 2012. Br J Sports Med. 2017;51(7):607–11.
87. Hielm N, Werner S, Renstrom P. Injury profile in junior tennis players: a prospective two year study. Knee Surg Sports Traumatol Arthrosc. 2010;18(6):845–50.
88. Campbell A, O'Sullivan P, Straker L, Elliott B, Reid M. Back pain in tennis players: a link with lumbar serve kinematics and range of motion. Med Sci Sports Exerc. 2014;46(2):351–7.
89. Campbell A, Straker L, O'Sullivan P, Elliott B, Reid M. Lumbar loading in the elite adolescent tennis serve: a link to low back pain. Med Sci Sports Exerc. 2013;45(8):1562–8.
90. Alyas F, Turner M, Connell D. MRI findings in the lumbar spine of asymptomatic adolescent elite tennis players. Br J Sports Med. 2007;41(11):836–41.
91. McBeth PB, Ball CG, Mulloy RH, Kirkpatrick AW. Alpine ski and snowboarding traumatic injuries: incidence, injury patterns, and risk factors for 10 years. Am J Surg. 2009;197(5):560–3.
92. Reid DC, Saboe L. Spine fractures in winter sports. Sports Med. 1989;7(6):393–9.
93. Boden BP, Prior C. Catastrophic spine injuries in sports. Curr Sports Med Rep. 2005;4(1):45–9.
94. Grabara M. Comparison of posture among adolescent male volleyball players and non-athletes. Biol Sport. 2015;32(1):79–85.
95. Kulling FA, Florianz H, Reepschläger B, Gasser J, Jost B, Lajtai G. High prevalence of disc degeneration and spondylolysis in the lumbar spine of professional beach volleyball players. Orthop J Sports Med. 2014;2(4):2325967114528862.
96. Hetsroni I, Mann G, Dolev E, Morgenstern D, Nyska M. Clay Shoveler's fracture in a volleyball player revealing an unusual source of pain. Phys Sports Med. 2005;33(7):38–42.
97. Slankamenac P, Jesic A, Avramov P, Zivanovis Z, Covic S, Till V. Multiple cervical artery dissection in a volleyball player. Arch Neurol. 2010;67(8):1024.
98. Purcell LK, Leblanc CM. Boxing participation by children and adolescents: a joint statement with the American Academy of Pediatrics. Paediatr Child Health. 2012;17:39–40.
99. Schwartz MB. Medical safety in boxing: administrative, ethical, legislative, and legal considerations. Clin Sports Med. 2009;28:505–14.

100. Scott I. Youth boxing ban in some Australian jurisdictions. Inj Prev. 1999;5:77.
101. Hart MG, Trivedi RA, Hutchinson PJ. Boxing sparring complicated by an acute subdural haematoma and brainstem haemorrhage. Br J Neurosurg. 2012;26:776–8.
102. Porter M, O'Brien M. Incidence and severity of injuries resulting from amateur boxing in Ireland. Clin J Sport Med. 1996;6:97–101.
103. Zazryn T, Cameron P, McCrory P. A prospective cohort study of injury in amateur and professional boxing. Br J Sports Med. 2006;40:670–4.
104. Siewe J, Rudat J, Zarghooni K, Sobottke R, Eysel P, Herren C, Knöll P, Illgner U, Michael J. Injuries in competitive boxing. A prospective study. Int J Sports Med. 2015;36(3):249–53.
105. Potter MR, Snyder AJ, Smith GA. Boxing injuries presenting to US emergency departments, 1990–2008. Am J Prev Med. 2011;40(4):462–7.
106. Schroeder GD, Vaccaro AR. Cervical spine injuries in the athlete. J Am Acad Orthop Surg. 2016;24(9):e122–33.
107. Donatelli R, Dimond D, Holland M. Sport-specific biomechanics of spinal injuries in the athlete (throwing athletes, rotational sports, and contact-collision sports). Clin Sports Med. 2012;31(3):381–96.
108. Posner M, Cameron KL, Wolf JM, Belmont PJ Jr, Owens BD. Epidemiology of major league baseball injuries. Am J Sports Med. 2011;39(8):1676–80.
109. Singh H, et al. Lumbar hyperextension in baseball pitching: a potential cause of spondylolysis. J Appl Biomech. 2018.
110. Wasser JG, Zaremski JL, Herman DC, Vincent HK. Assessment and rehabilitation of chronic low back pain in baseball: part II. Res Sports Med. 2017;25(2):231–43.
111. Selhorst M, Fischer A, MacDonald J. Prevalence of spondylolysis in symptomatic adolescent athletes: an assessment of sport risk in nonelite athletes. Clin J Sport Med. 2017.
112. Wasser JG, Zaremski JL, Herman DC, Vincent HK. Prevalence and proposed mechanisms of chronic low back pain in baseball: part I. Res Sports Med. 2017;25(2):219–30.
113. Garet M, Reiman MP, Mathers J, Sylvan J. Nonoperative treatment in lumbar spondylolysis and spondylolisthesis: a systematic review. Sports Health. 2013;5(3):225–32.
114. Panteliadis P, Nagra NS, Edwards KL, Behrbalk E, Boszczyk B. Athletic population with spondylolysis: review of outcomes following surgical repair or conservative management. Global Spine J. 2016;6(6):615–25.
115. Debnath UK, Freeman BJ, Gregory P, de la Harpe D, Kerslake RW, Webb JK. Clinical outcome and return to sport after the surgical treatment of spondylolysis in young athletes. J Bone Joint Surg Br. 2003;85(2):244–9.
116. Iwamoto J, Sato Y, Takeda T, Matsumoto H. Return to sports activity by athletes after treatment of spondylolysis. World J Orthop. 2010;1(1):26–30.
117. Arend JB, Borghuis J, Koen AP, et al. Core muscle response times and postural reactions in soccer players and nonplayers. Med Sci Sports Ex. 2010;10:108–14.
118. Shah T, Cloke DJ, Rushton S, Shirley MD, Deehan DJ. Lower back symptoms in adolescent soccer players. Predictors of functional recovery. Orthop J Sports Med. 2014;2(4):2325967114529703.
119. El Rassi G, Takemitsu M, Woratanarat P, Shah SA. Lumbar spondylolysis in pediatric and adolescent soccer players. Am J Sports Med. 2005;33(11):1688–93.
120. Aoki H, Kohno T, Fujiya H, Kato H, Yatabe K, Morikawa T, Seki J. Incidence of injury among adolescent soccer players: a comparative study of artificial and natural grass turfs. Clin J Sport Med. 2010;20(1):1–7.
121. Cassas KJ, Cassettari-Wayhs A. Childhood and adolescent sports-related overuse injuries. Am Fam Physician. 2006;73:1014–22.
122. Purcell L, Micheli LJ. Low back pain in young athletes. Sports Health. 2009;1:212–22.
123. Sakai T, Sairyo K, Suzue N, Kosaka H, Yasui N. Incidence and etiology of lumbar spondylolysis: review of the literature. J Orthop Sci. 2010;15(3):281–8.
124. Sys J, Michielsen J, Bracke P, Martens M, Verstreken J. Nonoperative treatment of active spondylolysis in elite athletes with normal X-ray findings: literature review and results of conservative treatment. Eur Spine J. 2001;10(6):498–504.
125. Herkowitz I, Harry N, et al. Rothman-Simeone the spine E-book: expert consult, vol. 1. Philadelphia: Elsevier Health Sciences; 2017.
126. Paulus S, Kennedy DJ. Return to play consideration for cervical spine injuries in athletes. Phys Med Rehabil Clin N Am. 2014;25:723–33.
127. Dailey A, Harrop JS, France JC. High-energy contact sports and cervical spine neuropraxia injuries. Spine. 2010;35:S193–201.
128. Kepler CK, Vaccaro AR. Injuries and abnormalities of the cervical spine and return to play criteria. Clin Sports Med. 2012;31:499–508.
129. Torg JS. Cervical spine injuries and the return to football. Sports Health. 2009;1(5):376–83.

Part IV

Sports Trauma

Facial Trauma

20

Sérgio Rocha Piedade, Leonardo Manoel Carvalho,
Luis António Mendes, Milton Possedente,
and Daniel Miranda Ferreira

20.1 Introduction

The facial skeleton is made up of 14 bones, which contain essential structures and sensory organs of the body responsible for sight, smell, hearing, taste, mastication, and teeth and oral cavity. Its bone architecture is well-organized with vertical and horizontal bone walls that allow protection to soft tissues and resistance against regular external and internal forces applied to the face. Besides that, it is one of the most vascularized regions in the body, where bleeding is a common clinical event, reinforcing the importance of the use of gloves and glasses when approaching these sports injuries.

In sports, the face is widely exposed and subject to traumas as it is located in the frontal region of the head [1]. In general, sports involve twisting movements, racing with acceleration and deceleration, ball launches, direct hits with the ball, and player-to-player contact. In boxing, taekwondo, karate, and other martial arts, facial trauma is a common event, while in soccer, rugby, and basketball, it is a result of the direct trauma from the opponent's head, elbow, knee, or even the ball [2, 3].

The magnitude of the injury is directed related to the trauma mechanism and energy as well as the type and size of sports material (ball, stick, racquet) involved [4]. In this context, small balls such as those used in squash or baseball concentrate kinetic energy when hitting the human body, potentializing tissue damage [5]. Therefore, the protective equipment plays a vital role in reducing the risk of facial injuries in sports. Although in some sports modalities the use of a mouthguard, eye protection, helmets, and headgear is recommended, educational interventions are still needed to raise the athletes' awareness and motivation of its use [6, 7].

Considering that the mechanisms of sports trauma to the face, head, and cervical spine have similarities between them, the managing of facial injuries should involve a careful assessment of the head and cervical spine status. This chapter aims to discuss and present the most common injuries reported on facial trauma in sports as well as the initial management of these injuries in the field or sports arena, minimizing the occurrence of significant injuries, establishing the adequate strategy according to the facial injury, and preventing injury.

S. R. Piedade (✉)
Department of Orthopedics and Traumatology, State University of Campinas—UNICAMP, Exercise and Sports Medicine, Campinas, SP, Brazil
e-mail: piedade@fcm.unicamp.br

L. M. Carvalho · L. A. Mendes · M. Possedente
State University of Campinas—UNICAMP, Exercise and Sports Medicine, Campinas, SP, Brazil
e-mail: luiz.mendes@hc.fm.usp.br; miltonpossedente@uol.com.br

D. M. Ferreira
Department of Radiology, State University of Campinas—UNICAMP, Exercise and Sports Medicine, Campinas, SP, Brazil

S. Rocha Piedade et al. (eds.), *The Sports Medicine Physician*,
https://doi.org/10.1007/978-3-030-10433-7_20

20.2 Facial Trauma Assessment in Sports

According to the mechanism of sports injury, part of the trauma energy is absorbed by the cervical spine or by the head. In such sports (motorcycle races, MMA), the higher trauma energy could produce substantial soft tissue and bone damage and critical bleeding and, thus, cause mechanical problems to the athlete's airway, especially when the athlete presents some neurological deficits or is in unconsciousness status [8].

In the field of play, the initial assessment starts with airway, breathing, circulation, and disability, but with particular attention to the need for prior cervical spine stabilization and neurological status when managing the facial trauma [9]. In most instances, the soft tissue bleeding is well-controlled by direct pressure with a sterile gauze, while ice is directly applied to minimize the tissue edema and swelling when the athlete is removed from the field [10].

In general, minor traumas present no obstacle to the athlete's prompt return to the game, whereas higher traumas require an accurate clinical evaluation, making the athlete leave the game. When the athlete is out of the game, the soft tissue damage can be assessed under adequate light and also under local anesthesia if necessary. Skin lacerations, deep abrasions, areas of active bleeding, or bruising can be well analyzed and approached, debrided, and sutured under sterile conditions. This apart, palpation allows precise information of the tissue consistency such as edema, hematomas, presence of bone crepitus, or depression that could suggest a bone fracture and the need for radiological evaluation (X-rays, CT, or MRI) [11].

The function of the temporomandibular joint, as well as the facial muscle activity, can be evaluated by asking the athlete to open and close his mouth and eyes actively, where the symmetry of muscle actions confirms its regular status. Considering that the most frequent orofacial lesions are dental ones and lacerations of soft tissues, the facial assessment involves an oral evaluation to identify internal and external injuries of the mouth. The following sections will approach the sports injuries to facial bones, teeth, eyes, and ears, separately.

20.3 Facial Bone Fractures

Facial bone fractures may be manifested by asymmetry, irregularity, instability, and deformity of bone edges detected during the physical assessment (inspection and palpation). Considering the complex facial bone anatomy, CT scanning is the imaging modality of choice as it offers images in tridimensional view of osseous structures and allows to rule out associated injuries (intracranial injuries), while X-ray can be inconclusive.

20.4 Orbital Fractures

Orbital fractures result from direct traumas to the periorbital regions due to a wrist, or ball, a list, or even player-to-player contact. The floor and the medial wall of the orbit are less thick and resistant and, therefore, more prone to fracture. Herniation of the orbit contents could happen through the fracture site causing functional deficit resulting in diplopia and loss of ocular motricity due to the entrapment of periocular muscles, mainly the rectus muscles. It could also be associated with a critical periorbital lesion, edema, ecchymosis, and crepitus. Paresthesia in the cheeks may indicate the involvement of the infraorbital nerve, and a radiological assessment by bird-eye plain radiography or CT should be ordered. An often-neglected orientation is that these athletes should not blow their nose because of the risk of nasal content herniation to the orbit [12, 13]. An orbital fracture should be promptly referred to an ophthalmologist's assessment, particularly in the presence of muscle entrapment or persistent oculocardiac reflex (vomiting, bradycardia, and hypotension).

The sports medicine physician in youth academies (i.e., with children) should be aware of a rare orbital fracture presentation consisting of a greenstick fracture that has spontaneously reduced but has caused a periorbital muscle entrapment

[14]. The patient may present with no apparent signs of injury, but ocular mobility dysfunction and persistent oculocardiac reflex are observed.

20.5 Maxillary Fractures

Maxillary fractures usually result from blunt trauma. An accurate reduction of the bone fracture is crucial for both function and facial aesthetics re-establishment. Maxillary fractures are often accompanied by cranial damage, nasal airway obstruction, soft palate edema, hemorrhage into the sinuses, disturbance of the orbit contents, cerebrospinal fluid rhinorrhea, and reduced sensation in the infraorbital region [15]. Maxillary fractures are classified as Le Fort I, II, and III (Fig. 20.1a, b).

20.6 Mandible Fractures

Sports-related accidents are the third major cause of maxilla and mandible fractures. Fractures can occur from contact between athletes, between athletes and their surroundings, and from falls and from direct blow. This type of fracture has been decreasing over time due to better preventive measures and equipment. The condyles and mandibular angle are the most common sites of fractures (Figs. 20.2a and 20.4b). Non-displaced fractures can be managed conservatively with analgesia, and displaced fractures need closed reduction and fixation.

20.7 Nasal Fractures

The nasal bones are at high risk of injury in any sports practice, and they are the most fractured facial bones, resulting in a common sequela of sports injuries (Fig. 20.3). Clinically, it is often manifested by heavy bleeding, and, therefore, the initial management in the field is controlling the nasal hemorrhage [10]. In such cases, epistaxis control or septal hematoma drainage are needed to avoid nasal obstruction or severe pain. Nasal fractures can often be addressed with closed reduction techniques if nasal obstruction or cosmetic deformity is present. In the setting of complex nasal trauma, an open approach may be indicated.

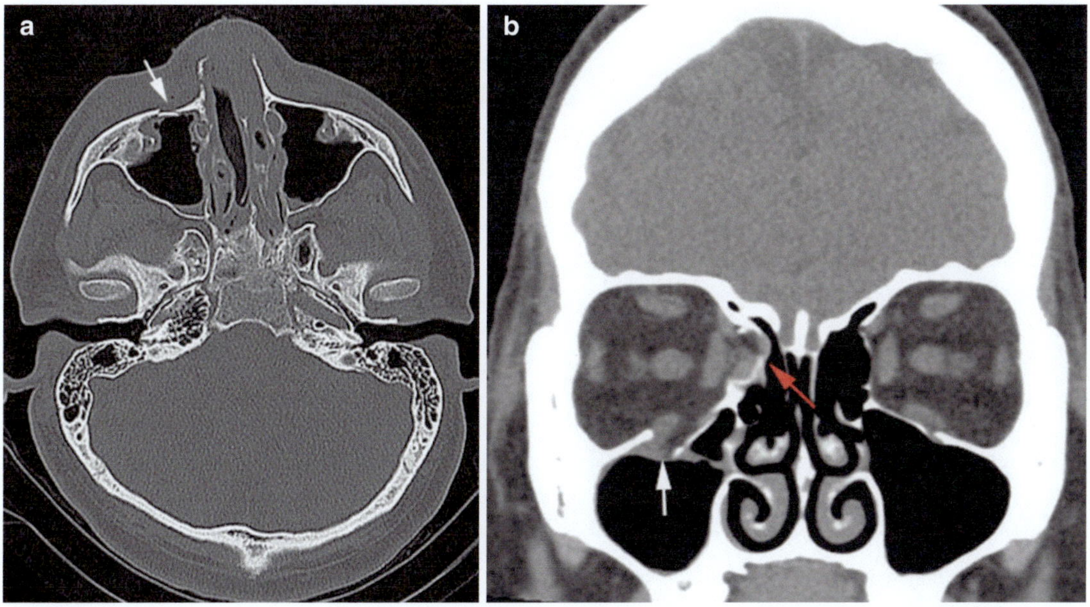

Fig. 20.1 (**a**) Axial CT scan. Fracture of the anterior wall of the maxillary sinus (white arrow). (**b**) Coronal CT scan—fracture of medial wall (white arrow) and floor (red arrow) of orbit, with herniation of the intra-orbital fat and medial rectus and inferior rectus muscles. Two cases

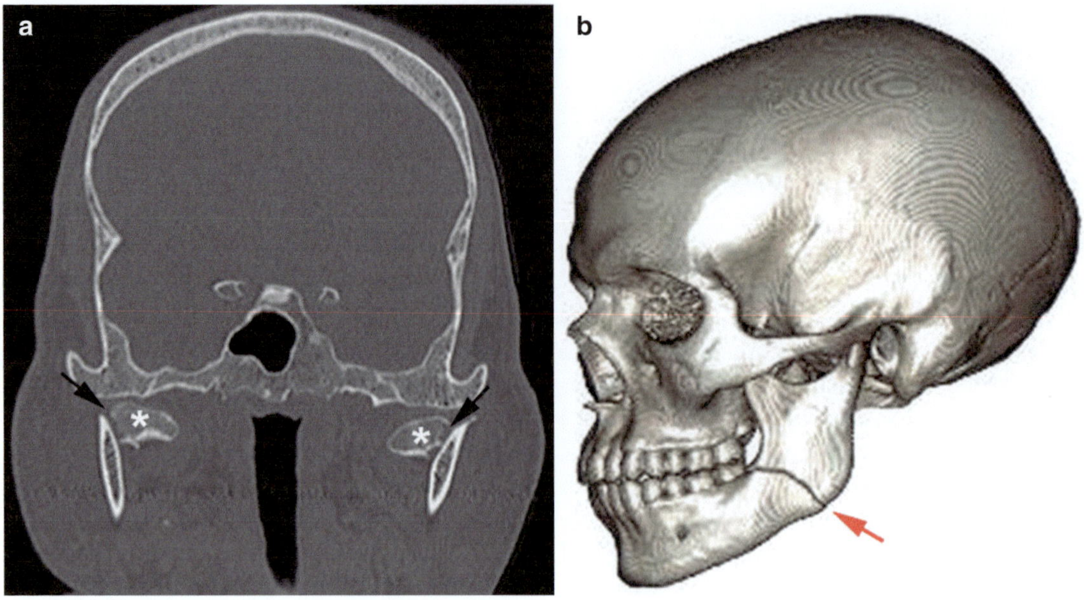

Fig. 20.2 (**a**) Coronal CT scan. Bicondylar fracture of the mandible (white arrows) with medial displacement of condyles (asterisk). (**b**) 3D CT reconstruction. Non-displaced complete fracture of the left mandible angle (red arrow)

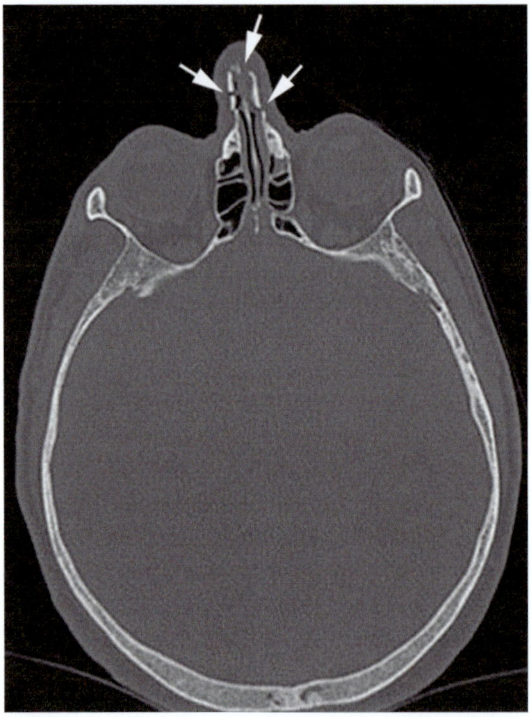

Fig. 20.3 Comminuted fracture of the nasal bone (white arrows), without the involvement of nasal septum (axial CT scan view)

20.8 Basilar Skull and Temporal Bone Fractures

These kinds of fractures result from direct trauma to the occipital skull and temporal bone. According to the fracture line toward the long axis of the bone, temporal fractures are classified as longitudinal, transversal, and oblique (Fig. 20.4).

Athletes involved in sports such as motorcycling, skateboarding, and bicycling have at higher risk than others are [16]. Usually, the most common symptoms are dizziness, vertigo, loss of consciousness, hemotympanum, and TM rupture. Signals of ecchymosis like Battle sign and raccoon eye can be present in the clinical evaluation (Fig. 20.5). This apart, cerebrospinal fluid rhinorrhea can also occur from fracture, and there is a higher risk of meningitis development. High-resolution head CT is the gold standard for diagnosis. MRI can be useful for defining vascular damaged.

The treatment depends on the clinical evaluation; if the athlete has a stable neurological state, an observation can be an option. The

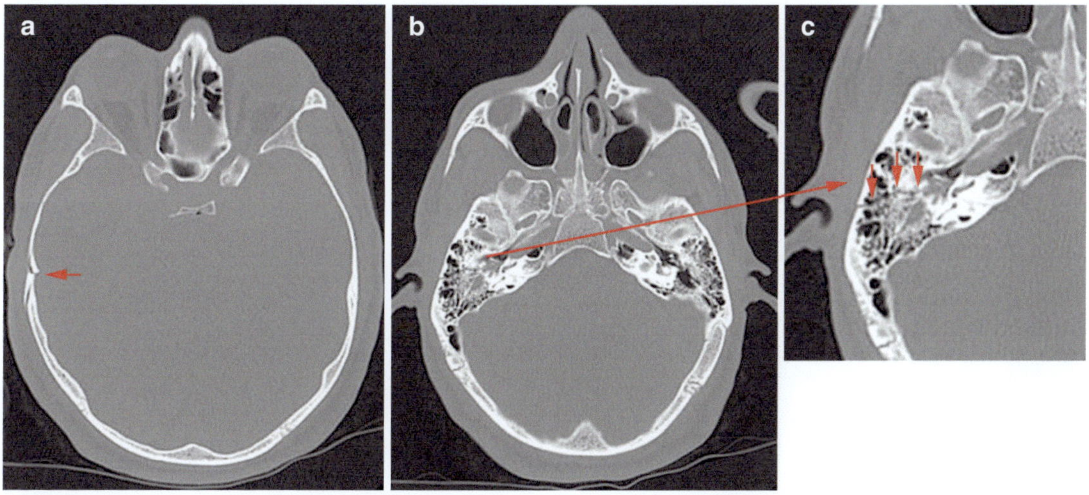

Fig. 20.4 Temporal bone fractures (axial CT scan view): (**a**) fracture of squamous portion of temporal bone (white arrow) and (**b**, **c**) fracture of petrous portion of temporal bone (red arrows in magnified image)

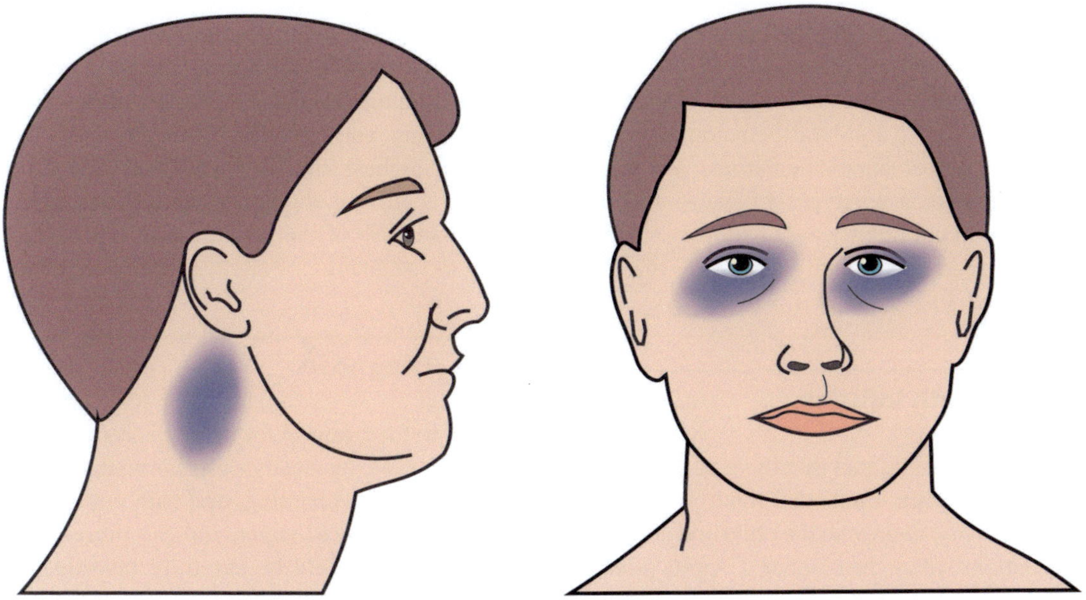

Fig. 20.5 Battle sign and raccoon eyes

athlete should be referred to a specialist for evaluation and discuss a surgical option In cases of brain herniation, intracranial bleeding, hearing loss and persistent cerebrospinal fluid (CSF) leak for more than two weeks [16]. Athletes who have sustained a temporal fracture must discuss with the surgeon an individualized approach about when to return to play. Bearing in mind, the athlete should not return to sports practice until the fracture has healed.

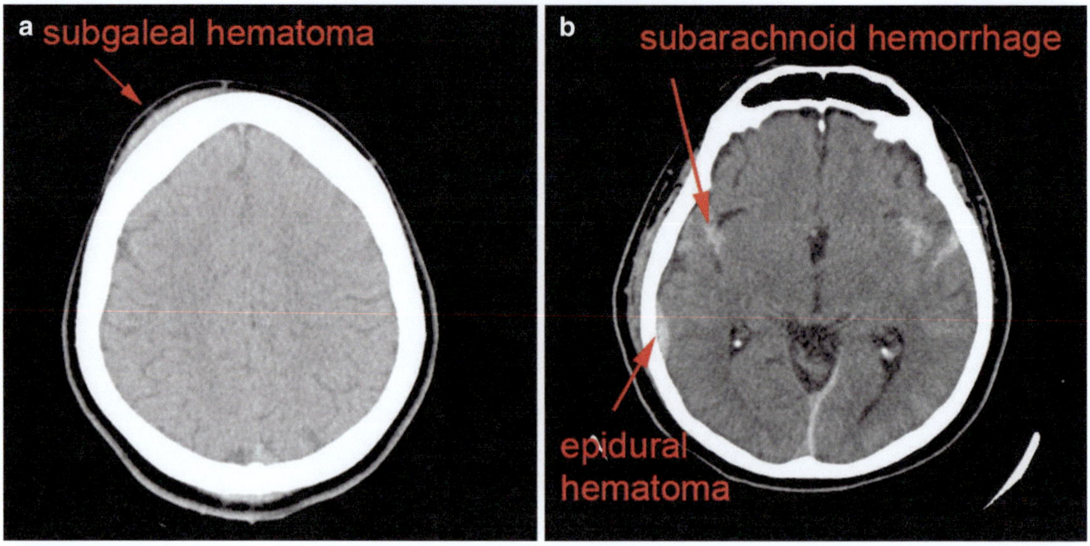

Fig. 20.6 (**a**,**b**) Intracranial hematomas

20.9 Intracranial Hematomas

Facial traumas are often associated with intracranial injuries [17]. Epidural hematoma, subdural hematoma, subarachnoid hematoma, and intracerebral hematoma are types of blood collection inside the skull. Subgaleal hematomas are blood collations in the small parts of the skull (Fig. 20.6a, b).

20.10 Tooth Injuries

It should be considered that there is a close relationship between traumatic tooth injuries and sports activity, mainly, in the child and adolescent populations where the number of sports practitioners has increased. Tooth injuries are commonly seen in contact sports, comprising falls and collisions. Basketball has shown a considerable tooth injury rate, because the high speed of the game, jumping and landing, and turns which predispose to the player-to-player collision. Moreover, soccer, rugby, wrestling, boxing, and martial arts also have higher-risk factors of dental injuries. During the Pan American Games held in Rio de Janeiro 2017 [18], a cross-sectional epidemiological survey was conducted to evaluate the prevalence of dental trauma in high-performance athletes from 42 countries. Prior dental trauma was reported in 49.6%, and most of these injuries had happened during training or games (63.5%), where wrestling, boxing, and basketball were the sports that had the highest injury prevalence. The most affected tooth was the upper central incisor, and more than 80% of the athletes have reported no use of mouthguard.

20.11 Diagnosis

Trauma to face, jaw, or, even, any part of head or neck followed by ecchymosis, bruising, facial swelling, mouth bleeding, and pain could present indirect clinical signs, and the presence of tooth injuries should be carefully investigated. In clinical practice, dental injuries may be presented as dentoalveolar, tooth fracture, displacement, or even tooth avulsion and fracture of the alveolar process (Fig. 20.7), which impacts negatively on the athletes' sports activity as it impairs the oral function. Due to their anatomical localization, the superior central incisor teeth are commonly affected by sports trauma. In most instances, a dental surgeon is not available in the field or sports arena, and therefore, the sports medicine physician should approach these injuries.

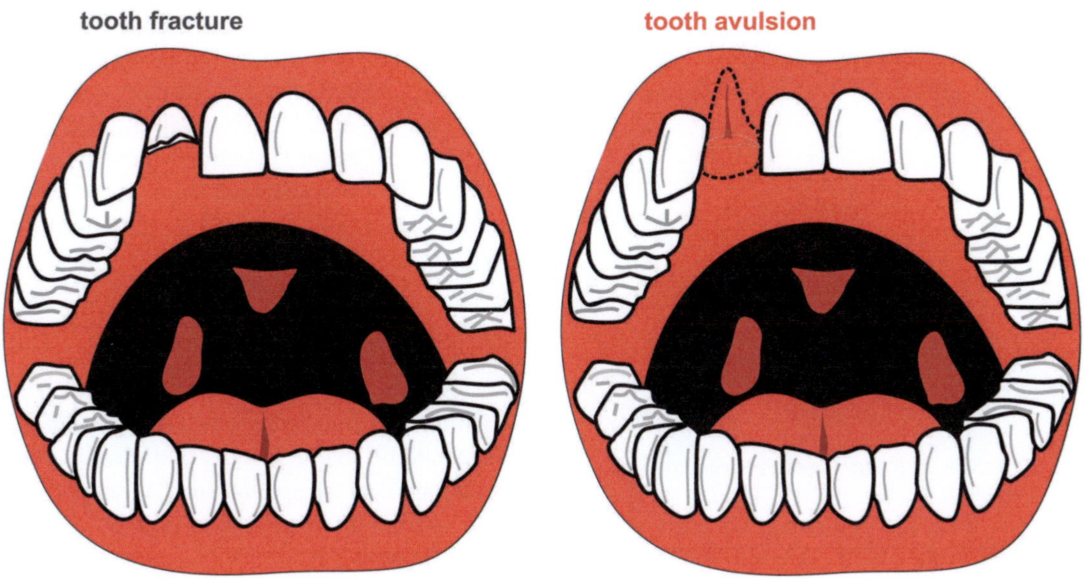

Fig. 20.7 Tooth fracture and tooth avulson

20.12 Managing Tooth Avulsion in the Field or Sports Arena

Tooth avulsion is a critical dental injury where the prognosis is strictly related to an adequate first aid. In these cases, the sports medicine physician should deal with it following some rules:

- After making the diagnosis of tooth avulsion and finding the tooth, keep it and mobilize it by its crown avoiding touching the root.
- When the tooth is dirty, it should be carefully cleaned with cold water.
- If possible, the tooth should be repositioned into its natural site (alveolar process), with no friction or resistance during the repositioning attempt.
- In cases where tooth repositioning is not possible, the tooth should be stored in a recipient with milk or patient's saliva (dry storage should be avoided), and the dentist's assessment should be performed during the first 30 min after trauma.

20.13 Prevention Measures

The protective equipment plays a vital role in reducing the risk of facial injuries in sports. In this context, an oral protector (mouthguards) significantly reduces the frequency and severity of orofacial injuries in sports, but their use is not uniform or mandatory in most modalities of sports. The use of a custom-made oral protector should be encouraged as it ensures a better fit and comfort, protecting and facilitating speech and breathing which has a direct impact on the athlete's sports performance.

The mouthguards are classified as stock mouthguard, mouth-formed protectors, and custom-made mouthguards.

Stock mouthguards have the advantages of oral adjustment and low cost, but the disadvantages are that they work only with closed mouth (there is no retention) and could also cause difficulties in speaking, breathing, and athlete's concentration.

Mouth-formed protectors are prefabricated protectors plasticized in hot water and molded in the mouth by the user. They are commercially available, but their quality and cost vary. Moreover, although they are the most used ones, they are not recommended for all sports because they have little retention, and there is the possibility of dislodging during sports activity and airway blockage.

Custom-made mouthguards are made according to the patient's personal measurements and customized in a dental office, using individual molding. They offer better protection, retention, comfort, fitting, speaking, and breathing easily

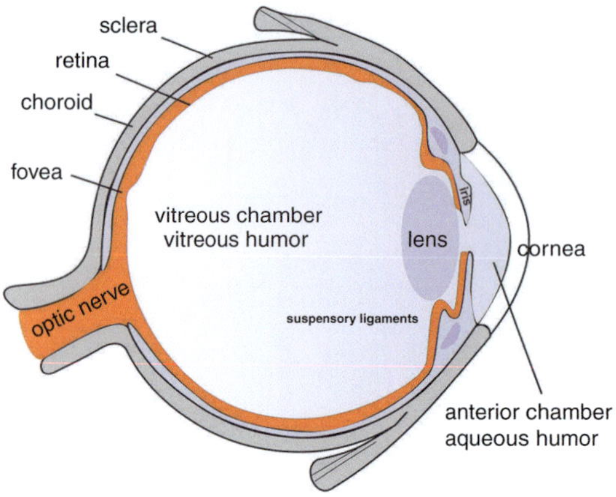

Fig. 20.8 Schematic drawing of eye anatomy

according to the sports. When evaluated in elite taekwondo athletes, they did not cause negative effects on the aerobic performance capacity. They are recommended for the successful prevention of tooth lesions, but their cost is higher.

20.14 Eye Injuries

The eye is composed of three spherical tunics, fibrous, vascular, and internal (Fig. 20.8). In the fibrous tunic there is the sclera, which is the external fibrous component of the bulb of the eyes, responsible for the eyes' shape and resistance due to the periocular muscle attachment, while the cornea is the transparent portion that covers the anterior chamber. The vascular tunic involves the choroid, ciliary body, and iris. The choroid is a vascular layer that is continuous with the ciliary body, joining the choroid to the iris and acting on the fixation and adjustment of the focus of the lens, where the iris is positioned anterior to the lens, a contractile diaphragm with a central opening, the pupil. The inner tunic is composed of the retina which is responsible for the luminous stimulus capture.

20.15 Epidemiology

Although eye injuries are relatively rare in sports, they cannot be neglected because of their potential to cause a significant functional impairment. In the United States, it is estimated that about 40% of eye injuries admitted to the hospital care were sports related, and 13% of them were penetrating ocular injuries. The majority (72%) of these lesions occur in young people under 25 years old. The most cited sports involved are baseball, basketball, hockey, soccer, and racquet sports [4, 19–22].

20.16 Ocular Evaluation

Regarding eye trauma, the sports medicine physician should be able to identify and rule out clinical findings and symptoms such as tearing and ocular fluid drainage, photophobia, blurred vision, diplopia, pain, nausea, scotomas, and flashes of light. Therefore, an ophthalmoscope and a slit lamp should be part of the equipment in sports medical bags, particularly in sports where these injuries are commonly seen. Visual acuity should be checked using the Snellen chart or written texts, and the visual field status, pupil symmetry and reflex, conjunctiva, cornea, and eyelids should be examined. Special attention should be given to the possibility of foreign bodies and any macroscopic evidence of bleeding in the anterior chamber. Whenever a possibility exists, fluoroscopy should be performed, and, in case of doubtful physical examination or insecurity of the professional, the athlete should be referred to an ophthalmologist.

20.17 Common Ophthalmologic Injuries

20.17.1 Eyelid Injuries

Direct trauma to the ocular region and also indirect trauma by means of a pair of broken glasses can cause lesions to the eyelids. Closed lesions should be treated with ice and analgesia, not forgetting to rule out possible associated with orbit fracture [23, 24]. Lacerations of the eyelids should be carefully evaluated, mainly when they occur in the medial region, due to the risk of injury to the lacrimal drainage system [25].

Lesions involving the tear duct, orbital fat exposure, and complete lacerations or involving the margin of the eyelid should be referred to evaluation by an ophthalmologist.

20.17.2 Foreign Bodies and Corneal Injuries

Foreign bodies are the most common sports-related eye injuries. In outdoor sports, the eyes have a higher risk of damage by exposition to foreign bodies produced by dust and debris. The athlete could present an acute complaint of pain and sensation of "sand in the eye" associated with conjunctival hyperemia. The eye should be carefully evaluated, everting the eyelid to find the foreign body. Removal can be performed with a swab soaked in saline solution. However, if the removal attempt is not successful, the athlete should be referred to an ophthalmologist [26].

In this context, corneal abrasions are one of the complications of foreign bodies resulting in pain, photophobia, tearing, and foreign body sensation [27]. An evaluation with cobalt blue light and fluorescein is recommended to identify the extent of the injury. The athlete should use a topical antibiotic and stay away from the sports activity until resolution (3–5 days) [28, 29]. Patching is currently avoided because it may not improve healing or reduce pain [30].

20.17.3 Subconjunctival Hemorrhage and Conjunctival Lacerations

The onset of this clinical symptom is quite common after blunt trauma, manifesting as a reddish region limited to a white portion of the sclera, not invading the cornea [31]. When isolated, this is not clinically significant; however, if there is no history of trauma, it is prudent to check blood pressure and investigate a history of excessive bleeding [32].

In the presence of subconjunctival hemorrhages, careful inspection of the eyeball should be performed to rule out other serious injuries due to a foreign body, conjunctival laceration, ocular penetration, and orbital fracture.

The presence of associated conjunctival lacerations requires the use of topical antibiotics and an overnight pressure patch. The athlete should return to training when there is evidence of re-epithelization. Lacerations larger than 1 cm may need to be sutured by an ophthalmologist.

20.17.4 Hyphema

It consists of bleeding in the anterior chamber due to a rupture of iris vessels. Heavy bleeding can be easily observed at clinical evaluation, while the slit lamp plays an essential role in detecting smaller volumes of blood. The athlete should be referred for daily ophthalmological evaluation, due to needing to monitor intraocular pressure. Anti-inflammatory drugs are not indicated, and topical corticosteroid is not efficient [33]. The athlete should not return to sports practice until resolution [34].

20.17.5 Traumatic Iris

It is an inflammatory reaction of the anterior chamber that occurs days or weeks after ocular trauma, manifested by eye pain, photophobia, and tearing. The use of slit lamp confirms the diagnosis, but an ophthalmologic evaluation is recommended. The treatment is done with topical corticosteroids, and return to sports is allowed when the athlete is asymptomatic.

20.17.6 Traumatic Iridodialysis

It is the detachment of the iris from the ciliary insertion, where small displacements may be asymptomatic and do not require treatment, while larger dialysis could result in monopolar diplopia and photophobia. A flattening of the outer iris circumference can be observed. An ophthalmologic evaluation is mandatory, and surgical correction may be necessary [35].

20.17.7 Lens Dislocation

Blunt trauma can cause tearing of the suspensory ligament of the lens. This injury could lead to a partial dislocation may cause few symptoms or a complete dislocation into the anterior chamber causing a permanently blurred vision. The complications of this pathology include secondary glaucoma, retinal detachment, cataract, and vision loss. Surgical repair is often the treatment of choice [36].

20.17.8 Retinal Detachment

It can be caused due to trauma to the eye and posterior trauma to the head or reported by intense Valsalva maneuvers, occurring hours or days after the trauma, manifested by blurred vision, flashes of light, and peripheral vision loss. Clinical causes include diabetes, sickle cell disease, and central retinal vein occlusion, and athletes with significant myopia are at higher risk as well as those with a positive family history and prior ocular surgeries. The diagnosis is based on fundoscopy but may be inaccurate in the initial setting. The treatment may be conservative or surgical, according to the extent of the injury [37], and requires withdrawal from the sports until ophthalmologic release.

20.17.9 Penetrating Injuries and Ruptured Globe

The presence of a flat chamber, black tissue exposure on the outer surface of the globe, subconjunctival hemorrhage of the entire globe, or drainage of gel or fluid may be signs of penetrating injuries and ruptured globe. In these cases, pressure on the eye and removal of penetrating foreign bodies should be avoided due to the risk of eye collapse. The athlete should be urgently forwarded to the hospital and be seen by an ophthalmologist to verify the need for surgery [38].

20.17.10 Ear Injuries

Although ear injuries are not common in sports, the sports physician must not be negligent because these injuries could result in some vital function impairment to the athlete such as hearing and balance [39, 40]. The knowledge on its diagnosis, treatment, and prevention plays a vital role for the sports medicine physician not only in the field of play or sports arena, but also in his office. Therefore, the sports medicine physician should be prepared to manage these injuries, making a careful clinical evaluation and avoiding bodily damages.

20.17.11 Anatomy

The ear has three compartments: the external ear involves the pinna, the external auditory canal that is responsible for collecting sound, and the tympanic membrane (or eardrum), which divides the external ear and the middle ear.

Behind the tympanic membrane, the middle ear is in the petrous portion of the temporal bone and consists of an auditory ossicle (malleus, incus, and staples) that helps to transmit wave sounds in the internal ear through the oval window. The internal ear comprises of the cochlea (sensorial hearing) and the labyrinth which is responsible for detecting linear and angular acceleration.

Due to these anatomical particularities, temporal bone fractures could produce lacerations and perforations of the tympanic membrane, and they could also impair the communication with the nasopharynx named Eustachian (auditory) tube, which equilizes the environmental air and medial air, affecting hearing and balance.

20.17.12 Auricular Hematoma

Considering that the external ear has thin skin and minimal subcutaneous tissue, blunt and repeated traumas (shearing forces) applied directly to it could disrupt the connections between the perichondrium and the cartilage, causing blood to accumulate in the subperichondral space and, consequently, resulting in an auricular hematoma. It is commonly seen in contact sports such as judo, jiu-jitsu, wrestling, boxing, rugby, and even water polo [40].

The most prevalent clinical signs and symptoms are swelling, pain, and pressure. The best approach for early drainage should be done within 1 or 2 days; however, this could also be possible 1 week later [40, 41]. Return to play after drainage can be immediate, and athletes at higher risk should wear protector gear to minimize the chance of an auricular hematoma [41]. Eventually, chronic swelling could be developed in cauliflower ear resulted from new fibrous cartilage and necrosis.

20.17.13 Ear Laceration

Ear laceration repair may be complicated due to its thin skin, although the auricle has good blood supply with low risk of infection. Primary repair is considered for smaller-than-2 cm laceration, while for bigger-than-3 cm lacerations, a graft could be necessary to close the wound. Complications involve chondrites, failure to cover cartilage with skin and blood loss as a result of significant lacerations.

Return to play depends on the size of the ear laceration. Good repair and homeostasis of small lacerations allow a prompt return to sports activity, while massive ear lacerations and avulsions will need soft tissue healing before returning to play. Athletes may wear adequate protection to minimize the risk of infection [41].

20.17.14 Otitis Externa

It is the inflammation or infection of the external auditory canal. It could occur due to the disruption of the cerumen (the natural first line of canal protection), water (aquatic) sports, high environmental temperatures, cotton tip applicators, and foreign objects such as earplugs [40, 41]. Discharged otalgia and otorrhea are common clinical symptoms. The discharge can be seen in varying colors between gray to green under an otoscopic exam. The treatment has the focus on external canal hygiene, topical antibiotics, and corticosteroid and pain control (NAISD). Fluoroquinolones and steroids cover most of the common pathogens. Usually, the treatment lasts 1 week, and the athlete should be away from sports practice until the end of the treatment. In the literature, prevention is still controversial, although swimmers have the best barrier to protect themselves when they wear a swim cap [39].

20.17.15 Tympanic Membrane (TM) Perforation

Barotrauma, acoustic trauma, temporal bone fracture, and penetrating trauma are possible causes of tympanic membrane perforation. Therefore, this kind of injury is most related to scuba diving, surfing, boxing, mixed martial arts, and diving. The athlete can complain of sudden hearing loss at first, and dizziness, pain, nausea, and tinnitus can also be associated with it. The sports medicine physician should be attentive to a Battle sign, a bruise behind the ear, which may occur 2–6 h after injury, indicating a possible skull fracture [41] (Fig. 20.4).

Most times, this lesion heals itself without intervention. The treatment initially comprises of pain management such as dry warm surroundings, and analgesics (e.g., acetaminophen). However, NSAID should be avoided due to a higher risk of intracranial bleeding. To prevent further infection, the following measures should be taken; ear protection when showering, no swimming until the tympanic membrane is completely healed, the wearing of headgear in high risk sports, and earplugs in certain sports. Adopted infection prevention measures are ear protection when showering, swimming prohibition until the complete healing of the tympanic membrane, and wearing of headgear in higher-risk sports and earplugs in sports event such as hunting. In case of a contained wound, ofloxacin otic drops can be used for 3 to 5 days.

An otolaryngologist evaluation should be asked in case of:

- Hearing loss greater than 40 dB in an audiometry testing or subjective decreased perception of speech, marked asymmetry in hearing or persisting feelings of ear fullness
- Vestibular symptoms, such as nausea, vomiting, nystagmus, and ataxia

- Otorrhea
- Rhinorrhea
- Facial nerve paralysis/paresis

Swimmers, divers, and surfers cannot return until the healing of TM, which heals in 4–8 weeks [40]. If the athlete has a temporal bone fracture or hearing loss, return to sports practice should be individualized.

20.17.16 Diving and Ear Barotrauma and Eustachian Tube Dysfunction

These are the most common complications related to scuba diving and flying (during descent especially) [16, 40–43], where quick changes of the pressure cause ear pain and traumatic injury. Usually, the pressure between the middle ear and the external environment should be equalized, but when the equilibrium is not kept, inflammation and rupture of the tympanic membrane could occur.

The patient can complain of pain or pressure, vertigo, tinnitus, and hearing loss, and blood can be observed in the otoscopic evaluation if the tympanic membrane is perforated. The injury classification should be defined toward treatment and prognosis [43] (Table 20.1). Grade 0 and 1 could be treated with education and medical therapy, for example, an oral or nasal decongestant. Grade 2 should be referred to an otolaryngologist for further evaluation.

When there are symptoms of nasal congestion, ear infection, or Eustachian tube dysfunction, air travel and diving should be avoided to prevent ear barotrauma. The athlete is allowed to return to sports practice when the tympanic membrane has been healed. The surgeon should be consulted in case of postsurgical event (i.e., myringoplasty).

Table 20.1 Classification and clinical findings

Classification	Clinical findings
Grade 0	Symptoms with no otologic signs of trauma
Grade 1	Any increased redness of TM when compared to baseline, serious, or slightly serosanguinous fluid and/or trapped air behind the TM
Grade 2	Profuse bleeding in any location and/or perforation of the TM

TM tympanic membrane

Take-Home Messages

- Knowledge of the dynamics of sports modality is helpful to identify the mechanism of facial trauma and associated injuries.
- Airway status, breathing, circulation, and care of cervical spine stabilization and neurological status comprise the initial assessment to facial trauma.
- Signs and symptoms for a referral to an ophthalmologist:

Altered fundoscopy	Hyphema	Penetrating foreign body	Severe eye pain
Blurred vision (persistent)	Irregular pupil	Perforated globe	Visual field loss
Diplopia	Laceration medial/ margin eyelid	Photophobia (persistent)	

- Tooth avulsion is a critical dental injury where the prognosis is strictly related to an adequate first aid—"don't touch the root!"
- Keep eyes open to indirect signs of basilar skull and temporal bone fractures such as raccoon eyes and Battle sign.
- Auricular hematoma is best approached for early drainage within the first 2 days after trauma.
- The protective equipment plays a vital role in reducing the risk of facial injuries in sports.

References

1. Murphy C, O'Connell JE, Kearns G, Stassen L. Sports-related maxillofacial injuries. J Craniofac Surg. 2015;26(7):2120–3.
2. Black AM, Eliason PH, Patton DA, Emery CA. Epidemiology of facial injuries in sport. Clin Sports Med. 2017;36(2):237–55.
3. Farrington T, Onambele-Pearson G, Taylor RL, Earl P, Winwood K. A review of facial protective equipment use in sport and the impact on injury incidence. Br J Oral Maxillofac Surg. 2012;50(3):233–8.
4. Boden BP, Pierpoint LA, Boden RG, Comstock RD, Kerr ZY. Eye injuries in high school and collegiate athletes. Sports Health. 2017;9(5):444–9.

5. Piccininni P, Clough A, Padilla R, Piccininni G. Dental and orofacial injuries. Clin Sports Med. 2017;36(2):369–405.
6. Green JI. The role of Mouthguards in preventing and reducing sports-related trauma. Prim Dent J. 2017;6(2):27–34.
7. Black AM, Patton DA, Eliason PH, Emery CA. Prevention of sport-related facial injuries. Clin Sports Med. 2017;36(2):257–78.
8. Rahman SA, Chandrasala S. When to suspect head injury or cervical spine injury in maxillofacial trauma? Dent Res J (Isfahan). 2014;11(3):336–44.
9. Bhamra J, Morar Y, Khan W, Deep K, Hammer A. Cervical spine immobilization in sports related injuries: review of current guidelines and a case study of an injured athlete. Open Orthop J. 2012;6:548–52.
10. Marston AP, O'Brien EK, Hamilton GS. Nasal injuries in sports. Clin Sports Med. 2017;36(2):337–53.
11. Patel Y, Goljan P, Pierce TP, Scillia A, Issa K, McInerney VK, et al. Management of nasal fractures in sports. Sports Med. 2017;47(10):1919–23.
12. Gart MS, Gosain AK. Evidence-based medicine: orbital floor fractures. Plast Reconstr Surg. 2014;134(6):1345–55.
13. Boyette JR, Pemberton JD, Bonilla-Velez J. Management of orbital fractures: challenges and solutions. Clin Ophthalmol. 2015;9:2127–37.
14. Wang NC, Ma L, Wu SY, Yang FR, Tsai YJ. Orbital blow-out fractures in children: characterization and surgical outcome. Chang Gung Med J. 2010;33(3):313–20.
15. Viozzi CF. Maxillofacial and mandibular fractures in sports. Clin Sports Med. 2017;36(2):355–68.
16. Cassaday K, Vazquez G, Wright JM. Ear problems and injuries in athletes. Curr Sports Med Rep. 2014;13(1):22–6.
17. Bailes JE, Hudson V. Classification of sport-related head trauma: a spectrum of mild to severe injury. J Athl Train. 2001;36(3):236–43.
18. Andrade RA, Evans PL, Almeida AL, da Silva JJ, Guedes AM, Guedes FR, et al. Prevalence of dental trauma in Pan American games athletes. Dent Traumatol. 2010;26(3):248–53.
19. Hoskin AK, Yardley AM, Hanman K, Lam G, Mackey DA. Sports-related eye and adnexal injuries in the Western Australian paediatric population. Acta Ophthalmol. 2016;94(6):e407–10.
20. Moon S, Ryoo HW, Ahn JY, Park JB, Seo KS, Shin SD, et al. Analysis on sports and recreation activity-related eye injuries presenting to the emergency department. Int J Ophthalmol. 2016;9(10):1499–505.
21. Leivo T, Haavisto AK, Sahraravand A. Sports-related eye injuries: the current picture. Acta Ophthalmol. 2015;93(3):224–31.
22. Gökçe G, Ceylan OM, Erdurman FC, Durukan AH, Sobacı G. Soccer ball related posterior segment closed-globe injuries in outdoor amateur players. Ulus Travma Acil Cerrahi Derg. 2013;19(3):219–22.
23. Pargament JM, Armenia J, Nerad JA. Physical and chemical injuries to eyes and eyelids. Clin Dermatol. 2015;33(2):234–7.
24. Murchison AP, Bilyk JR. Management of eyelid injuries. Facial Plast Surg. 2010;26(6):464–81.
25. Cohen NA, Antunes MB, Morgenstern KE. Prevention and management of lacrimal duct injury. Otolaryngol Clin North Am. 2010;43(4):781–8.
26. Ahmed F, House RJ, Feldman BH. Corneal abrasions and corneal foreign bodies. Prim Care. 2015;42(3):363–75.
27. Lin YB, Gardiner MF. Fingernail-induced corneal abrasions: case series from an ophthalmology emergency department. Cornea. 2014;33(7):691–5.
28. Saccomano SJ, Ferrara LR. Managing corneal abrasions in primary care. Nurse Pract. 2014;39(9):1–6.
29. Wipperman JL, Dorsch JN. Evaluation and management of corneal abrasions. Am Fam Physician. 2013;87(2):114–20.
30. Lim CH, Turner A, Lim BX. Patching for corneal abrasion. Cochrane Database Syst Rev. 2016;7:CD004764.
31. Hu DN, Mou CH, Chao SC, Lin CY, Nien CW, Kuan PT, et al. Incidence of non-traumatic subconjunctival hemorrhage in a nationwide study in Taiwan from 2000 to 2011. PLoS One. 2015;10(7):e0132762.
32. Tarlan B, Kiratli H. Subconjunctival hemorrhage: risk factors and potential indicators. Clin Ophthalmol. 2013;7:1163–70.
33. Türkoğlu EB, Celik T, Celik E, Ozkan N, Bursalı O, Coşkun SB, et al. Is topical corticosteroid necessary in traumatic hyphema? J Fr Ophtalmol. 2014;37(8):613–7.
34. Gharaibeh A, Savage HI, Scherer RW, Goldberg MF, Lindsley K. Medical interventions for traumatic hyphema. Cochrane Database Syst Rev. 2013;(12):CD005431.
35. Kenney KS, Fanciullo LM. Automobile air bags: friend or foe? A case of air bag-associated ocular trauma and a related literature review. Optometry. 2005;76(7):382–6.
36. Hoffman RS, Snyder ME, Devgan U, Allen QB, Yeoh R, Braga-Mele R, et al. Management of the subluxated crystalline lens. J Cataract Refract Surg. 2013;39(12):1904–15.
37. Steel D. Retinal detachment. BMJ Clin Evid. 2014;2014:0710.
38. Li X, Zarbin MA, Bhagat N. Pediatric open globe injury: a review of the literature. J Emerg Trauma Shock. 2015;8(4):216–23.
39. Hirose Y, Shikino K, Ikusaka M. Surfer's ear and external auditory canal exostoses. QJM. 2016;109(11):759.
40. Osetinsky LM, Hamilton GS, Carlson ML. Sport injuries of the ear and temporal bone. Clin Sports Med. 2017;36(2):315–35.
41. Eagles K, Fralich L, Stevenson JH. Ear trauma. Clin Sports Med. 2013;32(2):303–16.
42. Haik J, Givol O, Kornhaber R, Cleary M, Ofir H, Harats M. Cauliflower ear—a minimally invasive treatment method in a wrestling athlete: a case report. Int Med Case Rep J. 2018;11:5–7.
43. O'Neill OJ, Frank AJ. Diving, ear barotrauma. Treasure Island: StatPearls Publishing; 2018.

Thoracic

21

Ivan Felizardo Contrera Toro
and Ricardo Kalaf Mussi

21.1 Background

21.1.1 Sports Activities Related to Thoracic Trauma

Sports-related chest trauma most frequently affects osteomuscular structures of the thoracic cage, such as rib fractures associated or not with flail chest and sternum and fractures of the clavicle, sternum-clavicular joints, and sternal manubrium, aimed at protecting intrathoracic organs against more severe injuries. Injuries to structures that constitute the thoracic wall may be extremely painful and lead to morbidity, when not recognized and appropriately managed. In blunt high-energy trauma or even perforating trauma, intrathoracic structures may be affected. Despite the lower rate of these injuries, they may lead to fatal outcome. Surgical interventions in blunt thoracic trauma are required in less than 10% and in penetrating wounds 15–30%, according to the ATLS 9th edition.

When the event occurs in the prehospital setting, the athlete sustaining chest injury should be transferred as rapidly as possible to a trauma referral center where recognition of these injuries should include primarily the mechanism of injury; initial evaluation of the airway, ventilation, circulatory, and hemodynamic status; and level of consciousness. After initial care and appropriate resuscitation of vital organ functions when necessary, a second more detailed survey is required for planning definitive care. In cases of greater severity, practitioners should be diligent and prepared to manage cardiac emergencies with the use of automated external defibrillators, subsequently referring the patient to emergency units with more resources. Hypoxia is the most important factor in chest injuries. Therefore, this disturbance should be rapidly identified, providing adequate supplementation according to the severity and circumstances.

Every medical practitioner or paramedic involved in amateur or professional sports should be familiar with the initial evaluation and management of the main thoracic occurrences during sporting activities. It is fundamental to distinguish less severe injuries from those that pose an imminent risk of death, including tension pneumothorax, open pneumothorax, airway obstructions and injuries, flail chest, blunt cardiac injuries (commotio cordis), cardiac tamponade, and massive hemothorax.

Blunt chest trauma in sporting activities occur most frequently during sports on wheels, such as ice skates, roller skates, bicycles, motorcycles, and automobiles. Regarding winter sports, skiers, snowboarders, and particularly ice hockey athletes are the most frequently affected.

I. F. C. Toro · R. Kalaf Mussi (✉)
Thoracic Surgery Division, State University of Campinas—UNICAMP, Campinas, SP, Brazil
e-mail: rkalaf@fcm.unicamp.br

S. Rocha Piedade et al. (eds.), *The Sports Medicine Physician*,
https://doi.org/10.1007/978-3-030-10433-7_21

Sports with more intense individual physical contact that can cause a higher number of chest traumas are styles of wrestling, while team sports that can cause chest trauma include handball, basketball, football, and rugby.

21.2 Clavicle Fractures, Rib Fractures, and Flail Chest

Rib fractures may occur by forceful impact on the thoracic wall, such as a blow with a hockey stick during a hockey game in the grass, or result from a more generalized anteroposterior compression of the thoracic cage during sudden interruption of kinetics in a high-speed motor vehicle accident against a fixed fence. Rib fractures usually are single events but may be associated with other complicating factors of moderate to high risk, such as hemothorax, pneumothorax, and pulmonary contusion in the acute phase or with bronchopneumonic processes in the subacute phase.

The first three costal cartilages are relatively protected by the scapula, clavicle, and soft parts, while the lower ribs are relatively mobile. Blunt chest trauma of the first rib in general related to impact with great kinetic forces may be associated with potentially severe injuries to the subclavian artery, aorta, and pulmonary parenchyma. The most common fractures occur from the fourth to ninth ribs as we can in.

Anteroposterior compression of the cavity may cause fracture in the outer middle third of the chest cavity, while local force applied directly tends to direct bony fragments inside the thorax predisposing to pneumo- and/or hemothorax.

Clinical features (and findings): In general, intense chest pain with local hypersensitivity and crepitus are the most frequent findings. In cases of multiple fractures, chest deformity may occur.

Exams: Chest radiograph should be the initial imaging test. When clinical findings are very suggestive of fracture and the x-ray failed to show fractures, the specific rib view or ultrasound may be used, exceptionally complemented by computed tomography, which is the gold standard in bone injuries (Fig. 21.1). Nuclear magnetic resonance imaging is the method of choice in injuries where there is a suspicion of soft tissue injuries.

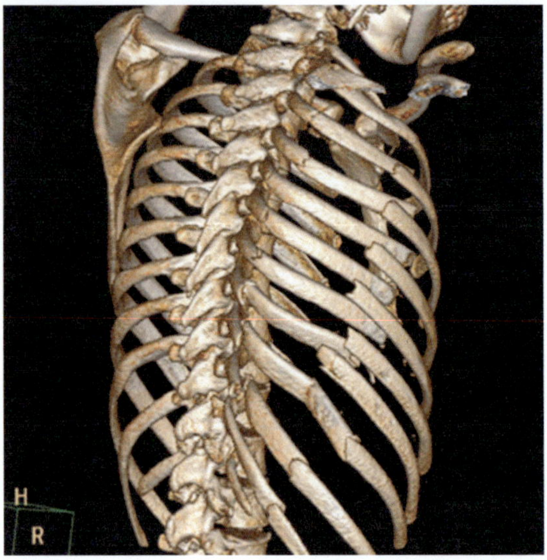

Fig. 21.1 CT scan shows various rib fractures on the right side of a woman after a fall during horseback riding

Blunt chest trauma of the first rib requires evaluation with angio-CT of the chest for a better investigation of suspected vascular injuries.

21.2.1 Treatment (Stable X Unstable Patient)

Analgesia is the main treatment of rib fractures without other comorbid conditions. In addition to greater comfort, it reduces the time to return to physical and work activities. There are a growing number of articles in the medical literature in the last years and various prospective and retrospective ongoing clinical studies listed in ClinicalTrials.gov evaluating surgical treatment in rib fractures. Surgical fixation with plates has been recommended in patients sustaining five or more fractures with flail chest, in incomplete bone repair, or marked fracture dislocation during thoracotomy. Furthermore, surgery should be considered when three or more fractures occur in patients under mechanical ventilation or there is intense fracture dislocation [3].

The **clavicle** connects the axial skeleton to the upper extremity. It contributes to movement and

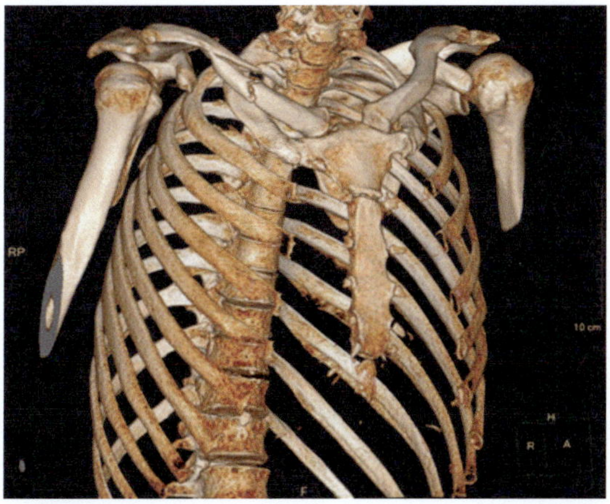

Fig. 21.2 CT scan shows a clavicle fracture in middle third on the right side

stability of the upper limbs and promotes protection of underlying neurovascular structures. The clavicle is the most commonly broken bone, and fractures occur in up to 15% of both children and adults [6] and account for up to 10% of all sports-related fractures.

Sporting activities with or without direct contact between athletes are the main cause of clavicle fractures, in around 45.3%, and bicycle activities correspond to 16% of cases and American football 12% and soccer 6%. The majority of fractures are located in the middle third (81%) (Fig. 21.2), lateral (17%), and medial (2%).

Approximately 85% of clavicle fractures that occur in the pediatric age group are related to sports or recreational activities. Nonsurgical treatment with a sling or figure-of-eight bandage is appropriate for this age group, since it is associated with excellent remodeling and bone repair.

Several studies have compared surgical and nonsurgical treatments in clavicle fractures in adult athletes with significant advantages in early return to competitions and a lower rate of refracture. Although a moderate reduction in shoulder function may be well tolerated, early return to sports activities even with compromised function is of great importance to athletes. It prevents the loss of training periods for both amateur and professional athletes [6]. Nevertheless, it is fundamental that patients be aware of the potential risks of complications, including neurovascular

Table 21.1 Main indications for surgical treatment of clavicle fractures

Absolute	Relative
• Open fractures	• Shortening of clavicle fracture >1.5 cm
• Marked angulation	• Comminuted fracture
• Separation with risk of skin perforation	• Floating shoulder
• Neurovascular compromise	• Deviation with cosmetic compromise
• Partial symptomatic consolidation	

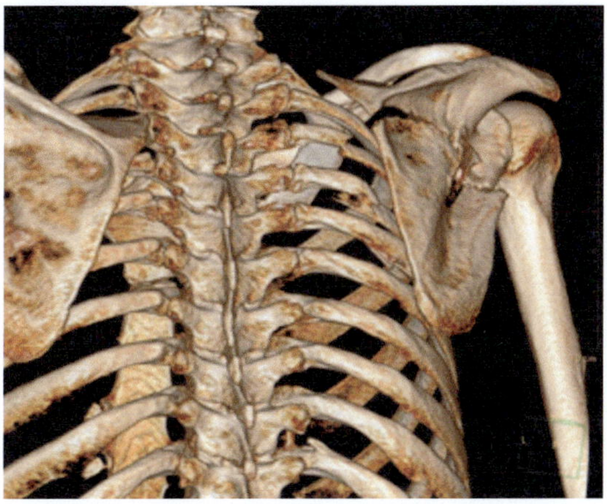

Fig. 21.3 CT scan shows a scapular fracture on the right side of a man after mountain biking fall

injuries and infection. The most adequate surgical technique has still not been well-established.

The main absolute and relative indications for surgical treatment of clavicle fractures are listed on Table 21.1.

Complications related to surgical treatment of the clavicle include infection which may range (0–18%) and nonunion (2–15%), neurovascular injury (0–5%), adhesive capsulitis (0–7%), refracture after removal of the plate (0–8%).

There are various methods for fracture fixation selected by the nature and location of the injury. For middle-third clavicle fractures, techniques include plate and intramedullary nail fixation. Lateral fractures are managed with techniques that involve acromioclavicular joint hooks (ACJ spanning hook), coracoclavicular suture, and screw fixation [18]. Sternal and scapular fractures (Fig. 21.3) are generally the results of a direct impact with high kinetic energy, and its repair occasionally is indicated.

21.2.2 Flail Chest

Flail chest occurs when three or more consecutive ribs are fractured in two or more locations, creating an independent segment of the chest wall that moves paradoxically. This may cause intense acute pain, pulmonary atelectasis, and alveolar collapse, with repercussions on ventilation and gas exchange. Furthermore, loss of chest wall integrity predisposes the patient to adult respiratory distress syndrome, which may require and/or prolong the need for mechanical ventilation. Mortality rates may range from 20 to 42%.

Conservative treatment is based on effective analgesia and mechanical ventilatory assistance to establish chest wall integrity. However, surgical management with rib fixation has become a more common option, and a number of systematic reviews have described better outcomes [14].

When isolated, this condition does not result in any major ventilatory or oxygenation disorder. Definitive treatment is vigorous opioid analgesia possibly using epidural blockade, fluidification of secretions, and physical therapy. Nevertheless, since it is mostly associated with some degree of underlying pulmonary contusion, severe hypoxia may occur requiring supplemental oxygen and even mechanical ventilation. Volume replacement with crystalloids may aggravate respiratory distress and warrants special attention.

Diagnosis is made by physical examination of the chest wall associated with adequate chest radiograph.

21.3 Pulmonary Contusion and Respiratory Distress Syndrome

Clinical features (and findings): It is the most common complication in blunt force trauma, typically resulting from trauma with elevated kinetic energy that may occur in motor vehicle accidents and falls. It is characterized by intraparenchymal hemorrhage, interstitial edema, and alveolar collapse which may impair respiratory function. It is rarely reported in association with sports, but some cases in the literature are related to injuries in football players.

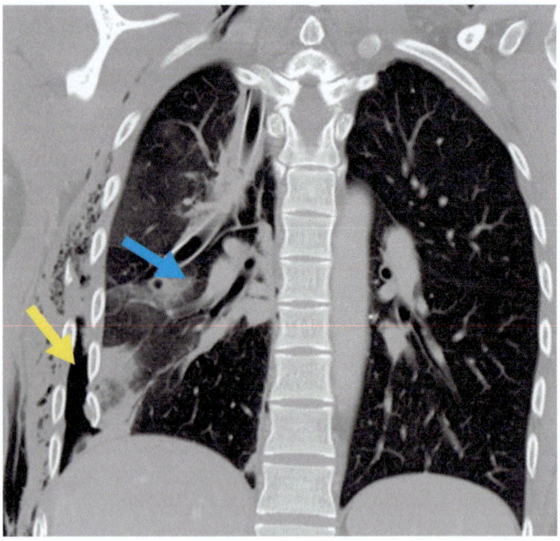

Fig. 21.4 CT scan shows a pulmonary contusion (blue arrow) and pneumothorax (yellow arrow) of a woman after fall during horseback riding

Physical examination (look, feel, listen, percuss): Clinical and radiological manifestations may occur immediately or later. Typical findings are dyspnea, hypoxia, tachypnea, blood-tinged sputum, and chest pain. Auscultation may reveal crackles or reduced breath sounds.

Exams: The initial exam is the chest radiograph. However, this exam frequently underestimates findings which may be absent in 10–36% of the cases. Focal or diffuse opacity affecting segments or even lobes may develop within 48 h. Computed tomography of the chest offers a greater sensitivity (Fig. 21.4), and it is the imaging method of choice for the evaluation of pulmonary contusion.

21.3.1 Treatment (Stable X Unstable Patient)

It depends directly on the extension of the injury. Management in minor sports-related injuries most frequently is supportive and includes oxygen supplementation, analgesia, pulmonary toilet, and judicious administration of endovenous fluids to avoid worsening of pulmonary edema that was initially developed. Orotracheal intubation with mechanical ventilation may be considered in cases of severe hypoxemia $PaO2 < 65$ mmHg or $SaO2 < 90$.

Complications of pulmonary contusion may range from pneumonia to adult respiratory distress syndrome and are related to greater severity and mortality higher than 20%. It is worth mentioning that pulmonary contusions in athletes occur at a low rate in healthy young individuals and are usually not associated with mortality.

We should never underestimate the severity of blunt lung injury, since there may be a broad range of clinical signs that do not always correlate with radiologic findings. When a contusion occurs without other complications, return to activities is usually after 7 days [7].

21.4 Pneumothorax and/or Hemothorax, Pneumomediastinum

21.4.1 Pneumothorax

Pneumothorax is the result of air entry into the pleural cavity due to both blunt and penetrating lung trauma. In sports-related chest trauma, collisions, falls, or frequently both are involved. Three mechanisms may cause pneumothorax in blunt lung trauma: spontaneous, barotrauma, or mechanical trauma. Pulmonary laceration with air leak is the most common cause of closed pneumothorax due to rib fracture during sporting activities. Although less frequent, these occurrences are more commonly related to contact and collision sports such as ice hockey, soccer, rugby, and American football. Other sports that involve high kinetic energy such as snowboarding, horseback riding, or skiing may also be associated with barotrauma. Barotrauma is more commonly related to diving and powerlifting. Spontaneous pneumothorax may occur in any circumstance independent of sporting activity, but there are reports in athletes during racing, tennis, golf, cycling, wrestling, and rowing [11, 22].

Clinical features (and findings): Irrespective of the mechanism, pneumothorax resulting from sporting activities must have an adequate initial evaluation since it may progress to situations of greater risk.

Diagnosis is commonly made by history and physical examination. Dyspnea, chest pain, and tachypnea are the most common clinical findings, eventually associated with subcutaneous emphysema. In more severe cases, tachypnea, anxiety, and loss of consciousness may occur. Eventually, traumatic pneumothorax may be asymptomatic and found on chest radiograph.

Physical examination (look, feel, listen, percuss): The most common findings in the physical examination are subcutaneous emphysema, crepitus, and hyperresonance with fremitus to percussion.

Exams: Whenever pneumothorax is suspected in an individual participating in a sporting event who sustains chest trauma, a chest radiograph should be ordered. In certain cases, small volumes of pneumothorax may not be seen in the imaging test with the athlete supine. We should bear in mind that athletes usually have a greater respiratory capacity and the adrenaline surge of competition that may mask intrathoracic injuries for prolonged periods due to minimization of their symptoms.

21.4.2 Hemothorax

Hemothorax in blunt chest trauma generally is related to contusion and laceration of the parenchyma and visceral pleura with bleeding into the pleural cavity. Penetrating wounds or multiple rib fractures may be associated with injuries to the intercostal or internal thoracic arteries. In situations that involve greater kinetic energy, aortic rupture should be considered. The most common site for aortic injuries is the isthmus (90%), ascending aorta (5–10%), and descending aorta at the level of the diaphragm (1–3%). In practice, around 50% of cases die at the scene of trauma. In general, these emergencies are related to sports with high kinetic energy and also after falls from considerable heights. When aortic rupture is suspected during clinical examination, diagnostic confirmation should be obtained by angiotomography of the chest and immediate surgery [19].

21.4.3 Treatment (Stable X Unstable Patient)

In the majority of cases, pneumothorax and hemothorax are present simultaneously and in distinct volumes in patients with blunt thoracic trauma. Management in blunt trauma is based on the magnitude of its components, in addition to clinical and hemodynamic aspects.

In cases of hemodynamically stable patients without respiratory distress, conservative management may be adopted in the presence of a small volume of hemothorax and/or pneumothorax. It is worth mentioning that when conservative treatment is the option, periodic clinical and radiologic observation is mandatory until discharge from outpatient facility.

In moderate or large volumes of hemothorax or pneumothorax, hemodynamic instability, or respiratory distress, underwater seal tube chest drainage is indicated at the level of the nipple region (fifth intercostal space) in the midaxillary line using a 36 or 38 French chest tube.

After chest drainage, initial blood loss that is higher than 1500 mL of blood or 1/3 or more of total blood volume of the patient or even a volume lower than 1.5 L but blood loss of more than 200 mL/h for a period of 2–4 h characterizes massive hemothorax. In these cases, rigorous attention is required with volume replacement and use of autotransfusion, when possible. These patients usually sustain injuries to systemic or hilar vessels. Exploratory thoracotomy is indicated for effective bleeding control.

Tension pneumothorax is a condition in which lung injury may cause airflow into the pleural cavity. In addition to causing pneumothorax, this flow may lead to total collapse of the homolateral lung. Continuous airflow without adequate drainage may progress to a condition of elevated intrathoracic pressure, shifting the mediastinum to the contralateral side, reducing venous return, and consequently leading to obstructive circulatory shock. This condition is characterized by the presence of some or all of the following signs or symptoms: chest pain, respiratory distress, tachycardia, hypotension, tracheal deviation contralateral to the injured site, absence of vesicular murmur, thoracic hyperinflation without movement, neck distension, and cyanosis. Signs of tension pneumothorax must be differentiated from cardiac tamponade, since the latter does not present with tracheal deviation, absence of vesicular murmur, and hyperresonance to percussion.

This condition causes imminent death risk and should be treated immediately with cavity decompression by a large-bore needle of sufficient length (e.g., >8 cm) to reach the pleural cavity. Initial management (needle decompression) is followed by chest tube drainage at the nipple level in the midaxillary line.

Open pneumothorax is a condition in which there was a significant loss of tissue with a great defect in the thoracic wall that causes increased intrathoracic pressure to levels of atmospheric pressure. If the defect of the thoracic wall is greater than or equal to 2/3 of the diameter of the trachea, the air passes inside the cavity causing pulmonary collapse with ventilatory compromise, resulting in hypoxia and hypercapnia.

Initial treatment consists of sterile dressing (plastic or gauze) that is applied to occlude the entire extension of the chest wall defect. Three of the four angles must be fixed as a flap valve system to allow air to escape from the cavity through a free angle during expiration. Meanwhile, during inspiration, the dressing will provide occlusion and not allow air to enter the thoracic cavity. Immediately afterward, a conventional chest tube drainage is performed until the defect in the thoracic wall is adequately corrected and also to prevent tension pneumothorax determined by the occlusive dressing.

21.5 Tracheobronchial Rupture

Main causes of airway injuries in sports are related to automobile accidents and sports that involve intense physical contact or high velocity with the possibility of abrupt thoracic compression, such as skiing, skating, car racing, cycling, etc. Other sports where darts, weights, and discs are thrown may be a risk for third parties (referees, aides, assistants, or the public) who are not minimally protected against these objects.

Professionals involved with the health and well-being of athletes must understand the meaning and potential severity of this type of injury, particularly to the larynx and trachea, since these are potentially major causes of death in trauma (80% at the scene of the accident) [1]. Early diagnosis may ensure effective management in these potentially fatal cases and reduce late complications. The majority of tracheobronchial injuries occur inside the thorax and most commonly in the distal third of the trachea.

Three mechanisms are responsible for tracheothoracic trauma: (1) anteroposterior compression of the thoracic cavity and/or neck, (2) deceleration or abrupt acceleration, and (3) increased intrathoracic pressure with closed vocal cords [17, 20].

Clinical features (and findings): The main physical signs of airway injury are respiratory failure, hoarseness, cervical crepitus, increased neck diameter, and subcutaneous emphysema. All patients with these symptoms must undergo bronchofibroscopy or CT with virtual bronchoscopy [15, 16]. Over time small lesions may lead to mediastinal infection or stricture of the trachea/affected bronchus [21]. Signs that may suggest greater severity include progressive edema, audible stridor with hemoptysis, dyspnea with change in position of the ictus cordis (tension pneumothorax), and hypoxia with a significant decrease in oxygen saturation. In a patient with tube drainage, escape of a large amount of air, without lung expansion, should alert to the possibility of injury to the trachea and/or bronchus. Whenever possible, diagnostic confirmation is obtained by bronchoscopy.

Due to the severity of the injuries, the majority of cases die at the scene of the accident, and diagnosis is confirmed at autopsy.

21.5.1 Treatment (Stable X Unstable Patient)

Initial treatment goal is to maintain life, primarily with oxygen supplementation and general measures [17]. Chest drainage is mandatory in cases of pneumothorax, in an attempt to expand the lung, increasing areas of gas exchange. However, adequate lung expansion may not occur due to the size of the injury to the tracheobronchial tree, and sometimes more than one chest tube is necessary.

When immediate obstruction is present, a fiber-optic bronchoscope is the gold standard for intubation (Fig. 21.5) [17]. Cricothyroidostomy is rarely indicated, since the injury may be located below the tip of the cannula. When necessary, tracheostomy should be performed at the site of the hissing wound in the trachea, if existent.

Definitive procedures for specific injuries may vary from clinical observation to surgical repair of the injury, mobilization, and/or resection of segments, lobes, or even the lung, in cases of injury to the main bronchus without the possibility of correction of the injuries and/or even application of ortheses for variable periods of time [15, 17, 21].

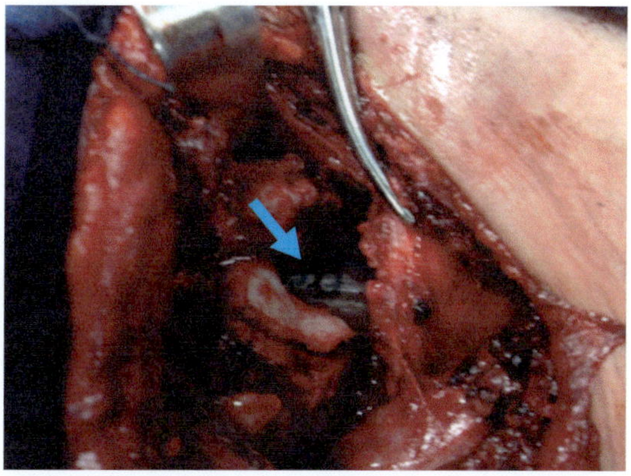

Fig. 21.5 Injury to the trachea with total separation from the larynx and inside orotracheal tube (blue arrow) (courtesy Fraga, G)

21.5.2 Prevention

Improvement in protective gear in sports that generate high kinetic velocity, such as cervical protectors, safety belts, and chest protection shirts, may reduce the chance of injuries. Other effective measures to decrease the risk of tracheobronchial injuries might improve isolation of areas of potential risk in sports where darts, discs, and weights are thrown, etc. However, only training paramedical and medical teams to suspect and identify possible victims of these injuries can reduce sequelae and mortality [5].

21.6 Blunt Aortic Injury

In all accidents with blunt chest trauma, around 1/6 are caused by aortic rupture. Calculating all deaths from accidents involving vascular injury, aortic injury accounts for 90%.

The mechanism of trauma in this type of injury was first described in 1557 by Andres Vesalius while studying the autopsy of an individual with sudden death after falling from a horse.

With a high mortality at the scene of the accident, survivors can also die after hospital admission, if aortic injury is not immediately recognized and investigated. Hospital death is due to rupture of the pseudoaneurysm, formed when bleeding is contained by the thoracic fascia and pleura (Fig. 21.6).

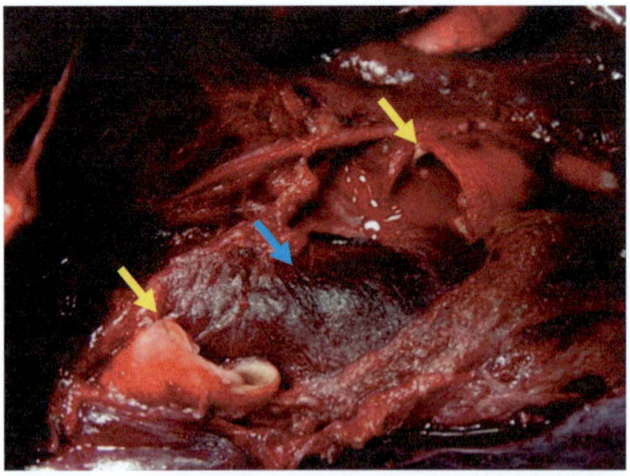

Fig. 21.6 Complete injury to the aorta. Note two stumps of retracted aorta (yellow arrows) and a large hematoma in the mediastinum (blue arrow) (courtesy Fraga, G)

Traumatic injury to the aorta occurs mainly (63%) in the aortic isthmus (Fig. 21.8), at 1 cm below the site where the left subclavian artery exits and the aorta remains fixed at the ligamentum arteriosum. Injuries to the ascending or low descending aorta are usually caused by bone fractures, primarily of the ribs or vertebrae.

All sports involved with the mechanism of velocity and abrupt deceleration may cause complete or partial rupture of the aorta. Automobile racing, motorcycling, cycling, horseback riding, mountaineering, parachute jumping, skiing (water or snow), jet skiing, snowboarding, and pole vaulting are the main examples. In pole vaulting, injury may occur when the athlete falls outside the protector landing mat.

The mechanism of injury is linked to stretching and torsion of the aorta in the zone of the isthmus, due to movement of the heart and ascending aorta, in addition to a phenomenon termed "water hammer effect." This effect results from increased hydrostatic pressure in blood vessels, due to thoracic compression. The aortic arch is elevated with partial obstruction of the descending aorta at the passage of the diaphragmatic hiatus, increasing pressure dramatically and producing fluid pressure waves.

Clinical features (and findings): To reduce mortality due to this injury, all accidents involving blunt chest trauma which are related to acceleration and deceleration must arouse suspicion and be investigated.

There are no specific signs and symptoms. However, interscapular pain, dyspnea, and hoarseness (injury to the left recurrent nerve that bypasses the aortic arch) may occur. It is important to bear in mind that the majority of patients sustain other associated injuries, e.g., craniocephalic, chest, or pelvic fractures, etc., which may mask symptoms.

Physical examination (look, feel, listen, percuss): On physical examination, the imprint of the steering wheel or sports-related object on the chest, heart murmurs that were nonexistent, interscapular murmur, extensive hemothorax, progressive supraclavicular hematoma, absence of left radial pulse, and paraplegia are alert signs for aortic injury.

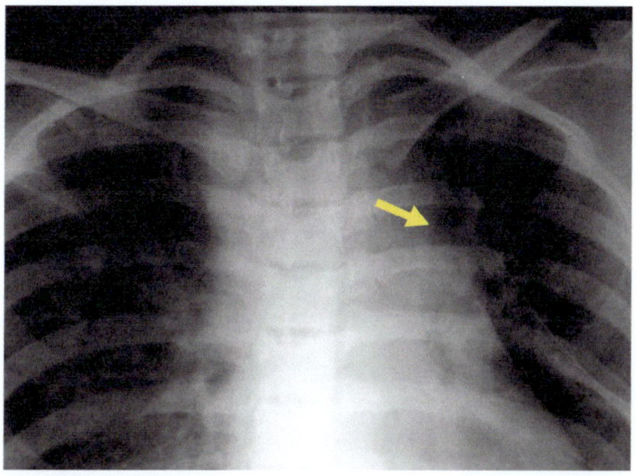

Fig. 21.7 Mediastinal widening (yellow arrow) (courtesy Fraga, G)

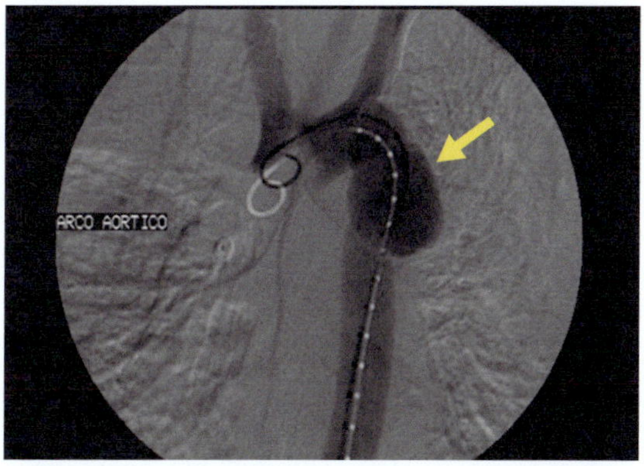

Fig. 21.8 Aneurysm in the isthmus region (courtesy Menezes, F)

Exams: Imaging tests are crucial for diagnostic confirmation and assist in the search for other concomitant injuries [10]. The main imaging methods that may aide in the diagnosis of aortic rupture are discussed, as follows:

Plain AP x-ray: The x-ray is part of standardized care in the chest trauma patient and is performed in the emergency room. It has a good sensitivity (62–90%) but low specificity. The main signs are mediastinal widening (Fig. 21.7), blurring of the aortic knob, tracheal deviation to the right, left apical hematoma, elevation of the left main bronchus, and extensive pleural effusion. All these signs are nonspecific and must be confirmed by other diagnostic methods. It is important to bear in mind that up to 7% of patients that sustain aortic injury may have a normal plain chest x-ray [8].

21.6.1 Computed Tomography

CT is currently the most widely used imaging test for the diagnosis of mediastinal trauma, such as injury to the aorta. The new generation multichannel CT technology through vascular reconstruction can locate the injury in a matter of minutes. Its sensitivity and negative predictive value are nearly 100% [8]. Helicoidal CT, more simple and rapid, with less contrast injection and lower renal damage than arteriography, is the method of choice for rapid diagnosis and surgical intervention in the majority of cases.

21.6.2 Aortography

Although it is not the gold standard for definition of aortic injury, aortography with catheter insertion through the femoral artery has lost ground for multichannel CT. The technique has a morbidity rate of 1% and mortality rate of 0.003%, which are much higher than those for CT scan. It is a more expensive imaging test. However, in large centers it permits endovascular intervention (Fig. 21.8) with placement of prostheses and may sometimes substitute for open surgery, which has higher morbidity and mortality rates [16].

Transesophageal echocardiogram: The use of transesophageal echocardiogram (TE) has limited indication in some unstable patients with suspected aortic injury on chest radiograph who should not be transported to the Radiology Division. Another indication is due to the current worldwide epidemic of obesity. It may be indicated in the morbidly obese patient who may not fit into a conventional tomography scanner [16].

Assessment at the bedside, it takes advantage of the proximity of the esophagus to the aorta at the area of highest incidence of injuries. It has a sensitivity of 86% and specificity of 92% and permits detection and location of the lesion. The method is operator-dependent and requires a trained team both in TE and trauma.

There are some blind spots in TE, the area of the aorta close to the carina, distal aorta, and branches of the aortic arch, where injuries occur in less than 10% of cases.

The main contraindications are patients with severe craniofacial injuries and esophageal injury due to trauma.

21.6.3 Nuclear Magnetic Resonance Imaging

It has a role only in chronic injuries and is not applied in the acute patient with a suspicion of aortic lesion close to the site of traumatic injury. Patient access to MRI is limited; the technique is time-consuming and requires total immobility of the patient. On initial evaluation, it has no advantages over computed tomography [16].

21.6.4 Treatment (Stable X Unstable Patient)

Although it may seem clear that aortic injury always requires correction, this is not always possible or recommended.

Patients with minor injuries, without large hematomas or more severe hemorrhage, should be controlled with medication using beta-blockers and hypotensive agents. Treatment goal is to decrease tension at the site of injury, maintaining maximum arterial pressure of 100 mmHg and heart rate of 80 bpm.

Surgery should also be avoided in patients sustaining other severe associated injuries such as severe traumatic brain injury, massive burns, pulmonary contusion with the impossibility of total pulmonary collapse during surgery, coagulopathy, and lack of an experienced surgical team.

In surgical patients sustaining major abdominal bleeding with a stable aorta, it is recommended to perform abdominal surgery for damage, followed by thoracotomy or placement of vascular endoprosthesis.

Endovascular surgery, also called minimally invasive corrective technique, has grown substantially (Fig. 21.9). When possible, it is currently the treatment of choice for aortic injuries. With stent placement through an artery (mostly the femoral artery), blood loss is minimum, and a change in ventilation is not necessary. Occlusion of the aorta does not occur, decreasing neurologic injuries due to spinal ischemia and renal injuries.

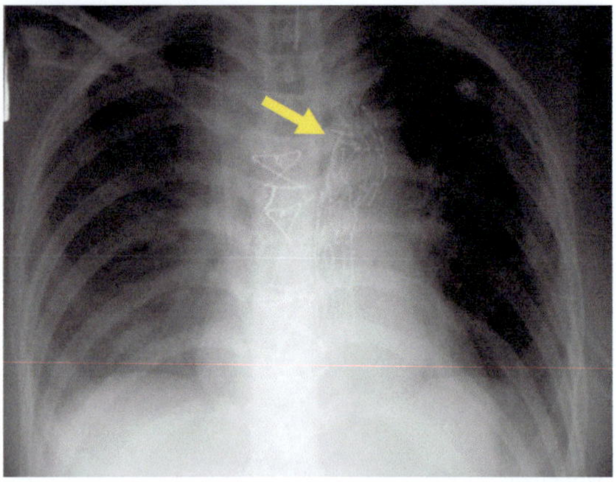

Fig. 21.9 Placement of endovascular stent during surgery (courtesy Menezes, F)

Traditional surgical technique is reserved for some special situations. Normally, a heart-lung machine is required to establish cardiopulmonary bypass and decrease the morbidity of the procedure.

21.6.5 Differential Diagnosis

Differential diagnosis includes trauma to other thoracic organs, e.g., the thyme, heart, and esophagus. Aortic lesion may also be minimized in massive hemothorax caused by pulmonary laceration or rupture of vessels such as pulmonary artery and vein, left hemi-azygos, and splenic rupture with injury to the diaphragm.

21.6.6 Prevention

Preventive factors are those that can decrease chest trauma but primarily reduce abrupt deceleration. Limiting the speed of sports on wheels, ski circuits with less ramps, and use of clothes that can help absorb impact may play a relevant role.

It is necessary to mention that in prehospital treatment of a patient suspected of aortic injury, the use of antishock pneumatic equipment is contraindicated, due to increase in peripheral vascular resistance and tension of the aortic wall.

21.7 Blunt Myocardial Injury: Commotio Cordis

Myocardial contusion may be defined as impact on the precordial region, with momentary decrease in the anteroposterior diameter, which can lead to the formation of hematoma of the cardiac wall until valvular rupture due to increased pressure.

Three mechanisms have been described for this type of injury: direct injury with a bony fragment (sternum or rib), compression of the heart full of blood, and increased pressure in the cardiac chambers due to abdominal compression with a closed glottis [2].

The presence of heart disease, especially one that progresses with increasing size of the heart, may predispose to contusion. Cardiac contusion is most prevalent in sports related to wrestling, with punches and kicks, high-velocity sports that may cause direct trauma to the sternum, and falls [9].

Autopsy findings ranged from petechiae and hematomas to myocardial rupture with pericardial tamponade.

Clinical features (and findings): Minor injuries may remain undetected, and the only symptom is cardiac arrhythmia, initiated by extranodal focus. In more severe cases, the clinical picture may simulate myocardial infarction. Patients have continuous precordial pain with or without irradiation. Ventricular arrhythmia and even sudden death may occur [9].

Exams: The electrocardiogram is mandatory for identification of myocardial ischemic zones and characterization of arrhythmia.

Cardiac enzymes are normally altered, and the CK-MB curve should be measured.

Transthoracic echocardiogram and/or transesophageal is of great help and may show the location and size of the injuries, repercussions on the cardiac chambers, and presence or absence of blood in the pericardium.

Chest CT scan is helpful particularly in alterations of the myocardial wall and in pericardial effusion.

21.7.1 Treatment (Stable X Unstable Patient)

In the majority of cases, treatment is clinical, with control of heart rate and rhythm. Even patients without any apparent injury on echocardiogram must be monitored, since arrhythmia may appear during the first 24 h.

Administration of antiarrhythmic drugs and maintenance of homeostasis are necessary in patients with symptomatic ventricular premature beats or those at risk of ventricular fibrillation.

Treatment is very similar to that of acute myocardial infarction. Absolute rest is required, in an attempt to decrease cardiac work.

In cases of rupture of the cardiac valves or septum, the clinical picture is dramatic, and intervention of the cardiac surgeon is often necessary [9].

21.7.2 Prevention

Prevention is similar to that of chest trauma in general: decrease the velocity of sports on wheels or skis, use of protective gear to reduce trauma, training of medical and paramedical teams in the identification of cardiac contusion risk.

21.8 Commotio Cordis

Commotio cordis is ventricular fibrillation that may or not be followed by sudden death due to *cardiac arrhythmia* produced by impact of an object against the left side of the chest, without the occurrence of rib fracture or fracture of the sternum and without direct heart damage [13].

This condition should not be confused with cardiac contusions resulting from accidental bone injury with bony fragments that damage the heart.

Known ever since the first reports of Chinese martial arts technique, in which a blow to the left side of the chest led to death, the first reports in the literature emerged in the nineteenth century.

It is a rare disorder. However, it is widely publicized since it affects healthy amateur or professional athletes, without any previous heart disease.

The majority of victims are men (95%) and young (only 9% over age 25 years) and 75% occur during professional (50%) or amateur (25%) games [12].

Most have been reported with sports that use blunt projectiles such as balls or discs (baseball, hockey, and lacrosse) or intense physical contact (American football, soccer, and hockey).

Mechanism: despite an apparent traumatic cause, cardiac arrest is due to an electrical event translated as ventricular fibrillation that occurs immediately after impact on the left thorax. In experimental studies, several critical events must occur to promote commotio cordis [13]. Two major events are (1) location of the crash in the left anterior region, in the area corresponding to the heart, and (2) it should occur at the peak of the T wave, an event that lasts 10–20 ms [12].

Clinical picture and therapy: the clinical picture is cardiac arrest with circulatory collapse. Patient outcome depends on promptness of resuscitation with the use of defibrillators. The success rate of CPR performed within 3 min of cardiac arrest was 25%. In contrast, the success rate in CPR initiated after 3 min was 3%. Ten to 15% of patients will live and receive hospital discharge [13].

Prevention: The use of protective gear for the left thoracic region is necessary, particularly in young individuals aged 25 or less who participate in the sports mentioned above [4]. Among the protective measures are the use of softer balls in softball and baseball, chest protectors in contact sports and sports with projectiles, and presence of automated defibrillators wherever sports are played with training of technicians and other staff members [13]. These measures may contribute to a decrease in cases and increase in survival of patients affected by this fatality [12].

21.9 Traumatic Diaphragmatic Hernia

Diaphragmatic injuries are uncommon and occur in approximately 3% of patients with thoracoabdominal trauma. Usually, these injuries do not cause acute morbidity in trauma patients and are frequently missed clinically. However, they are important to recognize due to the potential for late adverse outcomes related to hernia formation.

Traumatic diaphragmatic injuries may be penetrating or blunt, depending on the causal factor and sporting activity. Nevertheless, it has a relatively low rate in athletes in particular. Spontaneous ruptures have also been reported in the literature and are caused by a sudden increase in abdominal pressure resulting from a pressure gradient between abdominal and thoracic pressure through the diaphragm in very extenuating physical activities. Previous congenital lesions obviously cannot be ruled out in these cases.

In general, in penetrating injuries there is early suspicion and diagnosis. Nevertheless, blunt trauma lesions may go undetected in 10–20% of cases, due to difficulty in interpretation (as in cases of acute gastric dilatation after trauma, hemopneumothorax, and subpulmonary hematoma) making differentiation very difficult even with the use of computed tomography. Lesions may appear later as radiological findings or clinical manifestations related to alterations in intestinal transit time or indirect manifestations due to compression of the lung parenchyma. There is a greater incidence of left-sided blunt trauma, probably due to the obliterative or protective effect of the liver.

Upon diagnostic suspicion of left-sided injury which occurs in up to 90% of cases, a nasogastric tube should be inserted. When the tube appears in the thoracic cavity after radiographic control, there is no need for more complex contrast-enhanced imaging techniques.

When suspicion still remains and imaging tests are not fully elucidative, invasive diagnostic procedures may be required, including laparoscopy or thoracoscopy.

When acute injury has been identified, the abdominal approach for repair of the lesion is preferable. When it is a chronic lesion due to a number of adhesions in thoracic structures, a thoracic approach is recommended.

Direct repair of the lesions with primary suture is the best option whenever possible. In more chronic situations, the use of prosthetic materials may be necessary for adequate closure of the rupture.

21.9.1 Cardiac Tamponade

Cardiac trauma is identified in less than 10% of all trauma admissions. Due to its anterior position, the right ventricle is most easily affected, while the left atrium is less frequently affected.

More than 90% of cases occur in sports that involve great kinetic energy and high-speed events, including car racing and motorcycle sports. Among winter sports, there is a high risk for cardiac trauma in skiing and snowboarding.

Cardiac tamponade is a medical emergency that is more commonly related to perforating cardiac lesions. It is extremely rare as a result of blunt trauma and may be caused by direct injuries to the heart, great vessels of the base of the heart, or pericardial vessels.

Clinical course may be insidious in onset and slow or present rapid hemodynamic deterioration. Cardiac tamponade occurs when localized or distributed intrapericardial collection elevates pressure inside the pericardium causing hemodynamic impact due to restricted filling of the cardiac chambers.

The three principal features of cardiac tamponade (Beck's triad) may be clinically observed: (1) a rise in venous pressure, (2) decrease in arterial blood pressure, and (3) muffling of heart sounds. Sometimes these findings may also be present in cases of tension pneumothorax. Clinically, alert signs in differential diagnosis should include the absence of vesicular murmur on pulmonary auscultation in pneumothorax and Kussmaul's sign, which is a rise in venous pressure on inspiration during spontaneous respiration in cardiac tamponade (paradoxical venous pressure).

In massive pericardial effusions, T-wave inversion may occur in the electrocardiogram. When there is a large intrapericardial volume, generally above 200 mL, an enlarged cardiac silhouette is detected on chest x-ray. Echocardiogram has a diagnostic accuracy of up to 90–95%.

After diagnostic confirmation, provided the patient fails to respond to usual resuscitative measures for hemorrhagic shock, a procedure for adequate drainage of the pericardial content is necessary. Subxiphoid pericardiocentesis guided or not by echocardiography with aspiration of content should be the alternative in patients with severe hemodynamic instability, allowing relief until pericardiotomy via thoracotomy is available in a surgical theater for adequate evacuation of blood and blood clots and effective repair of the cardiac or vascular lesion.

Take-Home Messages

- Thoracic trauma most often involves bone structures.
- It needs an initial judicious evaluation due to more serious or life-threatening intrathoracic traumatic lesions.
- After initial evaluation and clinical stabilization, the patient should be removed as soon as possible to a trauma center for specific advanced radiologic exams and definitive therapy.

References

1. Al-Koudmani I, Darwish B, Al-Kateb K, Taifour Y. Chest trauma experience over eleven-year period at al-mouassat university teaching hospital-Damascus: a retrospective review of 888 cases. J Cardiothorac Surg. 2012;7:35.
2. Asensio JA, Petrone P, Toro IFC. Trauma cardiaco penetrante, Trauma edit Atheneu. p. 305–26. ISBN 978-85-388-0082-8.
3. de Moya M, Nirula R, Biffl W. Rib fixation: who, what, when? Trauma Surg Acute Care Open. 2017;2(1):e000059.
4. Doerer JJ, Haas TS, Estes NA, Link MS, Maron BJ. Evaluation of chest barriers for protection against

sudden death due to commotio cordis. Am J Cardiol. 2007;99(6):857–9.
5. Fabian RL. Sports injury to the larynx and trachea. Phys Sportsmed. 1989;17(2):111–8.
6. Fanter NJ, Kenny RM, Baker CL. Surgical treatment of clavicle fractures in the adolescent athlete. Sports Health. 2015;7(2):137–41.
7. Feden JP. Closed lung trauma. Clin Sports Med. 2013;32(2):255–65.
8. Harris JH, et al. To reduce routine computed tomographic angiography for thoracic aortic injury assessment in level II blunt trauma patients using three mediastinal signs on the initial chest radiograph: a preliminary report. Emerg Radiol. 2018;25:387–91.
9. Huis In 't Veld MA, Craft CA, Hood RE. Blunt cardiac trauma review. Cardiol Clin. 2018;36(1):183–91.
10. Keenan RJ, Van Deusen MA, Alegre RA, Normando Jr GR. Trauma Torácico, Trauma edit Atheneu. p. 245–56. ISBN 978-85-388-0082-8.
11. Kizer KW, MacQuarrie MB. Pulmonary air leaks resulting from outdoor sports. A clinical series and literature review. Am J Sports Med. 1999;27(4):517–20.
12. Link MS. Pathophysiology, prevention, and treatment of commotio cordis. Curr Cardiol Rep. 2014;16(6):495.
13. Menezes RG, Fatima H, Hussain SA, Ahmed S, Singh PK, Kharoshah MA, et al. Commotio cordis: a review. Med Sci Law. 2017;57(3):146–51.
14. Naidoo K, Hanbali L, Bates P. The natural history of flail chest injuries. Chin J Traumatol. 2017;20(5):293–6.
15. Noh D, Lee CK, Hwang JJ, Cho HM. Concomitant avulsion injury of the subclavian vessels and the main bronchus caused by blunt trauma. Korean J Thorac Cardiovasc Surg. 2018;51(2):153–5.
16. Patel N, Mansouri M, Shankar S, Singh A. Imaging of acute thoracic trauma. In: Emergency radiology: imaging of acute pathologies. 2nd ed. Springer International Publishing; 2017. p. 403–18. https://doi.org/10.1007/978-3-319-65397-6_24.
17. Prokakis C, Koletsis EN, Dedeilias P, Fligou F, Filos K, Dougenis D. Airway trauma: a review on epidemiology, mechanisms of injury, diagnosis and treatment. J Cardiothorac Surg. 2014;9:117.
18. Robertson GA, Wood AM, Oliver CW. Displaced middle-third clavicle fracture management in sport: still a challenge in 2018. Should you call the surgeon to speed return to play? Br J Sports Med. 2018;52(6):348–9.
19. Singhal P, Kejriwal N. Ascending aortic tear with severe aortic regurgitation following rugby injury. Heart Lung Circ. 2009;18(2):150–1.
20. Shorr RM, Crittenden M, Indeck M, Hartunian SL, Rodriguez A. Blunt thoracic trauma. Analysis of 515 patients. Ann Surg. 1987;206(2):200–5.
21. Symbas PN, Justicz AG, Ricketts RR. Rupture of the airways from blunt trauma: treatment of complex injuries. Ann Thorac Surg. 1992;54(1):177–83.
22. Wilkerson RG, Stone MB. Sensitivity of bedside ultrasound and supine anteroposterior chest radiographs for the identification of pneumothorax after blunt trauma. Acad Emerg Med. 2010;17(1):11–7.

22 Abdomen

Rui Pedro Borlido Escaleira

22.1 Evaluation of the Athlete with Abdominal Trauma: An Overview

Concerning trauma, athletes and coaches are extremely focused on those injuries that may compromise their performance and career, and therefore musculoskeletal/extremity trauma is subjectively assumed to be their principal concern. This reality can seriously affect their perception of other symptoms and signs related to trauma, distracting them and the sports physician that is proceeding to the primary survey from eventual abdominal trauma, which elevates the possibility of misdiagnosing rare but serious abdominal potentially life-threatening injuries.

Although abdominal muscle strains and contusions are the most common sports injuries and can be treated conservatively [1], abdominal trauma evaluation can be challenging and is extremely important in the sports trauma scenario, especially when significant kinetic energy is transferred to the torso from a direct blow, deceleration, or penetration injury.

Unrecognized abdominal and pelvic injuries continue to be a cause of preventable death. Intraperitoneal bleeding from a solid organ or a mesenteric laceration, a hollow viscus rupture with peritonitis, and retroperitoneal bleeding or bleeding from the bony pelvis may compromise the outcome if not diagnosed early. In the classic study of trauma centers versus non-trauma centers in California published in 1979, West et al. demonstrated that the majority of preventable deaths resulted from unrecognized, and therefore untreated, intra-abdominal hemorrhage [2].

According to Advanced Trauma Life Support (ATLS®) program of the American College of Surgeons [3], when we face an injured athlete, we must proceed to a primary systematic evaluation of the, airway (A), breathing (B), circulation (C), disability (D), and exposure (E) in a timely fashion (primary survey) and early identify and treat if possible (in the sideline or in the track) the life-threatening injuries. Even if we cannot treat the injuries promptly, their early recognition, report, and transfer to the emergency team in the hospital setting have a significant impact on the outcome [3–5].

Concerning to abdominal trauma, the early assessment of "circulation" in the primary survey is mandatory because of the possibility of hemorrhage in the abdomen and pelvis in any athlete who has sustained blunt trauma (more common in the sports setting) or victim of penetrating torso wounds between the nipple and perineum (less common).

In most cases, the sports medicine physician is the first health-care provider to arrive at the trauma scene, and the first survey will be of his responsibility.

R. P. B. Escaleira (✉)
General Surgery Department, Hospital de Santa Luzia—Alto Minho Health Care Unit, Viana do Castelo, Portugal

S. Rocha Piedade et al. (eds.), *The Sports Medicine Physician*, https://doi.org/10.1007/978-3-030-10433-7_22

There are some questions the sports medicine physician may ask, and we will try to answer in this chapter:

1. **When to suspect of abdominal trauma injury?**
2. **Which is the initial diagnostic workflow in the evaluation of the athlete with abdominal trauma?**
3. **Which athletes can immediately return to play and which athletes should be removed and transferred for further evaluation?**
4. **Which diagnostic techniques are used in patients with abdominal trauma?**
5. Although there are some issues regarding abdominal trauma that are very specific and from the responsibility of the trauma surgeon/general surgeon and therefore will not be discussed here, it is important for the sports medicine physician to have an **overview of the principal blunt traumatic abdominal injuries, their appropriate treatment, as well as particular concerns regarding return to play.**

All these issues will be discussed in this chapter.

22.2 When to Suspect of Abdominal Trauma Injury?

To answer this question, it is important to integrate the basic knowledge of the anatomy of the abdomen, mechanism of injury, and physical examination of the patient.

22.2.1 Anatomy of the Abdomen

For practical purposes as it has implications in the diagnosis and treatment strategy, it is essential to define three abdominopelvic compartments.

1. **The peritoneal cavity** that contains the majority of the hollow viscus (distal esophagus, stomach, the first portion of the duodenum, jejunum, ileum, transverse colon) and solid organs as the anterior, inferior, and superior face of the liver and the spleen.

   Problems occurring inside this cavity are mostly associated with blunt or penetrating trauma to the *anterior abdomen* which is defined topographically as the area between the costal margins superiorly, the inguinal ligaments and the symphysis pubis inferiorly, and the anterior axillary lines laterally. It is also important to know that trauma involving the *thoracoabdominal* transition area (inferiorly to the trans-nipple line anteriorly) may be associated with rib fractures, lung and pleura lesions, and concomitant lesion of abdominal organs as the spleen (left subcostal area), liver (right subcostal area), stomach (epigastric area), and diaphragm.
2. **The** retroperitoneal **space**, where we can find most of the duodenum, pancreas, kidneys, and ureters, the posterior aspects of the ascending and descending colon, abdominal aorta, inferior vena cava, and the retroperitoneal components of the pelvic cavity.

   Problems occurring in this space are usually associated with blunt or penetrating trauma to the *flank* (the area between the anterior and posterior axillary lines from the sixth intercostal space to the iliac crest) and to the back (the area located posterior to the posterior axillary lines from the tip of the scapula to the iliac crests).

   Chance fractures, especially in thoracolumbar spine vertebra, may also be associated with retroperitoneal and abdominal visceral injuries.

   As we will see later in this chapter, it is usually difficult to diagnose injuries in the retroperitoneal visceral structures earlier. The physical examination of this area has low sensibility and specificity.
3. **The** pelvic **cavity** is the most caudal portion of both peritoneal and retroperitoneal spaces and is structurally dependent on the pelvic bones. It contains the iliac vessels, rectum, bladder, and the internal reproductive organs in the female.

   If we suspect of pelvic fractures, we must always exclude injury of vascular, intestinal, and genitourinary structures. Misdiagnosis evolving those injuries may be problematic.

22.2.2 Mechanism of Injury

Abdominal trauma can be divided into blunt and penetrating subtypes. Differentiating into blunt or penetrating trauma has practical implications in the diagnosis and treatment [3]. Understanding the subjacent mechanism facilitates the interpretation of the initial evaluation and the stratification of trauma severity because it directs the identification of the potential injuries. Globally, blunt trauma is the cause of more than 80% of abdominal injuries, whereas penetrating injuries account for approximately 20% [6, 7]. Concerning sports injuries related to abdominal trauma, blunt trauma is even more frequent. Although the physical examination is fundamental in the initial evaluation of these patients, in the case of blunt trauma, the definition of the volume, localization, and extension of injury is more difficult when compared to penetrating trauma and is thus associated with higher morbidity and mortality due to delays in the diagnosis. Some studies have shown the sensitivity of physical examination in the range of only 55–65% in the setting of blunt abdominal trauma [8–10], and up to 20% of patients with hemoperitoneum may not manifest peritoneal signs [11]. These data support the importance of a good description of the trauma mechanism before starting the primary survey. The patient's ability to relate the course of events may be compromised by the head or spinal cord injury, and therefore witnesses at the scene, particularly paramedical personnel, often provide the most reliable data.

22.2.2.1 Blunt Trauma

This type of trauma results from a direct blow into the abdomen, the situation we may find in contact or collision sports, such as soccer, rugby, football, hockey, boxing, and martial arts, and also in noncontact sports such as bodyboarding, surfing, cycling, skiing, and snowboarding. Motorized sports must also be considered as they are ultimately related to accidents involving multisystem injuries.

The depth and the magnitude of the injury are proportional to the force transferred during the trauma. We can find *compression and crush injuries* to solid and hollow organs complicated with secondary hemorrhage, contamination with visceral contents, and associated peritonitis. *Shearing injuries* are a form of crushing injuries that can be associated with *acceleration/deceleration injuries* in which there is a differential movement of fixed and nonfixed segments and parts of the body. Lacerations of the spleen and liver, at the sites of their fixed supporting ligaments, and bucket handle injuries to the small bowel (a type of mesenteric injury) are examples.

The spleen is the most frequently injured abdominal organ in sports and the most common cause of death due to blunt abdominal trauma among athletes [12], followed by the liver and small bowel with less incidence. Retroperitoneal hematomas must also be considered although their presentation is less conspicuous.

It is important to remember that pilot restraint (in the case of motorized sports) can themselves cause blunt trauma to the liver, duodenum, and pancreas, and rib fractures can cause direct damage to the liver or spleen.

22.2.2.2 Penetrating Trauma

This type of trauma is rare in a sports setting. Stab wounds transfer less kinetic energy to the surrounding tissues and cause damage by lacerating and cutting. Unless you find an athlete with evisceration, it is usually difficult to understand on the sideline or track if the stab wound in the anterior abdomen, flank, or back penetrates the peritoneal cavity or the peritoneum.

Low-velocity gunshot wounds also induce a lacerating and cutting pattern, although associated with more kinetic energy transfer. Concerning high-velocity gunshot wounds can cause increased damaged surrounding the track of the projectile due to temporary cavitation. They also can cause additional intra-abdominal injuries based upon secondary bullet and bone fragmentation.

Injuries related to stab wounds most commonly involve the liver (40%), small bowel (30%), diaphragm (20%), and colon (15%). Gunshot wounds most commonly affect the small bowel (50%), colon (40%), liver (30%), and abdominal vascular structures (25%) [3].

22.3 Which Is the Initial Diagnostic Workflow in the Evaluation of the Athlete with Abdominal Trauma?

The evaluation and reanimation of trauma patients should respect the basic principles supported by Advanced Trauma Life Support (ATLS®) of the American College of Surgeons [3].

According to ATLS®, we must proceed to a primary survey in a timely fashion which implies the evaluation and correction of the problems encountered in the:

- Airway (A) with the protection of the cervical spine
- Breathing (B)
- Circulation (C)
- Disability (D)
- Exposure (E)

The early assessment of "circulation" in the first survey is mandatory in the athlete with abdominal trauma as it has practical implications in the definition of the hemodynamic status, helps the physician to suspect of an active intra-abdominal hemorrhage, and stratifies trauma severity and therefore the early need to transfer to a trauma care center. At this point, the recognition (or exclusion) of hemorrhagic shock is needed, while resuscitative measures are carried out.

The sports medicine physician must be able, after the integration of the mechanism of injury and the primary survey (focusing on hemodynamic and abdominal examination), to identify:

- The athlete suspected to have abdominal trauma with transient complaints that present with a normal abdomen, a normal hemodynamic status, and no other injuries and can return immediately to the field or track.
- The athlete with positive but equivocal findings in the physical examination that elevate the suspicion for intra-abdominal injuries and a normal hemodynamic status. These patients need to transfer to a trauma care center to continue the investigation.
- The athlete with an evident abdominal injury that needs urgent transfer to a trauma care center to continue the investigation and treatment. The hemodynamic status must always be the pacemaker of the transferring process.

22.3.1 Recognition of Shock

Recognizing (or excluding) shock must be the first step when it comes to "C" evaluation, simultaneously to the initiation of fluid resuscitation protocol with crystalloid solutions.

Although severe circulatory shock evidenced by inadequate perfusion of the skin, hypotension, tachycardia, elevated respiratory rate, and confusion is easy to recognize, it is crucial to recognize shock earlier. After the airway and adequate ventilation have been ensured, proceed to a careful evaluation of the circulatory status to identify the early manifestations of shock, especially tachycardia and cutaneous vasoconstriction, which are typical early physiologic responses to volume loss in most adults. Systolic blood pressure is not a sensible indicator, and exclusive reliance on this hemodynamic marker probably will result in delayed recognition of the shock state, especially in athletes.

Athletes have specific physiologic responses to hypovolemia because training induces chronic cardiovascular adaptations. Blood volume increases, cardiac output increases, stroke volume increases, and the resting pulse can average values under 60 bpm after years of endurance training [13]. Therefore the usual responses to hypovolemia may not be present even when a significant amount of blood is lost (compensatory mechanisms can preclude a measurable fall in systolic blood pressure until up to one-third of the patient's blood volume is lost).

In the athlete, we must look carefully to:

- Pulse rate: It can be a pitfall (as an example, 90 bpm in an athlete with a cardiac rest rate of 40 may be a compensatory mechanism for a depressed stroke volume and effectively is an "abnormal finding").
- Pulse character and pulse pressure: A narrow pulse pressure, which is the difference between systolic and diastolic pressure, in a hypovolemic shock patient indicates a decreasing cardiac output and an increased peripheral vascular resistance.
- Respiratory rate (increased initially and depressed lately).
- Skin circulation (compromised with vasoconstriction).

The current "gold standard" for assessment of perfusion following injury is a measurement of the serum lactate. Elevated lactate levels indicate organ dysfunction and failure in severely injured trauma patients and therefore reflect inadequate perfusion and oxygenation of ischemic tissues [8, 14]. Mackersie et al., in an evaluation of 3223 patients with blunt trauma, found that the risk of abdominal injury was significantly increased in the presence of an arterial base deficit of 3 mmol/L or more, the presence of significant chest trauma, the presence of pelvic fractures, or the presence of hypotension [8].

Be careful because the initial evaluation of the circulatory status based on physical examination and/or serum lactate may be compromised if the athlete was performing at high levels of intensity before the accident, but it is expected to become more reliable after a few minutes of immobilization and external warming.

Concluding, any injured athlete with suspicious for abdominal trauma who is cold and has tachycardia after a significant period (some minutes) of immobilization and warming is considered to be in shock until proven otherwise.

22.3.2 Causes of Shock: Differential Diagnosis

In trauma, the shock is classified as hemorrhagic (most frequent) or nonhemorrhagic. Shock in acute abdominal trauma is hemorrhagic until proven otherwise. Nonetheless it is also important to exclude nonhemorrhagic causes of shock, as tension pneumothorax, cardiac tamponade, cardiogenic shock (myocardial injury), and neurogenic shock. The work-up for the identification of these causes will not be explored in this chapter, but it is important to know that in the case of shock, multisystem trauma is not infrequent to the coexistence of more than one cause of shock.

Septic shock is not frequent immediately after injury but can also be the cause of shock in abdominal trauma patients if there was a delay in the diagnosis (hours to days). In this case, hollow viscus perforation with peritoneal or extraperitoneal contamination must be considered, especially but not exclusively in penetrating trauma.

22.3.3 Abdominal Examination

First of all…

- *"Positive clinical findings may be relevant. Negative ones are not!* [14]."
- When on the sideline or track, if the patient presents with a hemodynamic abnormality, a meticulous abdominal physical examination is not indicated. You must immediately get an IV access, start fluid resuscitation, and transfer the victim to a medical facility.

In trauma, it is challenging to assess the abdomen, as the history may not be available and all the available physical signs may be misleading. Blood is not initially a peritoneal irritant, and therefore it may be difficult to assess the presence or quantify the blood in the abdomen. Nevertheless, a physical examination is very important to drive our investigation and should be conducted in a systematic fashion respecting the classic sequence *inspection, auscultation, percussion, and palpation*. We must look for direct and/or indirect signs of anterior, flank, and back abdominal trauma, pelvic trauma, genitourinary trauma, as well as peritoneal signs. It is important to start with a good exposition although preventing from hypothermia.

Inspection: We must look for contusions and abrasions (especially in blunt trauma) and lacerations, penetrating wounds, the evisceration of peritoneal contents, and impaled foreign bodies in penetrating trauma. Blood at the urethral meatus, perineal hematoma, and vaginal or rectal hemorrhage are worrisome features related to pelvic trauma and must be carefully investigated.

Auscultation: In trauma, the setting is difficult to perform careful auscultation. However, the absence of bowel sounds may be an unspecific and late indirect sign of free peritoneal blood.

Percussion may elicit signs of peritoneal irritation. If we can exclude voluntary guarding during abdominal **palpation**, involuntary guarding must also be assumed as a sign of peritoneal irritation. If they are positive, we must admit the presence of an intraperitoneal lesion; if they are not, we cannot exclude it. In the case of evaluation of an abdominal wall hematoma, palpation and percussion may help us to define its boundaries although we cannot exclude an intraperitoneal origin.

There are some classic signs and symptoms that usually elevate the suspicion for specific abdominal lesions in blunt trauma:

- **Splenic injury** may cause left upper quadrant pain and referred pain to the left shoulder (Kerr's sign). Left thoracic trauma at the level of thoracoabdominal transition area may cause splenic injury, even without rib fractures (especially in younger athletes). Athletes with a recent history of infectious mononucleosis may be at a higher risk of splenic rupture due to splenomegaly [15].
- **Liver injury** is usually associated with right upper quadrant pain and tenderness, referred pain to the right shoulder. An ecchymosis around the umbilicus (Cullen's sign) may be present.
- **Kidney injury** is often caused by trauma to the back and flank and may also be associated with rib fractures. Hematuria, flank ecchymosis (Grey Turner's sign), and focal tenderness may be also present.

Mechanical instability of the pelvic ring must be tested if a pelvic fracture is suspected [16] by manually pushing inward and outward the iliac crests at the level of the anterior superior iliac spine (the compression-distraction maneuver). This procedure should be performed only once during the physical examination due to the risk of aggravating ongoing pelvic hemorrhage (remember that *"the first blood clot is the best clot…"*). Therefore, it should not be done in patients with shock and an evident pelvic fracture.

22.4 Which Athletes Can Immediately Return to Play and Which Athletes Should Be Removed and Transferred from Competition for Further Evaluation?

The following flowchart that correlates with abdominal trauma mechanism, hemodynamic status, and physical examination was made to help sports medicine physician to decide rapidly (in the sideline).

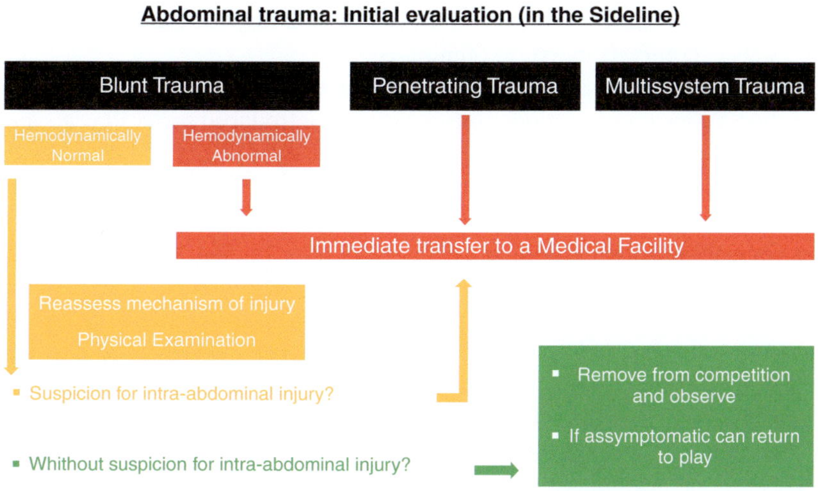

22.5 Which Diagnostic Procedures Are Useful in Patients with Abdominal Trauma?

The diagnostic work-up depends primarily on the hemodynamic status of the patient, as well on the mechanism of trauma, the abdominal region affected, and the type and localization of the suspected lesions. Selection of the diagnostic technique procedures should respect diagnostic accuracy and efficiency (regarding invasiveness, potential harms, time consumption, and resource use). We must remember that false-negative findings or delayed diagnoses increase the risk of severe complications, so it is important to know the specificity and sensibility of each type of diagnostic procedure.

Patients with abdominal trauma and *unstable* hemodynamic status non-responsive to fluid resuscitation may be (with high probability) candidates for a resuscitative laparotomy. In this case, identifying life-threatening injuries enables priority-oriented management and therefore *point-of-care* imaging (like FAST—focused assessment with sonography for trauma), or other procedures (like diagnostic peritoneal lavage) directed for the detection of free fluid in the abdominal cavity (blood) is mandatory in the emergency department.

Patients with abdominal trauma and are hemodynamically unstable, moreover, can be submitted to more accurate diagnostic procedures (like computed tomography) to define the best definitive treatment.

22.5.1 Focused Assessment of Sonography for Trauma (FAST)

Ultrasonography performed using a four-quadrant, focused assessment of sonography for trauma (FAST) is regarded as a critical instrument for the initial assessment of patients with suspected blunt abdominal and thoracoabdominal trauma in the emergency department setting [17–21] especially if the patient is in shock. FAST is a non-invasive, rapid, and inexpensive procedure with excellent specificity but rather low sensitivity (<90%) [22] in detecting and excluding free peritoneal blood as an indicator of organ injury.

A positive FAST in the athlete with unstable hemodynamic status non-responsive to fluid resuscitation is an indication for laparotomy.

A negative FAST does not exclude intra-abdominal lesions (the prevalence of organ injury without accompanying free fluid ranges from 5 to 37% [23]). In this case, if the athlete has a hemodynamic status compatible with performing a CT scan, it should be done.

In the hands of most operators, ultrasound will detect a minimum of 200 mL of fluid in the peritoneum [24]. Overall, FAST has a sensitivity between 73 and 88% and a specificity between 98 and 100% and is 96–98% accurate [21]. This level of accuracy is independent of the practitioner performing the study. Surgeons, emergency medicine physicians, ultrasound technicians, and radiologists have equivalent results [21]. The experience of sports medicine physicians with ultrasonography is increasing, especially in the musculoskeletal examination. It would be important to extend that experience to FAST so that in the future this procedure can be carried out on the sideline as an adjunct to physical examination. Nevertheless, if the sports medicine physician chooses to perform FAST on the sideline, evaluation should not delay the transfer of the patient to a medical facility if indicated.

Consider the advantages and disadvantages of FAST as follows:

Focused assessment with sonography for trauma	
Advantages	Disadvantages
Is portable: Can be done at the bedside in the emergency department or **on the sideline**	User dependent
Permits an early diagnosis	Unhelpful for diagnosing hollow viscus injury
Noninvasive, performed rapidly, and inexpensive	Misses diaphragm and retroperitoneal injuries
Repeatable and reproducible	Obesity, subcutaneous air, and previous abdominal operations can compromise the accuracy of ultrasound
Excellent specificity	Does not rule out organ injury in the absence of hemoperitoneum

Ultrasonography can also be used to diagnose post-traumatic abdominal wall hematomas or hernias.

22.5.2 Diagnostic Peritoneal Lavage

Diagnostic peritoneal lavage is an invasive procedure introduced some 50 years ago as a method of evaluation of the abdomen. Its use has markedly decreased because of advances in imaging technology and increased non-operative management after trauma. It allows investigation of the presence of blood in the peritoneal space with high sensitivity (>97%) [14] although with limited specificity (because of the significant false-positive rate of the technique), but it does not identify the organ of injury. It also has value in the diagnosis of a possible hollow viscus injury. The accuracy of DPL has been reported to be between 92 and 98% [21].

It should be performed by a surgical team in the emergency department (not in the sideline!) and is indicated in patients with hemodynamic abnormalities who sustain blunt or penetrating abdominal trauma. In this case, a **positive DPL is an indication for laparotomy.** Hemodynamically stable patients with equivocal results are best managed by additional diagnostic testing to avoid unnecessary laparotomies.

A DPL is generally considered as positive if:

- Gross blood (>10 mL) or gastrointestinal contents are easily aspirated from the peritoneal cavity

If this condition is not achieved, lavage is performed infusing saline into the peritoneum to mix with possible blood and/or gastrointestinal contents and then to recover the fluid for analysis. In this case, DPL is generally considered as positive if:

- Red cell count is >100,000 cells/mm^3.
- White cell count is >500/mm^3.
- There is amylase, bile, or gastrointestinal content in the lavage return.
- Gram stain with bacteria is present.

Consider the advantages and disadvantages of DPL as follows:

Diagnostic peritoneal lavage	
Advantages	Disadvantages
Permits an early diagnosis Performed rapidly and inexpensive High sensitivity Can detect bowel injury	Invasive **(not feasible in the sideline)** Limited specificity Misses injuries of the retroperitoneum and diaphragm False-positive results may occur in the presence of pelvis fractures

22.5.3 Computed Tomography

Computed tomography is the *gold standard* in the evaluation of abdominal trauma because intraperitoneal and retroperitoneal injuries can be detected, the amount of intra-abdominal blood loss can be estimated, and it is possible both to recognize the organ that is injured and to grade the severity of the injury. Nevertheless, CT is a diagnostic procedure that requires transport of the patient to the radiology suite, administration of contrast, and scanning, which is time-consuming. **Therefore this procedure should be used only in hemodynamically stable** patients. Allergy to the contrast agent when nonionic contrast is not available and an uncooperative patient who cannot be safely sedated are relative contraindications.

CT scanning has the unique ability to detect clinically unsuspected injuries, and therefore sensitivity between 92 and 97.6% and specificity as high as 98.7% have been reported in patients submitted to emergency CT scanning [25, 26]. When it comes to clinical decision-making in blunt abdominal trauma, CT scanning has proved to be superior to other methods in the diagnosis of injuries that require surgical intervention [27]. Negative predictive value of CT scanning in blunt abdominal trauma is high (99.63%), so a negative CT scan usually permits safe discharge of patients with blunt abdominal trauma [28]. Nevertheless, most authors still recommend admission and observation after a negative CT scan [29, 30] if the mechanism of injury is significant.

CT scanning is adequate for evaluation of penetrating back and flank trauma but may be inadequate for the diagnosis of some mesenteric injuries and miss hollow visceral injuries. In patients at high risk for mesenteric or hollow visceral injury (as in penetrating trauma), DPL is generally felt to be a more appropriate test [21]. CT can also miss some diaphragmatic and pancreatic injuries in the early phase.

Consider the advantages and disadvantages of CT as follows:

Computed tomography	
Advantages	Disadvantages
Most specific for diagnosing injury (organ-specific) High sensitive Can detect retroperitoneal lesions	The patient must be hemodynamically stable Need transport Misses diaphragm, bowel, and some pancreatic injuries Cost and time

22.5.4 Contrast Studies

Contrast studies can be helpful in the diagnosis of specifically suspected injuries if the hemodynamic status allows it:

- Specific **upper and lower gastrointestinal contrast studies**, as well as biliary-pancreatic contrast-enhanced imaging, may be indicated if a retroperitoneal-gastrointestinal structure-isolated injury is suspected and CT scans or DPL are equivocal.
- **Urethrography** must be performed if a urethral lesion is suspected. If we find a normal urethrogram, then we can exclude urethra disruption and can proceed to the insertion of an indwelling urinary catheter.
- **Cystography** is indicated if a bladder rupture is suspected. It can be achieved with a simple cystogram or with a more specific CT cystography.
- **Intravenous pyelography** is an alternative to contrast-enhanced CT to evaluate suspected urinary system injuries.

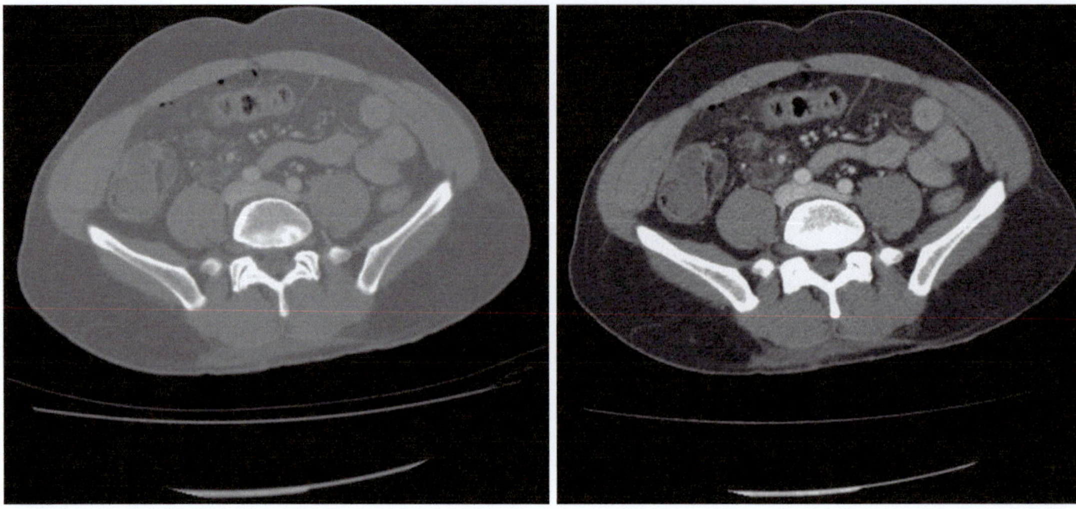

Images 22.1 and 22.2 Free peritoneal air

22.5.5 Routine Screening Radiographs

Abdominal films specifically oriented to diagnose intra-abdominal injury are not usually useful. Even when it comes to looking for infradiaphragmatic free air, an erect chest radiograph (if possible and safe to do it) will provide more information than an erect abdominal film.

Nevertheless, it is important to remember the importance of obtaining an anteroposterior chest film and a pelvic film, as preconized by Advanced Trauma Life Support (ATLS®) program of the American College of Surgeons as adjuncts to the primary survey.

22.6 Overview of the Principal Blunt Traumatic Abdominal Injuries, Their Appropriate Treatment, as well as Special Concerns Regarding Return to Play

22.6.1 Splenic Injury

The spleen is a very vascularized and delicate organ and can be damaged easily during blunt thoracoabdominal trauma, especially direct trauma to the left lower chest wall or left upper quadrant of the abdomen. The avascular suspensory ligaments of the spleen also place it at risk of avulsion during rapid deceleration. The presence of a splenic capsule makes it possible to occur a delayed splenic rupture which incidence ranges from 1 to 8% in adults and 0 to 7.5% in children [12]. Therefore the spleen is one of the most frequently injured abdominal organs in sports and the most common cause of death due to blunt abdominal trauma-related hemorrhagic shock among athletes [12]. Certain diseases increase the risk for complicated splenic trauma, like infectious mononucleosis [15, 31, 32].

The athlete with splenic injury may present left upper quadrant pain and referred pain to the left shoulder (Kerr's sign). Peritoneal signs may not be present. The assessment of signs of hypovolemia is mandatory, and the hemodynamic status will be the most important prognostic indicator when it comes to decision-making.

In the hemodynamically unstable patient, a FAST (or DPL) during resuscitation is indicated, and if positive, operative treatment is necessary.

In the hemodynamically stable patients, abdominal CT is the most reliable method to identify and assess the severity of injury to the spleen (evidence level II) [32] as well as identify the patients with active bleeding (presence of contrast blush on the CT scan). With contrast enhancement, a splenic laceration will be presented as an irregular, linear hypodensity, whereas an intrasplenic hematoma will appear as a hypodense area in a non-perfusing region of the spleen [33].

American Association for the Surgery of Trauma's Spleen injury scale [34] is an important tool for decision-making protocols:

American Association for the Surgery of Trauma's (AAST) Spleen injury scale [34]		
Grade[a]	Injury type	Description of injury
I	Hematoma	Subcapsular <10% surface area
	Laceration	Capsular tear <1 cm parenchymal depth
II	Hematoma	Subcapsular, 10–50% surface area Intraparenchymal, <5 cm in diameter
	Laceration	Capsular tear, 1–3 cm parenchymal depth that does not involve a trabecular vessel
III	Hematoma	Subcapsular, >50% surface area or expanding Ruptured subcapsular or parenchymal hematoma Intraparenchymal hematoma >5 cm or expanding
	Laceration	>3 cm parenchymal depth or involving trabecular vessels
IV	Laceration	Laceration involving segmental or hilar vessels producing major devascularization (>25% of the spleen)
V	Laceration	Completely shattered spleen
	Vascular	Hilar vascular injury with devascularized spleen

[a]Advance one grade for multiple injuries up to grade III

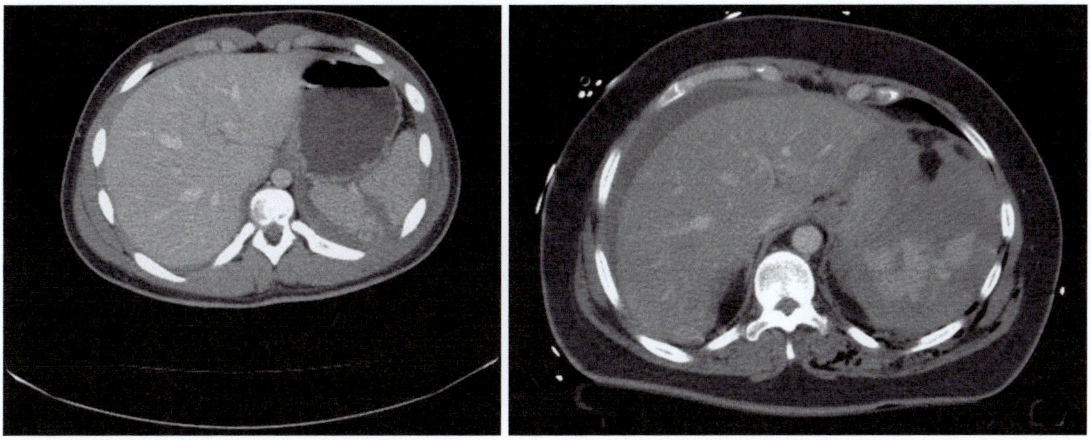

Images 22.3 and 22.4 Splenic laceration

Management of blunt splenic injuries has evolved during the past decade to more non-operative management due to the evolution of the critical care units, to the implementation of damage-control hemostatic resuscitation protocols [35–39] as well as to transvascular procedures [40] to stop the parenchymal bleeding. Splenic preservation is preferred over splenectomy because splenectomy is associated with overwhelming postsplenectomy infection (particularly from encapsulated organisms such as pneumococcus [41]) and with other general post-operative complications.

Hemodynamically stable patients with AAST grade I, II, or III splenic injuries with no other associated abdominal injuries requiring surgical intervention and who have no comorbidities to preclude close observation are candidates for non-operative management [42]. Given the current state of the interventional radiology (with the possibility of angiographic embolization), AAST grade IV or V splenic injuries in hemodynamically stable patients are not absolute contraindications for non-operative management [42]. Nevertheless, the risk of treatment failure is proportional to the injury scale grade [14]. The 2012 Eastern Association for the Surgery of Trauma (EAST) guidelines for the management of blunt splenic injury suggests non-operative management for the hemodynamically stable patient regardless of injury grade, patient age, or presence of associated injuries [43].

22.6.2 Hepatic Injury

Like the spleen, the liver is susceptible to injury during blunt thoracoabdominal trauma, especially when direct compressive or shear forces are applied to the right lower chest wall or right upper quadrant of the abdomen. Consequently the liver is also one of the most frequently injured abdominal organs in sports [44]. Although most injuries to the liver (like a subcapsular or intraparenchymal hematoma or low-grade lacerations) do not require surgical intervention, management of severe hepatic lesions can be challenging and disastrous because they may involve combined parenchymal, intrahepatic vascular, and biliary system injury.

The athlete with liver injury may present right upper quadrant pain and tenderness, referred pain to the right shoulder. An ecchymosis around the umbilicus (Cullen's sign) may be present, and peritoneal signs may not be present. The assessment of signs of hypovolemia is mandatory, and the hemodynamic status will be the most important prognostic indicator when it comes to decision-making.

In the hemodynamically unstable patient, a FAST (or DPL) during resuscitation is indicated, and if positive, surgical exploration is required to achieve hemostasis and exclude other sources of bleeding.

In the hemodynamically stable patients, abdominal CT scanning is an invaluable diagnostic aid to identify and assess the severity of injury to the liver and allows the surgeon to identify those patients who can be safely managed non-operatively, to assist decision-making in non-operative management, and to act as a baseline for comparison in future imaging studies [32, 42].

Patient with penetrating liver trauma and hemodynamically stable can also be managed non-operatively. Nevertheless, the risk of bile leakage is high, so the follow-up must be made closely.

American Association for the Surgery of Trauma's Liver injury scale [34] is an important tool for decision-making protocols:

American Association for the Surgery of Trauma's (AAST) Liver injury scale [34]

Grade[a]	Injury type	Description of injury
I	Hematoma	Subcapsular <10% surface area
	Laceration	Capsular tear <1 cm parenchymal depth
II	Hematoma	Subcapsular, 10–50% surface area Intraparenchymal, <10 cm in diameter
	Laceration	Capsular tear, 1–3 cm parenchymal depth, <10 cm in length
III	Hematoma	Subcapsular, >50% surface area of ruptured subcapsular or parenchymal hematoma Intraparenchymal hematoma >10 cm or expanding
	Laceration	>3 cm parenchymal depth
IV	Laceration	Parenchymal disruption involving 25–75% hepatic lobe or 1–3 Couinaud segments within a single lobe
V	Laceration	Parenchymal disruption involving >75% of a hepatic lobe or >3 Couinaud segments within a single lobe
	Vascular	Juxtahepatic venous injuries, i.e., retrohepatic vena cava/ central major hepatic veins
VI	Vascular	Hepatic avulsion

[a]Advance one grade for multiple injuries up to grade IV

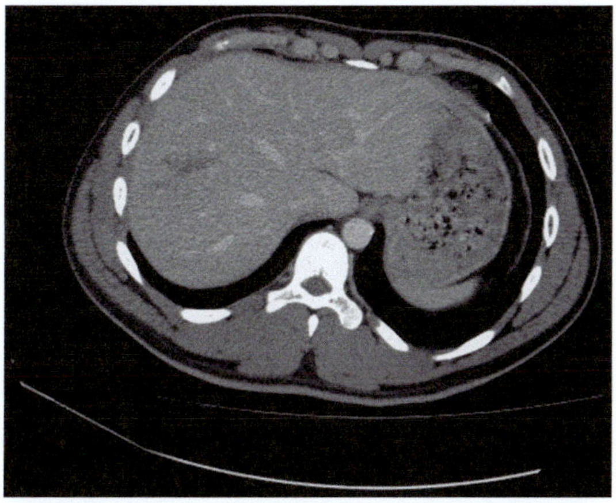

Image 22.5 Hepatic laceration

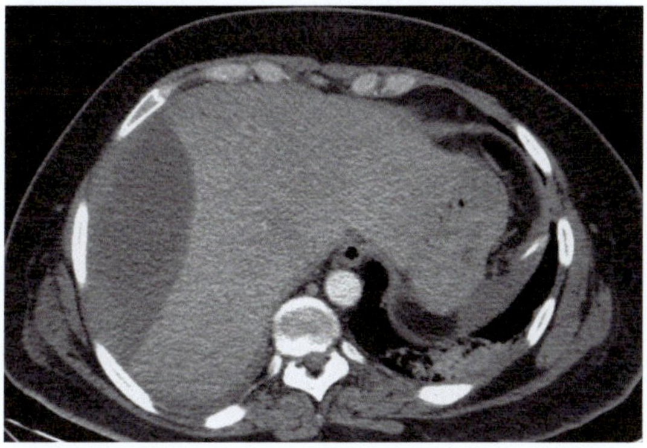

Image 22.6 Subcapsular hepatic hematoma

Management of blunt hepatic injuries has evolved during the past decade to more non-operative management due to the evolution of the critical care units, to the implementation of damage-control hemostatic resuscitation protocols [35–39] as well as to transvascular procedures [40] to stop the parenchymal bleeding. Actually, nearly all children and 50–80% of adults with blunt hepatic injuries can be treated non-operatively, because most liver injuries will stop bleeding spontaneously [12].

Isolated hepatic injuries that are not extensive (grades I–III) are usually managed non-operatively. Extensive parenchymal injuries and those involving the juxtahepatic veins (grades IV and V) may require complex maneuvers for successful treatment. Hepatic avulsion (grade VI) is usually lethal [42].

The 2012 EAST guidelines for the management of blunt hepatic injury are identical to those for blunt splenic injuries with adjunct interventions and include angiography, endoscopic retrograde cholangiopancreatography, endoscopy, and laparoscopy [43].

22.6.3 Renal Injury

The kidney is the most commonly injured genitourinary organ, occurring in 5% of all trauma cases [45]. The sports-related blunt renal injury is often isolated [46] and usually results from a solitary blow to the flank sustained during sports-related activities, such as skiing, contact sports, or biking [47]. Although most sports-related renal injuries are low-grade (AAST grades I–II), isolated blows to the flank sustained during sports-related activities can also produce high-grade renal injury (AAST grades III–V) [47–50].

The athlete with kidney injury may present hematuria (the best indicator of renal injury), flank ecchymosis (Grey Turner's sign), and focal tenderness. The European Association of Urology guidelines recommend imaging in all abdominal trauma patients with the presence of hematuria and shock or with major associated injuries [51]. The investigation of choice in an unstable patient is immediate surgery. Stable blunt abdominal trauma patients with gross hematuria generally need evaluation via a CT scan. However, the absence of hematuria does not preclude significant renal injury [52], and injuries such as renal artery laceration or avulsion may not present hematuria [53].

Contrast CT is the gold standard imaging modality. Also, to allow grading of renal injuries, it provides a proper evaluation of intra-abdominal and retroperitoneal structures, with an excellent sensitivity of detecting concomitant injuries. CT has a negative predictive value of 99.8% [54].

The AAST kidney injury score [55] both aids management and confers a prognostic element [56]. Furthermore, AAST scoring is the most important variable predicting the need for kidney repair or nephrectomy [57].

American Association for the Surgery of Trauma's (AAST) Kidney injury scale [55]		
Grade[a]	Injury type	Description of injury
I	Contusion	Microscopic or gross hematuria
	Hematoma	Subcapsular, non-expanding without parenchymal laceration
II	Hematoma	Non-expanding perirenal hematoma confined to renal retroperitoneum
	Laceration	<1 cm parenchymal depth of renal cortex without urinary extravasation
III	Laceration	>1 cm parenchymal depth of renal cortex without collecting system rupture or urinary extravasation
IV	Laceration	Parenchymal laceration extending through the renal cortex, medulla, collecting system
	Vascular	Main renal artery or vein injury with contained hemorrhage
V	Laceration	Completely shattered kidney
	Vascular	Avulsion of renal hilum which non-vascularized kidney

[a]Advance one grade for multiple or bilateral injuries up to grade III

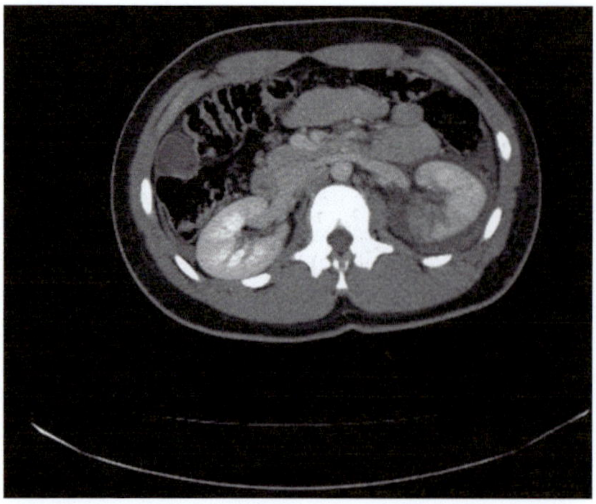

Image 22.7 Renal laceration

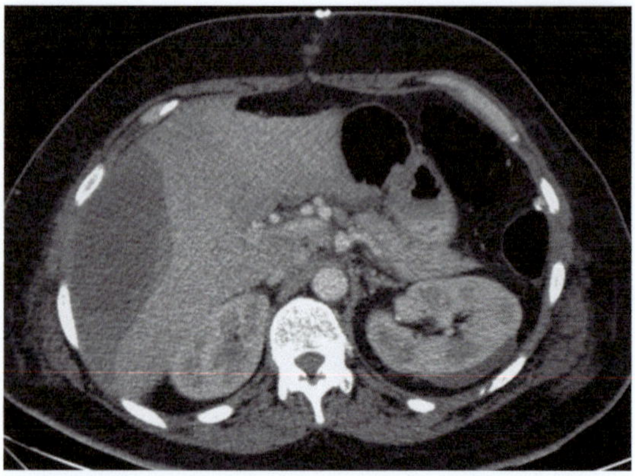

Image 22.8 Subcapsular hepatic hematoma and subcapsular renal hematoma in a splenectomized patient

The management of renal trauma can be divided into conservative, radiological (angioembolization), and surgical. Conservative management has become the preferred strategy in the acute management of renal trauma, consisting in admission with strict bed rest, clinical monitoring and serial examination, hematological and serological monitoring, and imaging assessment "on demand" until resolution of hematuria. Radiological approach (angiography and selective embolization) has been successful (83% success rates) for management of grade IV and V renal injuries with vascular complications [58]. Surgical exploration is reserved for those patients presenting with significant renal trauma with associated hemodynamic instability [59]. Absolute indications for laparotomy are persistent life-threatening hemorrhage, renal pedicle injury, and an expanding or pulsatile retroperitoneal hematoma (indicating a renal artery rupture).

When it comes to follow-up imaging, some authors suggest re-imaging upon resolution of microscopic hematuria, others before discharge, while some repeat CT scans 6–10 weeks after initial injury. The European Association of Urology recommends that long-term follow-up imaging should ultimately be decided on a case-by-case basis (level C evidence) [60].

22.6.4 Pancreatic Injury

Because of the frequently delayed diagnosis and the severity of pancreatic and combined pancreaticoduodenal injuries, the sports-related traumatic pancreatic injury is associated with high morbidity and mortality [61]. Pancreatic injuries usually result from a direct epigastric blow that compresses the organ against the vertebral column and must be suspected in all patients with abdominal injuries, even those who initially have few signs. Because of pancreatic retroperitoneal position, blunt pancreatic trauma can be subtle at presentation and consequently a high level of suspicion integrated with an aggressive imaging study is needed to early identify an injury. Serum amylase levels can be elevated in many abdominal injuries and are neither specific nor sensitive to pancreatic injury. Nevertheless, in a study by Takishima, serum amylase elevated in 84% of patients with pancreatic injury at presentation: elevated in 76% (<3 h postinjury) and 100% (>3 h postinjury) [62]. CT is 85% accurate but does not always help with the grading of the injury, and endoscopic retrograde cholangiopancreatography (ERCP) and magnetic resonance cholangiopancreatography (MRCP) can be helpful in selected stable patients [14].

Management of pancreatic injury is variable, depending on the severity, the site of the injury, and the integrity of the main pancreatic duct. In non-complicated cases, it can be done through a conservative approach associated or not to simple drainage procedures but in complicated cases may be necessary highly challenging surgical procedures.

22.6.5 Return-to-Play Decisions After Blunt Abdominal Trauma

Return-to-play decisions after blunt abdominal trauma should be individualized, and athletes must be fully nutritionally and metabolically recovered before engaging unrestricted activity. There is a lack of consensus on recommendations for resuming full activity after blunt abdominal trauma injuries (concerning to intensity and duration of restricted activity). Whether changing to a noncontact sport or being authorized by a physician for a contact sport, an athletic trainer or sports medicine physician should educate the athlete to engage in a progressive and gradual return to exercise and competition. The athlete must be also taught to monitor for red flags regarding signs and symptoms.

1. Recommendations for resuming unrestricted **activity after splenic injury** vary from 3 weeks to greater than 6 months for severe injury, depending on the injury grade score [44, 63, 64]. Athletes submitted to splenectomy return to play much sooner [44], and sometimes this fact is used as an indication for splenectomy in elite athletes (elective splenectomy for elite athletes in order to achieve a faster return to play should be reserved for exceptional situations). Postsplenectomy vaccination with pneumococcal and meningococcal vaccines is recommended [65].
2. Literature on **return to play after liver injury** is scarce, and recommendations for resuming unrestricted activity after hepatic injury are dependent on the type and severity of the injury. Although healing time for hepatic lacerations is different from subcapsular hematomas [66], it is estimated that healing from a laceration and subcapsular hematoma occurs in 2–4 months, whereas complex injuries require up to 6 months [67]. Although imaging follow-up (US or CT) of athletes with liver injury must be guided by symptoms, some authors recommend return to unrestricted activity only after a normal CT, usually 3–6 months after injury. This strategy may increase unnecessary radiation exposure on the athletes.

According to a review published by Juyia and Kerr in 2014 [44] concerning return to play after liver and spleen trauma:

- Athletes should only engage in a light activity for the first 3 months after traumatic liver or spleen injury and then gradually return to unrestricted activity as tolerated (SORT Evidence Rating C).
- Average healing times documented on CT and ultrasound can be a helpful guide to the length of activity restriction (SORT Evidence Rating C).
- Follow-up imaging is not recommended unless clinically indicated (SORT Evidence Rating C).

3. Decision-making about **return to play after kidney injury** is difficult due to the lack of specific international guidelines and consensus, and therefore the decision must be decided on an individual basis by the athlete and the sports medicine physician.

   Conservatively managed athletes with renal contusions should be observed until hematuria clears and should be excluded from contact sports for 6 weeks. More severe injuries may take 6–8 weeks to heal, and in this case, the athlete may have to wait for 6–12 months before a safe return to contact/collision sports [56, 68].

   The athlete with the solitary kidney appears to have a low risk for kidney loss with participation in both contact and noncontact sports, but it remains a controversial issue that requires patient education and an individualized approach [56].
4. Literature on **return to play after pancreatic injury** is scarce. It depends on the resolution of the disease process and symptoms and must be decided on an individual basis by the athlete and the sports medicine physician.

Take-Home Messages

- Unrecognized abdominal and pelvic injuries continue to be a cause of preventable death.
- We must exclude abdominal trauma when significant kinetic energy is transferred to the torso from a direct blow, deceleration, or penetration injury.
- Blunt trauma is by far more frequent than penetrating trauma.
- The spleen is the most frequently injured abdominal organ in sports and the most common cause of death due to blunt abdominal trauma, followed by the liver and small bowel with less incidence. Retroperitoneal hematomas must also be considered although their presentation is less conspicuous.
- The correlation between trauma mechanism, the abdominal area involved, and the hemodynamic status is mandatory, as it has practical implications in diagnostic and treatment strategies.
- When on the sideline or track, if the patient presents with a hemodynamic abnormality, a meticulous abdominal physical examination is not indicated. You must immediately get an IV access, start fluid resuscitation, and transfer the victim to a medical facility.
- If the athlete victim of abdominal trauma is hemodynamically unstable, *point-of-care* imaging (like FAST—focused assessment with sonography for trauma) or other procedures (like diagnostic peritoneal lavage) directed for the detection of free fluid in the abdominal cavity (blood) are mandatory in the emergency department.
- If the athlete victim of abdominal trauma is hemodynamically stable, we can proceed to more accurate diagnostic procedures (like computed tomography) to define the best definitive treatment.
- Management of blunt abdominal injuries has evolved during the past decade to more nonoperative management.
- Return-to-play decisions after blunt abdominal trauma should be individualized, and athletes must be fully nutritionally and metabolically recovered before engaging unrestricted activity.
- There is a lack of consensus on recommendations for resuming full activity after blunt abdominal trauma injuries (concerning to intensity and duration of restricted activity).
- Sports medicine physician should educate the athlete to engage in a progressive and gradual return to exercise and competition. The athlete must be also taught to monitor for red flags regarding signs and symptoms.

References

1. Johnson R. Abdominal wall injuries: rectus abdominis strains, oblique strains, rectus sheath hematoma. Curr Sports Med Rep. 2006;5:99–103. West JC, Trunkey DD, Lim RC. System of trauma care: a study of two counties. Arch Surg. 1979;114:455–60.
2. West JC, Trunkey DD, Lim RC. System of trauma care: a study of two counties. Arch Surg. 1979;114: 455–60.
3. ATLS Subcommittee, American College of Surgeons' Committee on Trauma, International ATLS Working Group. Advanced trauma and life support—ATLS 9th

ed. J Trauma Acute Care Surg. 2013;74(5):1363–6. https://doi.org/10.1097/TA.0b013e31828b82f5.
4. Thomas SH. Helicopter EMS transport outcomes literature: annotated review of articles published 2004–2006. Prehosp Emerg Care. 2007;11(4):477–88.
5. Sullivent EE, Faul M, Wald MM. Reduced mortality in injured adults transported by helicopter emergency medical services. Prehosp Emerg Care. 2011;15(3):295–302.
6. Haider AH, Chang DC, Haut ER, et al. Mechanism of injury predicts patient mortality and impairment after blunt trauma. J Surg Res. 2009;153:138–42.
7. Nishijima DK, Simel DL, Wisner DH, Holmes JF. Does this adult patient have a blunt intra-abdominal injury? JAMA. 2012;307:1517–27.
8. Mackersie RC, Tiwary AD, Shackford SR, Hoft DB. Intraabdominal injury following blunt trauma. Identifying the high-risk patient using objective risk factors. Arch Surg. 1989;124(7):809–13.
9. Brown CK, Dunn KA, Wilson K. Diagnostic evaluation of patients with blunt abdominal trauma: a decision analysis. Acad Emerg Med. 2000;7:385–96.
10. Isenhour J, Marx J. Abdominal trauma. In: Legome E, Shockley LW, editors. Trauma: a comprehensive emergency medicine approach. Cambridge: Cambridge University Press; 2011. p. 213.
11. American College of Surgeons Committee on Trauma. ATLS: Advanced Trauma Life Support for Doctors. 8th ed. Chicago, IL: American College of Surgeons; 2008.
12. Rifat SF, Gilvydis RP. Blunt abdominal trauma in sports. Curr Sports Med Rep. 2003;2(2):93–7.
13. Blomqvist CG, Saltin B. Cardiovascular adaptations to physical training. Annu Rev Physiol. 1983;45:169–89.
14. Boffard KD. Abdominal trauma. Core topics in general and emergency surgery. Vol. 13. p. 229–67.
15. Shephard RJ. Exercise and the athlete with infectious mononucleosis. Clin J Sport Med. 2017;27(2):168–78.
16. Coccolini F, et al. Pelvic trauma: WSES classification and guidelines. World J Emerg Surg. 2017;12:5.
17. Scalea TM, Rodriguez A, Chiu WC, Brenneman FD, Fallon WF Jr, Kato K, et al. Focused Assessment with Sonography for Trauma (FAST): results from an international consensus conference. J Trauma. 1999;46(3):466–72.
18. Kirkpatrick AW, Sustic A, Blaivas M. Introduction to the use of ultrasound in critical care medicine. Crit Care Med. 2007;35:S123–5.
19. Wherrett LJ, Boulanger BR, McLellan BA, Brenneman FD, Rizoli SB, Culhane J, Hamilton P. Hypotension after blunt abdominal trauma: the role of emergent abdominal sonography in surgical triage. J Trauma. 1996;41(5):815–20.
20. Rozycki GS, Ochsner MG, Schmidt JA, Frankel HL, Davis TP, Wang D, Champion HR. A prospective study of surgeon-performed ultrasound as the primary adjuvant modality for injured patient assessment. J Trauma. 1995;39(3):492–8; discussion 498–500.
21. Hoff WS, Holevar M, Nagy KK, Patterson L, Young JS, Arrillaga A, Najarian MP, Valenziano CP, Eastern Asociation for the Surgery of Trauma. Practice management guidelines for the evaluation of blunt abdominal trauma: the EAST practice management guidelines work group. J Trauma. 2002;53(3):602–15.
22. Stengel D, Bauwens K, Sehouli J, Porzsolt F, Rademacher G, Mutze S, et al. Systematic review and meta-analysis of emergency ultrasonography for blunt abdominal trauma. Br J Surg. 2001;88(7):901–12.
23. Yoshii H, Sato M, Yamamoto S, Motegi M, Okusawa S, Kitano M, et al. Usefulness and limitations of ultrasonography in the initial evaluation of blunt abdominal trauma. J Trauma. 1998;45(1):45–50.
24. Branney SW, Wolfe RE, Moore EE, et al. Quantitative sensitivity of ultrasound in detecting free intraperitoneal fluid. J Trauma. 1995;39:375–80.
25. Peitzman AB, Makaroun MS, Slasky BS, et al. Prospective study of computed tomography in initial management of blunt abdominal trauma. J Trauma. 1986;26:585–92.
26. Webster VJ. Abdominal trauma: pre-operative assessment and postoperative problems in intensive care. Anaesth Intensive Care. 1985;13:258–62.
27. Stengel D, Rademacher G, Ekkernkamp A, Güthoff C, Mutze S. Emergency ultrasound-based algorithms for diagnosing blunt abdominal trauma. Cochrane Database Syst Rev. 2015;(9):CD004446.
28. Livingston DH, Lavery RF, Passannante MR, et al. Admission or observation is not necessary after a negative abdominal computed tomographic scan in patients with suspected blunt abdominal trauma: results of a prospective, multi-institutional trial. J Trauma. 1998;44:272–82.
29. Lang EK. Intra-abdominal and retroperitoneal organ injuries diagnosed on dynamic computed tomograms obtained for assessment of renal trauma. J Trauma. 1990;30:1161–8.
30. Matsubara TK, Fong HM, Burns CM. Computed tomography of abdomen (CTA) in management of blunt abdominal trauma. J Trauma. 1990;30:410–4.
31. Becker J, Smith J. Return to play after infectious mononucleosis. Sports Health. 2014;6(3):232–8. https://doi.org/10.1177/1941738114521984.
32. Herring SA, Kibler WB, Putukian M. The team physician and the return-to-play decision: a consensus statement-2012 update. Med Sci Sports Exerc. 2012;44(12):2446–8.
33. Walter KD. Radiographic evaluation of the patient with sport-related abdominal trauma. Curr Sports Med Rep. 2007;6:115–9.
34. Moore EE, Cogbill TH, Jurkovich GJ, et al. Organ Injury Scaling: spleen and liver (1994 revision). J Trauma. 1995;38(3):323–4.
35. Cirocchi R, Montedori A, Farinella E, Bonacini I, Tagliabue L, Abraha I. Damage control surgery for abdominal trauma. Cochrane Database Syst Rev. 2013;(3):CD007438. https://doi.org/10.1002/14651858.CD007438.pub3.
36. Curry N, Hopewell S, Dorée C, Hyde C, Brohi K, Stanworth S. The acutemanagement of trauma hemor-

rhage: a systematic review of randomized controlled trials. Crit Care. 2011;15(2):R92.
37. Gruen RL, Brohi K, Schreiber M, Balogh ZJ, Pitt V, Narayan M, et al. Haemorrhage control in severely injured patients. Lancet. 2012;380(9847):1099–108.
38. Ker K, Kiriya J, Perel P, Edwards P, Shakur H, Roberts I. Avoidable mortality from giving tranexamic acid to bleeding trauma patients: an estimation based on WHO mortality data, a systematic literature review and data from the CRASH-2 trial. BMC Emerg Med. 2012;12(3):3.
39. Maegele M, Spinella PC, Schöchl H. The acute coagulopathy of trauma: mechanisms and tools for risk stratification. Shock. 2012;38(5):450–8.
40. Vam der Vlies CH, van Delden OM, Punt BJ, Ponsen KJ, Reekers JA, Goslings JC. Literature review of the role of ultrasound, computed tomography, and transcatheter arterial embolization for the treatment of traumatic splenic injuries. Cardiovasc Intervent Radiol. 2010;33(6):1079–87.
41. Peitzman AB, Ford HR, Harbrecht BG, et al. Injury to the spleen. Curr Prob Surg. 2001;38:921–1008.
42. Alonso M, Brathwaite C, Garcia V, et al. Practice Management Guidelines Work Group. Blunt liver and spleen injuries: non-operative management. http://www.east.org/tpg/livspleen.
43. Stassen NA, Bhullar I, Cheng JD, et al. Eastern Association for the Surgery of Trauma. Selective nonoperative management of blunt splenic injury: an Eastern Association for the Surgery of Trauma practice management guideline. J Trauma Acute Care Surg. 2012;73(Suppl 4):S294–300.
44. Juyia RF, Kerr HA. Return to play after liver and spleen trauma. Sports Health. 2014;6(3):239–45. https://doi.org/10.1177/1941738114528468.
45. Santucci RA, Wessells H, Bartsch G, Descotes J, Heyns CF, McAninch JW, Nash P, Schmidlin F. Evaluation and management of renal injuries: consensus statement of the renal trauma subcommittee. BJU Int. 2004;93:937–54.
46. Patel DP, et al. High-grade renal injuries are often isolated in sports-related trauma. Injury. 2015;46(7):1245–9.
47. Lloyd GL, Slack S, McWilliams KL, Black A, Nicholson TM. Renal trauma from recreational accidents manifests different injury patterns than urban renal trauma. J Urol. 2012;188:163–8. [PubMed: 22591969].
48. Fanning DM, Forde JC, Mohan P. A simple football injury leading to a grade 4 renal trauma. BMJ Case Rep. 2012;2012. pii: bcr1020114959 https://doi.org/10.1136/bcr.10.2011.4959.
49. Bjurlin MA, Zhao LC, Goble SM, Hollowell CM. Bicycle-related genitourinary injuries. Urology. 2011;78:1187–90. [PubMed: 21945282].
50. Brophy RH, Gamradt SC, Barnes RP, Powell JW, DelPizzo JJ, Rodeo SA, et al. Kidney injuries in professional American football: implications for management of an athlete with 1 functioning kidney. Am J Sports Med. 2008;36:85–90. [PubMed: 17986635].
51. Djakovic N, Plas E, Martinez-Pineiro L, Lynch T, Mor Y, Santucci RA, Serafetinidis E, Turkeri LN, Hohenfellner M. Guidelines on urological trauma. European Association of Urology; 2008.
52. Alsono RC, Nacenta SB, Martinez PD, Guerrero AS, Fuentes CG. Kidney in danger: CT findings of blunt and penetrating trauma. Radiographics. 2009;29:2033–53.
53. McAndrew JD, Corriere JN Jr. Radiographic evaluation of renal trauma: evaluation of 1103 consecutive patients. Br J Urol. 1994;73:352–4.
54. Bent C, Iyngkaran T, Power N, Matson M, Hajdinjak T, Buchholz N, Fotheringham T. Urological injuries following trauma. Clin Radiol. 2008;63:1361–71.
55. Moore EE, Shackford SR, Pachter HL, et al. Organ injury scaling: spleen, liver and kidney. J Trauma. 1989;29:1664–6.
56. Bernard JJ. Renal trauma: evaluation, management and return to play. Curr Sports Med Rep. 2009;8:98–103.
57. Santucci RA, Fisher MB. The literature increasingly supports expectant (conservative) management of renal trauma—a systematic review. J Trauma. 2005;59:491–503.
58. Hom J. The risk of intra abdominal injuries in pediatric patients with stable blunt abdominal trauma and negative abdominal computed tomography. Acad Emerg Med. 2010;17:469–75.
59. Hotaling JM, Sorensen MD, Smith TG 3rd, Rivara FP, Wessells H, Voelzke BB. Analysis of diagnostic angiography and angioembolisation in the acute management of renal trauma using a national data set. J Urol. 2011;185:1316–20.
60. Summerton DJ, Djakovic N, Kitrey ND, Kuehhas F, Lumen N, Serafetinidis E. Guidelines on urological trauma. European Association of Urology; 2013.
61. Echlin PS, Klein WB. Pancreatic injury in the athlete. Curr Sports Med Rep. 2005;4(2):96–101.
62. Takishima T. Serum amylase level on admission in the diagnosis of blunt injury to the pancreas. Ann Surg. 1997;226:70–6.
63. Fata P, Robinson L, Fakhry SM. A survey of EAST member practices in blunt splenic injury: a description of current trends and opportunities for improvement. J Trauma. 2005;59:836–42.
64. Gandhi RR, Keller MS, Schwab CW, Stafford PW. Pediatric splenic injury: pathway to play? J Pediatr Surg. 1999;34:55–9.
65. Di Sabatino A, Carsetti R, Corazza GR. Post-splenectomy and hyposplenic states. Lancet. 2011;378:86–97.
66. Tiberio GA, Portolani N, Coniglio A, et al. Evaluation of the healing time of nonoperatively managed liver injuries. Hepatogastroenterology. 2008;55:1010–2.
67. Karp MP, Cooney DR, Pros GA, et al. The nonoperative management of pediatric hepatic trauma. J Pediatr Surg. 1983;18:512–8.
68. Holmes FC, Hunt JJ, Sevier TL. Renal injury in sport. Curr Sports Med Rep. 2003;2:103–9.

23 Shoulder: The Thrower's Shoulder

Lukas N. Muench, Andreas B. Imhoff, and Sebastian Siebenlist

23.1 Introduction

Due to the specific motion pattern, overhead and throwing sports (e.g. javelin throwing, baseball, tennis or volleyball) result in high stress to the athlete's shoulder. Besides acute injuries (e.g. fractures or dislocation injuries), these sports show a higher incidence of long-term overload damage of the shoulder joint. Asymptomatic junior overhead athletes already present structural and biomechanical changes [1, 2].

In a long-term process, degenerative damage of the shoulder joint may occur with permanently limited functionality [3]. To avoid a progression with further structural damage and to restore the function of the shoulder joint at the same time, a complete evaluation of the relevant pathological factors is necessary. Moreover, the understanding of the underlying pathology is essential to initiate a differentiated therapy.

23.2 Evolution of the Human Throwing Movement

The knowledge of the changes during the Homo sapiens' evolution is the base to understand the underlying pathologies. When bipedalism freed the arms enabling the upper extremity for complex and specific motion sequences, the humans' unique throwing abilities were made possible. The position of the scapula varied to a more caudal and dorsal position resulting in a higher range of motion. Secondary, the glenoid level changed from a rather cranial to a more lateral orientation. In addition, the human's trunk flexibility allowed more torso rotation. Decreased humeral torsion increased the external rotation of the shoulder joint. These anatomical features make it possible to store and release more elastic energy at the shoulder. Thus, the Homo sapiens is able to throw projectiles with high speed and great accuracy [4].

However, biomechanical studies show that this unique throwing ability inevitably requires extreme abduction and external rotation of the glenohumeral joint, which may result in permanent overloading of the capsular and musculotendinous structures [5, 6].

L. N. Muench · A. B. Imhoff (✉) · S. Siebenlist
Department of Orthopaedic Sports Medicine,
Technical University of Munich, Munich, Germany
e-mail: lukasnawid.muench@mri.tum.de;
imhoff@tum.de; sebastian.siebenlist@tum.de

S. Rocha Piedade et al. (eds.), *The Sports Medicine Physician*,
https://doi.org/10.1007/978-3-030-10433-7_23

23.3 Biomechanics of the Human Throwing Movement

An effective throwing technique is based on the successive use of kinetic energy and is divided into six phases. The whole throwing motion usually takes less than 2 s to occur. The first three phases consist of wind-up, early cocking and late cocking. In the wind-up phase, there is a torsion of the whole body from the lower extremity up to the shoulders. In the early-cocking phase, the athlete begins to externally rotate the upper extremity with maximum external rotation of 165 ± 11° in the late-cocking phase. This generates maximum preload and storage of kinetic energy. The acceleration phase transfers the kinetic energy to the projectile followed by the final two phases of deceleration and follow-through [7, 8].

During the throwing motion, high peak loads are caused. The great angular velocity of the shoulder joint of up to 7000°/s and the transfer of kinetic energy during deceleration and follow-through generate an extreme joint distraction [9, 10]. Thus, a repetitive distention of the anterior joint capsule (increased external rotation in 90° abduction) and a simultaneous shortening of the dorsal capsular structures (decreased internal rotation in 90° abduction) occur [7].

The unequal distribution of training loads also leads to an imbalance of the muscular force couples. This presents itself especially in the relative strength of external and internal rotating muscles of the rotator cuff. Besides, the unilateral loading causes a dysfunctional coordination of the scapulothoracic muscles (M. rhomboidei, M. trapezius and M. serratus anterior), which may interrupt the kinetic chain between the scapula and trunk (scapula dyskinesia) [11].

23.4 Pathology of the Thrower's Shoulder

Several theories exist for the development of the complex pathology of a thrower's shoulder. Even if there is an enormous variance regarding the theoretical models, they can be generally combined to basic principles. Shortening of the dorsal capsular structures results in a decreased internal rotation in high abduction and appears already in early stages as a glenohumeral internal rotation deficit (GIRD). In addition, unequal distribution of training loads leads to weakening of the external rotating muscles of the rotator cuff [12].

Repetitive distention of the anterior capsule with simultaneous shortening of the dorsal capsular structures leads to a decentralization and posterosuperior translation of the humeral head in positions of external rotation and abduction. This probably results in an internal "impingement" in the area of the posterosuperior glenoid (PSI) with contact of the articular-sided insertion of the supraspinatus and infraspinatus tendon and the posterosuperior glenoid rim. Finally, this cascade leads to partial or complete ruptures of the rotator cuff. In combination with labral or pulley lesions or detachment of the long biceps tendon anchor (SLAP), the thrower's shoulder may have a poor prognosis [7, 12, 13].

23.5 The Keys for a Successful Treatment

The mentioned theoretical models are useful to understand the underlying pathology but are only of limited use in clinical practice. For this reason, it is helpful to classify the complex of problems of the athlete's shoulder into five underlying structures with a simple approach for a clinical evaluation. In addition to the clinical examination, X-rays of the shoulder and MR arthrography are useful. Moreover, specific examination using the ABER position (abduction external rotation) proved to be of value and allows to interpret the diagnostic findings more precisely.

Based on clinical examination and imaging, *the five-point check for the athlete's shoulder* was developed by our team including the joint capsule, scapula, joint stability, rotator cuff and biceps tendon complex [14].

23.5.1 Joint Capsule

Compared to the contralateral side, the mobility of the affected shoulder has to be examined with special regard to a glenohumeral internal rotation

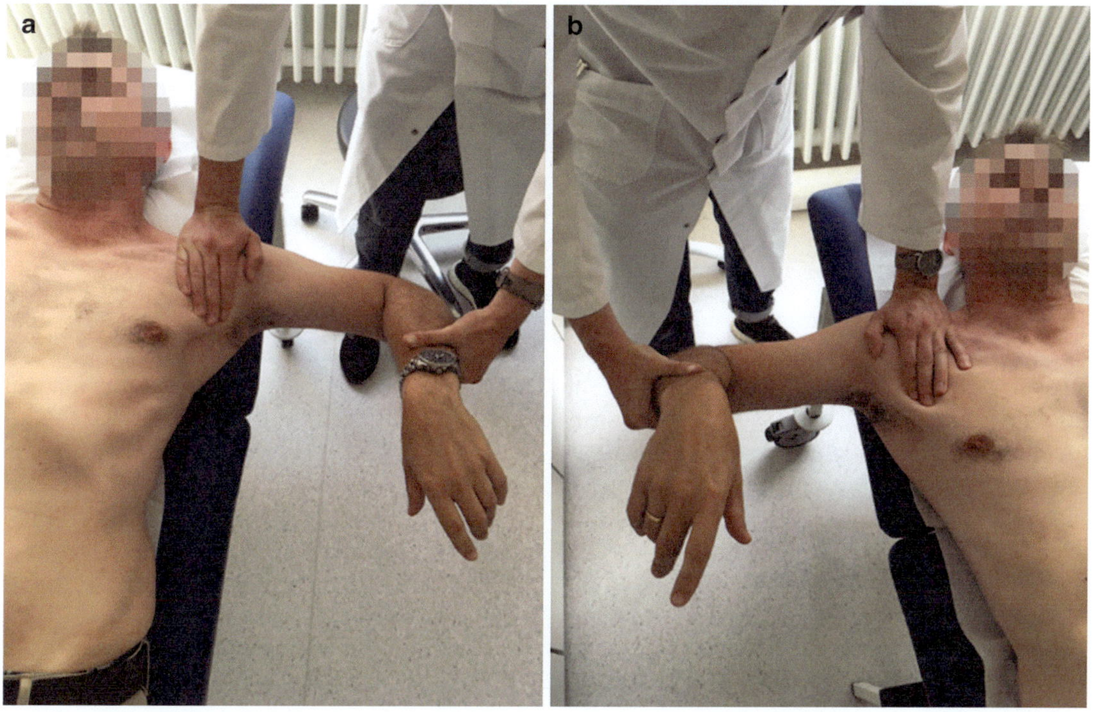

Fig. 23.1 Patient with GIRD. (**a**) The unaffected left shoulder; (**b**) GIRD of the right shoulder

deficit (GIRD). Burkhart et al. [11] defined the "shoulder at risk" as a shoulder with a decreased ability of internal rotation of 20° compared to the unaffected side. Essential for the evaluation is not the ability of internal rotation all alone but the total arc of rotation in 90° abduction and fixed scapula (Fig. 23.1).

In throwing athletes, the range of motion of the shoulder is shifted into external rotation. A deviation in rotational ability of more than 20° of the 180° arc of motion in this position is pathological. Moreover, some studies show that an increased humeral retrotorsion represents itself as a risk factor for the development of a glenohumeral internal rotation deficit [15].

For clinical evaluation, it is very important to examine the patient in supine position with 90° abduction and fixed scapula to avoid a compensatory scapula movement.

23.5.2 Scapula

Optimal glenoid position and transfer of kinetic energy require a precise and stable scapula alignment. During torsion of the torso, the scapula has to be moved dorsally in the axis between both shoulders. In case of a scapular dyskinesia (e.g. due to pathological scapula protraction), the development of a symptomatic posterosuperior impingement (PSI) is more likely [16]. During clinical examination, a possible contraction of the pectoralis minor muscle (leading to scapula protraction) has to be identified. Additionally, the amplitude of scapula movement as well as the scapulothoracic rhythm is examined while standing behind the patient with the patient repetitively raising both arms. The scapula assistance test (SAT) is also helpful to determine scapula dyskinesis.

23.5.3 Stability

In this context, stability of the capsular structures of the glenohumeral joint is of crucial relevance. Signs of instability as defined by a positive apprehension or relocation test and signs of hyperlaxity (sulcus sign, Gagey's test) have to be evaluated. Supplemental MRI scans detect labral lesions, an extended joint capsule or signs of a prior luxation (Hill-Sachs lesion). At the same time, core stability is an important factor. One-legged squads or jumping tests are useful to obtain principal orientation.

23.5.4 Rotator Cuff

Due to the contact of the articular-sided supraspinatus and infraspinatus tendon with the posterosuperior glenoid rim, the PSI leads to the development of cystic lesions at the footprint area. High-grade articular-sided partial tears of the rotator cuff result in a muscular imbalance of the force couples. Therefore, an exact clinical examination including common rotator cuff tests and provocation tests as the "thrower test" (pain in the posterosuperior area of the glenohumeral joint during high abduction and external rotation against resistance in throwing direction) is important (Fig. 23.2). In addition, MRI diagnostics may reveal articular-sided partial lesions (PASTA lesion) or complete ruptures of the rotator cuff. Moreover, the ABER position allows the identification of a pathological contact with the posterosuperior labrum.

23.5.5 Biceps Tendon Complex

Using specific tests for the biceps tendon complex (e.g. O'Brien test, Yergason test, Speed test, crank test), clinical examination focuses on pulley lesions, tendinitis of the long biceps tendon and detachment of the biceps tendon anchor (SLAP lesion) (Fig. 23.3). Especially, the O'Brien test is essential to rule out biceps tendon anchor pathology. Pulley lesions present pressure pain in the rotator interval and increasing pain during external rotation of the arm. For verification of SLAP lesions, the MR arthrography has a high diagnostic performance but is limited in the classification of different types of SLAP lesions [17]. Positioning the arm in abduction and external rotation (ABER) during MR arthrography is use-

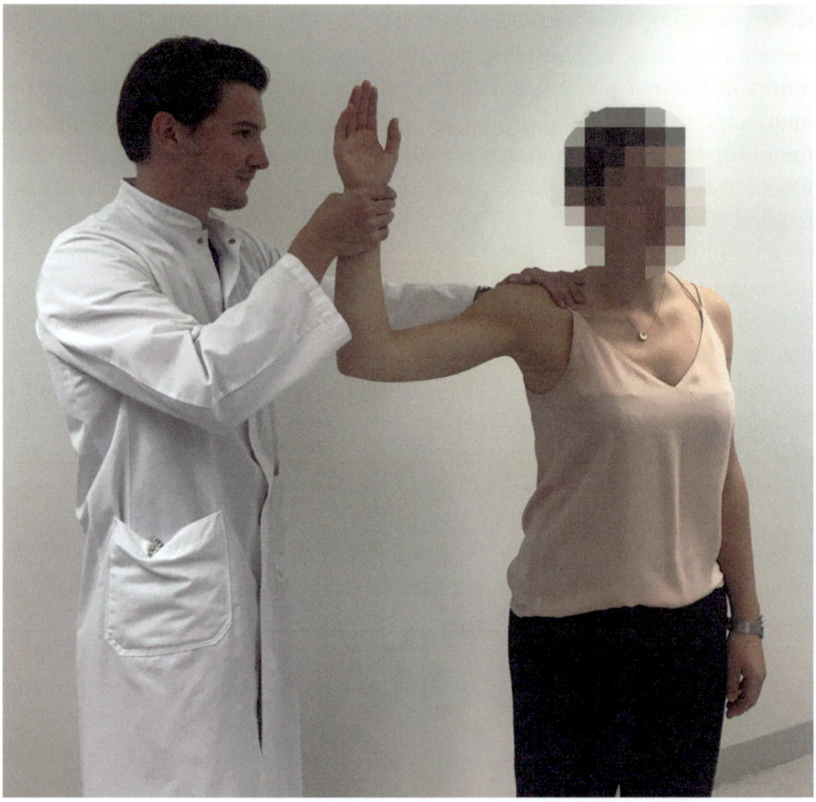

Fig. 23.2 Thrower test

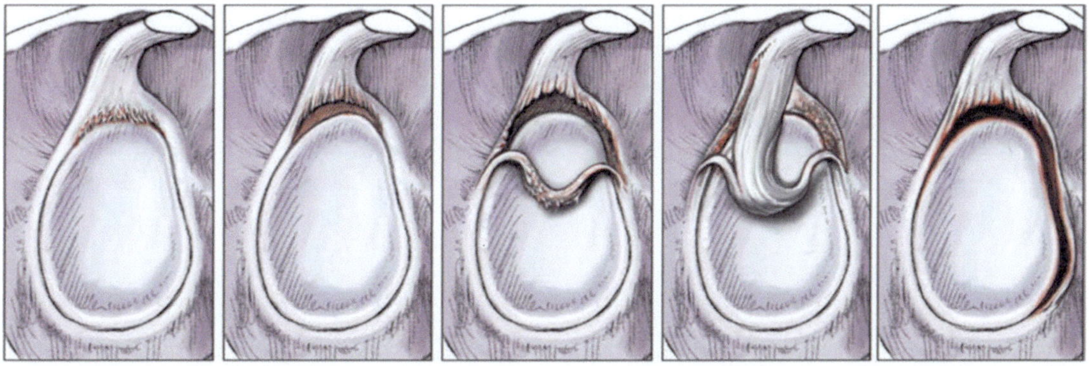

Fig. 23.3 Classification of SLAP lesions (type I–V). A. B. Imhoff, M. J. Feucht Atlas sportorthopädisch-sporttraumatologische Operationen. 2. Auflage; Springer. Kapitel 4: Instabilität; p. 104

ful to detect and characterize labroligamentous lesions as well as partial tears of the rotator cuff undersurface [18, 19].

Initially, Snyder et al. identified four different types of SLAP lesions [20] (Fig. 23.3). Type I presents fraying and degenerative appearance of the superior labrum with an intact attachment of the biceps tendon to the labrum. SLAP-II lesions show a detachment of the superior labrum and biceps tendon from the supraglenoid tubercle. Type III displays an into the joint displaceable bucket-handle tear of the superior labrum with an intact biceps tendon anchor. Type IV is a bucket-handle tear where the tear extends into the biceps tendon. Maffet et al. added three further subclasses of SLAP lesions, including type V, which is described as an anterior-inferior Bankart lesion continuing superiorly to the biceps tendon [21]. Currently, ten different types of SLAP lesions have been described in the literature [22].

23.6 Therapy

23.6.1 Conservative Treatment

The primary therapeutic approach is nonoperative, addressing the identified functional deficits. Initially, eccentric and concentric rotational strength of the shoulder, neuromuscular control, and functional capacity have to be analysed. Besides, an evaluation of the mobility of cervical and thoracic spine as well as mobility, stability, and strength of the trunk and lower extremity is necessary [23]. The athlete has to pass a graded rehabilitation programme to achieve full functional restoration. Based on the individual athlete's performance level, the complete kinetic chain, joint mobility, strength and endurance as well as neuromuscular control are trained with varying intensity [24]. The rehabilitation goes along with a clinical reasoning process and includes sport-specific requirements and evidence-based recommendations [25].

A GIRD is addressed by stretching the posterior capsular structures with the "cross-body stretch" or the "sleeper stretch" [26]. The "corner stretch" is used for relaxation of the pectoralis minor muscle. These stretching exercises decrease the athlete's pain and reduce the GIRD [27]. At first, neuromuscular control of the rotator cuff is trained concomitantly, followed by a specific strengthening of the rotator cuff muscles. Concomitant affection of the biceps tendon requires a dosed and adapted increase of load bearing. Therefore, flexion of the shoulder in supine position should be initially avoided, followed by eccentric and plyometric exercises according to the required sport-specific profile [28].

The treatment of scapular dyskinesia is essential for the shoulder function and is based on a progressive rehabilitation algorithm [29]. Training has to be focused on the restoration of flexibility of the periscapular muscles (pectoralis

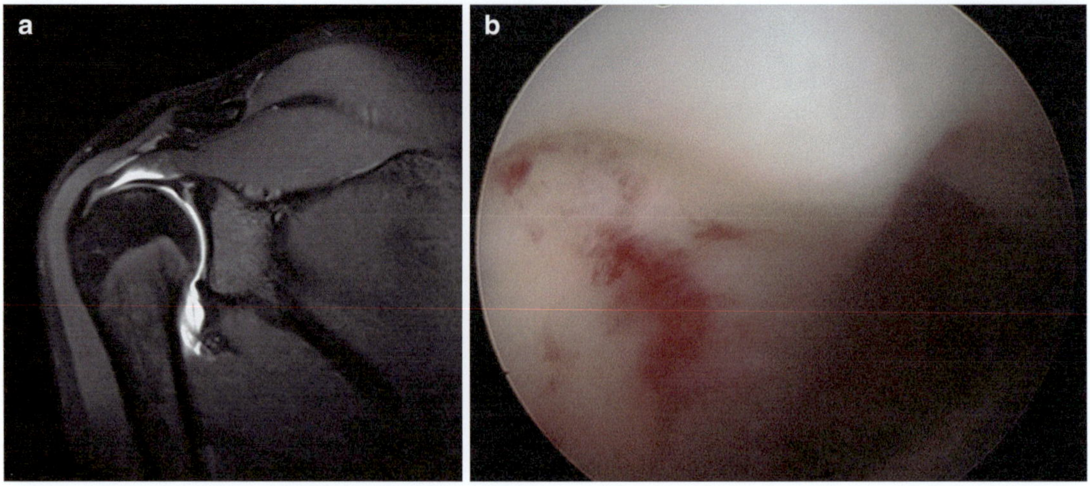

Fig. 23.4 SLAP-II lesion. (**a**) MRI scan; (**b**) arthroscopic view

minor, levator scapulae and rhomboidei muscles) and elimination of scapulothoracic muscular imbalances. In this context, the centralization of the humeral head deserves special consideration. Dynamic stabilization is trained by multidimensional concentric-eccentric and plyometric motion requests to avoid an excessive cranial migration of the joint centre [24].

Moreover, endurance of periscapular and rotator cuff muscles is part of the rehabilitation programme. During fatigue conditions, glenohumeral and scapulothoracic control is maintained and thus stabilizes the glenoid position and centralization of the humeral head. In addition, strength, stability and neuromuscular control of the trunk and lower extremity are essential for an optimal throwing technique and therefore should be improved [30].

Following a multistage model, the decision to return to play or not is made. According to this model, health status, participation risk, and decision modifiers are considered [31].

23.6.2 Surgical Treatment

Overhead athletes often present pathologies of the biceps tendon anchor (SLAP lesions) without any responsiveness to physiotherapeutic treatment. According to the existing type of lesion, different arthroscopic surgical approaches are evident. In case of a SLAP-II lesion, method of choice is the refixation of the SLAP complex to the superior glenoid rim using suture anchors (Fig. 23.4). In type III lesions, the displaced bucket-handle tear is resected. If the tear of the biceps tendon anchor is located in the vascularized area next to the bone at the supraglenoid tubercle, a refixation of the SLAP complex with suture anchors can be considered. In general, type IV lesions require biceps tenodesis. In SLAP-V lesions, an arthroscopic refixation of the SLAP complex together with the anterior capsule-labrum complex is mandatory. If there is a concomitant pulley lesion with a resulting instability of the biceps tendon, a biceps tenodesis is needed. In case of SLAP-III, SLAP-IV and SLAP-V lesions, a biceps tenodesis always should be considered because of inconsistent clinical results after SLAP repair described in the literature [32–35].

Over the past 10 years, the total number of biceps tenodeses has increased, whereas the number and relative percentage of SLAP repairs have decreased. Especially in overhead athletes and patients over 35 years of age, a biceps tenodesis should be preferred. Chalmers et al. found that pitchers who underwent a SLAP repair had altered patterns of thoracic rotation compared to the controls and pitchers who had undergone a biceps tenodesis [34]. Laughlin et al. found deficiencies in pitching biomechanics in collegiate and professional pitchers who underwent SLAP repair [36]. Even in SLAP-II lesions, only 50% of the overhead athletes return to pre-injury level of play [37]. Therefore, biceps tenodesis is a reliable option compared to SLAP repair [35].

After cutting the long head of the biceps tendon at its attachment, there is the possibility to perform either an intraarticular or subpectoral tenodesis. The intraarticular tenodesis is carried out entirely arthroscopically with tendon fixation right at the entry point to the sulcus bicipitalis. The disadvantage of this procedure may be sulcus bicipitalis-related pain due to remaining pain receptors. In case of a subpectoral tenodesis, the tendon is fixed at the distal part of the sulcus bicipitalis, 2 cm proximal to the caudal margin of the pectoralis major muscle. Therefore, an additional incision of 1.5–3 cm length is necessary [38, 39].

Author's preferred procedure represents the subpectoral tenodesis using all-suture soft anchors via a limited minimally invasive approach as shown in Fig. 23.5 [38, 40].

Nevertheless, overhead athletes often suffer from articular-sided partial lesions of the supraspinatus tendon. If an appropriate and complete rehabilitation has failed, indication for surgical approach is given. The size of the tear is essential for the kind of operative treatment. If over 50% of the supraspinatus tendon is ruptured, authors favour the completion of the rupture and refixation to the original footprint. In contrast to the transtendinous technique, the completion of the rupture minimizes the risk of a too medial refixation of the articular-sided tendon tissue. Especially in overhead athletes, this should be avoided because of the required range of motion. In case of lesions of under 50% of tendon thickness, a debridement is recommended [41].

Concerning return-to-play rates, the results of surgical treatment of partial-thickness rotator cuff tears are poor. In professional throwers, debridement shows inconsistent return-to-play rates from 16 to 76% [42]. Regarding the repair of articular-sided partial-thickness rotator cuff tears, the two techniques show no significant difference. Of the patients treated with the transtendinous technique, 75% returned to the same level of sport, compared to 67% of the patients who underwent a full-thickness conversion and repair [43]. Two recent reviews show an overall rate of return to sport of 79–84.7%, including 60.5–65.9% at an equivalent level of play. Nevertheless, only 49.9–54.5% of the professional athletes reached their pre-injury level [44, 45]. There is only a slight difference in the return-to-sport rate between debridement (53.7%) and repair (47.5%) [45]. The mean time for returning to sport following surgery was 8.3 months [45].

Fact Box 1: Pathology of the Thrower's Shoulder

- Shortening of the dorsal capsular structures results in GIRD.
- Repetitive distention of the anterior capsule.
- Decentralization and posterosuperior translation of the humeral head leads to PSI.
- Finally, lesions of the rotator cuff, biceps anchor complex and pulley system.

Fact Box 2: Therapy Essentials

- Graded rehabilitation programme to achieve full functional restoration.
- Training of complete kinetic chain, joint mobility, strength, endurance and neuromuscular control.
- Addressing GIRD and scapula dyskinesia by stretching and strengthening of periscapular muscles.
- Surgical treatment of SLAP lesions with SLAP repair or subpectoral biceps tenodesis.

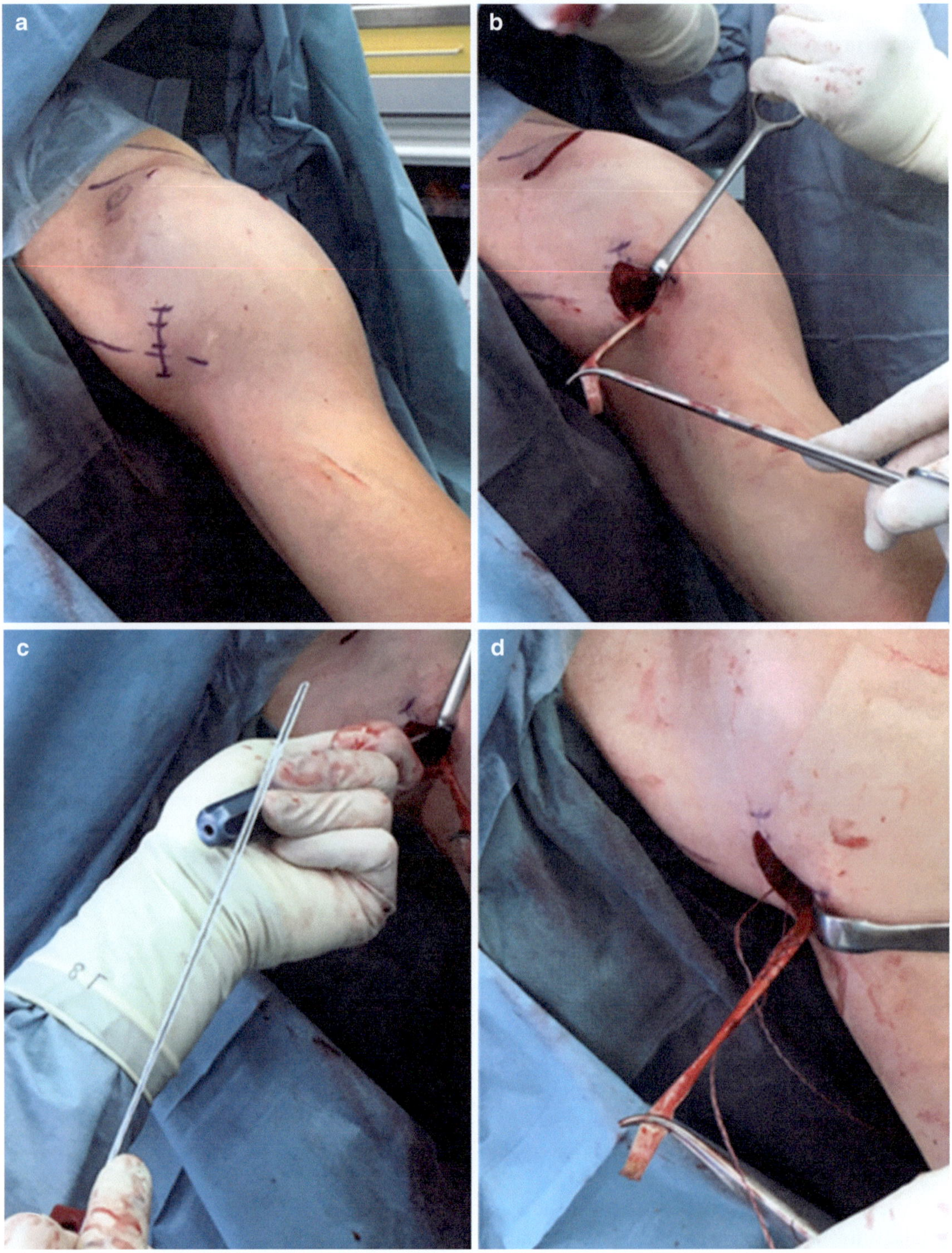

Fig. 23.5 Subpectoral biceps tenodesis. (**a**) Marking of the caudal margin of the pectoralis major muscle and 1.5–3 cm-long incision in the course of the axillary fold. (**b**) Identification of the myotendinous junction after pulling out the long-head biceps tendon. (**c**) Insertion of the all-suture soft anchor over the target device. (**d**) Stitching of the tendon at the myotendinous junction. Subsequently, tendon shortening and pulling in using the free suture limb

Take-Home Messages

- Due to the specific motion pattern, overhead and throwing sports result in high stress to the athlete's shoulder and therefore show a higher incidence of long-term overload damage.
- Understanding the pathology of the thrower's shoulder, several aspects have to be considered. Shortening of the dorsal capsular structures results in a GIRD. In combination with a repetitive distention of the anterior capsule, this leads to a decentralization and posterosuperior translation of the humeral head. Due to the contact of the articular-sided insertion of the supraspinatus and infraspinatus tendon and the posterosuperior glenoid rim, a PSI develops. Finally, rotator cuff tears as well as lesions of the biceps anchor complex and pulley system occur.
- Based on clinical examination and imaging, *the five-point check for the athlete's shoulder* was developed including the joint capsule, scapula, joint stability, rotator cuff and biceps tendon complex.
- Conservative therapy is based on a graded rehabilitation programme, including training of the complete kinetic chain, joint mobility, strength, endurance and neuromuscular control. A GIRD should be addressed by stretching, whereas a scapula dyskinesia requires intensive strengthening of the periscapular muscles.
- Surgical treatment includes SLAP repair, subpectoral biceps tenodesis or refixation of rotator cuff tears to the original footprint.

References

1. Beitzel K, Beitzel KI, Zandt JF, Buchmann S, Schwirtz A, Imhoff AB, Reiser M, Brucker PU. Premature cystic lesions in shoulders of elite junior javelin and volleyball athletes: a comparative evaluation using 3.0 Tesla MRI. J Shoulder Elbow Surg. 2013;22(6):792–9.
2. Beitzel K, Zandt JF, Buchmann S, Beitzel KI, Schwirtz A, Imhoff AB, Brucker PU. Structural and biomechanical changes in shoulders of junior javelin throwers: a comprehensive evaluation as a proof of concept for a preventive exercise protocol. Knee Surg Sports Traumatol Arthrosc. 2016;24(6):1931–42.
3. Schmitt H, Hansmann HJ, Brocai DR, Loew M. Long term changes of the throwing arm of former elite javelin throwers. Int J Sports Med. 2001;22(4):275–9.
4. Roach NT, Venkadesan M, Rainbow MJ, Lieberman DE. Elastic energy storage in the shoulder and the evolution of high-speed throwing in Homo. Nature. 2013;498(7455):483–6.
5. Burkhart SS, Morgan CD, Kibler WB. The disabled throwing shoulder: spectrum of pathology. Part II: evaluation and treatment of SLAP lesions in throwers. Arthroscopy. 2003;19(5):531–9.
6. Wilk KE, Meister K, Andrews JR. Current concepts in the rehabilitation of the overhead throwing athlete. Am J Sports Med. 2002;30(1):136–51.
7. Braun S, Kokmeyer D, Millett PJ. Shoulder injuries in the throwing athlete. J Bone Joint Surg Am. 2009;91(4):966–78.
8. Fleisig GS, Andrews JR, Dillman CJ, Escamilla RF. Kinetics of baseball pitching with implications about injury mechanisms. Am J Sports Med. 1995;23(2):233–9.
9. Fleisig GS, Barrentine SW, Escamilla RF, Andrews JR. Biomechanics of overhand throwing with implications for injuries. Sports Med. 1996;21(6):421–37.
10. Leonard J, Hutchinson MR. Shoulder injuries in skeletally immature throwers: review and current thoughts. Br J Sports Med. 2010;44(5):306–10.
11. Burkhart SS, Morgan CD, Kibler WB. The disabled throwing shoulder: spectrum of pathology Part III: the SICK scapula, scapular dyskinesis, the kinetic chain, and rehabilitation. Arthroscopy. 2003;19(6):641–61.
12. Burkhart SS, Morgan CD, Kibler WB. The disabled throwing shoulder: spectrum of pathology Part I: pathoanatomy and biomechanics. Arthroscopy. 2003;19(4):404–20.
13. Walch G, Boileau P, Noel E, Donell ST. Impingement of the deep surface of the supraspinatus tendon on the posterosuperior glenoid rim: an arthroscopic study. J Shoulder Elbow Surg. 1992;1(5):238–45.
14. Beitzel K, Reuter S, Imhoff A, Braun S. Die Sportlerschulter: Der 5-Punkte-Check zum Therapieerfolg. Dtsch Z Sportmed. 2016;67:103–10.
15. Noonan TJ, Shanley E, Bailey LB, Wyland DJ, Kissenberth MJ, Hawkins RJ, Thigpen CA. Professional pitchers with glenohumeral internal rotation deficit (GIRD) display greater humeral retrotorsion than pitchers without GIRD. Am J Sports Med. 2015;43(6):1448–54.
16. Laudner KG, Myers JB, Pasquale MR, Bradley JP, Lephart SM. Scapular dysfunction in throwers with pathologic internal impingement. J Orthop Sports Phys Ther. 2006;36(7):485–94.
17. Waldt S, Burkart A, Lange P, Imhoff AB, Rummeny EJ, Woertler K. Diagnostic performance of MR arthrography in the assessment of superior labral anteroposterior lesions of the shoulder. AJR Am J Roentgenol. 2004;182(5):1271–8.
18. Tirman PF, Bost FW, Steinbach LS, Mall JC, Peterfy CG, Sampson TG, Sheehan WE, Forbes JR, Genant HK. MR arthrographic depiction of tears of the rotator

cuff: benefit of abduction and external rotation of the arm. Radiology. 1994;192(3):851–6.
19. Tian CY, Cui GQ, Zheng ZZ, Ren AH. The added value of ABER position for the detection and classification of anteroinferior labroligamentous lesions in MR arthrography of the shoulder. Eur J Radiol. 2013;82(4):651–7.
20. Snyder SJ, Karzel RP, Del Pizzo W, Ferkel RD, Friedman MJ. SLAP lesions of the shoulder. Arthroscopy. 1990;6(4):274–9.
21. Maffet MW, Gartsman GM, Moseley B. Superior labrum-biceps tendon complex lesions of the shoulder. Am J Sports Med. 1995;23(1):93–8.
22. Powell SE, Nord KD, Ryu RKN. The diagnosis, classification and treatment of SLAP lesions. Oper Tech Sports Med. 2012;20:46–56.
23. van der Hoeven H, Kibler WB. Shoulder injuries in tennis players. Br J Sports Med. 2006;40(5):435–40; discussion 440.
24. Kibler WB, Kuhn JE, Wilk K, Sciascia A, Moore S, Laudner K, Ellenbecker T, Thigpen C, Uhl T. The disabled throwing shoulder: spectrum of pathology-10-year update. Arthroscopy. 2013;29(1):141–61.e126.
25. Cools AM, Borms D, Castelein B, Vanderstukken F, Johansson FR. Evidence-based rehabilitation of athletes with glenohumeral instability. Knee Surg Sports Traumatol Arthrosc. 2016;24(2):382–9.
26. McClure P, Balaicuis J, Heiland D, Broersma ME, Thorndike CK, Wood A. A randomized controlled comparison of stretching procedures for posterior shoulder tightness. J Orthop Sports Phys Ther. 2007;37(3):108–14.
27. Tyler TF, Nicholas SJ, Lee SJ, Mullaney M, McHugh MP. Correction of posterior shoulder tightness is associated with symptom resolution in patients with internal impingement. Am J Sports Med. 2010;38(1):114–9.
28. Cools AM, Borms D, Cottens S, Himpe M, Meersdom S, Cagnie B. Rehabilitation exercises for athletes with biceps disorders and SLAP lesions: a continuum of exercises with increasing loads on the biceps. Am J Sports Med. 2014;42(6):1315–22.
29. Ellenbecker TS, Cools A. Rehabilitation of shoulder impingement syndrome and rotator cuff injuries: an evidence-based review. Br J Sports Med. 2010;44(5):319–27.
30. Reinold MM, Gill TJ, Wilk KE, Andrews JR. Current concepts in the evaluation and treatment of the shoulder in overhead throwing athletes, part 2: injury prevention and treatment. Sports Health. 2010;2(2):101–15.
31. Creighton DW, Shrier I, Shultz R, Meeuwisse WH, Matheson GO. Return-to-play in sport: a decision-based model. Clin J Sport Med. 2010;20(5):379–85.
32. Barber A, Field LD, Ryu R. Biceps tendon and superior labrum injuries: decision-marking. J Bone Joint Surg Am. 2007;89(8):1844–55.
33. Linke RD, Burkart A, Imhoff AB. [The arthroscopic SLAP refixation]. Orthopade. 2003;32(7):627–31.
34. Chalmers PN, Trombley R, Cip J, Monson B, Forsythe B, Nicholson GP, Bush-Joseph CA, Cole BJ, Wimmer MA, Romeo AA, et al. Postoperative restoration of upper extremity motion and neuromuscular control during the overhand pitch: evaluation of tenodesis and repair for superior labral anterior-posterior tears. Am J Sports Med. 2014;42(12):2825–36.
35. Erickson BJ, Jain A, Abrams GD, Nicholson GP, Cole BJ, Romeo AA, Verma NN. SLAP lesions: trends in treatment. Arthroscopy. 2016;32(6):976–81.
36. Laughlin WA, Fleisig GS, Scillia AJ, Aune KT, Cain EL, Dugas JR. Deficiencies in pitching biomechanics in baseball players with a history of superior labrum anterior-posterior repair. Am J Sports Med. 2014;42(12):2837–41.
37. Park JY, Chung SW, Jeon SH, Lee JG, Oh KS. Clinical and radiological outcomes of type 2 superior labral anterior posterior repairs in elite overhead athletes. Am J Sports Med. 2013;41(6):1372–9.
38. Braun S, Imhoff AB. [Modern treatment strategies for the long head of the biceps tendon]. Orthopade. 2018;47(2):113–20.
39. Denard PJ, Dai X, Hanypsiak BT, Burkhart SS. Anatomy of the biceps tendon: implications for restoring physiological length-tension relation during biceps tenodesis with interference screw fixation. Arthroscopy. 2012;28(10):1352–8.
40. Braun S, Minzlaff P, Imhoff AB. [Subpectoral tenodesis of the long head of the biceps tendon for pathologies of the long head of the biceps tendon and the biceps pulley]. Oper Orthop Traumatol. 2012;24(6):479–85.
41. Willinger L, Beitzel K. Überlastung der Supraspinatussehne beim Überkopfsportler. Arthroskopie. 2017;30(3):173–8.
42. Kuhn JE. Current concepts: rotator cuff pathology in athletes—a source of pain or adaptive pathology? Curr Sports Med Rep. 2013;12(5):311–5.
43. Franceschi F, Papalia R, Del Buono A, Vasta S, Costa V, Maffulli N, Denaro V. Articular-sided rotator cuff tears: which is the best repair? A three-year prospective randomised controlled trial. Int Orthop. 2013;37(8):1487–93.
44. Klouche S, Lefevre N, Herman S, Gerometta A, Bohu Y. Return to sport after rotator cuff tear repair: a systematic review and meta-analysis. Am J Sports Med. 2016;44(7):1877–87.
45. Reuter S, Imhoff AB, Martetschläger F. Impact of rotator cuff surgery on postoperative sporting activity. J Sports Med Phys Fitness. 2018;58(4):480–8.

Sports Trauma: Elbow

24

Sebastian Siebenlist, Lucca Lacheta,
Christine L. Redmond, and Gregory I. Bain

24.1 Acute Elbow Injury: Simple Dislocation

24.1.1 Introduction

By definition the simple elbow dislocation is described as one without concomitant fractures with the exception of small avulsions of less than 2 mm [1, 2]. The incidence for simple elbow dislocation ranges from 3 to 9 per 100,000 individuals through different periods of life with male adults at highest risk especially following sports or accidents [1–4]. Up to date, no validated classification exists for simple elbow dislocations. A consensus to descriptively grade the injury according to direction of elbow dislocation exists. Posterior and posterolateral dislocations are most commonly observed, while anterior and divergent dislocations are rare, and their occurrence is limited to pediatric cases or with concomitant fractures. The exact injury mechanism is still subject of current debates in literature. O'Driscoll proposed the theory of the posterolateral rotation—so-called Horii circle—with soft tissue disruption from the lateral side to medial side caused by a fall on the outstretched forearm. This hypothesis is currently most cited and accepted trauma mechanism [5, 6].

S. Siebenlist · L. Lacheta
Department of Orthopaedic Sports Medicine, Technical University of Munich, Munich, Germany
e-mail: sebastian.siebenlist@tum.de; Lucca.Lacheta@mri.tum.de

C. L. Redmond
RAP Division, SALHN, SA Health, University of South Australia, Adelaide, SA, Australia

G. I. Bain (✉)
Department of Orthopaedic Surgery, Flinders University, Flinders Medical Centre, Adelaide, SA, Australia
e-mail: admin@gregbain.com.au

24.1.2 Clinical Findings

The key to diagnosis is in taking the history as precisely as possible to get information about the injury patterns and mechanism with special respect to arm position at the time of impact. In the absence of deformity, some patients report spontaneous or self-reduction, while others just complain of pain and swelling. These patients have to be asked about additional clicking events, feelings of instability, or deformity at the time of injury. An accurate physical examination and focused neurovascular evaluation should be performed. The patient should be instructed to actively move his injured elbow to grossly verify the muscular joint stabilization. During the first days after reduction, medial and/or lateral bruises can occur as a sign of soft tissue disruption including the muscular fascia.

Anteroposterior and lateral radiographs are obligatory to confirm dislocation and direction

S. Rocha Piedade et al. (eds.), *The Sports Medicine Physician*,
https://doi.org/10.1007/978-3-030-10433-7_24

as well as to determine or exclude associated fractures even in patients with already self- or spontaneous reduced elbow joint. Ligament integrity can be assessed by taking an X-ray while stress testing but is often difficult due to pain. Anteroposterior and lateral radiographs should be repeated within the first week after reduction to rule out secondary decentration with persistent drop sign (ulnohumeral distance >3–4 mm) as a sign for persistence instability [7].

To achieve a better overview of involved soft tissue structures and grade of injury, MRI examination is recommended (ideally within the first week post-injury). The MRI can illustrate the continuity of the static ligamentous constraints and the dynamic muscular stabilizers. To assess joint congruity, MRI should be performed with extended elbow (if possible). Radiocapitellar and axial ulnohumeral incongruity in patients with posterolateral rotatory instability can be detected by the use of specified cutoff points as described by Hackl et al. [8].

Ultrasound examination can help to assess the collateral ligaments and the common flexor and extensor origins by dynamic testing. However, in the acute injury, this examination is limited by patient compliance, pain, swelling, and investigator's experience.

24.1.3 Treatment Options

Most patients can be treated with non-operative management following closed reduction. Early mobilization does not increase the risk of re-dislocation and leads to improved functional outcomes. A rehabilitation program including active-assisted and active exercises is crucial to maintain concentric reduction while injured soft tissues are healing.

Operative management is indicated if a closed reduction is not possible or in case of open dislocations and vascular injuries and when recurrent instability occurs when the elbow is flexed to less than 30°.

24.1.4 Rehabilitation

Most simple elbow dislocation injuries are stable postreduction, and patients may return to sport in a hinged brace approximately within the first 2–4 weeks after injury. The criterion for return to sport is that the athlete has to demonstrate pain-free range of motion without neurologic dysfunction. There is a need for research on the optimal period of immobilization, but our protocol is that the brace protects the healing of soft tissue injury and has to be worn for at least 8 weeks for all athletic activities.

In the first few days postoperatively, the patient has a splint to protect the repair as swelling subsides. After the first week, the athlete will be fitted with a hinged brace. Early goals are to manage pain and inflammation and regain active elbow movement. Initially, range of motion is limited but is gradually increased over 3–6 weeks to full arc of motion. Strengthening of the shoulder, wrist, and hand can be initiated with isometric exercises through multiple joint angles. As pain and inflammation settle, goals are to restore pain-free movement and strengthen the upper limb to return to pre-injury function. Therapists should be aware of heterotopic ossification as a possible complication, if there are increasing pain and loss of movement of the elbow joint [9]. Most athletes return to sports in a brace within 3–6 weeks postoperatively and continue activities in a brace until 3–4 months, depending on surgical procedure, strength, and function.

The literature demonstrates clearly that conservative treatment for management of simple elbow dislocations leads to favorable outcomes [4, 10–14]. There is evidence that prolonged immobilization has detrimental effects, so cast immobilization should not exceed 2 weeks (flexion contractures of 20–30° seen in patients with immobilization beyond 3–4 weeks). There are benefits to early mobilization, and patients have returned to work and daily activities earlier, compared to cast immobilization, when managed with sling immobilization for 2 weeks and active range of motion within the first week—using an overhead motion protocol [11, 14].

24.2 Valgus Instability in Throwing Athletes

24.2.1 Introduction

Valgus injury is an uncommon injury that has been identified in athletes that throw repeatedly, especially baseball pitchers. It has also been identified in javelin throwers and tennis players and following trauma. Valgus instability develops from the tensile forces on the medial compartment and compression to the lateral compartment. The tensile forces are applied to the medial stabilizers, consisting of the medial ulnar collateral ligament (MUCL) and the common flexor origin (CFO). Compression and shear forces are applied to the radial head and capitellum.

The MUCL is protected by the stabilizing effects of the flexor and pronator muscles during the throwing action. When these muscles become fatigued from overtraining, the forces generated during throwing can exceed the maximum load capacity of the MUCL. Repeated microtrauma to the medial elbow compartment can result in elongation and structural weakness of the MUCL [15].

24.2.2 Clinical Findings

The diagnosis of valgus instability is primarily made by clinical findings. Range of motion may be increased in the throwing arm due to an elongated MCL. Pain is provoked by palpating the sublime tubercle or the medial epicondyle. Increased gapping of the joint can be observed when manual valgus stress is applied in 0° and 15° [15]. The milking maneuver test applies valgus stress especially to the anterior MUCL bundle and results in pain and/or gapping in patients with severe valgus instability. All tests are compared to the uninjured contralateral elbow, to rule out generalized laxity.

Plain radiographs are indicated and may identify intra-articular lesions, such as loose bodies or osteophytes. A dynamic X-ray examination can be performed to confirm the clinical diagnosis. A MRI scan can identify tendinosis, partial and complete rupture of the MUCL, as well as osteochondral defects in the lateral compartment. A CT scan can identify loose bodies and impingement due to osteophytes.

24.2.3 Treatment Options

Conservative treatment is indicated for MUCL strains and partial ruptures and where there are no intra-articular lesions. The initial management is rest from sport and pain management. A structured rehabilitation and return to sport program can be started when the symptoms have settled. An elbow orthosis may be prescribed to reduce valgus stress [14].

Surgical MUCL repair is indicated for acute MUCL rupture, within 3 weeks of injury. MUCL reconstruction is indicated for late presentations of MUCL rupture or chronic persistent strained MUCL that has failed conservative treatment (Fig. 24.1). The reconstruction involves inserting

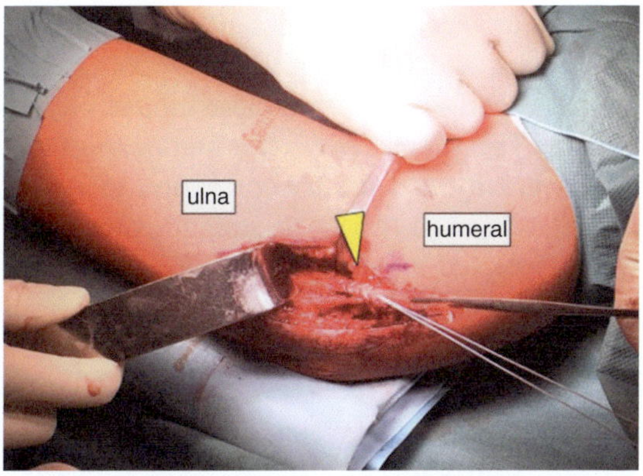

Fig. 24.1 Shuttled graft (yellow arrow) through the ulnar bone tunnels

a tendon graft, such as the palmaris longus, hamstring, or allograft.

24.2.4 Rehabilitation

The initial management for strains and partial ruptures is to moderate pain and modify activities, including resting from sport. When symptoms settle, physical conditioning and coaching the proper mechanics for the throwing action are part of a structured rehabilitation program. Guidelines on returning to sport and resuming throwing have been developed [16]. Strengthening, flexibility, dynamic stabilization, and plyometric exercises are used to retrain the throwing action, which involves the transfer of forces from the legs and trunk to the throwing arm, in a sequence of accelerating and decelerating movements.

Postoperative rehabilitation programs after ligament and tendon reconstruction are based on the intraoperative findings and the stages of tissue healing which predict the strength of repaired structures. Goals are established that are tailored to the symptoms and demands of the patient.

Rehabilitation commences after a period of immobilization. Following ligament or tendon reconstruction, a posterior cast is applied at 90° flexion for 3–4 days, followed by a removable elbow orthosis for 6 weeks. For MCL reconstruction, motion in the orthosis is limited to 20–60° for the first 2 weeks, then 10–110° at 3–4 weeks, and full range by 6 weeks. Active motion is performed within these limited arcs of motion. The supine, overhead motion protocol allows gravity and the triceps action to act as joint stabilizers [14]. Muscle strengthening starts when protected movement finishes and the athlete may be ready to return to sport from 12 weeks postoperatively.

24.2.5 Clinical Outcome

The success rate of the currently most common surgical procedures for MUCL reconstruction is up to 93% [17–20]. Athletes return to their original level of sports in 81–92% of cases [21–23].

24.3 Capitellar Osteochondritis Dissecans

24.3.1 Introduction

The capitellum begins ossification at the age of 1–2 years, and the process is completed between the ages of 14 and 17. Growing, young bones, which are highly vasculated, are thought not to resist compression well and can develop compression fractures. These subchondral compression (micro-)fractures present with bone edema on MRI, which compromises circulation, leading to avascular necrosis (AVN) and subsequent loose body formation. The AVN is characterized as posttraumatic and therefore is a different entity compared to the juvenile osteochondrosis of the capitellum, which has an atraumatic, asymptomatic onset in children under the age of 10 years.

24.3.2 Clinical Findings

The major complain in patients with OCD is lateral elbow pain while throwing, which may persist at rest. During physical examination, the radiocapitellar joint can be tender to palpation. Chronic OCD, with loose body formation, can present with loss of motion, pain aggravated by flexion, flexion contracture, and possible occasional snapping.

Simple radiographs can show osteopenia and chronic OCD changes, such as loose bodies. MRI can be used to stage the lesion and helps to decide whether to proceed with conservative or surgical treatment.

24.3.3 Treatment Options

Stable lesions (MRI grade 1 or 2) can be treated conservatively with relative rest. Healing might take up to 12 months. If symptoms do not change over this long period, drilling of the capitellum to stimulate healing can be discussed with the patient.

Our approach is to surgically debride the capitellar footprint, if the fragment is surrounded by fluid, and refix the fragment with screws or pins. Loose bodies are removed in chronic injuries.

24.3.4 Rehabilitation

Conservative treatment initially consists of a lengthy period of rest and avoiding the aggravating activity in sport. When the symptoms have settled, which is more likely in an early lesion, active therapy can commence. Rehabilitation progresses through restoring elbow range of motion and strength and undertaking an interval throwing program prior to returning to sport.

24.4 Valgus Extension Overload

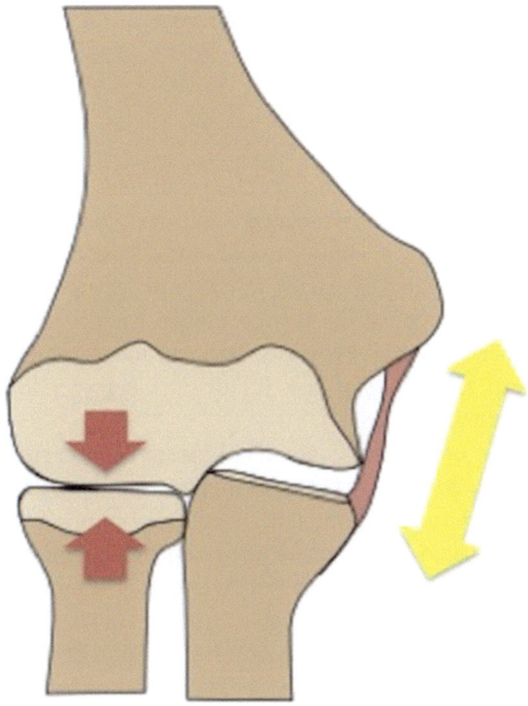

Fig. 24.2 Valgus extension overload (VEO) syndrome: overuse of the medial ligamentous stabilizers with increased compression load to the posterolateral part of the elbow from [24]

Valgus extension overload (VEO) is a syndrome of symptoms and physical findings associated with throwing activities and usually accompanied by valgus instability [24]. The ulnar collateral ligament (UCL) experiences an average of 64 Nm of valgus stress with each overhead throw, of which approximately 50% has to be taken by the UCL [25]. The ulnar collateral ligament (UCL) is the main ligamentous stabilizer to the medial part of the elbow. Repetitive overuse that increases UCL laxity will also result in increased compression to the lateral articular part of the elbow and the fossa olecrani (Fig. 24.2). Over time, degenerative changes such as osteophytes rise slowly in the posterolateral compartment [26]. The diagnosis of VEO can typically be made by a thorough history and physical examination. Additionally, simple radiographs or MRI can confirm degenerative changes. Typical complaints for VEO are medial pain at the onset of arm acceleration (UCL) and posterior pain at ball release when the elbow reaches full extension (posterolateral structures). Athletes with isolated VEO without structural UCL issues should be treated with active rest from throwing (approximately 10–14 days; in athletes with prolonged symptoms, 4–6 weeks; afterward, gradual return to sports) and start specific exercises to increase the flexor pronator strength and rotator cuff strength. Nonsteroidal anti-inflammatory medication may also be used in the acute stage for a short period.

24.5 Little Leaguer's Elbow

"Little leaguer's elbow" summarizes all possible overuse elbow injuries in young athletes and was first described by Brogan and Crow who reported radiographic changes occurring in young throwers' elbows. The most common injuries include medial epicondyle apophysitis, capitellar osteochondritis dissecans, radial head deformation, flexion contracture, and olecranon injury. Triceps apophysitis, posterior impingement, radiocapitellar meniscoid lesions, loose body formation, ulnar collateral ligament attenuation, and nerve disorders may also result from extensive throwing.

24.6 Distal Biceps Tendon Rupture

24.6.1 Introduction

An acute distal biceps tendon rupture is an injury that has been associated with weight lifting, smoking, or anabolic steroid abuse. The mechanism of injury is usually a sudden eccentric force applied against the flexing elbow. Men in their middle decades (40–60 years) and the dominant arm are at higher risk for distal biceps tendon ruptures [27, 28].

In contrast to acute distal biceps tendon ruptures, partial ruptures, chronic tendonopathies, and bicipitoradial bursitis are less common and associated with activities requiring repetitive movements, which occur without a traumatic event [29, 30].

The distal biceps tendon has an area of relatively poor vascularity, between the proximal supply by the brachial artery and the distal supply by the posterior recurrent artery. This hypovascularized zone may predispose the distal biceps tendon to rupture [31]. The distal biceps tendon can also be subjected to mechanical impingement from the ulna shaft during forearm rotation, which may predispose the tendon to degeneration, prior to rupture [31].

Several clinical tests that aid in the diagnosis of complete rupture have been described. O'Driscoll described the hook sign (Table 24.1), where the patient actively supinates and flexes the elbow to 90°. The examiner finger is hooked under the distal biceps tendon from the lateral side. In the complete tear, the hook test is considered the best test in making the diagnosis [27]. However, there are a number of cases where it can be difficult to interpret. These include presentations where:

1. The biceps sheath remains attached distally despite tendon retraction.
2. A pseudotendon bridges the gap in a chronic tear [33].
3. The partial or single head ruptures.

In these cases, we consider that the tendon is palpable, but will yield to pressure when performing the hook test [32] (Table 24.2).

24.6.2 Clinical Findings

The distal biceps tendon rupture is primarily a clinical diagnosis. The athlete will report sudden pain and loss of flexion and supination strength, sometimes accompanied by an audible "pop" while the flexed elbow is eccentrically loaded. With a complete rupture, the muscle belly will displace proximally, giving the appearance of a "pop-eyed" deformity. The hook test can confirm the discontinuity of the tendon in the antecubital fossa in case of complete ruptures [27].

MRI using the FABS view will allow assessment of the biceps tendon and its attachment [34]. Complete tears with retraction are usually easily identified with loss of continuity of the tendon to the radial tuberosity. Partial tears may have more subtle changes, including tendonitis, bursal effusion, and signal changes near the distal attachment. The partial ruptures can be graded (more or less than 50%) [35].

24.6.3 Treatment Options

The recommended treatment will depend upon the grade of biceps tear as defined by the clinical assessment, MRI, and operative findings. Tables 24.1 and 24.2 provide an assessment and algorithm.

Conservative treatment is indicated for partial tears and complete tears in low-demand individuals. Some athletes may elect to delay surgery until the end of the playing season; however, this

Table 24.1 Hook test: clinical assessment and interpretation (Modified from [32])

Hook test	Grade	Tendon
Normal	N	Taut, unyielding, symmetrical
Yielding	A1	Taut, but yielding, asymmetrical
Lax	A2	Complete tear
Absent	A3	Tendon retracted

Table 24.2 Distal biceps pathologies: classification, assessment, and management (Modified from [32])

Grade	Injury	Clinical	Hook test	MRI	Management
0	Tendinosis, bursitis	Atraumatic, tender, swollen	N	Bursitis, effusion, tendinosis	Non-operative, bursectomy, biopsy
1A	Low-grade partial tear (<50% footprint)	Pain, weakness against resistance	N, A1	Bursitis, effusion, footprint irregularity	Endoscopic debridement
1B	Isolated head rupture	Pain, weakness against resistance	A1	Isolated head avulsion	Repair isolated head
1C	High-grade partial tear (>50% footprint)	Pain and weakness	A1	Incomplete footprint detachment	Complete tear and repair
2	Complete tendon rupture, lacertus intact	Tendon medialized by lacertus, weak	A2	Detached tendon within sheath	Repair
3	Tendon and lacertus rupture retracted	Retracted muscle, marked weakness	A3	Retracted tendon and muscle	Repair
4A	Chronic rupture, lacertus intact	Marked weakness	A1, A2	Pseudotendon to footprint (A1) Contracted tendon in sheath (A2)	Repair
4B	Chronic tendon and lacertus rupture	Retracted muscle, marked weakness	A3	Retracted tendon within fibrous cocoon	Repair in flexion or use tendon graft

increases the risk of surgical complications and the need for a tendon graft [36].

For complete acute tears, the natural history is to continue to have weakness [37]. This reduces the ability to sustain supination power and presents as fatigue weakness, cramps, and pain with repetitive activities. Therefore for acute complete tears, early surgery is recommended, to restore strength and prevent these symptoms. Ideally, the procedure is done within 3 weeks to avoid scar formation [38].

Several fixation techniques are available for repair: extracortical button, intramedullary button, interference screw, and suture anchor [39–42]. There is a trend toward a two-point fixation, as there are two functional tendon bundles [43]. The single-incision approach is more commonly used now as there is less risk of synostosis and loss of forearm rotation (Fig. 24.3).

Schmitt has highlighted the importance of anatomic repairs of the distal biceps tendon [45]. For this reason, newer methods have been aimed at performing a true anatomic repair [46–49]. Comparative studies have demonstrated superior supination and flexion strength when an anatomical repair is performed [49].

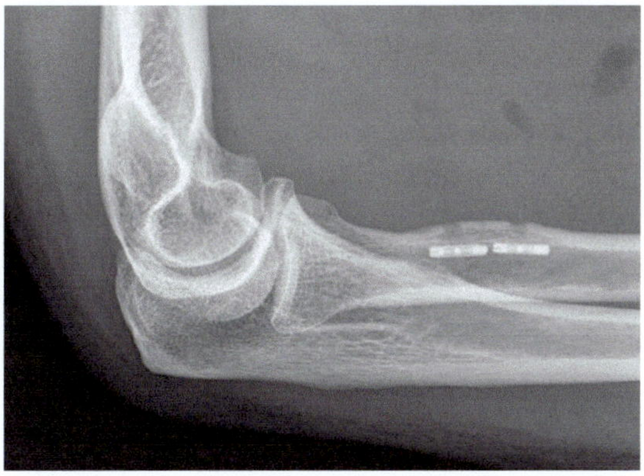

Fig. 24.3 Postoperative X-ray after distal biceps tendon repair with the double intramedullary button technique [42, 44]

Partial distal biceps tendon repairs are an area of interest. They can occur in the patient who has an eccentric load to the biceps, as seen in the complete tears. Repetitive activities can also cause bursitis and partial tear as the tendon impinges between the radius and ulna. Examination findings can be subtle, and as such, the diagnosis is often missed. Clinical findings of partial distal biceps tendon tears and bursitis include [32]:

1. Biceps muscle pistoning. During active forearm rotation, the biceps musculotendinous junction will normally migrate proximally and distally. In the complete tear, the muscle will retract and budge. In the partial tear, the muscle may be flatter due to atrophy and translate less.
2. Passive pronation is restricted and painful. There may also be crepitus.
3. Localized discomfort and tenderness over the radial tuberosity with 90° flexion and full supination against resistance.
4. Yielding hook test.
5. Weakness of supination in maximal elbow flexion.

Diagnostic endoscopy provides visualization of the tendon, bursa, and radial tuberosity [46, 47]. Therapeutic endoscopy includes bursectomy; release of the tendon and repair can be performed [46, 47, 49].

24.6.4 Rehabilitation

A posterior cast is applied at 90° flexion for 3–4 days, and then an elbow orthosis is worn for 6 weeks. In the first 2–4 weeks of rehabilitation, movement into the last 20° of extension is restricted, in order to protect the repair. Active supination is restricted by the orthosis for the first 6 weeks. Resistance training can start after the orthosis is removed and full active movement is achieved. Strengthening is progressed with functional training directed to the specific sport, and the athlete may be ready to return to sports at 12 weeks.

24.6.5 Clinical Outcome

Clinical outcomes are generally good following surgical repair of distal biceps tendons (Redmond, 2016 #382) [17, 18, 21–23, 50]. Anatomic repairs have been demonstrated to have better strength [51].

24.7 Lateral Epicondylitis

24.7.1 Introduction

Symptoms of lateral epicondylitis usually develop from activities that involve repetitive motions and overuse of the wrist extensors or supinator muscles. The most common affected muscle is the extensor carpi radialis brevis. Over time, a chronic tendonosis develops, and increased cross-linkage and collagen deposition can be seen within the tendon. Ongoing accumulation of load may then lead to structural failure of the tendon with partial or complete rupture.

24.7.2 Clinical Findings

Patients typically complain pain around the lateral epicondyle that radiates into the common extensor muscles of the forearm. Pain scale can vary from mild to severe with affection of daily activities. Tenderness is more likely to be found on palpation at the insertion site of the extensor carpi radialis brevis just anterior to the lateral epicondyle. A number of tests have been described to reproduce the pain. They all actively contract the wrist extensor muscle group against resistance to recreate the pain.

24.7.3 Treatment

First-line treatment is non-operative treatment consisting of rest, avoidance of aggravating activities, and modification of behavior during work, sport, and daily life accompanied by anti-inflammatory medication in the acute period. This should lead to a remission of the symptoms. Bisset et al. showed that non-operative treatment leads to similar results after 52 weeks compared to corticosteroid injections. Bisset et al. described a positive effect of physical therapy in reducing pain with focus on preserving range of motion and eccentric strengthening exercises. This treatment was found to be superior to conservative treatment alone at 6 weeks.

Epicondylar counterforce braces lead to a reduction of tension in the forearm extensors. Several studies have shown a positive effect on pain relief compared to placebo orthosis; however, meta-analysis did not find one type of brace to be better than others.

Surgery is preserved for patients who failed non-operative treatment or with complete tear of the common extensor origin.

24.8 Distal Triceps Tendon Rupture

24.8.1 Introduction

The distal triceps tendon rupture is a rare injury that has been reported in professional football players [52]. It can occur from a fall on the outstretched hand or direct trauma [53]. An eccentric loading of the contracting triceps muscle produces osseous avulsions of the bony insertion at the olecranon or occasionally at the musculotendinous junction [54–56].

Spontaneous ruptures have also been reported in weight lifters and following elbow arthroplasty [57, 58]. They have been associated with cortisone and steroid abuse and some systemic diseases [30, 59].

24.8.2 Clinical Findings

The diagnosis of a distal triceps tendon rupture can be made clinically. The tendon gap at the distal triceps may be difficult to palpate due to soft tissue swelling. Triceps strength can be tested against gravity by asking the patient to extend the elbow, with the arm overhead and the elbow at 90° of flexion. In case of partial ruptures, an active extension can be possible but with decreased strength compared to the uninjured contralateral site. Additionally, in complete ruptures, a manually applied compression of the muscle belly does not lead to elbow extension (equivalent to Thompson test for Achilles tendon).

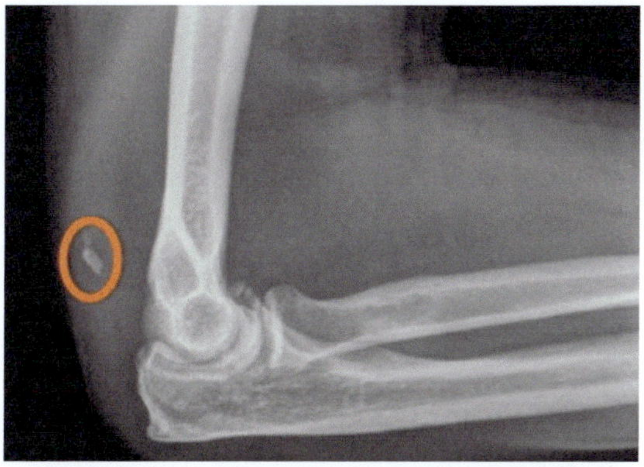

Fig. 24.4 Common bony distal triceps avulsion ("flake of bone") (orange circle)

Plain radiographs are needed to rule out common bony avulsion ("flake of bone") of the insertion (Fig. 24.4).

To grade partial or total rupture and assess retraction, an MRI scan or ultrasound examination should be performed. Especially in chronic cases, the MRI should be used to judge tendon retraction and muscle quality.

24.8.3 Treatment Options

Conservative management is indicated for partial distal triceps rupture (<50%), where some extension strength is maintained, and for musculotendinous ruptures [60]. Immobilization in a cast or orthosis with flexion is restricted to 30° for 4–6 weeks. Full motion may recover by 12 weeks and full extension strength by 6–9 months [60].

Surgery is indicated for complete ruptures and performed within 3 weeks to minimize scar formation. Techniques include transosseous cruciate repair technique [61], knotless suture-bridge repair technique [62], and V-shaped double-row repair technique [63] (Fig. 24.5).

24.8.4 Rehabilitation

There is insufficient evidence to determine the optimal position in which the elbow is immobilized, in order to protect the triceps repair.

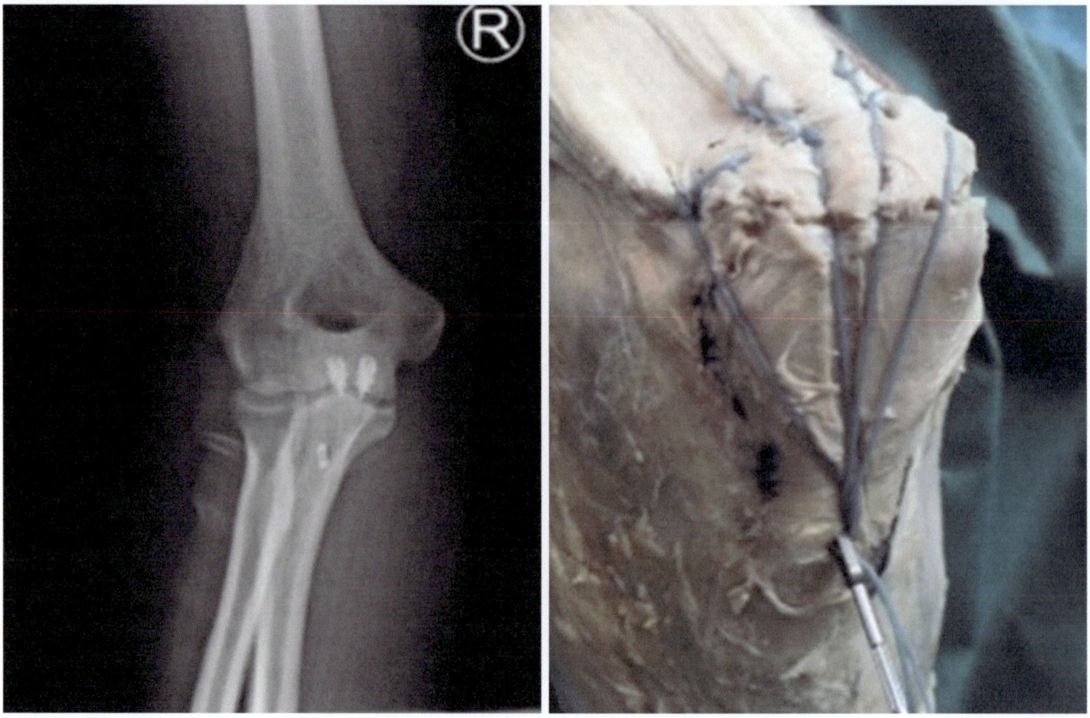

Fig. 24.5 Postoperative X-ray, two proximal suture anchors and one distal unicortical button (left); cadaver demonstration, V-shaped distal triceps reconstruction with intramedullary placed distal button (right)

A posterior cast is applied (in 90° flexion or near full extension, depending on surgeon preference) for 3–4 days, followed by a removable elbow orthosis for 6 weeks. Passive- and active-assisted therapy commences once the cast is removed. Active motion is limited to 0–60° of flexion for the first 6 weeks. Rehabilitation starts by controlling pain and swelling and gently moving the elbow through the available range. Active extension against resistance is then introduced when the orthosis is removed. A structured approach to strengthening the arm and returning to functional activities is advised, as the triceps muscle tends to be weaker than the biceps. Return to sports may be possible at week 12, if the athlete has recovered full strength.

24.8.5 Clinical Outcome

Surgical repairs have good functional outcomes with minimal re-ruptures [64] and high patient satisfaction [65].

24.9 Olecranon Stress Fracture

24.9.1 Introduction

Olecranon stress fractures are due to repetitive tensile forces generated by the triceps tendon or mechanical impingement. They are rare and usually in baseball pitchers, javelin throwers, weight lifters, or gymnasts [66–68].

24.9.2 Diagnosis

Athletes report a long-standing history of posterolateral elbow pain, aggravated by throwing. The clinical examination and plain radiographs may show no abnormal findings. MRI scan and/or CT scans usually demonstrate the stress fracture.

24.9.3 Treatment

Initial management is to avoid the aggravating activities, such as throwing. In addition, bone growth stimulation with calcium and vitamin D may be prescribed. Screw fixation is the preferred surgical procedure [66].

24.9.4 Clinical Outcome

A return to previous level of play was seen in most baseball pitchers (17/18, 93%). Hardware removal was required in 33% [66]. Average return to play was 21 weeks [68].

References

1. Josefsson PO, Nilsson BE. Incidence of elbow dislocation. Acta Orthop Scand. 1986;57(6):537–8.
2. Josefsson PO, Johnell O, Gentz CF. Long-term sequelae of simple dislocation of the elbow. J Bone Joint Surg Am. 1984;66(6):927–30.
3. Anakwe RE, Middleton SD, Jenkins PJ, McQueen MM, Court-Brown CM. Patient-reported outcomes after simple dislocation of the elbow. J Bone Joint Surg Am. 2011;93(13):1220–6. https://doi.org/10.2106/JBJS.J.00860.
4. Mehlhoff TL, Noble PC, Bennett JB, Tullos HS. Simple dislocation of the elbow in the adult. Results after closed treatment. J Bone Joint Surg Am. 1988;70(2):244–9.
5. O'Driscoll SW, Morrey BF, Korinek S, An KN. Elbow subluxation and dislocation. A spectrum of instability. Clin Orthop Relat Res. 1992;(280):186–97.
6. O'Driscoll SW, Bell DF, Morrey BF. Posterolateral rotatory instability of the elbow. J Bone Joint Surg Am. 1991;73(3):440–6.
7. Pipicelli JG, Chinchalkar SJ, Grewal R, King GJ. Therapeutic implications of the radiographic "drop sign" following elbow dislocation. J Hand Ther. 2012;25(3):346–53; quiz 354. https://doi.org/10.1016/j.jht.2012.03.003.
8. Hackl M, Wegmann K, Ries C, Leschinger T, Burkhart KJ, Muller LP. Reliability of magnetic resonance imaging signs of posterolateral rotatory instability of the elbow. J Hand Surg Am. 2015;40(7):1428–33. https://doi.org/10.1016/j.jhsa.2015.04.029.
9. Winkler S, Wagner F, Weber M, Matussek J, Craiovan B, Heers G, Springorum HR, Grifka J, Renkawitz T. Current therapeutic strategies of heterotopic ossification—a survey amongst orthopaedic and trauma departments in Germany. BMC Musculoskeletal Disord. 2015;16:313.
10. Cohen MS, Hastings H 2nd. Acute elbow dislocation: evaluation and management. J Am Acad Orthop Surg. 1998;6(1):15–23.
11. Protzman RR. Dislocation of the elbow joint. J Bone Joint Surg Am. 1978;60(4):539–41.
12. Royle SG. Posterior dislocation of the elbow. Clin Orthop Relat Res. 1991;(269):201–4.
13. Ross G, McDevitt ER, Chronister R, Ove PN. Treatment of simple elbow dislocation using an immediate motion protocol. Am J Sports Med. 1999;27(3):308–11. https://doi.org/10.1177/03635465990270030701.
14. Maripuri SN, Debnath UK, Rao P, Mohanty K. Simple elbow dislocation among adults: a comparative study of two different methods of treatment. Injury. 2007;38(11):1254–8. https://doi.org/10.1016/j.injury.2007.02.040.
15. Cain EL Jr, Dugas JR, Wolf RS, Andrews JR. Elbow injuries in throwing athletes: a current concepts review. Am J Sports Med. 2003;31(4):621–35. https://doi.org/10.1177/03635465030310042601.
16. Wilk KE, Meister K, Andrews JR. Current concepts in the rehabilitation of the overhead throwing athlete. Am J Sports Med. 2002;30(1):136–51.
17. Ahmad CS, Lee TQ, ElAttrache NS. Biomechanical evaluation of a new ulnar collateral ligament reconstruction technique with interference screw fixation. Am J Sports Med. 2003;31(3):332–7. https://doi.org/10.1177/03635465030310030201.
18. Dodson CC, Thomas A, Dines JS, Nho SJ, Williams RJ 3rd, Altchek DW. Medial ulnar collateral ligament reconstruction of the elbow in throwing athletes. Am J Sports Med. 2006;34(12):1926–32. https://doi.org/10.1177/0363546506290988.

19. Paletta GA Jr, Wright RW. The modified docking procedure for elbow ulnar collateral ligament reconstruction: 2-year follow-up in elite throwers. Am J Sports Med. 2006;34(10):1594–8. https://doi.org/10.1177/0363546506289884.
20. Thompson WH, Jobe FW, Yocum LA, Pink MM. Ulnar collateral ligament reconstruction in athletes: muscle-splitting approach without transposition of the ulnar nerve. J Shoulder Elbow Surg. 2001;10(2):152–7. https://doi.org/10.1067/mse.2001.112881.
21. Azar FM, Andrews JR, Wilk KE, Groh D. Operative treatment of ulnar collateral ligament injuries of the elbow in athletes. Am J Sports Med. 2000;28(1):16–23. https://doi.org/10.1177/03635465000280011401.
22. Erickson BJ, Bach BR Jr, Bush-Joseph CA, Verma NN, Romeo AA. Medial ulnar collateral ligament reconstruction of the elbow in major league baseball players: where do we stand? World J Orthop. 2016;7(6):355–60. https://doi.org/10.5312/wjo.v7.i6.355.
23. Rohrbough JT, Altchek DW, Hyman J, Williams RJ 3rd, Botts JD. Medial collateral ligament reconstruction of the elbow using the docking technique. Am J Sports Med. 2002;30(4):541–8. https://doi.org/10.1177/03635465020300041401.
24. Lacheta L, Scheiderer B, Diermeier T, Imhoff A, Siebenlist S. Valgus instability of the elbow in throwing athletes. MMW Fortschr Med. 2018;160(12):47–50. https://doi.org/10.1007/s15006-018-0707-6.
25. Fleisig GS, Andrews JR, Dillman CJ, Escamilla RF. Kinetics of baseball pitching with implications about injury mechanisms. Am J Sports Med. 1995;23(2):233–9. https://doi.org/10.1177/036354659502300218.
26. Dugas JR. Valgus extension overload: diagnosis and treatment. Clin Sports Med. 2010;29(4):645–54. https://doi.org/10.1016/j.csm.2010.07.001.
27. O'Driscoll SW, Goncalves LB, Dietz P. The hook test for distal biceps tendon avulsion. Am J Sports Med. 2007;35(11):1865–9. https://doi.org/10.1177/0363546507305016.
28. Safran MR, Graham SM. Distal biceps tendon ruptures: incidence, demographics, and the effect of smoking. Clin Orthop Relat Res. 2002;404:275–83.
29. Behun MA, Geeslin AG, O'Hagan EC, King JC. Partial tears of the distal biceps Brachii tendon: a systematic review of surgical outcomes. J Hand Surg Am. 2016;41(7):e175–89. https://doi.org/10.1016/j.jhsa.2016.04.019.
30. Yeh PC, Dodds SD, Smart LR, Mazzocca AD, Sethi PM. Distal triceps rupture. J Am Acad Orthop Surg. 2010;18(1):31–40.
31. Seiler JG 3rd, Parker LM, Chamberland PD, Sherbourne GM, Carpenter WA. The distal biceps tendon. Two potential mechanisms involved in its rupture: arterial supply and mechanical impingement. J Shoulder Elbow Surg. 1995;4(3):149–56.
32. Bain G, Phadnis J, Saeed H. Biceps tendon pathology. In: Pederzini L, Eygendaal D, Denti M, editors. Elbow and sport. 1st ed. New York: Springer; 2016. p. 143–52.
33. Phadnis J, Bain G. Distal biceps tendinopathy. In: Ring D, Steinmann S, editors. Advanced reconstruction: elbow. 2nd ed. Rosemont: American Academy of Orthopaedic Surgeons; 2017. p. 81–90.
34. Giuffre BM, Moss MJ. Optimal positioning for MRI of the distal biceps brachii tendon: flexed abducted supinated view. AJR Am J Roentgenol. 2004;182(4):944–6. https://doi.org/10.2214/ajr.182.4.1820944.
35. Bain GI, Johnson LJ, Turner PC. Treatment of partial distal biceps tendon tears. Sports Med Arthrosc Rev. 2008;16(3):154–61. https://doi.org/10.1097/JSA.0b013e318183eb60.
36. Hallam P, Bain GI. Repair of chronic distal biceps tendon ruptures using autologous hamstring graft and the endobutton. J Shoulder Elbow Surg. 2004;13(6):648–51. https://doi.org/10.1016/S1058274604000771.
37. Baker BE, Bierwagen D. Rupture of the distal tendon of the biceps brachii. Operative versus non-operative treatment. J Bone Joint Surg Am. 1985;67(3):414–7.
38. Stucken C, Ciccotti MG. Distal biceps and triceps injuries in athletes. Sports Med Arthrosc Rev. 2014;22(3):153–63. https://doi.org/10.1097/JSA.0000000000000030.
39. Bain GI, Prem H, Heptinstall RJ, Verhellen R, Paix D. Repair of distal biceps tendon rupture: a new technique using the Endobutton. J Shoulder Elbow Surg. 2000;9(2):120–6.
40. Barnes SJ, Coleman SG, Gilpin D. Repair of avulsed insertion of biceps. A new technique in four cases. J Bone Joint Surg Br. 1993;75(6):938–9.
41. Heinzelmann AD, Savoie FH 3rd, Ramsey JR, Field LD, Mazzocca AD. A combined technique for distal biceps repair using a soft tissue button and biotenodesis interference screw. Am J Sports Med. 2009;37(5):989–94. https://doi.org/10.1177/0363546508330130.
42. Siebenlist S, Elser F, Sandmann GH, Buchholz A, Martetschlager F, Stockle U, Lenich A. The double intramedullary cortical button fixation for distal biceps tendon repair. Knee Surg Sports Traumatol Arthrosc. 2011;19(11):1925–9. https://doi.org/10.1007/s00167-011-1569-y.
43. Eames MH, Bain GI, Fogg QA, van Riet RP. Distal biceps tendon anatomy: a cadaveric study. J Bone Joint Surg Am. 2007;89(5):1044–9. https://doi.org/10.2106/JBJS.D.02992.
44. Siebenlist S, Schmitt A, Imhoff AB, Lenich A, Sandmann GH, Braun KF, Kirchhoff C, Biberthaler P, Buchholz A. Intramedullary cortical button repair for distal biceps tendon rupture: a single-center experience. J Hand Surg Am. 2018.
45. Jarrett CD, Weir DM, Stuffmann ES, Jain S, Miller MC, Schmidt CC. Anatomic and biomechanical analysis of the short and long head components of the distal biceps tendon. J Shoulder Elbow Surg. 2012;21(7):942–8. https://doi.org/10.1016/j.jse.2011.04.030.

46. Phadnis J, Bain G. Endoscopic-assisted distal biceps footprint repair. Tech Hand Up Extrem Surg. 2015;19(2):55–9. https://doi.org/10.1097/BTH.0000000000000078.
47. Bhatia DN. Endoscopic distal biceps repair: endoscopic anatomy and dual-anchor repair using a proximal anterolateral "parabiceps portal". Arthrosc Tech. 2015;4(6):e785–93. https://doi.org/10.1016/j.eats.2015.07.031.
48. Tanner C, Toby Johnson T, Muradov P, Lisa Husak L. Single incision power optimizing cost-effective (SPOC) distal biceps repair. JSES. 2013;22(3):305–11.
49. Bellringer S, Phadnis J, Human T, Redmond C, Bain G. Biomechanical comparison of transosseous cortical button and footprint repair techniques for acute distal biceps tendon ruptures. Shoulder & Elbow. 2019; https://doi.org/10.1177/1758573218815312.
50. Redmond C. Functional outcomes after distal biceps brachii repair: A case series. Int J Sports Phys Ther. 2016;11:962.
51. Bellringer SF, et al. Biomechanical comparison of transosseous cortical button and Footprint repair techniques for acute distal biceps tendon ruptures. Shoulder Elbow. 2019; https://doi.org/10.1177/1758573218815312.
52. Mair SD, Isbell WM, Gill TJ, Schlegel TF, Hawkins RJ. Triceps tendon ruptures in professional football players. Am J Sports Med. 2004;32(2):431–4. https://doi.org/10.1177/0095399703258707.
53. Anzel SH, Covey KW, Weiner AD, Lipscomb PR. Disruption of muscles and tendons; an analysis of 1014 cases. Surgery. 1959;45(3):406–14.
54. Keener JD, Chafik D, Kim HM, Galatz LM, Yamaguchi K. Insertional anatomy of the triceps brachii tendon. J Shoulder Elbow Surg. 2010;19(3):399–405. https://doi.org/10.1016/j.jse.2009.10.008.
55. Madsen M, Marx RG, Millett PJ, Rodeo SA, Sperling JW, Warren RF. Surgical anatomy of the triceps brachii tendon: anatomical study and clinical correlation. Am J Sports Med. 2006;34(11):1839–43. https://doi.org/10.1177/0363546506288752.
56. O'Driscoll SW. Intramuscular triceps rupture. Can J Surg. 1992;35(2):203–7.
57. Sollender JL, Rayan GM, Barden GA. Triceps tendon rupture in weight lifters. J Shoulder Elbow Surg. 1998;7(2):151–3.
58. Dachs RP, Fleming MA, Chivers DA, Carrara HR, Du Plessis JP, Vrettos BC, Roche SJ. Total elbow arthroplasty: outcomes after triceps-detaching and triceps-sparing approaches. J Shoulder Elbow Surg. 2015;24(3):339–47. https://doi.org/10.1016/j.jse.2014.11.038.
59. Tsourvakas S, Gouvalas K, Gimtsas C, Tsianas N, Founta P, Ameridis N. Bilateral and simultaneous rupture of the triceps tendons in chronic renal failure and secondary hyperparathyroidism. Arch Orthop Trauma Surg. 2004;124(4):278–80. https://doi.org/10.1007/s00402-003-0628-3.
60. Demirhan M, Ersen A. Distal triceps ruptures. EFORT Open Rev. 2016;1(6):255–9. https://doi.org/10.1302/2058-5241.1.000038.
61. Scheiderer B, Imhoff FB, Morikawa D, Lacheta L, Obopilwe E, Cote MP, Imhoff AB, Mazzocca AD, Siebenlist S. The V-shaped distal triceps tendon repair: a comparative biomechanical analysis. Am J Sports Med. 2018;46(8):1952–8.
62. Yeh PC, Stephens KT, Solovyova O, Obopilwe E, Smart LR, Mazzocca AD, Sethi PM. The distal triceps tendon footprint and a biomechanical analysis of 3 repair techniques. Am J Sports Med. 2010;38(5):1025–33. https://doi.org/10.1177/0363546509358319.
63. Scheiderer B, Lacheta L, Imhoff AB, Siebenlist S. V-shaped double-row distal triceps tendon repair: a novel technique using unicortical button fixation. Eur J Med Res. 2017;22(1):9. https://doi.org/10.1186/s40001-017-0250-4.
64. Horneff JG 3rd, Aleem A, Nicholson T, Lervick G, Murthi A, Sethi P, Getz C, Lazarus MD, Ramsey ML, Abboud JA, Tashjian R. Functional outcomes of distal triceps tendon repair comparing transosseous bone tunnels with suture anchor constructs. J Shoulder Elbow Surg. 2017;26(12):2213–9. https://doi.org/10.1016/j.jse.2017.08.006.
65. Giannicola G, Bullitta G, Rotini R, Murena L, Blonna D, Iapicca M, Restuccia G, Merolla G, Fontana M, Greco A, Scacchi M, Cinotti G. Results of primary repair of distal triceps tendon ruptures in a general population. Bone Joint J. 2018;100-B(5):610–6. https://doi.org/10.1302/0301-620X.100B5.BJJ-2017-1057.R2.
66. Paci JM, Dugas JR, Guy JA, Cain EL Jr, Fleisig GS, Hurst C, Wilk KE, Andrews JR. Cannulated screw fixation of refractory olecranon stress fractures with and without associated injuries allows a return to baseball. Am J Sports Med. 2013;41(2):306–12. https://doi.org/10.1177/0363546512469089.
67. Nuber GW, Diment MT. Olecranon stress fractures in throwers. A report of two cases and a review of the literature. Clin Orthop Relat Res. 1992;(278):58–61.
68. Fujioka H, Tsunemi K, Takagi Y, Tanaka J. Treatment of stress fracture of the olecranon in throwing athletes with internal fixation through a small incision. Sports Med Arthrosc Rehabil Ther Technol. 2012;4(1):49. https://doi.org/10.1186/1758-2555-4-49.

Sports Trauma: Wrist and Hand 25

Margaret W. M. Fok, Christine L. Redmond, and Gregory I. Bain

25.1 Introduction

Wrist and hand injuries are common entities in many contact and ball sports [1, 2]. Wrist injuries often occur from a fall, and the finger can be injured attempting to catch a ball or from being caught in clothing. Early assessment and management provide the best outcome. But, referral to an experienced orthopedic hand surgeon is frequently delayed. The athlete continues to compete with a painful wrist or swollen finger, which can lead to further injury of the secondary stabilizers and articular surfaces. It is common for the athlete to present 6 months after a fall with a stiff, painful, unstable joint with degenerative arthritis. Unfortunately, these late presentations are a much greater challenge to manage. It is too late to simply reduce the joint or the fracture, so a salvage procedure such as a fusion may be required.

When the athlete "hangs up their boots," it is these hand and wrist injuries that continue to cause them ongoing pain and disability. It is common for the following conditions to present late:

- Wrist—scaphoid fractures, scapholunate (SL) instability, and TFCC tears
- Hand—PIP joint dislocations, FDP tendon ruptures, and skier's thumb

The role of the hand therapist is critical in rehabilitation following injury and surgery. They provide valuable education, splints, edema control, and exercises. The exercises are directed toward tendon guiding, joint mobility, strength, and sports-specific training drills.

25.2 Acute Wrist Injury

For the acute wrist injury, our clinical decisions are based on an algorithm (Fig. 25.1). When assessing a wrist, we start with a general history and examination. The swelling and tenderness on palpation can help localize injured structures. Physical examination can suggest whether the injury is a fracture or a soft tissue sprain. For example, displaced distal radius fracture and perilunate dislocation usually present with diffuse swelling, pain, and limited range of movement of the wrist. As there are many structures in the wrist that can be injured, it is common to

M. W. M. Fok
Department of Orthopaedics and Traumatology, Queen Mary Hospital, The University of Hong Kong, Hong Kong, China

C. L. Redmond
Flinders Medical Centre, Adelaide, SA, Australia
e-mail: Christine.redmond@sa.gov.au

G. I. Bain (✉)
Department of Orthopaedic Surgery, Flinders University, Flinders Medical Centre, Adelaide, SA, Australia
e-mail: admin@gregbain.com.au

S. Rocha Piedade et al. (eds.), *The Sports Medicine Physician*,
https://doi.org/10.1007/978-3-030-10433-7_25

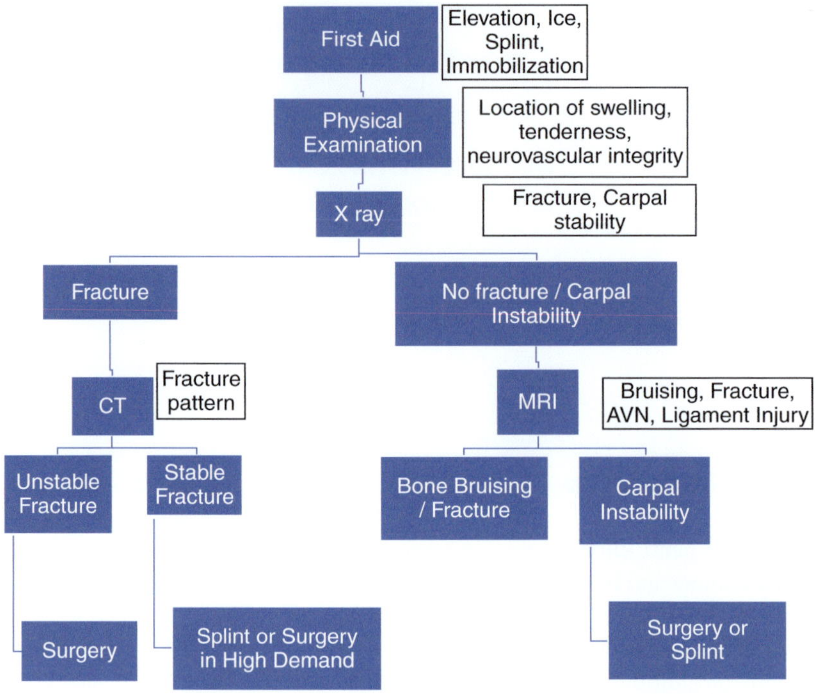

Fig. 25.1 Algorithm in managing acute wrist injuries

categorize presentations as either radial- or ulnar-sided disorders of the wrist.

25.2.1 Imaging

Standard radiographs (AP and lateral views) of the wrist are performed. Scaphoid radiological views are indicated if there is tenderness in the anatomic snuff box. In cases of suspected scapholunate instability and perilunate dislocation, the identification of a break in the Gilula lines [3] is helpful for diagnosis on an AP view of the wrist (Fig. 25.2). Lateral view is also used to assess the position of the lunate in cases of suspected carpal instability. Dorsal intercalated segmental instability (DISI), where the lunate tilts dorsally with respect to the axis of the radius and makes a scapholunate angle of >60°, suggests scapholunate dissociation. In contrast, volar intercalated segmental instability (VISI), where the lunate flexes with respect to the axis of the radius and makes a scapholunate angle of <30°, suggests an injury to the lunotriquetral ligament.

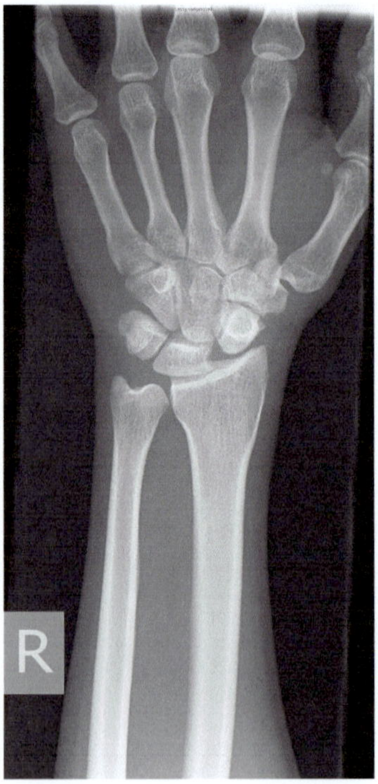

Fig. 25.2 AP radiograph wrist showing that the Gilula lines are broken

Further imaging includes computer tomography (CT), which allows better understanding of the osseous structures, and MRI which is useful for the soft tissues, especially the scapholunate ligament and the triangular fibrocartilage complex (TFCC).

Third-line investigations include a SPECT scan [4], which is a hybrid of bone scan and CT scan. It provides the very high specificity of the bone scan and the anatomic localization of the CT scan. The 4D CT scan is useful to assess the dynamic component of carpal instability [4].

25.2.2 Acute Carpal Tunnel Syndrome

Acute carpal tunnel syndrome can be a complication of a wrist injury [5, 6]. Symptoms include severe pain and paresthesia in the radial 3½ digits. This complication has been associated with distal radius fracture or perilunate dislocation and requires urgent surgery, to decompress the median nerve.

Depending on the expertise of the surgeon, one-stage (e.g., fracture and joint fixation and open carpal tunnel release) or two-stage operations (e.g., open carpal tunnel release and external fixator followed by internal fixation when the swelling has subsided) are indicated [1, 5, 7].

25.2.3 Radial Wrist Pain

For *acute radial wrist pain* and swelling, scaphoid fracture is the most common condition [1], followed by radial styloid fracture and scapholunate dissociation. A careful palpation to feel the exact location of tenderness, and knowing the underlying anatomical structures, assists in the diagnosis. (e.g., tenderness anatomical snuff box—*scaphoid fracture*). Dynamic tests of instability can provide additional information that may be missed by palpation alone. Pain and instability elicited on Watson test (i.e., compressing the scaphoid tubercle while bringing wrist from ulnar deviation to radial deviation) imply SL instability [8].

25.2.3.1 Scaphoid Fracture

Scaphoid fractures can be problematic as they can be difficult to diagnosis and are prone to malunion and non-union. If the scaphoid heals with a "humpback deformity," then it will affect the kinematics of the wrist. A delay in diagnosis increases the risk of scaphoid non-union, which predisposes the wrist to degenerative arthritis in the following 10–20 years [9]. Surgical management of non-union of the scaphoid, with wrist immobilization for 6–10 weeks, has about 85% success. Limited and full wrist fusions are indicated for patients with arthritis and for the non-unions which fail to heal with surgery.

Plain radiographs of the wrist (AP, lateral, and scaphoid views) are the initial imaging. In cases where an undisplaced fracture of the scaphoid is suspected, yet with a normal X-ray, a CT or MRI scan may be useful for diagnosis [10, 11]. If scans are not readily available, a short arm cast (including thumb immobilization of suspected scaphoid fracture) is applied for 2 weeks for temporary immobilization. An undisplaced fracture can be more readily seen on reassessment radiograph due to the bone resorption at the fracture site.

Undisplaced fractures can be managed with cast immobilization for 8 weeks, and 90% will unite [12]. Early mobilization can be permitted if internal fixation is performed [13–15]. Internal fixation is usually recommended for fractures in the proximal pole of the scaphoid, as they are associated with a non-union rate of 50% [16]. Displaced scaphoid should be managed with internal fixation to prevent non-union and deformity.

25.2.3.2 Radial Styloid Fractures

For radial styloid fracture, it is important to look for associated scapholunate dissociation and more importantly perilunate dissociation [17]. Surgical intervention with joint reduction and fracture fixation is indicated when carpal instability is part of the presentation.

25.2.3.3 Scapholunate Instability

Scapholunate (SL) instability is less commonly seen than scaphoid fracture but is often missed. The pain and swelling are usually less severe than the scaphoid fracture and are located more diffusely over the scapholunate region, rather than at the anatomical snuffbox. Static SL instability can be seen on AP or lateral views of the wrist. *SL dissociation* is diagnosed if SL gap is ≥3 mm on the AP view [18], and *dorsal intercalated segment instability* (*DISI*) is diagnosed when the scapholunate angle is greater than 60° on the lateral view of MRI (Fig. 25.3) [18]. Dynamic instability of the SL joint can be seen with clenched fist AP radiograph of the wrist (SL gap of ≥3 mm) [18, 19]. Magnetic resonance imaging (MRI) ± arthrogram or diagnostic wrist arthroscopy can also be performed to assess the integrity of the SL ligament.

Surgical treatment for scapholunate dissociation is achieved by ligament repair or debridement, Kirschner wires, or a temporary SL screw, followed by joint immobilization of at least 8–12 weeks [10, 19, 20]. If tenderness is elicited on palpating the SL junction but no obvious increase in SL gap is noted on radiograph, temporary immobilization with a removal wrist splint may be given for 2–3 weeks, before reassessing the wrist. For dynamic instability, both wrist immobilization of at least 8 weeks with splint and surgical repair or debridement are acceptable treatment options [19]. Exercises to strengthen the wrist that use a strong grip are not permitted for at least 12 weeks, as making a fist is the classic stress test for SL ligament tears.

25.2.4 Ulnar Wrist Pain

The common causes of acute ulnar wrist pain from a traumatic injury include the following: distal radioulnar joint subluxation/dislocation, ECU subluxation/dislocation, and hook of hamate fracture. It can be difficult to differentiate which structures are injured, but careful physical examination and imaging help in making the correct diagnosis.

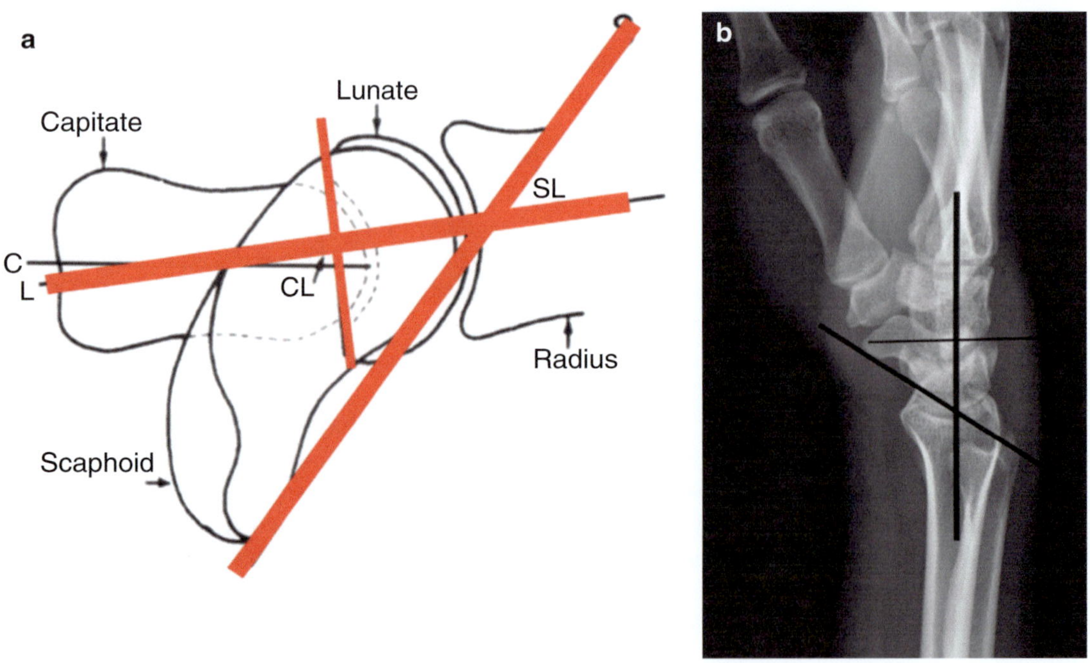

Fig. 25.3 Schematic drawing (**a**) and lateral radiograph wrist (**b**) on how to measure scapholunate angle to determine SL dissociation

25.2.4.1 Distal Radioulnar Joint Instability

Distal radioulnar joint (DRUJ) subluxation or dislocation can be the result of a fall on an outstretched hand in athletes, such as gymnasts, racquet players, hockey players, skiers, and pole vaulters [1]. In some instances, a "pop" may have been heard at the time of the injury. The joint may be dislocated or have spontaneously reduced. If the joint is dislocated, reduction is warranted under anesthesia.

The ballottement test can be used to elicit DRUJ instability. In this test, the amount of displacement of the ulnar head in supination, neutral, and pronation is compared to the contralateral wrist.

Distal radius fractures and basal ulnar styloid fractures are often associated with DRUJ instability [21–23]. DRUJ subluxation/dislocation is usually a result of a triangular fibrocartilage complex (TFCC) tear.

Conservative therapy with an above-elbow brace to keep the forearm in supination or pronation (depending on whether the DRUJ is stable at supination or pronation) for 6 weeks is well accepted [24]. Surgical repair or reconstruction with either arthroscopic or open technique is usually reserved when conservative therapy fails and instability persists [25, 26].

25.2.4.2 Extensor Carpi Ulnaris Subluxation/Dislocation

ECU subluxation/dislocation is a result of the disruption of its own fibro-osseous tunnel that lies over the distal ulna. A classic example is when a rugby player attempts to grip the ball tightly, with the wrist flexed and supinated, and the ECU tendon subluxates from the sudden increase in the isometric force [27]. The athlete would present with painful snapping or clicking sensation of the tendon during pronation and supination movements [25]. Ultrasound and MRI may be performed to support the diagnosis but is usually not necessary. Early diagnosis of ECU tendon subluxation can be treated with a short arm cast or split for 1–3 months [10, 28]. However, for cases with delayed presentation, surgical intervention to reconstruct the sheath and stabilize the ECU tendon is recommended [29, 30].

25.2.4.3 Hook of Hamate Fracture

Hook of hamate fracture can occur from the sudden impact when the golf club hits the ground or the baseball hits the very end of the bat [10]. There is pain and localized tenderness over the hook of the hamate. It is easily missed, as it may not be evident on plain radiographs. It is more easily seen in a carpal tunnel view or in the supinated oblique view (hook of hamate view). CT scan is preferred as it provided an excellent image of the fracture [10] (Fig. 25.4). Hook of hamate fracture can be managed conservatively, but it can remain painful, as there is a 50% rate of non-union [31, 32]. They can be internally fixed, but excision is usually preferred [32].

25.3 Chronic Wrist Pain

Chronic wrist pain in sport can develop from a past acute injury that may not have been investigated at the time or may develop through overuse. It can be classified by location similarly to acute wrist pain.

25.3.1 Radial Wrist Pain

Athletes may have persistent pain from *missed scaphoid fracture* or *scapholunate dissociation*. Patterns of posttraumatic wrist arthrosis may have developed, such as scaphoid non-union advanced collapse (*SNAC*) and scapholunate advanced collapse (*SLAC*) wrist. Imaging and wrist arthroscopy are useful to diagnose these conditions and to perform debridement of associated synovitis. Reconstructive wrist surgery or even limited wrist fusion may be required in advanced cases.

25.3.1.1 de Quervain's Disease

de Quervain's disease, stenosing tenosynovitis of the first extensor compartment, is caused by repeated movement of the thumb and wrist in

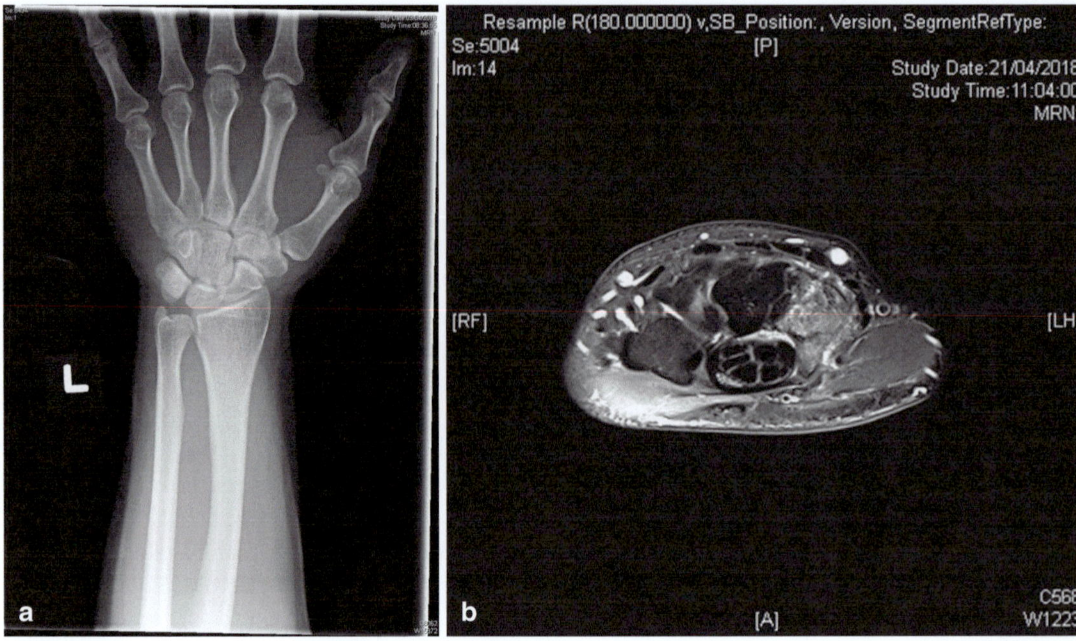

Fig. 25.4 Hook of hamate fracture: (**a**) AP radiograph wrist showing no obvious fracture of the carpal bone, (**b**) MRI axial cut of carpal bones showing hook of hamate fracture

racquet sports, rowing and golf [28]. There are pain and tenderness along the first extensor compartment of the wrist. Finkelstein's test is positive when pain is elicited by ulnar deviating a fisted wrist, with the thumb in the palm [33]. This diagnosis can be further confirmed when the test is negative with the thumb out of the fist. It is a clinical diagnosis, based on history and examination. Imaging is only used to rule out other diagnosis, e.g., missed scaphoid fracture or first carpal-metacarpal joint degeneration.

Treatment includes rest, NSAIDs, and forearm-based thumb splint [34]. Corticosteroid injection into the tendon sheath is often successful [35–37]. Surgical release is performed if non-operative treatment fails.

25.3.2 Ulnar Wrist Pain

ECU tendinopathy and TFCC tear resulting in DRUJ instability are the most common causes for ulnar wrist pain in athletes, especially for those playing golf, tennis, football, baseball, rugby, hockey, and basketball. Due to their similarity in symptoms, and their comparative prevalence in sports, it can be a diagnostic challenge. The other less common but frequently missed conditions are ulnar nerve irritation and ulnar artery thrombosis.

Like radial wrist pain, clinical assessment utilizes identification of localized tenderness. On examination, palpate for tenderness over the ulnar styloid, TFC, ulnar head, lunotriquetral ligament, and hook of hamate. Additional investigation like X-ray, CT, MRI, or nerve conduction study may be necessary.

25.3.2.1 Extensor Carpi Ulnaris Tendinopathy

ECU tendinopathy is a condition that results from chronic loading of the tendon, due to repetitive flexion and extension of the wrist, particularly in supination. This is most frequently seen in tennis players and golfers [10]. There will be swelling and a constant dull ache on the dorso-ulnar aspect of the wrist and sudden searing pain felt along the ECU tendon on active contraction of the muscle. The ECU synergy test is a sensitive and specific test for ECU tendinitis [38]. This test is performed with the wrist in supination and neutral flexion/extension. Pain is felt over the ECU tendon when the adducted and extended index and middle fingers are resisted. Ultrasound and MRI show a thickened tendon with increased fluid in the surrounding sheath [25]. Management is usually conservative with NSAIDs and a short arm splint to maintain the wrist at 30° extension and ulnar deviation for 3 weeks [10]. A corticosteroid injection may be given if conservative therapies fail. Surgical debridement of the tendon and release of the compartment are usually not necessary.

25.3.2.2 Triangular Fibrocartilage Complex Tear and Distal Radioulnar Joint Instability

For *TFCC tear with DRUJ instability*, patient usually complains of ulnar wrist pain following a fall. Pain may be precipitated by activities which require forceful wrist flexion and rotation (e.g., golf, racket sports, wringing dry a towel, or opening a jar). DRUJ ballottement test, ulnocarpal stress test, and press test are some of the common maneuvers to elicit DRUJ joint instability [25]. The movements need to be compared with the unaffected side to differentiate normal from pathological laxity.

First-line imaging are plain radiographs. Radiographs will identify fractures and positive ulnar variance (predisposes for ulnar impaction syndrome and TFCC degenerative tear) [25]. For patients with significant injuries or persistent pain, an MRI is commonly used to assess the integrity of TFCC. It has a sensitivity of 67–100% and specificity of 71–100% [39]. MRI arthrogram appears to be superior in the diagnosis but is a more uncomfortable investigation. Diagnostic wrist arthroscopy remains the gold standard in the assessment of TFCC.

In the acute case, the forearm is immobilized in an above-elbow splint in supination for 6 weeks. For chronic DRUJ instability, surgery is required [10, 25]. Arthroscopic repair and reconstruction have gained popularity over open surgery in recent years. In the setting of positive ulnar variance, concomitant ulnar shortening osteotomy or wafer procedure should be considered. Six weeks of immobilization is recommended postoperatively. Rehabilitation starts after this period, with the aim to return to sports after 3–6 months.

25.3.2.3 Ulnar Nerve Irritation

Ulnar nerve irritation at the wrist can be a result of hook of hamate fracture non-union, causing repetitive trauma to the nerve, or chronic pressure applied to the area of Guyon's canal, typically seen in cyclists with sustained gripping of the handlebars. Symptoms include pain felt in the hypothenar area and numbness of the ring and little finger, sparing the dorsum of the hand [40]. In chronic cases, weakness of the intrinsic muscle of the hand may be observed. While the diagnosis is mainly clinical, nerve conduction test can be used to confirm and to differentiate the diagnosis from cubital tunnel syndrome. Treatment is often conservative. Making recommendations to change hand positions on the handlebars and wearing cycling gloves with protective gel padding are strategies to reduce the chronic pressure. In some cases, a rest from cycling, prescribing nonsteroidal anti-inflammatory medication, and a period in a wrist splint may be appropriate. In cases of hook of hamate non-union, surgical excision of the hook of hamate may be performed if conservative therapy fails.

25.3.2.4 Ulnar Artery Thrombosis

Ulnar artery thrombosis, also known as hypothenar hammer syndrome, is a condition of which results from repetitive microtrauma to the ulnar artery at the level of Guyon's canal [41]. This can occur with baseball, badminton, handball, football, hockey, karate, and golf [42]. Patient complains of the presence of a tender mass in the

Fact Box: Wrist Injuries

- Often missed, produce early arthritis and persistent pain and stiffness
- **Diffused wrist pain and swelling**
  - Acute: distal radius fracture and perilunate dislocation
  - Chronic: wrist arthritis—posttraumatic

- **Radial wrist pain and swelling**
  - Acute: Fracture of scaphoid or radial styloid and SL dissociation
  - Chronic: SLAC, SNAC, and de Quervain's tenosynovitis
- **Ulnar wrist pain and swelling**
  - Acute: DRUJ instability, ECU instability, and hook of hamate fracture
  - Chronic: ECU tendinopathy, TFCC tear, DRUJ instability, ulnar nerve irritation, and ulnar artery thrombosis
- **Investigation**
  - X-ray first line
- If symptoms persist, CT for bone or MRI for soft tissue

hypothenar eminence, pain in the palm, ulnar nerve irritation, as well as ischemic changes to the ring finger and little finger. Ultrasound and MRI/MR angiography can be used to confirm the diagnosis [43]. Conservative management includes rest from aggravating activities, smoking cessation, and the use of vasodilators. Surgical management involves excising and reconstructing the thrombosed segment with a vein graft [42].

25.4 Acute Hand Injury

Unlike wrist injuries, where both acute and chronic injuries are common, most hand injuries in sports are caused by a single traumatic event. However, they are commonly missed and often present late.

25.4.1 Metacarpal and Phalangeal Fracture

Metacarpal and *phalangeal fractures* are the most common fractures of the upper extremity in athletes, especially those in contact and ball sports. Most of these fractures are low-energy trauma from a direct blow, twisting, or crush injury [1]. Closed, simple extra-articular, and undisplaced intra-articular phalangeal fractures with no rotational deformity can be managed with protected mobilization with buddy taping for 4 weeks.

Closed fractures of the proximal 2/3 of the proximal phalanx can be unstable, due to the intrinsic muscles flexing the proximal fragment and the extensor mechanism extending the distal fragment. After closed reduction, the MCPJ is splinted in 70° flexion for 4 weeks. Splinting in MCP joint flexion with PIP joint extension at rest allows the extension mechanism to provide a compressive force that stabilizes the fracture [44]. For fractures with rotational deformity, derotation taping can be used [45]. When a fifth metacarpal fracture has involved the ulnar nerve, the malrotation is reduced and then the Jahss maneuver performed. The finger is taped, so that the rotation is maintained and then an ulnar gutter is applied with the MCP in flexion. If there is marked flexion or shortening, then internal fixation with K wires, mini-screws or plates, and screws has been advocated [46–48]. In all cases, early mobilization is needed to prevent finger stiffness.

25.4.2 Fractures of the Metacarpal Neck

Fractures of the metacarpal neck are common in combat sports. *Boxer fracture*, a fracture of the fifth metacarpal neck, is the most prevalent of all, but it is not limited just to boxers. In fact, trained boxers typically punch with greater force at the second and third rays. When no rotational deformity is present, angulation is usually accepted, ranging from 10° in the second metacarpal up to 40° in the fifth ray. For the repeat offender, up to 70° of flexion can be tolerated in the fifth metacarpal neck [49]. In cases of rotational deformity, closed reduction and derotation taping can be performed [45]. Reduction and fixation may be required if the metacarpal head is flexed to the point that it is prominent in the hand and causes discomfort with gripping [50].

25.4.3 Proximal Interphalangeal Joint Injuries

Proximal interphalangeal joint (*PIPJ*) injuries are common in ball sports, when the finger is jammed at the time of catching a ball, causing a hyperextension injury. As they are often managed on field by the coach, they have been described as the "coach's finger" [51]. Unfortunately, these are often missed and can end up with a poor outcome [52]. This highlights the importance of professional assessment and management of these injuries, of which we follow an algorithm (Fig. 25.5).

It is critical to have good-quality AP and lateral radiographs of the injured finger. *Dorsal dislocation* is the most common and usually associated with an avulsion of the volar plate with a fracture of the volar rim of the middle phalanx (Fig. 25.6) [53]. The dislocation needs to be reduced in the acute setting, usually via a closed reduction under ring block. Traction together with pressure to the dorsal aspect of the base of the middle phalanx as the finger is brought into flexion is recommended for reduction. Postreduction radiograph of the finger is needed to confirm a congruent joint reduction. Stability and laxity should also be checked clinically.

On the lateral radiograph, the presence of dorsal displacement should be accurately assessed. Any dorsal subluxation of the middle phalanx on the lateral radiograph is abnormal. If the fracture is <33% of the articular surface, it is usually stable and can be treated with reduction of the dislocation and protected mobilization. Dorsal block splint with the PIPJ at 20–30° of flexion is given for 3 weeks and may be followed by a period of buddy splinting [54].

When the avulsion fracture is >33% of the articular surface, the construct is unstable because the collateral ligament is attached to the avulsed fragment [55]. This large fragment usually requires fixation to provide joint stability. If the joint remains subluxated or the volar fragment is comminuted, then surgical management can be difficult but is usually required.

Volar dislocation of the PIP joint is uncommon and has a poor prognosis as the central slip is usually involved [56]. Joint reduction is required, and the central slip either repaired or allowed to heal, but with the joint stabilization with a K wire [56].

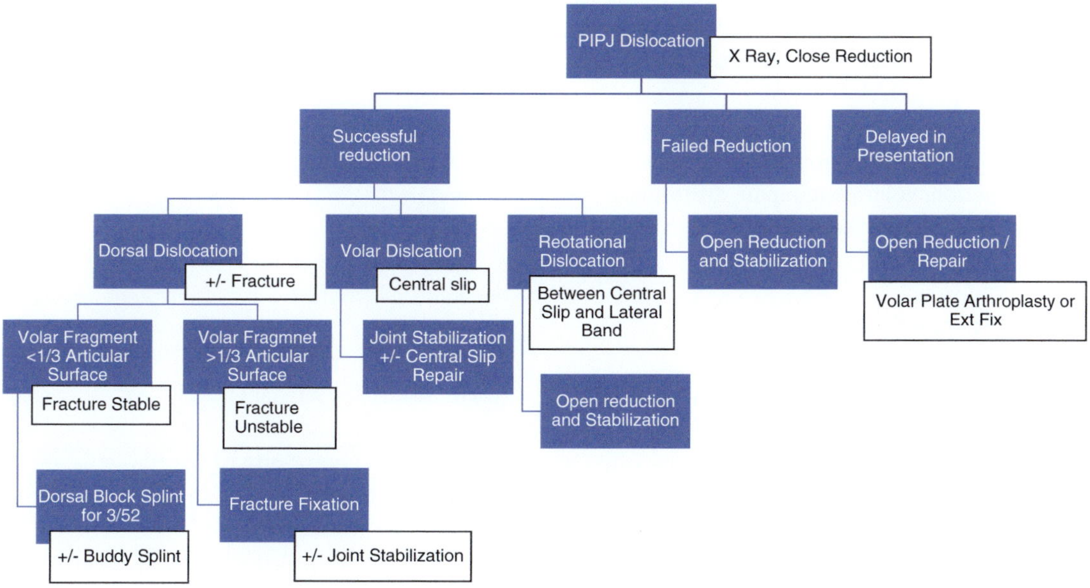

Fig. 25.5 Algorithm in managing PIPJ injuries

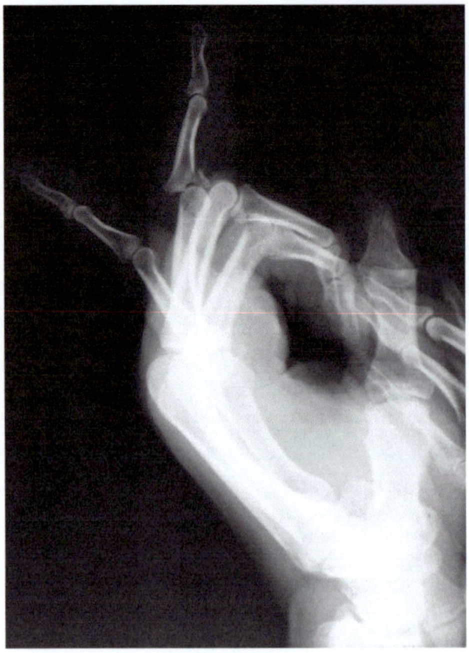

Fig. 25.6 Lateral radiograph of ring finger showing PIP joint fracture dislocation

If the PIP joint is malrotated on examination or the proximal and middle phalanx appear to have different rotations, then there is likely to be a *rotatory dislocation*. The condyle of proximal phalanx usually buttonholes between the central slip and lateral bands. Therefore open reduction, repair, and Kirchner wire pinning are recommended [57].

In cases of *delayed presentation* or failed closed reduction, surgical management including open reduction, volar plate repair, arthroplasty, or external fixation may be required [52, 57].

25.4.4 Jersey Finger

Jersey finger is an avulsion of the flexor digitorum profundus tendon (FDP) from the distal phalangeal joint, which usually occurs when a player grasps an opposition player's jersey [28]. There will be painful "pop," and the athlete will present with a stiff swollen finger and can't flex the DIPJ. Radiographs are required to identify any associated fracture. A three-level classification has prognostic value as it reflects the integrity of the nutrient support of the tendon (Fig. 25.7) [58–60]. Early surgical repair is recommended. In a delayed presentation or in a case where the patient refuses to undergo a prolonged tendon rehabilitation, excision of the stump may be performed if discomfort is experienced and the patient accepts the inability of flexing the DIPJ [28].

25.4.5 Mallet Finger

Mallet finger is the failure of the terminal extensor digitorum tendon which typically presents with a flexed DIPJ, as they are unable to actively extend the joint. Volar subluxation of the DIPJ is not uncommon on radiographs. The majority of mallet fingers can be satisfactorily treated with a short mallet splint, holding the DIPJ in full extension all of the time for 6–8 weeks [61]. Surgical Kirchner wire or screw fixation may be indicated if the fractures involve >30% of the articular surface and volar subluxation of the DIPJ [28].

Fact Box: Hand Injuries

Assessment

- Often misdiagnosed as just a finger sprain
- Most can be treated conservatively with a splint
- Most dislocations can be treated with reduction and splint
- Stability must be checked post reduction

Indications for surgery

- Open fractures
- Rotational deformity of the finger
- Joint incongruity
- Multiple fractures

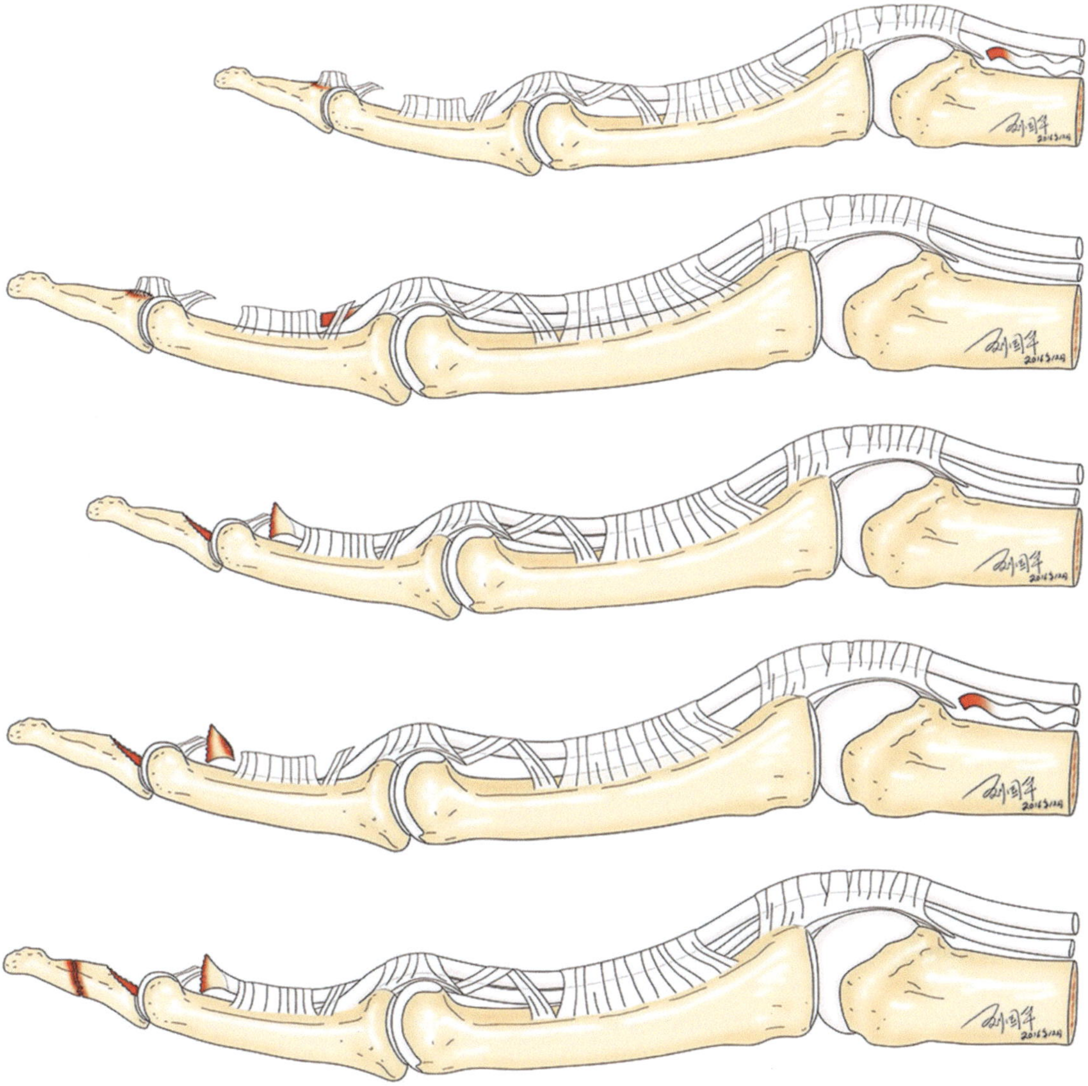

Fig. 25.7 Classification of jersey fingers (Copyright Dr. Margaret Fok)

25.4.6 Traumatic Subluxation of the Extensor Tendon/Sagittal Band Rupture

Traumatic subluxation of the extensor tendon at the metacarpophalangeal joint (MCPJ) is caused by rupture of the sagittal band (usually the radial side), which is the primary stabilizer of the extensor tendon at the MCPJ level (Fig. 25.8) [62]. There may be extensor tendon triggering, as the extensor tendon snaps over the metacarpal head during movement from flexion to extension. In acute (<3 weeks), a hand therapist should make a custom-made splint to block MCPJ from flexion while freeing PIPJ for 6–8 weeks. With a delayed presentation, a repair or reconstruction of the sagittal band is needed [28]. A splint is needed for protection for 6 weeks postoperatively.

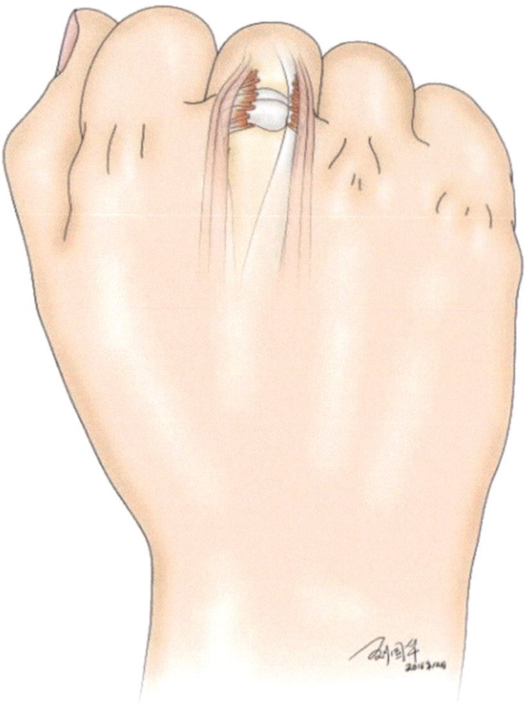

Fig. 25.8 Radial sagittal band rupture causing extensor tendon subluxation to the ulnar side (Copyright Dr. Margaret Fok)

25.4.7 Skier's or Gamekeeper's Thumb

Skier's thumb is a rupture of the ulnar collateral ligament (UCL) of the first MCPJ. It is common in recreational skiing, following a fall, and in ball sports [63]. There are pain, swelling, and weakness in pinch grip due to the instability of the MCP joint.

If the MCP joint is unstable in full extension, and in 30° flexion, then the UCL, accessory collateral ligaments, and the volar plate are disrupted [64]. Ultrasound or MRI can be performed in cases where complete ULC tear is suspected. A Stener lesion occurs when the ruptured UCL is displaced and the adductor pollicis muscle becomes interposed between the ruptured UCL and its insertion [65]. Immobilization in a thumb splint for 4–6 weeks is recommended with partial and complete UCL tear without Stener lesion. For the Stener lesion or gross instability, surgical repair is indicated. In cases of delayed presentation, i.e., after 3 months, UCL reconstruction may be necessary [63].

25.5 Rehabilitation for Hand and Wrist Injuries

The role of the hand therapist is critical in rehabilitation following wrist and hand injuries and surgery. Hand therapists provide valuable education, edema control, scar management, orthoses, and exercises.

Education is a key component to managing de Quervain's tendinopathy, as risk factors include poor skills in the sport, inadequate neuromuscular control, and increased time spent performing the sport. These factors can be addressed by patient education, skills acquisition, and activity modification [66].

Edema routinely occurs after injury, creating tension in tissues that can lead to predictable deformity. Hand swelling will limit finger joint and tendon motion, which can create permanent contractures and compromise function and performance. Wrist injuries often develop difficulty with supination and flexion. Finger injuries often develop difficulty with MCP flexion and PIP and DIP joint extension [67]. Methods to reduce edema include compression, elevation, exercise, and manual edema mobilization [68].

Static orthotics are used to immobilize healing tissues, to prevent deformity and to prevent contracture of soft tissue. Collateral ligament length is maintained by splinting the IP joints in extension and MCP joints in 70–90° of flexion [67]. A

Fact Box: Tendon and Ligament Injuries of the Digits

- Tendon/ligament injuries are often associated with a bony avulsion.
- Does the tendon/ligament avulsion affect joint stability or tendon function?
- **Indications for surgery**
  - FDP avulsion
  - Gamekeeper's thumb (UCL MCP joint)
  - Large bony mallet finger fractures

wrist extension immobilization orthotic can be used to treat wrist fractures and is often used for carpal instability, to relieve pain and prevent movements that aggravates symptoms, in conjunction with isometric exercises and advice on activity modification [69].

Uncertainty surrounds the optimal time frames to introduce exercises and limit the period of immobilization. Shorter immobilization periods, so that exercises are started earlier, have been found to be more effective than longer immobilization periods for some wrist fractures [70] and similarly effective for boxer's fractures [71] and wrist sprains [72].

Exercises are designed to restore passive or active limitations to specific structures. Movement can be isolated at specific joints, referred to as blocking exercises. Differential tendon gliding exercises promote full excursion of the flexor digitorum superficialis (FDS) and flexor digitorum profundus (FDP) tendons and are important for preventing hand or wrist stiffness. An active limitation, or lag, due to weakness can be addressed with place and hold exercises, which encourage maximal contraction required to achieve full active joint motion [67].

Specific exercises are progressed to retraining functional tasks needed for daily activities and sport. Sports-specific drills vary resistance, repetitions, speed, and volume of training to restore strength, coordination, and confidence before returning to competition.

Take-Home Messages

- Wrist and hand injuries are very common in sports trauma. However, they are often missed or treated as simple sprains. A high index of suspicion is needed when symptoms and signs persist. A thorough and detailed physical examination may suggest the structure(s) involved. Additional imaging, like CT scan and MRI scan, is recommended if X-ray is unremarkable or difficult to interpret.
- Most injuries can be treated conservatively with a satisfactory outcome. In contrast, when the presentation is delayed, early degenerative changes may have occurred, and a salvage procedure may be indicated instead. An example is an undisplaced fracture of the scaphoid, of which 90% will heal in a cast. Yet untreated is likely to result in a non-union and then a SNAC wrist in 10–15 years.
- Surgery is indicated for some presentations seen in acute settings. Examples are finger fractures with rotational deformity, PIPJ volar dislocation, and Stener lesion in a skier's thumb.
- Rehabilitation is an important part in the management of many wrist and hand injuries. Different kinds of exercise are recommended in different stages of the healing process. Patients and hand therapists need to work hand in hand to achieve the best outcomes.

Acknowledgment For assistance in preparation of this manuscript, Kimberley Ruxton, Research Manager, Department of Orthopaedic Surgery, Flinders University, and Flinders Medical Centre, Adelaide, Australia; upperlimb@flinders.edu.au; +61882044289.

References

1. Rettig AC. Athletic injuries of the wrist and hand. Part I: traumatic injuries of the wrist. Am J Sports Med. 2003;31:1038–48.
2. Rettig AC. Epidemiology of hand and wrist injuries in sports. Clin Sports Med. 1998;17:401–6.
3. Gilula LA, Weeks PM. Post-traumatic ligamentous instabilities of the wrist. Radiology. 1978;129:641–51.
4. Corre AL, Huynh KP, Dhaliwal RS, Bain GI. Development of a protocol for SPECT/CT in the assessment of wrist disorders. J Wrist Surg. 2016;5:297–305.
5. Green DP, O'Brien ET. Classification and management of carpal dislocations. Clin Orthop Relat Res. 1980;(149):55–72.
6. Dunn JC, Koehler LR, Kusnezov NA, Polfer E, Orr JD, Pirela-Cruz MA, Mitchell JS. Perilunate dislocations and perilunate fracture dislocations in the U.S. military. J Wrist Surg. 2018;7:57–65.
7. Woon CY-L, Baxamusa T. A stepwise approach to management of open radiocarpal fracture-dislocations: a case report. J Hand Surg Asian Pac Vol. 2017;22:366–70.
8. Watson HK, Ballet FL. The SLAC wrist: scapholunate advanced collapse pattern of degenerative arthritis. J Hand Surg Am. 1984;9:358–65.
9. Mack GR, Bosse MJ, Gelberman RH, Yu E. The natural history of scaphoid non-union. J Bone Joint Surg Am. 1984;66:504–9.

10. Fufa DT, Goldfarb CA. Sports injuries of the wrist. Curr Rev Musculoskelet Med. 2012;6:35–40.
11. Suh N, Grewal R. Controversies and best practices for acute scaphoid fracture management. J Hand Surg Eur Vol. 2018;43:4–12.
12. Grewal R, Suh N, MacDermid JC. Is casting for non-displaced simple scaphoid waist fracture effective? A CT based assessment of union. Open Orthop J. 2016;10:431–8.
13. Bond CD, Shin AY, McBride MT, Dao KD. Percutaneous screw fixation or cast immobilization for nondisplaced scaphoid fractures. J Bone Joint Surg Am. 2001;83:483–8.
14. Ram AN, Chung KC. Evidence-based management of acute nondisplaced scaphoid waist fractures. J Hand Surg Am. 2009;34:735–8.
15. Ibrahim T, Qureshi A, Sutton AJ, Dias JJ. Surgical versus nonsurgical treatment of acute minimally displaced and undisplaced scaphoid waist fractures: pairwise and network meta-analyses of randomized controlled trials. J Hand Surg Am. 2011;36:1759–1768.e1.
16. Düppe H, Johnell O, Lundborg G, Karlsson M, Redlund-Johnell I. Long-term results of fracture of the scaphoid. A follow-up study of more than thirty years. J Bone Joint Surg Am. 1994;76:249–52.
17. Helm RH, Tonkin MA. The Chauffeur's fracture: simple or complex? J Hand Surg Br. 2016;17:156–9.
18. Chennagiri RJR, Lindau TR. Assessment of scapholunate instability and review of evidence for management in the absence of arthritis. J Hand Surg Eur Vol. 2013;38:727–38.
19. Kitay A, Wolfe SW. Scapholunate instability: current concepts in diagnosis and management. J Hand Surg Am. 2012;37:2175–96.
20. Fok MWM, Fernandez DL. Chronic scapholunate instability treated with temporary screw fixation. J Hand Surg Am. 2015;40:752–8.
21. Fok MWM, Fang CX, Lau TW, Fung YKE, Fung BKK, Leung FKL. The status of triangular fibrocartilage complex after the union of distal radius fractures with internal plate fixation. Int Orthop. 2018;78:357–1922.
22. Kim JK, Yun Y-H, Kim DJ, Yun GU. Comparison of united and nonunited fractures of the ulnar styloid following volar-plate fixation of distal radius fractures. Injury. 2011;42:371–5.
23. Wijffels M, Ring D. The influence of non-union of the ulnar styloid on pain, wrist function and instability after distal radius fracture. J Hand Microsurg. 2011;3:11–4.
24. Minami A. Triangular fibrocartilage complex tears. Hand Surg. 2015;20:1–9.
25. Pang EQ, Yao J. Ulnar-sided wrist pain in the athlete (TFCC/DRUJ/ECU). Curr Rev Musculoskelet Med. 2017;10:53–61.
26. Henry MH. Management of acute triangular fibrocartilage complex injury of the wrist. J Am Acad Orthop Surg. 2008;16:320–9.
27. Campbell D, Campbell R, O'Connor P, Hawkes R. Sports-related extensor carpi ulnaris pathology: a review of functional anatomy, sports injury and management. Br J Sports Med. 2013;47:1105–11.
28. Fok MWM, Liu B, White J, Bain G. Hand and wrist tendinopathies. In: Muscle and tendon injuries. 5th ed. Berlin: Springer; 2017. p. 241–53.
29. Inoue G, Tamura Y. Surgical treatment for recurrent dislocation of the extensor carpi ulnaris tendon. J Hand Surg Br. 2001;26:556–9.
30. Burkhart SS, Wood MB, Linscheid RL. Posttraumatic recurrent subluxation of the extensor carpi ulnaris tendon. J Hand Surg Am. 1982;7:1–3.
31. Whalen JL, Bishop AT, Linscheid RL. Nonoperative treatment of acute hamate hook fractures. J Hand Surg Am. 1992;17:507–11.
32. Scheufler O, Kamusella P, Tadda L, Radmer S, Russo SG, Andresen R. High incidence of hamate hook fractures in underwater rugby players: diagnostic and therapeutic implications. Hand Surg. 2013;18:357–63.
33. Stein AH. Stenosing tendovaginitis at the radial styloid process (de Quervain's disease). Arch Surg. 1951;63:216–28.
34. Adams JE, Habbu R. Tendinopathies of the hand and wrist. J Am Acad Orthop Surg. 2015;23:741–50.
35. Jirarattanaphochai K, Saengnipanthkul S, Vipulakorn K, Jianmongkol S, Chatuparisute P, Jung S. Treatment of de Quervain disease with triamcinolone injection with or without nimesulide. J Bone Joint Surg Am. 2004;86:2700–6.
36. Peters-Veluthamaningal C, van der Windt DA, Winters JC, Meyboom-de Jong B. Corticosteroid injection for de Quervain's tenosynovitis. Cochrane Database Syst Rev. 2009;27A:322.
37. Richie CA, Briner WW. Corticosteroid injection for treatment of de Quervain's tenosynovitis: a pooled quantitative literature evaluation. J Am Board Fam Pract. 2003;16:102–6.
38. Ruland RT, Hogan CJ. The ECU synergy test: an aid to diagnose ECU tendonitis. J Hand Surg Am. 2008;33:1777–82.
39. Lee RKL, Ng AWH, Tong CSL, Griffith JF, Tse WL, Wong C, Ho PC. Intrinsic ligament and triangular fibrocartilage complex tears of the wrist: comparison of MDCT arthrography, conventional 3-T MRI, and MR arthrography. Skelet Radiol. 2013;42:1277–85.
40. Ruchelsman DE, Lee SK. Neurovascular injuries of the hand in athletes. Curr Orthop Prac. 2009;20:409–15.
41. Kumar Y, Hooda K, Lo L, Karol I. Ulnar artery aneurysm and hypothenar hammer syndrome. BMJ Case Rep. 2015;2015:bcr2015211444.
42. Müller LP, Rudig L, Kreitner KF, Degreif J. Hypothenar hammer syndrome in sports. Knee Surg Sports Traumatol Arthrosc. 1996;4:167–70.
43. Blum AG, Zabel J-P, Kohlmann R, Batch T, Barbara K, Zhu X, Dautel G, Dap F. Pathologic conditions of the hypothenar eminence: evaluation with multidetector CT and MR imaging. Radiographics. 2006;26:1021–44.

44. Fok MWM, Ip WY, Fung BKK, Chan RK, Chow SP. Ten-year results using a dynamic treatment for proximal phalangeal fractures of the hands. Orthopedics. 2013;36:e348–52.
45. Bain GI, Guy SD. Derotation taping for metacarpal and phalangeal fractures. Tech Hand Up Extrem Surg. 2003;7:130–2.
46. Carpenter S, Rohde RS. Treatment of phalangeal fractures. Hand Clin. 2013;29:519–34.
47. Gaston RG, Chadderdon C. Phalangeal fractures: displaced/nondisplaced. Hand Clin. 2012;28:395–401, x
48. Kollitz KM, Hammert WC, Vedder NB, Huang JI. Metacarpal fractures: treatment and complications. Hand (N Y). 2014;9:16–23.
49. Fufa DT, Goldfarb CA. Fractures of the thumb and finger metacarpals in athletes. Hand Clin. 2012;28:379–88, x
50. Goldfarb CA. Commentary metacarpal fracture in the professional baseball player. Hand Clin. 2012;28:389.
51. McCue FC, Andrews JR, Hakala M, Gieck JH. The coach's finger. J Sports Med. 1974;2:270–5.
52. Bain GI, Mehta JA, Heptinstall RJ, Bria M. Dynamic external fixation for injuries of the proximal interphalangeal joint. J Bone Joint Surg Br. 1998;80:1014–9.
53. Chen F, Kalainov DM. Phalanx fractures and dislocations in athletes. Curr Rev Musculoskelet Med. 2017;10:10–6.
54. Bain GI, Roth JH, Mehta JA. Injuries of the proximal interphalangeal joint. Br J Hand Ther. 2016;3:9–12.
55. de Haseth KB, Neuhaus V, Mudgal CS. Dorsal fracture-dislocations of the proximal interphalangeal joint: evaluation of closed reduction and percutaneous Kirschner wire pinning. Hand (N Y). 2014;10:88–93.
56. Bain GI, Mehta JA. The proximal interphalangeal joint: surgical and mobilisation options. Br J Hand Ther. 2016;3:13–8.
57. Rettig AC. Athletic injuries of the wrist and hand: part II: overuse injuries of the wrist and traumatic injuries to the hand. Am J Sports Med. 2004;32:262–73.
58. Leddy JP, Packer JW. Avulsion of the profundus tendon insertion in athletes. J Hand Surg Am. 1977;2:66–9.
59. Al-Qattan MM. Type 5 avulsion of the insertion of the flexor digitorum profundus tendon. J Hand Surg Br. 2001;26:427–31.
60. Smith JH. Avulsion of a profundus tendon with simultaneous intraarticular fracture of the distal phalanx–case report. J Hand Surg Am. 1981;6:600–1.
61. Garberman SF, Diao E, Peimer CA. Mallet finger: results of early versus delayed closed treatment. J Hand Surg Am. 1994;19:850–2.
62. Lin JD, Strauch RJ. Closed soft tissue extensor mechanism injuries (mallet, boutonniere, and sagittal band). J Hand Surg Am. 2014;39:1005–11.
63. Avery DM, Inkellis ER, Carlson MG. Thumb collateral ligament injuries in the athlete. Curr Rev Musculoskelet Med. 2017;10:28–37.
64. Malik AK, Morris T, Chou D, Sorene E, Taylor E. Clinical testing of ulnar collateral ligament injuries of the thumb. J Hand Surg Eur Vol. 2009;34:363–6.
65. Stener B. Displacement of the ruptured ulnar collateral ligament of the metacarpo-phalangeal joint of the thumb. J Bone Joint Surg Br. 1962;44-B:869–79.
66. Fedorczyk JM. Tendinopathies of the elbow, wrist, and hand: histopathology and clinical considerations. J Hand Ther. 2012;25:191–201.
67. Cooper C. Fundamentals of hand therapy. Amsterdam: Elsevier Health Sciences; 2013.
68. Knygsand-Roenhoej K, Maribo T. A randomized clinical controlled study comparing the effect of modified manual edema mobilization treatment with traditional edema technique in patients with a fracture of the distal radius. J Hand Ther. 2011;24:184–94.
69. Prosser R, Herbert R, LaStayo PC. Current practice in the diagnosis and treatment of carpal instability—results of a survey of Australian hand therapists. J Hand Ther. 2007;20:239–43.
70. Bruder AM, Shields N, Dodd KJ, Taylor NF. Prescribed exercise programs may not be effective in reducing impairments and improving activity during upper limb fracture rehabilitation: a systematic review. J Physiother. 2017;63:205–20.
71. Muller MGS, Poolman RW, van Hoogstraten MJ, Steller EP. Immediate mobilization gives good results in boxer's fractures with volar angulation up to 70 degrees: a prospective randomized trial comparing immediate mobilization with cast immobilization. Arch Orthop Trauma Surg. 2003;123:534–7.
72. Clementson M, Thomsen N, Jørgsholm P, Besjakov J, Björkman A. Is early mobilisation better than immobilisation in the treatment of wrist sprains? J Plast Surg Hand Surg. 2016;50:156–60.

26 Sports Trauma: The Hip

Molly C. Meadows and Marc R. Safran

26.1 Introduction

Hip injuries are common among athletes, representing approximately 6% of all sports injuries [1]. Furthermore, hip injuries have received increased attention in recent years as a result of identification of sources of non-arthritic hip pain and damage, improved evaluation techniques, such as physical examination and imaging, as well as less morbid approaches to evaluation and management of hip problems, such as hip arthroscopy.

The hip joint is a constrained synovial joint that functions to support the body in static and dynamic activities. The fibrous capsule with ligamentous thickenings and the acetabular labrum contribute to the inherent stability of the hip joint. Finally, the multiple muscles crossing the hip joint further contribute to dynamic stability of the hip throughout the physiologic range of motion. However, there is wide variability in the bony morphology of the hip, leading to predisposition to intra- and extra-articular hip pathology. Furthermore, multiple studies have demonstrated an increased prevalence of femoroacetabular impingement (FAI) anatomy in athletes as compared to the general population, leading to an increased risk of intra-articular injury to the hip joint.

Symptoms about the hip and groin in athletes can present a diagnostic challenge, as pain can be referred from multiple locations including the lumbar spine, genitourinary system, extra-articular musculature, and hip joint itself. Understanding the diagnosis and management of common hip injuries in athletes is essential to appropriate treatment, as well as to maximize outcomes and return to play.

26.2 Muscle Strains/Sprains

Muscle strains are the most common type of athletic injury to the hip and groin region. These injuries typically occur from an eccentric contraction in a muscle group crossing two joints. While strains most frequently occur at the myotendinous junction, they can occur anywhere along the muscle belly. The most common muscle strain injuries about the hip occur to the hip flexors, quadriceps, hamstrings, and adductor muscles [1]. These injuries can be classified as grade I, II, or III depending on the severity of the injury. Grade I strains involve tearing of a few muscle fibers with pain but minimal loss of strength. Grade II injuries involve more extensive partial tearing with some strength loss. Grade III injuries are complete tears with loss of function. In adolescent patients, the origin or insertion of

M. C. Meadows · M. R. Safran (✉)
Division of Sports Medicine, Department of Orthopaedic Surgery, Stanford University, Stanford, CA, USA
e-mail: Mollym2@stanford.edu; msafran@stanford.edu

S. Rocha Piedade et al. (eds.), *The Sports Medicine Physician*,
https://doi.org/10.1007/978-3-030-10433-7_26

the tendon may be avulsed with a bony fragment, and these are classified as grade IIIB injuries [2].

Quadriceps strains most commonly involve the rectus femoris, often in sports that emphasize sprinting or kicking (Fig. 26.1a). These injuries typically present as pain and swelling in the anterior thigh, with painful and potentially weak knee extension with the hip flexed. Iliopsoas strains are also common hip flexor strains, and athletes may complain of groin or lower abdominal pain that is worse with attempts at resisted hip flexion (Fig. 26.1b). Adductor strains result from an abduc-

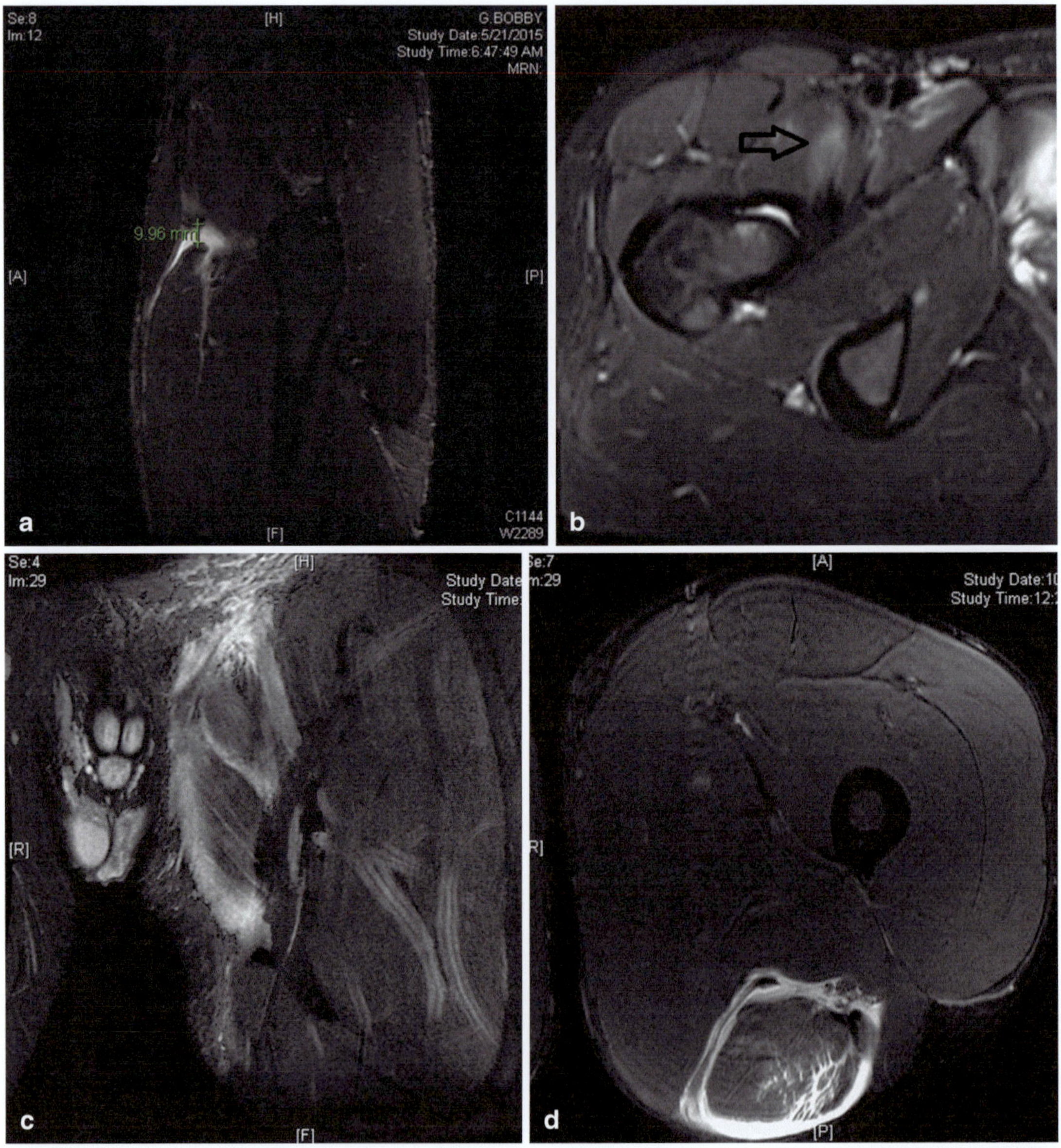

Fig. 26.1 Muscle strains. (**a**) Is an acute rectus femoris strain in an American professional football kicker seen on a sagittal view T2 MRI. The green line demonstrates the nearly 1 cm displacement of the tendon from the anterior inferior iliac spine. (**b**) Is a coronal T2 MRI of a professional tennis player with acute right iliopsoas strain. Arrow points to edema within the iliopsoas. (**c**) Demonstrates an acute adductor strain with diffuse edema in a male collegiate soccer player on coronal T2-weighted MRI. (**d**) Is an axial MRI (T2 weighted) of a 28-year-old professional American football player's thigh with an acute hamstring avulsion

tion force on the thigh during an attempted adduction movement, such as with kicking a soccer ball, but are also common during skating in ice hockey (Fig. 26.1c). As such, these are common injuries in American football, ice hockey, and soccer. They present as acute onset medial groin pain that is worse with resisted adduction [1]. Hip flexor injuries are the most common injury to the hip in NFL players, representing 63% of all muscle strains in this population. These injuries are also associated with cutting and pivoting maneuvers in sport. Hamstring injuries classically result from forced hip flexion with the knee in extension; however, any sport that involves rapid acceleration and deceleration puts the hamstring at risk for injury (Fig. 26.1d). Patients with a hamstring injury often describe a pop associated with pain and bruising at the posterior hip. In severe cases, a gap may be palpable at the posterior thigh. Functionally, there are two common main types of hamstring injury—injuries at the muscle-tendon junction, which are treated conservatively but have a high recurrence rate, and the hamstring avulsion from the ischial tuberosity, which may require surgery.

Radiographs in the setting of a suspected muscle strain are useful to assess for avulsion injury, particularly in skeletally immature patients. Additionally, MRI is a useful diagnostic and prognostic tool to evaluate the degree of muscle involvement or to distinguish a partial from a complete tear. The majority of muscle strains are treated non-operatively with rest, NSAIDs, and a progressive rehabilitation program. Rehabilitation should begin with gentle range of motion exercises and gradually progress to strengthening and sport-specific activity. In cases of complete tears, particularly of the hamstring tendon avulsion, surgical repair is recommended to return the athlete to their pre-injury level of function [1].

While typically amenable to nonsurgical management, muscle strains present a significant cause of disability in the athletic population. Indeed, among NFL players who sustained muscle strains, the overall mean playing time lost was 10.2 days, with a range of 1–197 days [3]. One study found that in a population of professional ice hockey players, a preseason exercise program was effective in reducing the incidence of adductor muscle strains [4]. Further studies are needed to identify athletes at risk for muscle strains and to develop effective exercise programs to mitigate these risks.

26.3 Hip Contusions

Contusions about the hip are common in contact sports, as they typically result from a collisions or falls to the ground [3]. Contusions range from superficial subcutaneous hematoma formation to more severe injuries involving subperiosteal edema. An iliac crest contusion, commonly referred to as a hip pointer, occurs from a direct blow to the iliac crest or a fall onto the anterior hip. These injuries present as acute pain over the iliac crest. Examination will often reveal an antalgic gait, tenderness to palpation, and decreased strength testing in any of the muscle groups that attach at the iliac crest [5]. Radiographs are obtained to rule out an iliac crest avulsion, as an apophysis may persist until age 25 (Fig. 26.2). Management of these injuries in the acute setting involves ice, compression, and a brief period of crutch use to reduce swelling and hematoma formation. As pain improves and bleeding subsides, typically around 3 days post-injury, a rehabilitation program can be initiated. In settings where immediate return to play is important, an injection of local anesthetic with or without corticosteroid can be performed to decrease pain. While

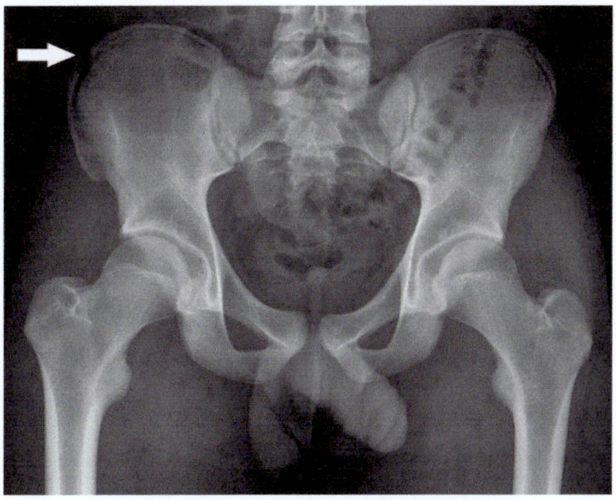

Fig. 26.2 Iliac crest avulsion fracture in a 19-year-old collegiate basketball player

there is no clear data to support this treatment option, reports demonstrate that elite athletes can often return to play immediately following injection with additional padding [6]. Aspiration of the lysed hematoma may also be attempted in high-level athletes to hasten return to sport.

Quadriceps contusions are another common injury in collision sports, typically as a result of a kick or direct helmet blow to the thigh. These injuries cause swelling and edema of the thigh and limited knee range of motion as a result of trauma to the muscle fibers. These injuries are classified based on knee range of motion at 12–24 h post-injury, with greater limitations in motion correlating with more severe injuries and prolonged recovery time [7]. Initial treatment involves immobilizing the knee at 120 degrees of flexion with compression and ice for the first 24 h post-injury, an algorithm that has been shown to decrease the time to return to full athletic activity, as the knee flexion limits hematoma formation [8]. While rare, very severe contusions should be monitored for anterior thigh compartment syndrome and managed accordingly. After the initial period of immobilization, unrestricted active range of motion exercises are initiated. Crutches are recommended until the athlete regains appropriate quadriceps muscle control, and gradual return to noncontact sport may begin when control and range of motion return. Contact is generally permitted at around the 3-week time point, provided the athlete has regained full strength. In collision sports, the use of a thigh pad may help reduce the risk of recurrent injury. Myositis ossificans is a late complication that can occur following a severe contusion, with reported occurrence rates of 9–14%, but may be avoided by early use of NSAIDS (started 48 h after injury). Myositis ossificans is self-limiting and typically does not require surgical treatment, but it can lead to a period of lost playing time secondary to pain [9].

26.4 Labral Tears/FAI

The acetabular labrum attaches to the bony rim and joins with the transverse acetabular ligament inferiorly to circumferentially cover the perimeter of the acetabulum. The anterior labrum typically has a smooth transition to articular cartilage at the chondral edge, whereas the posterior labrum is often separated from the underlying cartilage by a physiologic cleft [10]. The labrum serves to deepen the acetabular socket and provide a suction seal for the hip joint, thereby adding stability to the joint and protecting the articular cartilage [11, 12]. The strain along the acetabular labrum depends on the position of the lower extremity. The greatest strain at the posterior labrum results when the hip is flexed and adducted, whereas hyperextension and external rotation of the hip create strain at the anterior labrum [13].

Labral tears can result from an acute traumatic injury or more commonly from chronic repetitive microtrauma secondary to FAI or microinstability. FAI morphology includes CAM-type impingement from asphericity of the femoral head and pincer-type impingement from acetabular over-coverage. Both types of abnormal anatomy cause bony impingement against the acetabular rim and subsequent damage to the labrum. Multiple studies have demonstrated that participation in athletic activities is a risk factor for development of FAI, leading to increased prevalence of FAI and labral tears in the athletic population [14–17]. Patients with an acute labral tear will present with pain or catching in the groin area following a pivoting or cutting injury to the hip. However, in the setting of FAI and chronic labral injury, patients often cannot identify a specific inciting event. On physical examination, the flexion-adduction-internal rotation maneuver, often referred to as the impingement test, will elicit symptoms in patients with FAI. However, while very sensitive, this maneuver is not specific to impingement and may cause pain with any type of intra-articular pathology [18]. Additionally, a dynamic labral stress test taking the hip through a range of motion can be performed, which involves rotating and axially loading the hip in an impingement position, to elicit catching and pain from a torn labrum.

Radiographs, including a high-quality anteroposterior pelvis film and a lateral film of the affected hip, are essential in the setting of a suspected labral tear to evaluate for FAI anatomy (Fig. 26.3a). MRI with gadolinium can provide information regarding the presence of a labral tear or other intra-articular pathology, as well as further detail regarding the bony morphology of the hip and femur (Fig. 26.3b). While imaging is helpful to guide treatment, a diagnostic intra-articular injection of local anesthetic provides the most powerful tool to determine if intra-articular pathology is the cause of pain, as 70–90% of asymptomatic adults have labral tears on MRI [19]. Relief with an anesthetic can often be ascertained following an MR arthrography, as the contrast is combined with local anesthetic.

Treatment of labral tears and FAI typically begins with conservative measures such as activity modification, anti-inflammatory medications, and a focused physical therapy

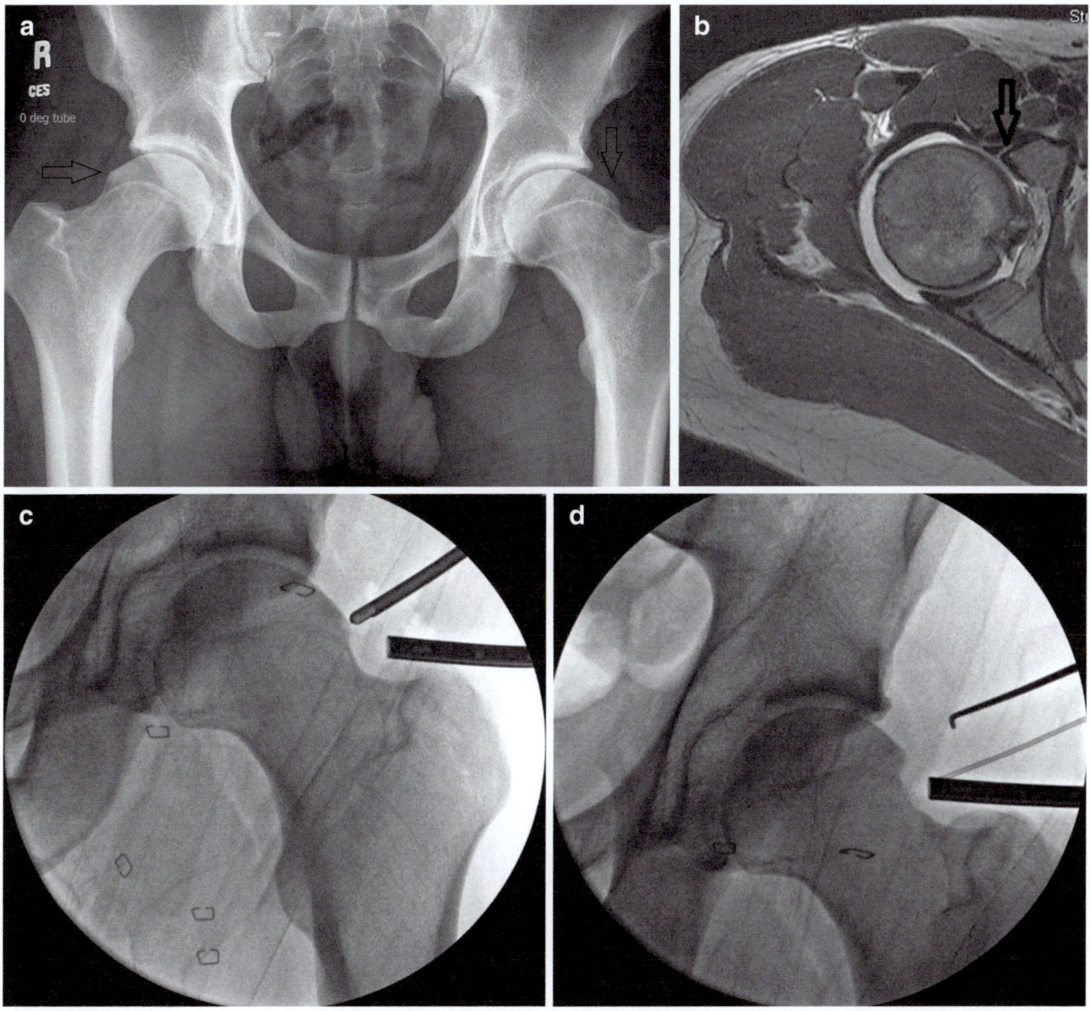

Fig. 26.3 FAI and labral tears. (**a**) Demonstrates an AP pelvis radiograph of an American professional ice hockey player with FAI. Arrows point to the cam lesion (asphericity of the femoral head). (**b**) Is a T1-weighted axial MRI of the right hip of a professional soccer player with the arrow pointing to the labrum separated from the acetabulum at the labral chondral junction. The labrum, to the left, looks homogeneous, while maintaining its triangular shape, while the acetabulum is to the right. (**c**) Is an intra-operative image of a collegiate basketball player with FAI—shaver is at the maximal offset of the cam lesion—while (**d**) is the same patient after resection of the cam lesion seen on intraoperative fluoroscopy

program. When symptoms persist despite conservative management, surgical management with hip arthroscopy is appropriate. In addition to addressing the labrum, acetabular rim resection, cheilectomy (femoral osteoplasty), chondroplasty, microfracture, debridement of ligamentum teres tears, and capsular plication can be performed to treat any additional pathology (Fig. 26.3c, d). With regard to management of the labrum at the time of arthroscopy, multiple studies have demonstrated superior outcomes following labral repair compared with debridement [20–22]. Thus, any unstable labrum amenable to repair should undergo refixation to recreate the suction seal. Selective debridement is an option in patients with irreparable labral tears and no evidence of instability. However, active athletes with significant labral deficiency or an irreparable labrum may be best treated with labral reconstruction to restore stability of the hip joint [23].

Outcomes of hip arthroscopy for athletes have been generally favorable, which high rates of return to play [24–26]. In a study of 98 elite-level athletes, 84.2% of female athletes and 83.3% of male athletes were able to return to their presurgery level of play at a mean age of 8.3 months for women and 8.8 months for men. A shorter duration of preoperative symptoms was predictive of return to baseline level of competition, suggesting that early intervention should be considered to optimize function and return to play [27].

Key Points

- Labral tears most commonly occur in the setting of FAI or hip instability.
- FAI is significantly more common in athletes than nonathletes.
- Intra-articular injection of anesthetic is a useful diagnostic tool.
- Hip arthroscopy is an effective treatment for symptomatic intra-articular pathology in the athletic population.
- Goals of arthroscopy should include labral repair, and management of chondral lesions, impingement, or capsular laxity as needed.

26.5 Hip Subluxation/Dislocation

While dislocation of the hip is a rare occurrence in sports, this injury is associated with significant morbidity, and timely recognition and management is paramount. Hip dislocation is more common in high-energy activities such as football [28]; however, it has been reported in a variety of different sports. While data regarding hip dislocations in athletes is limited, it has been estimated that approximately 2–5% of hip dislocations occur in the athletic setting [29]. Literature suggests that FAI anatomy places the hip at a higher risk for traumatic dislocation and subluxation in athletes [30, 31].

The direction of dislocation depends on the position of the hip at the time of impact. Posterior dislocations occur when a posterior force is directed against a flexed knee with the hip in a flexed, adducted, and internally rotated position. In sports, this occurs most frequently when an athlete's knee is forcefully directed against the field during a tackle. Anterior dislocations occur when the hip is forcefully flexed, abducted, and externally rotated. This typically occurs in sports such as gymnastics that involve split-type activities [32]. If hip dislocation is suspected, an on-field neurovascular examination should be performed, and urgent transport to a medical facility should be initiated. Minimizing time to reduction is essential to decrease the risk of avascular necrosis [33]. A single attempt at sideline reduction is appropriate, as the reduction can be easier prior to spasm of the surrounding muscles. However, multiple attempts should be avoided to minimize the risk of further damage to the articular cartilage. If a sideline reduction is successful, transfer to a medical facility is still required, as a postreduction CT scan is recommended to assess for associated fracture or presence of loose bodies within the joint (Fig. 26.4) [29]. While there is no clear consensus regarding management of simple dislocations without associated fracture, some authors recommend 6–8 weeks of toe touch weight-bearing, with gradual progressive return to full range of motion and athletic activity [33]. However, most high-level athletes who suffer a traumatic hip dislocation rarely return to the

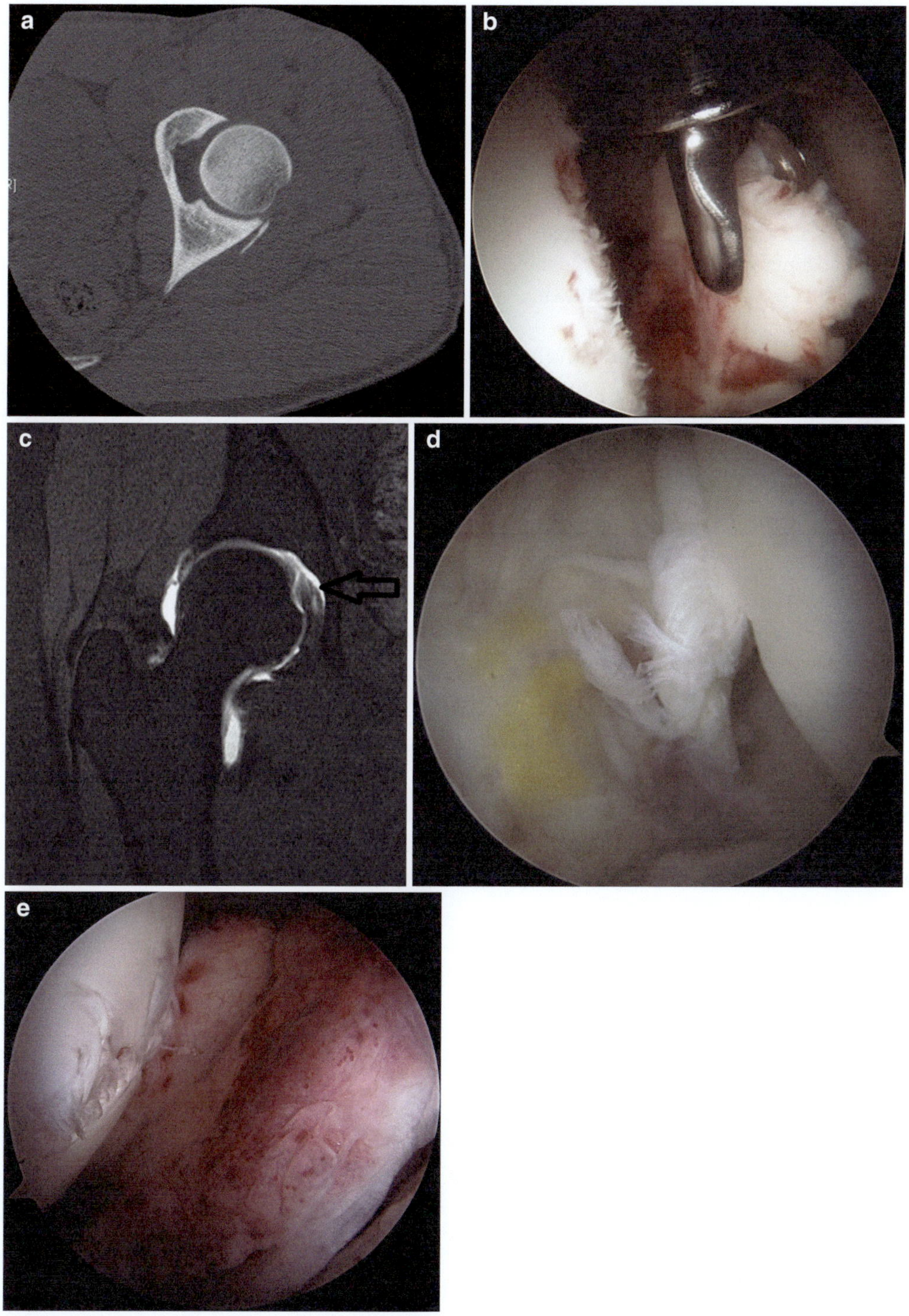

Fig. 26.4 Hip instability. Thirty-year-old male American professional football player following reduction of hip dislocation. (**a**) Is an axial cut of a CT scan demonstrating the lack of concentric reduction of the femoral head within the acetabulum. There is also a small posterior wall fracture seen. (**b**) Is an arthroscopic view demonstration of removal of a loose fragment of the femoral head articular cartilage that had sheared off. (**c**) Is a coronal MRI, T2 weighted, with an arrow pointing to a ligamentum teres tear in a competitive gymnast. (**d**) Is an arthroscopic view of a male martial artist with borderline dysplasia, demonstrating a ligamentum teres tear associated with hip instability. (**e**) is an arthroscopic picture from a female dancer with central femoral head chondromalacia as a result of microinstability

same level of play. Philippon et al. performed hip arthroscopy on 14 professional athletes following hip dislocation and noted labral tears and chondral defects in all patients, as well as loose bodies in 11 of 14 patients [34]. Despite these injuries, all 14 patients in this series returned to competitive sports at the professional level. However, these chondrolabral injuries, in addition to capsular laxity and microinstability, likely contribute to the overall poor outcomes following hip dislocation.

While hip dislocation is a relatively rare injury, hip subluxation is more common and less frequently recognized. A fall onto a flexed knee can cause a subluxation of the femoral head to the acetabular rim. Additionally, repetitive microtrauma can cause injury to the soft tissue structures about the hip, leading to instability [35]. Finally, generalized ligamentous laxity, particularly when combined with athletic activities that place the hip joint in supraphysiologic positions such as gymnastics and dance, can predispose the hip to anterior instability. Like dislocations, suspected traumatic hip subluxations should be evaluated with advanced imaging to rule out intra-articular loose bodies or acetabular rim fractures [28] and should be managed accordingly. Alternatively, chronic hip instability is initially managed non-operatively with physical therapy and rest from inciting activities. If symptoms persist despite non-operative measures, hip arthroscopy and capsular plication are recommended to stabilize the joint. Concomitant pathology associated with hip instability, such as chondral lesions (usually of the central femoral head), ligamentum teres hypertrophy or tears, and labral tears, should be addressed at the time of arthroscopy (Fig. 26.4c, d) [35, 36]. Isolated arthroscopic capsular plication has been shown to improve hip pain and function at 1-year follow-up [37]; however, further data is needed to assess the long-term results of this procedure.

Key Points

- While hip dislocations are rare injuries in sports, hip subluxation and chronic instability are more common entities.
- On field reduction of hip dislocations may be attempted, but transfer to a medical facility for postreduction imaging is required.
- Early reduction is the most important factor to reduce the risk of osteonecrosis.
- Chronic hip instability can be treated successfully with arthroscopic capsular plication.

26.6 Chondral Injuries

Chondral injuries of the hip most commonly develop as sequelae of chronic impingement or instability as previously described (Fig. 26.5). In addition, Byrd et al. described a lateral impact injury as a mechanism of cartilage injury. He reported four cases of male athletes who suffered a fall directly onto the lateral aspect of the hip and developed persistent pain in the groin. Initial radiographs in all cases were unremarkable. MRI in two of the four cases was normal, in one case revealed signal changes in the femoral head, and in the final case demonstrated an effusion of the hip joint. All patients ultimately underwent hip arthroscopy. Two of the patients were found to have a grade III chondral lesion of the weight-bearing portion of the acetabulum. One patient had two large loose bodies located just above the fossa, as well as damage to the femoral head car-

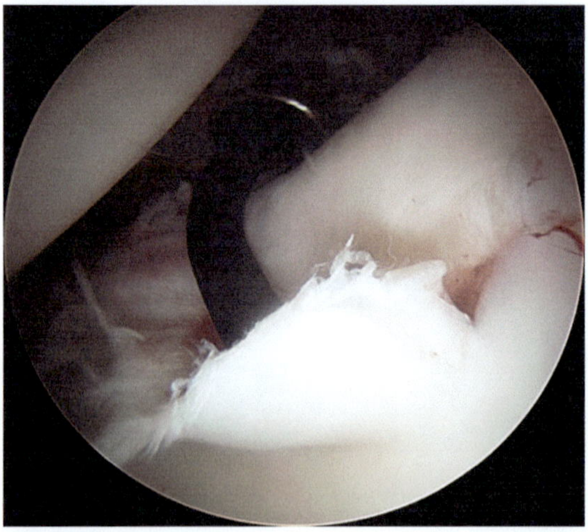

Fig. 26.5 Chondral delamination seen with FAI. Arthroscopic view of acetabular chondral delamination in the basketball player seen in Fig. 26.3c, d

tilage, thought to be secondary to third body wear. The patient with femoral head signal changes on his MRI was found to have an unstable grade IV chondral lesion of the medial femoral head superior to the fovea. All lesions were treated with debridement and/or removal of the fragments arthroscopically, with good short-term results in three of four patients. The author proposes that direct impact to the greater trochanter in patients with high bone density causes significant force transmission to the cartilage surfaces of the hip joint [38].

Regardless of mechanism, chondral injuries of the hip should be managed at the time of arthroscopy with debridement, with or without microfracture or autologous chondrocyte implantation. Additionally, large lesions may require open treatment with surgical hip dislocation and osteoarticular allograft. The literature supporting management strategies of hip chondral lesions varies widely, and further studies are required to determine the indications for each particular hip preservation technique [39].

26.7 Conclusion

Traumatic injuries of the hip and groin are common in athletes, particularly in sports that involve twisting, pivoting, and collision contact. Muscle strains and contusions represent the most common acute hip injuries in athletes. However, intra-articular pathology such as labral tears and FAI is increasingly recognized as our understanding of these conditions develops and the field of hip arthroscopy expands. Further research regarding prevention and management of specific intra-articular hip pathology will ideally decrease the incidence of hip injuries in athletes and allow for more reliable return to pre-injury level of play.

References

1. Anderson K, Strickland SM, Warren R. Hip and groin injuries in athletes. Am J Sports Med. 2001;29(4):521–33. https://doi.org/10.1177/03635465010290042501.
2. Zarins B, Ciullo JV. Acute muscle and tendon injuries in athletes. Clin Sports Med. 1983;2(1):167–82.
3. Feeley BT, Powell JW, Muller MS, Barnes RP, Warren RF, Kelly BT. Hip injuries and labral tears in the national football league. Am J Sports Med. 2008;36(11):2187–95. https://doi.org/10.1177/0363546508319898.
4. Tyler TF, Nicholas SJ, Campbell RJ, Donellan S, McHugh MP. The effectiveness of a preseason exercise program to prevent adductor muscle strains in professional ice hockey players. Am J Sports Med. 2002;30(5):680–3. https://doi.org/10.1177/03635465020300050801.
5. DeLee J. DeLee & Drez's orthopaedic sports medicine: principles and practice. Philadelphia: Saunders; 2003.
6. Hall M, Anderson J. Hip pointers. Clin Sports Med. 2013;32(2):325–30. https://doi.org/10.1016/j.csm.2012.12.010.
7. Jackson DW, Feagin JA. Quadriceps contusions in young athletes. Relation of severity of injury to treatment and prognosis. J Bone Joint Surg Am. 1973;55(1):95–105.
8. Aronen JG, Garrick JG, Chronister RD, McDevitt ER. Quadriceps contusions: clinical results of immediate immobilization in 120 degrees of knee flexion. Clin J Sport Med. 2006;16(5):383–7. https://doi.org/10.1097/01.jsm.0000244605.34283.94.
9. Walczak BE, Johnson CN, Howe BM. Myositis ossificans. J Am Acad Orthop Surg. 2015;23(10):612–22. https://doi.org/10.5435/JAAOS-D-14-00269.
10. Petersen W, Petersen F, Tillmann B. Structure and vascularization of the acetabular labrum with regard to the pathogenesis and healing of labral lesions. Arch Orthop Trauma Surg. 2003;123(6):283–8. https://doi.org/10.1007/s00402-003-0527-7.
11. Seldes RM, Tan V, Hunt J, Katz M, Winiarsky R, Fitzgerald RH. Anatomy, histologic features, and vascularity of the adult acetabular labrum. Clin Orthop Relat Res. 2001;382:232–40.
12. Myers CA, Register BC, Lertwanich P, et al. Role of the acetabular labrum and the iliofemoral ligament in hip stability: an in vitro biplane fluoroscopy study. Am J Sports Med. 2011;39(1_Suppl):85S–91S. https://doi.org/10.1177/0363546511412161.
13. Safran MR, Giordano G, Lindsey DP, et al. Strains across the acetabular labrum during hip motion: a cadaveric model. Am J Sports Med. 2011;39(Suppl(1_suppl)):92S–102S. https://doi.org/10.1177/0363546511414017.
14. Kapron AL, Peters CL, Aoki SK, et al. The prevalence of radiographic findings of structural hip deformities in female collegiate athletes. Am J Sports Med. 2015;43(6):1324–30. https://doi.org/10.1177/0363546515576908.
15. Agricola R, Bessems JHJM, Ginai AZ, et al. The development of Cam-type deformity in adolescent and young male soccer players. Am J Sports Med. 2012;40(5):1099–106. https://doi.org/10.1177/0363546512438381.
16. Agricola R, Heijboer MP, Ginai AZ, et al. A cam deformity is gradually acquired during skeletal maturation in adolescent and young male soccer players:

a prospective study with minimum 2-year follow-up. Am J Sports Med. 2014;42(4):798–806. https://doi.org/10.1177/0363546514524364.
17. Lerebours F, Robertson W, Neri B, Schulz B, Youm T, Limpisvasti O. Prevalence of Cam-type morphology in Elite ice hockey players. Am J Sports Med. 2016;44(4):1024–30. https://doi.org/10.1177/0363546515624671.
18. Trofa DP, Mayeux SE, Parisien RL, Ahmad CS, Lynch TS. Mastering the physical examination of the athlete's hip. Am J Orthop. 2017;46(1):10–6.
19. Byrd JWT, Jones KS. Diagnostic accuracy of clinical assessment, magnetic resonance imaging, magnetic resonance arthrography, and intra-articular injection in hip arthroscopy patients. Am J Sports Med. 2004;32(7):1668–74. https://doi.org/10.1177/0363546504266480.
20. Krych AJ, Thompson M, Knutson Z, Scoon J, Coleman SH. Arthroscopic labral repair versus selective labral debridement in female patients with femoroacetabular impingement: a prospective randomized study. Arthroscopy. 2013;29(1):46–53. https://doi.org/10.1016/j.arthro.2012.07.011.
21. Espinosa N, Beck M, Rothenfluh DA, Ganz R, Leunig M. Treatment of femoro-acetabular impingement: preliminary results of labral refixation. Surgical technique. J Bone Joint Surg Am. 2007;89 (Suppl 2 Pt.1):36–53. https://doi.org/10.2106/JBJS.F.01123.
22. Larson CM, Giveans MR. Arthroscopic debridement versus refixation of the acetabular labrum associated with femoroacetabular impingement. Arthroscopy. 2009;25(4):369–76. https://doi.org/10.1016/j.arthro.2008.12.014.
23. Domb BG, Hartigan DE, Perets I. Decision making for labral treatment in the hip: repair versus débridement versus reconstruction. J Am Acad Orthop Surg. 2017;25(3):e53–62. https://doi.org/10.5435/JAAOS-D-16-00144.
24. Nho SJ, Magennis EM, Singh CK, Kelly BT. Outcomes after the arthroscopic treatment of femoroacetabular impingement in a mixed group of high-level athletes. Am J Sports Med. 2011;39(Suppl):14S–9S. https://doi.org/10.1177/0363546511401900.
25. Alradwan H, Philippon MJ, Farrokhyar F, et al. Return to preinjury activity levels after surgical management of femoroacetabular impingement in athletes. Arthroscopy. 2012;28(10):1567–76. https://doi.org/10.1016/j.arthro.2012.03.016.
26. Nwachukwu BU, Bedi A, Premkumar A, Draovitch P, Kelly BT. Characteristics and outcomes of arthroscopic femoroacetabular impingement surgery in the National Football League. Am J Sports Med. 2018;46(1):144–8. https://doi.org/10.1177/0363546517729163.
27. Shibata KR, Matsuda S, Safran MR. Arthroscopic hip surgery in the Elite athlete: comparison of female and male competitive athletes. Am J Sports Med. 2017;45(8):1730–9. https://doi.org/10.1177/0363546517697296.
28. Moorman CT, Warren RF, Hershman EB, et al. Traumatic posterior hip subluxation in American football. J Bone Joint Surg Am. 2003;85-A(7):1190–6.
29. Pallia CS, Scott RE, Chao DJ. Traumatic hip dislocation in athletes. Curr Sports Med Rep. 2002;1(6):338–45.
30. Mayer SW, Abdo JCM, Hill MK, Kestel LA, Pan Z, Novais EN. Femoroacetabular impingement is associated with sports-related posterior hip instability in adolescents: a matched-cohort study. Am J Sports Med. 2016;44(9):2299–303. https://doi.org/10.1177/0363546516651119.
31. Berkes MB, Cross MB, Shindle MK, Bedi A, Kelly BT. Traumatic posterior hip instability and femoroacetabular impingement in athletes. Am J Orthop. 2012;41(4):166–71.
32. Paletta GA, Andrish JT. Injuries about the hip and pelvis in the young athlete. Clin Sports Med. 1995;14(3):591–628.
33. Foulk DM, Mullis BH. Hip dislocation: evaluation and management. J Am Acad Orthop Surg. 2010;18(4):199–209.
34. Philippon MJ, Kuppersmith DA, Wolff AB, Briggs KK. Arthroscopic findings following traumatic hip dislocation in 14 professional athletes. Arthroscopy. 2009;25(2):169–74. https://doi.org/10.1016/j.arthro.2008.09.013.
35. Boykin RE, Anz AW, Bushnell BD, Kocher MS, Stubbs AJ, Philippon MJ. Hip instability. J Am Acad Orthop Surg. 2011;19(6):340–9.
36. Shibata KR, Matsuda S, Safran MR. Is there a distinct pattern to the acetabular labrum and articular cartilage damage in the non-dysplastic hip with instability? Knee Surg Sports Traumatol Arthrosc. 2017;25(1):84–93. https://doi.org/10.1007/s00167-016-4342-4.
37. Kalisvaart MM, Safran MR. Hip instability treated with arthroscopic capsular plication. Knee Surg Sports Traumatol Arthrosc. 2017;25(1):24–30. https://doi.org/10.1007/s00167-016-4377-6.
38. Byrd JW. Lateral impact injury. A source of occult hip pathology. Clin Sports Med. 2001;20(4):801–15.
39. Marquez-Lara A, Mannava S, Howse EA, Stone AV, Stubbs AJ. Arthroscopic management of hip chondral defects: a systematic review of the literature. Arthroscopy. 2016;32(7):1435–43. https://doi.org/10.1016/j.arthro.2016.01.058.

Traumatic Knee Injuries

27

Steffen Sauer and Mark Clatworthy

27.1 Patella Dislocation

27.1.1 Background

The patella represents the largest sesamoid bone of the human body and is incorporated into the quadriceps tendon. Patella dislocations are a common sports-related knee injury and defined as the complete disengagement of the patella from the trochlear groove. According to the frequency and associated trauma mechanism, patella dislocations may be subdivided into traumatic, recurrent, and habitual dislocations. Traumatic (inaugural/single) dislocations are usually the result of a relevant trauma, typically a pivoting maneuver with a twisting movement about the flexed knee [1]. Recurrent (several) patella dislocations usually occur during normal activities and are facilitated by dysplastic changes in the patellofemoral joint [2, 3]. Habitual patella dislocation is defined as the consistent dislocation of the patella whenever the knee is flexed. Predisposing factors of patella dislocation include genu valgum, patella alta, increased distance between the tibial tuberosity and the trochlear groove (TTTG distance), as well as increased internal rotation and anteversion of the femur [1, 4]. The patella usually dislocates laterally, leading to a rupture of the medial patellofemoral ligament (MPFL). Subsequently, the lack of medial retrain provided by the MPFL may lead to patellar instability and recurrent dislocation, especially in cases with associated bony dysplasia or muscle weakness. Spontaneous relocation is usually seen; otherwise, emergency reduction is required.

27.1.2 Symptoms

Symptoms arising from patella dislocation are frequently related to the traumatic event and type of dislocation. Traumatic first-time patella dislocation usually provokes medial para-patellar pain as a result of capsular disruption which is often followed by rapid onset of effusion. However, effusion may be absent, especially in recurrent dislocations where giving way and locking may be the leading symptoms.

S. Sauer
Aarhus University Hospital / Aleris Hamlet Hospital, Aarhus, Denmark
e-mail: stefsaue@rm.dk

M. Clatworthy (✉)
Aarhus University Hospital / Aleris Hamlet Hospital, Aarhus, Denmark

ACL Study Group, Auckland, New Zealand

ISAKOS Knee Sports and Preservation Committee, ISAKOS Arthroscopy Committee, San Ramon, CA, USA

Herodicus Society, Opelousas, LA, USA
e-mail: markc@abjs.con.nz

S. Rocha Piedade et al. (eds.), *The Sports Medicine Physician*,
https://doi.org/10.1007/978-3-030-10433-7_27

27.1.3 Diagnosis

The diagnosis is typically made with the patella reduced as the vast majority of patella dislocations undergo spontaneous reduction. Clinical examination will usually reveal pain or a depression upon palpation of the medial retinaculum, usually disrupted during the dislocation. Pain during patellofemoral compression or palpation of the lateral condyle is usually present as a result of the patellofemoral collision during the dislocation. A positive apprehension sign when the examiner attempts to manually reproduce the luxation may be present and is thought to be pathognomonic for patella dislocation. In patients with recurrent patella luxation, patellar mal-tracking may become evident with a positive J-sign when the knee is extended. Massive effusion is typically seen in association with osteochondral lesions.

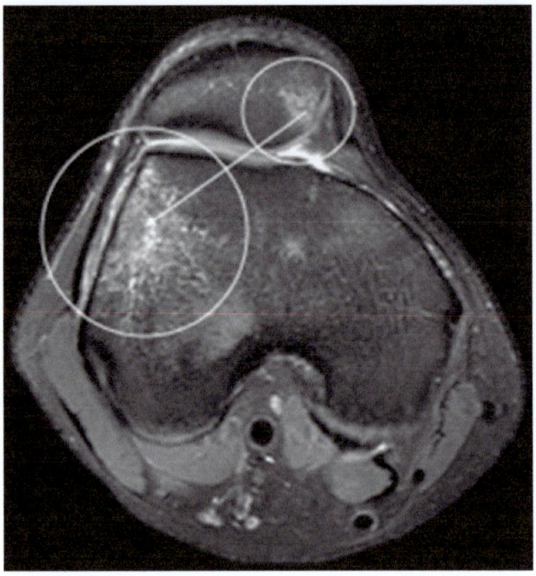

Fig. 27.1 Bone bruising following patellofemoral collision during luxation

27.1.4 Imaging

Radiographs may visualize irregularities in the contour of the lateral femoral condyle and/or the medial patella facet consistent with osteochondral fractures. MRI is used to determine whether there are any osteochondral lesions, visualize bone bruising as a result of the patellofemoral collision (Fig. 27.1) and identify eventual concomitant ligamentous or meniscal lesions. Furthermore, MRI is used to identify the degree of patellofemoral malalignment including the TTTG distance which has implications for the indication of surgical realignment procedures, such as tibial tubercle osteotomies.

27.1.5 Treatment

If the patella is dislocated, emergency reduction is indicated; the knee is hereby extended, and the patella is reduced by pushing the patella medially. Following spontaneous or manual reduction of first-time patella dislocation, a conservative treatment approach is indicated [4]. This may entail RICE (rest, ice, compression, elevation), initial knee immobilization, and progressive muscle strengthening. Knee arthroscopy may be indicated in the setting of chondral damage or osteochondral lesions that require re-fixation [1]. In recurrent cases of patella dislocation, surgical stabilization of the patella by either repairing or reconstructing the MPFL is indicated. However, there is no reliable data regarding joint stability or patient satisfaction after either conservative or operative treatment. Procedures that aim for correction of dysplasia as trochleoplasties should be reserved for cases in which initial surgery has failed.

Take-Home Message

The majority of first-time patella dislocations can be treated conservatively. However, acute MRI scan is indicated in cases with massive knee effusion to identify eventual osteochondral lesions which are suitable for subacute re-fixation [1].

Treatment Algorithm

- First-time patella dislocation → conservative treatment
- Recurrent patella dislocation → MPFL reconstruction
- First-time patella dislocation with osteochondral lesion → osteochondral re-fixation if possible and MPFL reconstruction

Facts

- Common injury.
- The vast majority of patella dislocations relocate spontaneously.
- MRI may be useful to identify typical bone bruising, osteochondral fractures and predisposing factors.

27.2 Meniscus Injury

27.2.1 Background

Meniscal lesions are among the most common injuries of the knee joint and the most frequent indication for knee arthroscopy. Meniscal lesions are more often degenerative than traumatic in origin and classified after location (medial/lateral, anterior/posterior) and by morphology (longitudinal, radial, horizontal, flap-tear-type, bucket-handle-type). Bucket-handle tears are further classified in accordance with location and associated meniscal blood supply from the geniculate artery which has implications for healing potential (white-white zone, red-white zone, red-red zone) [5]. Meniscal lesions of the menisco-capsular junction area (ramp lesions) and the meniscal root area are further classified in accordance with specific injury pattern, which has implications for treatment procedures [6]. The medial meniscus is more frequently injured than the lateral meniscus due to its more rigid tibial and capsular attachment [7]. However, in association with ACL injures, lateral meniscal tears including root injuries are reported to be more frequent compared to medial meniscal tears [8]. The latter, however, may be easily missed during arthroscopy if the posterior menisco-capsular junction area of the medial meniscus is not thoroughly inspected [6]. The medial meniscus does not only account for half of the shock capacity of the medial compartment but does also restrain the tibia from anterior translation [9]. This is the reason why a large number of patients with ACL injuries have concomitant tears of the medial meniscus [7]. The lateral meniscus is more mobile compared to the medial meniscus. As the knee moves, the lateral meniscus moves back and forth across the tibia and is hereby stabilized by menisco-femoral ligaments. As the lateral meniscus can absorb up to 70% of the shock to the lateral compartment of the knee, total lateral meniscectomy is commonly associated with rapid onset of OA. Recently, the role of the lateral meniscus for rotational knee stability has become more evident which has emphasized the importance of meniscal root repairs for better ACLR outcomes [10]. Over time, menisci become more rigid, and the incidence of degenerative meniscal tears increases. Especially in association with osteoarthritis, degenerative lesions of the posterior horn of the medial meniscus are frequently seen. There is an emerging body of literature challenging the beneficial effect of partial meniscectomy as a treatment strategy of these degenerative lesions [11, 12]. Traumatic meniscal lesions usually arise from a twisting movement about the flexed knee with the ipsilateral foot planted; the resulting compressive and rotational forces cause the meniscus to tear. Degenerative lesions are often not associated with a history of trauma.

27.2.2 Symptoms

Symptoms arising from meniscal tears are frequently related to location, morphology, and origin of the lesion. Purely traumatic meniscal lesions are associated with a sudden onset of focal pain after a rotational knee trauma. However, the degree of instant posttraumatic pain is variable. Patients sustaining small tears without tissue displacement usually proceed with sports activities. Severe tears are associated with more significant pain and, especially in bucket-handle meniscus lesions, with hemarthrosis and a fixed flexion deformity with the displaced meniscus preventing full extension. However, a complete bucket-handle lesion may be displaced anteriorly to the femoral condyle without compromising range of knee motion. Other symptoms of meniscal injury include click sensation, catching, and instability due to proprioceptive misinformation caused by the displacement of meniscal tissue. Degenerative lesions often show a subtle debut of diffuse pain without preceding trauma. The ability to squat is usually compromised. A serous effusion and quadriceps atrophy may be encountered.

27.2.3 Diagnosis

The diagnosis of meniscal tears is based on the history of injury followed by clinical examination. Partial, horizontal, and anterior meniscal tears without mechanical interference may present without clinical findings. Meniscal injuries are typically associated with pain upon palpation of the joint line and may be aggravated by a variety of meniscal provocation tests. The accuracy of the physical examination is dependent on the type of injury and the observer [13]. Among the most important tests are the McMurray's test (pain or popping sensation over the joint line during external tibial rotation under repeated passive flexion/extension) [13], the Steinmann I sign (pain during passive knee rotation), and the Thessaly test [14]. The latter has recently been popularized as loading forces on the menisci are simulated; the patient stands hereby on one leg with the knee flexed while actively rotating the knee and body. Pain and locking constitute a positive test. As no isolated test is highly conclusive, a combination of meniscal provocation tests is recommended, and multiple positive findings with a history of relevant trauma suggest a meniscal injury. A negative test does not exclude a meniscal lesion. Hemarthrosis and reduced range of motion are commonly seen in association with displaced meniscal tears.

27.2.4 Imaging

MRI represents the main imaging modality for the diagnosis of meniscal tears and shows high sensitivity and specificity. Especially when range of knee motion is compromised, MRI should be performed to visualize meniscal injuries that require immediate attention [15]. Generally, however, MRI findings need to be interpreted in relation to clinical findings. Mucoid degeneration of the meniscus, which is associated with an increased signal from the center of the meniscus, is a common finding and should not be misinterpreted as a traumatic tear.

27.2.5 Treatment

The treatment of meniscal tears should depend on location, morphology, origin, as well as the correlation of meniscal injuries with clinical symptoms and associated lesions. Other factors affecting treatment procedures include patient age and activity level. In general, treatment of meniscal lesions should always aim to restore the best possible function of the meniscus, consequently reducing pain [9]. Bucket-handle lesions with high healing potential should be repaired, regardless of patient age. Different methods are hereby used including all-inside, inside-out, and outside-in suturing techniques, which are mostly dependent on lesion accessibility [16, 17]. Isolated meniscal lesions without mechanical symptoms and chondral erosion may initially be treated conservatively. Partial meniscectomy is indicated for cases in which resection of dysfunctional meniscal tissue is believed to optimize meniscal pressure distribution by restoring a sharp meniscal rim, e.g., in flap-tear lesions or radial tears. However, it must be kept in mind that the loss of functional meniscal tissue may enhance chondral degeneration [18, 19]. Unstable meniscal lesions that affect the meniscal root or ramp areas should be addressed, especially in the setting of concomitant ACL injury. Meniscal root avulsions should be reattached through a transtibial tunnel [20, 21]. Unstable meniscal ramp lesions are best addressed with an all-inside or inside-out suturing technique through an additional posteromedial portal [22]. In contrast, degenerative lesions with underlying OA without meniscal displacement and mechanical symptoms should be treated conservatively as no evidence is supporting the beneficial effects of partial meniscectomy [5, 23–26]. Meniscus allograft transplantation is an option for young patients with extensive meniscal loss with pain and or early chondral loss.

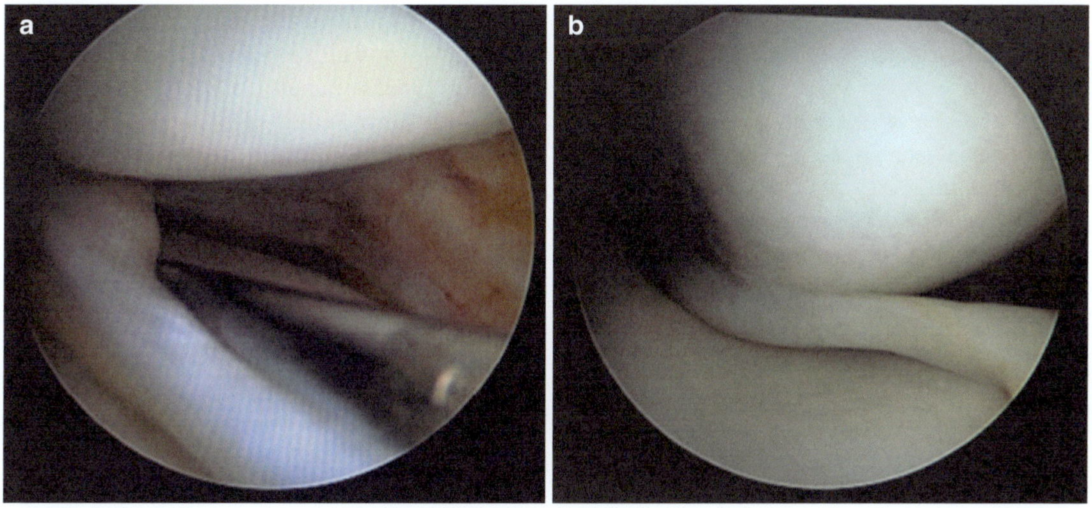

Fig. 27.2 Acute bucket-handle meniscus lesion. (**a**) (Left): a small meniscal rim can be seen where the meniscus has been detached from the capsule. (**b**) (right): interfering meniscal tissue lying between the femur and tibia may cause an extension deficit

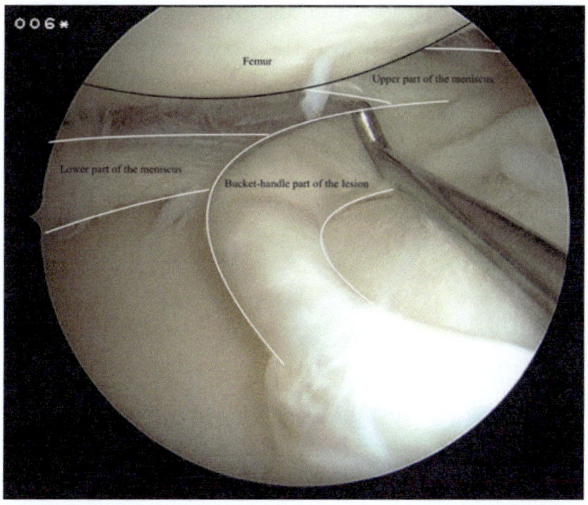

Fig. 27.3 Complex lateral meniscus injury. The central part of the meniscus lies between the femur and tibia as the bucket-handle part of the injury. The peripheral part of the meniscus is torn transversally leaving a lower and upper meniscal portion

Take-Home Message

Patients presenting with the inability to fully extend the knee after a relevant trauma should undergo subacute MRI to identify meniscal injuries that require immediate attention such as bucket-handle lesions.

Diagnosis Algorithm for Acute Meniscal Injuries

- Hemarthrosis and reduced range of knee motion → MRI to exclude fracture, patella dislocation, ligament lesions, and bucket-handle meniscus injury
- Normal range of motion without instability → RICE and reevaluation after 2–3 weeks

Diagnosis Algorithm for Chronic Meniscal Injuries

- Plain radiographs showing OA → conservative treatment
- Plain radiographs without OA → MRI to visualize meniscal injuries suitable for surgery

Treatment Algorithm

- Degenerative meniscal lesions → conservative treatment
- Degenerative meniscal lesions with locking/catching → arthroscopy and partial meniscectomy where indicated
- Bucket-handle meniscal lesions → subacute arthroscopy and meniscal repair
- RAMP lesions → Repair: Inside-out or all-inside suture where indicated
- Root lesions → Repair: Transtibial root re-fixation

Facts

- The meniscus should always be preserved if possible.
- Meniscal surgery is specialist surgery demanding special techniques, especially for root and ramp lesions.
- There is no evidence supporting the beneficial effect of partial meniscectomy for undisplaced tears in patients with underlying OA.

27.3 ACL Injury

27.3.1 Background

The anterior cruciate ligament (ACL) enables stable knee kinematics by limiting internal tibial rotation and anterior tibial translation. As the ACL has migrated anteriorly during embryologic development to its central position, it has preserved synovial coverage. The ACL has been thought to be comprised of two distinguishable bundles: an anteromedial and a posterolateral bundle. Recent anatomical studies, however, have emphasized the ribbonlike structure of the ACL [27]; rather than bundles the ACL is composed of direct and indirect fibers according to their insertional morphology [28]. Acute ACL ruptures are predominantly the result of a noncontact rotational or hyperextensional trauma [29, 30]. Altered biomechanics of the ACL-deficient knee may cause symptoms of instability, subsequent meniscal and chondral injury, as well as osteoarthritis [31, 32]. ACL reconstruction (ACLR) is preformed to improve knee stability and shows overall satisfactory results and low revision rates. The therapeutic approach to ACL injuries has historically been a dynamic process, entailing repair procedures, augmentations, open and arthroscopic reconstructions, as well as a variety of graft choices. Even though arthroscopic procedures are currently chosen over open approaches and reconstructions over repair procedures, the optimal graft choice is still controversially discussed. Meta-analysis of studies comparing the outcomes of ACLR depending on graft choice including auto- and allografts and bone-tendon-bone versus pure tendon grafts has not emerged a specific superior graft [33–40]. The reconstruction of both ACL bundles (double-bundle ACLR) has been proposed by some authors [41, 42]. However, its necessity has been challenged as the procedure is technically more demanding without clearly improving patient outcomes [43, 44]. In single-bundle ACLR, graft positioning has been a matter of debate, especially after the transportal ACLR technique has been established as the gold standard [45–47]. Patients with high-grade pivot-shift and habitual ligament laxity have shown higher ACL failure rates. In these patients, additional extra-articular stabilizing procedures such as the lateral tenodesis or anterior lateral ligament (ALL) reconstruction have currently been popularized and thought to lower ACLR failure and revision rates [48–51]. In general, the susceptibility of ACL lesions is higher among women compared to men engaged in the same pivoting sports [52–54]. Physiological factors such as neuromuscular control and quadriceps-dominant deceleration, the geometrical shape of the knee joint, and hormonal factors are thought to be the explanation of this disparity [46, 47, 55–60].

27.3.2 Symptoms

Symptoms associated with ACL injury include a audible pop at the time of injury followed by intense pain, rapid onset of knee effusion and a subsequent inability to continue with sports activity. Other symptoms including reduced range of knee motion may be present and are usually aggravated by concomitant meniscal injuries. Subjective instability with or without giving way phenomenon is usually reported. However, subjective instability may first be evident when pain is resolved and the knee is fully loaded.

27.3.3 Diagnosis

Clinical assessment of the knee is best performed shortly after ACL injury before the onset of muscular guarding and effusion. The Pivot shift test is considered the best test to determine an ACL injury as it replicates the subluxation of the ACL deficient knee. However, in the acute setting the test may be difficult to perform due to pain and muscular guarding. In this case, the Lachman´s test is preferred [61, 62]. The knee is hereby flexed 20–30°, and the amount of anterior tibial translation and the quality of the translation endpoint are evaluated by pulling the lower leg in a forward direction [63]. The test usually induces less pain and muscular guarding than the anterior drawers test in which the knee is flexed 90° or the pivot-shift test, in which a dynamic subluxation of the tibia is induced [64]. Meta-analysis of the efficacy of these tests finds the Lachman test to be the most useful with sensitivity and specificity of 85% and 94%, respectively [61]. Especially regarding the anterior drawers test, PCL injury may mimic ACL insufficiency as the posterior sag will give the impression of increased anterior tibial translation, when in fact the knee is reduced to its neutral position. The clinical examination should include assessment of concomitant injuries that require immediate attention such as meniscal lesions, MCL, LCL, PCL and posterolateral corner injuries as well as acute patellar dislocations. Hemarthrosis may be evacuated by percutaneous aspiration for pain relief.

27.3.4 Imaging

MRI is used to confirm the diagnosis and visualize concomitant injuries. Plain radiographs may visualize an avulsion fracture of the lateral tibial plateau referred to as the Segond fracture which is usually associated with ACL injury [65, 66]. In addition, plain radiographs may visualize an avulsion fracture of the tibial ACL insertion which may be suitable for ORIF.

27.3.5 Treatment

Acute management of ACL injury include RICE and oral analgesics. Crutches may initially be indicated to avoid full weight-bearing in cases of severe instability and extensive bone bruising. Further management including the necessity and timing of eventual ACL reconstruction is dependent on several factors such as patient age and functional level, degree of instability, the condition of the knee, and concomitant injuries. In general, patients with concomitant ligament injury or unstable meniscus lesions usually need surgical reconstruction due to increased instability of the knee [67]. Furthermore, patients who experience significant knee instability wishing to resume high-demand sports or occupation usually benefit from ACL reconstruction. Isolated ACL lesions with stable meniscal lesions may be treated conservatively, especially if return to pivoting sports is not desired [68]. As a general rule, ACL surgery is scheduled 6–8 weeks after the injury when normal range of motion is restored, swelling has gone and peripheral structures including MCL lesions have healed. Injuries that need immediate surgical attention (e.g., bucket-handle injuries) should be addressed subacutely. Even though evidence is inconclusive, ACL reconstruction is often postponed until normal range of knee motion is restored to avoid complications including arthrofibrosis [69, 70]. However, there is no consensus among knee surgeons regarding optimal timing of ACLR. According to a systematic review of 69 studies including 7556 participants, 90% of patients undergoing ACL reconstruction achieve normal or near-normal knee function. However, only 55% of patients resume their preinjury level of competition [71]. This suggests that psychological factors like fear of reinjury may play an important role in the treatment of ACL injury [71, 72]. There is no cutoff age for ACL reconstruction, and based on observational studies, it shows overall satisfactory results in patients over 40 years of age [73]. Even though rigorous prospective studies are rare, ACL deficiency is thought to be associated with increased risk of chondral and meniscal degeneration [74]. It remains a matter of debate how much the initial trauma itself contributes to progressive joint degeneration and to what extent ACL reconstruction may modulate this risk [75–77]. In addition, the severity of the initial trauma, extent of meniscal injury, knee biomechanics, and subsequent patient activity level may affect the development of joint degeneration (Fig. 27.4).

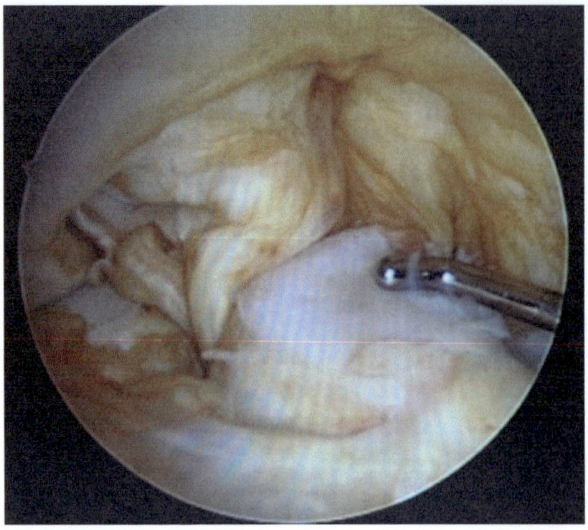

Fig. 27.4 ACL injury

Take-Home Message
A relevant knee trauma with early onset of effusion is highly suspicious for ACL injury. Muscular guarding may conceal instability, especially concerning the anterior drawers test.

Treatment Algorithm
- If ACLR is indicated → usually 6–8 weeks after injury when range of motion is normalized
- ACL rupture with concomitant bucket-handle meniscal injury and fixed flexion deformity → Subacute meniscal suture if indicated, delayed ACLR until range of motion is normalized

Facts
- Up to seventy-seven percent of patients presenting with traumatic knee hemarthrosis have an ACL injury.
- ACLR delay may enhance meniscus and chondral degeneration.
- ACL deficiency is associated with increased risk of further injury (e.g., meniscal tear), chronic pain, and decreased level of activity.
- OA may develop regardless of treatment approach.
- No graft choice has been shown to be superior.
- Geometrical features of the knee joint affect ACL injury and ACL graft failure risk.

27.4 PCL Injury

27.4.1 Background

The posterior cruciate ligament (PCL) is the strongest of the intra-capsular ligaments of the knee and primary restrain to posterior translation [78]. As the PCL has migrated anteriorly during embryologic development to its more central position, it has preserved synovial coverage. This extra-synovial location accounts for limited effusion in isolated PCL ruptures. The proximity to the posterior capsule, however, ensures blood supply to the PCL after complete rupture, which allows satisfactory results of primary PCL repair and conservative treatment in some cases [79–81]. The femoral and tibial insertion sites of the PCL are approximately three times larger than its midportion diameter. The PCL is inconsistently accompanied by two ligamentous structures that stretch between the medial condyle and posterior horn of the lateral meniscus, referred to as the Humphrey and Wrisberg ligament. PCL ruptures may be classified based on timing (acute versus chronic) and severity (isolated versus multi-ligament). Isolated PCL ruptures are usually the result of a fall onto the flexed knee or forced hyperextension. PCL lesions are more likely found in the setting of complex multi-ligament injuries after high-velocity trauma mechanisms. In these cases, thorough assessment of the knee including the neurovascular status is crucial for satisfactory outcomes [82]. Isolated PCL lesions usually show subtle clinical appearance and may therefore go frequently undetected, leading to chronic insufficiency, a flexion deficit or generalized anterior knee pain [83]. The majority of athletes with isolated PCL injuries may continue to function at a high level [79, 80].

27.4.2 Symptoms

Clinical findings of acute PCL ruptures are highly dependent on the preceding trauma and thereof resulting concomitant injuries. Especially lesions of the posterolateral corner may severely aggravate knee instability. In isolated PCL lesions, effusion is uncommon as the blood usually drains into the posterior soft tissues and lower leg. In addition, muscle guarding may conceal mild instability. Pain in the fossa poplitea may therefore be the only perceptible symptom. A popping sensation is rarely reported, and patients with isolated PCL lesions are usually able to instantly resume sporting activities. In contrast, PCL lesions in the setting of multi-ligament lesions are usually associated with hemarthrosis, severe instability, inability to bear weight, as well as reduced range of knee motion. Patients presenting with chronic PCL deficiency suffer from a fixed anterior subluxation of the medial femoral condyle in relation to the tibia, which may cause generalized anterior knee and symptoms related to degeneration of the medial tibiofemoral joint compartment [83, 84].

27.4.3 Diagnosis

Acute and especially isolated PCL lesions may be challenging to diagnose and are frequently overlooked. Spontaneous posterior drawer sign is rare and primarily present with concomitant injury of the posterolateral corner [85]. Anterior-posterior translation is frequently seen in the chronic phase when muscular guarding is overcome [86]. In these cases, a positive posterior drawer test is typically found. Lesions of the posterolateral corner with rotational instability are assessed with the dial test; the patient is hereby lying prone, and both knees are externally rotated and compared.

27.4.4 Imaging

Plain radiographs may visualize posterior tibial displacement or an avulsion fracture of the tibial PCL insertion site. Subacute MRI is indicated when PCL lesions are suspected. However, MRI does not reveal the functional status of the PCL and degree of instability of the lesion. In chronic injuries the PCL may heal in a lengthened position and appear normal on the MRI scan. Treatment is therefore based on symptoms and clinical findings including the degree of tibial displacement and associated functional instability.

27.4.5 Treatment

Displaced avulsion fractures of the tibial insertion should undergo ORIF to prevent PCL insufficiency. Arthroscopically assisted procedures and fracture fixation with suspension devices have also shown promising results. Ligamentous lesions should primarily undergo conservative treatment including rehabilitation with a dynamic brace that supports anterior reposition of the tibia during flexion [87]. Results after conservative treatment with mild instability are usually good [80, 88]. PCL reconstruction (PCLR) is indicated in cases of chronic instability [89, 90]. Surgical results after PCLR, especially after severe instability, are worse compared to ACLR outcomes [91–93]. PCL lesions in the setting of a multi-ligament injury should be treated operatively while addressing all injuries in a single operation to ensure early mobilization which is thought to be of paramount importance for satisfactory outcomes [94].

Take-Home Message
Isolated PCL lesions are easily overlooked. Pain in the fossa poplitea after a relevant trauma may be the only symptom.

Treatment Algorithm
- Acute isolated PCL → dynamic bracing
- Chronic PCL lesions with mild instability →physiotherapy
- Chronic PCL lesion with distinct instability → PCL reconstruction
- PCL injury in the setting of multi-ligament lesions (e.g., PLC) → multi-ligament reconstruction in a single operation

Facts

- PCL lesions with spontaneous posterior drawer sign are usually associated with lesions of the posterolateral corner (PLC) [85].

- Massive effusion after PCL injury is uncommon as the blood usually drains into the posterior soft tissues and lower leg.
- Isolated PCL lesions show good outcomes when treated conservatively.

27.5 MCL Injury

27.5.1 Background

The medial collateral ligament (MCL) is one of the most commonly injured structures of the knee joint [95, 96]. Partial or complete MCL ruptures are typically the result of a direct valgus trauma, less frequently the result of indirect injury mechanisms including abduction and rotation of the lower leg [97]. MCL injuries usually carry low morbidity, in spite of the complex three-layered medial anatomical structure of the knee [98–100]. The superficial MCL (sMCL) is located within the second layer between the deep MCL and the sartorial fascia. The superficial MCL is considered the main static retrain against valgus stress and rotational forces. The deep MCL lies in the third and deepest layer and forms the middle third of the medial capsule [100]. The deep MCL is not ascribed a significant joint stabilizing function [101]. From the second and third layer originates a conjoint ligamentous structure referred to as the posterior oblique ligament (POL). The deep MCL and posterior oblique ligament have attachments to the medial meniscus which explains why MCL injuries may be associated with medial meniscal tears. MCL injuries are classified into minor stable injuries (grade I), partial injuries with mild instability (grade II), and complete tears with severe instability (grade III). MCL injuries carry low morbidity and tend to heal without complications undergoing the following stages: hemorrhage, inflammation, repair, and remodeling. Most patients will resume preinjury level of competitive sports following conservative treatment. Even though most MCL injuries occur isolated, they may be associated with both ACL and medial meniscus injury, referred to as the unhappy triad. Patients with chronic symptomatic MCL insufficiency should undergo MCL reconstruction [102, 103]. Patients with acute MCL lesions in a severe multi-structural injury setting should undergo repair or reconstruction to ensure early mobilization [102, 104, 105].

27.5.2 Symptoms

Isolated MCL injury is usually associated with pain and periarticular swelling along the course of the MCL. Joint effusion is usually absent and typically indicates concurrent intra-articular structural injury. Concomitant ACL and meniscal injury may aggravate instability and impair range of motion.

27.5.3 Diagnosis

Clinical findings are tenderness along the MCL, predominantly at the femoral insertion site. Instability may be present in 20–30 degrees of flexion indicating MCL insufficiency. Instability in both 20–30 degrees of flexion and extension is usually a sign of combined MCL, posteromedial capsule and ACL injury.

27.5.4 Imaging

Plain radiographs may visualize a bony MCL avulsion. In chronic cases, an osseous irregularity at the femoral insertion site is seen as a result of repetitive trauma, referred to as the Pellegrini-Stieda complex [66, 106]. MRI and ultrasound are used to confirm the diagnosis. Stress radiographs comparing both knees where manual valgus stress is applied may be used to quantify the extent of instability [107, 108].

27.5.5 Treatment

Isolated MCL sprains without valgus instability may be treated conservatively after the RICE principle (rest, ice, compression, and elevation) [104]. Early remobilization is encouraged. Grade

II and III lesions associated with valgus instability require a coronal stabilizing brace for 5–6 weeks; free range of motion is usually granted. Surgical intervention is rarely indicated as conservative treatment usually shows good results [103]. However, a grade III lesion is often associated with multi-ligament lesions where repair procedures or reconstruction may be indicated in a multi-ligament reconstruction setting [104, 109, 110]. In chronic cases with ongoing instability, MCL reconstruction is usually indicated [96].

Take-Home Message
Even though isolated MCL injury is frequently seen, thorough assessment of the knee is crucial to correctly identify concomitant meniscal or ligamentous injury.

Treatment Algorithm
- Grade I → RICE following early remobilization
- Grade II → coronal stabilizing brace with free range of motion for 6 weeks
- Grade III → often associated with multi-ligament lesions where repair procedures or reconstruction may be indicated

27.6 LCL Injury/Posterolateral Corner Injury

27.6.1 Background

The lateral (fibular) collateral ligament (LCL) runs just proximal and posterior to the lateral femoral epicondyle to the anterolateral aspect of the fibular head. Due to its tubular shape and the fact that the axial rotational axis of the knee lies within the medial compartment [111], complete injuries of the LCL usually lead to significant instability and poor conservative healing potential. If undetected or untreated, chronic instability is usually seen, frequently associated with a thrust gait [112, 113]. Isolated LCL lesions are rare and the result of a direct varus trauma. Most frequently, LCL lesions are present in the setting of multi-ligament injuries following high-energy trauma mechanisms [114]. The most commonly associated injuries are the posterior cruciate ligament and the popliteus tendon and the popliteo-fibular ligament [115]. The latter are referred to as the main static stabilizing structures of the posterolateral corner (PLC) in conjunction with the LCL. Other structures forming the posterolateral corner include the lateral capsule and iliotibial band, the biceps tendon and lateral head of the gastrocnemius muscle, as well as variable structures such as the arcuate and fabellofibular ligament. Especially following high-energy trauma mechanisms, a fibular avulsion fracture (arcuate fracture) or a common peroneal nerve injury may be present [115].

27.6.2 Symptoms

Pain and swelling along the lateral aspect of the knee is usually found. Complete LCL lesions and associated ACL/PCL or PLC injuries lead to instability near full knee extension [116], typically compounding stair climbing and pivoting maneuvers.

27.6.3 Diagnosis

Ecchymosis and lateral joint line tenderness may be present and may be aggravated by concomitant meniscal injuries. Coronal stability of the knee is assessed in 20–30 degrees of flexion and extension. Instability in extension and 20–30 degrees of flexion is usually associated with injuries of the posterior capsule and cruciate ligaments. Rotational stability is assessed with the dial test; the patient is hereby lying prone, and both knees are externally rotated at 30 and 90 degrees of flexion. The extent of external rotation is compared to the non-affected side. Rotational asymmetry at 30° but not in 90° indicates an isolated PLC injury. Rotational asymmetry at 30 and 90° indicates a combined PLC and PCL injury. Chronic instability may become evident in a thrust gait.

27.6.4 Imaging

MRI is used to confirm the diagnosis. Plain radiographs may visualize a fibular avulsion fracture of the biceps tendon suitable for subacute refixation. Stress radiographs comparing both knees where manual varus stress is applied may be used to quantify the extent of joint opening and instability.

27.6.5 Treatment

Isolated partial LCL lesions with no varus instability in full knee extension may initially be treated conservatively. This entails RICE (rest, ice, compression, elevation) and functional rehabilitation with a coronal stabilizing brace for 6 weeks. Conservative treatment of complete LCL lesions may result in ongoing varus instability. In these cases, LCL reconstruction is usually indicated. Patients with rotational instability should undergo LCL/PLC reconstruction. Patients with combined ACL/PCL and LCL/PLC insufficiency should undergo multi-ligament reconstruction [114].

Take-Home Message
LCL lesions are frequently associated with lesions of the posterior cruciate ligament and structures of the posterolateral corner (PLC).

Treatment Algorithm
- Grade I and II LCL lesion → RICE and coronal stabilizing brace for 6 weeks
- Grade III LCL lesion with coronal instability → LCL reconstruction
- LCL/PLC lesion with rotational instability → LCL/PLC reconstruction
- Multi-ligament setting → acute reconstruction ±(ACL/PCL/LCL/PCL)

27.7 Multi-ligament Injury

Multi-ligament injuries are predominantly the result of high-energy trauma mechanisms, and their management requires specialist expertise [117]. Ongoing development in the field of sports traumatology has uncovered a much higher incidence of multi-ligament injuries than initially thought. Thorough assessment of the knee after relevant trauma is crucial to correctly identify the extent of complex multi-ligament injuries [82, 118]. Multi-ligament injuries are typically addressed in a single operation to ensure early mobilization which is thought to be of paramount importance for satisfactory outcomes. In chronic situations, malalignment of the lower limb needs to be addressed before collateral ligament reconstruction is performed. In acute initial management of multi-ligament injuries, the neurovascular status needs to be assessed in accordance with ATLS principles, and CT angiography should always be considered in order to identify vascular injury, especially after knee dislocation [119, 120]. Overlooked vascular injuries are associated with high morbidity and may lead to amputation of the lower limb [121].

27.8 Quadriceps Tendon and Patellar Ligament Rupture

27.8.1 Background

Quadriceps tendon and patellar ligament ruptures may be partial or complete and commonly affect the nondominant knee of male patients beyond 30 years of age. In younger patients, ruptures are usually the result of a direct trauma. In older patients, the rupture usually represents the final stage of prolonged underlying tendon degeneration. Associated factors which are thought to increase the susceptibility of these ruptures include diabetes, connective tissue disorders, renal failure, and the use of intra-articular injections or fluoroquinolone antibiotics [122, 123].

27.8.2 Symptoms

Patients with acute ruptures present with pain and swelling at the rupture site. A popping sensation may be noted at the time of injury, especially in complete ruptures, followed by the inability to continue with sports activity.

27.8.3 Diagnosis

Tenderness and a palpable defect at the rupture site of the quadriceps tendon or patellar ligament are usually found. Knee extension against resistance and a straight leg rise is usually not possible. Quadriceps tendon rupture is associated with reduction of the patella height, while patellar ligament rupture is associated with elevation of the patella height.

27.8.4 Imaging

Ultrasound and MRI are used to confirm the diagnosis. Plain radiographs may show patella alta in patellar ligament ruptures and patella baja in quadriceps tendon ruptures [124].

27.8.5 Treatment

Partial quadriceps tendon and patella ligament ruptures may be treated conservatively with short-term brace immobilization in full extension with a progressive range-of-motion and weight-bearing protocol. Complete quadriceps tendon and patellar ligament ruptures should undergo primary end to end, trans-osseous or suture-anchor repair depending on rupture site location. Tendon reconstruction with auto- or allografts may be necessary in special cases. The use of NSAID for pain management after acute tendon rupture is still a matter of controversy as both beneficial and deleterious effects of NSAID on tendon healing have been reported [125, 126].

Treatment Algorithm

- Partial ruptures → immobilization with progressive ROM and weight-bearing
- Complete ruptures → repair

References

1. Duthon VB. Acute traumatic patellar dislocation. Orthop Traumatol Surg Res. 2015;101:S59–67.
2. Arendt EA, Fithian DC, Cohen E. Current concepts of lateral patella dislocation. Clin Sports Med. 2002;21:499–519.
3. Zaffagnini S, et al. The patellofemoral joint: from dysplasia to dislocation. EFORT Open Rev. 2017;2:204–14.
4. Frosch, S. et al. [The treatment of patellar dislocation: a systematic review]. Z Orthop Unfall. 2011;149:630–45.
5. Mordecai SC, Al-Hadithy N, Ware HE, Gupte CM. Treatment of meniscal tears: an evidence based approach. World J Orthop. 2014;5:233–41.
6. Chahla J, Dean CS, Moatshe G, Mitchell JJ, Cram TR, Yacuzzi C, LaPrade RF. Meniscal Ramp Lesions. Orthop J Sports Med. 2016;4(7):2325967116657781.
7. Ahn JH, Bae TS, Kang K-S, Kang SY, Lee SH. Longitudinal tear of the medial meniscus posterior horn in the anterior cruciate ligament-deficient knee significantly influences anterior stability. Am J Sports Med. 2011;39:2187–93.
8. Nikolić DK. Lateral meniscal tears and their evolution in acute injuries of the anterior cruciate ligament of the knee. Knee Surg Sports Traumatol Arthrosc. 1998;6(1):26–30.
9. Tscholl PM, Duthon VB, Cavalier M, Menetrey J. Current treatment strategy of meniscal lesions in athletes. Rev Med Suisse. 2016;12:1284–7.
10. Shybut TB, et al. Effect of lateral meniscal root tear on the stability of the anterior cruciate ligament-deficient knee. Am J Sports Med. 2015;43:905–11.
11. Sihvonen R, et al. Arthroscopic partial meniscectomy versus placebo surgery for a degenerative meniscus tear: a 2-year follow-up of the randomised controlled trial. Ann Rheum Dis. 2018;77:188–95.
12. Thorlund JB, Juhl CB, Roos EM, Lohmander LS. Arthroscopic surgery for degenerative knee: systematic review and meta-analysis of benefits and harms. Br J Sports Med. 2015;49:1229–35.
13. Scholten RJ, et al. The accuracy of physical diagnostic tests for assessing meniscal lesions of the knee: a meta-analysis. J Fam Pract. 2001;50:938–44.
14. Karachalios T, Hantes M, Zibis AH, Zachos V, Karantanas AH, Malizos KN. Diagnostic accuracy of a new clinical test (the Thessaly Test) for early detection of meniscal tears. J Bone Joint Surg. 87(5):955–62.
15. Helmark IC, Neergaard K, Krogsgaard MR. Traumatic knee extension deficit (the locked knee): can MRI reduce the need for arthroscopy? Knee Surg Sports Traumatol Arthrosc. 2007;15:863–8.
16. Barber FA, McGarry JE. Meniscal repair techniques. Sports Med Arthrosc Rev. 2007;15:199–207.

17. Fok AWM, Yau WP. Early results of all-inside meniscal repairs using a pre-loaded suture anchor. Hong Kong Med J. 2013;19:124–8.
18. Roemer FW, et al. Partial meniscectomy is associated with increased risk of incident radiographic osteoarthritis and worsening cartilage damage in the following year. Eur Radiol. 2017;27:404–13.
19. van Meer BL, et al. Which determinants predict tibiofemoral and patellofemoral osteoarthritis after anterior cruciate ligament injury? A systematic review. Br J Sports Med. 2015;49:975–83.
20. Bhatia S, LaPrade CM, Ellman MB, LaPrade RF. Meniscal root tears: significance, diagnosis, and treatment. Am J Sports Med. 2014;42:3016–30.
21. LaPrade RF, Matheny LM, Moulton SG, James EW, Dean CS. Posterior meniscal root repairs: outcomes of an anatomic transtibial pull-out technique. Am J Sports Med. 2017;45:884–91.
22. DePhillipo NN, Cinque ME, Kennedy NI, Chahla J, Geeslin AG, Moatshe G, Engebretsen L, LaPrade RF. Inside-out repair of meniscal ramp lesions. Arthrosc Tech. 2017;6(4):e1315–20.
23. Herrlin S, Hållander M, Wange P, Weidenhielm L, Werner S. Arthroscopic or conservative treatment of degenerative medial meniscal tears: a prospective randomised trial. Knee Surg Sports Traumatol Arthrosc. 2007;15:393–401.
24. Khan M, Evaniew N, Bedi A, Ayeni OR, Bhandari M. Arthroscopic surgery for degenerative tears of the meniscus: a systematic review and meta-analysis. CMAJ. 2014;186:1057–64.
25. Kise NJ, et al. Exercise therapy versus arthroscopic partial meniscectomy for degenerative meniscal tear in middle aged patients: randomised controlled trial with two year follow-up. BMJ. 2016;354:i3740.
26. Ménétrey J, Siegrist O, Fritschy D. Medial meniscectomy in patients over the age of fifty: a six year follow-up study. Swiss Surg. 2002;8:113–9.
27. Śmigielski R, Zdanowicz U, Drwięga M, Ciszek B, Ciszkowska-Łysoń B, Siebold R. Ribbon like appearance of the midsubstance fibres of the anterior cruciate ligament close to its femoral insertion site: a cadaveric study including 111 knees. Knee Surg Sports Traumatol Arthrosc. 2015;23(11):3143–50.
28. Moulton SG, Steineman BD, Haut Donahue TL, Fontboté CA, Cram TR, LaPrade RF. Direct versus indirect ACL femoral attachment fibres and their implications on ACL graft placement. Knee Surg Sports Traumatol Arthrosc. 2017;25(1):165–71.
29. Alentorn-Geli E, et al. Prevention of non-contact anterior cruciate ligament injuries in soccer players. Part 1: mechanisms of injury and underlying risk factors. Knee Surg Sports Traumatol Arthrosc. 2009;17:705–29.
30. Koga H, et al. Mechanisms for noncontact anterior cruciate ligament injuries: knee joint kinematics in 10 injury situations from female team handball and basketball. Am J Sports Med. 2010;38:2218–25.
31. Lohmander LS, Englund PM, Dahl LL, Roos EM. The long-term consequence of anterior cruciate ligament and meniscus injuries: osteoarthritis. Am J Sports Med. 2007;35:1756–69.
32. Mihelic R, Jurdana H, Jotanovic Z, Madjarevic T, Tudor A. Long-term results of anterior cruciate ligament reconstruction: a comparison with non-operative treatment with a follow-up of 17–20 years. Int Orthop. 2011;35:1093–7.
33. Carey JL, Dunn WR, Dahm DL, Zeger SL, Spindler KP. A systematic review of anterior cruciate ligament reconstruction with autograft compared with allograft. J Bone Joint Surg Am. 2009;91:2242–50.
34. Cavaignac E, et al. Is quadriceps tendon autograft a better choice than hamstring autograft for anterior cruciate ligament reconstruction? A comparative study with a mean follow-up of 3.6 years. Am J Sports Med. 2017;45:1326–32.
35. Dopirak RM, Adamany DC, Steensen RN. A comparison of autogenous patellar tendon and hamstring tendon grafts for anterior cruciate ligament reconstruction. Orthopedics. 2004;27:837–42; quiz 843–844.
36. Foster TE, Wolfe BL, Ryan S, Silvestri L, Kaye EK. Does the graft source really matter in the outcome of patients undergoing anterior cruciate ligament reconstruction? An evaluation of autograft versus allograft reconstruction results: a systematic review. Am J Sports Med. 2010;38:189–99.
37. Goldblatt JP, Fitzsimmons SE, Balk E, Richmond JC. Reconstruction of the anterior cruciate ligament: meta-analysis of patellar tendon versus hamstring tendon autograft. Art Ther. 2005;21:791–803.
38. Hu J, Qu J, Xu D, Zhou J, Lu H. Allograft versus autograft for anterior cruciate ligament reconstruction: an up-to-date meta-analysis of prospective studies. Int Orthop. 2013;37:311–20.
39. Laoruengthana A, Pattayakorn S, Chotanaputhi T, Kosiyatrakul A. Clinical comparison between six-strand hamstring tendon and patellar tendon autograft in arthroscopic anterior cruciate ligament reconstruction: a prospective, randomized clinical trial. J Med Assoc Thai. 2009;92:491–7.
40. Xie X, et al. A meta-analysis of bone-patellar tendon-bone autograft versus four-strand hamstring tendon autograft for anterior cruciate ligament reconstruction. Knee. 2015;22:100–10.
41. Li X, Xu C, Song J, Jiang N, Yu B. Single-bundle versus double-bundle anterior cruciate ligament reconstruction: an up-to-date meta-analysis. Int Orthop. 2013;37:213–26.
42. Siebold R, Branch TP, Freedberg HI, Jacobs CA. A matched pairs comparison of single- versus double-bundle anterior cruciate ligament reconstructions, clinical results and manual laxity testing. Knee Surg Sports Traumatol Arthrosc. 2011;19(Suppl 1):S4–11.
43. Kondo E, Yasuda K, Azuma H, Tanabe Y, Yagi T. Prospective clinical comparisons of anatomic

double-bundle versus single-bundle anterior cruciate ligament reconstruction procedures in 328 consecutive patients. Am J Sports Med. 2008;36:1675–87.
44. Murawski CD, van Eck CF, Irrgang JJ, Tashman S, Fu FH. Operative treatment of primary anterior cruciate ligament rupture in adults. J Bone Joint Surg Am. 2014;96:685–94.
45. Brophy RH, et al. Changes in the length of virtual anterior cruciate ligament fibers during stability testing: a comparison of conventional single-bundle reconstruction and native anterior cruciate ligament. Am J Sports Med. 2008;36:2196–203.
46. Sauer S, English R, Clatworthy M. The ratio of tibial slope and meniscal bone angle for the prediction of ACL reconstruction failure risk. Surg J. 2018;4(3):e152–9.
47. Clatworthy M, Sauer S, Roberts T. Transportal central femoral tunnel placement has a significantly higher revision rate than transtibial AM femoral tunnel placement in hamstring ACL reconstruction. Knee Surg Sports Traumatol Arthrosc. https://doi.org/10.1007/s00167-018-5036-x.
48. Guenther D, et al. The role of extra-articular tenodesis in combined ACL and anterolateral capsular injury. J Bone Joint Surg Am. 2017;99:1654–60.
49. Ramesh R, Von Arx O, Azzopardi T, Schranz PJ. The risk of anterior cruciate ligament rupture with generalised joint laxity. J Bone Joint Surg Br. 2005;87:800–3.
50. Slette EL, et al. Biomechanical results of lateral extra-articular Tenodesis procedures of the knee: a systematic review. Art Ther. 2016;32:2592–611.
51. Weber AE, et al. Lateral augmentation procedures in anterior cruciate ligament reconstruction: anatomic, biomechanical, imaging, and clinical evidence. Am J Sports Med 2018:363546517751140. https://doi.org/10.1177/0363546517751140.
52. Mountcastle SB, Posner M, Kragh JF, Taylor DC. Gender differences in anterior cruciate ligament injury vary with activity: epidemiology of anterior cruciate ligament injuries in a young, athletic population. Am J Sports Med. 2007;35:1635–42.
53. Prodromos CC, Han Y, Rogowski J, Joyce B, Shi K. A meta-analysis of the incidence of anterior cruciate ligament tears as a function of gender, sport, and a knee injury-reduction regimen. Art Ther. 2007;23:1320–1325.e6.
54. Toth AP, Cordasco FA. Anterior cruciate ligament injuries in the female athlete. J Gend Specif Med. 2001;4:25–34.
55. Hewett TE, Myer GD, Zazulak BT. Hamstrings to quadriceps peak torque ratios diverge between sexes with increasing isokinetic angular velocity. J Sci Med Sport. 2008;11:452–9.
56. Hewett TE, Zazulak BT, Myer GD. Effects of the menstrual cycle on anterior cruciate ligament injury risk: a systematic review. Am J Sports Med. 2007;35:659–68.
57. LaPrade RF, Burnett QM. Femoral intercondylar notch stenosis and correlation to anterior cruciate ligament injuries. A prospective study. Am J Sports Med. 1994;22:198–202; discussion 203.
58. Shelbourne KD, Davis TJ, Klootwyk TE. The relationship between intercondylar notch width of the femur and the incidence of anterior cruciate ligament tears. A prospective study. Am J Sports Med. 1998;26:402–8.
59. Wordeman SC, Quatman CE, Kaeding CC, Hewett TE. In vivo evidence for tibial plateau slope as a risk factor for anterior cruciate ligament injury: a systematic review and meta-analysis. Am J Sports Med. 2012;40:1673–81.
60. Sauer S, Clatworthy M. The effect of medial tibial slope on anterior tibial translation and short-term ACL reconstruction outcome. Surg J. 2018;4(3):e160–3.
61. Benjaminse A, Gokeler A, van der Schans CP. Clinical diagnosis of an anterior cruciate ligament rupture: a meta-analysis. J Orthop Sports Phys Ther. 2006;36:267–88.
62. van Eck CF, van den Bekerom MPJ, Fu FH, Poolman RW, Kerkhoffs GMMJ. Methods to diagnose acute anterior cruciate ligament rupture: a meta-analysis of physical examinations with and without anaesthesia. Knee Surg Sports Traumatol Arthrosc. 2013;21:1895–903.
63. König DP, Rütt J, Kumm D, Breidenbach E. Diagnosis of anterior knee instability. Comparison between the Lachman test, the KT-1000 arthrometer and the ultrasound Lachman test. Unfallchirurg. 1998;101:209–13.
64. Lane CG, Warren R, Pearle AD. The pivot shift. J Am Acad Orthop Surg. 2008;16:679–88.
65. Goldman AB, Pavlov H, Rubenstein D. The Segond fracture of the proximal tibia: a small avulsion that reflects major ligamentous damage. AJR Am J Roentgenol. 1988;151:1163–7.
66. Lee CH, et al. Osseous injury associated with ligamentous tear of the knee. Can Assoc Radiol J. 2016;67:379–86.
67. Lorbach O, et al. The influence of the medial meniscus in different conditions on anterior tibial translation in the anterior cruciate deficient knee. Int Orthop. 2015;39:681–7.
68. Monk AP, et al. Surgical versus conservative interventions for treating anterior cruciate ligament injuries. Cochrane Database Syst Rev. 2016;4:CD011166.
69. Duquin TR, Wind WM, Fineberg MS, Smolinski RJ, Buyea CM. Current trends in anterior cruciate ligament reconstruction. J Knee Surg. 2009;22:7–12.
70. Mayr HO, Weig TG, Plitz W. Arthrofibrosis following ACL reconstruction—reasons and outcome. Arch Orthop Trauma Surg. 2004;124:518–22.
71. Ardern CL, Taylor NF, Feller JA, Webster KE. Fifty-five per cent return to competitive sport following anterior cruciate ligament reconstruction surgery: an updated systematic review and meta-analysis including aspects of physical functioning and contextual factors. Br J Sports Med. 2014;48:1543–52.

72. Czuppon S, Racette BA, Klein SE, Harris-Hayes M. Variables associated with return to sport following anterior cruciate ligament reconstruction: a systematic review. Br J Sports Med. 2014;48:356–64.
73. Legnani C, Terzaghi C, Borgo E, Ventura A. Management of anterior cruciate ligament rupture in patients aged 40 years and older. J Orthop Traumatol. 2011;12:177–84.
74. Sri-Ram K, Salmon LJ, Pinczewski LA, Roe JP. The incidence of secondary pathology after anterior cruciate ligament rupture in 5086 patients requiring ligament reconstruction. Bone Joint J. 2013;95-B:59–64.
75. Barenius B, et al. Increased risk of osteoarthritis after anterior cruciate ligament reconstruction: a 14-year follow-up study of a randomized controlled trial. Am J Sports Med. 2014;42:1049–57.
76. Frobell RB, et al. Treatment for acute anterior cruciate ligament tear: five year outcome of randomised trial. Br J Sports Med. 2015;49:700.
77. Gillquist J, Messner K. Anterior cruciate ligament reconstruction and the long-term incidence of gonarthrosis. Sports Med. 1999;27:143–56.
78. Wind WM, Bergfeld JA, Parker RD. Evaluation and treatment of posterior cruciate ligament injuries: revisited. Am J Sports Med. 2004;32:1765–75.
79. Agolley D, Gabr A, Benjamin-Laing H, Haddad FS. Successful return to sports in athletes following non-operative management of acute isolated posterior cruciate ligament injuries: medium-term follow-up. Bone Joint J. 2017;99-B:774–8.
80. Parolie JM, Bergfeld JA. Long-term results of nonoperative treatment of isolated posterior cruciate ligament injuries in the athlete. Am J Sports Med. 1986;14:35–8.
81. Patel DV, Allen AA, Warren RF, Wickiewicz TL, Simonian PT. The nonoperative treatment of acute, isolated (partial or complete) posterior cruciate ligament-deficient knees: an intermediate-term follow-up study. HSS J. 2007;3:137–46.
82. Woodmass JM, et al. Poly-traumatic multi-ligament knee injuries: is the knee the limiting factor? Knee Surg Sports Traumatol Arthrosc. 2018;26(9):2865–71. https://doi.org/10.1007/s00167-017-4784-3.
83. Logan M, Williams A, Lavelle J, Gedroyc W, Freeman M. The effect of posterior cruciate ligament deficiency on knee kinematics. Am J Sports Med. 2004;32:1915–22.
84. Allen CR, Kaplan LD, Fluhme DJ, Harner CD. Posterior cruciate ligament injuries. Curr Opin Rheumatol. 2002;14:142–9.
85. Sekiya JK, Whiddon DR, Zehms CT, Miller MD. A clinically relevant assessment of posterior cruciate ligament and posterolateral corner injuries. Evaluation of isolated and combined deficiency. J Bone Joint Surg Am. 2008;90:1621–7.
86. Rosenthal MD, Rainey CE, Tognoni A, Worms R. Evaluation and management of posterior cruciate ligament injuries. Phys Ther Sport. 2012;13:196–208.
87. Jansson KS, Costello KE, O'Brien L, Wijdicks CA, Laprade RF. A historical perspective of PCL bracing. Knee Surg Sports Traumatol Arthrosc. 2013;21:1064–70.
88. Fowler PJ, Messieh SS. Isolated posterior cruciate ligament injuries in athletes. Am J Sports Med. 1987;15:553–7.
89. Bedi A, Musahl V, Cowan JB. Management of posterior cruciate ligament injuries: an evidence-based review. J Am Acad Orthop Surg. 2016;24:277–89.
90. Lopez-Vidriero E, Simon DA, Johnson DH. Initial evaluation of posterior cruciate ligament injuries: history, physical examination, imaging studies, surgical and nonsurgical indications. Sports Med Arthrosc Rev. 2010;18:230–7.
91. Hammoud S, Reinhardt KR, Marx RG. Outcomes of posterior cruciate ligament treatment: a review of the evidence. Sports Med Arthrosc Rev. 2010;18:280–91.
92. Pierce CM, O'Brien L, Griffin LW, Laprade RF. Posterior cruciate ligament tears: functional and postoperative rehabilitation. Knee Surg Sports Traumatol Arthrosc. 2013;21:1071–84.
93. Voos JE, Mauro CS, Wente T, Warren RF, Wickiewicz TL. Posterior cruciate ligament: anatomy, biomechanics, and outcomes. Am J Sports Med. 2012;40:222–31.
94. Harner CD, Höher J. Evaluation and treatment of posterior cruciate ligament injuries. Am J Sports Med. 1998;26:471–82.
95. Craft JA, Kurzweil PR. Physical examination and imaging of medial collateral ligament and posteromedial corner of the knee. Sports Med Arthrosc Rev. 2015;23:e1–6.
96. Duffy PS, Miyamoto RG. Management of medial collateral ligament injuries in the knee: an update and review. Phys Sportsmed. 2010;38:48–54.
97. Schein A, et al. Structure and function, injury, pathology, and treatment of the medial collateral ligament of the knee. Emerg Radiol. 2012;19:489–98.
98. Lundberg M, Messner K. Long-term prognosis of isolated partial medial collateral ligament ruptures. A ten-year clinical and radiographic evaluation of a prospectively observed group of patients. Am J Sports Med. 1996;24:160–3.
99. Lundberg M, Messner K. Ten-year prognosis of isolated and combined medial collateral ligament ruptures. A matched comparison in 40 patients using clinical and radiographic evaluations. Am J Sports Med. 1997;25:2–6.
100. Warren LF, Marshall JL. The supporting structures and layers on the medial side of the knee: an anatomical analysis. J Bone Joint Surg Am. 1979;61:56–62.
101. Narvani A, Mahmud T, Lavelle J, Williams A. Injury to the proximal deep medial collateral ligament: a

problematical subgroup of injuries. J Bone Joint Surg Br. 2010;92:949–53.
102. Fanelli GC, Harris JD. Surgical treatment of acute medial collateral ligament and posteromedial corner injuries of the knee. Sports Med Arthrosc Rev. 2006;14:78–83.
103. Menzer H, Treme G, Wascher D. Surgical treatment of medial instability of the knee. Sports Med Arthrosc Rev. 2015;23:77–84.
104. Smyth MP, Koh JL. A review of surgical and nonsurgical outcomes of medial knee injuries. Sports Med Arthrosc Rev. 2015;23:e15–22.
105. Stannard JP. Medial and posteromedial instability of the knee: evaluation, treatment, and results. Sports Med Arthrosc Rev. 2010;18:263–8.
106. Wang JC, Shapiro MS. Pellegrini-Stieda syndrome. Am J Orthop. 1995;24:493–7.
107. Kurzweil PR, Kelley ST. Physical examination and imaging of the medial collateral ligament and posteromedial corner of the knee. Sports Med Arthrosc Rev. 2006;14:67–73.
108. Laprade RF, Bernhardson AS, Griffith CJ, Macalena JA, Wijdicks CA. Correlation of valgus stress radiographs with medial knee ligament injuries: an in vitro biomechanical study. Am J Sports Med. 2010;38:330–8.
109. Bollier M, Smith PA. Anterior cruciate ligament and medial collateral ligament injuries. J Knee Surg. 2014;27:359–68.
110. Jiang KN, West RV. Management of chronic combined ACL medial posteromedial instability of the knee. Sports Med Arthrosc Rev. 2015;23:85–90.
111. Blaha JD, Mancinelli CA, Simons WH, Kish VL, Thyagarajan G. Kinematics of the human knee using an open chain cadaver model. Clin Orthop Relat Res. 410:25–34.
112. Lunden JB, Bzdusek PJ, Monson JK, Malcomson KW, Laprade RF. Current concepts in the recognition and treatment of posterolateral corner injuries of the knee. J Orthop Sports Phys Ther. 2010;40:502–16.
113. Ranawat A, Baker CL, Henry S, Harner CD. Posterolateral corner injury of the knee: evaluation and management. J Am Acad Orthop Surg. 2008;16:506–18.
114. Malone AA, Dowd GSE, Saifuddin A. Injuries of the posterior cruciate ligament and posterolateral corner of the knee. Injury. 2006;37:485–501.
115. Davies H, Unwin A, Aichroth P. The posterolateral corner of the knee. Anatomy, biomechanics and management of injuries. Injury. 2004;35:68–75.
116. Frank JB, Youm T, Meislin RJ, Rokito AS. Posterolateral corner injuries of the knee. Bull NYU Hosp Jt Dis. 2007;65:106–14.
117. Helgeson MD, Lehman RA, Murphy KP. Initial evaluation of the acute and chronic multiple ligament injured knee. J Knee Surg. 2005;18:213–9.
118. Tay AKL, MacDonald PB. Complications associated with treatment of multiple ligament injured (dislocated) knee. Sports Med Arthrosc Rev. 2011;19:153–61.
119. Peskun CJ, et al. Diagnosis and management of knee dislocations. Phys Sportsmed. 2010;38:101–11.
120. Seroyer ST, Musahl V, Harner CD. Management of the acute knee dislocation: the Pittsburgh experience. Injury. 2008;39:710–8.
121. Johnson ME, Foster L, DeLee JC. Neurologic and vascular injuries associated with knee ligament injuries. Am J Sports Med. 2008;36:2448–62.
122. Kim BS, Kim YW, Song EK, Seon JK, Do Kang K, Kim HN. Simultaneous bilateral quadriceps tendon rupture in a patient with chronic renal failure. Knee Surg Relat Res. 2012;24(1):56–9.
123. Omar M, Haas P, Ettinger M, Krettek C, Petri M. Simultaneous bilateral quadriceps tendon rupture following long-term low-dose nasal corticosteroid application. Case Rep Orthop. 2013;2013:1–5.
124. Hockings M, Cameron JC. Patella baja following chronic quadriceps tendon rupture. Knee. 2004;11(2):95–7.
125. Hanson CA, Weinhold PS, Afshari HM, Dahners LE. The effect of analgesic agents on the healing rat medial collateral ligament. Am J Sports Med. 2005;33:674–9.
126. Warden SJ, et al. Low-intensity pulsed ultrasound accelerates and a nonsteroidal anti-inflammatory drug delays knee ligament healing. Am J Sports Med. 2006;34:1094–102.

Sports Trauma: Ankle and Foot

28

Bruno Silva Pereira and C. Niek van Dijk

28.1 Sports Injuries

Healthy, pain-free foot and ankle function is both essential for participation in most sports and, statistically, is also most frequently impaired in athletes. As the base of the lower quarter kinetic chain, the foot and ankle form a cornerstone of lower body biomechanics, ensuring efficient stabilization, movement, and power development. Injuries to this area must be properly managed to ensure a return to pre-injury status as well as avoid development of secondary injuries [1].

B. S. Pereira (✉)
Department of Orthopedic Surgery, Hospital de Braga, Braga, Portugal

Faculty of Medicine, University of Barcelona, Barcelona, Spain

Clínica do Dragão, Espregueira-Mendes Sports Center, FIFA Medical Centre of Excellence, Porto, Portugal

C. N. van Dijk
Clínica do Dragão, Espregueira-Mendes Sports Center, FIFA Medical Centre of Excellence, Porto, Portugal

Department Orthopedic Surgery, Academic Medical Center (AMC), Amsterdam, The Netherlands

FIFA Medical Centre of Excellence Ripoll De Prado & Van Dijk Sport Clinic, Madrid, Spain
e-mail: c.n.vandijk@amc.uva.nl

28.2 Epidemiology and Injuries

28.2.1 All Sports

Ankle sprains are the most common of the foot and ankle injuries affecting athletes, accounting for up to 21% of all sports injuries, with the most common mechanism being forced inversion and tearing of one or more lateral ligaments. In a review of injuries treated at a multispecialty sports clinic, 25% of injuries occurring in 19 of the most popular sports involved the foot and ankle [2].

28.2.2 Women's Gymnastics

Kerr et al. reported that data collected from 11 women's college gymnastic programs show that ankle sprains are the most common injuries and account for large proportions of injuries across all types of gymnastic equipment. Ankle and lower leg/Achilles tendon injuries have the highest rates of recurrence. Ankle injuries account for 17.9%, lower leg/Achilles tendon injuries account for 13.6%, and foot injuries account for 12.4% of all reported injuries. The majority of injuries occur in the preseason. Severe injuries—those resulting in more than 3 weeks of time loss—account for 12.4% of all injuries. Of these, 53.7% are season-ending injuries for the student-athlete. This data represents a reduced time-loss

S. Rocha Piedade et al. (eds.), *The Sports Medicine Physician*,
https://doi.org/10.1007/978-3-030-10433-7_28

injury rate compared to previous surveillance data. Addition of safety padding and equipment redesign is thought to have contributed to the injury reductions [3].

28.2.3 Pivotal Sports

In a prospective observational study, 35% of midtarsal joint injuries involved sports accidents. Midtarsal joint sprain (MJS), also referred to as Chopart's injury, occurs more commonly in pivoting sports such as soccer, rugby, basketball, and tennis. Chopart's injury presents a diagnostic and clinical challenge. When it occurs, it is often severe. Foot inversion accounted for 76% of all cases, followed by plantar flexion in 21% [4].

28.2.4 Running

Most running-related injuries are associated with repetitive microtrauma and arise from a combination of individual anatomical and biomechanical factors, training errors, and limited running experience. Ankle and Achilles tendon injuries are the most prevalent injuries of the foot and ankle. A survey of marathon race participants found 54% lifetime incidence of all running-related injuries among long-distance runners, with one-third of recreational runners affected by at least one minor injury of any kind per season. Risk factors include male gender, short running history of approximately 1–3 years, previous injuries, and BMI. Additionally, higher age and barefoot running are risk factors for lifetime running-related lower leg injuries. Training distances of 21–50 km per week increase a runner's risk for lifetime running-related injuries of the foot [5].

28.2.5 Soccer

Foot and ankle injuries are common in both amateur and semiprofessional soccer players. A newly developed standardized questionnaire revealed that 42% of all soccer injuries occur to the foot or ankle, with 61% of those being ankle injuries. Age, weight, height, and shorter warm-ups were significantly correlated. Players who had sustained five or more injuries were significantly older, heavier, and taller than those with fewer than five injuries. Amateur players reported a much higher rate of foot and ankle injuries than semiprofessional players, with rates of 64% and 40%, respectively. The vast majority (80%) of foot and ankle injuries occurred while playing in a match. However, the position played did not correlate with increased foot or ankle injury occurrence [6].

28.3 Most Common Injuries

28.3.1 Ankle Instability

Definition: Chronic ankle instability (CAI) is generally seen as having two potential etiologies: mechanical instability and functional instability. The term mechanical instability is often used synonymously with "laxity" to describe movement beyond the ankle's physiologic limit. However, laxity should be reserved to describe the pathologic movement beyond the ankle's physiologic limits. This can exist with or without complaints. Mechanical instability should be reserved for a patient with recurrent giving way due to an ankle with laxity. By contrast, functional instability is a subjective sensation of ankle giving way or history of recurrent ankle sprains arising from impaired proprioception and neuromuscular function. Tenen et al. found that high school athletes are more likely to experience chronic ankle instability than college athletes and women are more likely than men to have CAI at both the high school and college level [7, 8].

Biomechanically, the subtalar joint serves a critical function in ankle movement by acting as a hinge around which the leg rotates on the foot during weight-bearing. The muscles around the ankle together with the subtalar and talocrural joints determine the ankle's ability to counteract torque. The muscular imbalance has been shown to be a more significant contributing factor than muscle weakness in chronic ankle instability. In particular, smaller dorsiflexion-to-inversion strength ratio and greater eversion-to-inversion strength are predictors of ankle-inversion injury. The typical scenario in traumatic injuries is that the evertor muscles are unable to counteract external inversion torque [7].

Diagnosis: Consideration of ligament anatomy and anatomical variants can help with the precise diagnosis of ankle injuries. It is also the most important stabilizer of the ankle joint. The anterior talofibular ligament (ATFL), which limits anterior displacement of the talus and plantar ankle flexion, is the most commonly injured ankle ligament. It lies horizontal to the ankle in neutral position. However, in plantar flexion, it inclines downward and is subject to strain and injury, particularly during inversion [9]. ATFL lesions can be isolated or combined with calcaneofibular ligament (CFL) lesions.

Anatomic variants of the calcaneofibular ligament are common and should be considered in the diagnostic process. In 35% of the population, the ligament is reinforced by the lateral talocalcaneal ligament; in 23% a lateral talocalcaneal ligament is present anteriorly and is anatomically distinct from the calcaneofibular ligament. The lateral talocalcaneal ligament is absent in 42% of cases, with an anterior talocalcaneal ligament in its place. In these individuals, the calcaneofibular ligament becomes more important as a stabilizer of the subtalar joint [9].

A multidisciplinary clinical practice guideline has been proposed to improve diagnosis and treatment of acute lateral ankle ligament injuries and reduce societal costs associated with these injuries. Ottawa ankle rules for ruling out fracture after acute ankle injury should be performed as an emergency room evaluative tool. On physical examination, the presence of hematoma along with local pressure pain or positive anterior drawer test is a strong indicator of lateral ankle ligament rupture. Van Dijk has determined that the delayed physical examination of the ankle 4–7 days after trauma has the highest sensitivity and specificity for the diagnosis of an acute lateral ligament rupture [10]. This strategy was adopted by the ISAKOS consensus statement as the diagnostic strategy of choice. The Cumberland Ankle Instability Tool (CAIT) is a valid and reliable patient-reported outcome measure for assessing ankle instability. Its advantage is that it is short and concise thereby decreasing patient burden and increasing reliability. The CAIT also uses a numeric measuring scale and is completed for both ankles, allowing for separate assessment of each ankle. If the rupture is suspected, a repeat physical examination can be performed within a few days of the first examination, to allow time for pain, swelling, and muscle tension to subside [10–14].

Treatment of acute ruptures: Rehabilitation of athletes following lateral ankle injury should include varied exercises emphasizing maintenance of proprioception, strength, coordination, and function. The merits of cryotherapy for an acute ankle injury have not been definitively proven, though ice in combination with exercise is more effective than heat for reducing swelling. Ice combined with rest, compression, and elevation is also valuable during the acute phase. Prolonged immobilization of 4 weeks or more has been discredited in favor of shorter, 10-day periods with early initiation of functional treatments [15].

Interestingly, the number of ligaments injured does not seem to affect the prognosis for acute lateral ankle ligament injury. Acute pain and swelling can complicate the diagnostic and treatment process by delaying grade (I, II, III) assignment for the first 4–5 days. Three main treatment modalities include surgical, conservative via immobilization with cast or splint, and functional conservative via tape or brace [15].

Currently, functional treatment is favored over operative treatment. For athletes however operative treatment has been shown to result in a more stable ankle, while the rehab time is not longer when compared to functional treatment [16].

Outcomes: There is currently insufficient evidence in support of surgery over conservative treatment for acute lesions. For elite athletes surgery, however, it should be considered since surgery has shown to result in a more stable ankle. However, there is evidence supporting functional treatment over immobilization, with tape, semi-rigid brace, and lace-up brace producing equivalent results for treating acute lateral ankle ligament injuries within the 6-month recovery window. Kerkhoffs et al. note that 60–90% of athletes with acute ankle instability injuries can return to sports and can perform to pre-injury levels after 12 weeks [16–18].

Treatment of chronic instability: Before conducting any surgical procedure, nonsurgical management is highly recommended for patients with chronic ankle instability at least over the first 2-month period. During the rehabilitation stage, physiotherapy with neuromuscular and proprioceptive training should be provided. In case of functional instability, proprioceptive and neuromuscular deficits are probably important cause; a minimum period of 3–6 months of physiotherapist rehabilitation, consisting of strengthening exercises of the active stabilizers of the ankle and proprioceptive training, was recommended [14–17].

Surgical management is advised when chronic ankle instability is persistent, and other options are of no use. Operative procedures of chronically unstable ankles fall into anatomic repair, nonanatomic reconstruction, and anatomic reconstruction.

The anatomic repair is defined as suturing of the torn lateral ligaments. The classic Broström procedure is thus defined as a true repair of the lateral ligaments including the ATFL and CFL. However, it is rarely performed as a standalone procedure, because it is usually augmented with a transfer of the extensor retinaculum either as a proximal advancement—the Gould procedure. The Gould modification adds an augmentation with a transfer of the extensor retinaculum [14–17].

The reconstruction refers to the replacement of the chronically deficient lateral ligaments with local tissues or with autograft or allograft tissue. Reconstruction may be anatomical or nonanatomical.

Anatomic reconstruction with tendon graft or transfer was traditionally procedures that have been reserved for patients who have failed a prior Broström-Gould repair. However, patients who may stress their ankle to a greater degree than normal, including those with high body mass index, heavy labor occupation, or sports requirements, or patients with congenital ligament laxity may benefit from performing ligament reconstruction as the primary procedure. Although isometry of the lateral ankle ligaments has not been proven, placement of the tendon grafts at the ligaments' anatomical origin and insertion should be performed. The goal is to achieve good ankle stability without over-constraining the ankle or subtalar joints. The nonanatomic positioning of the graft may alter the biomechanics of the joints resulting in joint loading alterations which may lead to joint degeneration over time [19].

Nonanatomic reconstructions of the lateral ankle ligaments have a long track record in the orthopedic literature where they have been shown historically to work well to establish a stable hindfoot for functional activities. The long-term results in the ankle reveal an increased incidence of degenerative changes in the hindfoot. One of the options is by also applying a nonanatomic tenodesis, which is stabilizing the end of the tendon to a bone. Watson-Jones developed a procedure to limit rotation and interior subluxation: They used peroneus brevis and routed the tendon through anterior-to-posterior (distal-to-proximal) style passing through the fibula to be secured to the talar neck. Another option is the Chrisman-Snook reconstruction procedure; the peroneus brevis tendon is the first split and then driven into the fibula and then into the calcaneus. This procedure supports anatomic reconstruction, but some patients were reported to experience nonphysiological kinematics and subtalar stiffness. In our opinion consensus is that with modern fixation techniques and the known long-term degenerative sequelae associated with nonanatomic reconstruction, these procedures should be avoided [7, 10, 11, 14].

Because intra-articular conditions such as impingement, talus osteochondral lesions, osteophytes, and chondromalacia can accompany chronic ankle instability and can be factored in dysfunction and pain, arthroscopy is ready to lend a hand to diagnose and treat the ankle instability [17, 18].

In our opinion, Broström-Gould repair is still considered the gold standard treatment in patients with chronic lateral ankle ligament laxity requiring surgical treatment. However, in some patients, anatomic reconstruction may be preferred. Moreover, the use of arthroscopy to do or assist the surgery is mandatory.

28.3.2 Anterior and Posterior Impingement

Definition: Anterior and posterior impingement syndromes may include abnormal entrapment or contact of structures in the anterior, anterolateral, anteromedial, posterior, posteromedial, posterolateral, and syndesmotic structures of the ankle. Posterior ankle impingement syndrome is a common repetitive plantarflexion injury. It often occurs in dancers and soccer players but can occur in all sports. Posterior impingement most commonly stems from the pathology of the lateral process of the posterior talus or, less commonly, from tibiotalar or subtalar degenerative joint disease. Anterior impingement is the most common chronic injury in the ankle. Chronic lateral ankle instability has been identified as a possible contributing factor in anterior impingement, but it can occur in any sports with recurrent hyperdorsiflexion. The majority of cases (63% and above) involve synovitis in the anterior compartment, anterior lateral gutter, or other soft tissue lesions. Soft tissue hypertrophy or osteophyte growth encroaches upon the space between the anterior lip of the tibia and the dorsal talar neck. Anterior osteophytes are common and occur in 59% of dancers without impingement symptoms. Most professional soccer players have spurs at the end of their career (personal observation of the senior author) [20–22].

Diagnosis: Accurate diagnosis starts with a thorough physical exam including neurovascular evaluation, strength, and range of motion. Presentation in posterior impingement is generally a pain deep to the Achilles tendon, sometimes confused with Achilles or peroneal tendon pathology. Pain is aggravated by forced plantar flexion of the ankle. A negative plantarflexion test does rule out posterior impingement. Posterior impingement is often combined with flexor hallucis longus tendinitis. Active flexion and extension of the great toe can help localize the pain of such an FHL tendinitis [20, 22].

Diagnosis in anterior impingement is mainly clinical, though imaging is required to rule out other pathologies and locate osteophytes. Anterior impingement typically presents as pain during terminal dorsiflexion. History in anterior impingement often reveals multiple ankle sprains or pain that worsens through a training session or performance. Palpation elicits tenderness along the anterior joint line and thickening of the synovium. Recognizable tenderness on palpation confirms the diagnosis. Osteophytes may be palpable at the anterior lateral or anterior medical joint line. The classic anterior ankle impingement has four typical presentations: the lip of the tibia, neck of the talus, both, or secondary to frank osteoarthritis [21, 23].

X-ray, CT, and MRI are all useful imaging methods. An x-ray should include weight-bearing AP, lateral, and mortise views. The lateral view should be carefully analyzed for the presence of exostoses and posterior bony anomalies. Oblique views can help assess bony abnormalities. In the case of anteromedial recognizable tenderness on palpation, one should order an anteromedial impingement view (AMI view) like van Dijk described in 2002 [24]. This oblique view can help assess bony abnormalities on the medial side of the joint. Consider MRI in case osteochondral defects are part of the differential diagnosis. The posterior impingement x-ray view (PIM view) provides superior diagnostic accuracy over the lateral view for detecting os trigonum, while MRI can detect soft tissue anomalies, such as peroneus quartus. Soft tissue injuries associated with posterior impingement include posterior capsuloligamentous injury or flexor hallucis longus tendinopathy [20–22, 24].

Treatment: Physical therapy should focus on the entire kinetic chain. Night splint or removable walking brace can be used briefly. High-level athletes may benefit from ultrasound-guided injections. Surgery is indicated if symptoms persist after 3 months of conservative care. Arthroscopy is advantageous for the patient regarding smaller incisions and shorter recovery times. Surgery for anterior impingement may involve resection, debridement, or both. Surgery for posterior impingement involves resection of involved structures [21, 22].

Yasui, Hannon, et al. describe a four-stage arthroscopy that allows for full assessment of all posterior ankle and subtalar joint structures. The procedure involves dividing the hindfoot structures into four regions of interest: superolateral, superomedial, inferomedial, and inferolateral. Each region is methodically inspected and appropriately treated. This assessment has lost its use since diagnosis should not depend on arthroscopy. A diagnosis must be made before any surgery is performed. The arthroscope is used as a tool to perform the surgery and not as a diagnostic tool [22].

Baxter advises that exercising care while performing incisions can help reduce the risk of incisional neuromas. Anterior impingement spurs on the medial shoulder of the talus can be missed on lateral x-ray and may require nonweight-bearing, oblique views. To resect this "hidden" spur arthroscopically, the ankle must be held in dorsiflexion [25].

Outcomes: Conservative treatment has been shown to produce up to 60% success rates. Arthroscopy has resulted in high patient satisfaction rates and AOFAS scores, with low rates of complications. Tanawat et al. found that arthroscopic bony or soft tissue debridement each provide positive long-term outcomes where there are no arthritic changes, ligament laxity, or chondral lesions. Open treatment for posterior impingement using a lateral or medial approach produces good results but is associated with high rates of complications. Posterior endoscopy has shown significantly faster return to sports and lower complication rates; however, the technique is technically difficult. Yasui reports very good short-term results of the four-stage arthroscopy procedure, with low complication rates [20, 22, 23, 26, 27].

28.3.3 Osteochondral Lesions of the Talus

Definition: Osteochondral lesions of the talus (OLT) are the most common cartilage injury of the ankle, occurring in 50% of ankle sprains. Shimozono et al. report the rate of occurrence in athletes is five to nearly ten times that of the general population. Etiology is controversial and includes a diverse range of potential factors, such as acute or remote trauma, degenerative arthropathies, repetitive microtrauma, systemic metabolic disorders, genetic predisposition, abnormal vasculature, and systemic conditions. The talar dome is a common site for osteochondral lesions and is second to the knee in frequency. Posteromedial lesions tend to be deeper and cup-shaped, while anterolateral lesions tend to be shallow and wafer-shaped. Medial osteochondral lesions of the talus occur at a higher rate than lateral lesions. All lateral lesions and 36% of medial lesions are associated with trauma. These patients present with deep ankle pain. Van Dijk published on the cause of the pain in these lesions: that pain does not arise from the cartilage lesion but is most probably caused by repetitive high fluid pressure during walking, which results in stimulation of the highly innervated subchondral bone underneath the cartilage defect [28–31].

Diagnosis: The most important for the diagnosis is the history taking. A patient with an OLT has deep ankle pain. A thorough examination can sometimes reveal joint swelling, crepitus, reduced passive and active ranges of motion, and palpatory tenderness. Anterior drawer and talar tilt tests can assess laxity and help narrow the diagnosis; however, there are no confirming physical examination tests for osteochondral lesions. Physical exam signs may be absent, and the exam is often nondiagnostic. Most patients with an OLT will show a "normal ankle"; long-standing problems may involve compensatory contralateral knee, hip, and back pain [28, 32].

When symptoms persist after conservative management, imaging studies may be necessary to confirm the diagnosis. X-ray is the standard imaging method but misses up to 41% of OLT. The x-ray also lacks the personal ability to assess the integrity of the articular cartilage, and thus, its usefulness for accurately staging the disease process is limited. X-ray imaging should include weight-bearing, if tolerable. Mortise view is best for showing lateral lesions. Medial lesions are best viewed with anteroposterior views. Bilateral radiographs allow comparison of affected and non-affected sides, though contralateral lesions occur in up to 25%. MRI is better for evaluating cartilage and is 96% sensitive and 96% specific for diagnosing OLT. MRI is regarded as the gold standard for imaging pure cartilage lesions, with 100% specificity and 73–95% sensitivity. However, these lesions are seldom pure chondral injuries. Most symptomatic patients have osteochondral lesions. MRI and CT scan have shown similar diagnostic accuracy, but CT scan is preferred since it is much better for preoperative planning since it shows the exact extent and location of the lesion [28, 32–35].

SPECT/CT shows promise for improving treatment outcomes for OLT by improving the accuracy of disease staging. Morteza, Stuart, et al. reported that SPECT combined with multi-slice low-dose CT (MslCT) added clinical value in 89% of OLT patients with nonmalignant pathologies. Arthroscopy can also be used as a diagnostic tool when imaging is negative, and symptoms persist after conservative management has been tried. Arthroscopy offers the advantages of direct visualization and immediate treatment [36].

Treatment: Surgery is indicated in the event of failure of conservative therapy for chronic lesions and. Acute osteochondral fragments of >12 mm in size should be fixed (Figs. 28.1, 28.2, and 28.3). Concerning chronic lesions curettage, drilling, or microfracture techniques can be used on lesions <15 mm wide and <7 mm deep (Fig. 28.4). Larger lesions are candidates for fixation. Those which primary bone marrow stimulation surgery was tried and failed may be candidates for autologous chondrocyte implantation (ACI), osteochondral autograft transplantation (OATs or mosaicplasty), osteochondral allograft transplantation, or metal inlay implant. These secondary lesions can also benefit from a

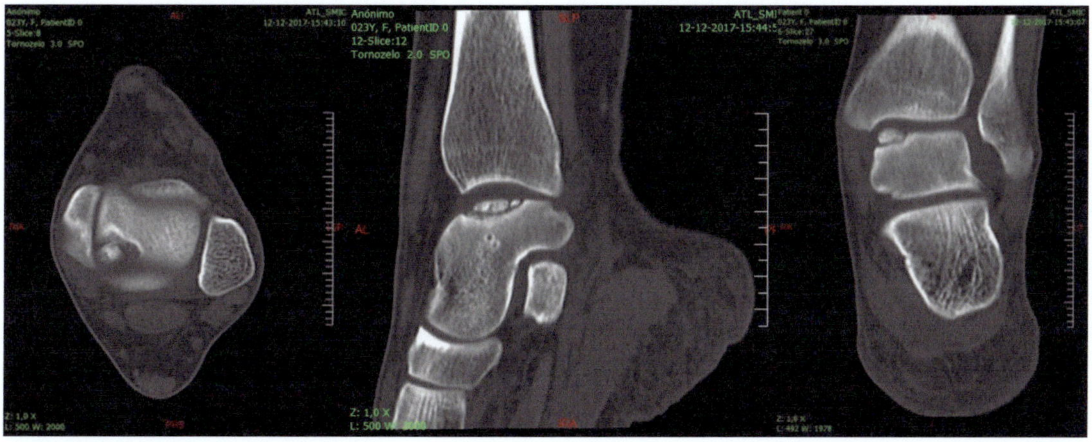

Fig. 28.1 OLT large defect

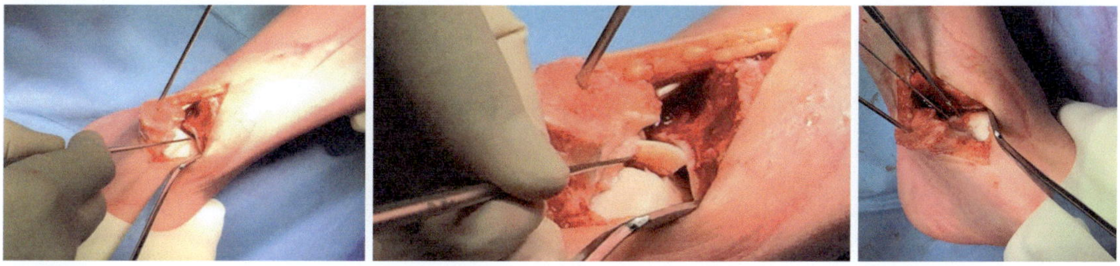

Fig. 28.2 Sequence of OLT larger lesion fixation

sliding calcaneal osteotomy in case of malalignment [28].

Spennacchio et al. reported that the 70° arthroscope could provide improved capabilities for visualizing for certain lesions involving the borders of the talar dome when compared to the 30° arthroscope. This method is particularly useful for uncontained lesions as it provides visualization of "hidden" portions of the lesions in the joint gutters. Successful treatment of a large talar dome defect, refractory to two previous arthroscopic procedures, using a novel contoured metal implant was reported by van Bergen et al. The technique uses an oblique osteotomy of the medial malleolus in order to provide adequate exposure to ensure accurate implantation [32, 37, 38].

Outcomes: Conservative treatment including weight-bearing tolerance has been reported by Zengerink et al. to produce successful outcomes in 45% of patients.

The operative treatment produces good-to-excellent outcomes in up to 85% of patients. For larger lesions or where previous bone marrow stimulation techniques have failed, there is evidence supporting autogenous chondrocyte implantation and osteochondral autograft or allograft transplantation [29, 32].

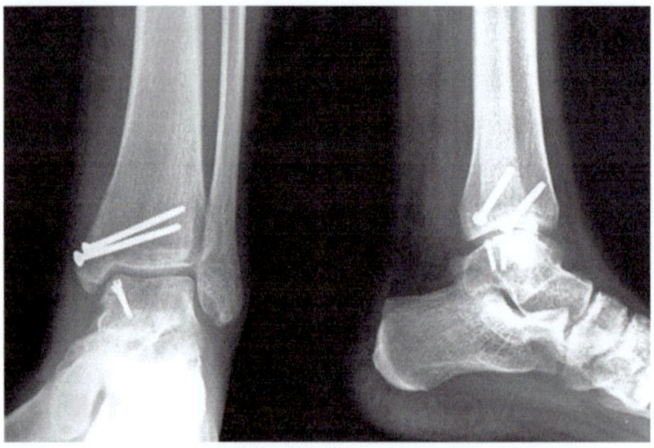

Fig. 28.3 Post-op x-ray

Microfracture arthroscopy for treatment of osteochondral defects of the talus is less effective for larger lesions. Tissue-engineered scaffolds have shown promising results in a single-step arthroscopic procedure that does not require traction, fibrin glue, or pins for scaffold stabilization. This procedure is shorter in duration and simpler to perform and eliminates neurapraxia risk associated with traction. However, the absence of tracks restricts access to anterior lesions from posterior portals, making the preoperative location of the lesion mandatory. Additionally, without gluing or pinning, it is imperative that the patient maintains neutral ankle position meticulously for 3 weeks following surgery [39].

28.3.4 Achilles Tendon Injuries

Definition: The terminology of Achilles tendon pathology has become inconsistent and confusing throughout the years. We use the terminology adapted from KSSTA: midportion Achilles tendinopathy, Achilles paratendinopathy, insertional Achilles tendinopathy retrocalcaneal bursitis, and superficial calcaneal bursitis [39–41].

Midportion Achilles tendinopathy is a clinical syndrome characterized by a combination of pain, swelling, and impaired performance. It includes, but is not limited to, the histopathological diagnosis of tendinosis. *Achilles paratendinopathy* is an acute or chronic inflammation and/or degenera-

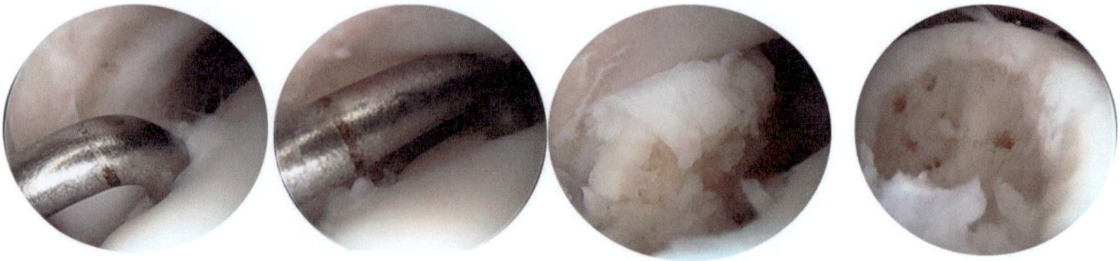

Fig. 28.4 Microfracture arthroscopy for treatment of osteochondral defects of the talus

tion of the thin membrane around the Achilles tendon. There are clear distinctions between acute paratendinopathy and chronic paratendinopathy, both in symptoms and in histopathology. *Insertional Achilles tendinopathy* is located at the insertion of the Achilles tendon onto the calcaneus; bone spurs and calcifications in the tendon proper at the insertion site may exist. *Retrocalcaneal bursitis* is an inflammation of the bursa in the recess between the anterior-inferior side of the Achilles tendon and the posterosuperior aspect of the calcaneus (retrocalcaneal recess). *Superficial calcaneal bursitis* is an inflammation of the bursa located between a calcaneal prominence or the Achilles tendon and the skin. Overuse injuries of the Achilles tendon can be either insertional or non-insertional based on anatomical location [31, 40–43].

Non-insertional Achilles tendinopathy occurs disproportionately in athletes compared to the general population, particularly affecting middle- and long-distance runners. Roche and Calder estimate that 9% of recreational athletes are affected and that chronic Achilles tendinopathy becomes a career-ending condition for up to 5% of professional runners. Concerning the non-insertional problems, van Dijk postulated that the pain does not originate from the tendon itself but from the nerves in the paratenon. The process starts within the tendon with local degeneration or microrupture. Since there are hardly vessels and nerves within the tendon by means of cytokines, a neurogenic response is induced with neovascularization and neoinnervation in the paratenon. It is these neonerves which cause the pain in these patients. Treatment originally addressed the tendon proper itself. Van Dijk, however, proposed endoscopic denervation of the painful area with excellent results. He also postulated the role of the plantaris tendon that may contribute to symptoms in some midportion Achilles tendinopathy patients. Anatomical studies have found firm connections between the plantaris and calcaneal tendons at the level of the midportion of the Achilles tendon. Plantaris excision has revealed the absence of tendinopathic changes; however, the majority of patients who clinically improve following surgery show presence of inflammatory changes in the peritendinous connective tissue surrounding the plantaris tendon, indicating that the pathologic process may involve a compressive or frictional component [39–46].

Concerning insertional Achilles tendinopathy is a distinct clinical entity from midportion/non-insertional Achilles tendinopathy or retrocalcaneal bursitis. It appears in the insertion of AT onto the calcaneus, most often with the formation of bone spurs and calcifications in the tendon proper at the insertion site. The patient has pain, stiffness, and sometimes a (solid) swelling.

Diagnosis: The condition can usually be diagnosed clinically via history and presentation. Tests for non-insertional Achilles tendinopathy include palpation for thickening, crepitus, and pain and tendon loading tests to elicit pain on passive dorsiflexion, single heel raise, and hopping. The painful arc sign, characterized by movement of the swollen tissue concurrently with ankle movement, can be used as an indication of tendinopathy but not paratendinopathy. Ultrasound and MRI are of equivalent accuracy in diagnosing this condition. Ultrasound tissue characterization and sonoelastography show promise for improving sensitivity and accuracy. Bloodwork may reveal the decreased activity of matrix metalloproteinases (MMPs), particularly MMP3 [39, 40, 42, 46].

Treatment: Conservative management with rest, activity modification, orthotics, and eccentric stretching is often recommended, initially. NSAIDs may have detrimental effects by inhibiting tendon cell migration and proliferation and by increasing leukotriene levels. Extracorporeal shockwave therapy (ESWT) has been used in conjunction with rehabilitative protocols [39, 40, 42, 46].

Injection therapies such as platelet-rich plasma are currently in wide use. Ultrasound-guided dry needling combined with high-volume image-guided injection has also been used. Dry needling involves repeated needling to the affected tendon to cause localized trauma and induce inflammation and formation of granulation tissue, which strengthens the tendon. High-volume image-guided injection (HVIGI) uses normal saline, local anesthetic, and corticosteroids. A mixture of 10 mL 0.5% bupivacaine hydrochloride and 25 mg of hydrocortisone acetate is injected between the anterior Achilles tendon and Kager's fat pad at the area of maximal neovascularization. This procedure works well in conjunction with eccentric exercises [39, 46, 47].

Limited understanding of the pathophysiology underlying chronic Achilles pain has resulted in a variety of surgical approaches. It has been postulated that intratendinous degeneration is the cause and that performing multiple tenotomies should increase blood supply and speed healing. Others theorize that neurovascular ingrowth is responsible for chronic pain in Achilles tendinopathy and that release of the paratenon helps resolve pain by its denervating effects. Multiple percutaneous longitudinal tenotomies using ultrasound guidance can be performed under local anesthesia as outpatient procedures [48–50].

Outcomes: Roche and Calder report that nonoperative management is successful long term in approximately 70% of cases. Pearce notes that eccentric stretching is the most effective conservative treatment. Ultrasound-guided dry needling combined with high-volume image-guided injection have produced good short- and medium-term symptom relief. Platelet-rich plasma has shown some improved healing in acute rupture but no improvement in symptoms over saline injection for chronic Achilles tendinopathy [39, 40, 47].

For recalcitrant cases, minimally invasive and tendinoscopic treatments show promising results. Baxter notes that operative treatment is 70–90% successful, provided a 3- to 6-month healing period before return to athletic participation is observed. With the exception of multiple percutaneous tenotomies, minimally invasive and endoscopic procedures for treatment of midportion Achilles tendinopathy are associated with lower complication rates than open procedures and produce similar rates of patient satisfaction [25, 39, 40].

A retrospective study by Opdam, Baltes, et al. found that endoscopic treatment of midportion Achilles tendinopathy using paratenon release combined with plantaris tendon resection produces high patient satisfaction rates and good functional outcomes. Cychosz, Phisitkul, et al. report weak evidence in the current literature for the use of tendoscopy for Achilles tendinopathy but add that the limited number of high-level studies speaks to the need for more studies and does not equate to a recommendation against the use of tendoscopy [25, 48, 49].

28.3.5 Plantar Fasciitis

Definition: A common overuse injury of the plantar fascia, which provides static support and dynamic shock absorption to the medial longitudinal arch. The condition is usually a result of repetitive microtrauma, causing microtears that lead to degeneration and inflammation. Plantar fasciitis affects elite as well as recreational athletes. It is common in runners and accounts for 10% of all running-related injuries. Women are slightly more prone than men. Pes planus and pes cavus are both risk factors, as are reduced ankle dorsiflexion and excessive pronation [51, 52].

Diagnosis: There is not a separate algorithm for athletes vs. nonathletes for diagnosing plantar fasciitis. Intense, acute heel pain at the anterior calcaneal insertions is a cardinal sign. History generally reveals the onset of pain upon first walking in the morning or after rest, though pain can also occur after prolonged walking, standing, or intense training. Palpation of the medial tubercle of the calcaneus and proximal plantar fascia assist with diagnosis. Ankle passive dorsiflexion and ankle dorsiflexion/eversion can be performed to rule out tarsal tunnel syndrome. Melvin notes that plantar fasciitis commonly occurs concurrently with heel spurs but that 50–75% of all heel pain patients have heel spurs, indicating that heel spurs may not be a cause of pain in plantar fasciitis [51, 52].

Diagnostic imaging should be performed in persistent cases in which symptoms remain after 4–6 months of conservative care or when signs and symptoms are atypical. X-ray and bone scans are used primarily to rule out a tumor or fracture. MRI and diagnostic ultrasound can be used to evaluate plantar fascia thickness, to confirm the diagnosis, and to evaluate the inflammatory process. Petraglia notes that nerve conduction studies can be also helpful in diagnosis [52].

Treatment: Treatment options for plantar fasciitis are numerous and varied. Conservative options include activity modification, night splints, and NSAIDS. Instrumental modalities may include laser, extracorporeal shock wave therapy, iontophoresis, ultrasound, cryoultrasound, and low-dose radiotherapy. Physical therapy may include massage, manipulative therapy, stretching, orthotic devices, low-dye taping, and kinesiotaping. Stretching exercises yield the most statistically significant long-term results. NSAIDs are not indicated as plantar fasciitis is considered a degenerative and not an inflammatory process. As an alternative therapy, injection of platelet-rich plasma can be used to promote healing. A minimally invasive surgical procedure called radiofrequency microtenotomy uses radiofrequency energy to improve blood flow and promote healing. This procedure allows more precision while preserving the plantar aponeurosis [51, 53].

Outcomes: Conservative therapy is successful in 90% of cases. A meta-analysis of randomized clinical trials revealed focused shock wave (FSW) therapy to be effective for relieving pain in chronic plantar fasciitis, with the advantages of fast recovery and patient convenience. Effectiveness was not confirmed for general extracorporeal shock wave therapy (ESWT) or radial shockwave (RSW) therapy. FSW concentrates waves on the tissue, while RSW disperses waves rather than concentrating them. Osman et al. report that pulsed radiofrequency to the medial calcaneal nerve is safe and effective for reducing pain and achieves analgesia in less time than thermal radiofrequency. The pauses between pulses allow heat to dissipate resulting in less risk of damage to surrounding nerves compared to thermal radiofrequency [53, 54].

Among injection therapies, botulinum toxin injections produce better results than corticosteroid injections. Corticosteroid injections produce short-lasting benefits that are superior to autologous blood but with the potential risk of fascia rupture and infection. PRP therapy has shown superior long-term pain relief and similar functional improvement compared to steroid injections, which carry the risk of abscess, osteomyelitis, fat pad atrophy, and plantar fascia tears. In the chronic phases of the condition, normal fascia is replaced by angiofibroblastic hyperplastic tissue, with no inflammation present. PRP supplies cytokines and growth factors as well as anti-inflammatory components that, in combination, initiate healing and halt degenerative changes [52, 55].

Surgery is recommended after 6–12 months of failed conservative treatment. Minimally invasive radiofrequency microtenotomy has produced promising results in refractory plantar fasciitis [47].

28.3.6 Lisfranc Sprain

Definition: The Lisfranc ligament spans the medial cuneiform and second metatarsal base. The tarsometatarsal articulation is supported by the "keystone" wedging of the second metatarsal into the cuneiform and vulnerable to injury when stressed. Damage may involve ligaments, fractures, or fracture-dislocations. Injury occurs via direct force from an external source or, most commonly, indirect force, whereby the foot is stationary, and the body exerts torque, rotation, or compression. Indirect injuries occur in equestrian sports in which the foot becomes caught in a stirrup and is forced into external rotation or twisting. Soccer and rugby players experience direct-force trauma from contact with another athlete landing on the heel during kneeling or lying prone. Statistically, 87.5% of Lisfranc injuries are closed and up to one-third involve low-energy trauma in athletes. Fracture of the base of the second metatarsal of often the only positive finding. This however represents a Lisfranc dislocation [56–59].

Diagnosis: Fracture dislocations can result in residual malunion and loss of function, making early diagnosis imperative. Midfoot swelling and loss of weight-bearing ability, particularly on tiptoe, may be the only physical exam findings. History will indicate injury mechanism consistent with a Lisfranc injury. Direct palpatory pain will localize to the medial or lateral foot at the tarsometatarsal area. Abduction and pronation of

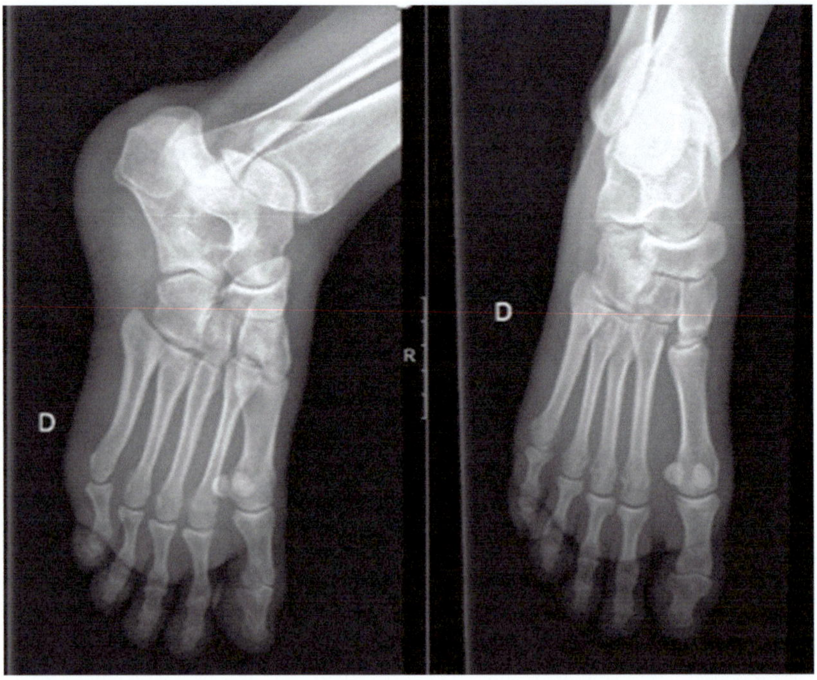

Fig. 28.5 Lisfranc fracture right foot

the forefoot with fixed hindfoot will also elicit pain [56, 60].

Plain radiographs are highly useful for diagnosis and postoperative assessment (Fig. 28.5). Weight-bearing dorsal anteroposterior, lateral, and 30° oblique views should be obtained and will commonly reveal diastasis between the first and second metatarsal bases. X-ray is potentially limited in precision due to swelling, projection angle, or image overlap. CT offers greater detail of small fractures and deviations but is limited in postoperative assessment due to interference from metal implants. Bone scans and MRI can detect occult fractures earlier than radiographs. Woodward et al. report characteristic sonographic findings indicating Lisfranc ligament tear [58–61].

Treatment: Stable injuries can be treated conservatively with a CAM boot for 6–10 weeks followed by physical therapy to restore strength, balance, and ROM [56, 58].

Treatment of fractures and fracture-dislocations is controversial, with some researchers asserting that nonoperative management is ineffective due to loss of alignment during casting. Particularly in athletes, displacement greater than 2 mm may require open reduction and internal fixation to ensure good outcomes. Procedural preference varies, with some orthopedists preferring closed fixation with percutaneous K-wires and others open reduction and internal fixation with AO screw fixation. Precise postoperative assessment allows for early intervention should complications arise [56, 62].

Following open reduction and fixation, the foot should be cast for 8–12 weeks. Full, non-casted weight-bearing should be avoided until the plates are removed at 8–12 weeks. A protective shoe should be worn for 3 months after cast removal [56].

Outcomes: Incidence of acute complications is high and results in lengthy hospitalizations. Three factors serve as important predictors of complications: the extent of local trauma, delay in diagnosis, and degree of displacement. Posttraumatic arthritis is common and usually requires a subsequent arthrodesis. Li et al. reported that CT imaging easier identification of nonanatomic reduction and poor internal fixation compared to radiographs [56, 59–61].

28.3.7 Stress Fractures

Definition: Stress fractures account for 10% of all sports-related injuries and occur as a result of repeated submaximal loads whereby shear forces, which stimulate osteoclast activity, exceed compressive forces, which stimulate osteoblast activity, ultimately exceeding the bone's ability to adapt. Lower limbs are most affected, with 25% of stress fractures occurring in the tarsals and 9% in the metatarsals. The incidence of stress fractures in military recruits varies from 5 to 30% per year, being higher in female recruits. The incidence in the nonmilitary athletic population varies from 1.1 to 31% per year, the highest being the incidence noted in track and field athletes. Retrospective studies in ballet dancers have shown the incidence of stress fractures to be between 22.2 and 31.5%, the most common location being the metatarsals. In a questionnaire-based survey by Pecina et al., 21.5% of elite figure skaters reported a stress fracture during their career; the most common site was the lumbosacral spine. Gymnasts showed an incidence of 16% stress fractures for men and 24% stress fractures for women [63–67].

Intrinsic risk factors include lack of physical activity, low body mass index, age (in males, incidence decreases after 17 years of age; in females, it increases after menarche), decreased muscle strength, and anatomical factors: low cross-sectional area, leg-length discrepancy, menstrual dysfunction, low bone mineral density, and eating disorders. Extrinsic risk factors include activity type, changes to training techniques or intensity, improper equipment or training surfaces, suboptimal nutrition, long-distance runners, alcohol, smoking, and low vitamin D levels [66].

Locations vary by sports; runners are prone to stress fractures of the medial malleolus, distal fibula, calcaneus, lesser metatarsal, and medial sesamoid bones. Ballet dancers, gymnasts, and tennis and volleyball players commonly experience fractures of the navicular and sesamoids. Basketball players are prone to the medial malleolus, navicular, and metatarsal fractures. Soccer players are prone to metatarsal V fractures [63, 66].

Diagnosis: Initial diagnosis is largely clinical and relies on history and physical examination. Typically, patients describe the insidious initial onset of pain, associated with a recent increase in training intensity with pain occurring toward the end of training sessions and intensifying gradually over weeks to become constant. The absence of rest pain helps to differentiate stress fractures from a variety of other conditions, including inflammatory pathologies and bone tumors. Usually, there is no history of trauma. Physical examination reveals pain on weight-bearing or range of motion and palpatory tenderness. Edema, ecchymosis, or a palpable callus may also be present [63, 64, 66].

Due to the nature of the healing process, stress fractures commonly evade x-ray diagnosis for the first 2 weeks until sufficient sclerosis and callus formation occur. These statistics range from 40 to 95% of cases, depending on location.

Cases with a high suspicion of a stress fracture and negative radiographs should be evaluated by alternative imaging techniques, such as an MRI, which provides high sensitivity and specificity, and CT, which is useful for evaluating for signs of periostitis and assessing fracture union in conservative management [17, 63, 65–67].

Treatment: Management varies with the sports, severity, and athletic level. Most stress fractures can be treated conservatively using boot immobilization for 6–8 weeks, followed by 6 weeks partial weight-bearing in a functional splint, followed by gradual return to sports. Low-impact activities can be maintained throughout. Asano et al. report that surgery should be considered early for elite athletes due to higher risk for dislocation and non-consolidation and for fractures of the navicular, which has a poor blood supply, and medial malleolus, which is prone to dislocation and non-consolidation. Van den Bekerom et al. caution that, in medial malleolus fractures, complete rest can lead to atrophy and deconditioning and should be avoided [63, 65].

Outcomes: Low-risk fractures usually heal within 4–8 weeks of limited activity. Surgical treatment in athletes is advantageous in that it speeds healing and allows a faster return to sports. For surgically treated navicular fractures, Asano et al. report an average time of 4 months for full healing and return to sports. For fifth metatarsal fractures, Robertson and Wood report a minimum of 75% return times within 13.8 weeks for surgical management and minimum of 33% return times within 19.2 weeks for conservative management. Conservative management of medial malleolus fractures has been found to take three times longer for a return to sports compared to surgical management [63, 65–68].

28.3.8 Posterior Tibial Tendinitis

Definition: Posterior tibial tendinitis is progressive, beginning with tendon dysfunction and progressing to ligamentous dysfunction and ultimately leading to flatfoot deformity. The tendon's sheath is unique in that the mesotenon layer lacks complete blood supply, particularly between the musculotendinous and osseous-tendinous junctions, and this is where most tendinopathy occurs. Anatomically, the posterior tibial tendon lies near the medial malleolus and beneath the flexor retinaculum and is vulnerable to injury in ankle fractures. Other risk factors include impingement at the fibro-osseous groove and insertion abnormalities. Posterior tibial tendinitis is three times more common in women [69–71].

Primarily a soft tissue tendinopathy results in altered biomechanics. Four stages are described. Stages 1 and 2 involve only soft tissues. In stage 2, permanent changes in the tendon have occurred. Development of subtalar arthritis defines stage 3. Involvement of the ankle joint defines stage 4. Van Dijk confirmed the presence of thickened vincula following trauma that, when released, provided symptom relief. Gody-Santos et al. report the presence of a polymorphism in the MMP-1 promoter gene, leading to degradation and removal of collagen from the extracellular matrix [70–72].

Diagnosis: Early diagnosis and intervention can help stop progression. Stage 1: Symptoms include pain over the medial foot and decreased endurance. Physical examination will reveal erythema, swelling, and tenderness. The medial arch is intact, and foot alignment is normal. Radiographs show normal foot and ankle alignment. MRI distinguishes normal and abnormal anatomy of the tendon sheath and provides superior visualization of abnormalities of the spring and deltoid ligaments [69, 70, 72].

Stage 2: Irreversible tendon changes may lead to rupture. Radiographs should be examined for talar-first metatarsal (Meary) angle, calcaneal pitch, talocalcaneal angle, and medial and lateral column heights on lateral weight-bearing views. Stage 3: Possibly fixed, non-flexible subtalar joint arthropathy is evident on x-ray, along with arthritic symptoms. Stage 4: Radiographs reveal fixed deformity with valgus ankle, calcaneal valgus, midfoot planus, and forefoot abduction with supination [70, 72].

Pain at the posterior margin of the medial malleolus without intra-articular pathology can signify adhesions and irregularities in the tendon sliding channel [73].

Treatment: Stage 1: Conservative treatment with immobilization, rest, and plaster cast or walker boot. Orthotics can reduce forefoot pronation and reduce stress on the tendon. Physiotherapy decreases acute swelling and strengthens the posterior tibialis muscle. Steroids should be avoided due to the risk of tendon rupture and fat atrophy. Ribbans and Garde report good results using saline infiltration of the sheath combined with physiotherapy. Synovectomy should be considered for nonresponsive cases after 3 months. Wake and Martin report that endoscopy is becoming the standard in stages 1 and 2 [61, 69, 72].

Stage 2: Soft tissue reconstructive procedures are preferable to bone or joint reconstruction [49]. Return to elite sports performance is unlikely without surgical intervention. Surgery should address lateral column lengthening and stabilizing medial column fusion [72].

Stages 3 and 4: Arthrodesis is usually required and may be single or multiple. Open or minimally invasive procedures can be used. Nishimura reports that ultrasonographic guidance can be used to assist with the insertion of an endoscope into the tendon sheath [70, 73].

Outcomes: Endoscopy offers shorter postoperative periods and smaller scars with equivalent results and greater patient satisfaction compared to open procedures. However, there is a risk of injury to the medial plantar nerve. Rehabilitation is lengthy, taking at least 12 months, with a return to high-impact elite sports not advised [69, 72].

28.3.9 Turf Toe

Definition: Turf toe was originally described as a hyperextension injury to the hallux metatarsophalangeal joint (MTPJ) resulting from overly flexible shoes on insufficiently flexible artificial turf. The condition is now recognized in a number of sports played on artificial turf as well as in sports requiring repetitive loading of the hallux, such as wrestling, basketball, and dancing. It encompasses a variety of injury mechanisms affecting the hallux plantar capsule, plantar muscles, and sesamoid complex [74–76].

The hallux MTPJ is inherently unstable and must withstand as much as eight times body weight during a running jump. The injury typically occurs when the foot receives an axial load while in a fixed equinus position at the ankle and the great toe in extension at the MTP joint. Waldrop et al. demonstrated that an increase of 3 mm between the sesamoids and the proximal phalanx increases the risk for severe injury to the plantar plate, with a likelihood of involving three ligaments [77, 78].

Diagnosis: Physical examination must include a comparison to the unaffected side. The drawer test for the first MTPJ is conducted by stabilizing the first metatarsal superiorly and inferiorly with one hand while applying an anterior and posterior translational force to the proximal phalanx to feel for dorsal or plantar subluxation. A positive test demonstrates anteroposterior instability. Stress and instability testing determines the need for surgery. Plantar plate rupture can be easily overlooked during a physical examination in severe injuries. Grade I injury involves sprain of the plantar capsular ligamentous complex. Grade II involves partial rupture of the plantar soft tissue structures. Grade III involves complete rupture and may require surgery [74, 78, 79].

Weight-bearing and stress AP, lateral, and axial sesamoid radiographs should be obtained for both feet. Fluoroscopy can help detect valgus instability and plantar plate integrity. Drakos et al. define stable injuries as a change of less than 2 mm on dorsiflexion stress radiographs in proximal retraction of the sesamoids compared with the unaffected side. MRI can provide detail regarding associated osseous, intra-articular, and soft tissue injuries and is preferable to CT [74, 79].

Treatment: Stable injuries can be treated with conservative treatment with casting or a stiff-soled shoe, gradual weight-bearing, orthotics, and physical therapy. Substantial but stable capsule injuries can be cast for 4–6 weeks [79].

Grade I injuries do not require the loss of playing time. After the acute phase, the toe can be taped in slight plantar flexion, and a toe separator can be used in medial injuries. Grade II injuries will require at least 2-week cessation of sports participation with a gradual progression from low- to high-impact exercises. Grade III injuries may require 8 weeks of immobilization and can take up to 6 months for resolution [78].

Waldrop et al. recommend surgery for injuries involving at least three of the four ligaments in athletes. For displaced fractures, excision of the smaller fragment with plantar plate repair has been done with and without augmentation. Open reduction and internal fixation can be accomplished using small screws [77, 79].

Outcomes: Accurate and early diagnosis is essential for successful outcomes and can result in full recovery and return to pre-injury activity for many patients, though McCormick et al. note persistence of residual or chronic symptoms in up to 50% of patients at 5-year follow-up in one study and persistent loss of range of motion in other studies. Covell et al. report 74% return to pre-injury playing level and average 3- to 4-month recovery time for surgical treatment of traumatic hallux valgus. A multidisciplinary team approach can help ensure optimal results [74, 76].

28.4 Conclusion

Worldwide, sports participation has increased substantially over the past few decades. In addition to increasing participation among youth, particularly girls, as the global population ages, older adults are also continuing to be active or choosing to begin sports participation at advance ages. As a result, sports medicine specialists are experiencing new diagnostic and treatment challenges. To meet those challenges, orthopedists, surgeons, and other orthopedic professionals are responding with innovative approaches to surgery and other management techniques. In the surgical realm, arthroscopy is finding increased utilization, often with excellent results, though, in some procedures, with certain attendant risks. Overall, the orthopedic professions are well-positioned to serve the changing needs of the sports community [80, 81].

References

1. Rehabilitation of ankle and foot injuries in athletes. https://www.ncbi.nlm.nih.gov/pmc/articles/PMC2786815/.
2. Saluta J, Nunley JA. Managing foot and ankle injuries in athletes. J Musculoskelet Med. 2010;27:355–63.
3. Epidemiology of National Collegiate Athletic Association women's gymnastics injuries, 2009–2010 through 2013–2014. https://www.ncbi.nlm.nih.gov/pmc/articles/PMC4629945/.
4. Prospective observational study of midtarsal joint sprain: epidemiological and ultrasonographic analysis. https://www.sciencedirect.com/science/article/pii/S1877056816300561?
5. Running injuries in the participants of Ljubljana Marathon. https://www.ncbi.nlm.nih.gov/pmc/articles/PMC5639808/.
6. Evaluating a standardized tool to explore the nature and extent of foot and ankle injuries in amateur and semi-professional footballers. https://www.ncbi.nlm.nih.gov/pmc/articles/PMC4864468/.
7. Commentary: functional ankle instability revisited. https://www.ncbi.nlm.nih.gov/pmc/articles/PMC164386/.
8. Prevalence of chronic ankle instability in high school and Division I athletes. https://www.ncbi.nlm.nih.gov/pubmed/24287210.
9. Anatomy of the ankle ligaments: a pictorial essay. https://www.ncbi.nlm.nih.gov/pmc/articles/PMC2855022/.
10. Diagnosis of ligament rupture of the ankle joint. Physical examination, arthrography, stress radiography and sonography compared in 160 patients after inversion trauma. https://www.ncbi.nlm.nih.gov/pubmed/9065068.
11. Diagnosis, treatment and prevention of ankle sprains: an evidence-based clinical guideline. http://bjsm.bmj.com/content/46/12/854.
12. The Cumberland Ankle Instability Tool (CAIT) in the Dutch population with and without complaints of ankle instability. https://www.ncbi.nlm.nih.gov/pmc/articles/PMC5847203/.
13. The ANKLE TRIAL (ANKLE treatment after injuries of the ankle ligaments): what is the benefit of external support devices in the functional treatment of acute ankle sprain?: a randomised controlled trial. https://www.ncbi.nlm.nih.gov/pmc/articles/PMC3306273/.
14. Van Dijk CN. Diagnosis of ankle sprain: history and physical examination. ISAKOS—FIMS World Consensus Conference on Ankle Instability. 2005. p. 21–2.
15. Randomized comparison of tape versus semi-rigid and versus lace-up ankle support in the treatment of acute lateral ankle ligament injury. https://www.ncbi.nlm.nih.gov/pmc/articles/PMC4823346/.
16. Van Dijk CN. The athletes' ankle: lateral ligament injury. Consensus Meeting ESSKA-AFAS. Warsaw; 2011.
17. Arthroscopic capsular shrinkage for treatment of chronic lateral ankle instability. https://www.ncbi.nlm.nih.gov/pmc/articles/PMC5794102/.
18. Arthroscopic repair of ankle instability with all-soft knotless anchors. https://www.ncbi.nlm.nih.gov/pmc/articles/PMC4811205/.
19. Consensus in chronic ankle instability: aetiology, assessment, surgical indications and place for arthroscopy. https://www.sciencedirect.com/science/article/pii/S187705681300234X.
20. Ankle impingement lavery. https://josr-online.biomedcentral.com/articles/10.1186/s13018-016-0430-x.
21. Anterior impingement syndrome in dancers OKane. https://www.ncbi.nlm.nih.gov/pmc/articles/PMC2684147/.
22. Posterior ankle impingement syndrome: a systematic four-stage approach Yasui. https://www.ncbi.nlm.nih.gov/pmc/articles/PMC5065672/.
23. Update on anterior ankle impingement. https://www.ncbi.nlm.nih.gov/pmc/articles/PMC3535150/.
24. Oblique radiograph for the detection of bone spurs in anterior ankle impingement. https://www.ncbi.nlm.nih.gov/pubmed/11904689.
25. Baxter's foot and ankle in sports. https://www.sciencedirect.com/science/book/9780323023580.
26. Hindfoot endoscopy for posterior ankle impingement. Surgical technique. https://www.ncbi.nlm.nih.gov/pubmed/19805591.
27. Posterior hindfoot arthroscopy: a review. https://www.ncbi.nlm.nih.gov/pubmed/23868522.
28. Management of osteochondral lesions of the Talar Dome Chamnanni. https://www.ncbi.nlm.nih.gov/pmc/articles/PMC5620407/.
29. Osteochondral lesions of the talus in the athlete: up to date review. https://www.ncbi.nlm.nih.gov/pmc/articles/PMC5344864/.

30. Osteochondral lesions of the talus: localization and morphologic data from 424 patients using a novel anatomical grid scheme. http://citeseerx.ist.psu.edu/viewdoc/download?doi=10.1.1.854.9808&rep=rep1&type=pdf.
31. Osteochondral defects in the ankle: why painful? https://www.ncbi.nlm.nih.gov/pmc/articles/PMC2855020/.
32. Osteochondral defects of the talus with a focus on platelet-rich plasma as a potential treatment option: a review. https://www.ncbi.nlm.nih.gov/pmc/articles/PMC5812391/.
33. Bilateral osteochondral lesions of the talus. http://citeseerx.ist.psu.edu/viewdoc/download?doi=10.1.1.887.1419&rep=rep1&type=pdf.
34. Prospective study on diagnostic strategies in osteochondral lesions of the talus. https://online.boneandjoint.org.uk/doi/full/10.1302/0301-620X.87B1.14702.
35. Ankle arthroscopy. https://www.springer.com/gp/book/9783642359880. ISBN 978-3-642-35989-7.
36. SPECT/CT in the management of osteochondral lesions of the talus. http://citeseerx.ist.psu.edu/viewdoc/download?doi=10.1.1.910.971&rep=rep1&type=pdf.
37. Improved visualization of the 70° arthroscope in the treatment of Talar osteochondral defects. https://www.ncbi.nlm.nih.gov/pmc/articles/PMC3716212/.
38. Tertiary osteochondral defect of the talus treated by a novel contoured metal implant. https://www.ncbi.nlm.nih.gov/pmc/articles/PMC3096766/.
39. Achilles tendinopathy. A REVIEW OF THE CURRENT CONCEPTS OF TREATMENT. http://citeseerx.ist.psu.edu/viewdoc/download?doi=10.1.1.859.8265&rep=rep1&type=pdf.
40. Non-insertional Achilles tendinopathy. https://online.boneandjoint.org.uk/doi/full/10.1302/2058-5241.1.160024.
41. Terminology for Achilles tendon related disorders. https://www.ncbi.nlm.nih.gov/pmc/articles/PMC3076576/pdf/167_2010_Article_1374.pdf.
42. Treatment of midportion Achilles tendinopathy: an evidence-based overview. https://doi.org/10.1007/s00167-014-3407-5. https://www.ncbi.nlm.nih.gov/pubmed/?term=10.1007%2Fs00167-014-3407-5.
43. Mid-portion Achilles tendinopathy: why painful? An evidence-based philosophy. https://doi.org/10.1007/s00167-011-1535-8. https://www.ncbi.nlm.nih.gov/pubmed/?term=10.1007%2Fs00167-011-1535-8.
44. Plantaris excision reduces pain in midportion Achilles tendinopathy even in the absence of plantaris tendinosis. https://www.ncbi.nlm.nih.gov/pmc/articles/PMC5298419/.
45. The plantaris tendon and a potential role in midportion Achilles tendinopathy: an observational anatomical study. https://www.ncbi.nlm.nih.gov/pmc/articles/PMC3058219/.
46. Treatment for insertional Achilles tendinopathy: a systematic review. https://www.ncbi.nlm.nih.gov/pubmed/23052113.
47. Effectiveness of dry needling and high-volume image-guided injection in the management of chronic mid-portion Achilles tendinopathy in adult population: a literature review. https://www.ncbi.nlm.nih.gov/pmc/articles/PMC5403875/.
48. Opdam KTM, Baltes TPA, et al. Endoscopic treatment of mid-portion Achilles tendinopathy: a retrospective case series of patient satisfaction and functional outcome at a 2- to 8-year follow-up. Arthroscopy. 2018;34(1):264–9.
49. Cychosz CC, Phisitkul P, et al. Foot and ankle tendoscopy: evidence-based recommendations. Arthroscopy. 2014;30(6):755–65.
50. Surgical treatment for midportion Achilles tendinopathy: a systematic review. https://www.ncbi.nlm.nih.gov/pmc/articles/PMC5487601/.
51. Primary care management of plantar fasciitis. http://mds.marshall.edu/cgi/viewcontent.cgi?article=1024&context=sm_orthopaedics.
52. Plantar fasciitis in athletes: diagnostic and treatment strategies. A systematic review. https://www.ncbi.nlm.nih.gov/pmc/articles/PMC5505577/.
53. Extracorporeal shock wave therapy is effective in treating chronic plantar fasciitis. https://www.ncbi.nlm.nih.gov/pmc/articles/PMC5403108/.
54. Pulsed compared to thermal radiofrequency to the medial calcaneal nerve for management of chronic refractory plantar fasciitis: a prospective comparative study. http://www.painphysicianjournal.com/current/pdf?article=MzExOA%3D%3D&journal=100.
55. Platelet-rich plasma as a treatment for plantar fasciitis. https://www.ncbi.nlm.nih.gov/pmc/articles/PMC5682822/.
56. Lisfranc injury of the foot: a commonly missed diagnosis. https://www.aafp.org/afp/1998/0701/p118.html.
57. Return to training and playing after acute Lisfranc injuries in elite professional soccer and Rugby players. http://journals.sagepub.com/doi/pdf/10.1177/0363546515616814.
58. Diagnosis and management of Lisfranc injuries and metatarsal fractures. http://citeseerx.ist.psu.edu/viewdoc/download?doi=10.1.1.919.4519&rep=rep1&type=pdf.
59. EPIDEMIOLOGICAL STUDY ON LISFRANC INJURIES. https://www.ncbi.nlm.nih.gov/pmc/articles/PMC5474402/.
60. Staged management of open Lisfranc injury experience from 14 patients. https://www.ncbi.nlm.nih.gov/pmc/articles/PMC5413238/.
61. Sonographic evaluation of Lisfranc ligament injuries. https://deepblue.lib.umich.edu/bitstream/handle/2027.42/135195/jum2009283351.pdf?sequence=1&isAllowed=y.
62. Evaluation of computed tomography post-processing images in postoperative assessment of Lisfranc injuries compared with plain radiographs. https://www.ncbi.nlm.nih.gov/pmc/articles/PMC5471664/.
63. Stress fractures in the foot and ankle of athletes. http://www.scielo.br/scielo.php?script=sci_arttext&pid=S0104-42302014000600512&lng=en&nrm=iso&tlng=en.
64. Stress fractures of the foot and ankle in athletes. https://www.ncbi.nlm.nih.gov/pmc/articles/PMC4212349/.

65. Lower limb stress fractures in sport: optimising their management and outcome. https://www.ncbi.nlm.nih.gov/pmc/articles/PMC5359760/.
66. Stress fractures in football. http://jisakos.bmj.com/content/early/2016/06/23/jisakos-2015-000010.info.
67. Fifth metatarsal fractures among male professional footballers: a potential career-ending disease. https://www.ncbi.nlm.nih.gov/pubmed/23467966.
68. Kerkhoffs GM. Treatment of proximal metatarsal V fractures in athletes and non-athletes. Br J Sports Med. 2012;46:644–8. https://doi.org/10.1136/bjsports-2011-090389.
69. Posterior tibial tendon endoscopic debridement for stage I and II posterior tibial tendon dysfunction. https://www.ncbi.nlm.nih.gov/pmc/articles/PMC5797905/.
70. Posterior tibial tendon dysfunction: an overview. https://www.ncbi.nlm.nih.gov/pmc/articles/PMC5620404/.
71. MMP-1 promoter polymorphism is associated with primary tendinopathy of the posterior tibial tendon. https://onlinelibrary.wiley.com/doi/abs/10.1002/jor.22321.
72. Tibialis posterior tendon and deltoid and spring ligament injuries in the elite athlete. https://www.academia.edu/24565882/Tibialis_Posterior_Tendon_and_Deltoid_and_Spring_Ligament_Injuries_in_the_Elite_Athlete?auto=download.
73. Ultrasound guidance in performing a tendoscopic surgery to treat posterior tibial tendinitis: a useful tool? https://www.ncbi.nlm.nih.gov/pmc/articles/PMC4960336/.
74. Operative treatment of traumatic hallux valgus in elite athletes. http://journals.sagepub.com/doi/pdf/10.1177/1071100717697961.
75. Incidence and risk factors for turf toe injuries in intercollegiate football: data from the National Collegiate Athletic Association Injury Surveillance System. http://journals.sagepub.com/doi/pdf/10.1177/1071100713514038.
76. Case series of first metatarsophalangeal joint injuries in division 1 college athletes. https://www.ncbi.nlm.nih.gov/pmc/articles/PMC4212353/.
77. Radiographic evaluation of plantar plate injury: an in vitro biomechanical study. http://journals.sagepub.com/doi/pdf/10.1177/1071100712464953.
78. Turf toe anatomy, diagnosis, and treatment. https://www.ncbi.nlm.nih.gov/pmc/articles/PMC3438874/.
79. Plantar-plate disruptions: "the severe turf-toe injury." Three cases in contact athletes. https://www.ncbi.nlm.nih.gov/pmc/articles/PMC4560019/.
80. Sports team participation among US high school girls, 1999-2015. http://journals.sagepub.com/doi/pdf/10.1177/0009922817732145.
81. Sport and ageing: a systematic review of the determinants and trends of participation in sport for older adults. https://www.ncbi.nlm.nih.gov/pmc/articles/PMC5741887/.

Part V

Special Conditions

29 Female Athlete Triad and RED-S

Samantha Tayne, Melody Hrubes,
Mark R. Hutchinson, and Margo Mountjoy

29.1 Overview

The appreciation and understanding of energy deficiency as it relates to the athlete population have evolved over time. The Female Athlete Triad was a phrase originally coined in 1993 to describe a phenomenon noted in female athletes experiencing a metabolic energy deficit leading to pathologic findings [1]. The Triad was described as disordered eating, osteoporosis, and amenorrhea (Fig. 29.1). As further research and consideration were given to this diagnosis, clinicians and researchers discovered that the original criteria defining the Triad were too narrow. The term was expanded and revised to low energy availability (with or without disordered eating), low bone mineral density, and menstrual dysfunction. In 2014, the International Olympic Committee released a consensus statement defining a new term, Relative Energy Deficiency in Sport (RED-S), expanding the diagnosis beyond just female participants to include all athletes, and allowing for a broader definition of energy deficiency in athletes that includes any physiologic and pathologic effects [2].

S. Tayne · M. Hrubes · M. R. Hutchinson (✉)
University of Illinois at Chicago, Chicago, IL, USA
e-mail: mhutch@uic.edu

M. Mountjoy
University of Guelph, Guelph, ON, Canada
e-mail: mountjm@mcmaster.com

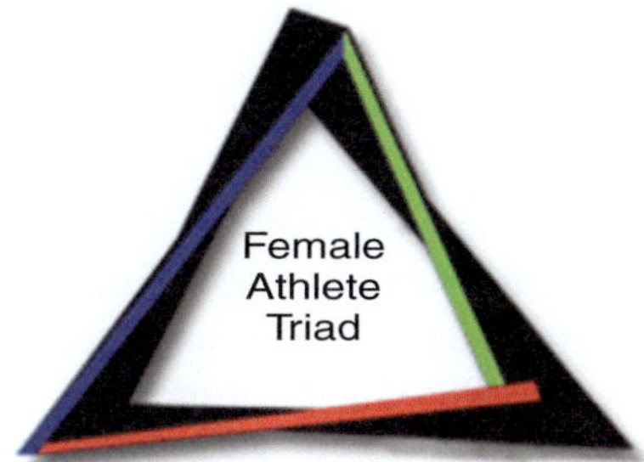

Fig. 29.1 The Female Athlete Triad

29.1.1 Key Definitions

The diagnoses of the Female Athlete Triad and RED-S require an understanding of several key definitions. Energy availability is defined as energy intake minus energy expenditure during exercise adjusted for fat-free mass (Eq. 29.1). Low energy availability (LEA) is when the equation falls into negative territory for an extended period of time, the absolute assessment that the reduction in energy availability below a specific threshold (30 kcal/kg of fast free mass per day) has recently been challenged. While these definitions are quite specific, there is no gold standard to measure energy availability, and it may be particularly difficult to measure in athletes with varied exercise regimens. Providers may attempt to measure energy availability through self-reported

S. Rocha Piedade et al. (eds.), *The Sports Medicine Physician*,
https://doi.org/10.1007/978-3-030-10433-7_29

food and exercises logs, or more often various tools are utilized to assess the outcomes of LEA, such as the Low Energy Availability in Females Questionnaire (LEAF-Q) and Female Athlete Screening Tool (FAST). These tools are typically used to screen for LEA in athletes, but are also imperfect and imprecise. Further, LEA can occur with or without disordered eating or eating disorders. Eating disorders include those with clinical criteria consistent with DSM-V definitions such as anorexia nervosa, bulimia nervosa, and unspecified feeding or eating disorder, while disordered eating includes a broader spectrum of pathologic eating behaviors and weight control.

$$\mathrm{EA}(\mathrm{kcal}/\mathrm{kg}) = \mathrm{EI}(\mathrm{kcal}) - \mathrm{EEE}(\mathrm{kcal}) / \mathrm{FFM}(\mathrm{kg}) \qquad (29.1)$$

Low energy availability may result in decreased bone mineral density, more specifically defined as osteoporosis and osteopenia. As defined by the World Health Organization, osteoporosis involves a *T* score of −2.5 and below and osteopenia a *T* score between −1.5 and −2.5. However, the *T* score assesses bone density as compared to the average healthy adult and was created to assess for risk of pathologic fracture in postmenopausal women, not premenopausal female athletes nor young male athletes. There is no standard to adjust bone mineral density for bone size, skeletal maturity, or body composition. Therefore, the applicability of the *T* score to the athlete population is limited. A *Z* score, which compares bone mineral density to the average for age, sex, weight, and ethnicity, may provide a better diagnostic measure, recognizing that elite athletes may still be inadequately measured or diagnosed when comparing to the average in a general population. Studies have indicated that athletes in weight-bearing sports typically have a bone mineral density *Z* score of 5–15% higher than nonathletes, suggesting that a *Z* score of anything less than −1.0 in an athlete participating in a weight-bearing sport should prompt further evaluation for osteopenia and energy deficiency [3].

Menstrual dysfunction related to LEA may include primary amenorrhea, secondary amenorrhea, and/or oligomenorrhea. Primary amenorrhea is failure of menses to occur by age 16 years, while secondary amenorrhea is a loss of menses for 3 or more months. Oligomenorrhea is infrequent menstruation, often going 35 days or greater between menses. In athletes, any of these forms of amenorrhea typically are due to functional hypothalamic amenorrhea, a disruption of pulsatile, hypothalamic gonadotropin-releasing hormone (GnRH) secretion caused by relative energy deficiency. Males may experience a similar phenomenon, known as male hypogonadism, a decrease in one or both of the functions of the testes—sperm production and testosterone formation. Low energy availability may result in secondary hypogonadism again due to disruption of release of GnRH and may relate to symptoms of androgen deficiency [4].

The pathophysiology of energy deficiency is still incompletely understood. There are many biomarkers of energy deficiency, including leptin, ghrelin, triiodothyronine, cortisol, insulin-like growth factor-1, insulin, and glucose. Leptin and ghrelin are regulators of appetite. Triiodothyronine is a regulator of metabolism through the hypothalamus-pituitary-thyroid axis. Cortisol is steroid hormone released in response to stress, and IGF-1 is a growth hormone that supports cell division and growth and may also be associated with systemic inflammation. Yet the appropriate method of measuring and utilizing these biomarkers is still an area requiring further study.

29.1.2 Epidemiology

The epidemiology of LEA in both female and male athletes has been hard to determine, especially given the difficulty in assessing LEA. However, studies have shown a higher frequency of pathologic eating behavior in athletes [5, 6], with 25% of female elite athletes in endurance sports, aesthetic sports, and weight-class sports showing evidence of clinical eating disorders compared to 9% of the general population [7]. Another study showed eating disorders in 31% of elite female athletes in "thin-build" sports compared to 5.5% of the control population [8].

This issue is not limited to female athletes, as studies have demonstrated increased disordered eating in mass-dependent sports in male athletes [6, 9, 10] and evidence of low energy availability in male endurance runners, jockeys, triathletes, and cyclists [11, 12].

Primary amenorrhea exists in less than 1% in girls over 15 years old in the United States; however one study indicates that this prevalence jumps to 7.4% in collegiate athletes and 22% in athletes competing in aesthetic sports [13]. The percentage of female athletes with secondary amenorrhea or oligomenorrhea is even higher; studies show numbers ranging from 31 to 44% in athletes, particularly those participating in lean sports, such as dancing and long distance running [13–15].

There is a lack of epidemiologic data relating bone mineral density to fractures in adolescents and premenopausal women, let alone to the athlete population. A systematic review that used WHO *T* scores found a prevalence of osteopenia ranging from 22% to 50% and a prevalence of osteoporosis ranging from 0% to 13% in female athletes, compared to 12% and 2.3% in a normal population, respectively [16]. As discussed previously, these numbers likely underestimate the relative loss of bone mineral density. More recently, studies including male athletes involved in mass-dependent or endurance sports are also at increased risk for decreased bone mineral density [4, 9, 11, 12].

Several studies have shown a prevalence of 1.2–4.3% of the complete Female Athlete Triad in college athletes [17–19]. However, these studies have used the narrowly defined parameters of the original Female Athlete Triad. More recent studies utilizing the broader definition of relative energy deficiency or LEA show a much higher prevalence, anywhere from 6 to 100% depending on the sport [20].

29.2 Background and History

The tradition of female athletic competition can trace its roots into antiquity. While ancient Greece is famous for establishing the Olympic Games (776 BC) where only male athletes were allowed to compete, the Heraean Games were established in the sixth century BC and involved competitions of young, unmarried women. In the fourth century BC, the rules were more lenient at the Olympic Games, and Cynisca became the first female Olympic champion in the four-horse chariot race. Unfortunately, continued advancement of women's participation in elite support was delayed for centuries. Medical care of female athletes has long been shrouded in the misconception that women are "more frail" and therefore at greater risk of injury compared to their male counterparts. Indeed, this misconception persisted during the establishment of the modern Olympic Games in 1896 as Baron de Coubertin felt the inclusion of women was "impractical, uninteresting, unaesthetic, and incorrect." In 1900, 22 women out of 997 athletes participated in the Paris Olympic Games but were restricted to tennis, sailing, croquet, equestrian, and golf. It was not until the 1984 Olympic Games in Los Angeles that women were allowed to run the marathon.

With societal changes in the late 1960s and early 1970s, a federal law in the United States, Title IX, was established that assured equal access to women for all facets of education including sports participation. Title IX led to an expansive growth in the number of female athletes participating in sports in the United States and a renewed focus on their health. As one might expect, early interest focused on factors that were uniquely female such as gynecology, hormones, and menstrual cycles [21–24, 41]. Subsequently, key researchers including Barbara Drinkwater began to recognize a correlation of pathologies with abnormal menses related to athletic participation. Menstrual dysfunction appeared to be directly related to decreased bone mineral density in these athletes [25–27]. Pathogenic weight control behaviors especially disordered eating also appeared to be directly related to abnormal menses ([28]). In response to this growing concern in 1992, the American College of Sports Medicine (ACSM) brought together a group of leading experts to discuss issues of defining the problem, create diagnostic parameters, develop screening and prevention protocols, as well as identify knowledge gaps and directions for future research [1]. Based on their observations and correlations of clinical findings, the group coined the term the Female Athlete Triad to define the apparent link between disordered eating, amenorrhea, and osteoporosis (Fig. 29.1) that were more common in female athletes. It is important to note that this first group of experts recognized that poor nutritional factors, i.e., decreased energy intake, and the psychological and social pressures of sport were the critical cause of the subsequent symptom trilogy. Over time, continued study and research have led to further understanding of the problem. In 1997, ACSM created a position stand on the Female Athlete Triad [29], which was updated in 2007 [3]. The core concepts of the interrelationship between energy balance, hormonal health, and bone health remain unchanged with the key philosophical update being that each of these facets was on a continuum from normal to pathologic that varies from individual to individual (Fig. 29.2). The updated position statement once again emphasized that the foundational trigger leading down the pathway to disease was poor energy availability.

Due to guideline and page count restrictions of ACSM position statements, the 2007 Position stand was not able to go as into as much depth regarding screening, management, and return to play as the authors would have liked. Subsequently, these weaknesses have been addressed via position stands and consensus statements by the National Athletic Trainers Association [30], by the Female Athlete Triad Coalition, [31], and by the International Olympic Committee (IOC) [2]. In addition to providing guidelines regarding screening, management, and return to play, the IOC consensus statement emphasized the underlying trigger pathophysiology of energy deficiency, by coining the term Relative Energy Deficiency in Sport or RED-S. While including the trilogy of the female athlete triad within the framework of RED-S, the expanded concept targets any pathophysiology, not limited to endocrine and bone metabolism, regardless of gender (Fig. 29.3).

29.3 Clinical Presentation and Diagnosis

As a provider caring for the athlete population, it is important to recognize those at risk for relative energy deficiency and the impact that might have on the athlete's performance and overall health. There are several sports that lend themselves to higher-risk athletes, including aesthetic, lean, and endurance sports. However, there is emerg-

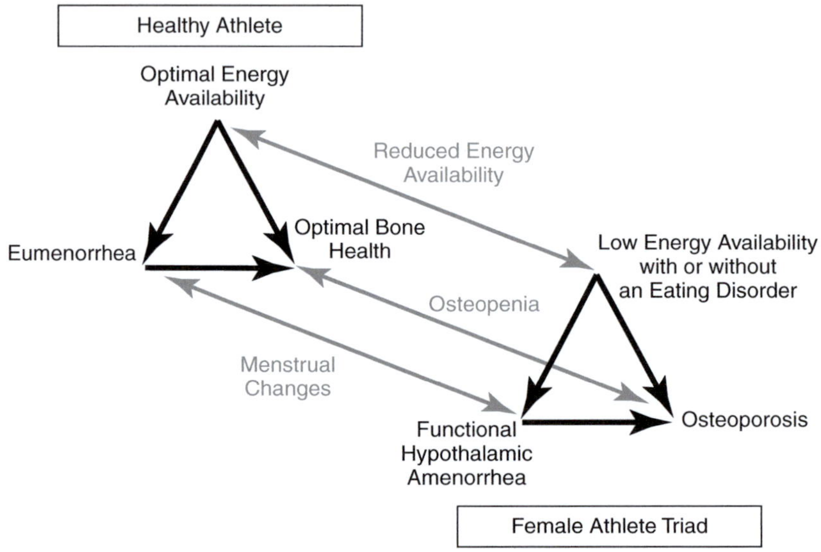

Fig. 29.2 Continuum of the Female Athlete Triad

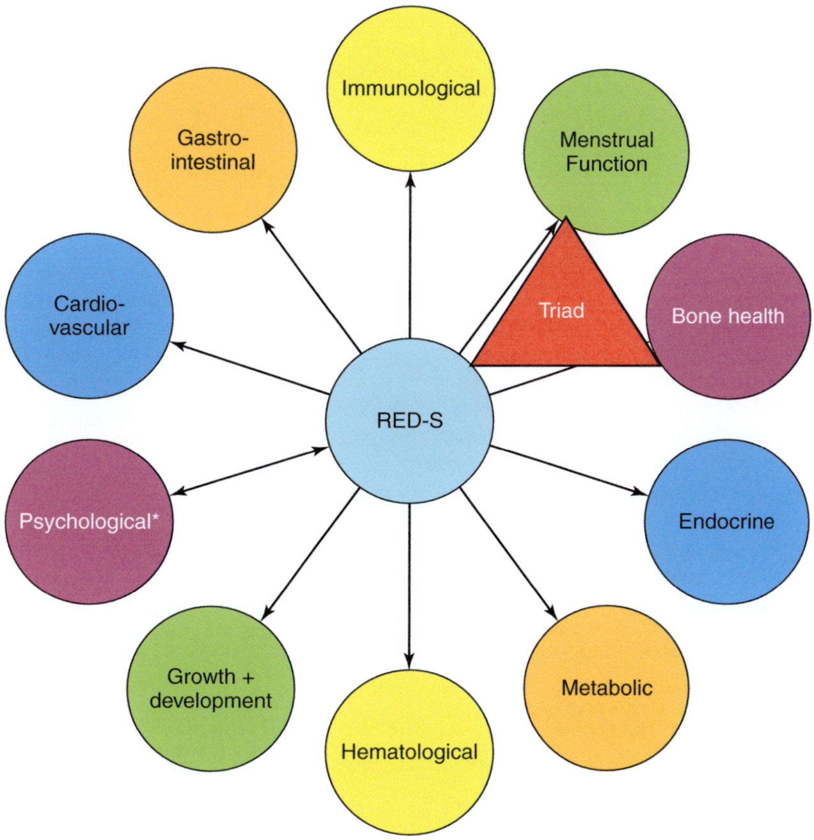

Fig. 29.3 Relative energy deficiency in sport. The effect of energy deficiency on various physiological functions. The original Female Triad is also incorporated into the RED-S framework (Reproduced from Mountjoy et al. [2])

ing evidence that RED-S is also present in sprint and power sports [32].

> While sports that emphasize aesthetic, leanness, and endurance are at elevated risk, relative energy deficiency may also be a problem in sprint and power sports.

As previously mentioned, there are limitations in measuring energy availability and deficiency; however there are multiple screening tools available, and they should be utilized during athlete pre-participation physical and annual physical examinations. Examples of such screening tools include Female Athlete Screening Tool (FAST) (Fig. 29.4), Brief Eating Disorder in Athletes Questionnaire (BEDA-Q) (Fig. 29.5), Low Energy Availability in Females Questionnaire (LEAF-Q) (Fig. 29.6), Eating Disorder Screen for Primary Care (ESP), and Disordered Eating Questionnaire. Similar screening tools specific to male athletes are being developed, including the Low Energy Availability in Males Questionnaire (LEAM-Q) [35]. The pre-participation physical examinations are a provider's best chance of detecting a problem before the athlete develops more severe pathology or injury or before there is a negative impact on performance. Athletes should be questioned regarding menses, a history of stress fractures, cardiac events, and a history of depression or insomnia. If the provider notes one component of RED-S in an athlete, the provider should continue a further, more in-depth evaluation of history, physical examination, and laboratory investigations.

Every female athlete should be asked about her menstrual function. Reports of amenorrhea or oligomenorrhea require further workup to exclude other physiologic and pathologic causes before diagnosing functional hypothalamic

Please answer as completely as possibly:

Key[a]: Exercise = Physical activity $\geq$ 20 minutes
Practice = Scheduled time allotted by coach to work as a team or individually in order to improve performance.
Training = Intense physical activity. The goal is to improve fitness level in order to perform optimally.

1. I participate in additional physical activity $\geq$ 20 minutes in length on days that I have practice or competition.
1)Frequently 2)Sometimes 3)Rarely 4)Never

2. If I cannot exercise, I find myself worrying that I will gain weight.
1)Frequently 2)Sometimes 3)Rarely 4)Never

3. I believe that most female athletes have some form of disordered eating habits.
1)Strongly Agree 2)Agree 3)Disagree 4)Strongly Disagree

4. During training, I control my fat and calorie intake carefully.
1)Frequently 2)Sometimes 3)Rarely 4)Never

5. I do not eat foods that have more than 3 grams of fat.
1)Strongly Agree 2)Agree 3)Disagree 4)Strongly Disagree

6. My performance would improve if I lost weight.
1)Strongly Agree 2)Agree 3)Disagree 4)Strongly Disagree

7. If I got on the scale tomorrow and gained 2 pounds, I would practice or exercise harder or longer than usual.
1)Frequently 2)Sometimes 3)Rarely 4)Never

8. I weigh myself__________.
1)Daily 2)2 or more times a week
3)Weekly 4)Monthly or less

9. If I chose to exercise on the day of competition (game/meet), I exercise for
1)2 or more hours 2)45 minutes to 1 hour
3)30 to 45 minutes 4)Less than 30 minutes

10. If I know that I will be consuming alcoholic beverages, I will skip meals on that day or the following day.
1)Frequently 2)Sometimes 3)Rarely 4)Never

11. I feel guilty if I choose fried foods for a meal.
1)Frequently 2)Sometimes 3)Rarely 4)Never

12. If I were to be injured, I would still exercise even if I was instructed not to do so by my athletic trainer or physician.
1)Strongly Agree 2)Agree 3)Disagree 4)Strongly Disagree

13. I take dietary or herbal supplements in order to increase my metabolism and/or to assist in burning fat.
1)Frequently 2)Sometimes 3)Rarely 4)Never

14. I am concerned about my percent body fat.
1)Frequently 2)Sometimes 3)Rarely 4)Never

15. Being an athlete, I am very conscious about consuming adequate calories and nutrients on a daily basis.
1)Frequently 2)Sometimes 3)Rarely 4)Never

16. I am worried that if I were to gain weight, my performance would decrease.
1)Strongly Agree 2)Agree 3)Disagree 4)Strongly Disagree

17. I think that being thin is associated with winning.
1)Strongly Agree 2)Agree 3)Disagree 4)Strongly Disagree

18. I train intensely for my sport so I will not gain weight.
1)Frequently 2)Sometimes 3)Rarely 4)Never

19. During season, I choose to exercise on my one day off from practice or competition.
1)Frequently 2)Sometimes 3)Rarely 4)Never

20. My friends tell me that I am thin but I feel fat.
1)Frequently 2)Sometimes 3)Rarely 4)Never

21. I feel uncomfortable eating around others.
1)Frequently 2)Sometimes 3)Rarely 4)Never

22. I limit the amount of carbohydrates that I eat.
1)Frequently 2)Sometimes 3)Rarely 4)Never

23. I try to lose weight to please others.
1)Frequently 2)Sometimes 3)Rarely 4)Never

24. If I were unable to compete in my sport, I would not feel good about myself.
1)Strongly Agree 2)Agree 3)Disagree 4)Strongly Disagree

25. If I were injured and unable to exercise, I would restrict my calorie intake.
1)Strongly Agree 2)Agree 3)Disagree 4)Strongly Disagree

26. In the past 2 years I have been unable to compete due to an injury.
1)7 or more times 2)4 to 6 times
3)1 to 3 times 4)No significant injuries

27. During practice I have trouble concentrating due to feelings of guilt about what I have eaten that day.
1)Frequently 2)Sometimes 3)Rarely 4)Never

28. I feel that I have a lot of good qualities.
1)Strongly Agree 2)Agree 3)Disagree 4)Strongly Disagree

29. At times I feel that I am no good at all.
1)Strongly Agree 2)Agree 3)Disagree 4)Strongly Disagree

30. I strive for perfection in all aspects of my life.
1)Strongly Agree 2)Agree 3)Disagree 4)Strongly Disagree

31. I avoid eating meat in order to stay thin.
1)Strongly Agree 2)Agree 3)Disagree 4)Strongly Disagree

32. I am happy with my present weight.
1)Yes 2)No

33. I have done things to keep my weight down that I believe are unhealthy.
1)Frequently 2)Sometimes 3)Rarely 4)Never

FIG. Female Athlete Assessment Tool (FAST)[b]
[a]*Initial validation studies have been conducted on the FAST. Future research wilt attempt to further validate the questionnaire.*
[b]*The key is used to quantify and define activity level for further clarification of the questions.*

Fig. 29.4 Female athlete screening tool (Reproduced from McNulty et al. [33])

amenorrhea due to low energy availability. Importantly, oral contraceptive pills (OCPs) and hormonal intrauterine devices (IUDs) may affect menstrual cycles such that it is no longer an appropriate assessment for normal menses or energy availability. Therefore, athlete use of OCPs and IUDs must also be ascertained. The counterpart to menstrual dysfunction in male athletes may not be as easily recognized; however male athletes with low testosterone may present

Items
1
I feel extremely guilty after overeating
☐always ☐usually ☐often ☐sometimes ☐rarely ☐never
2
I am preoccupied with the desire to be thinner
☐always ☐usually ☐often ☐sometimes ☐rarely ☐never
3
I think that my stomach is too big
☐always ☐usually ☐often ☐sometimes ☐rarely ☐never
4
I feel satisfied with the shape of my body
☐always ☐usually ☐often ☐sometimes ☐rarely ☐never
5
My parents have expected excellence of me
☐always ☐usually ☐often ☐sometimes ☐rarely ☐never
6
As a child, I tried very hard to avoid disappointing my parents and teachers
☐always ☐usually ☐often ☐sometimes ☐rarely ☐never
7
Are you trying to lose weight now?
☐Yes ☐No
8
Have you tried to lose weight?
☐Yes ☐No
9
If yes, how many times have you tried to lose weight?
☐1–2 ☐3–5 ☐>5 times
Dieting (trying to lose weight now and/or tried before ≥3 times)

Fig. 29.5 Brief Eating Disorder in Athletes Questionnaire (BEDA-Q). Positive scores are weighted as follows: 3, always; 2, usually; 1, often; 0, sometimes; 0, rarely; and 0, never, and reverse-scored items are weighted in the opposite manner (Reproduced from Martinsen et al. [34])

with symptoms of androgen deficiency warranting further workup [42]. Symptoms of androgen deficiency include lethargy, fatigue, depression, reduced muscle mass and strength, loss of body hair, hot flashes, increased sweating, reduced sexual desire, and sexual dysfunction. Workup of athletes with symptoms of androgen deficiency may include testosterone levels drawn in the morning and evening, luteinizing hormone and follicle-stimulating hormone levels, as well as further evaluation of eating behaviors and psychological assessment.

During pre-participation physical examinations, athletes should also undergo a cardiovascular examination and laboratory testing. All athletes should be questioned about a history of palpitations, lightheadedness, or dizziness occurring during exercise or while at rest. These symptoms may indicate bradycardia or orthostatic hypotension, which certainly require further cardiac testing to rule out a cardiac cause. However, providers should also realize that bradycardia and orthostatic hypotension, and even an arrhythmia, may indicate low energy availability in athletes with a negative cardiac workup, possibly due to an eating disorder or disordered eating. A prolonged QTc on EKG can also be a result of energy deficiency due to electrolyte imbalance. Laboratory testing can reveal anemia, altered electrolytes, low vitamin B12, folate, iron, magnesium, phosphorus, calcium, or albumin all due to relative energy deficiency. Electrolyte imbalances need to be corrected urgently to prevent a potentially catastrophic event. Indeed, based on the recommendations of the IOC [2], clinicians should be observant of a broad differential diagnosis of pathophysiologies that may be related to low energy availability.

Many athletes first present to a physician provider or orthopedic surgeon with symptoms of a stress fracture, which should immediately prompt further evaluation for LEA, including an evaluation for disordered eating, amenorrhea, and other markers of RED-S. These patients should also

Injuries	
Have you had absences from your training or participation from competition during the last year due to injuries?	☐ No, not at all ☐ Yes, once or twice ☐ Yes, three or four times ☐ Yes, five times or more
If yes, for how many days absence from training or participation in competition due to injuries have you had in the last year?	☐ 1–7 days ☐ 8–14 days ☐ 15–21 days ☐ 22 days or more
If yes, what kind of injuries have you had in the last year?	☐ Accidental ☐ Overload
Comments or further information regarding injuries:	

Illnesses	
Have you had absences from your training or participation from competition during the last year due to illness?	☐ No, not at all ☐ Yes, once or twice ☐ Yes, three or four times ☐ Yes, five times or more
If yes, for how many days absence from training or participation in competition due to have you had in the last year?	☐ 1–7 days ☐ 8–14 days ☐ 15–21 days ☐ 22 days or more
If yes, what kind of injuries have you had in the last year?	
Comments or further information regarding injuries:	

Dizziness	
Do you experience dizziness or lightheadedness?	☐ Yes, several times a day ☐ Yes, several times a week ☐ Yes, once or twice a week or more seldom ☐ Rarely or never

Cold sensitivity	
Do you experience sensitivity to cold?	☐ Yes, several times a day ☐ Yes, several times a week ☐ Yes, once or twice a week or more seldom ☐ Rarely or never

Gastrointestinal symptoms	
Do you feel gaseous or bloated in the abdomen, also when you do not have your period?	☐ Yes, several times a day ☐ Yes, several times a week ☐ Yes, once or twice a week or more seldom ☐ Rarely or never
Do you get cramps or which cannot be related to your menstruation?	☐ Yes, several times a day ☐ Yes, several times a week ☐ Yes, once or twice a week or more seldom ☐ Rarely or never

Fig. 29.6 Low Energy Availability in Females Questionnaire (LEAF-Q)

How often do you have bowel movements on average?	☐ Several times a day ☐ Once a day ☐ Every second day ☐ Twice a week ☐ Once a week or more rarely
How would you describe your normal stool?	☐ Normal (soft) ☐ Diarrhea-like (watery) ☐ Hard and dry
Comments regarding gastrointestinal function:	

Contraceptives	
Do you use oral contraceptives?	☐ Yes ☐ No
If yes, why do you use oral contraceptives?	☐ Contraception ☐ Reduce menstruation pains ☐ Reduction of bleeding ☐ To regulate menstrual cycle in relation performances etc ☐ Otherwise menstruation stops ☐ Other
If no, have you use oral contraceptives earlier?	☐ Yes ☐ No
If yes, when and for how long?	
Do you use any other kind of hormonal contraceptives (e.g, hormonal implant or coil)?	☐ Yes ☐ No
If yes, what kind?	☐ Hormonal patches ☐ Hormonal ring ☐ Hormonal coil ☐ Hormonal implant ☐ Other
Menstrual function	
How old were you when you had your first period?	☐ 11 years or younger ☐ 12–14 years ☐ 15 years or older ☐ I don't remember ☐ I have never menstruated
Did your first menstruation come naturally?	☐ Yes ☐ No ☐ I don't remember
If no, what kind of treatment was used to start your menstrual cycle?	☐ Hormonal treatment ☐ Reduced amount of exercise ☐ Weight gain ☐ Other
Do you have normal menstruation?	☐ Yes ☐ No ☐ I don't know
When was your last period?	☐ 0–4 weeks ago ☐ 1–2 months ago ☐ 3–4 months ago ☐ 5 months ago or more
Do you have normal menstruation?	☐ Yes ☐ No ☐ I don't know
When was your last period?	☐ 0–4 weeks ago ☐ 1–2 months ago ☐ 3–4 months ago ☐ 5 months ago or more
Are your periods regular?	☐ Yes, most of the time ☐ No, mostly not

Fig. 29.6 (continued)

For how many days do you normally bleed?	☐ 1–2 days ☐ 3–4 days ☐ 5–6 days ☐ 7–8 days ☐ 9 days or more
Have you ever had problems with menstrual bleeding?	☐ Yes ☐ No
How many periods have you had in the past year?	☐ 12 or more ☐ 9–11 ☐ 6–8 ☐ 3–5 ☐ 0–2
Have your periods ever stopped for 3 consecutive months or longer (besides pregnancy)?	☐ No, never ☐ Yes, it has happened before ☐ Yes, that's the situation now
Do you experience that your menstruation changes when you increase your exercise intensity, frequency or duration?	☐ Yes ☐ No
If yes, how?	☐ I bleed less ☐ I bleed more ☐ I bleed fewer days ☐ I bleed more days ☐ My menstruation stops

Fig. 29.6 (continued)

undergo evaluation of bone mineral density, specifically using the *Z* scores rather than *T* scores. *Z* scores, as discussed previously, provide a better assessment of bone mineral density in an athlete population than *T* scores, as *Z* scores compare the bone mineral density to an average for age, sex, weight, and ethnicity. Yet even the use of *Z* scores may be limited for evaluation of athletes, and providers should have a high suspicion for low BMD even when evaluation results place the athlete in the normal range compared to the general population.

Ultimately, LEA has effects on physical and mental health, as well as athlete performance. One study demonstrated that compared to athletes with adequate energy availability, those with low energy availability were 2.1 times more likely to report increased recovery time, 4.3 times more likely to report judgment impairments, 1.6 times more likely to report feeling uncoordinated, and 2 times more likely to report difficulty concentrating [36]. Those with low energy availability were further 1.6 times more likely to report feelings of irritability, 2.3 times more likely to report feelings of depression, and 1.5 times more likely to report a decrease in endurance during training or competition [36]. One study in junior elite female swimmers demonstrated a substantial effect of LEA; those athletes with energy deficit demonstrated a 9.8% regression in their 400-m swim over 12 weeks, as compared to those athletes without an energy deficit who experienced an 8.2% improvement [37]. These numbers indicate while athlete performance is impacted by many variables, a decline in performance should alert a coach or sport medicine/sport science specialist of possible energy deficiency (Fig. 29.7).

Low energy availability increases recovery time, decreases focus, decreases judgment, increases risk of depression, and reduces performance.

The most recent work from the IOC [35] suggests that measuring the *effects* of LEA may prove to be clinically more relevant than the *actual* measurements of energy availability (EA) due to the considerable effort needed to accurately assess EA and its frailties as a stand-alone diagnostic tool. They strongly suggest that this is true for both male and female athletes. Furthermore, they suggest that since cultural, social, psychological, and financial factors contribute to low energy

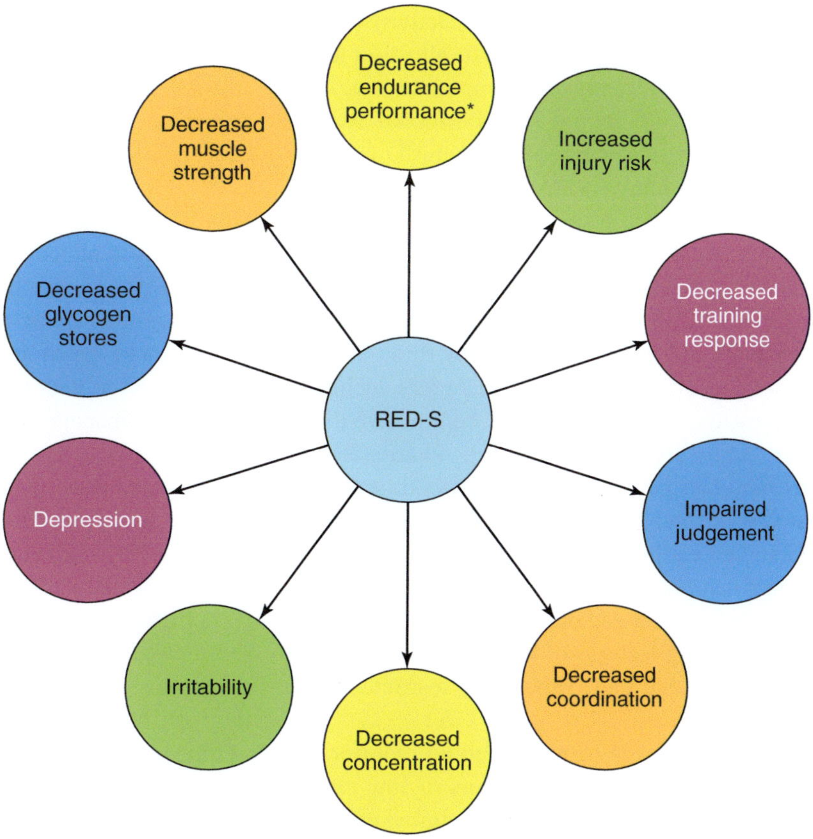

Fig. 29.7 Effects of LEA on athlete performance (Reproduced from Mountjoy et al. [2])

availability, all of these would have to be addressed for a holistic approach or prevention.

29.4 Therapeutic Interventions

Recognizing athletes with an energy deficit is an important initial step toward recovery and should trigger a team of medical professionals experienced in the unique demands of sport to initiate appropriate treatment. The importance of early intervention cannot be overstated given the potential irreversibility of some of the physiologic effects, such as lost opportunity for optimal bone mineral density accrual during adolescence. Once an athlete is identified as having, or at risk for having, relative energy deficiency, interventions for amelioration can begin. Effective treatment must address both the immediate issue of relative energy deficiency and the cause, which is often multifactorial.

Initially, the appropriate setting for treatment must be assessed. Depending on medical or psychiatric stability, an inpatient setting might be required for unstable vital signs or inability to ensure safety. Most often, treatment can be initiated and continued on an outpatient basis. Following the determination of the appropriate treatment setting, diet and/or exercise modification is the next step in order to improve energy availability. This occurs via increased oral energy intake, decreased energy expenditure through activity restriction, or more often a combination of both. Although the immediate goal is to prevent further injury, this also serves to establish a quantifiable assessment tool that can be regularly assessed by the athlete and members of the treatment team.

A registered dietician, ideally one with experience in the unique demands of sport, should meet with the athlete to assess current nutritional status through energy intake and macro-/micronutrient requirements based on activity level. Appointments at regular intervals allow for nutrition education, implementation, monitoring, and adjustments of oral intake. Nutritional supplementation with calcium and vitamin D for bone health or protein for intense exercise [38] might be necessary.

When disordered eating behavior contributes to energy deficiency, a mental health practitioner can address the underlying mental health disorder as well as the psychiatric comorbidities commonly occurring with eating disorders, including depression, anxiety, obsessive-compulsive disorder, and substance abuse [6]. Pharmacologic therapy can be considered, discussed, and initiated if deemed appropriate. In the absence of an identified eating disorder, a mental health practitioner can help the athlete develop strategies for healthy behavior and problem-solving in addition to addressing feelings of frustration, isolation, or depression that can come from restricted sport participation.

A primary care provider should monitor and treat other medical implications of low energy availability such as electrolyte imbalance and low bone mineral density. Laboratory testing can assess for nutritional status or other etiologies of menstrual dysfunction or amenorrhea. It should be noted that hormone replacement therapy has not been found to improve bone mineral density, and the oral contraceptive pill can delay and reduce menstrual cycle restoration [39]. The use of bisphosphonates and selective estrogen receptor modulators is not recommended [5]. The use of DEXA scans for the ongoing monitoring of bone mineral density is a multifactorial consideration based on the athlete's history and physical exam. Pharmacological intervention for low bone mineral density should be considered if there is no response after 1 year of non-pharmacologic therapy or if new fractures occur despite addressing energy deficiency [31].

In order to achieve a healthy energy balance, sports participation may need to be initially restricted in order to decrease energy expenditures. The athlete's level of activity should be regularly assessed by the treating physician and advanced as appropriate. Establishing a treatment contract and return-to-play expectations early in treatment can give the athlete control and context through specific expectations for treatment and recovery while establishing the goal of full return to sport. Progressive return to sport is an indication of a successful treatment strategy for energy deficiency. Given the multifactorial nature of energy deficiency, many considerations should be taken into account when considering return to play. When involved with the athlete's team, an athletic trainer can manage return to play on day-to-day basis, monitor for adverse effects or non-compliance, and update the coaching staff as appropriate. Establishing the importance and necessity for adherence to the treatment plan and treatment contract (Fig. 29.8) is critical to the compliance of the athlete. For female athletes, resumption of menses can be a reliable sign of adequate nutrition provided the absence of OCP or IUD use, however, should not be used as a marker of time to return to play, as resumption of menses is often delayed once energy balance is achieved.

Return to play is a decision process with participation of healthcare providers, coaches, and athletes based on continuous assessment of the athlete and the competitive environment. There are several tools available for risk stratification to guide safe return to sport, including a return-to-play model (Fig. 29.9) developed by the Female Athlete Triad Coalition [40] and a cumulative risk assessment model (Fig. 29.10), which incorporates evidence-based risk factors and designates a point value for each factor [31]. Similarly, the IOC created a "red light, yellow light, green light" clinical guidelines (Fig. 29.11) that can assist the clinician in determining when an athlete should be allowed to participate with or without restrictions [2]. Once an athlete has been returned to full sport, periodic weights can monitor for continued adequate nutritional status. More recently, the IOC has written an update on RED-S [35] which continues to emphasize the need to create a more practical tool to identify athletes at risk of relative energy deficits, the

____________________(Athlete Name)

The following items are mandatory and must be completed as prescribed. Failure to do so will result in the consequence listed below the requirements. All benefits and consequence are subject to change at any time and at the discretion of the Multidisciplinary Team. Multidisciplinary Team:

______________(Physician), _____________ (Psychotherapist), _____________(Dietitian)

Requirements:

☐ Meet with _______________ (therapist) 1x per week, or as recommended by therapist.
☐ Meet with _______________ (dietitian) 1x per week, or as recommended by dietitian.
☐ Meet with Dr. ____________ 1-2x per month, or as recommended by Dr. ____________.
☐ Follow daily meal plan set forth by sports dietitian.
☐ Keep daily workout log updated with specific type, length, and effort.
☐ Weight gain of _____ lbs per week.
☐ Weekly weigh-in with ____________(name team member), or at time intervals of ___weeks.
☐ Must achieve minimal acceptable body weight of___ lbs by______ (date).
☐ After this data, must maintain weight at or above minimal acceptable body weight.
☐ Limit of _____workout sessions per week with no one session being more than _____ minutes in length.
All activity counts (e.g., biking running, weight lifing, and swimming).

Benefits:

If ALL requirements are met then clearance to participate in team activities and use of athletic facilities will:
☐ be granted ☐ continue.

Consequences:

If ANY requirements(s) are not met then clearance to participate in team activities and use of athletic facilities will be revoked, and re-instatement will be at the discretion of the team physician and multidisciplinary team

I, ________________________have read this contract and all of my questions were answered.

______________________	______________________	___________
Athlete Name	Athlete Signature	Date
______________________	______________________	___________
Team Physician Name	Team Physician Signature	Date

Fig. 29.8 Example athlete treatment contract (Reproduced from Joy et al. [6])

need for increased awareness of the broad spectrum of pathophysiologic impact of low energy availability regardless of gender, and the need for more practical guidelines regarding return to play.

> Return-to-play decisions in more severe cases are complex and require a team approach that includes healthcare providers, nutritionists, coaches, and the athlete.

Multidisciplinary team members are required for comprehensive treatment of energy deficiency, and communication between treating team members is critical to athlete success. When the athlete involved is an adolescent, parental involvement is necessary. In addition to assisting with complex treatment plan compliance and implementation, families should be encouraged to participate in family therapy if appropriate. Although not required, family involvement in the treatment of energy deficiency can be an option for any athlete regardless of age.

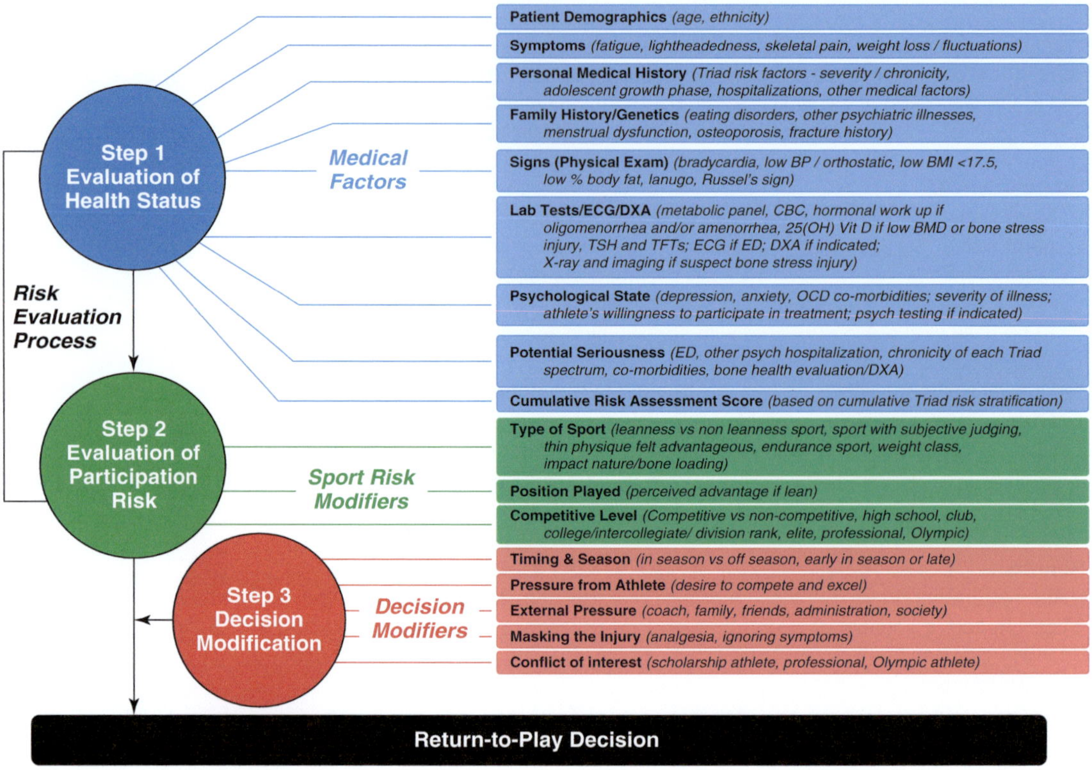

Fig. 29.9 Decision-based return-to-play model from the Female Athlete Triad Coalition Statement (Reproduced from Joy et al. [40])

29.5 Prevention

Prevention of relative energy deficiency, and the associated pathology, could be considered the most effective treatment. Coaches, parents, athletic administrators, judges/officials, and teammates can influence an athlete and help identify early signs of intentional or unintentional poor energy availability in an athlete. Negative comments on body size can lead to poor body image and eating disorders; therefore education on healthy feedback and support is important. Loss of menstruation is a sign of poor energy availability and should not be dismissed. Education regarding prevention and identification can come from the medical team caring for an athletic team, along with governing organizations and federations, such as the NCAA, through publications and conferences [3, 5, 6], or even peers [43]. Primary prevention strategies include educating athletes on healthy eating and the cost of poor nutrition, along with teaching teammates, to identify warning signs of an eating disorder. Teaching athletes methods to nourish their bodies correctly allows for a positive relationship with food, while educating about the harm to bodily a

Risk Factors	Magnitude of Risk Low Risk = 0 points each	 Moderate Risk = 1 point each	 High Risk = 2 points each
Low EA with or without DE/ED	☐ No dietary restriction	☐ Some dietary restriction‡; current/past history of DE;	☐ Meets DSM V criteria for ED*
Low BMI	☐ BMI ≥ 18.5 **or** ≥ 90% EW** or weight stable	☐ BMI 17.5 < 18.5 **or** < 90% EW **or** 5 to < 10% weight loss/month	☐ BMI ≤17.5 **or** < 85% EW **or** ≥ 10% weight loss/month
Delayed Menarche	☐ Menarche < 15 years	☐ Menarche 15 to < 16 years	☐ Menarche ≥16 years
Oligomenorrhea and/or Amenorrhea	☐ > 9 menses in 12 months*	☐ 6-9 menses in 12 months*	☐ < 6 menses in 12 months*
Low BMD	☐ Z-score ≥ -1.0	☐ Z-score -1.0*** < -2.0	☐ Z-score ≤ -2.0
Stree Reaction/Fracture	☐ None	☐ 1	☐ ≥ 2; ≥ 1 high risk or of trabecular bone sites†
Cumulative Risk (total each column, then add for total score)	**____ points +**	**____ points +**	**____ points = ____Total Score**

b

	Cumulative Risk Score*	Low Risk	Moderate Risk	High Risk
Full Clearance	0 – 1 point	☐		
Provisional/Limited Clearance	2 – 5 points		☐ Provisional Clearance ☐ Limited Clearance	
Restricted from Training and Competition	≥ 6 points			☐ Restricted from Training/ Competition-Provisional ☐ Disqualified

Fig. 29.10 (**a**) Cumulative risk assessment tool. (**b**) Clearance and return to play using cumulative risk assessment (Reproduced from DeSouza et al. [31])

health and athletic performance can provide motivation to achieve or maintain an adequate nutrition status.

Identifying the early signs of relative energy deficiency can prevent harmful habits and thought processes involved from becoming ingrained in the athlete's identity and approach to the sport. Teaching those in authority, peers, and the athletes themselves can prevent or identify relative energy deficiency in the early states.

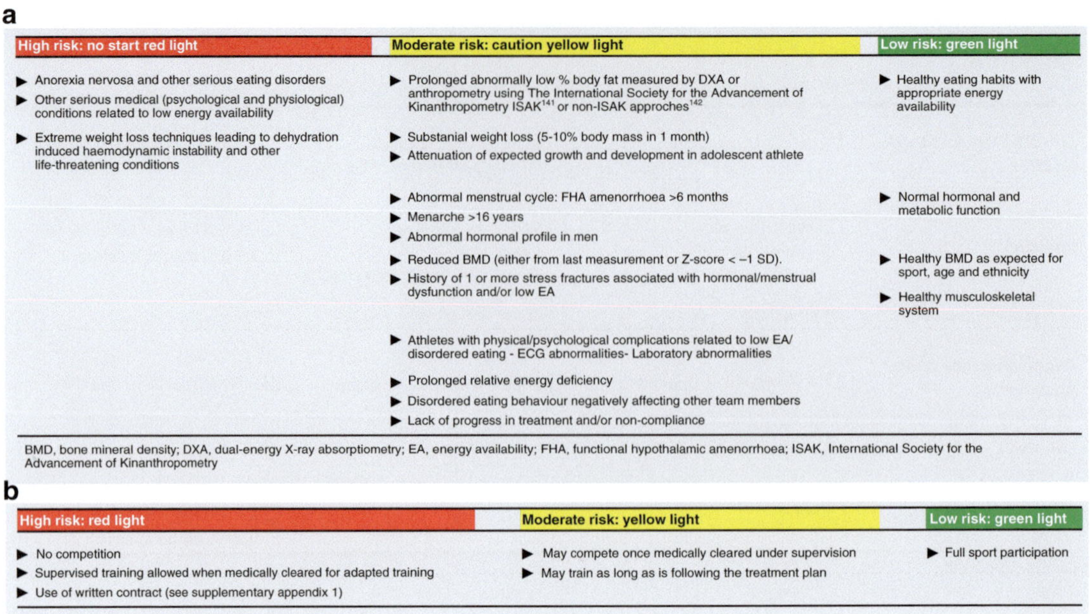

Fig. 29.11 (**a**) The Relative Energy Deficiency in Sport risk assessment model for sport participation. (**b**) The Relative Energy Deficiency in Sport return-to-play model (Reproduced from Mountjoy et al. [2])

Take-Home Messages

- Relative Energy Deficit Syndrome and the Female Athlete Triad are a complex group of pathologies usually triggered by low energy availability. Low energy availability can have negative effects on both males and females.
- Low energy availability predisposes athletes to possible physical injury, systemic pathology, psychological stress, and poor athletic performance.
- Early recognition and a team-based approach are the most effective interventions to optimize the health of the athlete and prevent more severe complications.

References

1. Yeager KK, Agostini R, Nattiv A, et al. The female athlete triad: disordered eating, amenorrhea, and osteoporosis. Med Sci Sports Exerc. 1993;25(7):775–7.
2. Mountjoy M, Sundgot-Borgen J, Burke L, et al. The IOC consensus statement: beyond the female athlete triad—relative energy deficiency in sport (RED-S). Br J Sports Med. 2014;48:491–7.
3. Nattiv A, Loucks AB, Manore MM, et al. American College of Sports Medicine position stand: the female athlete triad. Med Sci Sports Exerc. 2007;39(10):1867–82.
4. Hooper DR, Kraemer WJ, Saenz C, et al. The presence of symptoms of testosterone deficiency in the exercise-hypogonadal male condition and the role of nutrition. Eur J Appl Physiol. 2017;117:1349–75.
5. Drinkwater BL, Loucks A, Sherman RT, et al. IOC medical commission position stand on the female athlete triad. Medical and Scientific Commission, International Olympic Committee; 2005. https://www.olympic.org/news/consensus-statement-adopted-on-the-female-athlete-triad. Accessed 4 Mar 2018.
6. Joy E, Kussman A, Nattiv A. 2016 update on eating disorders in athletes: a comprehensive narrative review with a focus on clinical assessment and management. Br J Sports Med. 2016;50:154–62.
7. Sundgot-Borgen J, Torstveit MK. Prevalence of eating disorders in elite athletes is higher than in the general population. Clin J Sport Med. 2004;14:25–32.
8. Byrne S, Mclean N. Elite athletes: effects of the pressure to be thin. J Sci Med Sport. 2002;5:80–94.
9. Berkovich BE, Eliakim A, Nemet D, et al. Rapid weight loss among adolescents participating in competitive judo. Int J Sport Nutr Exerc Metab. 2016;26:276–84.
10. Chapman J, Woodman T. Disordered eating in male athletes: a meta-analysis. J Sports Sci. 2016;34(2):101–9.

11. Barrack MT, Fredericson M, Tenforde A, et al. Evidence of a cumulative effect for risk factors predicting low bone mass among male adolescent athletes. Br J Sports Med. 2017;51:200–5.
12. Viner RT, Harris M, Berning JR, et al. Energy availability and dietary patterns of adult male and female competitive cyclists with lower than expected bone mineral density. Int J Sport Nutr Exerc Metab. 2015;25:594–602.
13. Beals KA, Manore MM. Disorders of the female athlete triad among collegiate athletes. Int J Sport Nutr Exerc Metab. 2002;12:281–93.
14. Doyle-Lucas AF, Akers JD, Davy BM. Energetic efficiency, menstrual irregularity, and bone mineral density in elite professional female ballet dancers. J Dance Med Sci. 2010;4:146–54.
15. Dusek T. Influence of high intensity training on menstrual cycle disorders in athletes. Croat Med J. 2001;42:79–82.
16. Khan KM, Liu-Ambrose T, Sran MM, et al. New criteria for female athlete triad syndrome? As osteoporosis is rare, should osteopenia be among the criteria for defining the female athlete triad syndrome? Br J Sports Med. 2002;36:10–3.
17. Beals KA, Hill AK. The prevalence of disordered eating, menstrual dysfunction, and low bone mineral density among US collegiate athletes. Int J Sport Nutr Exerc Metab. 2006;16:1–23.
18. Nichols JF, Rauh MJ, Lawson MJ, et al. Prevalence of the female athlete triad syndrome among high school athletes. Arch Pediatr Adolesc Med. 2006;160:137–42.
19. Torstveit MK, Sundgot-Borgen J. The female athlete triad exists in both elite athletes and controls. Med Sci Sports Exerc. 2005;37:1449–59.
20. Logue D, Madigan MM, Delahunt E, et al. Low energy availability in athletes: a review of prevalence, dietary patterns, physiological health, and sports performance. Sports Med. 2018;48:73–96.
21. Erdelyi GJ. Gynecological survey of female athletes. J Sports Med Phys Fitness. 1962;2:174–9.
22. Prior JC, Yuen BH, Clement P, et al. Reversible luteal phase changes and infertility associated with marathon training. Lancet. 1982;2:269–79.
23. Puhl JL, Brown C, editors. The menstrual cycle and physical activity. Champaign: Human Kinetics, Inc.; 1986. p. 1–164.
24. Schwartz B, Cummings DC, Riordan E, et al. Exercise-associated amenorrhea: a distinct entity? Am J Obstet Gynecol. 1981;141:662–70.
25. Drinkwater BL, Nilson KM, Chestnut CH, et al. Bone mineral content of amenorrheic and eumenorrheic athletes. N Engl J Med. 1984;311:277–81.
26. Drinkwater BL, Nilson KM, Ott S, et al. Bone mineral density after resumption of menses in amenorrheic women. JAMA. 1986;256:380–2.
27. Marcus R, Cann C, Madvig P. Menstrual function and bone mass in elite women distance runners. Ann Intern Med. 1985;102:158–63.
28. Rosen LW, Hough DO. Pathogenic weight control behavior of female college gymnasts. Phys Sportsmed. 1988;16:141–6.
29. Otis CL, Drinkwater B, Johnson M, et al. American College of Sports Medicine Position Stand: the female athlete triad. Med Sci Sports Exerc. 1997;29(5): i–ix.
30. Bonci CM, Bonci LJ, Granger LR, et al. National Athletic Trainers' association position statement: preventing, detecting, and managing disordered eating in athletes. J Athl Train. 2008;43(1):80–108.
31. DeSouza MJ, Nattiv A, Joy E, et al. 2014 female athlete triad coalition consensus statement on treatment and return to play of the female athlete triad. Clin J Sport Med. 2014;24(2):96–119.
32. Sygo J, Coates A, Sesbreno E, Mountjoy M, Burr J. Prevalence of indicators of low energy availability in elite female sprinters. Int J Sport Nutr Exerc Metab. 2018;28(5):490–6.
33. McNulty KY, Adams CH, Anderson JM, et al. Development and validation of a screening tool to identify eating disorders in female athletes. J Am Diet Assoc. 2001;101:886–92.
34. Martinsen M, Holme I, Pensgaard AM, et al. The development of the brief eating disorder in athletes questionnaire. Med Sci Sports Exerc. 2014;46:1666–75.
35. Mountjoy M, Sundgot-Borgen J, Burke L, et al. The IOC consensus statement update: relative energy deficiency in sport (RED-S). Br J Sports Med. 2018;52(11):687–97; personal communication.
36. Ackerman K, Holtzman B, Cooper K, et al. Low energy availability surrogates correlate with health and performance consequences of relative energy deficiency in sport (RED-S). Br J Sports Med. Published online first: 02 Jun 2018. doi:10.1136/bjsports-2017-098958
37. Vanheest JL, Rodgers CD, Mahoney CE, et al. Ovarian suppression impairs sport performance in junior elite female swimmers. Med Sci Sports Exerc. 2014;46(1):156–66.
38. Manore MM, Barr SI, Butterfield GA. Nutrition and athletic performance. A joint position statement of the American Dietetic Association, the Dietitians of Canada, and the American College of Sports Medicine. Med Sci Sports Exerc. 2000;32: 2130–45.
39. Falsetti L, Gambera A, Barbetti L, et al. Long-term follow-up of functional hypothalamic amenorrhea and prognostic factors. J Clin Endocrinol Metab. 2002;87:500–5.
40. Joy E, De Souza MJ, Nattiv A. 2014 female athlete triad coalition consensus statement on treatment and return to play of the female athlete triad. Curr Sports Med Rep. 2014;12:219–32.
41. Dale E, Gerlack DH, Wilhite AL. Menstrual dysfunction in distance runners. Obstet Gynecol. 1979;54(1):47–53.
42. Tenforde AS, Barrack MT, Nattiv A, et al. Parallels with the female athlete triad in male athletes. Sports Med. 2016;46:171–82.
43. Becker CA, McDaniel, L, Bull S, Powell M, McIntyre K. Can we reduce eating disorder risk factors in female college athletes? A randomized exploratory investigation of two peer-led interventions. Body Image. 2012;9(1):31–42.

Sudden Cardiac Arrest

30

Clea Simone S. S. Colombo, Michael Papadakis, and Nabil Ghorayeb

30.1 Introduction

Sudden cardiac arrest (SCA) is defined as an unexpected cessation or severe malfunction of heart function followed by loss of consciousness due to haemodynamic collapse [1, 2]. Unfortunately, most SCAs progress to sudden cardiac death (SCD) [3]. SCA is responsible for 50% of cardiovascular mortality, and it is the third leading cause of death in the United States [1]. It is the end result of a heterogeneous group of conditions, the majority due to primary intrinsic cardiac abnormalities [4].

It is well established that regular exercise promotes health and prolongs life [5, 6]. Therefore, the athlete is considered not just a symbol of good health but also an invulnerable hero. Consequently, SCA in an athletic individual is always a tragic event and devastating for their families and the wider society.

SCA/SCD is often the first clinical manifestation of underlying cardiovascular disease. Most individuals with inherited cardiac diseases are asymptomatic, and therefore most individuals are unaware they harbour a substrate to malignant arrhythmias. Approximately 60% of SCDs occur during exertion [7, 8]. The adrenergic stimulus of exercise causes cardiovascular responses, which result to an increase of heart rate, stroke volume and blood pressure. Intense exercise during competitive sports may promote lethal arrhythmias in the presence of an abnormal substrate. Consequently, intense exercise is not the primary cause of the SCA but acts as a trigger in predisposed individuals [9].

Prevention of SCA/SCD encompasses a number of complementary strategies including the recognition of high-risk individuals, pre-participation cardiovascular evaluation and early defibrillation. The presence of quiescent cardiac disease has brought pre-participation cardiovascular evaluation of athletes at the forefront of preventative strategies for SCD. The aim is to identify athletes at potential risk of exercise-

C. S. S. S. Colombo (✉)
Cardiology Clinical Academic Group, St. George's University of London, London, UK

Department of Ergometry, Exercise, Nuclear Cardiology and Cardiovascular Rehabilitation (DERC), Brazilian Society of Cardiology (SBC), Rio de Janeiro, Brazil

Cuore Dello Sport, São Paulo, Brazil

M. Papadakis
Cardiology Clinical Academic Group, St. George's University of London, London, UK

European Section of Sports Cardiology and Exercise of the EAPC, Sophia Antipolis Cedex, France
e-mail: michael.papadakis@sgul.ac.uk

N. Ghorayeb
Institute Dante Pazzanese of Cardiology—Universidade São Paulo, São Paulo, Brazil

Heart Hospital (Hospital do Coração—HCor), São Paulo, Brazil
e-mail: ghorayeb@cardiol.br

S. Rocha Piedade et al. (eds.), *The Sports Medicine Physician*,
https://doi.org/10.1007/978-3-030-10433-7_30

induced fatal arrhythmias and through a number of life-style and medical interventions, including restriction from competition, to minimise their risk [10, 11]. The early recognition of a SCA and prompt emergency care during sports activity are essential to minimise SCD or serious brain damage [3, 12]. Data report that there is still a lack of trained personnel and proper emergency action plans, causing a delay to start cardiopulmonary resuscitation (CPR) and a negative impact on survival rate [13].

30.2 Epidemiology

The incidence of SCD in athletes varies depending on the age, gender, ethnicity, sports modality and the methodology used to acquire the data [14]. In addition, there is lack of systematic registries of SCD in athletes in most countries, and data are often based on media reports.

The rate of SCD among young athletes (<35 years) is reported as 2.1 per 100,000 athletes/year (a/y) in the Veneto region of Italy, approximately 2.8-fold greater compared to nonathletes (0.7 in 100,000 a/y). Women athletes are at lower risk with a reported ratio of female to male of 1:10 [9]. Black athletes seem to have a higher risk than white athletes, with a reported incidence rate of 4.7 per 100,000 a/y [15]. The sports modalities with highest rates of SCD reported are basketball and soccer [9, 15]. Among young athletes of the National Collegiate Athletic Association (NCAA) in the United States, the incidence rate of SCD was 1.9 per 100,000 a/y, but considerably higher, 19.2/100,000 a/y, in Division I male basketball players [15]. During long-distance running races, the incidence of SCA is reported as 1:184,000 runners (0.54 per 100,000 runners), and the incidence is higher during marathons (1.0 per 100,000 runners) than half-marathon (0.27 per 100,000 runners) whereas among triathlon participants is 1:52,630 participants (1.9 per 100,000 runners) [16].

30.3 Common Causes of SCD During Exercise

30.3.1 Noncardiac

Climate conditions and poorly regulated body temperature, inadequate electrolyte and fluid replacement or overhydration can trigger fatal arrhythmias and SCA. Hyperthermia and resultant rhabdomyolysis, renal failure and electrolyte disturbances are increasingly recognised as an important substrate for arrhythmias. Dehydration may also predispose to hyperkalaemia and hypernatraemia which in turn may result to SCA. Excessive water intake can cause significant hyponatraemia, leading to cerebral oedema, seizures, coma and respiratory and cardiac arrest.

Some drugs, illicit or not, can contribute as an arrhythmogenic substrate.

The use of diuretics and stimulants such as amphetamines and ephedrine is not uncommon, predisposing to hypokalaemia and tachycardia, especially in sports modalities where weight control is an important issue. The chronic use of anabolic-androgenic steroids to gain muscle mass and power may increase the risk of myocardial infarction and arrhythmias due to electrolyte imbalance or atherosclerosis. Other performance enhancement substances, such as recombinant human erythropoietin, can predispose to thromboembolic events and SCA [17]. The increasing use of supplements by both professional and recreational athletes poses a new challenge. Drinks and other supplements, often considered innocent, must be evaluated carefully, as they may contain electrolyte concentrations or other substances that in predisposed individuals may result to severe metabolic imbalance and SCA. "Contamination" of dietary supplements with anabolic steroids has also been reported [18, 19].

30.3.2 Cardiac

30.3.2.1 Inherited or Congenital

Structural

Hypertrophic Cardiomyopathy

Hypertrophic cardiomyopathy (HCM) has been reported as a major cause of SCD in young athletes, accounting for up to one third of deaths in some cohorts [8]. The prevalence of HCM is reported as 1:500 young individuals. It is an inherited myocardial disorder, most frequently transmitted in an autosomal-dominant mode. In up to 60% of cases is caused by mutations in cardiac sarcomere protein genes, most commonly beta-myosin heavy chain (MYH7) and myosin-binding protein C (MYBPC3). It is characterised by the presence of left ventricular hypertrophy (LVH), defined as a left ventricular wall thickness (LVWT) ≥ 15 mm in one or more left ventricular myocardial segments, in the absence of abnormal loading conditions, such as hypertension or valve disease. Microvascular dysfunction, mitral valve abnormalities and myocardial fibrosis are associated with the phenotypic expression of the disease.

The ECG is abnormal in more than 90% of HCM patients and is an early marker of disease, often predating structural changes by many years. The most common findings are left ventricular hypertrophy (LVH) associated with T-wave inversion (TWI) in lateral and/or inferior leads (81%), ST-segment depression and pathological Q waves (Fig. 30.1), [20]. Echocardiography can be used to confirm the diagnosis of HCM. Cardiac magnetic resonance (CMR) imaging can better delineate

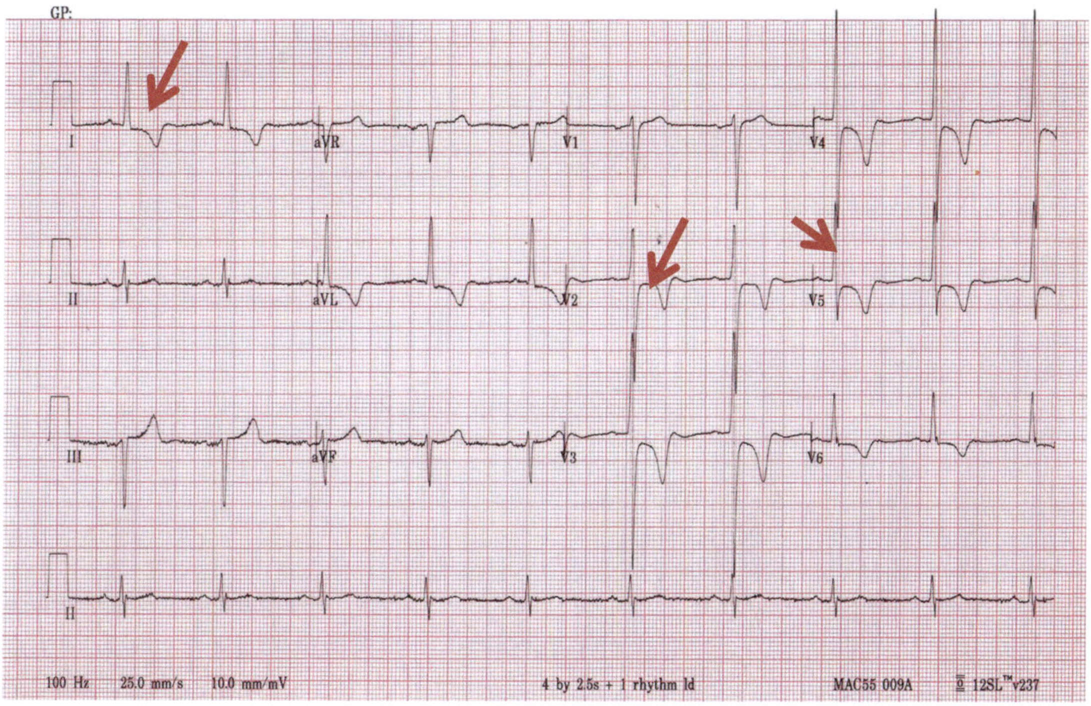

Fig. 30.1 Athlete's ECG with HCM. LVH associated with deep anterolateral TWI, ST-segment depression

localised or subtle hypertrophy, can detect microvascular disease and can identify myocardial fibrosis, which is present in 65% of patients and has been associated to an increased risk of SCD [21].

Athletes with HCM are more frequent in start-stop sports modalities, such as soccer, rugby and basketball [22]. This occurs probably due to their incapacity to sustain a prolonged augmentation of stroke volume, being more difficult to compete in endurance sports.

Cardiac physiological adaptation to exercise poses a challenge to differentiate HCM from athlete's heart in some athletes. Physiological LVH in athletes can overlap a mild HCM phenotype (LVWT = 13–15 mm), referred to as the "grey zone". The diagnostic conundrum is more frequent in black males and athletes involved in endurance sports. To differentiate physiology from pathology, it is essential to do a comprehensive assessment of the athlete, which in addition to a comprehensive history may include cardiopulmonary exercise testing (CPET), ECG monitoring, CMR and even familial evaluation. Detraining to assess resolution of the ECG changes and LV hypertrophy can also be of incremental value. Once the diagnosis of HCM is established, expert consensus recommendations advise against participation in competitive sports, with the possible exception of those of low intensity (class IA sports) [23].

Arrhythmogenic Right Ventricular Cardiomyopathy

Arrhythmogenic right ventricular cardiomyopathy (ARVC) is also an important cause of SCD in young athletes, accounting for 4–5% of deaths. The prevalence is 1:1000 in the general population, but can be as high as 0.4–0.8% in Italy (Veneto) and Greece (Naxos) [24]. It is transmitted as an autosomal-dominant trait with variable penetrance, caused by mutations in genes encoding cardiac desmosomal proteins. There is progressive replacement of the myocardium by fibrofatty tissue, from epicardium or mid-myocardium, extending to transmural, resulting in thinning of the wall and aneurysms. This interferes with electrical impulse conduction and leads to life-threatening arrhythmias. The risk of SCD is fivefold higher during competitive sports, and accumulating evidence suggests that intense exercise practice accelerates the progression of the disease [7, 23, 25].

The clinical diagnostic criteria include the presence of functional and structural changes of the right ventricle depolarisation and repolarisation ECG abnormalities and ventricular arrhythmias [25]. The left ventricle is also affected in the majority of cases, and the condition is more appropriately referred to as arrhythmogenic cardiomyopathy (ACM).

The ECG is abnormal in up to 80% of patients, with TWI in the right precordial leads (V1–3), prolonged QRS duration (>110 ms), epsilon wave (small amplitude potentials after QRS and before the onset of T wave), premature ventricular contractions (PVC) with left bundle branch block pattern and ventricular tachycardia (VT) (Fig. 30.2). Diastolic dilation of right ventricular outflow tract (>30 mm) and wall motion abnormalities are frequent findings in echocardiography [26].

The early disease process of ARVC can also overlap with physiological cardiac adaptation to exercise and represents another "grey zone" (Fig. 30.3). Recent studies have demonstrated that up to 30% of athletes exhibit right ventricular cavity dimensions which overlap with the dimensions suggested as part of the ARVC diagnosis criteria [27, 28].

Athletes with ARVC should be advised against participation in competitive sports (with the possible exception of class IA sports). Studies indicate that individuals with positive genotype and negative phenotype can develop the disease with intensive exercise; therefore, they should follow the same recommendations [29].

Congenital Coronary Artery Anomalies (CAA)

Coronary arteries present anomalous origin from sinus of Valsalva in 0.5–1.0% of individuals and are reported as the second most common cause of

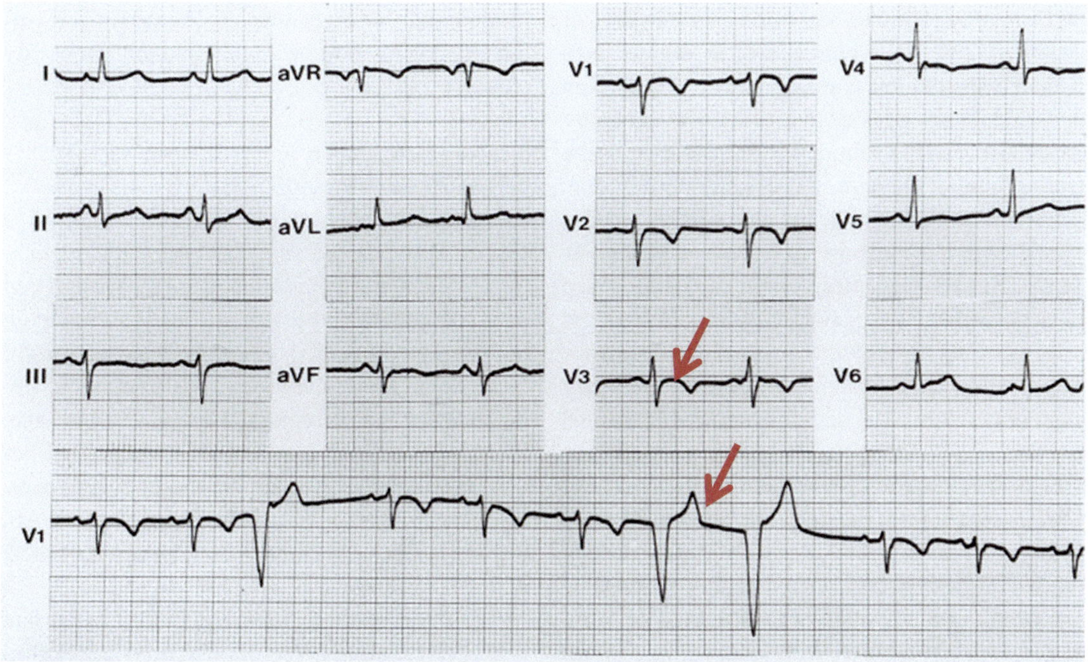

Fig. 30.2 Athlete's ECG with ARVC. Right precordial TWI (V1–3), isolated VE and couplets with LBBB morphology

Fig. 30.3 Specific and overlapping features of athlete's heart and cardiomyopathies. *ARVC* arrhytmogenic right ventricular cardiomyopathy; *HCM* hypertrophic cardiomyopathy; *IRBBB* incomplete right bundle branch block; *LV* left ventricle; *LVH* left ventricular hypertrophy; *LVWT* left ventricular wall thickness; *NSVT* non-sustained ventricular tachycardia; *QW* Q waves; *RV* right ventricle; *TWI* T wave inversion

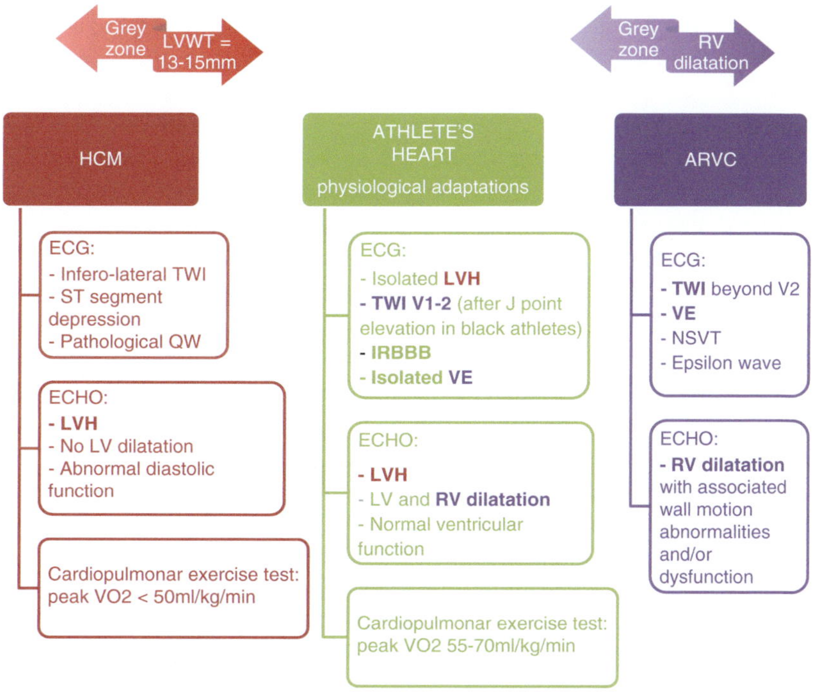

SCD in young athletes accounting for 17–24% of deaths [8, 26]. The higher risk of SCD is in individuals with the left coronary artery origin from the right sinus of Valsalva, with the coronary course between the pulmonary artery and the aorta. During intense exercise, the coronary artery may get compressed between the big vessels leading to myocardial ischaemia, ventricular arrhythmias and SCA. Coronary artery origin can be localised by echocardiography; however, the gold standard imaging tests are cardiac magnetic resonance angiography or computed tomography coronary angiography [30]. The demonstration of exertional ischaemia is challenging, and usual tests such as exercise testing, exercise echocardiography, stress CMR and nuclear imaging can be falsely reassuring. The recommendations for sports depend on the coronary artery anatomy, the presence of symptoms and the presence of inducible ischaemia. Usually, athletes with left coronary origin from right sinus or anomalies traversing between the great vessels should be restricted from participating in all competitive sports (with the possible exception of class IA sports). After surgical repair the decision depends on the results from the reassessment of the athlete [31].

Marfan Syndrome

Marfan syndrome (MS) accounts for 3% of SCD in young athletes [8]. It is an autosomal-dominant inherited disease of the connective tissue, caused by mutations in the fibrillin-1 (FBN1) gene with a prevalence of 1:5000 individuals. Multiple organs are affected with skeletal, cardiovascular, ocular, skin, lungs and nerve abnormalities. Cardiovascular abnormalities include aorta dilatation, dissection or rupture. Intense exercise increases the pressure in the aorta and can accelerate the progression. Tall athletes with hypermobility of the joints are common in some sports such as volleyball and basketball and should be evaluated carefully, especially if aortic root diameter enlargement is present (>40 mm in males and >34 mm in females) [32]. The diagnosis is done based on clinical features, family history, imaging and genetic testing, following the Ghent criteria [33]. Recommendations suggest that athletes diagnosed with MS should not participate in moderate- to high-intensity isometric and isotonic sports or sports with the potential for bodily collision [34].

Bicuspid Aortic Valve, Aortic Stenosis and Mitral Valve Prolapse

Bicuspid aortic valve (BAV) is a congenital valve abnormality that affects 1.5–2% of the population, with a male predominance of 3:1, and can be associated with thoracic aortic dilatation in up to 50% of adults [35]. Commonly, degenerative changes of the leaflets can result to aortic stenosis (AS) and/or regurgitation at a young age. Ventricular arrhythmias and ventricular dysfunction, with inadequate cardiac output during exercise, can be present in athletes with severe AS, leading to SCA. Aortic stenosis is a cause of SCD in 2–4% of young athletes [8].

Pre-participation evaluation has an important role because clinical history and physical examination can identify AS, usually presenting an aortic systolic murmur and symptoms of dyspnea and angina during exercise. Echocardiography can confirm the diagnosis and determine the severity of AS, and exercise testing is useful for risk stratification [26]. Athletes with AS should undergo regular evaluation. In the presence of moderate AS, they can participate in low- and moderate-intensity static or dynamic competitive sports, if asymptomatic and with normal response to exercise testing. Athletes with severe AS should not participate in competitive sports (with the possible exception of class IA sports, if they are asymptomatic) [36].

Mitral valve prolapse (MVP) is relatively common in the general population, with a prevalence of 3–5%. Despite the association of MVP and SCD is controversial, few cases of SCD have been reported in which MVP was the only abnormality identified, including in young athletes. Some patients with MVP can present ventricular fibrillation (VF) leading to SCA, but rarely during exercise [37]. MVP is considered a benign condition, and competitive athletes can participate in all sports unless it is associated with significant mitral regurgitation; with symptoms, such as severe chest pain or exertional syncope; or with documented ventricular tachycardia (VT) [37].

Electrical

Wolff-Parkinson-White Syndrome

Wolff-Parkinson-White (WPW) is a syndrome with paroxysmal arrhythmias due to an accessory pathway in a re-entrant circuit involving AV node-His axis. Approximately one third of the patients can develop atrial fibrillation, and there is a risk of VF secondary to rapid anterograde conduction via the accessory pathway in these individuals [38]. SCD can be the first manifestation in up to half of the patients, the majority during exercise or stress-induced, and it accounts for 1% of deaths in athletes [39, 40]. The prevalence in the general population is 0.1–0.3%. The patients may present with symptoms of palpitations and/or syncope, but 65% of adolescents and 40% of individuals >30 years with a typical ECG are asymptomatic. The ECG pattern includes delta wave, short P-R interval and prolonged QRS duration (Fig. 30.4). Structural cardiac diseases such as HCM and Ebstein anomaly can be associated with pre-excitation, and patients should undergo echocardiography to confirm a structurally normal heart [38, 39]. An ECG monitor and exercise testing may be helpful with risk stratification, as the presence of intermittent pre-excitation is considered a low-risk feature. The electrophysiological study is mandatory for symptomatic individuals and advisable in asymptomatic competitive athletes to evaluate the risk of sudden death. Catheter ablation is the treatment of choice for symptomatic athletes, athletes with documented arrhythmias or individuals with high-risk pathways [41]. The procedure is curative, with a high success rate, and permits return to competitive sports within 3 months.

Channelopathies

Inherited ion channel diseases are associated with life-threatening arrhythmias that can lead to SCA/SCD in a structurally normal heart, termed sudden arrhythmic death syndrome (SADS). Contemporary publications from the United Kingdom, United States of America and Australia have reported SADS as the most frequent cause of SCD in young and athletic individuals [7].

Long QT Syndrome

Individuals with long QT syndrome (LQTS) present loss- or gain-of-function mutations in genes encoding ion channels that cause cardiac repolarisation abnormalities and can lead to polymorphic VT. The estimated prevalence in the general population is 1:2500 [8]. Most of the clinically and genetically identified cases (up to 75% and 95%, respectively) are related to mutations in three genes, KCNQ1, KCNH2 (potassium ion channel) and SCN5A (sodium ion channel), determined as genotypes LQT1, LQT2 and LQT3. Adrenaline surges, such as during intense exercise, can trigger arrhythmias in LQT1 and LQT2, whereas in LQT3 SCD occurs more frequently at rest or during sleep. Swimming and diving are reported as specific triggers for SCA in LQT1 [42], while loud noises can trigger arrhythmias in LQT2 patients. Symptoms include palpitations, seizures and syncope. The diagnosis is based on a score with clinical and ECG evaluation. When evaluating the QT interval, the measurement should use the "Teach the tangent" method and be corrected for the respective heart rate (QTc), usually calculated by Bazett's formula (Fig. 30.5). Normal QTc values are <440 ms for males and <460 ms for females in the general population, in the absence of use of QT-prolonging drugs or electrolytes imbalance. Athletes tend to exhibit longer QT intervals, and a QTc value is considered abnormal when $\geq$ 470 ms for male and $\geq$480 ms for female athletes [43]. Therapy with beta-blockers is effective in LQT1 and LQT2 and is recommended as first-line treatment. Athletes with suspected/diagnosed LQTS should be advised to avoid QT-prolonging drugs, hyperthermia, dehydration and conditions predisposing to electrolytes imbalance. Competitive sports participation can be considered for asymptomatic athletes in places with an emergency plan and AED availability, with the exception of swimming in LQT1 [44].

Brugada Syndrome

Brugada syndrome (BrS) is a sodium ion channelopathy that accounts for a large proportion of SADS deaths. Its prevalence in the general population is estimated at 1:2000. The presumed

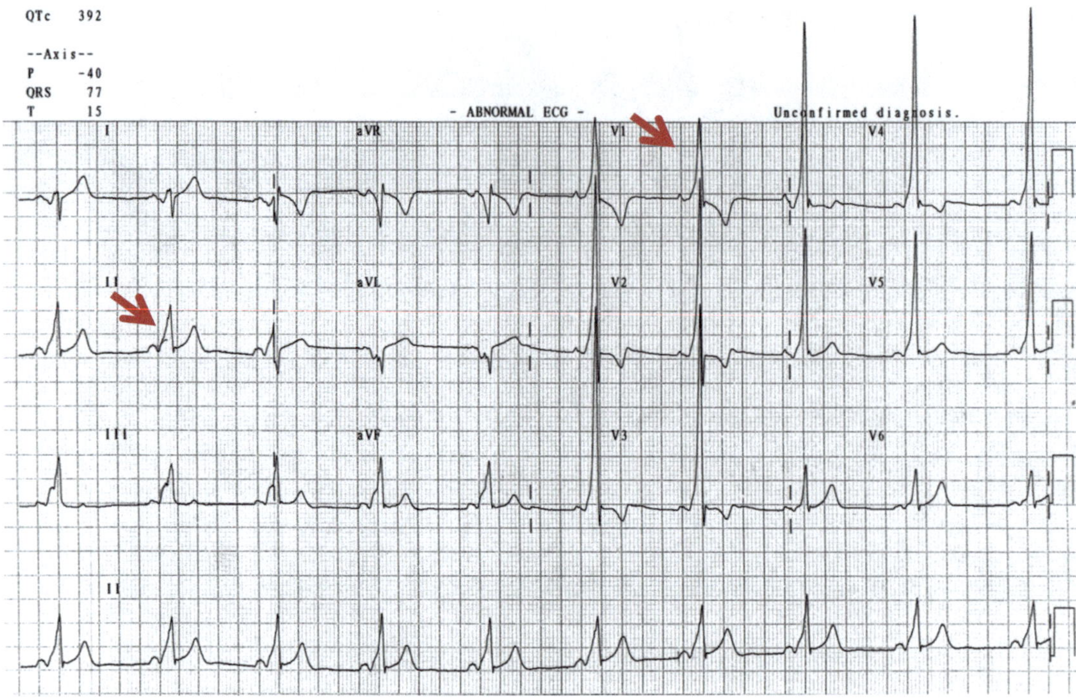

Type A – left sided accessory pathway – Delta wave and RBBB

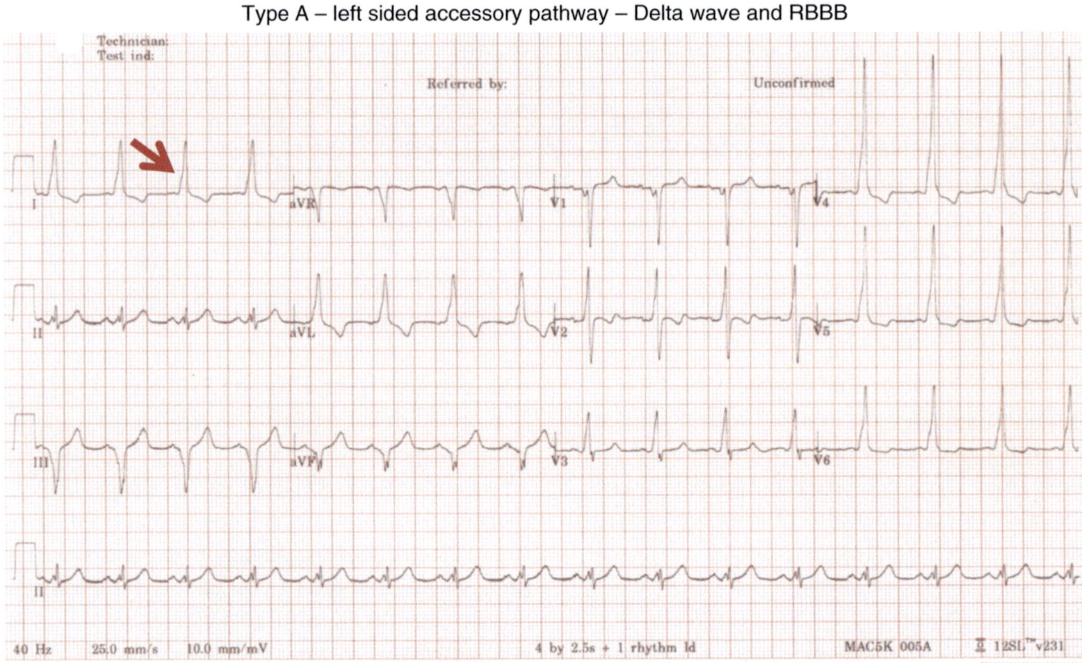

Type B – Right sided accessory pathway – Delta wave LBBB morphology

Fig. 30.4 WPW-ECG patterns. Type A—left-sided accessory pathway—delta wave and RBBB. Type B—right-sided accessory pathway—delta wave LBBB morphology

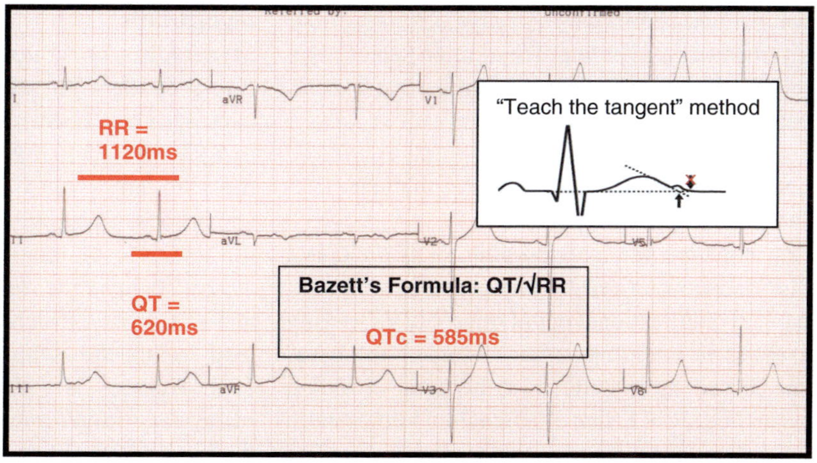

Fig. 30.5 LQTS-ECG and QT measurement

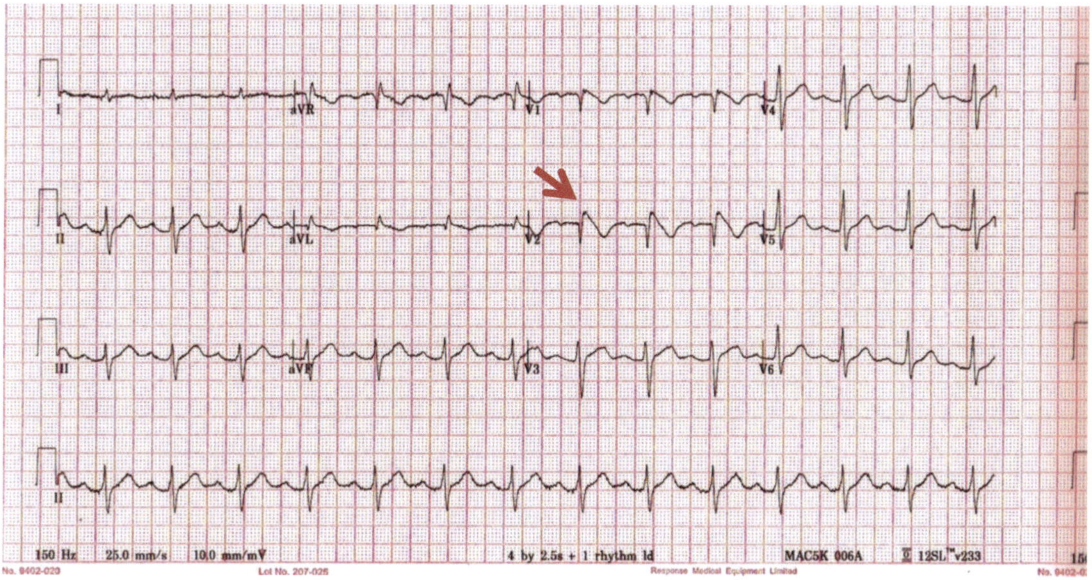

Fig. 30.6 Brugada syndrome—ECG type 1 pattern

mode of transmission is autosomal dominant, and the main identified gene linked to BrS is SCN5A, accounting for only 18–30% of cases. Although SCD typically occurs during rest, in athletes with BrS, the elevation of body temperature caused by high-intensity effort can trigger arrhythmias during exercise, and the increased vagal activity secondary to athletic conditioning may predispose to SCD at rest or the recovery phase of exercise. The typical ECG (type 1) shows a specific repolarisation pattern, characterised by a coved ST-segment elevation ≥2 mm followed by a negative T wave in right precordial leads (Fig. 30.6). The diagnostic pattern is typically dynamic and often concealed [45]. Athletes with BrS may be considered to participate in competitive sports with appropriate precautionary measures, avoiding dehydration, electrolyte imbalance, hyperthermia and drugs that exacerbate the BrS [44].

Catecholaminergic Polymorphic Ventricular Tachycardia

Catecholaminergic polymorphic VT (CPVT) is a disease characterised by malignant arrhythmias, typically bidirectional or polymorphic VT, during exercise or emotional stress. Most of the cases are caused by mutations in the gene encoding ryanodine (RyR2) that alter calcium homeostasis in cardiac myocytes triggering arrhythmias. The prevalence is estimated around 1:10,000. Usually, the symptom is stress-induced syncope starting in childhood, but SCD can be the first manifestation. A family history of syncope, seizures and SCD is present in 30% of patients. The resting ECG is normal. Exercise stress testing can induce premature ventricular complexes at the beginning that increase in frequency and complexity at progressive workloads. Beta-blocker therapy reduces VT occurrence, but 30% of patients still present with cardiac events [46, 47]. Competitive sports are not recommended to athletes with previously symptomatic CPVT or asymptomatic CPVT with documented exercise-induced arrhythmias [44].

30.3.2.2 Acquired

Atherosclerotic Coronary Artery Disease (CAD)

The major cause of SCD in older athletes (>35 years) is CAD, accounting up to 80% of cases [48]. Acute ischaemic events can initiate VT or VF. Even in athletes cardiovascular risk factors must be monitored, including periodic control of blood pressure, cholesterol and glucose levels, aiming at the prevention of atherosclerosis. Clinicians should maintain a high index of suspicion as athletes may present with atypical or minimal symptoms of ischaemia due to conditioning and the presence of collateral circulation and, in some cases, subconsciously underreport their symptoms.

Myocarditis

Myocarditis is an inflammatory cardiomyopathy, secondary to infective and non-infective causes. It has been reported to account for up to 13% of SCD in young athletes [10, 49]. The most common cause is a viral infection and sometimes can be subclinical [49]. Despite this, the presence of inflammatory infiltrate associated with myocyte degeneration and non-ischaemic necrosis, which are its characteristics can lead to life-threatening arrhythmias and SCA [50]. Athletes are more susceptible to upper respiratory infections, and it is described that the viral replication rate, myocardial inflammation and necrosis may be increased by exercise during the early phase of myocarditis [51, 52]. The inflammation usually completely resolves within 6 months but, occasionally, can progress to a chronic phase, with permanent myocardial dysfunction and arrhythmogenic scar. In order to prevent SCD, the athlete should return to exercise training after complete resolution of the disease, confirmed by a comprehensive medical re-evaluation [23].

Commotio Cordis

From the Latin, "agitation of the heart", it accounts for 2–3% of SCDs in young athletes. It refers to blunt, non-penetrating blow to the chest wall that causes VF and SCD and is different from cardiac contusion because there is no myocardial injury [53]. Animal models have demonstrated that the trauma must occur perpendicular to the chest, over the cardiac silhouette and during a specific 1% of the cardiac cycle, just before the T-wave peak [54]. Sports implicated include those using hard spherical objects such as hockey, lacrosse and baseball, as well as sports involving body collision and martial arts. The most important thing is to recognise *commotio cordis* and initiate prompt defibrillation. Previously, survival rates among *commotio cordis* victims were low, probably due to the lack of identification and late defibrillation. Fortunately, this has changed, and contemporary reports quote a survival rate in excess of 50% [55].

Box 30.1: Causes of Sudden Cardiac Death

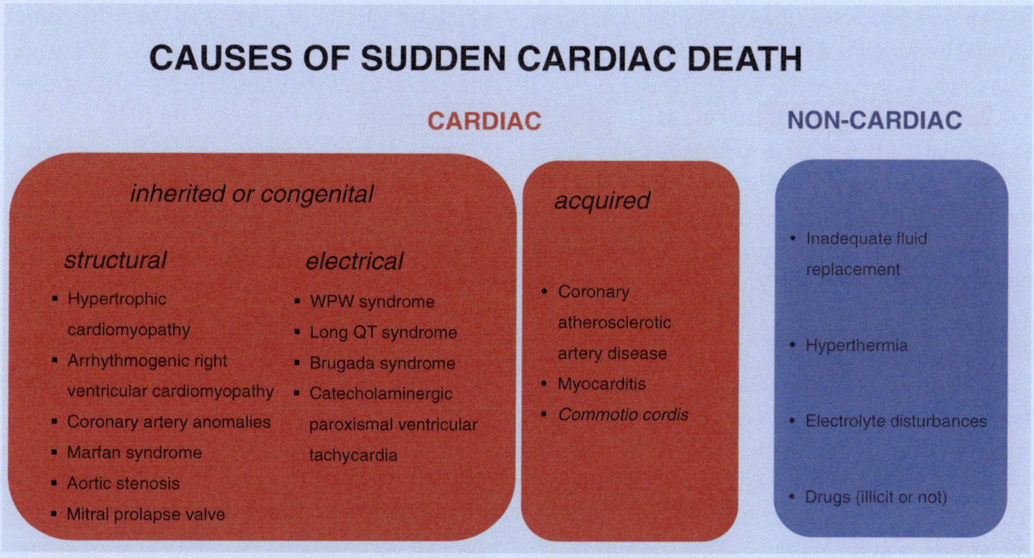

30.4 Prevention

30.4.1 Pre-participation Cardiovascular Evaluation (PPE)

The aim of PPE is to detect athletes with quiescent cardiac disease at potential risk of SCA and SCD. The medical evaluation includes a detailed history including symptoms and personal and family history and physical examination. In Italy, where PPE has been mandatory for competitive athletes since 1982, a 12-lead ECG is also included. The 26-year Veneto experience reported in a study showed a sharp decline of the incidence rate of SCD in young athletes after the introduction of systematic screening [10]. Among the screened athletes, the annual rate of death dropped from 3.6 to 0.43 per 100,000 person-years (86%), whereas it remained almost the same in the unscreened nonathletic population during the same period. A considerable proportion of the causes of SCD in athletes can be identified by the ECG, while history and physical examination have a very poor yield [56]. Despite the fact that inclusion of ECG in PPE increases more than fourfold the sensitivity of detecting cardiac disease, its inclusion remains controversial [11, 57, 58]. The European Society of Cardiology (ESC), the International Olympic Committee (IOC) and the *Fédération Internationale de Football Association* (FIFA) recommend PPE with ECG for all athletes [59, 60]. However, the American Heart Association supports just clinical questionnaire and physical examination as a routine evaluation, due to concerns relating predominantly to high false-positive rates, lack of expertise and associated costs [61]. Indeed, ECG interpretation can be challenging because athletes may exhibit ECG patterns caused by physiological adaptation to exercise that can overlap with the ECG phenotypes present in cardiac disease. Appropriate evaluation of the ECG by physicians trained in the field of sports cardiology improves the results [43, 62, 63].

30.4.2 Emergency Care

A well-established emergency response plan is extremely important in the sports arena. Time response is crucial to positive results. In the presence of SCA, the ideal target is to start cardiopulmonary resuscitation (CPR) in less than 1 min and defibrillation by 3–5 min. For each 1 min of delay, the chance of survival decreases by 10%

[64]. Unfortunately, the average survival rate of out-of-hospital SCA (OHCA), outside the context of a sports arena, is less than 10%, and it has not improved in 30 years, despite the medical advance.

30.4.2.1 Predictors of Survival

The survival rate after SCA to hospital admission is 23.8% but to hospital discharge is 7.6% [13]. Four clinical criteria have been identified as important predictors of survival from OHCA: (1) SCA witnessed by a bystander or emergency services, (2) provision of early CPR, (3) presence of shockable cardiac rhythm (VT or VF) and (4) return to spontaneous circulation in the local setting [13]. Based on this the "Chain of survival" was established which includes immediate recognition of SCA, early initiation of CPR, rapid defibrillation, effective advanced cardiac life support (ACLS) and good integration with post-SCA care [65].

Recognition

Any athlete who collapses and is unresponsive should be considered as SCA. Sometimes they can exhibit seizure-like activity and agonal breathing that causes confusion and delays the diagnosis of SCA. Assessment of the presence of a pulse can also cause delay. Thus, any unheralded syncope should be assumed as SCA, call for help and activate the emergency system.

Early CPR

Chest compressions should be initiated immediately. The last Basic Life Support (BLS) Guidelines changed the previous sequence "A-B-C" to "C-A-B" recommending chest compression before breath rescue (hands only) [66]. The focus is on the high quality of compressions to guarantee coronary and brain perfusion. The compressions should have an adequate rate (100/min) and depth (2 in or 5 cm), allowing full chest recoil in between, and must continue until the victim becomes responsive.

Rapid Defibrillation

This is a powerful predictor of success of resuscitation. An automated external defibrillator (AED) is the best strategy. High survival rate (71%) has been demonstrated in school-based AED programmes in the United States [67]. AED is able to identify the heart rhythm and to deliver a shock when indicated. The time of pause compressions pre shock should be minimum, and the compressions should resume immediately after shock. The cardiac rhythm should be checked and the procedure repeated every 2 min [66].

Once a trained rescuer is present, breath rescue should be delivered (by mouth to mouth or bag mask), with the ratio of 30 compressions to 2 ventilations (breath over 1 s, 8–10/min) [66].

30.4.2.2 Emergency Planning and Practice

The key to a good outcome is planning and practice.

Every venue of training and competition must have a written medical action plan (MAP), available to all staff, referees and visiting team. This is essential to guarantee the efficiency of the emergency responses. The MAP should name a medical director, who is responsible to coordinate and assign roles. First responders should be clearly defined and trained. Basic life support training should be done for all staff (including coaches, physiotherapists, referees, officials and administrators) and, ideally, ACLS certification for at least one physician. Personnel training and practice is the most important part of a successful plan. For rapid defibrillation, the access to AED should be within 3 min from anywhere in the arena. The number of AEDs may be calculated based on proposed algorithms (average velocity to cross a distance in the place, number of people) and have a mapping distribution [68, 69]. Emergency medication, oxygen and transport equipment must be available. It is recommended that 1–2 physicians are present per 50,000 spectators (not including the team physicians) and 1 nurse and 2 emergency responders per 10,000 spectators.

The collaboration with the local emergency services defining the place of transportation, the best way to go, time to arrive, number and location of ambulances and alertness of the nearest hospital should be planned in detail, aiming for a coordinated and integrated response. The medical director must ensure the documentation of all emergency care provided [2, 70].

Regular practice for the team and periodic review of the plan are parts of a good emergency response.

Box 30.2: SCD- Prevention Keys
- PRE-PARTICIPATION CARDIAC EVALUATION
- Investigation of individuals with cardiac symptoms
- FAMILY SCREENING AFTER SCD at a specialist centre
- ADEQUATE TREATMENT and recommendations relating to sport participation
- EMERGENCY response PLAN to facilitate EARLY CPR and defibrillation

30.4.2.3 Special Events and Venues

Some events such as marathons and Olympic Games need special planning.

Running events in open areas should have medical coverage along the way; 1–5 first-aid personnel per 1000 runners is recommended and at least 1 ACLS medical provider per 2500 and 1 BLS and 1 ACLS ambulance per 500 runners, being most of them on the latter half of the course and near the finish line. One AED should be available less than 1 mile away from any participant [71].

The challenge in Olympics is to coordinate the multiple events and teamwork, providing good communication and plan to multisport venues. During the competition in the venue area, the host medical staff is responsible for emergency care, whereas in the training area, visiting medical staff should assume their athlete's care [71].

30.4.3 Family Screening After SCD

Evaluation of the families is essential after a SCD to prevent other cases of SCD. It is reported that an initial clinical evaluation with rest ECG and echocardiogram can identify an inherited cardiac disease in 22% of families [72]. A more comprehensive evaluation is recommended for all first-degree relatives of victims with a normal post-mortem (SADS), since over half of the evaluated families have been identified with a channelopathy or cardiomyopathy. The investigation may include exercise testing, 24 h holter, CMR, drug provocation testing or other tests, depending on the suspicion [72, 73].

30.5 Conclusion

The occurrence of SCD in sports is always a tragic event, with a high impact on the wider society. Exercise is health, and people should be stimulated to be physically active. However, some predisposal individuals can present life-threatening arrhythmias triggered by sports. Pre-participation cardiovascular evaluation is effective to identify a great part of these individuals and is recommended to prevent SCD in all athletes. The assessment of athletes including clinical and family history, physical examination and 12-lead rest ECG done with expertise is very useful. Cardiomyopathies such as HCM and ARVC frequently present ECG abnormalities and can be identified in the screenings. Previous syncope episodes and family history of SCD at a young age associated with specific ECG abnormalities can also raise the suspicion of channelopathies such as LQTS and BRs.

In the presence of SCA, prompt recognition and early CPR and defibrillation are keys to survival. An emergency plan with personal training and regular practice is essential to a successful outcome.

Take-Home Messages
- **SCD IN SPORTS** is a relatively rare event but more frequent than previously thought with male athletes and athletes of African/Afro-Caribbean descent competing in high-intensity start-stop sports being at increased risk.
- Most athletes (80%) are asymptomatic with no known family history and SCA is the first clinical symptom.
- Most SCA (60–80%) occur either during or shortly after exertion but a significant proportion occurs at rest, outside the sporting arena.
- Most conditions predisposing young (<35 years) athletes to SCA are either congenital or inherited. In contrast, coronary atherosclerosis predominates in the older athletes.
- **PPE WITH ECG CAN PREVENT SCD IN ATHLETES** although significant concerns remain regarding false-negative and false-positive rates as well as cost implications and lack of expertise.

- **SCA RESCUE AND GOOD OUTCOME:**
  - IMMEDIATE initiation of CHEST COMPRESSION
  - DEFIBRILLATION within 3–5min
  - EMERGENCY response PLAN with trained personnel and regular practice

References

1. Graham R, McCoy MA, Schultz AM. Strategies to improve cardiac arrest survival: a time to act [Internet]. 2015. 456p. https://www.ncbi.nlm.nih.gov/books/NBK305685/pdf/Bookshelf_NBK305685.pdf.
2. Panhuyzen-Goedkoop NM, Wellens HJ, Piek JJ. Early recognition of sudden cardiac arrest in athletes during sports activity. Neth Heart J. 2018;26(1):21–5. https://doi.org/10.1007/s12471-017-1061-5.
3. Drezner JA, Rogers KJ. Sudden cardiac arrest in intercollegiate athletes: detailed analysis and outcomes of resuscitation in nine cases. Heart Rhythm. 2006;3(7):755–9.
4. Papadakis M, Sharma S, Cox S, et al. The magnitude of sudden cardiac death in the young: a death certificate-based review in England and Wales. Europace. 2009;11(10):1353–8.
5. Kokkinos P. Physical activity, health benefits, and mortality risk. ISRN Cardiol. 2012;2012:1–14.
6. Paffenbarger RS, Blair SN, Lee I-M. A history of physical activity, cardiovascular health and longevity: the scientific contributions of Jeremy N Morris, DSc, DPH, FRCP. Int J Epidemiol. 2001;30(5):1184–92. https://doi.org/10.1093/ije/30.5.1184.
7. Finocchiaro G, Papadakis M, Robertus JL, et al. Etiology of sudden death in sports insights from a United Kingdom Regional Registry. J Am Coll Cardiol. 2016;67(18):2108–15.
8. Maron BJ, Doerer JJ, Haas TS, et al. Sudden deaths in young competitive athletes analysis of 1866 deaths in the United States, 1980–2006. Circulation. 2009;119(8):1085–92.
9. Corrado D, Basso C, Rizzoli G, et al. Does sports activity enhance the risk of sudden death in adolescents and young adults? J Am Coll Cardiol. 2003;42(11):1959–63. https://doi.org/10.1016/j.jacc.2003.03.002.
10. Corrado D, Basso C, Pavei A, et al. Trends in sudden cardiovascular death in young competitive athletes. JAMA. 2006;296(13):1593–601.
11. Pelliccia A, Maron B. Preparticipation cardiovascular evaluation of the competitive athlete: perspectives from the 30-year Italian experience. Am J Cardiol. 1995;75(12):827–9.
12. Harmon KG, Asif IM, Maleszewski JJ, et al. Incidence and etiology of sudden cardiac arrest and death in high school athletes in the United States. Mayo Clin Proc. 2016;91(11):1493–502. https://doi.org/10.1016/j.mayocp.2016.07.021.
13. Sasson C, Rogers MAM, Dahl J, et al. Predictors of survival from out-of-hospital cardiac arrest: a systematic review and meta-analysis. Circ Cardiovasc Qual Outcomes. 2010;3(1):63–81. https://doi.org/10.1161/CIRCOUTCOMES.109.889576.
14. Asif IM, Harmon KG. Incidence and etiology of sudden cardiac death: new updates for athletic departments. Sport Health. 2017 May;9(3):268–79. https://doi.org/10.1177/1941738117694153.
15. Harmon KG, Asif IM, Maleszewski JJ, et al. Incidence, cause, and comparative frequency of sudden cardiac death in National Collegiate Athletic Association athletes—clinical perspective. Circulation. 2015;132(1):10–9. https://doi.org/10.1161/CIRCULATIONAHA.115.015431.
16. Kim JH, Malhotra R, Chiampas G, et al. Cardiac arrest during long-distance running races. N Engl J Med. 2012;366(2):130–40.
17. Dhar R, Stout CW, Link MS, et al. Cardiovascular toxicities of performance-enhancing substances in sports. Mayo Clin Proc. 2005;80(10):1307–15.
18. Abbate V, Kicman AT, Evans-Brown M, et al. Anabolic steroids detected in bodybuilding dietary supplements—a significant risk to public health. Drug Test Anal. 2015;7(7):609–18.
19. Cho SH, Park HJ, Lee JH, Kim HJ, et al. Monitoring of 35 illegally added steroid compounds in foods and dietary supplements. Food Addit Contam Part A Chem Anal Control Expo Risk Assess. 2014;31(9):1470–5.
20. Calore C, Zorzi A, Corrado D. Clinical meaning of isolated increase of QRS voltages in hypertrophic cardiomyopathy versus athlete's heart. J Electrocardiol. 2015;48(3):373–9. https://doi.org/10.1016/j.jelectrocard.2014.12.016.
21. Puntmann VO, Gebker R, Duckett S, et al. Left ventricular chamber dimensions and wall thickness by cardiovascular magnetic resonance: comparison with transthoracic echocardiography. Eur Heart J Cardiovasc Imaging. 2013;14(3):240–6.
22. Sheikh N, Papadakis M, Schnell F, et al. Clinical profile of athletes with hypertrophic cardiomyopathy. Circ Cardiovasc Imaging. 2015;8(7):1–11.
23. Maron BJ, Udelson JE, Bonow RO, et al. Eligibility and disqualification recommendations for competitive athletes with cardiovascular abnormalities: task force 3: hypertrophic cardiomyopathy, arrhythmogenic right ventricular cardiomyopathy and other cardiomyopathies, and myocarditis: a Scientific. J Am Coll Cardiol. 2015;66(21):2362–71.
24. McNally E, MacLeod H, Dellefave-Castillo L. Arrhythmogenic right ventricular cardiomyopathy. In: Adam MP, Ardinger HH, Pagon RA et al., editors. GeneReviews® [Internet]. Seattle: University of Washington; 2015. [Updated 2017 May 25].
25. Basso C, Corrado D, Marcus FI, et al. Arrhythmogenic right ventricular cardiomyopathy. Lancet. 2009; 373(9671):1289–300. https://doi.org/10.1016/S0140-6736(09)60256-7.
26. Mont L, Pelliccia A, Sharma S, et al. Pre-participation cardiovascular evaluation for athletic participants to

prevent sudden death: position paper from the EHRA and the EACPR, branches of the ESC. Endorsed by APHRS, HRS, and SOLAECE. Europace. 2017;19(1):139–63.
27. D'Ascenzi F, Pisicchio C, Caselli S, et al. RV remodeling in olympic athletes. JACC Cardiovasc Imaging. 2017;10(4):385–93.
28. Oxborough D, Sharma S, Shave R, et al. The right ventricle of the endurance athlete: the relationship between morphology and deformation. J Am Soc Echocardiogr. 2012;25(3):263–71. https://doi.org/10.1016/j.echo.2011.11.017.
29. D'Silva A, Sharma S. Management of young competitive athletes with cardiovascular conditions. Heart. 2017;103(6):463–73. https://doi.org/10.1136/heartjnl-2016-309435.
30. Chandra N, Bastiaenen R, Papadakis M, et al. Sudden cardiac death in young athletes. J Am Coll Cardiol. 2013;61(10):1027–40.
31. Van Hare GF, Ackerman MJ, Evangelista JK, et al. Eligibility and disqualification recommendations for competitive athletes with cardiovascular abnormalities: task force 4: congenital heart disease. Circulation. 2015;132(22):e281–91. https://doi.org/10.1161/CIR.0000000000000240.
32. Pelliccia A, Di Paolo FM, De Blasiis E, et al. Prevalence and clinical significance of aortic root dilation in highly trained competitive athletes. Circulation. 2010;122:698–706.
33. Loeys BL, Dietz HC, Braverman AC, et al. The revised Ghent nosology for the Marfan syndrome. J Med Genet. 2010;47(7):476–85.
34. Braverman AC, Harris K, Kovacs R, et al. Eligibility and disqualification recommendations for competitive athletes with cardiovascular abnormalities: task force 7: aortic diseases, including Marfan syndrome. J Am Coll Cardiol. 2015;6(21):2398–245.
35. Siu SC, Silversides CK. Bicuspid aortic valve disease. J Am Coll Cardiol. 2010;55(25):2789–800. https://doi.org/10.1016/j.jacc.2009.12.068.
36. Bonow RO, Nishimura RA, Thompson PD, et al. Eligibility and disqualification recommendations for competitive athletes with cardiovascular abnormalities: task force 5: valvular heart disease. J Am Coll Cardiol. 2015;66(21):2385–92.
37. Jeresaty RM. Mitral valve prolapse: definition and implications in athletes. J Am Coll Cardiol. 1986;7(1):231–6. https://doi.org/10.1016/S0735-1097(86)80286-8.
38. Cohen MI, Triedman JK, Cannon BC, et al. PACES/HRS expert consensus statement on the management of the asymptomatic young patient with a Wolff-Parkinson-White (WPW, ventricular preexcitation) electrocardiographic pattern: developed in partnership between the pediatric and congenital electrophysi. Heart Rhythm. 2012;9(6):1006–24. https://doi.org/10.1016/j.hrthm.2012.03.050.
39. Heidbuchel H, Panhuyzen-Goedkoop N, Corrado D, et al. Recommendations for participation in leisure-time physical activity and competitive sports in patients with arrhythmias and potentially arrhythmogenic conditions part I: supraventricular arrhythmias and pacemakers of the study group on sports cardiology. Eur J Cardiovasc Prev Rehabil. 2006;13(4):475–84.
40. Timmermans C, Smeets JLRM, Rodriguez LM, et al. Aborted sudden death in the Wolff-Parkinson-White syndrome. Am J Cardiol. 1995;76(7):492–4.
41. Link MS, Ackerman MJ, Kovacs RJ, et al. Eligibility and disqualification recommendations for competitive athletes with cardiovascular abnormalities: task force 9: arrhythmias and conduction defects. J Am Coll Cardiol. 2015;66(21):2412–23.
42. Ackerman MJ, Khositseth A, Tester DJ, et al. Congenital long QT syndrome in electrical diseases of the heart; genetics mechanisms, treatment, prevention. New York: Springer; 2008. p. 462–82.
43. Sharma S, Drezner JA, Baggish A, et al. International recommendations for electrocardiographic interpretation in athletes. Eur Heart J. 2017;69(8):1057–75. https://doi.org/10.1016/j.jacc.2017.01.015.
44. Ackerman MJ, Zipes DP, Kovacs RJ, et al. Eligibility and disqualification recommendations for competitive athletes with cardiovascular abnormalities: task force 10: the cardiac channelopathies: a scientific statement from the American Heart Association and American College of Cardiology. J Am Coll Cardiol. 2015;66(21):2124–8.
45. Antzelevitch C, Brugada P, Borggrefe M, et al. Brugada syndrome: report of the second consensus conference. Circulation. 2005;111(5):659–70.
46. Liu N, Ruan Y, Priori SG. Catecholaminergic polymorphic ventricular tachycardia. Prog Cardiovasc Dis. 2008;51(1):23–30.
47. Priori SG, Napolitano C, Tiso N, et al. Mutations in the cardiac ryanodine receptor gene (hRyR2) underlie catecholaminergic polymorphic ventricular tachycardia. Circulation. 2001;103(2):196–200.
48. Marijon E, Uy-Evanado A, Reinier K, et al. Sudden cardiac arrest during sports activity in middle age. Circulation. 2015;131(16):1384–91.
49. Basso C, Carturan E, Corrado D, et al. Myocarditis and dilated cardiomyopathy in athletes: diagnosis, management, and recommendations for sport activity. Cardiol Clin. 2007;25(3):423–9.
50. Aretz HT, Billingham ME, Edwards WD, et al. Myocarditis: a histopathologic definition and classification. Am J Cardiovasc Pathol. 1987;1:3–14.
51. Gatmaitan BG, Chason JL, Lerner AM. Augmentation of the virulence of murine coxsackievirus B3 myocardiopathy by exercise. J Exp Med. 1970;131:1121–36.
52. Friman G, Wesslen L. Special feature for the olympics. Effects of exercise on the immune system: infections and exercise in high performance athletes. Immunol Cell Biol. 2000;78:510–22.
53. Maron B, Estes N. Commotio cordis. N Engl J Med. 2010;362(10):917–27. https://doi.org/10.1056/NEJMra0910111.
54. Link MS, Wang PJ, Pandian NG, et al. An experimental model of sudden death due to low-energy chest-wall impact (commotio cordis). N Engl J Med.

1998;338(25):1805–11. https://doi.org/10.1056/NEJM199806183382504.
55. Link MS, Estes NAM, Maron BJ. Eligibility and disqualification recommendations for competitive athletes with cardiovascular abnormalities: task force 13: commotio cordis: a scientific statement from the American Heart Association and American College of Cardiology. J Am Coll Cardiol. 2015;66(21):2439–43.
56. Harmon KG, Zigman M, Drezner JA. The effectiveness of screening history, physical exam, and ECG to detect potentially lethal cardiac disorders in athletes: a systematic review/meta-analysis. J Electrocardiol. 2015;48(3):329–38. https://doi.org/10.1016/j.jelectrocard.2015.02.001.
57. Corrado D, Basso C, Schiavon M, et al. Screening for hypertrophic cardiomyopathy in young athletes. N Engl J Med. 1998;339(6):364–9. https://doi.org/10.1056/NEJM199808063390602.
58. Pelliccia A, Caselli S, Sharma S, et al. European Association of Preventive Cardiology (EAPC) and European Association of Cardiovascular Imaging (EACVI) joint position statement: recommendations for the indication and interpretation of cardiovascular imaging in the evaluation of the athlete's heart. Eur Heart J. 2018;39(21):1949–69. https://doi.org/10.1093/eurheartj/ehx532.
59. Pelliccia A, Fagard R, Bjornstad H, et al. Recommendations for competitive sports participation in athletes with cardiovascular disease: a consensus document from the Study Group of Sports Cardiology of the Working Group of Cardiac Rehabilitation and Exercise Physiology and the Working Group of Myocardial and Pericardial Diseases of the European Society of Cardiology. Eur Heart J. 2005;26(14):1422–45. https://doi.org/10.1093/eurheartj/ehi325.
60. International Olympic Committee Medical Commission. Sudden Cardiovascular Death in Sport—THE LAUSANNE RECOMMENDATIONS [Internet]. 2004 [cited 2018 Feb 2]. p. 10–3. Available from: https://www.olympic.org/news/sudden-cardio-vascular-death-in-sport-lausanne-recommendations-adopted.
61. Maron BJ, Friedman RA, Kligfield P, et al. Assessment of the 12-lead ECG as a screening test for detection of cardiovascular disease in healthy general populations of young people (12–25 years of age) a scientific statement from the American Heart Association and the American College of Cardiology. Circulation. 2014;130(15):1303–34.
62. Dhutia H, Malhotra A, Gabus V, et al. Cost implications of using different ECG criteria for screening young athletes in the United Kingdom. J Am Coll Cardiol. 2016;68(7):702–11.
63. Sheikh N, Papadakis M, Ghani S, et al. Comparison of electrocardiographic criteria for the detection of cardiac abnormalities in elite black and white athletes. Circulation. 2014;129(16):1637–49.
64. Marenco JP, Wang PJ, Link MS, et al. Improving survival from sudden cardiac arrest. JAMA. 2001;285(9):1193–200.
65. Field JM, Hazinski MF, Sayre MR, et al. Part 1: executive summary: 2010 American Heart Association guidelines for cardiopulmonary resuscitation and emergency cardiovascular care. Circulation. 2010;122(Suppl 3):640–57.
66. Berg RA, Hemphill R, Abella BS, et al. Part 5: adult basic life support: 2010 American Heart Association guidelines for cardiopulmonary resuscitation and emergency cardiovascular care. Circulation. 2010;122(Suppl. 3):S685–705.
67. Drezner JA, Toresdahl BG, Rao AL, et al. Outcomes from sudden cardiac arrest in US high schools: a 2-year prospective study from the national registry for AED use in sports. Br J Sports Med. 2013;47(18):1179–83.
68. Crocco TJ, Sayre MR, Liu T, et al. Mathematical determination of external defibrillators needed at mass gatherings. Prehosp Emerg Care. 2004;8(3):292–7. https://doi.org/10.1080/312703004295.
69. Motyka TM, Winslow JE, Newton K, et al. Method for determining automatic external defibrillator need at mass gatherings. Resuscitation. 2005;65(3):309–14.
70. Borjesson M, Serratosa L, Carre F, et al. Consensus document regarding cardiovascular safety at sports arenas. Eur Heart J. 2011;32(17):2119–24.
71. Toresdahl B, Courson R, Börjesson M, et al. Emergency cardiac care in the athletic setting: from schools to the Olympics. Br J Sports Med. 2012;46(Suppl 1):i85–9.
72. Behr ER, Dalageorgou C, Christiansen M, et al. Sudden arrhythmic death syndrome: familial evaluation identifies inheritable heart disease in the majority of families. Eur Heart J. 2008;29(13):1670–80.
73. Tan HL, Hofman N, Van Langen IM, et al. Sudden unexplained death: heritability and diagnostic yield of cardiological and genetic examination in surviving relatives. Circulation. 2005;112(2):207–13.

Concussion

31

Natalie Sherry and Michael W. Collins

31.1 Introduction

An estimated 1.6–3.8 million sport-related concussions (SRCs) occur annually in the United States [1], and there has been a rise in the number of athletes seeking treatment for this injury in recent years [2]. A concussion is defined as a transient neurometabolic crisis in the brain that is induced by a traumatic biomechanical force to the head or body. The mechanical trauma to the brain results in a distortion and stretching of neuronal structures allowing for unregulated ionic fluctuations that initiate a series of complex neurometabolic events disruptive to brain function [3, 4]. These pathophysiological changes are not detectable with conventional neuroimaging techniques (e.g., computed tomography [CT], magnetic resonance imaging [MRI]) [5] but can result in a myriad of neurological signs (e.g., loss of consciousness [LOC], posttraumatic amnesia [PTA]), symptoms (e.g., headache, blurred vision), and impairments (e.g., cognitive deficits, oculomotor abnormalities).

Several advancements have been made in the clinical evaluation, management, and treatment of SRC. In the past, sports medicine practitioners were forced to rely primarily on athletes' self-report of symptoms for diagnosing and managing SRC, but there are now empirically derived tools that can detect SRC using objective measures [6, 7]. A reliance on self-reported symptoms for the diagnosis and management of SRC is now criticized by the International Consensus Statements on Concussion in Sport [8, 9] due to the tendency for athletes to underreport their symptoms [10, 11]. The advancement of assessment tools for evaluating SRC has led to a shift in the field in which concussion experts now believe there are different subtypes or clinical profiles that occur after SRC, and each athlete must be treated in an individualized manner [12–14]. Given the heterogeneity in clinical presentations after SRC among athletes, a multimodal assessment of neurological functions is warranted. Furthermore, treatment of the injury may require a multidisciplinary approach that includes a dependence upon the expertise of multiple healthcare providers in order for the athlete to achieve a full recovery. This overview provides a framework for the clinical management of SRC based on the current trends in the assessment and treatment of the injury.

N. Sherry · M. W. Collins (✉)
Sports Medicine Concussion Program, Department of Orthopaedic Surgery, University of Pittsburgh Medical Center, Pittsburgh, PA, USA
e-mail: sherrynk@upmc.edu; collinsmw@upmc.edu

S. Rocha Piedade et al. (eds.), *The Sports Medicine Physician*,
https://doi.org/10.1007/978-3-030-10433-7_31

31.2 Clinical Management of Sport-Related Concussion

Sport organizations have started to implement standardized protocols for improving the identification and treatment of SRC. Although each injury is managed on an individual basis, some organizations have implemented guidelines for assisting sports medicine physicians, particularly team physicians, in diagnosing and managing SRC among athletes. Protocols may include guidelines for preseason (i.e., baseline) testing, sideline assessment of SRC, specialty management of SRC, and determining return to play status, as outlined in Fig. 31.1.

31.2.1 Preseason (i.e., Baseline) Testing

Prior to the beginning of the season, athletes are often required to undergo a preseason physical examination to ensure their medical readiness to play. Teams have started to utilize the preseason physical examination to incorporate concussion assessment tools, in which athletes are tested on concussion assessments when non-injured to allow for later comparison should an athlete sustain an SRC in the future. This baseline assessment model may be especially useful for evaluating the subtle cognitive deficits than can occur after SRC [15], particularly among athletes with a history of a neurodevelopmental condition (e.g., attention deficit hyperactivity disorder) [16, 17] or who exhibit above average intelligence [18]. It is recommended that all baseline testing utilizing functional assessment tools include validity indicators to prevent from attempted "sandbagging" (i.e., intentionally performing poorly) on their testing [19].

31.2.2 Sideline Assessment and Management

The goal of sideline assessment and management is to properly identify when an SRC has occurred and conduct an evaluation to determine whether a return to play is contraindicated. When there is any unusual neurological sign or symptom after a significant blow to the head or body, an athlete is prohibited from a return to sport participation within 24 h of injury [8]. Athletes suspected of sustaining an SRC must be removed from sport participation immediately and avoid activities with a risk of head injury, due to the risk of potential catastrophic outcome should an athlete sustain a second insult to the head when actively concussed [20, 21]. Recent research indicates that athletes who are not removed from play immediately after sustaining an SRC may double their recovery time [22].

Detection. Detection of SRC on-field or during sport can be difficult for the sports medicine physician given that not all SRCs result in observable signs of injury. More obvious signs of neurologic injury include the presence of LOC, PTA, incoordination/imbalance, vomiting, appearing dazed/confused, disorientation, or physical slowness after a blow to the head or body. However, many athletes who sustain an SRC will not exhibit any of these acute markers of injury. For instance, most athletes diagnosed with an SRC will have no accompanying LOC, and contrary to popular belief, the presence of LOC and other traditional markers of traumatic brain injury (TBI) is not considered to be a reliable predictor of the severity of SRC [23–25]. Other symptoms that are indicative of SRC, but cannot be readily observed and require questioning of the athlete, include complaints of headache, nausea, dizziness, tinnitus, visual disturbances, photo- and phonophobia, mental slowness, and sense of

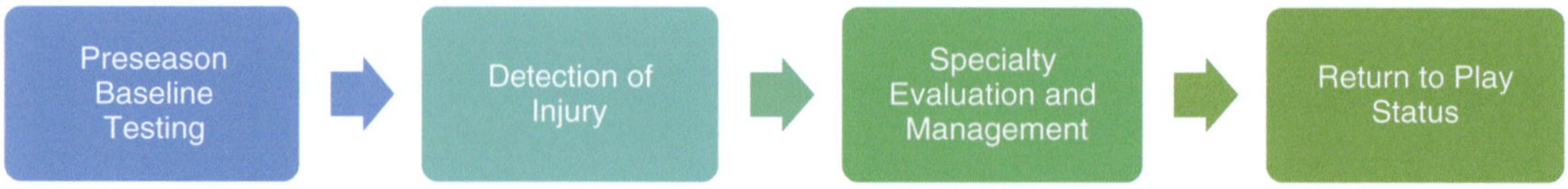

Fig. 31.1 Guidelines for the clinical management of sport-related concussion

imbalance. Detection of the injury requires vigilance of observable signs of injury as well as direct questioning of the athlete.

> **Fact Box**
> A loss of consciousness is not required for the diagnosis of concussion, and losing consciousness does not predict recovery from or the severity of the concussion.

Sideline assessment. Athletes suspected of sustaining an SRC are removed from play and further evaluated on the sideline. A standard sideline evaluation includes questioning of concussion signs and symptoms, a focused neurological examination, and mental status testing [26]. The sideline evaluation should incorporate athletes' self-report of symptoms in conjunction with objective tools to prevent athletes from minimizing their SRC symptoms in attempt to expedite their return to play [8, 27]. Questioning of signs and symptoms of SRC provides information to the sports medicine practitioner on subjective complaints of the athlete. A focused neurological examination must be conducted to rule out potentially emergent neurological sequelae (e.g., intracranial bleed, skull fracture) and evaluate neuromotor functions affected by SRC (e.g., vestibular function, oculomotor function). And lastly, mental status testing should include questions to determine if the athlete is oriented and cognitive screening for testing attentional and memory functions [28]. Unlike more severe TBIs, athletes with an SRC may be able to correctly answer traditional orientation questions (i.e., person, place, and time), and therefore, questions of recent memory (e.g., "what is the score of the game?" "what is the name of the opposing team?") may be more effective [29].

Results of all sideline assessments may be compared with baseline testing when possible to facilitate intraindividual interpretation. Any positive finding on sideline evaluation precludes a return to play based on international criteria [8]. Some governing bodies require further evaluation by a healthcare professional prior to allowing athletes to return to sport. For instance, all 50 states in the United States have legislation requiring that athletes participating in organized sports must receive clearance from a designated sports medicine practitioner prior to being permitted to return to full sport participation [30]. There is a call to action around the world to adopt such policies for management of SRC to protect the health of athletes [8].

31.2.3 Specialty Evaluation and Management of Concussion

The goal of outpatient or specialty management of SRC is to conduct a thorough assessment of the injury and develop an individualized treatment plan for rehabilitation. Some deficits of SRC may require formal treatment, and through a comprehensive, multimodal assessment, specific impairments and complicating factors related to the injury can be identified and addressed to potentially avoid the development of post-concussion syndrome (PCS). Identification of the specific impairments of the athlete [12] can assist in the development of a targeted treatment plan, rather than a one-size-fits-all approach to injury management. Emerging trends in research suggest there may be distinct clinical profiles that occur after an SRC. Proposed clinical profiles, or presentations after SRC, include posttraumatic migraine, ocular, vestibular, anxiety/mood, and cognitive fatigue [14]. Some athletes may exhibit signs of multiple clinical profiles, and each of these clinical profiles may require different types of treatment. Concussion experts advocate for a comprehensive assessment [26] to elucidate the clinical profile(s) and develop a patient-centered treatment plan after SRC [13, 14].

Comprehensive assessment. Traditional imaging for detecting acquired neurological injury (e.g., MRI, CT scan) is usually unremarkable following SRC. Structural neuroimaging is often not sensitive to the neurometabolic cascade following an uncomplicated concussion [5], and therefore, clinicians must rely on empirically derived, functional assessment tools for diagnosis and management of SRC. Standardized evaluation of SRC should include a thorough clinical interview, supported with information gathered from symptom inventories, neurocognitive testing, and vestibular/oculomotor screening [26], as displayed in Fig. 31.2.

31.2.3.1 Clinical Interview

Sports medicine physicians should aim to establish a rapport with athletes through a comprehensive clinical interview that details the nature of the injury and prior medical history. Essential components of the clinical interview include establishing the mechanism of injury (e.g., helmet-to-helmet hit), identifying immediate signs and acute markers of injury (e.g., LOC, dizziness), identifying potential medical or psychiatric risk factors for complicated recovery (e.g., major depressive disorder), detailing prior treatments and current symptoms (e.g., medications), and obtaining a psychosocial history (e.g., education level, employment) [14]. Through the clinical interview, hypotheses regarding the clinical profile can be established and tested with objective assessment tools sensitive to concussion.

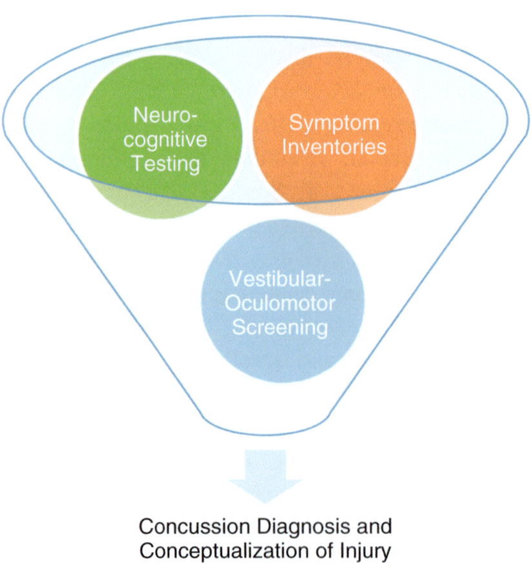

Fig. 31.2 Comprehensive evaluation of sport-related concussion

31.2.3.2 Symptom Inventories

Structured questionnaires designed to evaluate the specific symptoms and functional impairments after SRC provide an indication of the severity and nature of the injury. Athletes can experience a wide range of symptoms including physical, cognitive, mood, and sleep-related disturbances. Evaluating symptoms using a structured questionnaire, such as the Post-Concussion Symptom Scale (PCSS), provides a more comprehensive clinical profile than asking about symptoms using an open-ended interview approach [31]. Symptom questionnaires also allow for serial tracking of symptoms over time and are useful for prognosticating recovery time. Symptom severity at initial evaluation is a robust predictor of recovery time [32–34].

31.2.3.3 Neurocognitive Testing

Standardized neurocognitive testing provides an objective evaluation of brain impairment after SRC. Neurocognitive testing evaluates brain functions such as attention, reaction time, and memory that are commonly affected after SRC. Athletes who are reportedly asymptomatic may still demonstrate deficits on objective neurocognitive testing [6, 10, 35], and performance on neurocognitive testing can be compared to clinical cutoffs to prognosticate recovery time from the injury [32, 33]. Computerized neurocognitive testing may be more practical in the evaluation of SRC rather than traditional paper-and-pencil neuropsychological testing given its feasibility of use. Specifically, computerized neurocognitive testing allows for randomization of test stimuli to mitigate practice effects with serial test administration, an accurate measure of reaction time, and immediate scoring of performance to make expedited clinical decisions [36, 37]. Patterns of performance on neurocognitive testing can yield information on the type of clinical profile an athlete is demonstrating and determine the ability of an athlete to function in the school or occupational environment [14, 26]. Performance on neurocognitive testing can be compared to an athlete's baseline (i.e., preseason evaluation) for intraindividual comparison or using normative data; baseline comparison may be beneficial for nontraditional athletes or athletes with above/below average intelligence [16, 18, 38]. Performance validity indicators should additionally be utilized as part of cognitive testing to evaluate effort, which is important when there is concern of malingering or issues of secondary gain associated with the injury [26].

Fact Box
Athletes who deny symptoms may still demonstrate impairments from concussion on objective testing.

31.2.3.4 Vestibular/Oculomotor Screening

Focused neuromotor screening is an important aspect of a multimodal evaluation of SRC [26]. Over half of athletes will report dizziness or imbalance after an SRC [32, 39], which is suggestive of an underlying decompensation of the central vestibular system. The vestibular system is a multipart sensorimotor system that allows for neural control of postural stability (i.e., balance) and stabilization of vision during movement. Balance testing is useful in the acute phase of the injury, but such vestibulospinal impairments typically resolve within the first 72 h of injury [40, 41]. In contrast, deficits in vestibular and oculomotor functions (e.g., vestibular-ocular reflex [VOR], visual motion sensitivity, convergence) after SRC may persist much longer. Recent research indicates that a positive finding on vestibular-oculomotor screening [7] after SRC is predictive of a prolonged recovery time among athletes [42, 43]. Incorporating vestibular-oculomotor screening provides useful information to help delineate the athlete's clinical presentation after injury. Deficits in vestibular dysfunction can cause symptoms of motion sickness, which can become an obstacle for athletes trying to return to sport given the demand for dynamic movement in physical activity [14, 44].

Clinical profiles of concussion. Leading experts investigating concussion agree that not all concussions are the same. Athletes demonstrate an individualized constellation of different symptoms and deficits and may require different treatment approaches depending on the nature of their injury [13]. Sports practitioners advocate for an individualized, patient-centered treatment approach tailored to the athlete given the heterogeneity of clinical presentations and outcomes after SRC [8, 13]. Recent research indicates that there may be distinct clinical profiles after SRC that are associated with specific symptoms and impairments [12, 14, 45]. Some athletes may be more predisposed to a certain phenotype depending on risk factors in their medical history [46]. Proposed clinical profiles are displayed in Fig. 31.3 and include posttraumatic migraine, vestibular, ocular, anxiety/mood, and cognitive fatigue. Cervical involvement may be considered as a separate clinical profile, as some athletes' symptomology (e.g., headache) may be multifactorial and related to both head and neck injury [14]. These clinical profiles are not considered mutually exclusive, and athletes may exhibit symptomology from more than one clinical profile. Specialty management of SRC involves a comprehensive assessment to determine the specific clinical profile of the athlete and develop a targeted treatment plan to promote recovery and attempt to expedite return to play.

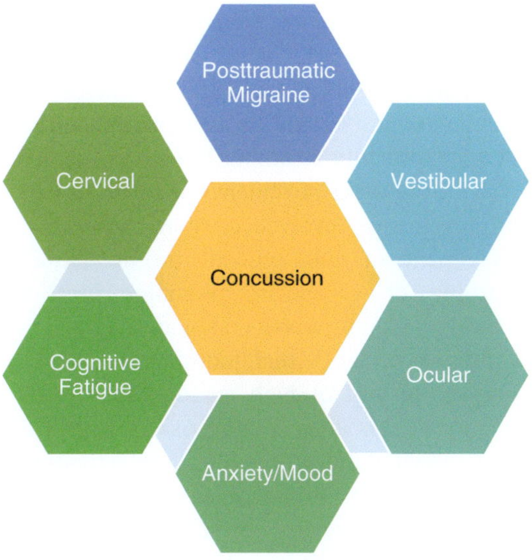

Fig. 31.3 Clinical profiles of sport-related concussion

31.2.3.5 Posttraumatic Migraine

Posttraumatic migraine is the onset of a headache with accompanying nausea and photosensitivity and/or phonosensitivity [47]. Athletes demonstrating this clinical profile report a headache of moderate-to-severe intensity, with a pulsating quality that lasts hours. Most athletes report headaches immediately after injury [39], but the persistence of migraine headaches may be a risk factor for a prolonged recovery [48, 49]. To evaluate the presence of this clinical profile, a thorough interview of headache characteristics, symptom inventories, and performance on neurocognitive testing should be considered. Athletes with posttraumatic migraine may perform more poorly on neurocognitive testing of verbal and visual memory [48]. Potential treatments for this clinical profile include behavioral management strategies (i.e., regulated sleep schedule, healthy diet, stress management, physical activity, and hydration) [50, 51], nutritional supplements [52, 53], and/or pharmacological intervention with a migraine preventative, abortive, and/or rescue medication [54, 55].

31.2.3.6 Vestibular

Vestibular dysfunction is associated with symptoms characteristic of motion sickness. Specifically, athletes may report sensations of dizziness, fogginess, unsteadiness, lightheadedness, and nausea when engaged in head and eye movements and/or when in complex/busy environments [14, 42, 56]. Athletes with this clinical profile may be asymptomatic at rest but have difficulty returning to physical activity given the dynamic movement (e.g., lateral or planar movements) involved in sport participation. Assessment of this clinical profile requires screening of vestibular/oculomotor functions including smooth pursuits, saccades, vestibular-ocular reflex, and visual motion sensitivity. A preinjury history of high susceptibility toward motion sickness is a potential risk factor for the development of this profile [46]. Active treatment of this clinical profile involves the development of a structured physical therapy plan tailored to the individual athlete in order to rehabilitate the vestibular system [43, 57, 58], and in protracted injuries pharmacological intervention may be warranted [54, 55].

31.2.3.7 Ocular

Athletes may experience posttraumatic vision changes after sustaining an SRC. Potential visual disturbances include blurred or double vision, trouble focusing eyes, asthenopia or fatigue with visually demanding activities, and/or headache/pressure behind the eyes [14]. The most common oculomotor problems after SRC are related to decompensation of convergence and accommodative functions [59, 60]. Clinical markers of this profile include a lowered performance on computerized neurocognitive testing [61, 62] and abnormalities on oculomotor screening of near point of convergence, accommodation, smooth pursuits, and/or saccades [7]. There is limited research on the potential risk factors associated with this clinical profile, but perhaps a history of developmental oculomotor abnormalities (e.g., strabismus) may render some athletes more vulnerable to posttraumatic vision disturbances after SRC [14]. The presence of oculomotor abnormalities after SRC is associated with a prolonged recovery time [42, 63]. Potential treatments may include vision therapy, vestibular-ocular therapy, and/or specialty eyeglasses [64, 65].

31.2.3.8 Anxiety/Mood

Athletes may experience a myriad of mood and emotional changes after sustaining an SRC. In addition to the psychological factors associated with the injury, there are several physiological changes in limbic-cortical circuitry secondary to the metabolic disturbance from SRC [3, 39, 66, 67]. Emotional changes may include feelings of anxiety, panic attacks, sadness, ruminative thinking, irritability, agitation, and mood lability. Some athletes may also have accompanying sleep dysregulation (e.g., trouble falling asleep) and engage in avoidant coping to prevent from emotionally triggering stimuli [68]. To determine if anxiety or mood factors are present after SRC, a thorough clinical interview utilizing a functional behavioral assessment approach, symptom inventories, and comparison of subjective complaints to objective test results is warranted to elucidate if there may be a psychological basis to reported symptoms [68]. A preinjury history of a mental health condition is a risk factor for the development of this clinical profile and one of the strongest predictors of a prolonged recovery from SRC [69, 70]. To treat the anxiety/mood clinical profile in the acute phase of injury, psychoeducation [71, 72] and a gradual return to functional activities [73, 74] are recommended. Protracted mental health complications after SRC may require psychotherapy [75–77] and/or psychotropic medications [78, 79].

31.2.3.9 Cognitive Fatigue

The cognitive fatigue clinical profile is characterized by complaints of difficulty with thinking skills (e.g., attention, processing speed, memory) and overwhelming fatigue. Functional complaints associated with this clinical profile may include feeling mentally slow, difficulty multitasking or retaining information, or exhaustion after engaging in cognitively demanding activity. Assessment of this clinical profile hinges on the athletes' pattern of symptom report and performance on objective neurocognitive testing [14]. A potential risk factor for the development of this clinical profile is a history of preinjury sleep difficulties [80]. Limited research has been conducted for the treatment of this clinical profile, but this is some preliminary evidence for the use of cognitive therapy [72] or pharmacological intervention [81].

Return to play criteria. To protect the safety of athletes, there are established international guidelines standardizing the protocol for determining readiness of an athlete to return to sport after sustaining an SRC [8]. When an athlete is suspected or diagnosed with an SRC, they are never to returned to play on the same day as the injury [8]. The goal of these established guidelines is to prevent an athlete from returning to play prematurely and suffering a second insult to the head when actively concussed. There are three major conditions that must be met prior to considering clearance of an athlete back to contact sports: (1) athletes must be symptom-free from concussion at rest, (2) athletes must be

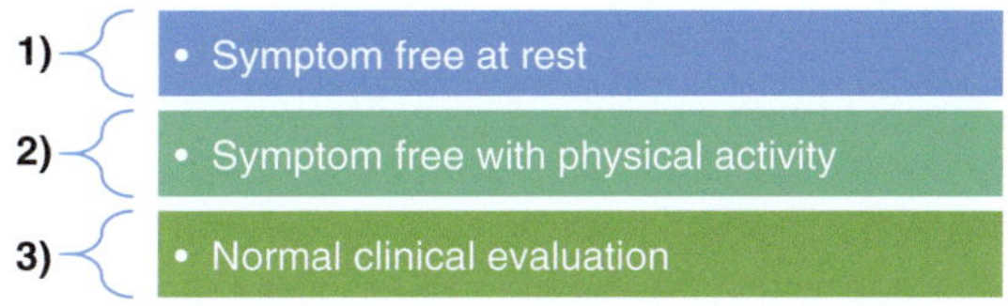

Fig. 31.4 Return to play criteria based on international guidelines

symptom-free from concussion with physical activity, and (3) athletes must demonstrate a normal clinical evaluation. Figure 31.4 provides an outline of criteria. Evaluation of tolerance of physical activity should incorporate a combination of both aerobic activity and dynamic movement. The current international guidelines for exertion protocols after SRC do not specify the necessity of incorporating dynamic movement in return to play evaluation, but given the prevalence of vestibular dysfunction after SRC, this may be an important assessment tool [8, 12]. If the criteria in Fig. 31.4 are not met, then the athlete should be held from play and receive further treatment. Making return to play decisions should always involve a multimodal assessment that incorporates both subjective and objective measures.

Fact Box

International guidelines require the following criteria to be met prior to returning an athlete to full sport participation after concussion: (1) athletes must be symptom-free from concussion at rest, (2) athletes must be symptom-free from concussion with physical activity, and (3) athletes must demonstrate a normal clinical evaluation.

Take-Home Message

Concussion is an individualized injury that requires a comprehensive assessment and targeted treatment approach. A multimodal evaluation of concussion sequelae allows for the determination of the clinical profile from the injury and a treatment plan tailored to the individual athlete. There have been several advancements in the tools available for evaluating concussion, and sports medicine practitioners should rely on a combination of subjective symptoms and performance on objective testing for clinical decision-making. There are established international guidelines for returning athletes to sport participation after sustaining a concussion.

References

1. Langlois JA, Rutland-Brown W, Wald MM. The epidemiology and impact of traumatic brain injury: a brief overview. J Head Trauma Rehabil. 2006;21(5):375–8.
2. Bakhos LL, Lockhart GR, Myers R, Linakis JG. Emergency department visits for concussion in young child athletes. Pediatrics. 2010;126(3):e550–6.
3. Barkhoudarian G, Hovda DA, Giza CC. The molecular pathophysiology of concussive brain injury. Clin Sports Med. 2011;30(1):33–48, iii–vii.
4. Giza CC, Hovda DA. The neurometabolic cascade of concussion. J Athl Train. 2001;36(3):228–35.
5. Haydel MJ, Preston CA, Mills TJ, Luber S, Blaudeau E, DeBlieux PM. Indications for computed tomography in patients with minor head injury. N Engl J Med. 2000;343(2):100–5.
6. Schatz P, Sandel N. Sensitivity and specificity of the online version of ImPACT in high school and collegiate athletes. Am J Sports Med. 2013;41(2):321–6.
7. Mucha A, Collins MW, Elbin RJ, et al. A Brief Vestibular/Ocular Motor Screening (VOMS) assessment to evaluate concussions: preliminary findings. Am J Sports Med. 2014;42(10):2479–86.
8. McCrory P, Meeuwisse W, Dvorak J, et al. Consensus statement on concussion in sport—the 5th international conference on concussion in sport held in Berlin, October 2016. Br J Sports Med. 2017;51(11):838–47. https://doi.org/10.1136/bjsports-2017-097699.
9. McCrory P, Meeuwisse W, Johnston K, et al. Consensus statement on concussion in sport: the 3rd international conference on concussion in sport held in Zurich, November 2008. Br J Sports Med. 2009;43(Suppl 1):i76–90.
10. Van Kampen DA, Lovell MR, Pardini JE, Collins MW, Fu FH. The "value added" of neurocognitive testing after sports-related concussion. Am J Sports Med. 2006;34(10):1630–5.
11. Delaney JS, Lacroix VJ, Leclerc S, Johnston KM. Concussions among university football and soccer players. Clin J Sport Med. 2002;12(6):331–8.
12. Henry LC, Elbin RJ, Collins MW, Marchetti G, Kontos AP. Examining recovery trajectories after sport-related concussion with a multimodal clinical assessment approach. Neurosurgery. 2016;78(2):232–41.
13. Collins MW, Kontos AP, Okonkwo DO, et al. Statements of agreement from the Targeted Evaluation and Active Management (TEAM) approaches to treating concussion meeting held in Pittsburgh, October 15–16, 2015. Neurosurgery. 2016;79(6):912–29.
14. Collins MW, Kontos AP, Reynolds E, Murawski CD, Fu FH. A comprehensive, targeted approach to the clinical care of athletes following sport-related concussion. Knee Surg Sports Traumatol Arthrosc. 2014;22(2):235–46.
15. Barth JT, Alves W, Ryan T, Macciocchi SN, Rimel RW, Nelson WE. Mild head injury in sports: neuropsychological sequelae and recovery of function. Mild head injury. New York: Oxford University Press; 1989. p. 257–75.
16. Elbin RJ, Kontos AP, Kegel N, Johnson E, Burkhart S, Schatz P. Individual and combined effects of LD and ADHD on computerized neurocognitive concussion test performance: evidence for separate norms. Arch Clin Neuropsychol. 2013;28(5):476–84.
17. Zuckerman SL, Lee YM, Odom MJ, Solomon GS, Sills AK. Baseline neurocognitive scores in athletes with attention deficit-spectrum disorders and/or learning disability. J Neurosurg Pediatr. 2013;12(2):103–9.
18. Schatz P, Robertshaw S. Comparing post-concussive neurocognitive test data to normative data presents risks for under-classifying "above average" athletes. Arch Clin Neuropsychol. 2014;29(7):625–32.
19. Schatz P, Glatts C. "Sandbagging" baseline test performance on ImPACT, without detection, is more difficult than it appears. Arch Clin Neuropsychol. 2013;28(3):236–44.
20. Cantu RC, Gean AD. Second-impact syndrome and a small subdural hematoma: an uncommon catastrophic result of repetitive head injury with a characteristic imaging appearance. J Neurotrauma. 2010;27(9):1557–64.
21. McCrory P, Davis G, Makdissi M. Second impact syndrome or cerebral swelling after sporting head injury. Curr Sports Med Rep. 2012;11(1):21–3.
22. Elbin R, Sufrinko A, Schatz P, et al. Removal from play after concussion and recovery time. Pediatrics. 2016:e20160910.
23. Collins MW, Iverson GL, Lovell MR, McKeag DB, Norwig J, Maroon J. On-field predictors of neuropsychological and symptom deficit following sports-related concussion. Clin J Sport Med. 2003;13(4):222–9.
24. Meehan WP 3rd, Mannix RC, Stracciolini A, Elbin RJ, Collins MW. Symptom severity predicts prolonged recovery after sport-related concussion, but age and amnesia do not. J Pediatr. 2013;163(3):721–5.
25. Lau BC, Kontos AP, Collins MW, Mucha A, Lovell MR. Which on-field signs/symptoms predict protracted recovery from sport-related concussion among high school football players? Am J Sports Med. 2011;39(11):2311–8.
26. National Institute of Neurological Disorders and Stroke. Sport-related concussion common data elements. 2017. https://www.commondataelements.

ninds.nih.gov/SRC.aspx#tab=Data_Standards. Accessed 27 Mar 2017.
27. McCrory P, Meeuwisse W, Aubry M, et al. Consensus statement on concussion in sport—the 4th international conference on concussion in sport held in Zurich, November 2012. J Sci Med Sport. 2013;16(3):178–89.
28. McCrea M, Kelly JP, Randolph C, et al. Standardized assessment of concussion (SAC): on-site mental status evaluation of the athlete. J Head Trauma Rehabil. 1998;13(2):27–35.
29. Maddocks DL, Dicker GD, Saling MM. The assessment of orientation following concussion in athletes. Clin J Sport Med. 1995;5(1):32–5.
30. National Conference of State Legislatures (2014) Traumatic brain injuries among youth athletes. Retrieved Februrary 14, 2019, from http://www.ncsl.org/research/health/traumatic-brain-injuries-among-youth-athletes.aspx
31. Elbin R, Knox J, Kegel N, et al. Assessing symptoms in adolescents following sport-related concussion: a comparison of four different approaches. Appl Neuropsychol Child. 2016;5(4):294–302.
32. Lau B, Lovell MR, Collins MW, Pardini J. Neurocognitive and symptom predictors of recovery in high school athletes. Clin J Sport Med. 2009;19(3):216–21.
33. Lau BC, Collins MW, Lovell MR. Cutoff scores in neurocognitive testing and symptom clusters that predict protracted recovery from concussions in high school athletes. Neurosurgery. 2012;70(2):371–9; discussion 379.
34. Meehan WP, Mannix R, Monuteaux MC, Stein CJ, Bachur RG. Early symptom burden predicts recovery after sport-related concussion. Neurology. 2014;83(24):2204–10.
35. Fazio VC, Lovell MR, Pardini JE, Collins MW. The relation between post concussion symptoms and neurocognitive performance in concussed athletes. NeuroRehabilitation. 2007;22(3):207–16.
36. Collins M, Lovell MR, Iverson GL, Ide T, Maroon J. Examining concussion rates and return to play in high school football players wearing newer helmet technology: a three-year prospective cohort study. Neurosurgery. 2006;58(2):275–86; discussion 275–286.
37. Cole WR, Arrieux JP, Schwab K, Ivins BJ, Qashu FM, Lewis SC. Test-retest reliability of four computerized neurocognitive assessment tools in an active duty military population. Arch Clin Neuropsychol. 2013;28(7):732–42.
38. Sandel NK, Worts PR, Burkhart S, Henry L. Comparison of baseline ImPACT performance in amateur motocross riders to football and basketball athletes. Brain Inj. 2018;32(4):493–7.
39. Kontos AP, Elbin RJ, Schatz P, Covassin T, Henry L, Pardini J, Collins MW. A revised factor structure for the post-concussion symptom scale: baseline and postconcussion factors. Am J Sports Med. 2012;40(10):2375–84.
40. Guskiewicz KM. Balance assessment in the management of sport-related concussion. Clin Sports Med. 2011;30(1):89–102.
41. Guskiewicz KM. Postural stability assessment following concussion: one piece of the puzzle. Clin J Sport Med. 2001;11(3):182–9.
42. Anzalone AJ, Blueitt D, Case T, et al. A positive vestibular/ocular motor screening (VOMS) is associated with increased recovery time after sports-related concussion in youth and adolescent athletes. Am J Sports Med. 2017;45(2):474–9.
43. Alsalaheen BA, Mucha A, Morris LO, et al. Vestibular rehabilitation for dizziness and balance disorders after concussion. J Neurol Phys Ther. 2010;34(2):87–93.
44. Alsalaheen BA, Whitney SL, Mucha A, Morris LO, Furman JM, Sparto PJ. Exercise prescription patterns in patients treated with vestibular rehabilitation after concussion. Physiother Res Int. 2013;18(2):100–8.
45. Ellis MJ, Leddy JJ, Willer B. Physiological, vestibulo-ocular and cervicogenic post-concussion disorders: an evidence-based classification system with directions for treatment. Brain Inj. 2015;29(2):238–48.
46. Sufrinko AM, Kegel NE, Mucha A, Collins MW, Kontos AP. History of high motion sickness susceptibility predicts vestibular dysfunction following sport/recreation-related concussion. Clin J Sport Med. 2017.
47. Headache Classification Committee of the International Headache Society (IHS). The international classification of headache disorders 2013. Cephalalgia 33(9):629–808.
48. Kontos AP, Elbin RJ, Lau B, et al. Posttraumatic migraine as a predictor of recovery and cognitive impairment after sport-related concussion. Am J Sports Med. 2013;41(7):1497–504.
49. Mihalik JP, Stump JE, Collins MW, Lovell MR, Field M, Maroon JC. Posttraumatic migraine characteristics in athletes following sports-related concussion. J Neurosurg. 2005;102(5):850–5.
50. Rains JC, Poceta JS. Headache and sleep disorders: review and clinical implications for headache management. Headache. 2006;46(9):1344–63.
51. Spierings EL, Ranke AH, Honkoop PC. Precipitating and aggravating factors of migraine versus tension-type headache. Headache. 2001;41(6):554–8.
52. Maizels M, Blumenfeld A, Burchette R. A combination of riboflavin, magnesium, and feverfew for migraine prophylaxis: a randomized trial. Headache. 2004;44(9):885–90.
53. Peikert A, Wilimzig C, Köhne-Volland R. Prophylaxis of migraine with oral magnesium: results from a prospective, multi-center, placebo-controlled and double-blind randomized study. Cephalalgia. 1996;16(4):257–63.
54. Snow V, Weiss K, Wall EM, Mottur-Pilson C. Pharmacologic management of acute attacks of migraine and prevention of migraine headache. Ann Intern Med. 2002;137(10):840–9.
55. Leddy JJ, Sandhu H, Sodhi V, Baker JG, Willer B. Rehabilitation of concussion and post-concussion syndrome. Sports health. 2012;4(2):147–54.

56. Goldberg JM, et al. The vestibular system: a sixth sense. New York: Oxford University Press; 2012.
57. Aligene K, Lin E. Vestibular and balance treatment of the concussed athlete. NeuroRehabilitation. 2013;32(3):543–53.
58. Gurley JM, Hujsak BD, Kelly JL. Vestibular rehabilitation following mild traumatic brain injury. NeuroRehabilitation. 2013;32(3):519–28.
59. Ciuffreda KJ, Kapoor N, Rutner D, Suchoff IB, Han ME, Craig S. Occurrence of oculomotor dysfunctions in acquired brain injury: a retrospective analysis. Optometry. 2007;78(4):155–61.
60. Capó-Aponte JE, Urosevich TG, Temme LA, Tarbett AK, Sanghera NK. Visual dysfunctions and symptoms during the subacute stage of blast-induced mild traumatic brain injury. Mil Med. 2012;177(7):804–13.
61. Master CL, Scheiman M, Gallaway M, et al. Vision diagnoses are common after concussion in adolescents. Clin Pediatr. 2016;55(3):260–7.
62. Pearce KL, Sufrinko A, Lau BC, Henry L, Collins MW, Kontos AP. Near point of convergence after a sport-related concussion: measurement reliability and relationship to neurocognitive impairment and symptoms. Am J Sports Med. 2015;43(12):3055–61.
63. Master CL, Master SR, Wiebe DJ, et al. Vision and vestibular system dysfunction predicts prolonged concussion recovery in children. Clin J Sport Med. 2018;28(2):139–45.
64. Ellis MJ, Cordingley D, Vis S, Reimer K, Leiter J, Russell K. Vestibulo-ocular dysfunction in pediatric sports-related concussion. J Neurosurg Pediatr. 2015;16(3):248–55.
65. Thiagarajan P, Ciuffreda KJ, Capo-Aponte JE, Ludlam DP, Kapoor N. Oculomotor neurorehabilitation for reading in mild traumatic brain injury (mTBI): an integrative approach. NeuroRehabilitation. 2014;34(1):129–46.
66. Smyth K, Sandhu SS, Crawford S, Dewey D, Parboosingh J, Barlow KM. The role of serotonin receptor alleles and environmental stressors in the development of post-concussive symptoms after pediatric mild traumatic brain injury. Dev Med Child Neurol. 2014;56(1):73–7.
67. Chen J-K, Johnston KM, Petrides M, Ptito A. Neural substrates of symptoms of depression following concussion in male athletes with persisting postconcussion symptoms. Arch Gen Psychiatry. 2008;65(1):81–9.
68. Sandel N, Reynolds E, Cohen PE, Gillie BL, Kontos AP. Anxiety and mood clinical profile following sport-related concussion: From risk factors to treatment. Sport Exerc Perform Psychol. 2017;6(3):304.
69. Ponsford J, Cameron P, Fitzgerald M, Grant M, Mikocka-Walus A, Schonberger M. Predictors of postconcussive symptoms 3 months after mild traumatic brain injury. Neuropsychology. 2012;26(3):304–13.
70. Carroll LJ, Cassidy JD, Peloso PM, et al. Prognosis for mild traumatic brain injury: results of the WHO Collaborating Centre Task Force on Mild Traumatic Brain Injury. J Rehabil Med. 2004;(43 Suppl):84–105.
71. Comper P, Bisschop S, Carnide N, Tricco A. A systematic review of treatments for mild traumatic brain injury. Brain Inj. 2005;19(11):863–80.
72. Cooper DB, Bunner AE, Kennedy JE, et al. Treatment of persistent post-concussive symptoms after mild traumatic brain injury: a systematic review of cognitive rehabilitation and behavioral health interventions in military service members and veterans. Brain Imaging Behav. 2015;9(3):403–20.
73. Hopko DR, Lejuez CW, Hopko SD. Behavioral activation as an intervention for coexistent depressive and anxiety symptoms. Clin Case Stud. 2004;3(1):37–48.
74. Mazzucchelli T, Kane R, Rees C. Behavioral activation treatments for depression in adults: a meta-analysis and review. Clin Psychol Sci Pract. 2009;16(4):383–411.
75. Mittenberg W, Canyock EM, Condit D, Patton C. Treatment of post-concussion syndrome following mild head injury. J Clin Exp Neuropsychol. 2001;23(6):829–36.
76. Hsieh M-Y, Ponsford J, Wong D, Schönberger M, Taffe J, Mckay A. Motivational interviewing and cognitive behaviour therapy for anxiety following traumatic brain injury: a pilot randomised controlled trial. Neuropsychol Rehabil. 2012;22(4):585–608.
77. Ponsford J, Lee N, Wong D, et al. Efficacy of motivational interviewing and cognitive behavioral therapy for anxiety and depression symptoms following traumatic brain injury. Psychol Med. 2016;46(5):1079–90.
78. Jorge RE, Acion L, Burin DI, Robinson RG. Sertraline for preventing mood disorders following traumatic brain injury: a randomized clinical trial. JAMA Psychiat. 2016;73(10):1041–7.
79. Fann JR, Uomoto JM, Katon WJ. Sertraline in the treatment of major depression following mild traumatic brain injury. J Neuropsychiatry Clin Neurosci. 2000;12(2):226–32.
80. Sufrinko A, Johnson EW, Henry LC. The influence of sleep duration and sleep-related symptoms on baseline neurocognitive performance among male and female high school athletes. Neuropsychology. 2016;30(4):484.
81. Reddy CC, Collins M, Lovell M, Kontos AP. Efficacy of amantadine treatment on symptoms and neurocognitive performance among adolescents following sports-related concussion. J Head Trauma Rehabil. 2013;28(4):260–5.

Doping

32

Maria João Cascais

32.1 Background

The concept of doping is old as sport itself. In an ideal world, this chapter would not be necessary, only in the historic concept. Unfortunately, here we are, providing some information for the sports medicine clinician, hoping that this text will guide him through these always changing issues. The changes are the essence of doping because there are new methods and rearrangement of old ones every day.

Doping is described at least since the Old Greece (Fig. 32.1) [1]; it was used by the Romans and the ancient tribes of Norway [2]. In the explosive growing of sport in the early twentieth century, all the issues came back from the past and were enhanced with the light of science.

The actual organization in terms of doping, education, and fair play is the WADA [World Anti-Doping Agency]. "The World Anti-Doping Agency [WADA] was established in 1999 as an independent international agency composed and funded equally by the sports movement and governments of the world. The key activities include scientific research, education, development of anti-doping capacities, and monitoring of the World Anti-Doping Code [Code]—the document harmonizing anti-doping policies in all sports and all countries" (https://www.wada-ama.org/en/who-we-are).

Having this in view, the rules of what athletes can take or do about doping do not leave any doubts as this cited site of WADA is available for every sport-concerned entity.

The List is updated every year and has started with the Olympic Committee "Under the leadership of the International Olympic Committee, the Prohibited List [List] was first published in 1963. Since 2004, as mandated by the World Anti-Doping Code [Code], the World Anti-Doping Agency [WADA] is responsible for the preparation and publication of the List (Fig. 32.2)" (www.usada.org/when-was-the-first-prohibited-list-created-and-how-does-a-substance-get-on-the-prohibited-list/).

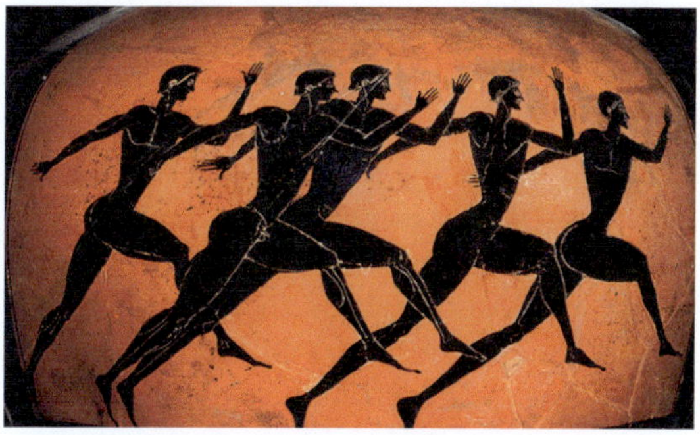

Fig. 32.1 Athletics in ancient Greece

M. J. Cascais (✉)
NOVA Medical School Lisbon, Lisboa, Portugal

Sports Medicine College, Medical Portuguese Order, Lisboa, Portugal

S. Rocha Piedade et al. (eds.), *The Sports Medicine Physician*,
https://doi.org/10.1007/978-3-030-10433-7_32

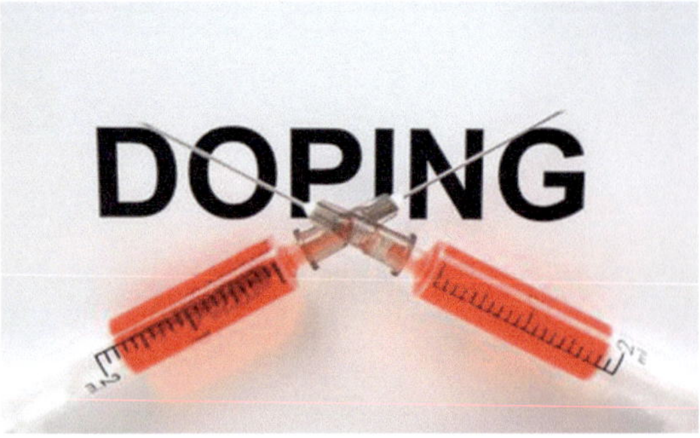

Fig. 32.2 Doping means many threats

The First World Conference on Doping in Sport held in Lausanne, Switzerland, on February 2–4, 1999, produced the Lausanne Declaration on Doping in Sport. This document provided for the creation of an independent international anti-doping agency to be operational for the Games of the XXVII Olympiad in Sydney in 2000 (https://www.wada-ama.org/en/who-we-are).

As the Olympic Movement governing body, the **IOC** makes the Code mandatory for the entire Movement. During the Olympic Games, it oversees all doping control and testing processes in compliance with the Code regulations. However, the IOC is striving to make all these processes independent. Since the Olympic Games Rio 2016, sanctioning has been handled by the **Court of Arbitration for Sport [CAS] and its Anti-Doping Division**. The creation of an **independent testing agency** is also underway (https://www.olympic.org/fight-against-doping).

WADA convenes an independent panel of international experts to consider the composition of the List on an annual basis. A substance or method will be considered for the List if it meets any two of the following three criteria: it has the potential to enhance sports performance; it represents an actual or potential health risk to the athlete; or it violates the spirit of sport (Fig. 32.2). After the List is drafted for any year, it is sent to stakeholders for comment and finally approved by the WADA Executive Committee. A new List is approved each October for implementation the following January to give athletes an opportunity to make the appropriate changes in medications.

32.2 The List: WADA

Reading the list is an important step not to be overwhelmed by all the chemical compounds inside it. This List has the first step to consider, the division between substances and methods **prohibited at all times** and the other refers to the substances and methods **prohibited only in competition.** The **Monitoring Program** is another chapter and finally the one called **The Summary of Major Modifications and Explanatory Notes.** With these tools that are published every year by the WADA, all the medical community and the athletes have a source of information that is the key to maintain the health of athletes and a clean sport.

Having the WADA List as a starting point becomes easier to go through all the doping issues nowadays, keeping in mind that this List is revised every year. Each individual has different genetic endowments, and this is translated in a more or less performance in sports [3]. Natural genetic advantages are, for example, the eight for sports like basketball, the predisposition for anaerobic explosive power like the deletion of alpha-actinin 3 [4], and many others that wore born with the athlete. In the future, modifications of genetic expression will be the ultimate goal of doping agents.

32.3 Prohibited Substances and Methods

32.3.1 Prohibited Substances and Methods at All Times

32.3.1.1 Non-approved Substances: SO

In this category fall all the substances that are not in the world pharmacopeia and so can include every new drug, coming from labs as a new molecule. Before as it was not referred in the list, athletes claimed that "what is not in the List is not banned."

32.3.1.2 S1 Anabolic Agents

This includes anabolic-androgen steroids, endogenous and exogenous, and other anabolic agents. The ergogenic effects of androgen steroids have been brought to light before the Second World War [5] were referred as noxious and dangerous but used without restrictions in the times of the Cold War [6]. Only in 1990, all was explained in a scientific way [7] and some people were convinced.

The anabolic-androgen steroid abuse gives an increase in muscle mass and circulating hemoglobin and has other deleterious effects like the depression of spermatogenesis and fertility, gynecomastia, and hepatotoxicity, just to cite some (Table 32.1). They are divided into endogenous and exogenous and the list you can find in WADA shows almost all the more used.

Different laboratory methods are used to isolate them in the urine, and today we have the Steroidal Passport that will be treated later in this chapter. The athletes consume androgens from many sources, including veterinary, counterfeit preparations; almost all are bought in illegal websites and labs.

There are other types of anabolic drugs, not steroidal, that you can find in the same chapter but in another division, like clenbuterol. These drugs are used for asthma and have similar effects to the anabolic steroid androgens.

Table 32.1 Effects of the misuse of anabolic steroids

Fluid retention
Acne
Increased blood pressure and cholesterol levels
Headaches
Reduced sexual functioning
Increase in muscle size
Swelling of feet and ankles
Insomnia
Rapid weight gain
Increased appetite
Improved healing

32.3.1.3 S2 Peptide Hormones, Growth Factors, Related Substances, and Mimetics

Under this complicated title are listed the hormones EPO, mimetics, and receptor agonists, the HIF [hypoxia-inducible factor], that have in common the same goal, to raise the level of hemoglobin by stimulating erythropoiesis. High levels of hemoglobin are useful in aerobic endurance sports, and it has been proved that these levels increase maximal exercise-induced oxygen consumption.

The HIF stabilizers and related small molecules interfere with molecular oxygen sensing mechanisms to simulate hypoxia leading to a release of red blood precursor cells [8]. Adverse effects include cardiovascular complications due to high blood viscosity [thromboembolism, hypertension, stroke, and, in the extreme, sudden death] and immune reactivity to the compounds injected [9].

Here in S2, we can also find hormones like chorionic gonadotropin [CG], luteinizing hormone [LH], growth hormone [GH], and corticotrophins and their releasing factors. The CG hormone binds to LH receptors and stimulates Leydig cells to secrete testosterone simulating the endogenous secretion. Side effects include edema and gynecomastia.

GH has been linked to athletes in sports like baseball, swimming, and cycling and is used out of the sport by high school students in the USA. It can cause insulin resistance, hyperglycemia, diabetes, and premature epiphyseal closure, for example [10].

Growth factors and growth factor modulators, like IGF-1 and VEGF [vascular endothelial growth factor], affect protein synthesis, and tissue regeneration has been used too [11].

32.3.1.4 S3 Beta-2 Agonists

All the medicaments for asthma with action like beta-2 agonists are prohibited except salbutamol, salmeterol, and formoterol in the doses indicated in the List [see the List for exact thresholds]. The asthmatic athlete is always a concern for the physician and coach, and all the beta-2 agonists outside the three cited here need authorization for therapeutic use.

32.3.1.5 S4 Hormone and Metabolic Modulators

In this chapter are listed the hormone and metabolic modulators used to treat diseases like prostatic cancer and breast cancer but are used by athletes to make a sustained rise in testosterone and hide the use of exogenous testosterone and other steroids.

Aromatase inhibitors block the "enzyme" aromatase which converts androgens [e.g., testosterone] into estrogens by a process called aromatization. Consequently, aromatase inhibitors lower estrogen levels in the blood or in tumor "tissues" by preventing the formation of estradiol [12]. Forbidden aromatase inhibitors are, but not limited to, anastrozole and letrozole.

Selective estrogen receptor modulators [SERMs] are compounds that bind with estrogen receptors and exhibit estrogen action in some tissues and antiestrogen action in other tissues. Forbidden SERMs are, but not limited to, raloxifene, tamoxifen, and toremifene. The abuse is just based on the suppression of biomedical side effects caused by an abuse of anabolic-androgenic steroids in males [13].

Myostatin or growth differentiation factor 8 is a "protein" of the skeletal muscle cells regulating the size of muscles by blocking extensive growth. Agents modifying the myostatin function, especially inhibiting the myostatin gene, are growth-regulating by apparently accelerating the development of muscle stem cells. In this context, the agents are forbidden, but not limited to myostatin inhibitors [14]. In metabolic modulators, the list has the hormone for diabetes like insulin, but it includes the famous meldonium that gave rise to the media case with Sharapova and other athletes in 2016.

Mildronate [3-[2,2,2-trimethylhydrazinium] propionate] (Fig. 32.3) was originally developed in the late 1970s as a growth-promoting agent for animals in the Latvian Institute of Organic Synthesis. Most of Mildronate's clinical benefits are mediated through its modulation of the carnitine metabolism, which is the essential factor in

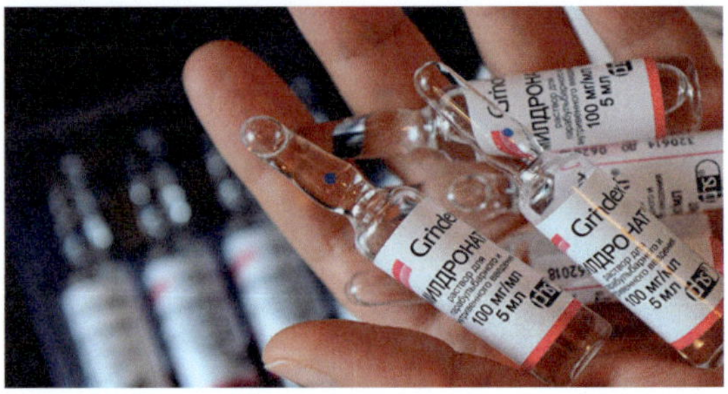

Fig. 32.3 Mildronate (meldonium)

regulating the cellular energy metabolism through fatty acid β-oxidation and glycolysis in the myocardium, as carnitine is the key molecule in fatty acid metabolism in mitochondrial membrane. Under aerobic conditions, carnitine improves myocardial functioning through enhancement of fatty acid β-oxidation that supplies about 80% of myocardial ATP generation. However, under oxygen deficiency, cytotoxic intermediates can accumulate in the cell due to an insufficient oxygen supply. Under sport-physiological aspects, reports on positive effects on the physical working capacity of elite athletes were published. Moreover, mildronate shows mood-improving effects, as well as an increased learning and memory performance, which are properties athletes may also benefit from [15].

32.3.1.6 S5 Diuretics and Masking Agents

These substances are used to eliminate fluid from the body and are used by athletes for two main purposes: one, to keep weight in the limits required, for example, in Judo, and the other, to mask the forbidden substances that they have been taken. The physician should be aware of the diseases, which require a diuretic because it will be necessary a TUE [Therapeutic Use Exemption].

32.4 Prohibited Methods

These methods include manipulation of blood and blood components, chemical and physical manipulation, and gene doping. Here are referred the blood transfusions autologous or heterologous, and it is set the limit of endovenous replacement outside hospital treatment, surgical procedures, or clinical diagnostic investigations, in 2018 no more than 100 mL in 12-h periods.

Gene Doping

> "the non-therapeutic use of cells, genes, genetic elements, or of the modulation of gene expression, having the capacity to enhance athletic performance" [16]. This kind of doping is obviously a product that has to be granted to the athlete by medical professionals.

There are four endurance genes that can match the needs of endurance sports: (1) erythropoietin [EPO] stimulating erythropoiesis, (2) peroxisome proliferator-activated receptor [PPAR] encoding enzymes of fatty acid oxidation, (3) hypoxia-inducible factors [HIF], and (4) angiotensin-converting enzyme [ACE] being a vasoconstrictor or vasodilator.

Some muscle genes are listed too like the myostatin, as negative muscle regulator; mechano growth factor [MGF], insulin-like growth factor-1 [IGF-1], and insulin-like growth factor-binding protein [IGFBP] for the control of muscle growth; and growth hormone [GH] for the control of muscle mass.

32.5 Substances and Methods Prohibited in Competition

Additionally, to all these groups, in competition, the following substances are prohibited.

32.5.1 S6 Stimulants

In this group of drugs, there are differences between specified and nonspecified substances.

The denomination concerns the stimulants that can be found in many medications for upper respiratory pathologies and cough syrups, and so the athlete could have taken them without the intention of doping, e.g., ephedrine and methylephedrine, which are positive when their concentration in urine is greater than 10 μg per mL.

The nonspecified substances include the medicaments used for ADHA [attention deficit hyperactivity disorder] that had explosive growth in the last 5 years. Therefore they require a TUE and other stimulants that have been abused, for improving mood and arousal and masking fatigue.

32.5.2 S7 Narcotics

These drugs are forbidden not because of the enhancement in performance, but because being pain killers, they would allow athletes to compete without an important mechanism of defense and survival—the pain.

By their structure, they cause addiction and mood alterations, and they are opioid-related molecules.

32.5.3 S8 Cannabinoids

They are a group of substances present in the plant *Cannabis sativa*; THC [tetrahydrocannabinol] is the main psychoactive component and binds to cannabinoid receptors in the brain. They cause euphoria, relaxation, and visual and auditory amplified perceptions. This THC is a social drug and should be treated like that because it has no improvement in performance in most of the sports.

32.5.4 S9 Glucocorticoids

Glucocorticoids are used to treat the inflammation process. The inflammatory process in the body has evolved for a useful purpose, namely, as a defensive reaction to the damage or injury of the tissues. Inflammation is designed to isolate the cause of the irritation, to eradicate the presumed invader, and to repair the surrounding damaged tissues, so using them in the sport without medical indication can lead to serious damage. They are prohibited in oral, intravenous, intramuscular, or rectal administration. All the other forms of administration are allowed.

They stand for a large percentage of TUEs in all countries and sports, but they are used by inhalation by many asthmatic or allergic athletes which do not need authorization.

32.6 Substances Prohibited in Particular Sports

This section has only one group of substances: the beta-blockers. Norepinephrine is the major neurotransmitter of the sympathetic nervous system, and it is released into the periphery upon activation of the sympathetic nervous system. Beta-blockers are drugs that bind to beta-adrenoceptors and thereby block the binding of norepinephrine and epinephrine to these receptors. That is, beta-blockers avoid the activation of these receptors, and in consequence catecholamines cannot carry out their function, and anxiety is reduced.

In archery and shooting, they are prohibited in and out of the competition. In automobile, golf, billiards, darts, skiing/snowboard, and some underwater sports, they are prohibited only in competition. Every year the agency releases another chapter that concerns the substances that are not forbidden yet but are being monitored in the anti-doping labs.

That group of substances could be part of the List next year or not. Anyway, sports medicine doctors should be aware of this chapter, so in the forthcoming season, they would not be surprised. All the changes from the anterior list are in a special chapter too.

32.7 Biological Passport

The new substances available for doping that mimic physiologic molecules produced by the body itself make detection very difficult. In order to keep sport clean, and to ensure the protection of the athlete's health, the WADA has developed with the collaboration of medical specialists the program of ABP [Athlete Biological Passport] (Fig. 32.4), which uses several physiologic results, that together in a computerized program [17] can produce a display of graphics and calculate the odds of a positive result, with a percentage of 99% of suspicion.

The action after this result can be taking other samples or calling the athlete because he can have a specific clinical situation that explains the results. Making it simpler, there are three modules of ABP: the Hematological, Steroidal, and subsidiary to this module the Endocrinological passport [18]. The Hematological profile is aimed to detect any form of blood doping or rEpo [19]. The Steroidal module aims to detect direct and indirect forms of doping with anabolic agents [20]. The endocrinological module doping is used to detect growth hormone factors and insulin growth factors [21].

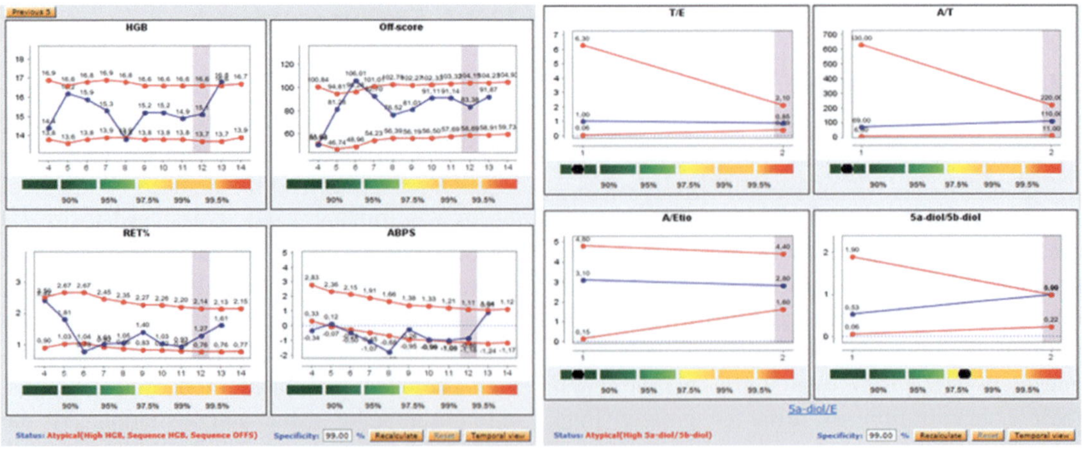

Fig. 32.4 Some aspects of the biological passport

In the definition of WADA: "The fundamental principle of the Athlete Biological Passport [ABP] is to monitor selected biological variables over time that indirectly reveal the effects of doping rather than attempting to detect the doping substance or method itself."

Finally, all the athletes have their data and special ID and number in a global system of registration and identification: the ADAMS, anti-doping administration, and management system, web-based data management system developed and administered by the World Anti-Doping Agency ["WADA"] in its role as a central clearinghouse for anti-doping information.

32.8 TUE [Therapeutic Use Exemptions]

When an athlete needs to be treated for the acute or chronic disease, he has the right to the treatment, no matter if it is a prohibited substance because health care comes first. Nevertheless, if it is a lifesaving issue or has to be medicated in a hospital or any kind of ER, the application form that exists in WADA must be sent to de ADO of the athlete, and it will be authorized retroactively. If it is a condition that is part of the athlete's life, like insulin for diabetes type 1, it will be sent a request to the ADO, together with a small clinical history and complimentary exams.

In any other cases, there must be submitted an application form with all the information about the disease, the athlete and the physician contact, that will go directly to the TUE Committee [TUEC] of each ADO. This TUEC will decide to authorize or not or to ask more details to the doctor. This procedure must be completed in 21 days, but as a rule, it only takes 3–5 days.

32.9 Conclusion

All that text is based in experience and documents available for every doctor. However, we must keep in mind that the best politics to avoid this "disease" [doping] is prevention. In this matter, all the society has a responsibility, and all that contact directly or indirectly must give their contribution to educate the young children in an early stage of the competition, because when they arrive at a big association, club, or federation it is already too late sometimes. An effort should be made by all governments and each individual that deal with sport, at all levels making prevention of misbehavior a very important goal to achieve.

Take-Home Messages

- Consult the list every year at January, because there are changes to be implemented and you should be acquainted with them.
- Check every medication of your athletes, even if it seems simple and comes from a respected clinician—you are the sports medicine doctor, it is your call.
- Prevention and education are the best methods to achieve a sport without doping.
- Anti-doping became a specialized process that moves thousands of people all around the world, doctors, lawyers, economists, athletes, etc.

References

1. Pausanias. Descriptions of Greece, a second century A.D. (Translated by W.H.S. Jones). Cambridge: Loeb Classical Library; 1959.
2. Voy R. Drugs, sport, and politics. Champaign: Leisure Press; 1991 (OR by the tribes of actual Norway).
3. Eynon N, et al. Genes and elite athletes: a roadmap for future research. J Physiol. 2011;589:3063–70.
4. Berman Y, North KN. A gene for speed: the emerging role of alpha-actinin-3 in muscle metabolism. Physiology (Bethesda). 2010;25:250–9.
5. David K, Dingemanse E, Freud J, Laqueur E. Uber krystallinisches mannliches Hormon aus Hoden,[Testosteron], wirksamer als aus Harn oder aus Cholestrin bereitetes Androsteron. Hoppe Seylers Zeischrift Physiologische Chemie. 1935;233:281–2.
6. Wade N. Anabolic steroids: doctors denounce them, but athletes aren't listening. Science. 1972;176:1399–403.
7. Bhasin S, et al. The effects of supraphysiologic doses of testosterone on muscle size and strength in normal men. N Engl J Med. 1996;335:1–7.
8. Beuck S, Schanzer W, Thevis M. Hypoxia-inducible factor stabilizers and other small-molecule erythropoiesis-stimulating agents in current and preventive doping analysis. Drug Test Anal. 2012;4:830–45.
9. Bennett CL, et al. Venous thromboembolism and mortality associated with recombinant erythropoietin

and darbepoetin administration for the treatment of cancer-associated anemia. JAMA. 2008;299:914–24.
10. Thieme D, Hemmersbach P, editors. Doping in sports. In: Handbook of experimental pharmacology, Vol. 195. Berlin: Springer; 2010. https://doi.org/10.1007/978-3-540-79088-4_8.
11. Guha N, et al. Biochemical markers of recombinant human insulin-like growth factor-I [rhIGF-I]/rhIGF binding protein-3 [rhIGFBP-3] misuse in athletes. Drug Test Anal. 2013;5:843–9.
12. Selective estrogen-receptor modulators — mechanisms of action and application to clinical practice. N Engl J Med. 2003;348(7):618–29.
13. Handelsman DJ. Indirect androgen doping by oestrogen blockade in sports. Br J Pharmacol. 2008;154:598–605.. [PMC free article]
14. Yamada AK, Verlengia R, Bueno Junior CR. Myostatin: genetic variants, therapy andgene doping. Braz J Pharm Sci. 2012;48(3):369–77.
15. Dzintare M, Kalvins I. Mildronate increases aerobic capabilities of athletes through carnitine-lowering effect. In: 5th Baltic sport science conference: current issues and new ideas in sports science, Kaunas, Lithuania, 18–19 April 2012. Lithuania: Lithuanian Academy of Physical Education; 2012. p. 59.
16. Pray L. Sports, gene doping, and WADA. Nature Education. 2008;1(1):77.
17. Taroni F, Aitken C, Garbolino P, Biedermann A. Bayesian networks and probabilistic inference in forensic science. Chichester: Wiley; 2006. 372p.
18. WADA. Athlete Biological Passport operating guidelines and compilation of required elements. Montreal: WADA; 2009.
19. Sottas PE, Robinson N, Saugy M. The athlete's biological passport and indirect markers of blood doping. Handb Exp Pharmacol. 2010;195:305–26.
20. Sottas PE, Saugy M, Saudan C. Endogenous steroid profiling in the Athlete Biological Passport. Endocrinol Metab Clin North Am. 2010;39:59–73.
21. Holt RI, Sönksen PH. Growth hormone, IGF-I and insulin and their abuse in sport. Br J Pharmacol. 2008;154:542–56.

33 Dermatological Injuries

Margarida Gonçalo and Luis Santiago

33.1 Introduction

Sports practice can be good to your body but is not completely safe to your skin. As the body's first line of defence to exogenous aggressors, the skin can suffer acute or chronic traumatic lesions and be more prone to cutaneous infections and allergic contact dermatitis due to sports equipment, and, on long term, outdoor sports activities with high sun exposure are associated with an increased risk of skin cancer. Although not life-threatening, these cutaneous lesions may have a significant impact on athletic performance, may need several hours/days away from training for recovery [1] and, therefore, need particular attention by the sports medicine physician or the dermatologist.

Some cutaneous lesions are acute, often self-limiting, and the diagnosis is obvious, like in frictional bullae or callosities. Others occur after some time in practice, like allergic contact dermatitis. Then the relation with sports may be less obvious, and additional tests may be necessary to confirm the diagnosis.

M. Gonçalo (✉)
Clinic of Dermatology, University Hospital and Faculty of Medicine, University of Coimbra, Coimbra, Portugal
e-mail: mgoncalo@fmed.uc.pt

L. Santiago
Clinic of Dermatology, University Hospital, Coimbra, Portugal

Some manifestations are common to all sports, but some are very particular to some modalities (like jogger's nipples, basketball pebble fingers, the ball site sign in table tennis [2], herpes or tinea gladiatorum in wrestlers [3]) or acquire particular aspects dependent on the sports activity (different types of callosities, chilblains and other cold-induced skin disorders in sports on ice or cold water, watersports hands or aquagenic syringeal acrokeratoderma [4]). Topical or systemic medication used by the patient, eventually to treat sports injuries, may also cause allergic contact or photoallergic contact dermatitis. Moreover some chronic skin diseases, e.g. atopic dermatitis or psoriasis, may interfere with sports, and a special attention should be given to these athletes to allow them enjoy the sports and achieve the best performances, but this is outside the scope of this chapter.

33.2 Acute and Chronic Traumatic Lesions

33.2.1 Skin Blisters

Repeated friction or mechanical tension can cause painful dermo-epidermal blistering particularly when the equipment is not very well fitted to the athlete's body, when there is excessive moisture or previous skin fragility (e.g. epidermolysis bullosa simplex) or when the skin is not

S. Rocha Piedade et al. (eds.), *The Sports Medicine Physician*,
https://doi.org/10.1007/978-3-030-10433-7_33

yet trained to stand this tension, namely, in young athletes beginning their training [5]. These serous or haemorrhagic blisters, which usually have a competent rooftop, should be drained on the more dependent area by a small sterile puncture to reduce tension and pain. The blister roof should be kept on site, as it is the best biological dressing that reduces pain and allows quick and complete healing. If rupture occurs and the lesion is painful due to dermal exposure, a simple dressing with sterile greasy gauze or hydrocolloid dressing left in place for a few days will control pain, prevent secondary infection and allow quick resolution. Friction blisters can be prevented by good skin hydration (applying a good emollient before sports activities), reducing skin moisture (use of antiperspirants or adequate clothing) and best adaptation of the equipment to the body, especially over bony prominences or where friction is higher.

33.2.2 Friction Dermatitis: Callosities and Corns

Acute exposure to friction without previous skin hardening or in more fragile areas can cause erythema, minor erosions and fissures with pain. "Jogger's nipples" occur after long runs or jogging that present as painful erythema with fissures, erosions and crusts on the nipples due to friction of the shirt [6]. "Pool toes" occur due to friction with the cement in the bottom or border of the swimming pool usually at the beginning of the swimming season [7]. "Basketball pebble fingers" present as purpura, erosions and fissures on the fingertips due to rotation and contact with the pebbled surface of the basketball [8]. "Canyoning hands" are characterized by fissuring and abrasion of the fingertips and hands due to exposure to cold water and contact with rocks during descent of the rapids [9].

Chronic repeated friction on the same area may be responsible for friction dermatitis [10], callosities and corns, knuckle pads or sports nodules [5].

Friction dermatitis can present as erythematous papules or plaques with hyperkeratosis and scaling or lichenification in an area of chronic friction. It has been described in sumo wrestlers localized to the knee/leg or the knuckles [10]; in baseball pitchers in the ankle and knee, known as "baseball pitcher's friction dermatitis"; and in rower's gluteal area, known as "rower's rump", which is due to friction in an unpadded seat or the metal training machines [8, 11].

Callosities represent an area of thickened skin, particularly dependent on the stratum corneum, formed as an asymptomatic protective reaction pattern to chronic and repetitive friction. They occur more commonly over the bony prominences of the feet, toes and hands or in weight-bearing areas (Fig. 33.1a).

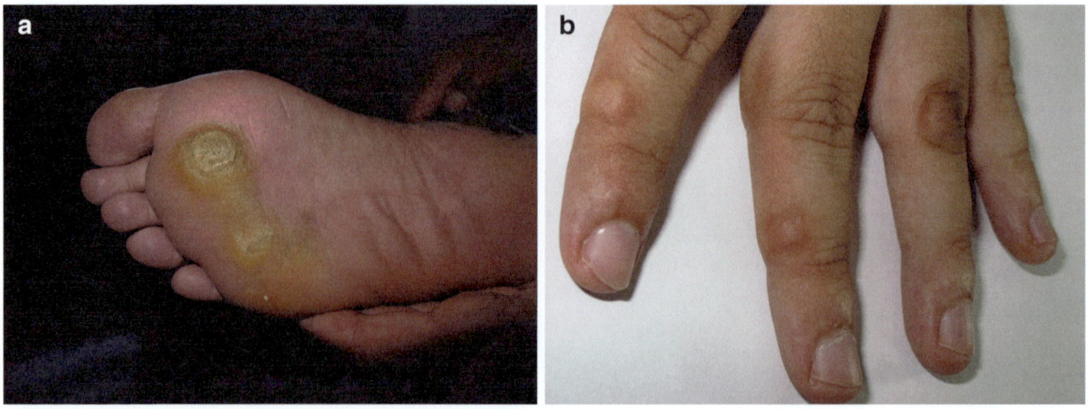

Fig. 33.1 Traumatic lesions due to chronic friction. Callosities in weight-bearing areas of the feet (**a**) and knuckle pads in a boxer (**b**)

"Pump bumps" are particularly frequent among ice skaters who use badly fitting skates [12].

Corns can be clinically similar to callosities, but they are painful and can become inflammatory, and they are associated with a small, 1–2 mm translucent central core within the base of the lesion, which is easily observed after curettage of the superficial keratosis. These corns need to be distinguished from plantar warts (no pinpoint black dots and persistence of dermatoglyphics), and treatment is required as they may limit sports activities. Warm soaking baths, curettage and keratolytics (urea, salicylic acid, retinoids) or more aggressive measures may be needed along with protection from friction.

Due to friction and pressure, some athletes also develop benign, asymptomatic, well-circumscribed, smooth, firm, skin-colour papules, nodules or plaques over the dorsal aspect of the proximal interphalangeal joints of the fingers or the dorsal aspects of the foot over joints, known as "knuckle pads" or sports-associated pads (Fig. 33.1b). They can be related to shoes but seem to be more frequent in the fingers, namely, in boxers [5]. Similar nodular lesions on chronic frictional areas—athlete's nodules—commonly observed in similar locations in surfers, boxers, skaters and football and hockey players, are also associated with epidermal thickening, but increased dermal collagen bundles or granulomatous reactions from exogenous material can co-exist [5].

Repeated friction, for instance, by the use of helmets, may cause mechanical acne localized to the area of contact. Acne in sports has also been associated with the high consumption of anabolic steroids, but more recently the use of milk-derived products and whey protein, particularly in body building sports, has been associated with more severe acne [13].

33.2.3 Cutaneous Haemorrhage

Abrupt tension or strong contact with the working surface or the equipment can cause superficial dermal haemorrhage, but red blood cells may further progress to the epidermis where they will persist until full epidermal renewal. Petechiae or a black macule on the plantar or posterolateral aspect of the heel, also known as "black heel" or "talon noir", is seen mostly in young athletic individuals who practice sports associated with quick starts and stops, particularly in harder surfaces, such as tennis, squash, football, ice skaters or gymnastics [14]. Similar lesions occur less frequently in the palms, particularly in the thenar eminence, namely, in weightlifters, gymnasts, golfers, tennis players, skiers and mountain climbers, as these athletes apply pressure to their hands (Fig. 33.2a) [5]. Although asymptomatic, these lesions may last for more than a month, especially in the feet and palms where the epidermis and stratum corneum are thicker, and they may be confused with pigmented lesions.

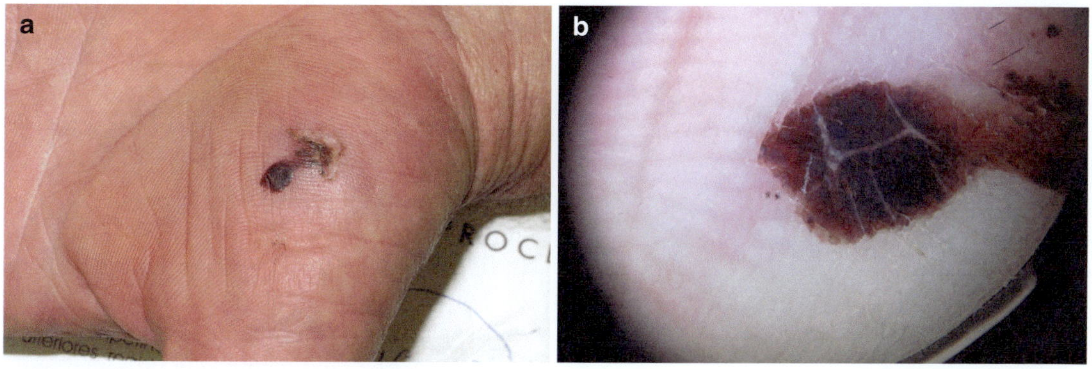

Fig. 33.2 Cutaneous haemorrhage on the thenar region of a tennis player (**a**), with the typical dermatoscopic aspect, showing blood within the stratum corneum (**b**)

Dermatoscopy allows a correct distinction between skin haemorrhage and melanoma or other pigmented lesion due to the "red-wine" colour of the blood and absence of the pigmented network (Fig. 33.2b) [15]. Moreover, skin curettage removes the pigmented stratum corneum, immediately confirms the diagnosis and resolves the "black heel".

When similar tension affects the toenails, particularly the hallux, subungueal and periungueal haematoma can occur. It is frequently associated with badly fitting shoes during long walks, namely, in marathon runners, or in sports associated with quick starts and stops [16]. An acute traumatic subungueal hematoma can be painful due to high tension under the nail plate. Immediate drainage by a small hole in the nail plate, performed, for instance, with a 2-mm biopsy punch before the hematoma gets organized, is advised. A smaller subungueal haematoma or chronic and repetitive haemorrhage into the nail apparatus with incorporation of the blood in the nail plate can be asymptomatic and go unnoticed (Fig. 33.3), but the dark colour that persists for months may be mistaken for subungueal melanoma. Dermatoscopy with the red/violet colour of the blood within the nail plate or nail bed may allow a correct distinction. Distal progression of the coloured lesion accompanying nail growth, which is nevertheless slow (>6 months in the hallux), also supports the diagnosis, but in case of doubt, a skin biopsy can establish the correct diagnosis.

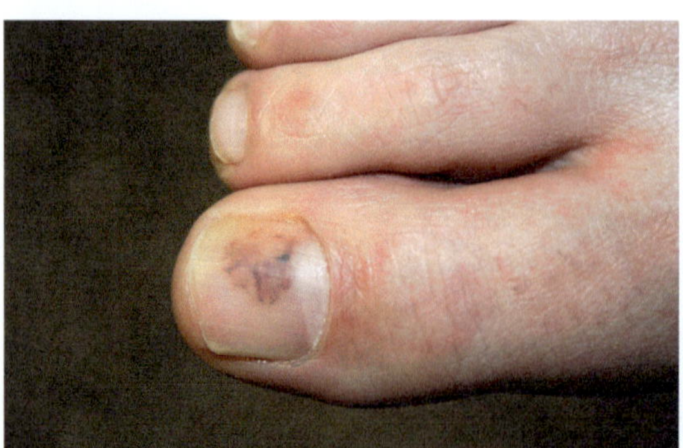

Fig. 33.3 Chronic subungueal haemorrhage at the middle portion of the nail, as it progressed distally with nail growth

In sports that involve high velocity balls, the unexpected impact of the ball on the skin—a paintball, a ping pong ball, a racquetball or a squash ball—may result either in erythema or petechial purpura or both. Lesions typically appear as a round or mostly as an annular ring of erythema or petechiae with or without accompanying ecchymosis and a clear centre, forming a targetoid lesion, known as the "ball site sign" or ball sports-induced targetoid erythema [2].

After a marathon, especially in hot temperatures, oedema of the lower limbs and feet can occur and be associated with petechial or more palpable purpura due to venous insufficiency and inflammatory capillaritis [16].

33.2.4 Onychocryptosis, Retronychia and Distrophic Toenails

Trauma, ill-fitting footwear, incorrect toenail trimming and malalignment of the toenail are concurrent factors for ingrown toenails (onychocryptosis), a painful disorder that may have a negative impact on athlete's performance. As the nail plate penetrates the dermis on the lateral nailfold, there is inflammation, often associated with bacterial infection and purulent discharge, granulation tissue and persistent oedema of the lateral nailfolds, which further predisposes to onychocryptosis (Fig. 33.4a). It affects mostly the inner lateral nailfold but can affect both nailfolds and both toes. If onychocryptosis does not resolve with simple measures like antiseptics, topical antibiotics and corticosteroids and correct nail trimming (strait cutting of the distal nail border), partial chemical or surgical matricectomy to reduce the width of the nail plate is advised.

Following trauma, mainly in runners or ballet dancers, painful retronychia can occur especially in the great toe (Fig. 33.4b). This situation that is often under-diagnosed consists on embedding of the nail plate into the proximal nailfold with separation from the nail matrix, followed by inflammation and pain of the proximal nailfold and the formation of a new nail plate under the detached one. The "old" nail plate will stop

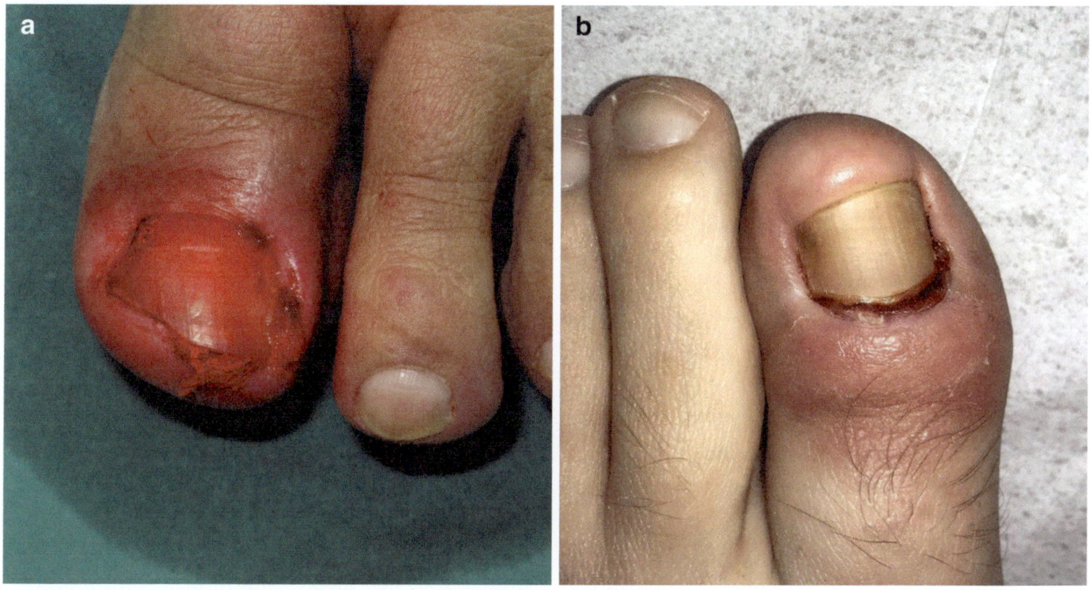

Fig. 33.4 Nail disorders in athletes. Ingrown toenails (onychocryptosis) with inflammation and granulation tissue on the lateral nailfold (**a**) and retronychia, with inflammation and haemorrhage on the proximal nailfold in a ballet dancer (**b**)

or reduce growing and detaches from the nail bed, and a new nail plate will form under it often in association with granulation tissue. Surgical nail avulsion confirms the diagnosis and is therapeutic [17].

Iterative trauma on the nail plate may favour distal and/or lateral onycholysis (detachment of the nail plate from the nail bed, with loss of transparency of the nail plate). It also predisposes to nail dystrophy, with hyperkeratosis, discolouration and thickening of the nail plate, which further disturbs shoe fitting, causes pain and predisposes to onychomycosis.

33.2.5 Piezogenic Papules

Piezogenic papules are multiple small subdermal fat herniations observed in weight-bearing areas, such as the lateral, posterior or medical surface of the heel. They present as small (1–5 mm), skin- or yellow-coloured papules that are usually painless and are most noticeable after standing and prolonged exercise or when pressure is applied to the affected area [18, 19]. Apart from the more frequent pedal piezogenic papules often found in long-distance runners, bilateral and multiple wrist and palmar papules can also be observed in sports where constant pressure around the hand may cause subdermal fat herniation, such as boxing or gymnastics [5].

33.3 Environment-Induced Cutaneous Lesions

Practising winter sports with inadequate protection or in very extreme conditions (high-mountain trekking, ice skaters) or watersports in cold water may induce cold-related dermatoses, like frostbite, chilblains (perniosis), Raynaud phenomenon, *Livedo reticularis*, cold-induced urticaria or cold panniculitis. Chilblains or frostbite affect mainly fingers and toes, but ears and nose can also suffer from cold-induced inflammation. Chilblains and cold-induced panniculitis have also been described in external surface of the arms and thighs in equestrian athletes in France [20]. Apart from adequate protection against the cold and wet, smoking should be discouraged, and calcium channel blockers can be used in more severe cases [21].

Heat exposure occurs mostly from hot treatments for sports lesions and can induce acute burns. *Erythema ab igne* with the typical reticulate erythematous and telangiectatic or pigmented pattern occurs in areas of chronic contact with hot compresses or other sources of heat. Exercising under high temperature with heavy sweating can induce miliaria rubra, presenting with asymptomatic tiny red superficial vesicles that correspond to sweat accumulation within the eccrine ducts and the epidermis. Moreover, exercising in a hot environment may enhance cholinergic urticaria, a transient but highly pruritic reaction that impairs physical activity for a few minutes to more than half an hour and is not often completely prevented by the use of oral H1-anti-histamines (Fig. 33.5).

Exposure to water in susceptible individuals can induce "watersports hands" or aquagenic syringeal acrokeratoderma. This condition affects the palms and soles and is characterized by hyperkeratotic hypopigmented papules and plaques, elicited after submersion in water. Symptoms include a burning pain and a tightening sensation in the palms, as well as hyperhidrosis, but symptoms resolve upon skin drying. It occurs mainly in females and patients with cystic fibrosis, but anyone can be affected [4].

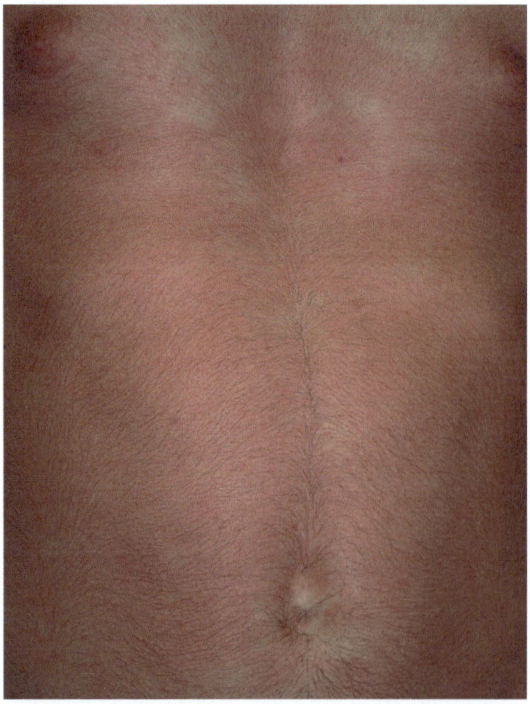

Fig. 33.5 Cholinergic urticaria with highly pruritic confluent erythema on the trunk with many small urticarial papular lesions that develops after increased body temperature during physical training and resolves in less than 30 min

Practising outdoor sports in areas of high ultraviolet (UV) radiation (beaches, sea, mountains, snow) during long sun exposure with no protection can induce an acute sunburn, with well-demarcated painful erythema, eventually with bullae. A sunburn-like reaction—phototoxicity—can occur in athletes with lower phototypes and with vitiligo or those exposed to plants containing phototoxic chemicals (fig trees, *Ruta graveolens*) during outdoor activities or under treatment with topical or systemic phototoxic drugs (tetracyclines, quinolones, amiodarone, phenothiazines, psoralens) [22]. Moreover, athletes can become sensitized and develop eczematous lesions as a manifestation of systemic photoallergy from drugs with known photosensitizing potential (piroxicam, fenofibrate, fluoroquinolones, thiazides) or photoallergic contact dermatitis, mostly from non-steroidal anti-inflammatory drugs (NSAID) used to treat skeletal/muscle pain (ketoprofen, piketoprofen, etofenamate), H1-anti-histamines to treat reactions to mosquito bites (promethazine) or even from UV filters used for their photoprotection (oxybenzone, octocrylene, butyl methoxydibenzoylmethane, cinnamates) [23, 24].

Athletes performing regular outdoor activities under high sun exposure (cycling, marathon running, tennis, sailing) who are chronically exposed to UV light have an increased risk of skin cancer, mostly squamous cell carcinoma but also basal cell carcinoma and melanoma, the latter associated with a poor prognosis. Athletes, particularly from older age groups, repeatedly show little knowledge on the increased skin cancer risk and, consequently, use inadequate or incomplete sun-protective measures [25, 26]. Organizers of competitions in many outdoor sports also demonstrate unawareness of this risk, even in more advanced countries, as they keep performing these activities at hours with high UV index, like cycling tours that usually oblige athletes to cycle at the most harmful hours. Apart from avoiding the hours of the day with higher UV light (11–16 h) and favouring shaded zones, athletes should choose adequate clothing and apply regularly waterproof sunscreens composed mainly of photostable filters. A single application of a sunscreen, particularly in watersports or in situations with heavy sweating, is certainly inadequate as some of the creams will be removed with water/sweating and many filters lose their effective UV protection after some time of irradiation.

33.4 Skin Infections

Cutaneous infections occur in several sports activities, by transfer of the pathogen between athletes by direct contact (wrestling, judo) and by fomites (sharing equipment or facilities) or because the activities modify the skin environment, disturb the protective skin barrier and/or change the skin microbiome favouring cutaneous infections (sweating, occlusion, friction, erosions and blisters). Some bacterial, viral and particularly cutaneous fungal infections have been reported more frequently in athletes [1].

Staphylococcus aureus causes infection of the hair follicles, folliculitis that occur mostly in areas of terminal body hair, of higher sweating and occlusion by equipment or clothing (thighs and buttocks in cyclists), or in athletes who perform regular shaving, therefore facilitating the penetration of the *S. aureus* into the hair follicle. Follicular *S. aureus* infections can sometimes be complicated with furunculosis or carbuncles (agglomeration of furuncules), which can be painful and leave cutaneous depressed scars even if treated correctly or progresses to cutaneous abscesses. These bacterial infections, particularly if caused by methicillin-resistant *S. aureus* (MRSA), can be transferred to other athletes who may develop active lesions or become asymptomatic MSRA carriers, harbouring the bacteria in their nares [11].

Impetigo, with weeping erosions and honey-coloured crusts, can also be transferred among athletes in sports activities with direct skin-to-skin contact (wrestling, judo). Apart from local antiseptics and topical antibiotics, oral antibiotics as well as eradication of *S. aureus* from the nares with local mupirocin may be necessary. Use of soaps with antibacterial agents, skin hydration and breathable clothing are among preventive measures that can be used in recurring lesions.

Prolonged footwear occlusion in athletes with hyperhidrosis can facilitate plantar skin infection by *Kytococcus sedentarius,* formerly known as *Micrococcus sedentarius*. This bacteria degrades keratin of the thicker stratum corneum on the weight-bearing areas of the feet causing small whitish crater-like depressions that may coalesce forming annular lesions—pitted keratolysis or *keratolysis plantare sulcatum* (Fig. 33.6a, b). It is asymptomatic but causes significant malodour. Treatment includes reduction of hyperhidrosis (aluminium salts), topical antibacterials (benzoyl

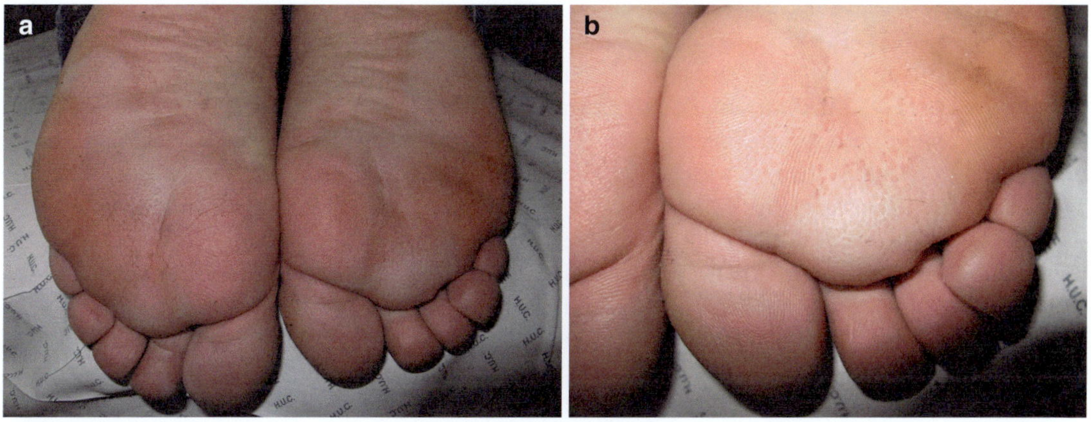

Fig. 33.6 Pitted keratolysis or keratolysis plantare sulcatum (**a**, **b**)

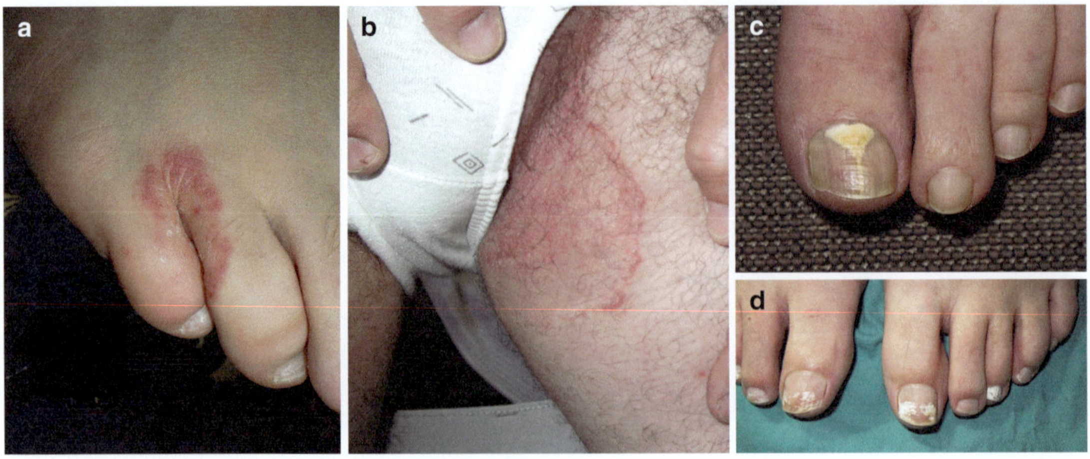

Fig. 33.7 Dermatophyte infections with lesions with an active border in the dorsum of the feet (*tinea pedis*) (**a**) and groin (*tinea cruris*) (**b**) and onychomycosis of the hallux with the yellowish colour of the nail plate progressing from the distal to the proximal nail plate (**c**) and white superficial onychomycosis of several toenails (**d**)

peroxide, erythromycin or clindamycin) and keratolytics (urea or topical retinoids).

Superficial dermatophyte infections, namely, *tinea pedis* and *tinea cruris* (Fig. 33.7a, b) caused mostly by *Trichophyton rubrum* and *T. mentagrophytes*, are more frequent in athletes who share equipment or facilities with no protection (swimming pools or showers with no slippers). *Tinea pedis* presents with different aspects: interdigital tinea with maceration, erythema, scaling and fissures, mostly on the fourth webspace; the vesicular type with pruritic erythema and vesicles in the fingers and soles, which mimics dyshidrotic eczema (pompholyx); and moccasin-type tinea, with slight erythema and scaling in the plantar and lateral skin of the feet—all of them occasionally with a typical active border on the dorsum of the feet (Fig. 33.7a) [11]. Occlusion and sweating of the feet facilitate *tinea pedis* and also toenail onychomycosis (Fig. 33.7c), a situation that can cause severe nail dystrophy and need prolonged oral treatment, except in the rare variant of white superficial onychomycosis (Fig. 33.7d).

Tinea gladiatorum, usually with an active papular and squamous or vesicular border and central lesional clearing, occurs in exposed skin areas due to infection by direct contact among athletes. Epidemics of *tinea gladiatorum* have been described in several teams of judo, wrestling and sumo wrestling, with studies confirming inter-athlete contagiousness, as the same fungus affects the athletes of the same team [1, 27].

Herpes simplex virus (HSV) can cause *herpes gladiatorum,* which develops 3–7 days after contact with an active lesion in another athlete. Grouped vesicles with a tendency to central umbilication occur on an erythematous base and progress to pustules, erosions and crusts before clearing within 10–14 days.

HPV (human papilloma virus) can cause cutaneous lesions transmissible among athletes, particularly plantar warts. These lesions present as firm skin-coloured keratotic papules, often with a clear rim separating them from normal skin and black dots that correspond to dermal vessel thrombosis within the hyperkeratotic verrucae. They may be asymptomatic, but when localized in weight-bearing areas of the body, they cause pain when walking or practising sports activities. Treatment with curettage and topical application of salicylic acid or 5-fluorouracile under occlusion or cryotherapy can resolve most situations.

Molluscum contagiosum, another viral skin infection, is frequently observed in atopic young swimmers as dome-shaped skin-coloured, pink or whitish 1–5 mm asymptomatic papules. They are more frequent in areas of atopic eczema and can also aggravate eczema around them. Curettage or application of a caustic liquid on the top of each lesion may resolve, but recurrence is frequent.

33.5 Allergic Contact Dermatitis

Repeated contact with sports equipment (clothing or devices) usually in association with heat and sweating may enhance liberation of allergens from the equipment to the athlete's skin and induce sensitization and, on further exposure, allergic contact dermatitis (ACD).

Immediate reactions with urticaria or angioedema have been described, mostly related with latex-derived equipment (rubber suits, elastic bandages) [28], but most cases of ACD are due to T-cell-mediated reactions to small chemicals (nickel, rubber chemicals, resins, fragrances, preservatives, etc.). ACD does not occur on first exposure, as previous sensitization to the chemical is necessary to generate enough specific T cells that recognize the chemical. In sensitized individuals, it takes several hours or days after contact with the culprit until lesions become clinically visible. The allergen has to penetrate the skin to be presented by skin epidermal and dermal dendritic cells to the specific T cells that will migrate to the skin and cause dermal and epidermal inflammation.

ACD presents as an acute or subacute eczematous reaction, with pruritic erythema and vesicles or desquamation or with chronic eczema and lichenification in cases of repeated exposure. It is localized in the area of skin contact with the culprit and can even have the form of the contacting object. Acute lesions may resolve within days after eviction of the causative allergen, but topical or systemic steroids are frequently necessary to clear the reaction. ACD can significantly impair sports performance; therefore, it is important to determine the causative allergen and explain how to avoid it, which is the only curative treatment for ACD.

Footwear can be a frequent cause of ACD presenting with lesions that localize mostly on the soles or the dorsum of the feet and spare interdigital spaces (Fig. 33.6a) but can have particular distribution depending on the special footwear piece that causes the reaction. The main allergens are chromium from natural leather, rubber chemicals (thiuram, carbamates, mercapto and thiourea derivatives, *para*-phenylenediamine (PPD) and other *para*-amino compounds) or glues (*p*-tertiary butyl phenol-formaldehyde resin) [9, 11, 29].

Thiourea derivatives in rubber are the main allergens in neoprene-derived swimming and diving suits and other protective equipment, namely, in swim goggles (Fig. 33.8). PPD derivatives from black rubber have been reported as a cause of ACD in hand grips in cycling [30] and swim fins [31]. In these settings ACD can occasionally be followed by long-lasting leukoderma, simulating vitiligo [32].

Recently a new allergen—acetophenone azine—has been identified in shin guards causing ACD in the anterior shins mainly of young football players (Fig. 33.9b) [33]. In occasional situations these athletes have experienced also footwear and widespread dermatitis and leukoderma [34].

Colophony, previously used in the powder/chalk for improving the grip in the gymnasium, was a cause of hand dermatitis and airborne

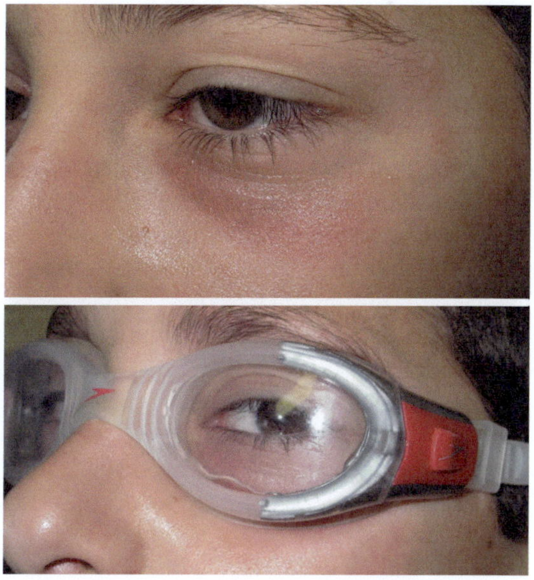

Fig. 33.8 Dermatitis with erythema and inflammation in the areas of contact with the rubber part of the swim goggles

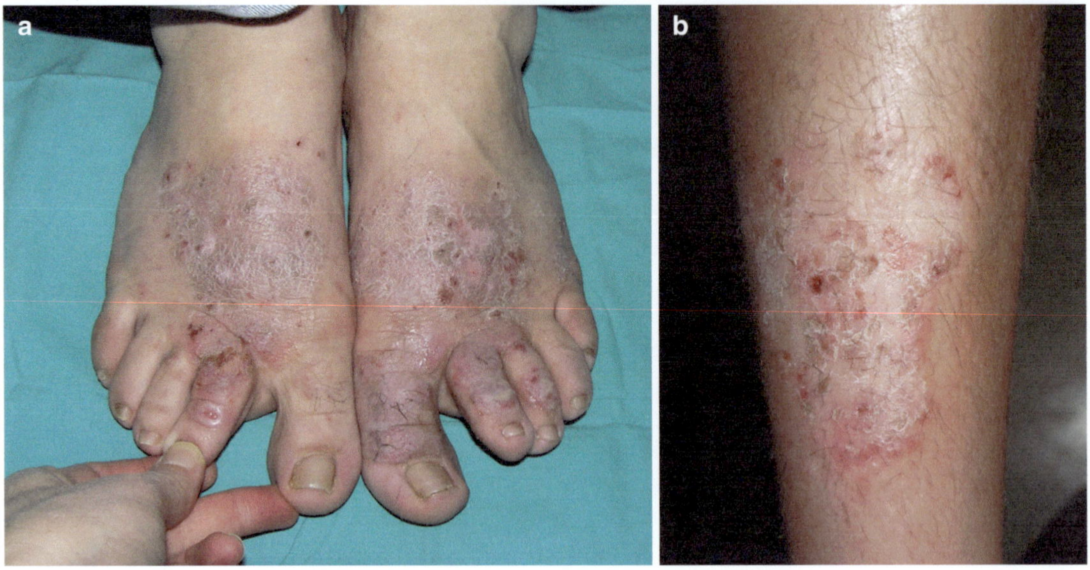

Fig. 33.9 Allergic contact dermatitis from tennis shoes, with chronic eczema involving the dorsum of the feet but sparing the digital webspaces (**a**) and eczema in a young football player localized in the shins and with the format of the shin guards responsible for the lesions (**b**)

eczema in gymnastics. Epoxy resin, used in the manufacture of tennis rackets and as a varnish protection in a billiard cue, was occasionally reported as a cause of hand ACD [35]. Nickel, a very frequent allergen in most populations, was recently found in many tools in the gym, and during 1-h training, it was shown that nickel can accumulate in the skin in amounts able to induce hand eczema [36]. Nickel and other metals have been reported as a cause of ACD particularly in weightlifters, with lesions localized also on the shoulders, arms and neck [11].

Topical drugs, namely, NSAIDs, antibiotics and antiseptics used to treat skin or muscle-skeletal injuries or skin care products used during sports activities, can also cause ACD by direct application on the skin, exposure to contaminated clothing or contact with the treated skin of a colleague [9].

Patch testing with delayed reading (Fig. 33.10a, b) using the baseline and additional series of allergens (rubber chemicals, footwear, topical drugs, sunscreens, cosmetics or fragrances), chosen according to the individual's exposure history, is the mainstay for the etiologic diagnosis of ACD. In many cases, it is very important to patch test additionally with fragments of the equipment or products to which the athlete has been exposed [29], as new allergens may be involved, as recently shown in the case of shin guard dermatitis [33].

33.6 Conclusion

Acute dermatological injuries and sports-related cutaneous diseases need to be prevented, properly recognized and treated in order to prevent impairing athlete's performance. Often a clinical dermatological observation is enough for the correct diagnosis, but additional studies, like patch testing, may be necessary to establish a correct diagnosis and therapy.

The sports medicine doctor/dermatologist should be able to diagnose lesions resulting from the direct effect of sports activities to which the athlete is exposed, but the doctor should be aware of the drugs used for other diseases, therapies used for sports injuries and special diets that may cause or favour skin diseases and could easily go unnoticed (e.g. drug photosensitivity or acne from whey protein). Special attention should be paid to differential diagnosis of sports-induced

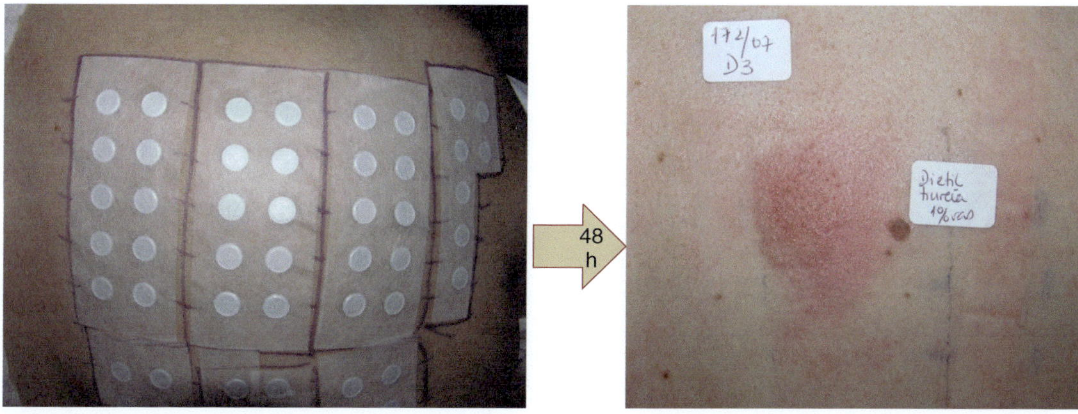

Fig. 33.10 Patch testing technique and a delayed (48 h) positive reaction with erythema, infiltration and papules (++) from diethylthiourea present in a neoprene swimsuit

pigmented cutaneous lesions, namely, the "black heel" or subungueal haematoma that can mimic acromelanoma/subungueal melanoma. Previous skin disease (atopic dermatitis, chronic urticaria) and their aggravation by sports should also be taken into account to advise the patients concerning the more adequate leisure/sports activities.

General doctors, dermatologists and sports medicine doctors should be able to prevent, recognize and treat sports-related/aggravated skin diseases. Doctors should be suspctious and perform correct diagnosis and treatments, in order to allow patients enjoy practising sports free of skin problems.

References

1. Herzog MM, Fraser MA, Register-Mihalik JK, Kerr ZY. Epidemiology of skin infections in men's wrestling: analysis of 2009–2010 through 2013–2014 National Collegiate Athletic Association Surveillance Data. J Athl Train. 2017;52(5):457–63.. http://natajournals.org/doi/10.4085/1062-6050-52.2.16
2. Cohen P. The ball SITE sign: ball sports-induced targetoid erythema in a racquetball player. Dermatol Pract Concept. 2015;5(3):47–52.
3. McClanahan C, Wanat K. Tinea corporis in a wrestling team cheerleader. Int J Women's Dermatol. 2016;2(4):143–4.
4. Kent JB, Statuta SM, Greer KE, MacKnight JM. Watersport hands. Sports Health. 2014;6(4): 360–2.
5. Emer JJ, Sivek R, Marciniak B. Sports dermatology: part 1 of 2 traumatic or mechanical injuries, inflammatory conditions, and exacerbations of pre-existing conditions. J Clin Aesthet Dermatol. 2015;8(4):31–43.
6. Kluger N, Francès P. Mamelon du jogger. Presse Med. 2013;42(6):1066–7.
7. Cohen P. Pool toes: a sports-related dermatosis of swimmers. Int J Dermatol. 2005;44:794–5.
8. Veien N. Clinical features In: Johansen J, Frosch P, Leppoittevin J-P, editors. Contact Dermatitis. 5th ed. Berlin: Springer; 2011. p. 255–303.
9. Kockentiet B, Adams BB. Contact dermatitis in athletes. J Am Acad Dermatol. 2007;56(6):1048–55.
10. Inui S, Itami S. 2 Cases of sumo wrestlers' friction dermatitis. Contact Dermatitis. 2008;58(6):374–5.
11. Farhadian JA, Tlougan BE, Adams BB, Leventhal JS, Sanchez MR. Skin conditions of baseball, cricket, and softball players. Sports Med. 2013;43(7):575–89.
12. Tlougan B, Mancini A, Mandell J, Cohen D, Sanchez M. Skin conditions in figure skaters, ice-hockey players and speed skaters: part I - mechanical dermatoses. Sport Med. 2011;41(9):709–19.
13. Simonart T. Acne and whey protein supplementation among bodybuilders. Dermatology. 2012;225(3):256–8.
14. Tammaro A, Magri F, Moliterni E, Parisella F, Mondello M, Persechino S. An uncommon localization of black heels in a free climbing instructor. Int Wound J. 2018;15(2):313–5.
15. Rubegni P, Feci L, Fimiani M. Talon Noir: utility of dermoscopy for differential diagnosis with respect to other acral skin growths. G Ital Dermatol Venerol. 2012;147(1):133–4.
16. Descamps V, Claessens YE, Doumenc B. Skin manifestations in ultramarathon runners: experience in the Marathon des Sables 2014. Br J Dermatol. 2017;177(2):562–3.
17. Campos M, Santos A. Retronychia: clinical diagnosis and surgical treatment. BMJ Case Rep. 2017;2(2017):bcr2016218758.

18. Rocha Bde O, Fernandes JD, Prates FV de O. Piezogenic pedal papules. An Bras Dermatol. 2015;90(6):928–9.
19. Turkmani MG. Piezogenic pedal papules treated successfully with deoxycholic acid injection. JAAD Case Rep. 2018;4(6):582–3.
20. Kluger N, Marty L, Bourseau-Quetier C, Blum M, Camus M. Perniosis/cold panniculitis in French equestrians: four cases. Int J Dermatol. 2016;55(12):e618–20.
21. Tlougan B, Mancini A, Mandell J, Cohen D, Sanchez M. kin conditions in figure skaters, ice-hockey players and speed skaters: part II - cold-induced, infectious and inflammatory dermatoses. Sports Med. 2011;41(11):967–84.
22. Gonçalo M, Giménez-Arnau AM. Drug photosensitivity. In: Katsambas A, Lotti T, Dessinioti C, D'Erme A, editors. European handbook of dermatological treatments. 3rd ed. Berlin: Springer; 2015. p. 233–51.
23. Gonçalo M, Ruas E, Figueiredo A, Gonçalo S. Contact and photocontact sensitivity to sunscreens. Contact Dermatitis. 1995;33(4):278–80.
24. Kerr AC, Ferguson J, Ibbotson SH, Dawe RS, Haylett AK, Rhodes LE, et al. A European multicentre photopatch test study. Br J Dermatol. 2012;166(5):1002–9.
25. Christoph S, Cazzaniga S, Hunger RE, Naldi L, Borradori L, Oberholzer PA. Ultraviolet radiation protection and skin cancer awareness in recreational athletes: a survey among participants in a running event. Swiss Med Wkly. 2016;146(March):w14297.
26. Ally M, Swetter S, Hirotsu K, Gordon J, Kim D, Wysong A, et al. Promoting sunscreen use and sunprotective practices in NCAA athletes: impact of SUNSPORT educational intervention for student-athletes, athletic trainers, and coaches. J Am Acad Dermatol. 2018;78(2):289–92.
27. Sakata Y, Ushigami T, Anzawa K, Mochizuki T. Molecular epidemiology of Trichophyton tonsurans, the causative dermatophyte of the epidemic of tinea gladiatorum in Japan between 2011 and 2015. Jpn J Infect Dis. 2018;71:140–4. https://www.jstage.jst.go.jp/article/yoken/advpub/0/advpub_JJID.2017.449/_article.
28. Buzzacott P, Dolen WK, Chimiak J. Case report: acute facial swelling in a recreational technical diver. Physiol Rep. 2017;5(7):5–8.
29. Marzario B, Burrows D, Skotnicki S. Contact dermatitis to personal sporting equipment in youth. J Cutan Med Surg. 2016;20(4):323–6.
30. Ozkaya E, Elinç-Aslan M. Black rubber sensitization by bicycle handgrips in a child with palmar hyperhidrosis. Dermatitis. 2011;22(4):E10–1.
31. Seyfarth F, Krautheim A, Schliemann S, Elsner P. Sensitization to para-amino compounds in swim fins in a 10-year-old boy. J Dtsch Dermatol Ges. 2009;7(9):770–2.
32. Sakuragi Y, Sawada Y, Nakamura M. Leukoderma following allergic contact dermatitis caused by the silicone component silprene-30A/B in swimming goggles. Contact Dermatitis. 2017;77(6):418–9.
33. Raison-Peyron N, Bergendorff O, Bourrain JL, Bruze M. Acetophenone azine: a new allergen responsible for severe contact dermatitis from shin pads. Contact Dermatitis. 2016;75(2):106–10.
34. Raison-Peyron N, Bergendorff O, Du-Thanh A, Bourrain J, Bruze M. Two new cases of severe allergic contact dermatitis caused by acetophenone azine. Contact Dermatitis. 2017;76(6):380–1.
35. Gonçalo S, Gonçalo M, Matos J, Marçues C. Contact dermatitis from a billiard cue. Contact Dermatitis. 1992;26(4):263.
36. Gumulka M, Matura M, Lidén C, Kettelarij JAB, Julander A. Nickel exposure when working out in the gym. Acta Derm Venereol. 2015;95(2):247–9.

Oral Health

34

Silvia Maria Rocha Piedade Damasceno, Marly Kimie Sonohara Gonzalez, Renata Bastos Del Hoyo Fernandes, and Vera Lucia Gramuglia

34.1 Background

For many years in sports, oral cavity care was limited to the prevention of traumatic lesions. The first records of actions involving odontological practice and sports date back to 1891 when mouthguards were utilized to protect British boxers' teeth [1].

Over the years, knowledge on the close relationship between oral health and general health has changed the focus and attention given to the oral cavity and its clinical manifestations. Besides contributing to an athlete's well-being, life quality, and self-esteem, a healthy mouth is essential to ensure efficient mastication and the ideal use of nutrients, resulting in energy to supply the high demands of trainings and competitions, positively reflecting on athletic performance.

Since the 19th Olympic Games in Mexico, in 1968, it has been reported that elite athletes present poor oral health conditions. Unfortunately, this clinical condition is still true nowadays, and a rising increase in the amount of dental care is mostly observed in main sports events [2]. Although oral problems are still part of elite athletes' reality, in amateur sports [3], this health condition tends to be even worse, partially due to the athlete's lack of orientation and lower economic condition.

During the 30th Olympic Games in London, in 2012, odontological care represented 30% of the total treatments in the health area, and it was only lower than the percentage of treatments related to the musculoskeletal system [4]. The athletes presented low oral health levels mainly related to periodontal diseases (gingivitis 76% and periodontitis 15%), dental caries (55%), dental erosion (45%), pain and discomfort in the oral mucosa (12%), and pericoronitis (9.9%), besides orofacial traumas (18%). These rates resulted in a negative impact on the athletes' quality of life (28%) and training or performance (18%).

In the 31st Olympiads in Rio de Janeiro, in 2016, a record of 1600 odontological treatments, besides 600 image exams and the making of 350 mouthguards [5], was reported. One important consideration is that the treatment of oral diseases and alterations is costly and a lot of times it is not affordable to a great number of athletes. Therefore, many of them take the opportunity to assess their oral health and treat preexisting oral problems using the facilities of the Olympic Games and other major sports events.

S. M. R. P. Damasceno (✉)
Odontology Center, Maringá, Parana, Brazil

M. K. S. Gonzalez
Odontology Center, Rosario, Santa Fe, Argentina

R. B. Del Hoyo Fernandes . V. L. Gramuglia
Odontology Center, Botucatu, Sao Paulo, Brazil

S. Rocha Piedade et al. (eds.), *The Sports Medicine Physician*,
https://doi.org/10.1007/978-3-030-10433-7_34

Considering that dental caries and periodontal diseases are preventable and that certain oral manifestations may be related to systemic diseases and conditions, the importance of the athletes' periodical oral health assessment is undeniable.

34.2 Seven Oral Health Assessment Points in Athletes (7 OHAPA)

In athletes, the oral health assessment periodicity is flexible according to the intensity of the training and competition schedule because it helps monitor an athlete's global health. Thus, for elite athletes, the oral health assessment must be carried out every 3 months or anticipated when it is necessary.

It is important to point out that the systematic assessment of an athlete's oral health allows uniformity and reproducibility to the process. In our clinical practice, we consider Seven Oral Health Assessment Points in Athletes (**7 OHAPA**), because they cover the entire oral cavity topography (Fig. 34.1): extra oral region (1st), lips (2nd), teeth (3rd), gingiva (gums) (4th), tongue and oropharynx (5th), other mucosae (6th), and saliva (7th).

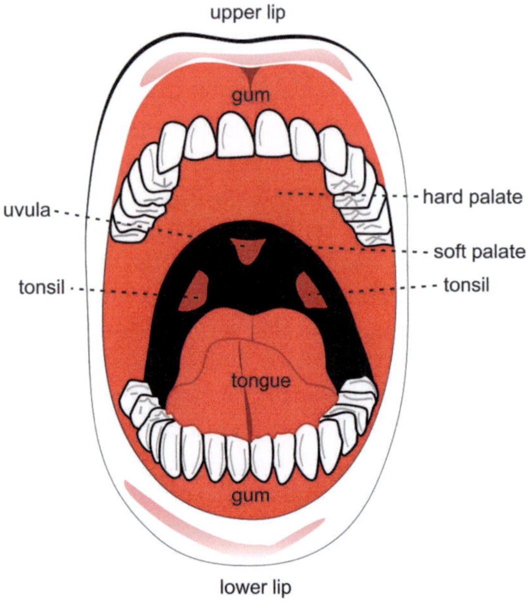

Fig. 34.1 Oral cavity topography, showing the structures of points 2–6

34.2.1 Extra Oral Region (First OHAPA)

34.2.1.1 Face and Neck

When examining the extra oral region, the presence of an increased volume in the medium and/or inferior third of the face can be related to different clinical disorders involving teeth, salivary glands, and lymph nodes.

Acute infectious dental abscess can evolve to other areas and result in posterior facial edema.

Alterations of greater salivary glands (SG) can have inflammatory, infectious, obstructive, or neoplastic nature. The infectious processes of SG are frequently caused by bacteria and viruses; present quick volumetric increase, pain, and salivary secretion reduction; and most of the times affect the parotid gland. Malignant tumors of SG represent only 3% of head and neck tumors, but 95% of palpable nodes in the parotid region have tumoral origin [6].

The examination and palpation of parotid, sublingual, submandibular, and cervical lymph nodes usually make easy to tell apart an inflammatory/infectious process (pain, heat, elasticity, and preservation of the shape with hyperemia on the skin) from a neoplastic one (painless, asymmetric shape, and loss of elasticity). In infectious processes of the oral cavity, the submandibular and sublingual chains are the most impaired (Fig. 34.2).

34.2.1.2 Temporomandibular Joint

A practical and functional assessment of temporomandibular joints (TMJs) can be done by placing two folded fingers (index and medium) at the proximal interphalangeal joints in the mouth. If there is a limitation to mouth opening, an athlete will not be able to perform this test [7] (Fig. 34.3). The limitation and deviation of mandibular movement as well as pain in TMJ may be a signal of temporomandibular disorders (TMDs).

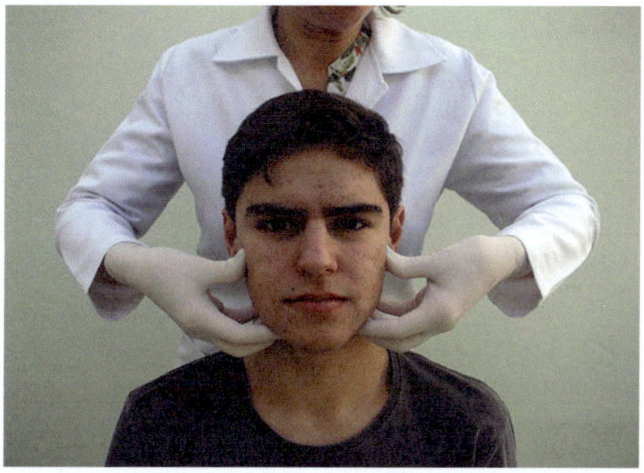

Fig. 34.2 Examination and palpation of submandibular and sublingual lymph nodes

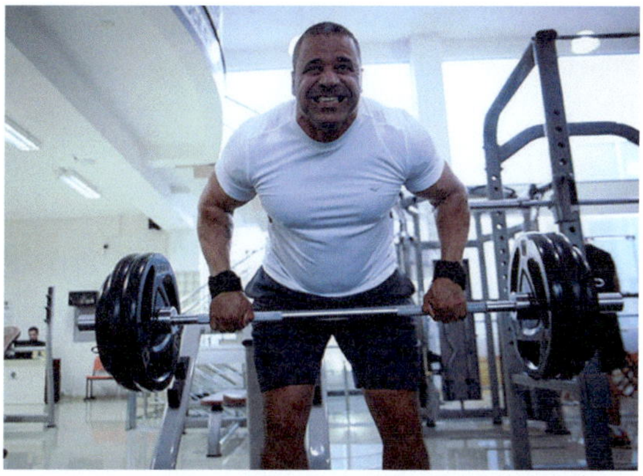

Fig. 34.4 Facial effort expression during weightlifting

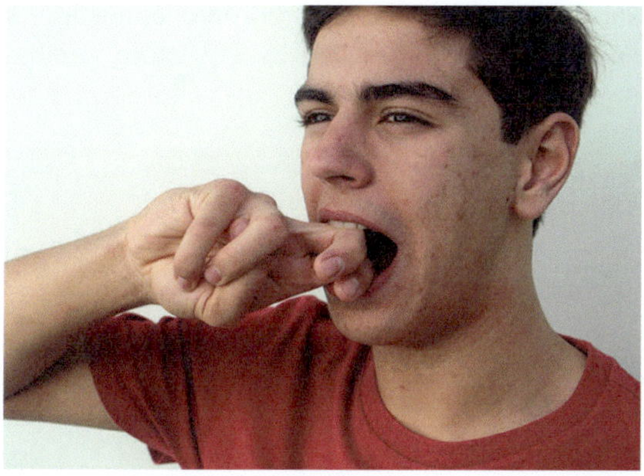

Fig. 34.3 Joint movement test showing an athlete's normal mouth opening

Athletes belong to the risk group for the development of TMDs because they are likely to have physical traumas in the middle third and inferior part of the face, and often live in situations involving anxiety, depression, or stress, which are common to the competitive environment, mainly when an athlete is recovering from lesions (convalescence) [8]. In this context, bruxism is one of the most frequently observed clinical problems. It is characterized by repetitive nonfunctional mandibular movements, mainly regulated by the central nervous system [9] and influenced by factors such as stress, anxiety, and traumas, besides drugs and diseases [10]. Bruxism causes microtraumas that can result in abrasion, cracks, and fractures of teeth and fillings besides muscular discomfort.

Another clinical picture that involves TMDs is the facial effort expression. Under this condition, athletes increase the frequency of involuntary mandibular clenching during vigorous physical exercising which involves muscles from the legs, arms, and back [11]. This involuntary masseter contraction has a positive correlation with cardiac frequency [12] (Fig. 34.4). In weightlifting, it is also observed that voluntary mandibular clenching increases body stability [13].

34.2.1.3 Breathing Pattern

Oral breathing (OB) pattern has been associated with posture alterations. Forward head posture in relation to shoulders, associated with elongated face, dark undereye circles, and lack of labial sealing, is a characteristic observed in individuals that use the oral cavity as their main respiratory route.

When OB is established, the most common oral alterations are malocclusion (posterior crossbite and anterior open bite), xerostomia, and gingivitis in upper anterior teeth as well as a greater risk of dental caries. Besides altering posture, OB reduces the diaphragmatic work, limits thoracic expansion, and decreases pulmonary ventilation, negatively impacting on oxygen absorption capacity and intake to produce energy during physical exercises [14]. Early treatment is fundamental especially for younger athletes, because it allows to easily establish physiological breathing through the nose as well as the harmonious facial growth, free from physiological and psychosocial discomfort of OB. On the other hand, in an adult athlete, a multidisciplinary approach is needed for the oral breather syndrome.

34.2.2 Lips (Second OHAPA)

Color alteration in lips can signal nutritional deficiencies, anemia or low blood pressure (pale), heart and lung diseases or hypothermia (purple), and liver disease (yellowish). In red lips—as well as in the palate, gingiva, and other mucosae—hyperpigmented lesions are generally benign (e.g., physiological melanoplasia) and can be related to diseases (e.g., Addison's disease) and use of medications (e.g., ketoconazole), or can be neoplastic (e.g., malignant melanoma), to name but a few [15].

34.2.2.1 Cheilitis

Angular cheilitis is a unilateral or bilateral chronic lesion with painful fissures in labial commissure and can be associated with atrophy, ulceration, candidiasis, and bacterial infection (Fig. 34.5a, b). Nutritional deficiencies, lip biting or lip licking habits, and loss of the vertical dimension of occlusion, which predisposes to saliva accumulation in labial commissures, are common risk factors for the development of angular cheilitis.

Actinic cheilitis is a potentially malignant condition in which lip redness, mainly in the inferior one, presents atrophy, pale areas, ulcerations, or crusting with characteristic blur demarcation of the lip, with or without pain. In sports in which there is chronic exposure to sunlight, pale-skin athletes are more predisposed to it [16].

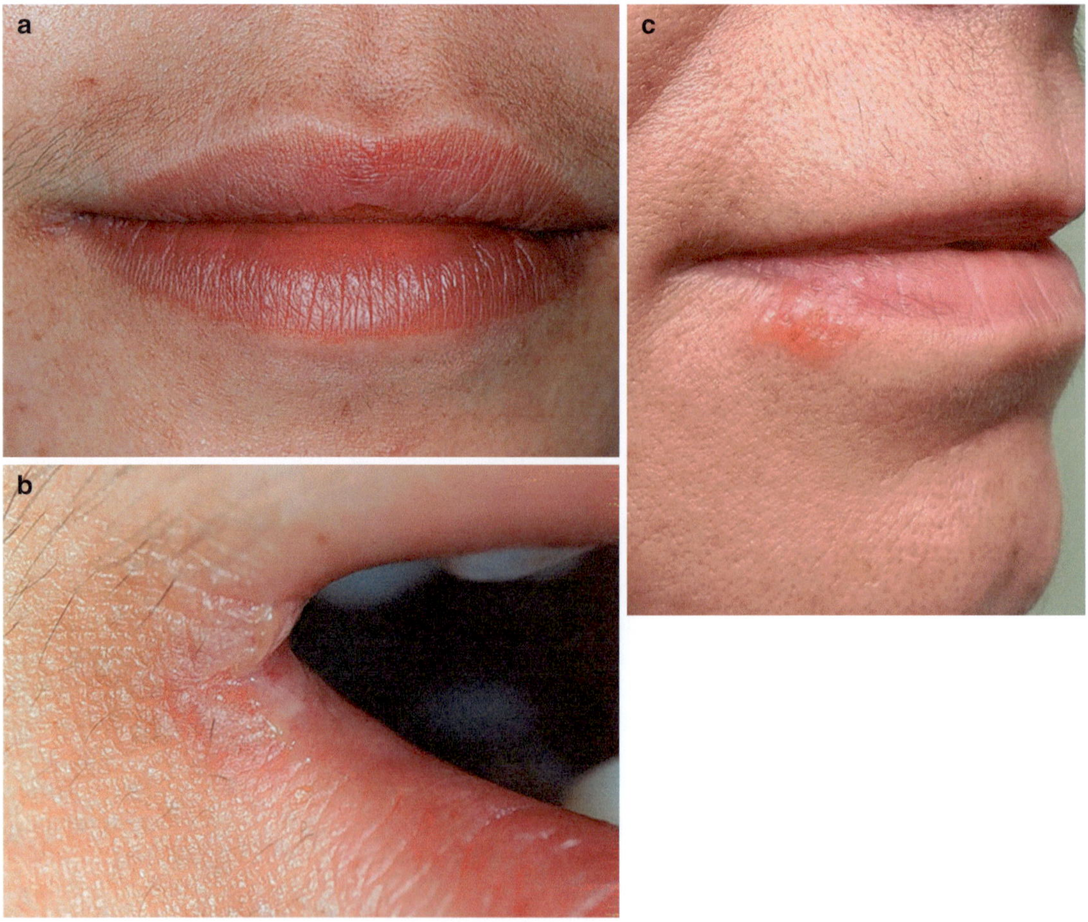

Fig. 34.5 Right unilateral angular cheilitis (**a**) with proximal view (**b**). Recurrent herpes simplex with vesicle and beginning of crust formation (**c**) on the border between lower lip and skin

34.2.2.2 Ulcers

Ulcers are the most common lesions of the oral mucosa. Painful ulcers are generally associated with mechanical, chemical, or thermal trauma.

34.2.2.3 Aphthous Ulcer

Recurrent aphthous ulcer (RAS), with an incidence of 20–60% [17], is among the most common non-traumatic ulcers in the oral cavity. It is characterized by the emergence of one or more small and very painful shallow ulcers in the nonkeratinized mucosa of the lips (also in the tongue, jugal mucosa, and mouth floor) and is frequently white or yellow with reddish borders and oval shape. They heal themselves spontaneously after some days and are recurrent. The bigger lesions reach up to 3 cm and are less prevalent and more persistent. The predisposing factors are deficiency of iron, vitamin B12, and folic acid; and the triggering factors are hormonal alterations, psychological stress, and immune system depression [18].

34.2.2.4 Painless Ulcers

Painless ulcers can indicate chronic trauma (e.g., parafunctional habits or poorly adapted prosthesis), syphilitic cancer, oral squamous cell carcinoma (OSCC), and non-Hodgkin lymphoma, among others [19]. OSCC represents 90% of malignant oral neoplasias, and the lower lip is one of the most affected areas [20]. This kind of ulcer is painless, hard, and white or red, does not heal [21], and is frequently associated with actinic cheilitis [20].

34.2.2.5 Herpes Simplex

Vesicles in the lip vermilion and the border with the skin frequently show recurrent herpes simplex (Fig. 34.5c), also frequent in the gingiva and palate. The primary infection by herpes simplex virus type 1 (HSV-1) usually occurs during childhood, followed by a latent period. In an athlete, the exposure to sunlight, wind, cold, physical or mental stress, and anxiety are factors associated with HSV-1 reactivation. Vesicles break up forming crusts that spontaneously heal from 7 to 14 days without leaving scars. Recurrences happen once or twice a year and are more frequent and serious in AIDS due to immunosuppression [22].

34.2.2.6 Labial Edema

Labial edema can be a result of immunological mechanisms (hereditary angioedema) and non-immunological ones (allergy), among others [23]. In cases of anaphylaxis, immediate therapeutic intervention is necessary.

Benign labial lesions may cause a dryness sensation, pain, itching, and others. On the other hand, neoplastic processes may be asymptomatic with discrete alterations. Labial lesions, including the malignant ones, are treatable when diagnosed early.

34.2.3 Teeth (Third OHAPA)

During tooth examination, it is essential to observe alterations in their integrity, biofilm stagnation (bacterial plaque), presence of calculus (tartar), and dental losses while evaluating the level of an athlete's awareness on the importance of oral health hygiene and maintenance.

34.2.3.1 Oral Hygiene and Carbohydrate Intake

Poor oral hygiene combined with high carbohydrate intake, which is commonly associated to athletes' nutrition, causes the proliferation of cariogenic microorganisms and formation of dental caries (Fig. 34.6a). During their progression, provoked pain (by hot, cold, sweet, and acid foods) may occur and evolve to spontaneous pain (pulpitis) and pulp necrosis, resulting in chronic or acute infections. In chronic infections, the formation of fistula in the region of the alveolar mucosa is usually observed, whereas in acute infections periapical abscess and posterior edema in the medium and/or inferior third of the face are formed. In the long run, the lack of dental caries treatment makes mastication and the ideal utilization of nutrients difficult by the athlete, increasing the risk of dental losses, occlusal maladjustments, and functional, aesthetic, and psychological damages, besides being a risk factor for systemic diseases.

34.2.3.2 Sports Drinks

Commercially available sports drinks have pH lower than the one considered critical (5.2–5.5)

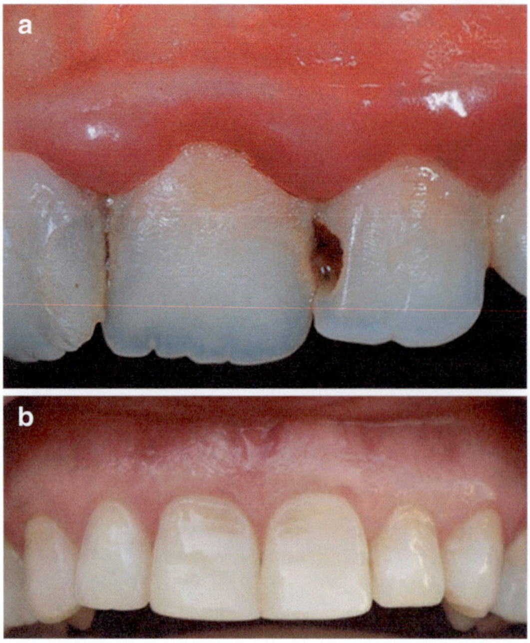

Fig. 34.6 Dental caries in upper lateral incisor and biofilm stagnation associated with chronic gingivitis (**a**). Dental corrosion in vestibular surface of upper central incisors due to consumption of sports drinks (**b**)

for dental enamel and can have a corrosive effect (erosion) on this surface [24] (Fig. 34.6b). A study carried out with college athletes in Ohio, USA [25], reported that 36.5% of the athletes presented dental corrosion and that 91.8% of the athletes with corrosion used to drink sports drinks. The dental corrosion risk is likely to be greater when associated with salivary flow reduction, observed after long exercising [26], due to the limitation of lubricant protective functions of saliva. In water sports, dental corrosion can be related to the frequent long activity in pools with chlorine water when pH monitoring is not adequate [27].

34.2.4 Gingiva (Fourth OHAPA)

34.2.4.1 Gingivitis

Chronic gingivitis affects more than 90% of the population, is painless with red swollen appearance, and presents gingival bleeding during dental brushing. In an examination, normal gingiva present pale pink color, scalloped contour, and absence of bleeding, whereas in periodontal diseases (gingivitis and periodontitis), a chronic bacterial inflammatory process in the tissues that surround the teeth is observed as a response to biofilm accumulation (bacterial plaque) [28].

If poor oral hygiene conditions persist, chronic gingivitis can evolve to periodontitis which is an infectious disease associated with predominantly gram-negative bacteria, mainly in the presence of a susceptible host (Fig. 34.7a). In the periodontal disease, the accumulation of suppuration may lead the formation of abscesses that cause gingival edema, pain, and dental mobility [29] (Fig. 34.7b). When a periodontal abscess occurs during competitions, it may affect the athlete's concentration and performance [30].

34.2.4.2 Pericoronaritis

Pericoronaritis is an acute infection around the crown of the third molars (Fig. 34.7c). It is characterized by pain, edema, and abscesses in the retromolar region and, in more severe cases, trismus, fever, and dysphagia with mastication difficulty. It is highly prevalent in young athletes from 17 to 26 years old [31] and represented 9.9% of the odontological treatments carried out during the 30th Olympic Games in London, in 2012 [4].

34.2.4.3 Necrotizing Ulcerative Gingivitis

Necrotizing ulcerative gingivitis (NUG) is a specific acute periodontal disease, commonly observed in younger athletes [28]. It presents papillae necrosis, pain, bleeding, and halitosis associated with predisposing factors that alter the individual's response such as stress, nutritional deficiencies, and immunological system disorders, particularly HIV infection [32], smoking, preexisting gingivitis, and trauma [33].

34.2.4.4 Hyperplasia and Bleeding

Gingival hyperplasia and bleeding are frequently observed as local inflammatory response to the presence of biofilm (periodontal disease). When these alterations occur in the absence of biofilm, associated with petechiae and ulcerations, they may represent the first signs of leu-

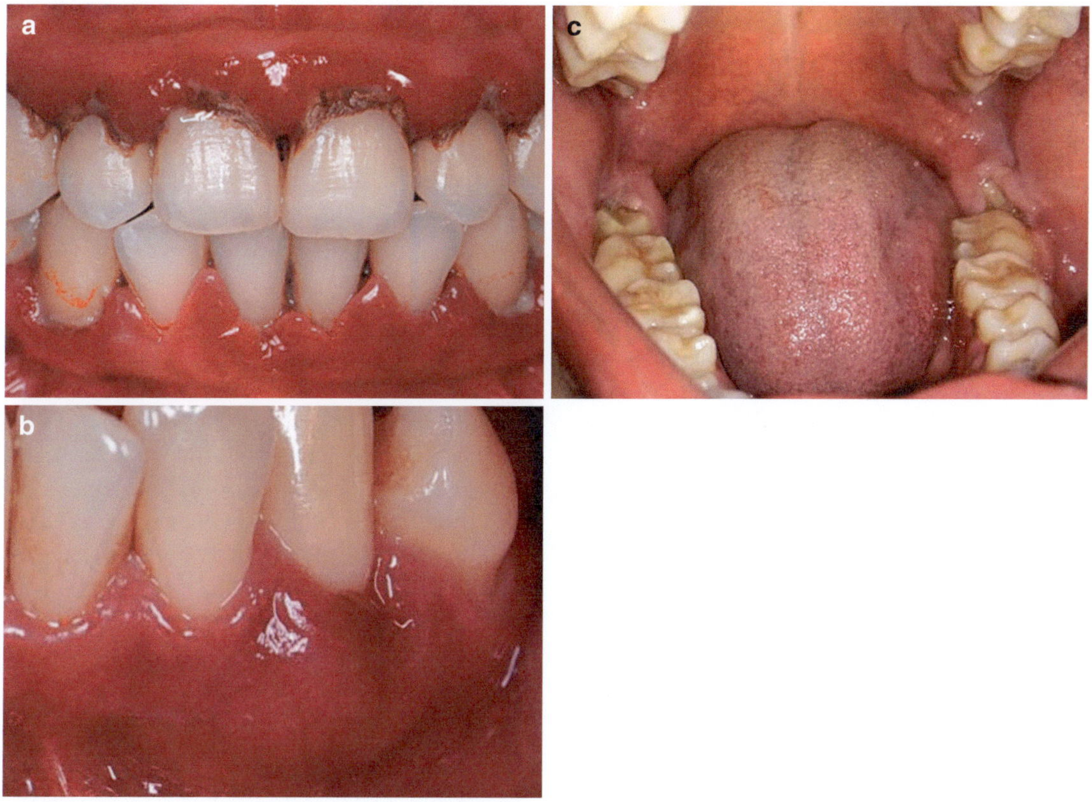

Fig. 34.7 Chronic periodontitis in the anterior region with the presence of calculus and biofilm (**a**). Acute periodontal abscess between lower left lateral incisor and canine (**b**). Pericoronitis in the region of the lower right and left third molars (**c**)

kemia [34]. The early leukemia diagnosis is important because it determines favorable prognostics.

34.2.5 Tongue and Oropharynx (Fifth OHAPA)

The examination of the tongue includes the dorsum, ventral surface, and lateral edges. When the tongue is sticking out, other parts of the oropharynx (soft palate, uvula, tonsils, and lateral and posterior part of the throat) can be examined.

The presence of pus in the tonsils and oropharynx associated with palpable painful cervical lymph nodes indicates bacterial pharyngotonsillitis. It is important to point out that rheumatic fever is a complication of pharyngotonsillitis caused by Group A beta hemolytic streptococcus and that may result in heart valve lesions, mainly in children and teenagers. This sequela is a risk factor for infectious endocarditis in the occurrence of bacteremias that can come from oral infection focus, invasive odontological procedures, or recurrent pharyngotonsillitis, among others. Therefore, a detailed anamnesis has an important role in the treatment because it may signal the need of preventive measures, such as antibiotic therapy, in patients with a history of repeated throat infections who are submitted to odontological procedures.

The tongue ventral surface and the mouth floor can be examined when the tip of the tongue is raised toward the palate, whereas the tongue root and lateral edges are examined with right-to-left sideways movement.

A scalloped tongue presents tooth marks on the edges and may indicate parafunctional habits (e.g., clenching bruxism).

Halitosis and keratin accumulation on the tongue dorsum are generally associated with poor oral hygiene, xerostomia, and others. Clinically, keratin accumulation looks like a white-yellowish plaque (coated tongue—Fig. 34.8a), and when hyperplasia of filiform papillae occurs (hairy tongue—Fig. 34.8b), the plaque becomes brown or black, and it is commonly associated with smoking.

Color variations from pale to intense red, almost purple, with papillae atrophy, sensitivity increase, and taste alteration can be related to nutritional deficiencies, anemias, and immunosuppression. In these cases, the development of oral candidiasis, an opportunistic fungal infection, usually occurs. Oral candidiasis is also commonly associated with other debilitating diseases such as AIDS.

Benign migratory glossitis is a common lesion among non-smoking allergic youngsters with unknown etiology. It presents atrophic reddish areas and white edges that migrate to the dorsum or the lateral region of the tongue and is asymptomatic or eventually painful [19] (Fig. 34.8c).

Hairy leukoplakia, related to the presence of Epstein-Barr virus (EBV), is a benign, usually asymptomatic lesion and more frequently occurs in the tongue edge, unilaterally or bilaterally. It looks like a white non-scrapable plaque with vertical rugged hyperplastic pattern and well-defined edges. It is almost exclusively related to HIV infection and observed in 16% of the infected individuals [35].

Idiopathic leukoplakia presents white, asymptomatic, non-scrapable plaque and is the most common potentially malignant lesion in the oral cavity (potential of malignant transformation of 5–10%) [19] (Fig. 34.8d).

34.2.6 Other Mucosae (Sixth OHAPA)

Besides the lips, gingiva, retromolar area, tongue, oropharynx, and mouth floor, the examination of oral mucosae also includes the alveolar and jugal mucosae and hard palate, which can reveal many other alterations besides the ones described before.

Crohn's disease has specific oral manifestations such as cobblestone mucosa (rigid plaques with hyperplastic, swollen, and cracked appearance) in the oral and palate mucosae [36]; hardened lesions like tag, generally in the labial vestibule and retromolar region; deep linear ulcerations; mucogingivitis; edema; and labial fissures, besides other non-specific lesions such as RAS, which is its most common oral manifestation. Oral lesions in Crohn's disease have a prevalence of 0.5–20% [37]. The oral symptoms precede the intestinal ones in 60% of the individuals [38].

Squamous cell papilloma, condylomata acuminata, and oral verrucas are the most prevalent lesions caused by human papilloma virus (HPV) in individuals with HIV/AIDS [39]. They are painless, exophytic, white, and rigid lesions with well-defined borders [40] and similar clinical appearance. They occur in any region of the mucosa, preferably where epithelium keratinization looks like the skin (e.g., hard palate and gingiva).

Kaposi's sarcoma corresponds to a malignant vascular neoplasia represented by maculae or nodes that vary from red to blue and mostly frequently observed on the palate, gingiva, and tongue dorsum [41]. It occurs in approximately 8% of individuals infected by HIV [35] and is considered the neoplasia that defines AIDS [18].

Non-Hodgkin lymphoma is heterogeneous with tissue masses with or without ulceration and tissue necrosis in which immunodeficiency is an important risk factor. The most affected regions are tonsils, palate, and gingiva [19]. It is the second most frequent neoplasia (4%) in individuals with HIV/AIDS [35], and its occurrence indicates a late complication of the disease.

34.2.7 Saliva (Seventh OHAPA)

Saliva is a biological fluid of compounds produced in the salivary glands (alpha amylase and immunoglobulin A [IgA-s]) and compounds disseminated in the plasma (water, metabolites, hormones, electrolytes, and proteins); its production and compo-

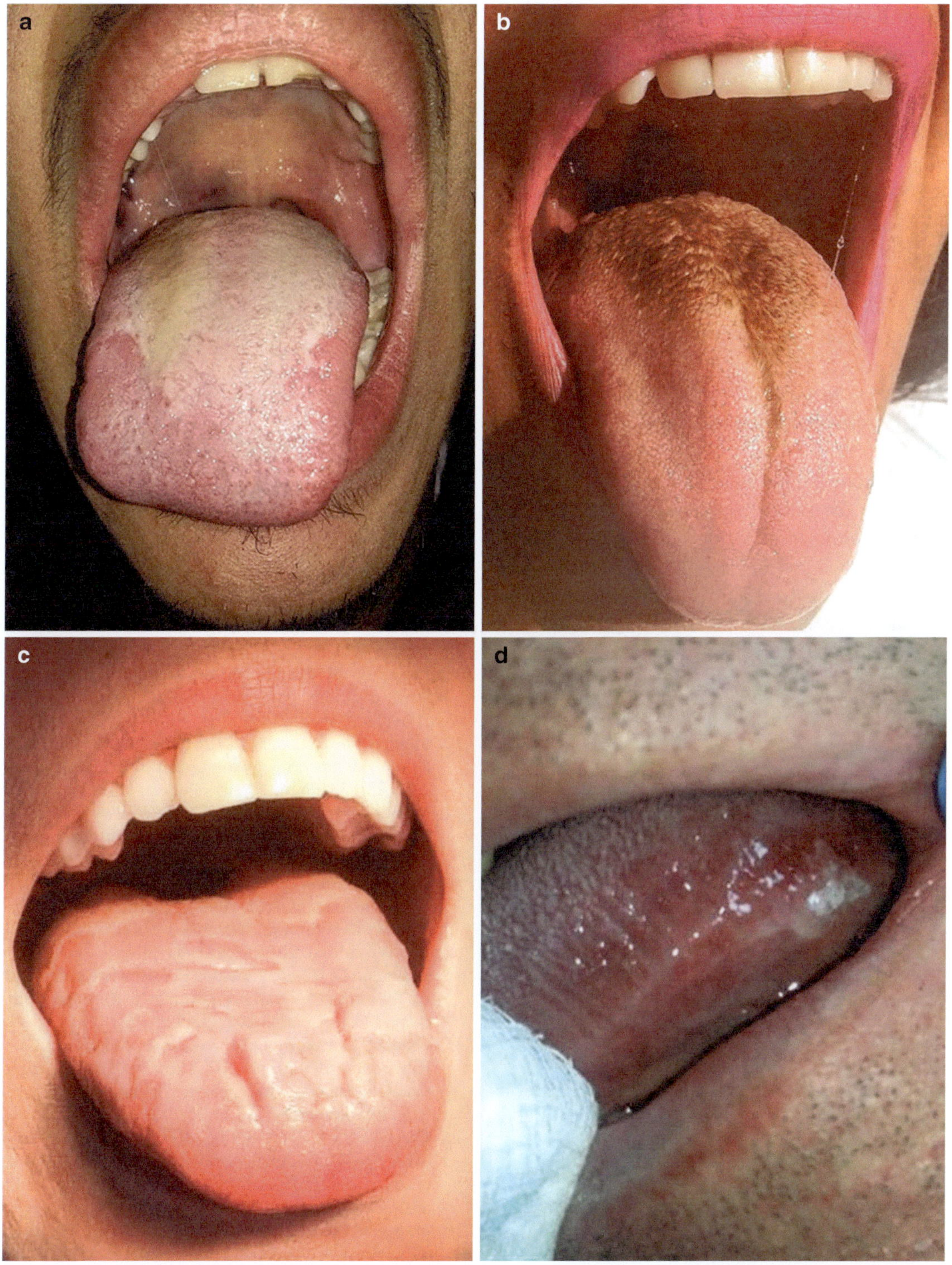

Fig. 34.8 Alterations in the tongue dorsum: coated tongue (**a**), hairy tongue (**b**), and benign migratory glossitis (**c**). Idiopathic leukoplakia on the lateral edge of the tongue with carcinoma diagnosis *in situ* (**d**)

sition depend on the activity of the sympathetic and parasympathetic nervous systems [42].

Sports activities cause systemic biochemical alterations that modify the composition of certain saliva components, which is a reflex of the physiological response of several systems. Thus, saliva analysis is a promising tool for diagnosis in sports (e.g., doping), monitoring athletes, while it helps a sports physician to evaluate and define training strategies as well as the appropriate exercise load and frequency, directly influencing an athlete's health and performance [43].

Therefore, saliva analysis may help identify positive potentially adverse clinical conditions like the ones described below:

- The concentrations of cortisol and testosterone in the saliva are related to physiological indexes of sports performance.
- Salivary alpha amylase is considered a biomarker of physical stress because under this condition their levels increase considerably [44].
- Reduction of IgA-s concentrations during and soon after intense exercising may make athletes more susceptible to infections. If the athletes are well conditioned, this variable becomes normal after a 48-h rest. IgA-s is an immunoglobulin that protects the upper respiratory tract, and a follow-up of its levels may help prevent these infections during competition and game periods [45].

Take-Home Messages

- Periodical assessment of athletes' oral health is fundamental to evaluate and monitor oral hygiene quality and also to verify the presence of local oral lesions and secondary oral lesions caused by nutritional deficiencies and systemic diseases.
- **The seven OHAPA** allows uniformity and reproducibility to the process because they approach the whole oral cavity topography adequately and consistently.
- Making athletes' aware that the oral health quality directly interferes in the athletic performance is a key point of this process.

References

1. Reed RV. Origin and early history of the dental mouthpiece. Br Dent J. 1994;176:478–80.
2. Needleman I, Ashley P, Fine P, Haddad F, Loosemore M, de Medici A, et al. Consensus statement: oral health and elite sport performance. Br Dent J. 2014;217:587–90.
3. Rosa AF, Costa SB, Silva PRS, Roxo CDMN, Machado GS, Teixeira AAA, et al. Estudo descritivo de alterações odontológicas verificadas em 400 jogadores de futebol. Rev Bras Med Esporte. 1999;5:55–8.
4. Needleman I, Ashley P, Petri A, Fortune F, Turner W, Jones J, et al. Oral health and impact on performance of athletes participating in the London 2012 Olympic Games: a cross-sectional study. Br J Sports Med. 2013;47:1054–8.
5. Manir M. Nações de IDH mais baixo aproveitam a policlínica do Rio-2016. 2016. http://esportes.estadao.com.br. Accessed 7 May 2018.
6. Condutas do Inca. Salivary gland tumors. Rev Bras Cancerologia. 2002;48:9–12.
7. Sailors ME. Evaluation of sports-related temporomandibular dysfunctions. J Athl Train. 1996;31:346–50.
8. Badel T, Jerolimov V, Pandurić J. Dental/orofacial trauma. Kinesiology. 2007;39:97–105.
9. Lobbezoo F, Naeije M. Bruxism is mainly regulated centrally, not peripherally. J Oral Rehabil. 2001;28:1085–91.
10. Manfredini D, Lobbezoo F. Role of psychosocial factors in the etiology of bruxism. J Orofac Pain. 2009;23:153–66.
11. Morree HM, Marcora SM. The face of effort: frowning muscle activity reflects effort during a physical task. Biol Psychol. 2010;85:377–82.
12. Huang D, Chou S, Chen Y, Chiou W. Frowning and jaw clenching muscle. Activity reflects the perception of effort during incremental workload cycling. J Sports Sci Med. 2014;13:921–8.
13. Hellmann D, Giannakopoulos NN, Blaser R, Eberhard L. The effect of various jaw motor tasks on body sway. J Oral Rehabil. 2011;38:729–36.
14. Okuro RT, Morcillo AM, Sakano E, Schivinski CIS, Ribeiro MAGO, Ribeiro JD. Exercise capacity, respiratory mechanics and posture in mouth breathers. Braz J Otorhinolaryngol. 2011;77:656–62.
15. Greenberg VA, Schlosser BJ, Mirowski GW. Diseases of the lips. Clin Dermatol 2017;35:e1–14. https://www.cidjournal.com/article/S0738-081X(17)30239-0/abstract. Accessed 20 May 2018.
16. De Souza Lucena EE, Costa DC, Da Silveira EJ, Lima KC. Prevalence and factors associated to actinic cheilitis in beach workers. Oral Dis. 2012;18:575–9.
17. Jurge S, Kuffer R, Scully C, Porter SR. Mucosal disease series. Number VI. Recurrent aphthous stomatitis. Oral Dis. 2006;12:1–21.

18. Patton LL. Oral lesions associated with human immunodeficiency virus disease. Dent Clin N Am. 2013;57:673–98.
19. Regezi J, Sciubba JJ, Jordan RCK. Patologia oral, correlações clinicopatológicas. 7th ed. Amsterdam: Elsevier; 2017. https://www.elsevier.com/books/patologia-oral/regezi/978-85-352-8705-9.
20. Moretti A, Vitullo F, Augurio A, Pacella A. Surgical management of lip cancer. Acta Otorhinolaryngol Ital. 2011;31:5–10.
21. Abreu L, Kruger E, Tennant M. Lip cancer in Western Australia, 1982-2006: a 25-year retrospective epidemiological study. Aust Dent J. 2009;54:130–5.
22. Balasubramaniam R, Kuperstein AS, Stoopler ET. Update on oral herpes virus infections. Dent Clin N Am. 2014;58:265–80.
23. Medeiros M Jr, Ml A, Bacellar O, ACS B, Pereira CB, Guimarães NS. Clinical evaluation of the lip swelling. Rev Bras Alerg Imunopatol. 2000;23:92–8.
24. Vasconcelos FMN, Vieira SCM, Colares V. Erosão dental: diagnóstico, prevenção e tratamento no âmbito da saúde bucal. Rev Bras Ciências Saúde. 2010;14:59–64.
25. Mathew T, Casamassimo PS, Hayes JR. Relationship between sports drinks and dental erosion in 304 university athletes in Columbus, Ohio, USA. Caries Res. 2002;36:281–7.
26. Walsh NP, Bishop NC, Blackwell J, Wierzbicki SG, Montague JC. Salivary IgA response to prolonged exercise in a cold environment in trained cyclists. Med Sci Sports Exerc. 2002;34:1632–7.
27. Milosevic A, O'Sullivan E. Diagnosis, prevention and management of dental erosion: summary of an updated national guideline. Prim Dent Care. 2008;15:11–2.
28. Piccininni P, Clough A, Padilla R, Piccininni G. Dental and orofacial injuries. Clin Sports Med. 2017;36:369–405.
29. Herrera, et al. The periodontal abscess: a review. J Clin Periodontol. 2000;27:377–86.
30. Amy E. Oro-facial injuries in Central American and Caribbean sports games: a 20 year experience. Dent Traumatol. 2005;21:127–30.
31. McNutt M, Partrick M, Shugars DA, Phillips C, White RP Jr. Impact of symptomatic pericoronitis on health-related quality of life. J Oral Maxillofac Surg. 2008;66:2482–7.
32. Malek R, Gharibi A, Khlil N, Kissa J. Necrotizing ulcerative gingivitis. Contemp Clin Dent. 2017;8:496–500.
33. Rowland RW. Necrotizing ulcerative gingivitis. Ann Periodontol. 1999;4:65–73.
34. McCord C, Johnson L. Oral manifestations of hematologic disease. Atlas Oral Maxillofac Surg Clin N Am. 2017;25:149–62.
35. Berberi A, Aoun G. Oral lesions associated with human immunodeficiency virus in 75 adult patients: a clinical study. J Korean Assoc Oral Maxillofac Surg. 2017;43:388–94.
36. Lankarani KB, Sivandzadeh GR, Hassanpour S. Oral manifestation in inflammatory bowel disease: a review. World J Gastroenterol. 2013;19:8571–9.
37. Mejia LM. Oral manifestations of gastrointestinal disorders. Atlas Oral Maxillofac Surg Clin N Am. 2017;25:93–104.
38. Vasovic M, Gajovic N, Brajkovic D. The relationship between the immune system and oral manifestations of inflammatory bowel disease: a review. Cent Eur J Immunol. 2016;41:302–10.
39. Danoso-Hofer F. Oral lesions associated with human immunodeficiency virus disease in adult patients, a clinical perspective. Rev Chilena Infectol. 2016;33:27–35.
40. Kumaraswamy KL, Vidhya M. Human papilloma virus and oral infections: an update. J Cancer Res Ther. 2011;7:120–7.
41. Feller L, Lemmer J, Wood NH, Jadwat Y, Raubenheimer EJ. HIV-associated oral Kaposi sarcoma and HHV-8: a review. J Int Acad Periodontol. 2007;9:129–36.
42. Nunes LAS, Macedo DV. Saliva as a diagnostic fluid in sports medicine: potential and limitations. J Bras Patol Med Lab. 2013;49:247–55.
43. Ueda AJZ. Determination of testosterone and cortisol levels in the saliva of high performance athletes. 2017. http://www.teses.usp.br/teses/disponiveis/23/23140/tde-07062017-150233/pt-br.php. Accessed 20 May 2018.
44. Koibuchi E, Suzuki Y. Exercise upregulates salivary amylase in humans (Review). Exp Ther Med. 2014;7:773–7.
45. Pastore GU, Moreira M, Bastos R, Galotti M, Leonardi MFP. Sports dentistry – an innovative proposal. Rev Bras Med Esporte. 2017;23:147–51.

35 Traveling Management

Steven R. Joseph

35.1 Introduction

Providing medical support to a traveling sports team offers an exciting but often challenging opportunity [1]. Depending on the sport and travel destination, astute management is required for the athletes to perform to their potential.

Variables such as climate (heat, cold, humidity), altitude, time zone changes, and travel time may offer significant obstacles to sport performance [2]. Sound strategies to minimize the impact on performance are necessary. Also, differences in culture including food, laws, and language may pose a challenge.

The role, type, scope, and number of medical practitioners will vary depending on overall team size, type of sport, available resources, and medical services provided by the host country or city. While multiday and multisport games such as the Olympics or FIFA World Cup require significant preparation, the same principles apply to single-day or single-event games and competitions.

Ideally, a sports governing body (i.e., a National Olympic Committee) will provide support structures and a planning framework. Once a chief medical officer (CMO) or medical director is appointed, they can provide input and direction. There may exist a formula for the number and type of practitioners required to care for a specific number of athletes and team officials. Common practitioners include athletic therapists, physiotherapists, sport medicine physicians, and orthopedic surgeons. The national organizations for each sport should provide input for selection as relevant.

Many recreational and sub-elite athletes are pursuing international competition and training without pre-existing support frameworks or national organizations. In these cases, a solo practitioner may have to take responsibility for all medical support and administration.

Regardless of scope, preparation is the key to successful traveling management and athlete performance, and it is the focus of our overview.

35.2 Preparation

35.2.1 Location

If possible, advanced scouting of the location or obtaining information from those who have been there prior is recommended. A site visit well in advance of the event is fruitful for the CMO. This visit may or may not be in conjunction with administrative staff visits. Visits to local medical

S. R. Joseph (✉)
Department of Family Medicine, Western University, London, ON, Canada

Fowler Kennedy Sports Medicine Clinic, London, ON, Canada

Roth McFarlane Hand and Upper Limb Centre (HULC), London, ON, Canada
e-mail: steven.joseph@lhsc.on.ca

S. Rocha Piedade et al. (eds.), *The Sports Medicine Physician*, https://doi.org/10.1007/978-3-030-10433-7_35

facilities, athletes' accommodations, and training and competition venues should be arranged. Meeting any local organizing personal can provide insight into potential challenges. Any advanced information will give the practitioner time to address nutrition, training, and local medical coverage concerns before team arrival or the start of the event.

35.2.1.1 Food

Proper nutrition is vital to athlete training and performance. Practitioners should identify local food sources and availability where possible [3]. Are there contamination concerns? Is high-quality nutritious food that meets the athlete's needs and performance regimen part of the local cuisine and food customs? Is the local water supply safe? If not is bottled water easily attainable?

If there are food and water concerns, athletes and the team may consider supplying their own. This can include at destination and during travel itself. Quality food choices are not generally numerous in airports or on planes [4]. Bringing food and nutritional supplements can be helpful but potentially problematic. Always ensure there are no concerns importing these items into a country. Customs and immigration websites should be referenced prior to travel.

Athletes and support staff should be educated on the risks of foodborne illnesses including food intoxication, hepatitis, and traveler's diarrhea. Many foodborne illnesses can be prevented by properly storing, cooking, cleaning, and handling foods [5]. General guidelines are outlined in Table 35.1. Hepatitis (vaccinations) and traveler's diarrhea will be covered in more detail later in the chapter.

35.2.1.2 Climate/Altitude

One must study the predicted weather patterns for the competition time frame. Many athletes are exposed to significant temperature and altitude extremes. The World Cup in 2022 is being played in Qatar, where the average temperature will be between 25 and 30 °C despite being scheduled over the winter (average daily temp over the summer is 42 °C!). Practitioners should

Table 35.1 General guidelines to reduce the risk of foodborne illness

• Refrigerate or freeze raw/cooked perishable foods promptly • Fruits and vegetables should be washed under running water before eating, cutting, or cooking • Raw meat, poultry, seafood, and their juices should be kept away from other foods • People should wash their hands for at least 20 s with warm, soapy water before and after handling raw meat, poultry, fish, shellfish, produce, or eggs	Avoid • Drinking tap water, using tap water to brush their teeth, or using ice made from tap water • Drinking unpasteurized milk or milk products • Eating raw fruits and vegetables, including lettuce and fruit salads, unless they peel the fruits or vegetables themselves • Eating raw or rare meat and fish • Eating meat or shellfish that is not hot when served • Eating food from street vendors

be familiar with related health issues and illnesses associated with extreme heat, cold, humidity, and altitude [6, 7]. Destination environment factors should be considered when identifying experienced support staff and medical kit selection.

Consider training at the altitude and climate conditions similar to event conditions to reduce the environmental health risks of athletes [8]. If unable to train in venue climate conditions, arranging to arrive early to acclimatize is a consideration. Identify athletes who have disease concerns specific to extreme climate conditions (i.e., sickle cell disease and altitude), and ensure medical staff are aware of initial symptoms and management.

For severe heat and humidity, athletes' instructions include limiting exposure and proper hydration. This includes arranging for access to water and electrolytes at accommodation, training, and competition sites. Proper cold weather clothing and training gear during winter exposure are required [9]. Teaching athletes' signs of frostbite is also appropriate. A summary of climate- and altitude-specific considerations outlined above should be disseminated to the team as part of the safety brief.

35.2.1.3 Local Medical Coverage

One should obtain knowledge of the local medical coverage at competition venues, athletic village, and local hospital and emergency facilities. Local medical authorities should be aware of the event (generally not an issue for major games) and be involved in the planning as necessary. Depending on the size of the event, the local medical coverage planning piece will be to simply be aware of the games, organizing body's medical support. Local resource availability will directly impact composition of the supporting medical kit and any necessary portable equipment. Where serious illness or injuries should be treated should be discussed pending local support. Are there concerns with time-sensitive repatriation planning? Further details will be discussed in emergency action plan (EAP) development. Important local medical contact numbers and addresses should be communicated to the team as required.

35.2.1.4 Accommodations

There are many facets to consider when finding or reviewing athlete accommodations. Are they in a safe area of the city? Proximity to venues? Is it difficult to find adequate transportation? Food, climate, and exposure risks discussed in prior sections also apply to accommodation selection and planning. It is ideal to have a dedicated medical room for athlete privacy and confidentiality. Long beds for tall athletes and accessible rooms for disabled athletes are considerations that should not be overlooked. Isolation rooms for sick athletes can reduce cross infection rates between teammates. If part of an athlete's village, ensure you have the appropriate contact and administration information if there are concerns.

35.2.2 Personnel

Personnel planning involves medical records, administration, travel documents, travel insurance, and drug testing considerations. Don't forget to include coaching, medical, and other support personnel when reviewing travel documents and administration. Review medical requirements, and ensure suitable medical staff with appropriate qualifications are available.

35.2.2.1 Medical Records

Ensure up-to-date medical records are available prior to and during the event. If not the normal team medical practitioner contacts coaches, officials, and team medical staff to identify any athletes that may have significant or ongoing medical concerns. It is important to address injuries prior to departure if possible. Some athletes will be undergoing specific rehab or therapy; if this should be continued during travel communication with rehabilitation staff who may not be traveling with the team is necessary. Often team officials and coaches can cause anxiety for the traveling practitioner due to underlying medical conditions such as coronary artery disease [10]. Records are to be kept secure. This may lead to additional travel challenges as electronic and mobile records are beginning to replace hard charts. There is ongoing concern with hacking into private medical files. The World Anti-Doping Agency (WADA) confirmed a cyber espionage group illegally gained access to confidential medical files in 2016 [11].

35.2.2.2 PPE (Pre-participation Examination)

The pre-participation examination (assessment) was covered in Chap. 2. Most teams and athletes will have some form of a PPE as part of their own program's medical requirements before training. There is ongoing research and debate to the effectiveness of a PPE [12]. Regardless, it is reasonable for the medical practitioner to attend pre-travel/competition camps to perform their own comprehensive medical assessments. Ensure there are no specific PPE requirements for the competition/event; if so be sure to allocate enough time and resources to complete.

35.2.2.3 Travel Documents

Obtaining and confirming travel documents such as visas and passports is generally not the responsibility of the medical staff. However, this may be an additional administrative role depending on team size and scope. Having this part of your checklist is never a poor idea (redundancy in travel preparation is not a concern). Some practitioners include this as part of the vaccination and medical record checklist. Travel insurance including medical coverage should be arranged for the team and support staff. Inquire early if this is part of the medical staff responsibility.

35.2.2.4 Drug Testing

This function is administrative and educational and can be taxing for both athletes and medical practitioners. Drug testing is undertaken at many international competitions; athletes and medical staff must be reminded about common over-the-counter (OTC) medications that are on the prohibited list. Providing a short reference sheet that lists these to athletes can be helpful though the best advice is to ensure athletes don't take any medication without reviewing with a qualified clinician.

If an athlete is required to take a medication to treat an illness or condition that happens to fall under the WADA prohibited list, a Therapeutic Use Exemption (TUE) may give that athlete the authorization to take the needed medicine [13]. TUEs should be completed at least 30 days prior to an athlete's next competition for in-competition prohibited substances; applications are required as soon as possible if the medical condition diagnosed requires a substance that is prohibited at all times [14]. Communicate with officials, athletes, and team staff to determine existing TUEs and any required TUEs not in place.

There are many resources that are helpful in navigating drug testing, prohibited medications, methods, and supplements. A great place to start is the World Anti-Doping Agency website (https://www.wada-ama.org/). It includes the prohibited list and TUE application process and identifies anti-doping organizations by country. Other initial resources to consider are the IOC Anti-Doping Rules and GlobalDRO (https://globaldro.com/Home).

35.2.2.5 Medical Staff

Depending on team composition, size, and local and event medical support, ensure you have adequate medical staff. This includes qualifications and number of personnel. Small teams traveling to a well-supported event may only require a qualified athletic therapist for medical support. Larger teams or less supported events may require multiple providers including athletic therapists, physiotherapists, nutritionists, sport med physicians, and orthopedic surgeons.

35.2.3 Equipment

Timely availability of proper medical equipment is an essential component of medical care while traveling. Equipment includes personal and team medications, clinician medical kit, and event coverage medical bag and supplies.

35.2.3.1 Medications

Ensure athlete's required medications are confirmed and transported. In some cases, the athlete themselves will pack it; other times it may be more feasible to keep the team medications together. General medications to bring can vary, and a reasonable starting point is included in Table 35.2. The quality of local pharmacies and availability of reputable medications will factor into medication planning. It is a good practice to bring all the medications you anticipate the team will need. Contact airlines or other travel providers beforehand to ensure appropriate documentation is prepared for

Table 35.2 Common travel medications

• Analgesics (acetaminophen) • Antibiotics (amoxicillin, doxycycline, Keflex, ciprofloxacin) • Epinephrine/EpiPen • Antidiarrheal (loperamide) • Antacid (Tums/Rolaids) • Eye/ear drops (tears, antibiotic) • Glucose tabs • ASA • Throat lozenges	• NSAIDS (ibuprofen, naproxen) • Topical (antibiotic ointment, antifungal, steroid, anti-inflammatory) • Antiemetic (Gravol) • Antihistamines (Benadryl, second generation) • Bronchodilators (salbutamol, beclomethasone, Atrovent) • Nitro spray • Sedatives (zopiclone, zolpidem)

transport of medications if required. This is often applied to syringes, needles, and controlled substances such as narcotics and benzodiazepines (these medications should rarely be included).

35.2.3.2 Medical Kit

Each clinician should carry a small kit while traveling to attend to common and minor medical issues that may occur. This should include Band-Aids, athletic tape, eye drops, antibiotic ointment, acetaminophen, ibuprofen, throat lozenges, dimenhydrinate, antihistamines, and gauze among others [1, 15].

35.2.3.3 Event Medical Bag and Supplies

In addition to the medications and clinician medical kit discussed above, an event medical bag and other supplies are often required. In practice medications and clinician medical kit are often included within the medical bag. While the contents will vary depending on local resources, common supplies include laceration equipment (sutures, Steri-Strips, lidocaine, instruments), SAM splints, tensor bandages, BP cuff, portable O_2 monitor, AED, airway equipment, pocket masks, stethoscope, ophthalmoscope, otoscope, penlight, scalpel, wound dressings, gloves, and a portable examining table.

35.2.4 Preventive Medicine

Health and safety concerns are not always related to specific injury risks involved in a sport. Communicable disease, insect-borne illnesses, and cultural-related incidents can also prove dangerous to the health and safety of the traveling team.

35.2.4.1 Vaccines

Common vaccines for athletes and staff are outlined in Table 35.3. Most of these vaccines are recommended as part of the public healthcare plans in some countries. If athletes are not up-to-date, these routine vaccinations are the recommended minimum. Depending on the location (host country) of the event, other vaccinations may be required. Some vaccines are even required to transit through a country while traveling; ensure these issues are identified well in advance. The Centers for Disease Control and Prevention travel website (https://wwwnc.cdc.gov/travel) and World Health Organization (http://www.who.int/) are sites to bookmark for related information. Other vaccines that may be considered or required include Japanese encephalitis, rabies, typhoid, cholera, and yellow fever.

35.2.4.2 Malaria

Insect-borne diseases are common in many parts of the world and have impacted large athletic events in the past. The most recent is the Zika virus and the 2016 Rio Summer Olympics [16, 17]. Mosquitos are the best-known disease vector and can transmit chikungunya, dengue fever, and malaria among others [18]. Preventive measures for insect-borne diseases include limiting outside exposure, using nets, wearing protective clothing, and using repellant. Review signs and symptoms of relevant insect-borne diseases with the team and medical staff.

Malaria, which is endemic in parts of Africa, Southeast Asia, and South America, can result in significant morbidity and mortality. Unlike dengue and chikungunya, there are prophylactic medications available when traveling. Websites such as the CDC or WHO can assist with identifying endemic areas and recommend specific prophylactic medications.

Interestingly, there are no consistent studies on ability to work, athletic performance, and chemo-

Table 35.3 Common vaccinations

• Hepatitis A
• Hepatitis B
• Measles, mumps, rubella
• Diphtheria
• Tetanus
• Pertussis
• *Haemophilus* influenza type B
• Human papillomavirus (HPV)
• Influenza
• Pneumococcal
• Meningococcal
• Varicella
• Polio

prophylaxis [19]. If choosing to use prophylactic medications, consider taking the medicine before starting extensive training and competition to identify any difficulties. Common side effects of the medication should factor into chemoprophylaxis decisions (i.e., doxycycline and photosensitivity not ideal for summer events). Timing of medication can be scheduled (i.e., weekly dosed medications can be planned around events—take as far away as actual event as possible).

35.2.4.3 Safety Brief

Prepare a safety brief to be given to the athletes and staff just prior to travel or at arrival. The safety brief includes team rules and regulations governing the event. Unsafe areas, times of day, and transportation routes should be reviewed. Specific laws or bylaws that are not common to the athletes' home country or unique to the destination are to be outlined. The brief should include food safety, the use and dangers of alcohol and illicit drugs, and caution with sexual activity. Sexually transmitted infections such as gonorrhea, chlamydia, HIV, syphilis, and hepatitis are concerns and should be discussed. Condoms should be readily available although abstinence is the ideal preventive measure. A buddy system or call out list can be developed to assist with safety and team communication. The safety brief can be published on a team dedicated website if available.

35.2.4.4 Culture Brief

Similar in nature to the structure of the safety brief, the culture brief is to review specific cultural norms and practices at destination. This includes language, greetings, physical contact, and customs. Review common local food, emphasize food safety, and be wary of food intoxication if local cuisine is not familiar. If possible, the brief should be given by someone local to the area upon arrival.

35.2.5 Emergency Planning

Although true sports emergencies are rare, it is essential to be prepared for the worst-case scenario. Despite proper planning, tragic outcomes can occur. Recent examples include (1) the death of Bahman Golbarnezhad, a paralympic athlete who died during a cycling event at the 2016 Summer Olympics in Rio De Janeiro, and (2) Nodar Kumaritashvii who died during luge practice and the 2010 Winter Olympics in Vancouver. However, in most cases advanced emergency planning can reduce morbidity and mortality during athletic events. Specific considerations are outlined below.

35.2.5.1 Emergency Action Plan (EAP)

A predetermined emergency action plan (EAP) allows for the proper assessment and care of athletes who have suffered injury or sudden illness [20]. An EAP should provide a team- and venue-specific framework outlining personnel roles and responsibilities in case of a significant medical event. These can be developed by the advanced medical scouting team if there is one. Depending on the structure of the event or games, EAPs may have been developed by the overarching organization (i.e., IOC) or local medical support. Obtaining and understanding any EAPs is a responsibility for the medical, admin, and coaching staff.

35.2.5.2 Repatriation

It is unlikely that there will be inadequate local resources to provide the required level of care for medical emergencies and critical illness. However, if local resources are not adequate, adequate medical facilities and appropriate transportation should be located. A plan should be in place for transportation home of injured or ill athletes for medical care as required (during or after the competition). Medical practitioners that are familiar with aeromedical transportation considerations are an asset [21, 22]. Some relative contraindications for air travel include an athlete with a pneumothorax, recent eye surgery, or fractures with circumferential casting.

35.2.5.3 Emergency Contacts

Emergency contacts for the team and local resources should be included and dispersed to the medical staff, coaches, athletes, and administrators. This should include local medical facilities, police, fire, ambulance, and national team or games liaisons depending on the athletic event.

It should also include national team personnel and/or games personnel depending on the athletic event. Each member of the team should have an emergency home contact number available beforehand. This information can be complied by the medical or admin staff.

35.2.6 Travel Fatigue

It is well documented that travel of any kind can affect natural circadian rhythm and athlete performance [23]. Considerable research is being undertaken to develop strategies to mitigate performance deficits in athlete populations that are required to travel prior to competitions.

35.2.6.1 Time Zone

Time zone changes can affect athletes' performance [24]. Eastward travel affects athletes more than westward [25]. A general rule of thumb is to allow one whole day of adjustment per hour of time zone change, although westward travel adjustment may be 1.5–2 h per day [10]. Recognizing time zone differences (especially multiple changes during an event or season) is important for medical planning. There are a variety of strategies to address this, and they will be discussed later in the section.

35.2.6.2 Sleep

Sleep can affect athlete performance in many domains [26]. Recent studies show that athletes do not get enough sleep or overrepresent the amount of quality sleep they achieve [27]. This is compounded during travel, especially travel that includes multiple time zone changes. Given the relationship of sleep and performance, significant attention needs to be given to travel fatigue management.

35.2.6.3 Hydration

Maintaining proper hydration during air travel is an often-overlooked aspect of travel fatigue and athletic performance [4]. Aviation guidelines suggest people can lose 2–4% of total body water during a 10-h flight. These losses can be further exacerbated with consumption of alcoholic beverages on the plane or during layovers. Adequate hydration in hot climates is important; arriving with a fluid deficit from travel can increase the risks of heat-related illness unless careful rehydration strategies are incorporated [28, 29].

35.2.6.4 Strategies

Speeding up the athletes' biological clock adaptation to the new time zone can reduce symptoms of travel fatigue and jet lag [30]. There are a variety of strategies to consider if planned length of stay is more than 5 days and at least three times zones away. A practical recommendation is to arrive 96 h before competition especially if traveling east [25]. This of course is not always feasible.

An alternate strategy is to adjust the sleep schedule gradually to the next time zone prior to departure. This should occur over a minimum of 2 days, more depending on how many time zones are to be crossed. If possible, the adjusted sleep schedule should match the destination schedule; however, even partial adjustment can help with adaptation at destination. Traveling eastward requires advancing the athlete's circadian clock (i.e., going to sleep earlier); westward requires circadian clock delay (going to sleep later).

Other strategies to assist in adaptation include the use of light exposure and exogenous melatonin (pills). Scheduled bright light in the early morning (i.e., using a light visor) to simulate an eastward destination wake-up time can assist with advancing a circadian clock; using sunglasses or dark rooms to avoid bright light in the afternoon can do the same. Melatonin pills signal darkness and can advance the circadian clock, promoting earlier sleep onset and morning awakening [31]. To be effective light exposure and melatonin strategies should be gradual and specific. It is recommended someone on the support team with appropriate experience and knowledge assist in planning any related sleep strategies. Combining light exposure and melatonin strategies with pre-travel sleep scheduling offers a synergistic and efficient approach to reducing the effects of travel fatigue.

If length of stay is short or there are minimal changes in time zone (1 or 2 h), short-term strategies can be used in lieu of the comprehensive strategies above. This can include ensuring adequate sleep the week before departure, avoiding work during destination sleep times, and scheduling important activities in the daytime of the home time zone. Light exposure strategies should be used on the airplane as warranted. Sleeping on flights is reasonable if it is during the night according to destination time; otherwise, it should be avoided [32].

35.3 Event/Onsite

While preparation before traveling is the key to successful travel management, onsite medical considerations and treatment plans for travel-related illness, symptoms, and environmental challenges are important aspects to consider once on the ground.

35.3.1 Traveler's Diarrhea

Quality and availability of water supplies will have been covered in the preparatory stage; however, it is a good practice to remind all athletes and support staff to avoid tap water and ice if there are any quality or source concerns. Always be prepared for last minute changes in plans or incorrect advanced planning information. Guidelines outlined in Table 35.1 above are helpful for reducing the risk of traveler's diarrhea.

Traveler's diarrhea is the most common illness to affect the traveling athlete [33]. It is frequently caused by exposure to *Escherichia coli*, although *Salmonella*, *Campylobacter*, *Shigella*, or *Giardia* are common. Although antimicrobial prophylaxis can be very effective, recent guidelines recommend leaving this approach on the sidelines. This recommendation is due to increasing antibiotic resistance and the rapid improvement of symptoms when treated with antibiotics with or without loperamide [34]. Fluoroquinolones remain the antibiotic class of choice although azithromycin is a strong alternative if there are concerns with resistance [34, 35]. Colitis-like symptoms or persistent diarrhea should not be ignored; the patient should be referred to an appropriate specialist [2].

35.3.2 Upper Respiratory Tract Illness

The incidence of upper respiratory tract illness (URTI) is higher in elite athletes during training and competitions [36]. URTIs are also common in air travelers [37]. Athletes and staff should be reminded about handwashing, care handling bottles and towels, adequate sleep, and maintaining hydration. A team member with respiratory symptoms should notify the medical staff immediately to address possible treatment and isolation. Care should be taken in treating URTI symptoms as many over-the-counter medications contain banned substances. Athletes with prolonged symptoms, fever, or productive cough may benefit from antibiotic intervention.

35.3.3 Jet Lag

Individual biological clock adaptation can vary widely, so despite adequate planning and pre-travel sleep practices, some athletes will undoubtedly have symptoms of jet lag post arrival. Symptoms can include poor sleep, daytime fatigue, impaired concentration, general malaise, headache, and poor performance.

Treatment considerations for those experiencing the effects of jet lag can include caffeine and hypnotics such as zolpidem (to address daytime function and insomnia, respectively). Other stimulants and sleep aids should be avoided in athletes as most of these substances are banned in competition. These alternate substances such as modafinil (to address daytime somnolence) can be considered for coaching or support staff traveling with the team [38].

35.3.4 Environment

35.3.4.1 Insects

Review timing and dose of any required prophylactic medications for vector-borne illness. Remind the team about proper personal protective equipment (netting, long clothes, repellant), exposure risks, and symptoms of insect-related illness [39]. Advise athletes to avoid or protect themselves during peak biting periods. For example, mosquito vectors of malaria are most active at dawn and dusk; mosquito vectors of Zika, dengue fever, and chikungunya are most active during the day.

35.3.4.2 Climate/Exposure

Climate-related illness and risks are further outlined in Chaps. 36 and 40. Upon arrival at destination, identify any further athletes at increased risk due to travel-related difficulties or illness. Take the opportunity to debrief the team if there are unexpected weather or venue changes that could lead to increased risk factors. Have team members and staff check gear and related performance equipment to identify any shortfalls prior to practice or competition.

35.4 Post

Congratulations, you've had a successful trip and have made it home with hopefully no major medical concerns or issues.

It is prudent to remind athletes and team members that travel-related fatigue and illness are relevant at this end. Proper planning related to returning to work and training should include integration strategies around sleep and nutrition. Athlete education will assist with injury prevention and fatigue on the return trip home.

35.4.1 Injury Surveillance

Tracking illness and injury during travel and competition is helpful for future planning and management. Were there any illnesses or injuries that could or should have been prevented? Any pattern that was surprising or unexpected? Consider creating a database to document injury patterns.

35.4.2 Review

An after-action review should be completed with medical staff, coaching staff, and sport officials as appropriate post travel and competition. Are there lessons to be learned related to communicable disease, environmental factors, travel, or performance? Was communication between the medical team, athletes, and staff effective? Lessons learned related to travel, performance, or location can be collated and kept in a running file. This information can be used for future traveling management by medical practitioners and administrators.

References

1. Kary JM, Lavallee M. Travel medicine and the international athlete. Clin Sports Med. 2007;26:489–503.
2. Pipe AL. International travel and the elite athlete. Clin J Sport Med. 2011;21:62–6.
3. Reilly T, Waterhouse J, Burke LM, Alonso JM, et al. Nutrition for travel. J Sports Sci. 2007;25(Suppl 1):S125–34.
4. British Journal of Sports Medicine (UK). How to keep athletes healthy when travelling [podcast on the internet]. Br J Sports Med. 2017 [cited 2018 Jun 18]. https://soundcloud.com/bmjpodcasts/sets/bjsm-1.
5. National Institute of Diabetes and Digestive and Kidney Diseases (US). Foodborne illnesses [Internet]. US Department of Health and Human Services; 2018 [cited 2018 May 25]. https://www.niddk.nih.gov/health-information/digestive-diseases/foodborne-illnesses.
6. Seto CK, Way D, O'Connor N. Environmental illness in athletes. Clin Sports Med. 2005;24:695–718.
7. Biem J, Koehncke N, Classen D, Dosman J. Out of the cold: management of hypothermia and frostbite. CMAJ. 2003;168:305–11.
8. Racinais S, Alonso JM, Coutts AJ, et al. Consensus recommendations on training and competing in the heat. Br J Sports Med. 2015;49:1164–73.
9. Noakes TD. Exercise and the cold. Ergonomics. 2000;43:1461–79.
10. Cook J, Harcourt P, Milne C, Al-Tunaiji H. Traveling with a team. In: Bruckner P, Khan K, editors. Clinical

sports medicine. 4th ed. Sydney: McGraw-Hill; 2012. p. 1208–20.

11. World Anti-Doping Agency (CA). WADA confirms attack by Russian Cyber Espionage Group [Internet]. World Anti-Doping Agency; 2016 [cited 2018 Jul 3]. https://www.wada-ama.org/en/media/news/2016-09/wada-confirms-attack-by-russian-cyber-espionage-group.
12. Wingfield K, Matheson GO, Meeuwisse WH. Preparticipation evaluation: an evidence-based review. Clin J Sport Med. 2004;14:109–22.
13. World Anti-Doping Agency (CA). The prohibited list [Internet]. World Anti-Doping Agency; 2018 [cited 2018 Jul 8]. https://www.wada-ama.org/en/what-we-do/the-prohibited-list.
14. World Anti-Doping Agency (CA). Guidelines – Therapeutic Use Exemptions (TUE) [Internet]. World Anti-Doping Agency; 2016 [cited 2018 Jul 8]. https://www.wada-ama.org/en/resources/therapeutic-use-exemption-tue/guidelines-therapeutic-use-exemptions-tue.
15. Buettner CM. The team physician's bag. Clin Sports Med. 1998;17:365–73.
16. Petersen E, Wilson ME, Touch S, et al. Rapid spread of zika virus in The Americas--implications for public health preparedness for mass gatherings at the 2016 Brazil Olympic Games. Int J Infect Dis. 2016;44:11–5.
17. Hamilton B, Exeter D, Beable S, Coleman L, Milne C. Zika Virus and the Rio Olympic Games. Clin J Sport Med. 2017; https://doi.org/10.1097/JSM.0000000000000551.
18. World Health Organization (CE). Vector-borne disease [Internet]. World Health Organization; 2017 [cited 2018 Jun 9]. http://www.who.int/news-room/fact-sheets/detail/vector-borne-diseases.
19. Terrell AG, Forde ME, Firth R, Ross DA. Malaria chemoprophylaxis and self-reported impact on ability to work: mefloquine versus doxycycline. J Travel Med. 2015;22:383–8.
20. Sport Med BC (CA). Emergency action plan [Internet]. Sport Med BC; 2017 [cited 2018 Jun 28]. https://sportmedbc.com/article/emergency-action-plan.
21. Parsons CJ, Bobechko WP. Aeromedical transport: its hidden problems. CMAJ. 1982;126:237–43.
22. Teichman PG, Donchin Y, Kot RJ. International aeromedical evacuation. N Engl J Med. 2007;356:262–70.
23. Reilly T, Edwards B. Altered sleep-wake cycles and physical performance in athletes. Physiol Behav. 2007;90:274–84.
24. Reilly T, Waterhouse J, Edwards B. Jet lag and air travel: implications for performance. Clin Sports Med. 2005;24:367–80.
25. Fowler PM, Knez W, Crowcroft S, et al. Greater effect of east versus west travel on jet lag, sleep, and team sport performance. Med Sci Sports Exerc. 2017;49:2548–61.
26. Simpson NS, Gibbs EL, Matheson GO. Optimizing sleep to maximize performance: implications and recommendations for elite athletes. Scand J Med Sci Sports. 2017;27:266–74.
27. Watson AM. Sleep and athletic performance. Curr Sports Med Rep. 2017;16:413–8.
28. Maughan R, Shirreffs S. Exercise in the heat: challenges and opportunities. J Sports Sci. 2004;22:917–27.
29. Wendt D, van Loon LJC, van Marken Lichtenbelt WD. Thermoregulation during exercise in the heat. Strategies for maintaining health and performance. Sports Med. 2007;37:669–82.
30. Arendt J. Managing jet lag: some of the problems and possible new solutions. Sleep Med Rev. 2009;13:249–56.
31. Eastman CI, Burgess HJ. How to travel the world without jet lag. Sleep Med Clin. 2009;4:241–55.
32. Waterhouse J, Reilly T, Atkinson G, Edwards B. Jet lag: trends and coping strategies. Lancet. 2007;369:1117–29.
33. Rendi-Wagner P, Kollaritsch H. Drug prophylaxis for traveler's diarrhea. Clin Infect Dis. 2002;34:628–33.
34. Riddle MS, et al. Guidelines for the prevention and treatment of travelers' diarrhea. J Travel Med. 2017;24:S57–74.
35. Riddle M, Arnold S, Tribble D. Effect of adjunctive loperamide in combination with antibiotics on treatment outcomes in traveler's diarrhea: a systematic review and meta-analysis. Clin Infect Dis. 2008;47:1007–14.
36. Spence L, Brown WJ, Pyne DB, et al. Incidence, etiology, and symptomatology of upper respiratory illness in elite athletes. Med Sci Sports Exerc. 2007;39:577–86.
37. Leder K, Newman D. Respiratory infections during air travel. Intern Med J. 2005;35:50–5.
38. Lee A, Galvez JC. Jet lag in athletes. Sports Health. 2012;4:211–6.
39. Igreja RP. Olympics in the tropics and infectious diseases. Clin Infect Dis. 2010;50:616–7.

Sports Under Extreme Conditions

36

Helge Krusemark and Annika Hackemann

36.1 Sports in the Heat

36.1.1 Overview

At high temperatures, a physical activity is a special physical stress for athletes. The loss of fluids and minerals due to increased sweating results in a limited performance. Acutely, the plasma volume decreases, and the concentration of the electrolytes in the plasma changes. The heat also leads to an increased anaerobic energy production with accelerated depletion of glycogen storage. Clinical signs, starting from a fluid loss of 2% of body weight, are weakness, headache, and tachycardia to confusion symptoms [1].

36.1.2 Regulation of Temperature

The body's own thermoregulation is subject to only slight fluctuations and ensures a largely constant body temperature in a range of 36.5–37.5 °C. This is achieved through a complex system of thermoreceptors in the central nervous system, visceral organs, musculature, and skin. When the body temperature increases, for example, more heat is released into the environment in order to maintain the temperature equilibrium (temperature homeostasis). The heat emission can be made by several mechanisms: convection, conduction, evaporation, and radiation [2].

At rest, the radiation ensures the majority of heat emission. In convection, heat is emitted by flowing liquids such as blood or gases (air, respiration). Conduction means the transfer of heat energy through direct contact with another solid or liquid medium. Evaporation (in the form of sweat production) represents the main part of the heat release under physical stress. However, as the outside temperature increases, this mechanism gets exhausted, causing an increased risk of overheating dependent on temperature and humidity [2, 3].

In order to achieve physiological adaptation, regular physical stress under appropriate climatic conditions is required. For a complete adaptation, up to 14 days are necessary. An increased concentration of plasma proteins initially leads to an increase in plasma volume, because the osmotic pressure of the proteins leads to an increased amount of fluid being transferred from the tissue into the vascular system. The increased blood volume reduces the heart rate required to maintain cardiac output. Furthermore, the quality of sweating is adjusted. The concentration of electrolytes of the sweat is reduced in order to prevent excessive electrolyte loss. These adaptions result in improved physical performance under these temperature conditions [4].

H. Krusemark (✉) · A. Hackemann
Department of Prevention and Sports Medicine, Technical University Munich, Munich, Germany
e-mail: Helge.Krusemark@mri.tum.de; Annika.Hackemann@mri.tum.de

S. Rocha Piedade et al. (eds.), *The Sports Medicine Physician*,
https://doi.org/10.1007/978-3-030-10433-7_36

The following recommendations can be derived from these findings. Before sports competitions, a sufficiently long stay in appropriate climate is recommended. In addition, care should be taken to ensure a sufficient supply of fluids and electrolytes and also carbohydrate intake if the exercise lasts longer than 1 h. It is also important to have adequate sun protection through appropriate, light, and bright clothing, headgear, and sun cream [4].

36.1.3 Risks of Physical Exertion in the Heat

There are six different types of heat damage.

1. Heat Exhaustion
   The increased fluid loss under heat conditions leads to dehydration with fatigue, dizziness, headache, and increased thirst. The body temperature can still be normal. The athlete should be carried to a cool place and lie flat or with slightly raised legs in case of circulatory instability. Tight-fitting clothes should be opened or removed and cool air supplied to the body if possible. Furthermore, sufficient hydration should be achieved (referable by ingestion of sodium-containing drinks) [5].
2. Heat Stroke
   A heat stroke is a life-threatening form of heat exhaustion with body temperature rising to over 40 °C. Additionally severe neurological and cardiovascular symptoms such as dizziness, cramps, cardiovascular instability, vomiting, or even coma can occur. In addition to the measures of heat exhaustion, medication has to be intervened in most cases in the sense of shock therapy. The fluid intake is usually intravenous [5].
3. Heat Cramps
   They occur mainly in heavy physical stress combined with a greatly increased loss of sweat. Due to the liquid and electrolyte shift, there is an impairment of the membrane stability of the cells, and this leads to muscle cramps. New explanations suggest that muscle fatigue is a reason for the onset of muscle cramps. This fatigue results in increased afferent activity of muscle spindles with reduced inhibitory afferent activity of Golgi tendon organs, both together cause an increased excitability of the muscle cell membrane and muscle cramps [6]. The administration of saline-enriched liquid usually leads quickly to an improvement of these symptoms.
4. Heat Collapse
   The heat collapse is usually triggered by standing for a long time in a hot environment after increased peripheral vasodilatation and an orthostatic shift of the blood into the legs have led to a reduced cerebral blood flow. However, heat collapse can also occur after physical exertion such as a marathon run. Therapy is similar to heat exhaustion (point 1) [7].
5. Sunstroke
   The sunstroke is caused by direct sunlight on the head and neck area, which leads to irritation of the meninges. It manifests in dizziness, nausea, vomiting, headache, ear noises, disturbances of consciousness, stiff neck up to cramps, and coma. Worth mentioning is the frequent delay between sun exposure and the appearance of symptoms. Depending on the severity of symptoms, treatment measures are similar to the measures at heat exhaustion (in addition, attention should be paid to slight lifting of the head), or a drug therapy should be administered. This includes the treatment with electrolyte drinks or in severe cases with an infusion (Ringer solution, about 500–1000 mL) [8].
6. Hyponatremia
   In association with long time exercising, excessive intake fluids low in electrolytes (and hereby especially sodium) and/or increased loss of sweat, thus electrolyte, can result in an imbalance of sodium-deficient electrolytes. The symptoms are weakness, nausea with vomiting, muscle spasms, disorientation, and swollen extremities. In severe cases, it can lead to brain or pulmonary edema. The therapy is carried out with medication through careful fluid administration and further in the hospital, because of potential serious complications. It is important that the hyponatremia is treated slowly and in a controlled

manner. In case of hyponatremia with moderate symptoms, causes are medicated; in severe symptoms, an infusion of 150 mL of 3% saline solution should be administered over 20 min [9].

36.2 Sports in the Cold

Physical activity at low temperatures also represents a particular stress for the athlete, as processes that consume a lot of energy and can severely restrict performance are necessary to maintain heat. Extreme cold leads to an increased release of stress hormones. These cause among other things a constriction of the vessels (vasoconstriction) and muscle tremors [2]. Due to the reduced blood circulation of the muscles, there is a faster consumption of energy sources (glucose and glycogen) and consecutively increased lactate production. At the heart, extreme cold leads to a peripheral vasoconstriction and thus to an increase in cardiac preload, stroke volume, and cardiac output. The stimulation of stretch receptors located in the atrium leads to the release of a diuresis-promoting hormone (ANP). With regard to breathing, there is an increased respiratory rate and increased oxygen uptake. Furthermore, the thickness of the subcutaneous fatty tissue and the influence of wind and humidity are decisive for the perception of cold. When moving in cold water, considerably more heat energy is lost than when moving in air at the same temperature. For the exercise in cold weather, it is important to do a sufficiently long warm-up and wear appropriate clothing in order to avoid strong energy-consuming shivering and thus ultimately a drop in core body temperature [2].

36.2.1 Cold Damage

Skin temperatures in the range of 0 °C may result in a local frostbite of exposed skin areas on the body. There are three different stages: superficial frostbite, blistering, and necrosis. For treatment the damaged areas should be warmed up, e.g., by a water bath with increasing temperatures. Depending on the degree of severity, drug (including analgesics, antibiotics) or surgical therapy may also be necessary [8].

36.2.2 Hypothermia

Hypothermia occurs when the body temperature falls below 35 °C. When practicing sports, particularly swimmers, tired endurance athletes, and athletes under alpine conditions have a high risk of hypothermia. There are four stages of hypothermia [10]:

- Stage I (mild hypothermia): Core temperature 35–32 °C. Symptoms: shivering.
- Stage II (moderate hypothermia): Core temperature 32–28 °C. Symptoms: no more shivering; the consciousness is increasingly clouded.
- Stage III (severe hypothermia): Core temperature 28–24 °C. Symptoms: no or only weak vital signs, cardiac arrest or minimal circulation, and unconsciousness.
- Stage IV: Core temperature <15 °C. Symptoms: death.

In mild and moderate hypothermia, passive reheating measures (wrapping in warm blankets) should be carried out. In addition, an improvement in environmental conditions must be considered (placing the supercooled person in a warm, wind-protected environment, taking off wet clothing). In severe hypothermia, there is an increased risk that the cold blood from the body periphery will be mobilized into the core of the body through movement during the rescue of the unconscious patient. This can lead immediately to cardiac arrhythmia which is difficult to treat and possibly even fatal (afterdrop) [10]. This is because a hypothermic heart has a lower fibrillation threshold, which means that cold blood can be a stimulus to trigger ventricular fibrillation (when warm and cold blood mix). Therefore, a very careful rescue in a horizontal position is important. Reheating then takes place in the ambulance or hospital. If this is not possible, a combination of internal (warm infusion solutions and warm peritoneal lavage) and external (warm air blankets) reheating has to be carried out [11]. With regard to resuscitation measures, it must be taken into account that severe hypothermia significantly reduces metabolic activity, especially in the brain, so that a longer circulatory arrest can be more likely to be survived than at normal temperatures. Thus, the brain can endure a ten times longer cardiac arrest at 18 °C than at 37 °C. Resuscitation should not be stopped until a body temperature of at least 36 °C is reached ("Nobody is dead until he is warm and dead") [11].

36.3 Sports at Altitude

When staying at altitude, the organism must adapt to many different environmental conditions compared to staying at normal altitudes. The increased radiation intensity and the reduced outside temperature require, in particular with regard to the equipment, adequate clothing and correspondingly a high sun protection factor [12].

With increasing altitude, the air pressure drops. However, with a constant percentage composition of the gas components in the air (Dalton's law), this corresponds to an increasingly reduced oxygen partial pressure. This means that the oxygen content in the inhaled air and, thus, also in the blood is reduced. This leads to different adaptive reactions in the organism. Acutely, there is an increase in heart rate, blood pressure, and increase in respiratory activity. In addition, due to the drop in oxygen partial pressure, hyperventilation occurs which leads to respiratory alkalosis. The alkalosis causes a left shift of the oxygen binding curve, which leads to an improved oxygen uptake in the lung and a poorer delivery into peripheral tissues. This increases the affinity of hemoglobin for oxygen and reduces physical performance [12].

Even after a few days, there is no complete adaptation of the cardiac-circulatory system. The performance and the oxygen saturation at rest and under load remain below the initial values at sea level. The heart rate at rest and during exercise is also higher than at the sea level (Fig. 36.1) [13].

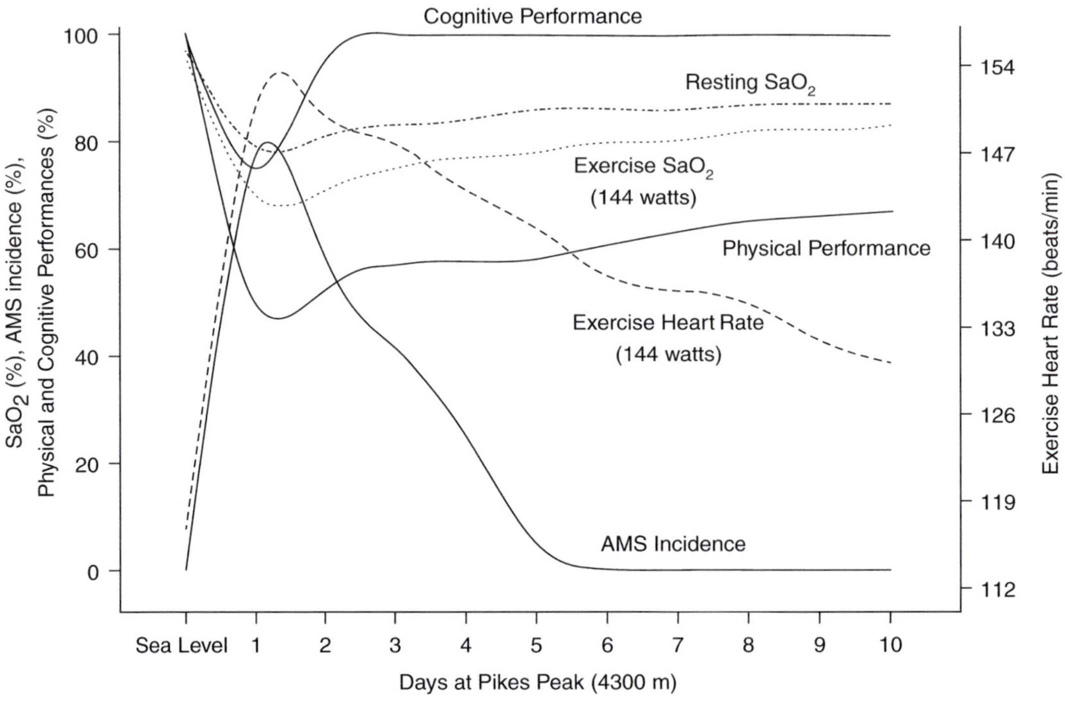

Fig. 36.1 Representative time course for altitude acclimatization of low-altitude residents directly ascending to 4300 m (Muza, Beidlemann et al. 2010) [13]

Oxygen deficiency leads to a stimulation of the hormone erythropoietin (EPO), which is predominantly produced in the kidney, and consequently to an increased and accelerated formation of new erythrocytes. Thus, the oxygen transport can be further improved.

36.3.1 Altitude Sickness

The changes mentioned under altitude conditions can lead to so-called altitude sickness. There are three different forms which occur individually or in combination and can typically manifest at a height of 3000–4500 m, but occasionally at a height of 2500 m:

1. Acute mountain sickness (AMS)
2. High-altitude cerebral edema (HACE)
3. High-altitude pulmonary edema (HAPE)

For the prevention of altitude sickness, it is advised that an ascent from 2500 m should not be higher than 400 m per day. In addition, acetazolamide (at least 250 mg/day) can be taken to prevent altitude sickness [14].

36.3.1.1 Acute Mountain Sickness (AMS)

Typical symptoms include headache, nausea/vomiting, loss of appetite, weakness, dizziness, and sleep disturbances. The symptoms often appear only a few hours after the start of the stay in the altitude and can increase to even higher amounts on further ascent. If the above symptoms did not improve, the affected person should descend 500–1000 m. Patients suffering from AMS are typically treated by halting ascent and using nonsteroidal anti-inflammatory drugs such as acetaminophen or aspirin for headache and, in some cases, antiemetic drugs for nausea [8].

36.3.1.2 High-Altitude Cerebral Edema (HACE)

The symptoms are similar to those of AMS, but also consciousness and balance disorders and particularly severe headache can occur. An immediate descent of at least 1000 m is recommended, possibly with oxygen intake. A further medicinal and decongestant therapy is also necessary. In severe AMS or incipient HACE, an intake of 8 mg of dexamethasone, followed by 4 mg every 6 h, is recommended [8]. If it is left untreated, the increased brain swelling can lead to a coma or death.

36.3.1.3 High-Altitude Pulmonary Edema (HAPE)

When a HAPE occurs, it comes to a dry cough, dyspnea already at rest, and possibly rattling sounds in the lungs with bloody-foamy phlegm. An immediate descent of at least 1000 m is recommended, as well as the administration of oxygen and other drugs that reduce the pulmonary hypertension. To reduce pulmonary pressure, 10–20 mg nifedipine and 2 × 50 mg sildenafil are prescribed [8].

36.4 Diving

Diving has become increasingly popular. However, not only healthy persons but also persons with, e.g., determined cardiovascular diseases can participate in this sport under certain conditions. Therefore, certain physical parameters must be taken into account, and any risks must be clarified by a medical eligibility test for diving.

The law of Dalton states that the total pressure of a gas is composed of the partial pressures of all gases contained in the gas mixture. Therefore, not the percentage of the gas but its partial pressure is crucial. Under physiological conditions, the percentage, thus, remains the same, but the level of the ambient pressure has a significant influence on the partial pressure. When diving the ambient pressure increases with increasing depth of water and thus the partial pressure of the individual gases. In general, the total pressure increases by 1 bar per 10 m depth. Dives deeper than 40 m are the absolute limit for the scuba diver [15].

36.4.1 Diving Conditions

The increase in the oxygen partial pressure can lead to a toxic effect of the oxygen at very great depths (Paul-Bert effect). However, larger problems are caused by the increase in nitrogen partial pressure. When diving with so-called compressed air, i.e., using a breathing mixture which has the same composition as the ambient air, there is a particularly strong increase in nitrogen partial pressure, as nitrogen physiologically has a proportion of 79% of the respiratory mixture.

Therefore, gas mixtures are used for diving which have an altered percentage of the individual gases. In these gas mixtures, the oxygen content is increased and the nitrogen content reduced. This may reduce the incidence of decompression sickness (see below), but it also carries the risk of increased oxygen toxicity. Hence, meticulous calculations are necessary to plan a dive.

36.4.2 Nitrogen Intoxication (Rapture of the Deep)

An increased ambient pressure may lead to an intoxication with nitrogen, also called a rapture of the deep. Depending on depth and nitrogen pressure, symptoms range from mild euphoria to severe dysregulation with hallucinations and coma to death. If the first symptoms of nitrogen intoxication occur, the partial pressure must be reduced by emerging slowly [15].

36.4.3 Barotrauma

Due to the strong pressure fluctuations during diving, injuries can occur to air-filled cavities that are connected to the surrounding atmosphere (middle ear, paranasal sinuses, lungs). This can happen both during the dive and reappearance. Barotrauma of the ear, nose, and throat can cause hearing loss, nausea, vomiting, dizziness, nosebleeds, and pain. The treatment is usually symptomatic. Pneumothorax is a severe form of barotrauma. This can evolve during rapid emergence while holding one's breath. There is a significant increased pressure within the lungs, which can lead to a rupture of the tissue and vessels and also to the passage of gas bubbles into the bloodstream (gas embolism). Typical symptoms of pneumothorax include coughing and dyspnea. The particularly severe form, the tension pneumothorax, can quickly lead to a life-threatening situation with circulatory failure. An immediate medical therapy is necessary. Depending on its location in the vascular system, gas embolism can cause various mild neurological as well as life-threatening symptoms. The first-line therapy is the administration of oxygen and when necessary also in a pressure chamber (hyperbaric therapy) [15].

36.4.4 Decompression Sickness

Under the increased ambient pressure during diving, the respiratory gases in the lungs increasingly dissolve into solution and accumulate in the tissue. When the ambient pressure is reduced, i.e., when emerging, the opposite happens: dissolved gases coming out of solution. This can result in damage to various tissues. Frequently affected are the musculoskeletal system (muscle and bone pain), the skin (itching), and the nervous system (numbness, balance disorders). Severe courses with circulatory disorders, pulmonary embolism, and neurological deficits are also possible. A medical therapy is immediately necessary. For this purpose, the patient must be placed in a pressure chamber. There, the patient is first exposed to a pressure corresponding to diving, and then a slow decompression is started [8].

References

1. Dickhuth H-H. Einführung in die Sport- und Leistungsmedizin. Schorndorf: Hofmann; 2016.
2. Birnesser H, et al. Praxiswissen Sportmedizin. Münster: Philippka-Sportverlag; 2008.
3. Raschka C, Nitsche L. Praktische Sportmedizin. Köln: Georg Thieme Verlag KG; 2016.

4. Racinais S, et al. Consensus recommendations on training and competing in the heat. Scand J Med Sci Sports. 2015;25:6–19.
5. Wonisch M, et al. Kompendium der Sportmedizin. Wien: Springer; 2017.
6. Qiu J, Kang J. Exercise associated muscle cramps—a current perspective. Sci Page Sports Med. 2017;1(1):3–14.
7. Dickhuth H-H, et al. Sport unter besonderen klimatischen Bedingungen—am Beispiel der Olympischen Spiele und der Paralympics in Athen. Schorndorf: Hofmann; 2004.
8. Müller S. Memorix Notfallmedizin. Stuttgart: Georg Thieme Verlag KG; 2017.
9. Bullmann C. Hyponatriämie. Arzneiverordnung in der Praxis. 2016;43(4):7.
10. Förster H. Sport und Umweltbedingungen. In: Wonisch M, Hofmann P, Förster H, Hörtnagl H, Ledl-Kurkowski E, editors. Kompendium der Sportmedizin. Wien: Springer; 2017.
11. Resuscitation G. Reanimation 2015. Leitlinien kompakt. A. Ulm; 2015.
12. Luks AM, et al. Acute high-altitude sickness. Eur Respir Rev. 2017;26(143):160096.
13. Muza SR, et al. Altitude preexposure recommendations for inducing acclimatization. High Alt Med Biol. 2010;11(2):87–92.
14. Low EV, et al. Identifying the lowest effective dose of acetazolamide for the prophylaxis of acute mountain sickness: systematic review and meta-analysis. BMJ. 2012;345:e6779.
15. Heitkamp H-C, Tetzlaff K. Sportmedizinische Aspekte des Tauchsports. In: Dickhuth H-H, Mayer F, Röcker K, Berg A, editors. Sportmedizin für Ärzte. Köln: Deutscher Ärzte Verlag; 2007.

37 Sports After Knee Arthroplasty

Bujar Shabani, Dafina Bytyqi, Cécile Batailler, Elvire Servien, and Sébastien Lustig

37.1 Introduction

> Life expectancy changed because people changed the way they lived.
> Lauren Carstensen, PhD.

People wish to stay more and more active, and as a consequence physical activity can ameliorate affluence-related chronic disease such as cardiovascular disease, diabetes mellitus, and cancer [1].

On the other hand, the prevalence of osteoarthritis affecting the knee is rising. Consequently, individuals with osteoarthritis have lower physical activity comparing their fellows [2]. In a national US survey, 44% of persons with arthritis were classified as inactive compared to 36% of adults without arthritis [3].

But, is the joint replacement a solution for this?

According to AJRR (American Joint Replacement Registry), 480,581 primary total knee arthroplasty were performed during 2017. In addition, in the United States, the demand for primary total knee arthroplasty is estimated to grow by 673% from 2005 to 2030, leading to 3.5 million annual procedures [4], while UKA is approximately 5% of all knee arthroplasty in AJRR.

The aim of this chapter is to discuss the key points about returning to sports after TKA and UKA.

37.2 Patient Expectations

Patients' expectations are particularly important because they are linked to request for elective and possibly costly treatments and are strongly related to patients' assessments of outcome [5]. Moreover, the patient expectations are strongly associated with patient satisfaction. The more exigent the patients, the greater is the risk of dissatisfaction after surgery. Therefore, it is crucial for surgeons to thoroughly explain to patients not only the benefits but also the risks and limitations of the total knee arthroplasty.

The primary goals of knee arthroplasty have traditionally been pain relief, regain range of motion, and restoration of daily living activities, with patients commonly discouraged from

Illustrations by Rosa Ballis

B. Shabani
Heimerer College, Prishtinë, Kosovo

Orthopedic Department, University Clinical Center of Kosovo, Prishtinë, Kosovo

D. Bytyqi
Orthopedic Department, University Clinical Center of Kosovo, Prishtinë, Kosovo

C. Batailler · E. Servien · S. Lustig (✉)
Albert Trillat Center, Lyon University Hospital, Lyon, France
e-mail: cecile.batailler@chu-lyon.fr; elvire.servien@chu-lyon.fr

S. Rocha Piedade et al. (eds.), *The Sports Medicine Physician*, https://doi.org/10.1007/978-3-030-10433-7_37

participating in high-activity athletics. However, nowadays patients' expectations regarding the procedure have increased; they expect to restore their "before osteoarthritis" activities including athletic activity.

De Achaval et al. found that not all patients have similar expectations [6]. Patients' expectations are formed by many factors, including their personality characteristics, social class, interactions with health professionals, and information obtained through their individual research [7]. In addition, a multicenter cohort study found that younger patients, male patients, and those with better preoperative health status had higher expectations regarding postoperative outcomes [8]. Older age, being female, and worse pain predicted longer recovery expectations [6].

- Explain thoroughly to patients the benefits but also the risks of surgery.
- More exigent the patients the greater is the risk of dissatisfaction.
- Older age, being female, and worse pain predicted longer recovery expectations.

37.3 Return to Sports

Due to the improvement of surgical technique and design of the implants, surgeons may now recommend participation in more demanding physical activities. However, the level of physical activity can be influenced by multiple factors including sociodemographic characteristics, postoperative pain, and functional status [9]. In addition, being active before operation plays a very important role. Sixty-five percent of patients participated in sports before surgery, respectively, and 77% who had participated in regular exercise in the year before surgery returned to sports, compared to 35% who had been inactive in the year before surgery [10]. Naal et al. demonstrated that patients treated with UKA are generally very active before the operation. The proportion of patients able to return to sports was 95% following UKA and 34–88% following TKA [11].

Identification and selection of patient are very important, especially for UKA. Geller et al. have shown that proper selection in accordance with the indications and contraindications for UKA is the important factors for the success of UKA in regard to returning to sport [12].

What is considered "safe" athletic activity and what constitutes "excessive" and therefore dangerous athletic activity that may threaten the integrity of the implant?

Swanson et al. have shown that physical activity helps patients after total joint arthroplasty (TJA) enhance the quality of the interface between the bone and prosthesis [13]. On the other hand, the surgeon concerns that participation in sporting activities following TJA increased joint load and consequently higher joint load can result in increased implant wear, periprosthetic osteolysis, and eventual prosthetic failure [14, 15].

Huch et al. in their study advise against high-impact sports activities after total joint replacement, in order to protect the life span of the prostheses [16]. In contrast, because of increasing patient desires to engage in a highly active lifestyle, especially young patients, many surgeons now promote a more liberal level of athletic activity after TJA. Survey data from Knee Society found that the number of "not recommended" sports decreased from 1999 to 2005 while activities that were "allowed with experienced" or "allowed" increased [7, 17].

While sport activities after total joint replacement remain a debated topic, surgeons should give to patients the best postoperative instructions on returning to sports based on existing evidence, and not based on patient desires [17].

- Being active before surgery plays a very important role.
- Physical activity enhances the quality of the interface between the bone and prosthesis.
- From 1999 to 2005 sports that were "allowed" or "allowed with experienced" increased.

37.4 How Long Does It Take to Return to Sports?

Patients after joint replacement want to go back to sports as soon as possible. Concerning the timing, UKA is superior to TKA. Lombardi et al. suggested that minimally invasive UKA using a rapid recovery protocol allows patients a faster return to a more functional level than TKA [18]. Munk et al. have shown that leg extension power reached preoperative levels after 1 month [19]. Similarly, DeClaire proved that most patients will return to normal daily activities within 10–14 days and can be relatively active within 4–6 weeks after surgery [20].

Patients also seem to be able to maintain these activity levels. Walton noted that 67% of their patients returned to and maintained the same or an increased level of activity at a minimum follow-up of 12 months after UKA [21]. In addition, Canetti et al. reported that robotic-assisted surgery for lateral UKA reduces the time to return to sports at a patient's pre-symptomatic level. This robotic tool permits surgeons to be less invasive regarding soft tissues and bony resection, which may lead to a shorter recovery [21].

On the other hand, return time to sport after TKA is longer. A study by Argenson et al. has shown that patients after TKA need 6 months to return to mainly low-impact sports [22]. Hopper and Leach reported a mean time of 4.1 months to return to low-impact sports [23], while Bock et al. reported an overall mean time of 4–7 months to return to both low- and higher-impact sports [24].

37.5 Biomechanical Consideration

Knee forces across the knee are very important after knee arthroplasty because unlike biological tissues, the material used in knee replacement do not regenerate or remodel [25].

In a study, Argenson et al. have found that subjects with UKA experienced kinematic patterns similar to those of the normal knee [26]. On the other hand, other studies conclude that despite improvements, the knee kinematics in TKA group differed from healthy control group. TKA group had a lower extension and lower range of axial rotation and an increased tibial posterior displacement [27]. Also, many TKA exhibit a mismatch between the femoral and tibial radius with high peak pressures on the polyethylene inlay [28].

There is a correlation between the angle of the load on the knee joint and polyethylene wear. Kuster et al. demonstrated that jogging and downhill walking produced large areas of overload polyethylene. Most knee implants have a higher congruency near extension, which decreases with increasing flexion, leading to a smaller contact area between femoral and tibial component. Therefore, activities with peak loads near extension, such as walking (20°), produce less stress on the polyethylene than activities with peak loads in more flexion, such as jogging (60°). A patient after TKA participated in a marathon run despite being discouraged by the surgeon. The polyethylene inlay broke at the 35-km mark due to severe delamination and destruction. Differently, cycling and power walking seem to be suitable activities while mountain hiking; patients are advised to avoid descents or at least use ski poles and walk slowly downhill to reduce the load on the knee joint. So, it is very important to consider both the load and the knee flexion regarding recommendation suitable for physical activities [28, 29].

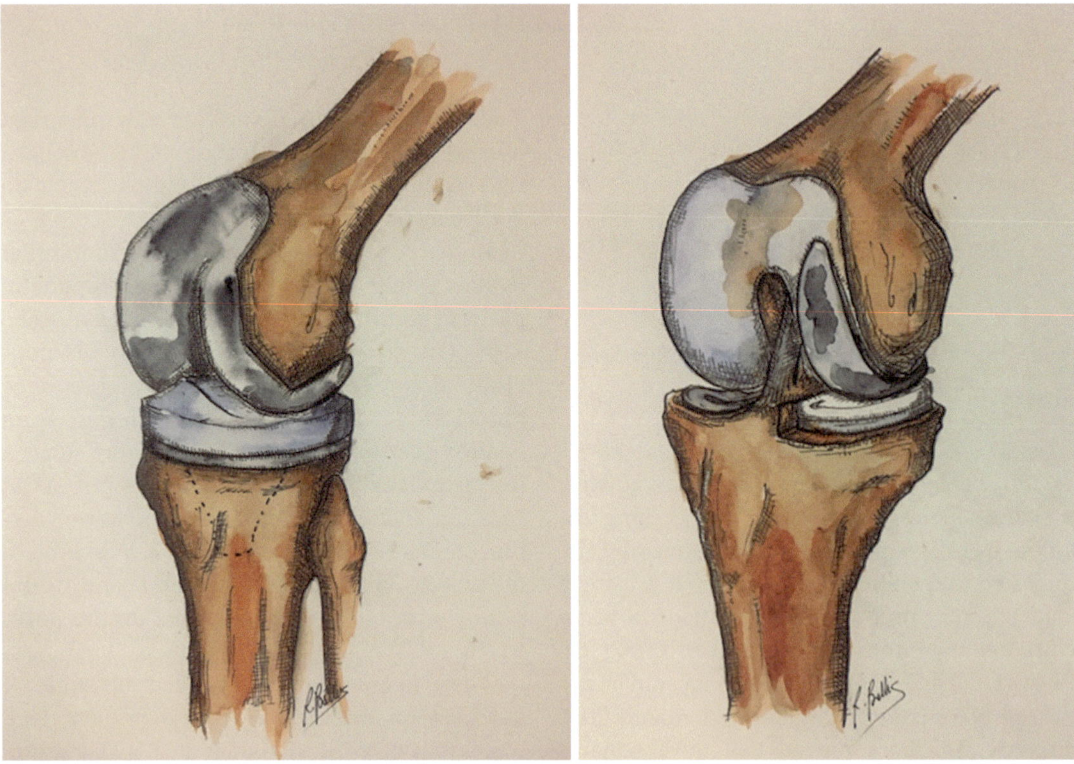

37.6 Sports Recommendations

Waldstein et al. demonstrated in a systematic review that 8 out of 17 studies showed a significant decrease returning in high-impact activities and a significant increase in low-impact activities [30].

A guideline developed by Clifford and Mallon recommends [31]:

- Low-impact activities like golf, swimming, walking, stationary bike, treadmill, and elliptical machines are recommended activities to all patients.
- Potentially low activities like bicycling, speed walking, cross-country skiing, dancing, Pilates, and rowing are recommended to patients with good balance and proprioception. In addition, these patients should be monitored by their surgeon regularly.
- Intermediate-impact activities like tennis, hiking, downhill skiing and snowboarding, weightlifting, ice skating, rollerblading, and low-impact aerobics are recommended to patients with experience in these sports in order to minimize risk of injury and accelerated implant wear.
- Very high-impact activities like racquetball, running, high-impact aerobics, most ball sports, martial arts, and rock climbing should be discouraged because of higher-risk injury.

Vogel et al. in their study have more or less the same recommendations (Table 37.1) [17].

Golf is very popular among older adults, but loss of motion in arthritic knee makes it difficult to play. So, many golfers see the TKA as a solution in order to be able to continue playing golf.

Mallon and Callaghan reported on the largest group of patients undergoing TKA in active players and defined playing golf as greater than three times per week. Eighty-four percent of the golfers reported no knee pain during the activity, while 62% reported no pain and 35% reported mild knee pain after the activity [32]. This pain is more common in the leading knee and has been

Table 37.1 Activity recommendations after TKA [17]

Recommended	Recommended with experience	Not recommended
Low-impact aerobics	Cycling	Racquetball/squash
Bowling	Hiking	Contact sports (football, hockey, soccer)
Golf	Rowing	Rock climbing
Dancing	Cross-country skiing	Jogging/running
Walking	Stationary skiing	Single tennis
Swimming	Speed walking	Waterskiing
	Doubles tennis	Baseball/softball
	Ice skating	Handball
		Martial arts

attributed to increased torque. In addition, D'Lima et al. demonstrated that increased loading in the leading knee during golf swing may also be a contributing factor of pain [32, 33]. Moreover, the length of the drive was reduced by 12 yd following knee replacement [32].

Regarding if the golf is recommended or not, a 2009 survey of members of the American Association of Hip and Knee Surgeons found that over 95% of members do not restrict patients undergoing TKA from playing golf [13]. Furthermore, golf is part of the recommended/allowed sports after TKA.

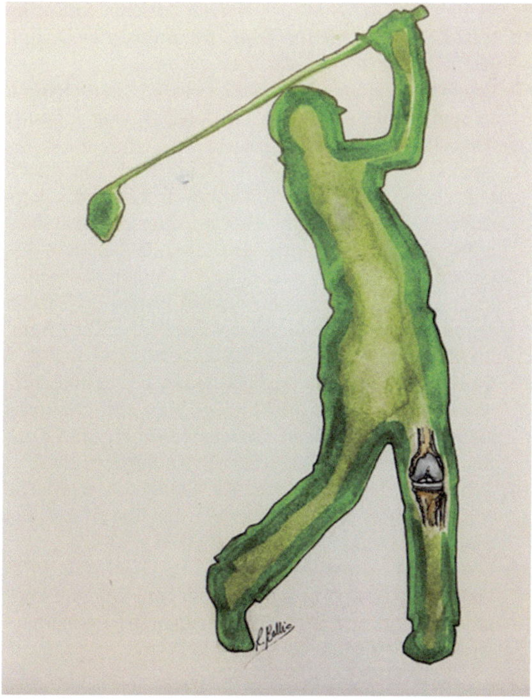

Judo is a contact sport, in which opponents use balance and body weight, with minimal physical effort, to throw or pin each other down or hold each other in a lock.

Lefevre et al. have shown that 62.5% of patients return to practice noncompetitive judo, 5.2 months (mean) after total knee replacement [34]. It is important to note that this was not the recommendation of the surgeons. This was the desire of the patients, because it is difficult for a judoka to give up practicing this sport because Judo is also a life philosophy [34]. However, patients must be informed of the higher risk of complication if they practice intensively.

It should be considered that in our knowledge, this is the only study about "Judo after TKA" and this study has a selection bias because it only included subjects practicing high-level judo who were still licensed at the French Judo Federation [34].

Tennis has a long history, and nowadays more and more people are choosing it as a way to maintain their fitness. Playing tennis can vary from high-impacted singles play to low-impacted social doubles play. Vogel et al. in their study have included doubles tennis as recommended with experience [17]. Playing doubles than singles is recommended, since it gives you a smaller court area to cover and is less physically demanding. It is also recommended a clay court surface, since it is softer and slower than hard courts. Also, wet surfaces should be avoided.

Mont et al. have shown that competitive tennis players were able to perform at a high level in their tennis activity after total knee arthroplasty as they were in their preoperative state. These players were able to play competitive singles and doubles tennis almost three times a week [35]. Similar result was reported also by LaPorte et al., who showed that patients were satisfied with their recovery even though they played at a lower level [36]. However, Mont et al. in their study found also that most of the surgeons did not advise playing tennis after TKA. They were reluctant in recommending playing tennis to their patients after TKA [35].

It is important also to note that tennis serve and forehand stroke generate greater forces than the backhand stroke [33]. After all, the Knee Society consensus recommendations permit doubles tennis but do not allow singles tennis [7].

- Eighty-four percent of the golfers reported no knee pain during playing.
- Ninety-five percent of the members of the American Association of the Hip and Knee surgeons do not restrict their patients from playing golf.
- The Knee Society permits doubles tennis but does not allow singles tennis.

37.7 Conclusion

Today patients' expectations have increased regarding knee replacement surgery. The activities that were "allowed with experience" or "allowed" increased as well. However, recommendation about returning to sports should be based on existing evidence and surgeons' experience, especially on intermediate- and high-impact activities.

Patients after UKA have shown faster returning to activities compared to those after TKA. Further work is required to evaluate the kinetic and kinematic of UKA and TKA in different sports in order to accurately describe the risks of these patients in returning to particular activities, even in the high-impact activities.

References

1. Haskell WL, Lee IM, Pate RR, et al. Physical activity and public health: updated recommendation for adults from the American College of Sports Medicine and the American Heart Association. Circulation. 2007;116:1081–93.
2. Dunlop DD, Song J, Semanik PA, et al. Objective physical activity measurement in the osteoarthritis initiative: are guidelines being met? Arthritis Rheum. 2011;63(11):3372–82.
3. Shih M, Hootman JM, Kruger J, Helmick CG. Physical activity in men and women with arthritis National Health Interview Survey. Am J Prev Med. 2002;30:385–93.
4. Kurtz S, Ong K, Lau E, et al. Projections of primary and revision hip and knee arthroplasty in the United States from 2005 to 2030. J Bone Joint Surg Am. 2007;89:780–5.
5. Uhlmann RF, Inui TS, Carter WB. Patient requests and expectations. Definitions and clinical applications. Med Care. 1984;22:681–5.
6. De Achaval S, et al. Patients' expectations about total knee arthroplasty outcomes. Health Expect. 2016;19(2):299–308.
7. Healy WL, Sharma S, Schwartz B, et al. Athletic activity after total joint arthroplasty. J Bone Joint Surg Am. 2008;90:2245–52.
8. Lingard EA, Sledge CB, Learmonth ID. Patient expectations regarding total knee arthroplasty: differences among the United States, United Kingdom, and Australia. J Bone Joint Surg Am. 2006;88:1201–7.
9. Chang MJ, et al. Activity levels and participation in physical activities by Korean patients following total knee arthroplasty. BMC Musculoskelet Disord. 2014;17(15):240.
10. Bradbury N, Borton D, Spoo G, Cross MJ. Participation in sports after total knee replacement. Am J Sports Med. 1998;26(4):530–5.
11. Naal F, Fischer M, Preuss A, Goldhahn J, von Knoch F, Preiss S, Munzinger U, Drobny T. Return to sports and recreational activity after unicompartmental knee arthroplasty. Am J Sports Med. 2007;35(10):1688–95.
12. Geller JA, Yoon RS, Macaulay W. Unicompartmental knee arthroplasty: a controversial history 177 and a rationale for contemporary resurgence. J Knee Surg. 2008;21(1):7–14.
13. Swanson EA, Schmalzried TP, Dorey FJ. Activity recommendations after total hip and knee arthroplasty: a survey of the American Association for Hip and Knee Surgeons. J Arthroplasty. 2009;24(6 Suppl):120–6.
14. Schmalzried TP, Shepherd EF, Dorey FJ, et al. The John Charnley Award: wear is a function of use, not time. Clin Orthop Relat Res. 2000;381:36–46.
15. Seyler TM, Mont MA, Ragland PS, Kachwala MM, Delanois RE. Sports activity after total hip and knee arthroplasty: specific recommendations concerning tennis. Sports Med. 2006;36(7):571–83.

16. Huch K, Muller KA, Sturmer T, Brenner H, Puhl W, Gunther KP. Sports activities 5 years after total knee or hip arthroplasty: the Ulm Osteoarthritis Study. Ann Rheum Dis. 2005;64(12):1715–20.
17. Vogel LA, Carotenuto G, Basti JJ, Levine WN. Physical activity after total joint arthroplasty. Sports Health. 2011;3(5):441–50.
18. Lombardi A, Berend K, Walter C, Aziz-Jacobo J, Cheney N. Is recovery faster for mobile-bearing 181 unicompartmental than total knee arthroplasty? Clin Orthop Relat Res. 2009;467(6):1450–7.
19. Munk S, Dalsgaard J, Kehlet H. Early recovery after fast-track Oxford unicompartmental knee 185 arthroplasty. Acta Orthop. 2012;83(1):41–5.
20. DeClaire J. Post-op rehabilitation protocols for the uni patient and recommended activity level. 173 partial knee arthroplasty: indications, technique and controversies (EE). 2012. http://www.aaosnotice.org/174 2012_Proceedings/adult-knee-Post-op.html.
21. Canetti R, Batailler C, Bankhead C, Neyret P, Servien E, Lustig S. Faster return to sport after robotic-assisted lateral unicompartmental knee arthroplasty: a comparative study. Arch Orthop Trauma Surg. 2018;138(12):1765–71. https://doi.org/10.1007/s00402-018-3042-6.
22. Argenson JN, Parratte S, Ashour A, et al. Patient-reported outcome correlates with knee function after a single-design mobile-bearing TKA. Clin Orthop Relat Res. 2008;466:2669–76.
23. Hopper GP, Leach WJ. Participation in sporting activities following knee replacement: total versus unicompartmental. Knee Surg Sports Traumatol Arthrosc. 2008;16:973–9.
24. Bock P, Schatz K, Wurnig C. Körperliche aktivität nach knietotalprothesenimplantation. Z Orthop Ihre Grenzgeb. 2003;141:272–6. https://doi.org/10.1055/s-2003-40081.
25. D'Lima DD, Chen PC, Colwell CW Jr. Polyethylene contact stresses, articular congruity, and knee alignment. Clin Orthop Relat Res. 2001;392:232–8.
26. Argenson JN, Komistek RD, Dennis DA. Kinematic characteristics of the unicompartmental knee. In: Total knee arthroplasty. New York: Springer; 2005. p. 148–51.
27. Bytyqi D, Shabani B, Cheze L, Neyret P, Lustig S. Does a third condyle TKA restore normal gait kinematics in varus knees? In vivo knee kinematic analysis. Arch Orthop Trauma Surg. 2017;137:409–16.
28. Kuster MS, Spalinger E, Blanksby BA, Gächter A. Endurance sports after total knee replacement: a biomechanical investigation. Med Sci Sports Exerc. 2000;32(4):721–4.
29. Lustig S, Magnussen R, Kacmaz E, Servien E, Neyret P. Unicompartmental knee replacement and return to sports. In: Sports injuries. Berlin: Springer; 2015. p. 2541–7.
30. Waldstein W, Kolbitsch P, Koller U, Boettner F, Windhager R. Sport and physical activity following unicompartmental knee arthroplasty: a systematic review. Knee Surg Sports Traumatol Arthrosc. 2016;25(3):717–28.
31. Clifford PE, Mallon WJ. Sports after total joint replacement. Clin Sports Med. 2005;24(1):175–86.
32. Mallon WJ, Callaghan JJ. Total knee arthroplasty in active golfers. J Arthroplast. 1993;8:299–306.
33. D'Lima DD, Steklov N, Patil S, Colwell CW Jr. The Mark Coventry Award: in vivo knee forces during recreation and exercise after knee arthroplasty. Clin Orthop Relat Res. 2008;466(11):2605–11.
34. Lefevre N, Rousseau D, Bohu Y, et al. Return to judo after joint replacement. Knee Surg Sports Traumatol Arthrosc. 2013;21:2889–94.
35. Mont MA, Rajadhyaksha AD, Marxen JL, Silberstein CE, Hungerford DS. Tennis after total knee arthroplasty. Am J Sports Med. 2002;30:163–6.
36. Cerciello S, et al. A review of sport recovery after total knee replacement. J Nov Physiother. 2013;S3:002.

Ringside Medicine

38

Joseph John Estwanik

38.1 Background

Ringside Medicine has now approached the distinction of becoming a subspecialty within medicine! OK, sub subspecialty. The physician attending to these dedicated athletes within the combat arts provides an array of services that blend expertise within many medical subspecialties for this subset of athletes [1]. We as physicians are obligated to create safety for those dedicated athletes who train and compete within their sport. They have earned the right to equal application of sports medicine technology and standards of care. The awareness of distinct mechanisms of injury allows predictive and then accurate diagnoses [2]. The demands of these combat sports (more than a contact sport) must be grasped so as to provide sports-specific rehabilitation and safely efficient return to play expectations. Ringside Medicine [3] provides a broad expanse of responsibility as its physicians must be knowledgeable and then respected by those competing within:

1. Amateur boxing
2. Pro boxing
3. Mixed martial arts
4. Innumerable disciplines to include judo, jiu-jitsu, tae kwon do, and so many others
5. Wrestling
6. Men/women
7. Youth/adult
8. Diverse venues: indoors, outdoors, large, and small
9. The "alphabet soup" of various ruling bodies, state/federal oversight, and sanctioning bodies
10. Multiple countries of origin with their cultural traditions

Virtually every country for many centuries has evolved their uniquely named and highly specific martial arts style: Kung Fu, China; Muay Thai, Thailand; Arnis, the Philippines; etc.

Boxing has become the adopted style for the United States. An awareness of customs goes a long way in developing rapport and trust within this community. Fellowship, mutual respect, and an understanding of rules, regulations, and protocol are critical. Period!!!

When a fighter suddenly goes down, ringside duties do not fall under "first aid" but truly "immediate" aid, with many people watching. There is no locker room present for privacy, no team of athletes to shield one by other activities, no half times, no braces, and no substitutions. The clock is often still running.

In reality, the physician for large pay-per-view televised events as well as small local

J. J. Estwanik (✉)
USA Boxing, US Olympic Training Center, Colorado Springs, CO, USA

Metrolina Orthopedic and SportsMedicine Clinic, Cornelius, NC, USA

S. Rocha Piedade et al. (eds.), *The Sports Medicine Physician*,
https://doi.org/10.1007/978-3-030-10433-7_38

shows must be proactive and realize that he too is a member of a team with the obligation to manage his doctorly duties just as others professionally allow "the show to go on!" Just as the sound, lighting, TV, and all other technical aspects are professional and highly synchronized, the ringside doctor assumes the **role of the physician producer**. Success measured in safety outcomes doesn't just happen, and a Ringside Physician should create an agenda for success. You cannot just show up at your seat as the bell rings and the show goes live. Nor can you exit as the lights dim with last bout! There are multiple segments for a Ringside Physician agenda and checklist [3].

38.2 Early

1. Review and discuss your expected and contractual obligations regarding salary and arrival dates/times for the various functions including physicals.
2. Analyze the credibility/reputation of the promoter.
3. Confirm the promoter's duties to obtain support services such as a dedicated ambulance, oxygen, stretcher, and cervical collar.
4. Know the calculated distance/transport time to emergency rooms with neurosurgery services.
5. Walk the facility and be sure that there is telephone or cellular signal.
6. Confirm the presence of proper support staff based on the event size and magnitude. A "team" approach with assisting medics, nurses, and physician assistants creates efficiencies. Create teams A and B to simultaneously cover the ring as well as locker rooms.

38.3 Prebout

1. Hand out the history questionnaires. Preferred are those created by the Association of Ringside Physicians available within their website.
2. Perform physicals. Important questions to ask for predicting fitness and preparation are:
   - What is your fight record?
   - How many miles/week do you run?
   - How many weeks of training for this event?
   - How much weight did you lose?
3. Utilize the pre-printed forms for the history, physical exam, and injury reports.
4. Perform a facility walk-thru:
   - Meet the referee.
   - Claim your location at ringside.
   - Meet security, introduce yourself, and plan ingress/egress and crowd control.
   - Find the treatment rooms.
   - Find all of the athlete locker rooms labeling each athlete's name on the doors.
   - Examine the ring for cleanliness, ropes, apron size, and ring ties (2/each side of ring ropes).
   - Evaluate lighting and obstructions for vision or entry.
   - Timekeeper's location to possibly communicate a rapid time-out.
   - Exact rescue squad location and introduce yourself with proper protocol.

38.4 Intrabout

1. Review Dr E's ten rules for ringside observation.
2. Basic tools of the trade: gloves, sponges, flashlight (torch), and oral airway.

38.5 Ring Responses

38.5.1 Short of a Knockout

The referee, the **"third man" in the ring**, usually and customarily stops a bout. The boxer is dependent upon intervention by a neutral party, the referee. In case you are summoned by the referee to evaluate a fighter, ascend the steps or have the cage door opened near your seat [1, 2].

Actually, your seating for a MMA event should be very close to the door so that you may respond to emergencies or enter for your opinion. In the majority of cases, your evaluation and grasp of the ongoing scenario are not a surprise. By alertly observing the circumstances within each round, your analysis is in evolution at all times, and your response and decision are anticipated rather than a surprise. I highly prefer that the doctors, if two, are seated together rather than opposing corners. Separating the physician robs the advantage of scholarly discussion and shared opinion. Most usually, assigned Ringside Physicians are of differing subspecialties. The ability to learn from each other and share input always benefits those athletes competing! Have your "tools of the trade" already open and avoid wasting time. Hygienic gloves, sponges, and a flashlight should be ready to go.

Once requested, enter the ring with composure. The referee will usually bring the athlete to you if possible, or you may need to travel to a more compromised or fallen athlete. So many times, your opinion as to a cut, eye poke, or sore rib pertains to your monitoring, not necessarily an emergency. The ref just wants your input as a situation is evolving. At this time, take your time. Speaking to the athlete, more closely evaluating a cut, checking vision, or palpating tender ribs can be performed in an unstressed manner. Just remember, during a bout, the doctor is not allowed to treat an injury. You are simply assessing for the ability for this one athlete to safely continue. To be fair, there is another athlete standing across the ring. Therefore, a lengthy and inefficient exam disadvantages the opponent unfairly. You can always be called to reevaluate this same athlete in question later within this round or in a subsequent round. In my past, as I allowed a fight to continue based on a cut, a second inter-fight viewing that confirmed lengthening or deepening of a cut or progressive decline of skills or alertness prompts my advice to stop the bout based on accumulating evidence. If you do decide that a bout must end, do so with decisive authority and self-confidence. A wishy-washy demeanor lacking confidence will only invite questions and second guessing. A firm non-subtle waving an end to the bout makes your life so much easier.

One of my professors from London once quoted "Decisive hesitation is far preferred to hesitative indecision." If you OK a bout to continue, do so with authority. If you end a bout, do so with authority. Do not leave room for ongoing scrutiny or it will go on and on. But, if allowed by your commission, answer questions based on medical science. No one knows more about sports medicine than an ARP-certified Ringside Physician. Simply explain the science without emotion. The undisputed fact is when a boxer is no longer able to defend himself, the bout must end. An early fight physician, Dr. McGown, states, "A bout must be stopped minutes early, rather than seconds late." Remember: **the rules, tradition, and protocol do not provide a mechanism to "quit" in traditional boxing or martial arts**. Mixed martial arts does uniquely employ the "tap out" as a safety mechanism, if the competitor wisely opts to do so. If, upon examining an athlete either during the physicals or within the heat of a bout, you sense their broken spirit, you must be the one who provides their honorable way out. Accept this gift and responsibility to represent your patient. You can be the bad guy! You take the blame. This has happened to me on many occasions. Once I have formally advised the bout to cease, with the athlete non-verbally or verbally asking me quietly to stop the bout, they will often put on a show complaining of the decision. They have to save face. Most usually, latter during the show, he/she returns and sincerely thanks me for helping and protecting them. That's our job.

38.6 The Sliding Scale of Tolerance

Just this year during a presentation to the World Boxing Association international meeting [1, 2], I mentioned that I make different decisions during amateur, pro, and championship events.

Remarks emanating from an individual within the audience focused upon a doctor's adherence to the Hippocratic Oath and rendering equal treatment to all. My precipitated remarks centered upon the topic of cuts and other injuries in general. Be it a facial cut, a bloody nose, a hand injury, fatigue, and others, yes, I let the pro fight go longer than the amateur.

Within an entire career of practicing medicine, we advise individuals differently based upon circumstances. I actually used the knee example of a torn anterior cruciate ligament. In patient A who is a healthy athletic 25-year-old, I would repair/reconstruct. In patient B who is a wheelchair-bound 80-year-old, I would not. A story was shared with me in my early residency days by a mentor, Art Steffie, MD. He, of spinal Steffie plate fame, was given advice in his early training days by George Phalen, MD, of the carpal tunnel Phalen's sign fame, "Art, I can teach you HOW to do surgery and WHY to do surgery, but I can never teach you WHEN to do surgery." This wisdom applies to Ringside Medicine. There are absolutes but there also exists a sliding scale of tolerance for circumstances and wise decision-making. This defines the SCIENCE of medicine balanced with the ART of medicine. By gaining experience within this sport and subculture of combat sports, an ability to properly navigate among science and rules/regulations will allow proper decisions to prevail [3].

38.6.1 Full Knockout

1. Observe how he falls: from an accumulation of blows, fatigue, or one solid punch?
2. Where did the blow land: head or body?
3. Was there a second injury mechanism of the head hitting the canvas or the neck in ropes?

If a knockout (Fig. 38.1):

- Maintain the airway.
- Protect the neck and assume a fracture until proven otherwise.
- Do not remove mouthpiece unless grossly obstructing; it can be useful.
- Initiate verbal questions and commands.
- A flashlight exam may or may not be useful but displays concern and buys time.
- Look busy and concerned.
- Be time efficient but do not showboat. "COMING AROUND" STAGE

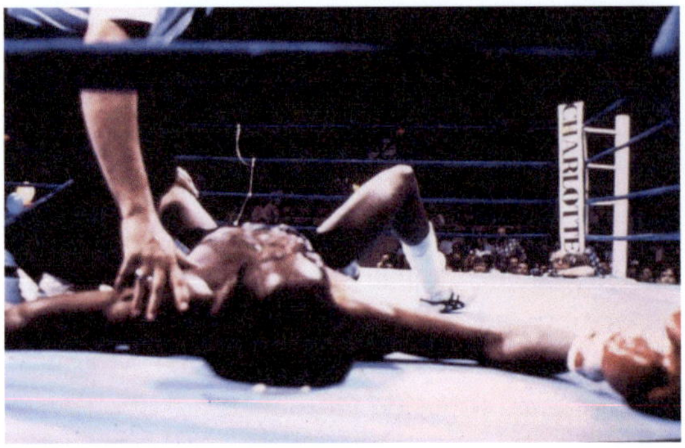

Fig. 38.1 A knockout in boxing

1. Continue protecting the cervical spine.
2. Control random movements with the help from docs, referee, or EMTs.
3. Don't get punched. I often kneel on the closest arm while ready to block a blow.
4. Reassure the awakening and often disoriented fighter.
5. Provide commands to test awareness.
6. Allow sitting on the canvas.
7. Allow sitting on a stool.
8. Allow standing.
9. Accompany the fighter to her corner.
10. Resume a more complete examination in the privacy of a locker room.
11. Report findings, diagnoses, and follow-up needs to the coach and family.

Severe acute brain injury can create a subdural hematoma related to athletic injury. These brain compressing bleeds are the most common form of catastrophic brain injury within boxing and martial arts. Epidural bleeds are far less common. Rapid recognition and urgent transfer efficiency to emergency facilities equipped for neurotrauma are paramount to successful outcome! As we know in all sports, brain acceleration and deceleration create the resultant forces. In boxing, the uppercut vertically and the cross punch horizontally form the coup and contrecoup pathology in addition to the other expected multi-axis forces involved (Fig. 38.2a–c). Subdural hematomas can viciously and rapidly occur but may also more subtly and stealthfully expand into increasingly recognizable symptoms. Within the ring, recognize degrading skills unrelated to exhaustion

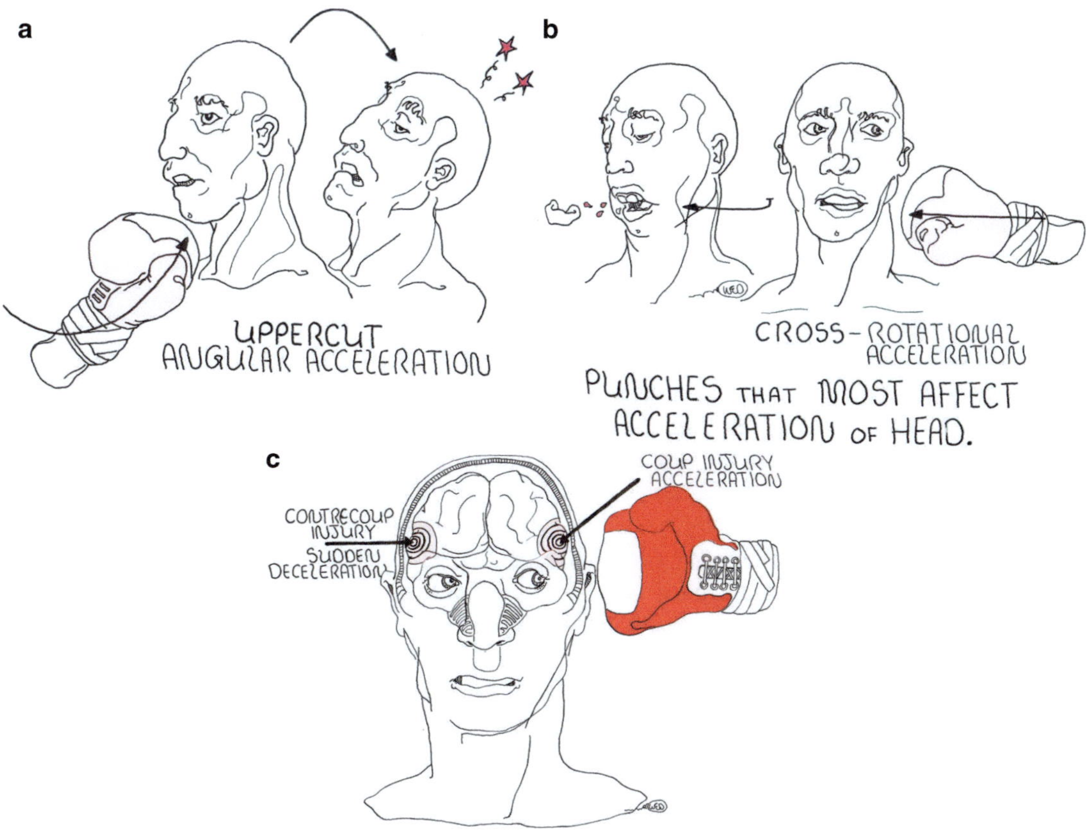

Fig. 38.2 Boxing blows: uppercut (**a**), punches (**b**), and contrecoup (**c**)

or dehydration. After a bout, instruct the athlete in question (and his coach) that they return to your position at ringside at stated intervals for the duration of the event so that you can monitor. You do not want to lose track of questionable but currently safe athletes. In impacted athletes who are properly recovering with normal exams but witnessed "tough bouts," discuss with athlete, family, friends, or coach their responsibility for monitoring that night and that limited sparring and alcohol are common sense. In questionable circumstances, send them to the hospital. Any criticism for an ambulance request will be weak and easily argued. Second-impact syndrome occurs soon after a seemingly minor head injury is suffered by an individual who is still experiencing symptoms from a prior concussion. This syndrome, which involves rapid swelling of the brain, has a 50% fatality rate. Younger individuals seem more exposed. Thus, our honestly gathered history during the physical exams required by all participants in the combat arts is of paramount importance. Remember, within boxing and martial arts, each athlete must be examined every day before every bout [2, 3].

38.7 Postbout

1. Examine ALL fighters. Repeat evaluations as needed throughout the event either as they return to the ring for a quick check-in or more formally in the locker room.
2. Complete all injury forms.
3. The doctor is the LAST to leave. Perform a final "sweep" of all locker rooms.

In serving as a Ringside Physician, the good news is that you possess the best location in the house with unobstructed view and rapid access to the excitement. The bad news is that this privilege carries with it the significant responsibility! You are sitting in the "hot seat."

I will have to admit that when at ringside, I wish for a boring fight although as a fan, I want action and excitement. The goal of a Ringside Physician is really not to be seen or needed. In reality, the embellished duties of ringside have been inflated by a description often utilized within the specialty of anesthesia—"hours of boredom, and moments of terror." A fight doc must demand the optimal visibility or leave the event. Be sure that access includes availability to rapidly ascend the steps to enter the ring and mat or open your Octagon gates (see diagram of ring setup, Fig. 38.3).

On one occasion, despite arriving early and "claiming" my seat for optimal visual surveillance and rapid access to the fighters, upon return, three ring girls had been placed in these doctor seats by the promoter. It was only when he understood that I was leaving for home and these three would now serve as his doctors; the seats were returned. On another occasion while serving with four or five international physicians for an Olympic Qualifying America's tournament finals, our immediate ringside seats, from this week-long tournament, were suddenly delegated to the international press and VIPs. We, docs, were allocated seats several rows distant and remote from rapid response, vision, and access. As a unified and bonded group of friends, we took seats with the audience. As the TV cameras were about to go live, a loudspeaker announcement sought our attention. Our group waving from this remote location caught their attention and rapid relocation ensued. I guess this is termed "stand your ground" for athlete safety. On many occasions, signage, advertising, and photographers can obstruct your critical view (Fig. 38.4).

Polite request for their relocation routinely allows cooperation in the name of athlete health. When at cage side or within a high-intensity crowded event, it is so helpful to introduce yourself as the Doc to the security staff who control access. The team concept immensely enhances all agendas and efficiencies. While at ringside, do not use your cell phone. A prominent fatality included audience video of the "unconcerned, inattentive" assigned physician constantly on the phone, ignoring the final round and collapse of the staggering athlete. Even after the unconscious fall to the canvas, the phone calls remained a priority. Yes, this is on YouTube. If it is very important to use my phone, I step away from ringside, while a fellow physician takes over. Or, I will wait until between bouts and step away, while an associate covers you. I never want to be witnessed with the phone near the active competition.

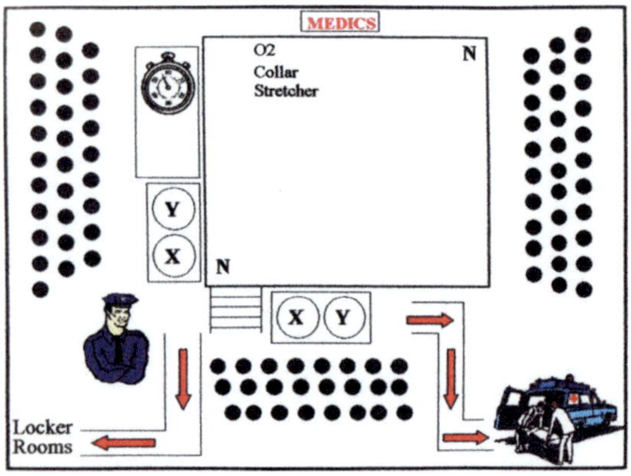

Fig. 38.3 Diagram of availability to rapidly ascend the steps to enter the ring, mat, or open your Octagon gates

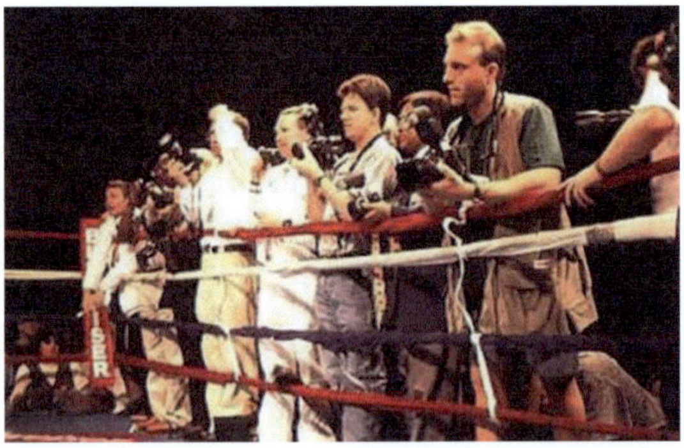

Fig. 38.4 Obstruction of the Ringside Physician's critical view by press photographers

38.7.1 The Ten Rules for Ringside Observation (Monitoring Safety)

Many years of observing the ups and downs of competition from ringside have allowed me to establish ten practical monitoring hints. All of my comments may not be based on researched, academic calculations but with real-life basics [3].

I Can't See His Eyes, but I Can Watch His Feet

1. **Stance**—A confident stance directly relates to that participant's skill level and training efforts. Balance means everything! A flat-footed, wide-based posture infers either an inadequately prepared novice or an injured fighter. The progression to a staggering stance denotes head injury or other major problems. Early in the event, a confident stance with eyes on the opponent confirms skill and training. Mid bout, stance relates to balance. Late within a fight, a flat-footed, wide-based, or staggering stance confirms problems.
2. **Ring movement**—Here's our chance to view "poetry in motion." The art and grace of athletics are no more evident than the floating, skillful movements of a dominant athlete. Without consulting scoreboards, computers, or bout sheets, the winner can be reliably predicted by who "dominates" the action. The "running" boxer is the defeated boxer (unless far ahead on points and purposely avoiding the taking of risks). You can just base your score on the gross positioning of the competitors.

I Can't See Her Eyes, but I Can Watch Her Hands

3. **Defense—The big "D."** This third principle actually occupies the #1 safety priority and reigns supreme for safe and timely cessation of competition. An effective defense is the ultimate determinate for combat safety. When defense is absent, the bout, match, or contest must cease. A winner has already emerged. In 1979, Dr. I. A. McCown wisely stated, "A one-sided contest should be halted minutes early, rather than seconds late." This mirrors my mindset and is readily quoted when potentially opening myself to criticism for demanding that a bout be stopped.
4. **Punch count**—The active and busy competitor is rarely in trouble. When a boxer is throwing punches, a wrestler working for the pin, or a martial artist creating combinations, we know that they remain healthy. Again, a winner can be predicted merely by "Who is throwing?" and "Who is busy?" This is not to say that the winner cannot also be hurt.
5. **Lowered arms**—Unless one possesses a very unconventional style, the sign of lowered arms means trouble. Fatigue and accumulated body blows will take their toll and drop the arms, thus opening the athlete to dangerous head blows. Boxing coaches urge patience and instruct the following pattern of attack to their athletes: "Go to the body and the head will follow." Knowledgeable audiences also understand the concept of "working the body" as I have amusingly heard them shout "Take the tires off that truck." Sometimes elbows are lowered to protect injured ribs. At times an injured extremity necessitates a one-armed contest. More than once, I have intensely followed, for a round or two, a boxer who slyly shields an injured shoulder, elbow, or hand as he protects his lead to hang on for the win. If his defense remains adequate, I'll hang on to the edge of my seat with him.

Fatigue Factors

6. **Clinches**—It is no surprise that tired athletes "tie up" an opponent to slow the flow of action. A tired, winning wrestler will ride his opponent while failing to work for additional points or a pin. Out of interest, I have counted the number of tie-ups or clinches within boxing events. In martial arts events, these five or ten situations per round would have provided excellent opportunities for a grappler to bring the boxer to the ground and into unfamiliar territory.
7. **"Bruise news"—accumulated trauma**—If an athlete is just plainly getting "beat up" and accumulating facial swelling, small cuts, bloody nose, etc., the writing is on the wall.

Usually, the winners stay pretty, but extremely competitive bouts may equally dole out punishment. Even the winner may appropriately be given a suspension in some circumstances.

8. **Number of standing "8" counts**—The "standing 8 count" is utilized in all amateur and some professional events. Amateur boxing rules stipulate defeat when a boxer receives three "8s" in a single round or a total of four "8s" at any time within the ensuing rounds. This is a good rule as it forces and ends to a noncompetitive situation. This ceases one-sided contests. The argument against this states that an "8 count" scenario allows the injured boxer unfair rest advantage and if the bout were allowed to continue slightly more, the bout would be officially ended, thus preventing the further accumulation of trauma to the looser. I have mixed opinion without a firm favoring conclusion. In the end, if the referee performs his duty for the overall safety of the boxer, then either scenario allows for this conclusion.

Extraneous Factors

9. **Referee level of attentiveness**—If a competent referee is handling the bout, the worries of the doctor, coach, parent, and athlete can be eased. If a skilled referee is hyperalert to one athlete, hovering close to break up the action, moving in tight to peer into his eyes, watch out! If good referees are nervous, I am nervous. If bad referees aren't nervous, I am nervous. Their level of activity and attentive focus mirror the flow of action and concern.
10. **Corner activity**—Nobody should know their athlete better than his personal coach. Focusing on the coach's facial grimaces, smiles, intense posture, or relaxed body imaging tells the tale of the tape. If they are happy, I'm usually happy. If they focus hyperactive attention to a cut or an extremity during the 1-min rest periods between rounds, I have an insider's hint on what stock to buy and where the money is. I am forewarned as to what area to observe during the next round. If you get to know the coaches, you will better learn to accurately read their body language. A ringside doctor must know that the 1-min "time-out" is NOT their time-out but a highly profitable and telltale 60 s for predictive information gathering.

By understanding and utilizing my ten rules of ringside observation, you'll accurately predict winners, losers, and importantly injuries. By alertly following a bout, I estimate a 90% plus accuracy level in predicting the injuries that will be present as competitors exit from the ring. However, sports and the art of medicine will be forever humbling. Just when you think that you know it all, the ever-motivated loser lands a lucky punch and knocks out his overwhelmingly superior opponent or the wrestler quickly reverses and pins his opponent. Do not forget the critical follow-up exam in the locker room after the session or during breaks during the event. I have picked up many injuries and complaints after the action and adrenaline subside.

38.8 Medical-Legal Implications of Ringside Duties

The sobering thought for ALL doctors covering ALL athlete events focuses our concentration on DEFENSIVE AWARENESS—yes, defense of our athlete's right to safe and fair competition but also the safety of our medical careers and licenses [3]. My past duties have included the comprehensive review of multiple catastrophic or fatal combat sports deaths. Additional to these reviews, testimony on several occasions further substantiate my gained perspective.

Should an untoward event occur, are many actions triggered? What are they looking for? Legal review and scrutiny will fully access all records of the event: pre, intra, and post. For us that translates into prebout exams, prebout history forms, environmental conditions, ring/cage setup and lighting, referee duties, efficiency of response, equipment, ambulance availability, and post bout exam performance (to name a few). The written interview and recorded records will be subpoenaed and meticulously dissected. Those records investigated within cases to which I have been authorized for review are of many and varied sources:

1. *Everyone now has a camera, video, or smartphone*. These recordings by passionate family, friends, televised events, or other athletes provide undeniable fact.

   The efficiency of response will be scrutinized second by second with an "attorney-grade" stopwatch and microscope. Formal depositions will in fact check claims and opinions. Be sure that you as a team physician attend and supervise only sanctioned events whether they be within the guidelines of USA Boxing as an amateur event or professional events approved and supervised by relevant state, tribal, or national government institutions.
2. Any waivers or releases signed by participants will be reviewed for declared facts or facts omitted by the athlete. A physician should expect accurate historical information. Athletes who deceive may have short and eternal consequences for their declarations. Always require athletes to sign your history forms to impress and assure full cooperation. Circumstances and cases have shown that athletes sustain a prebout head injury in the gym while sparring for the competition but have denied or failed to disclose that fact. In later interviews with teammates, the wife or family reveals headache, loss of appetite, or personality variance. Several personal physical exams or review of records have picked up recent head injury mechanisms from fights at school, auto accidents, hitting the windshield, or street fights not recognized by the athlete as a declarable prebout historical event. It wasn't in boxing, they say! Thus, I always ask: Have you EVER been knocked out or unconscious or had a concussion for any reason, at any time?
3. The individual passbooks or fight records of athletes can assist in identifying the risk factors of injury pattern, inactivity, losing streaks, sanction periods, win/loss record, recent competitions, or outright falsification.
4. Our physical exams should be standardized as an efficient checkoff form so that pertinent and sports-specific focuses are documented. The Association of Ringside Physicians and Association of Boxing Commissions websites provide these forms.
5. The promoter and facility contracts will be reviewed. One fatality case disclosed that no ambulance and oxygen source were available because within remote pages of the event contract, the responsibility (and cost) was marked out but unnoticed until the emergency occurred. This unnoticed cost savings did indeed not go unnoticed. The value of that athlete's life was beyond financial. Indeed, a Ringside Physician must demand dedicated ambulance and spine board, O2, and cervical collar at ringside. Check the facility O2 canister. I well remember being shown the "product" but felt thankfully compelled to check it myself, and, yes, it was "dead." The ambulance company did provide a full tank at ringside. Extremity splints are very appropriate articles to be demanded when covering mixed martial arts events. The splinting of extremities in a boxing competition is rare. Within a large venue, clearly and at all times, know the position of the EMT/ambulance team. On one occasion at a massive globally televised MMA event, these individuals with stretcher and supplies were moved from their original position. In an urgent injury scenario, the doctor must be able to initiate quick response verbal or visual contact with his "team." I have very definitely delayed events until the proper components are in place. Once, the event attended by 5000 paying customers was delayed for 2 h on a Saturday night because the promoter failed to make arrangements for ambulance service. Despite the city mayor and sheriff in attendance, the crowd was informed that fighter safety was the preeminent concern. Actually, they understood, and it was exhibited that safety is a dominant factor in boxing.
6. Efficiency of care is paramount. The seconds/minutes for physician entrance, evaluation, action, administration of oxygen, airway positioning, neck positioning with cervical stabilization, splinting, evacuation from the ring, and transport will all be mapped out and quantified.

7. Beyond your control, the emergency room, admission, and operating room records will be viewed. Subsequent laboratory reports have in my reviews confirmed the existence of illicit drugs present during the bout and obviously undeclared by the combatant. Neuroimaging and X-rays could disclose unhealed fractures or unhealed brain contusions/hemorrhage.
8. Several cases have disclosed at autopsy, findings of preexisting but unresolved brain bleeds that predisposed to the ultimate disaster of second-impact syndrome. Imaging and autopsy have also shifted the neuropathology from a fatal subdural to concurrent damage related to anoxia and probable lack of supportive care at ringside and transport.

   Ring/cage integrity and setup should be at least peripherally a concern to the physician as he evaluates the venue pre-completion. Having the ropes tight, two properly located spacer ties between the ropes on all four sides of the ring, hygienic and clean mats, safe stairs into the ring, and an adequately wide ring apron (the area of padding outside of the ropes) assure improved safety. I have studied two cases in which the athlete fell outside of the ring sustaining catastrophic injury in part due to hitting their head on hard surfaces. While sitting at ringside, I have witnessed my ring actually collapse. The slow-motion earthquake sensation of having the ring creak and groan as this sinking ship tipped on its side was surreal. The athletes clung to the ropes to avoid shipwreck. Fortunately, no crush injuries were sustained.

   To prevent disasters, ringside doctors must make a "sweep" of all locker rooms and athlete areas before leaving the venue. An athlete was found dead in the abandoned locker room.

38.9 To Prevent Catastrophe

The doctor is the last to leave!

Concerned physicians should "right" the wrongs that can be observed at ringside. If not, litigators will "write" the wrongs they observe at courtside.

38.10 Defensive Awareness Summary

Based upon my medical legal experiences related to ringside tragedy, the following summary provides previous factors of contention and medical concern.

Salient points:

1. No oxygen at ringside or a delay in administration.
2. No ambulance on site or significant delay in response to time, no prearrangement.
3. Improper ring/cage setup:
   - Too few ropes
   - No spacer ties
   - Ropes too loose
   - Padded obstacles near ring (stage or floor—two deaths resulting)
4. Inattention to altered details in event contracts.
5. No ringside doctor in attendance.
6. Physician assistant substituting for MD/DO.
7. Second-impact syndrome due to preexisting head blows sustained and unreported prior to the bout.
8. Undisclosed medication or illicit drug abuse.
9. Two fights in 1 day.
10. No post bout exam given.
11. Inappropriate length of rounds as surfacing on home video evidence. Straying from the rules.
12. Failure to respond to a crisis in a humanitarian, concerned manner.
13. The responsibility of all parties including the referee will be scrutinized.

Actual quotes from legal documents:

The valve for the oxygen tank at ringside did not work and O2 could not be administered.

"X's girlfriend commented to numerous individuals that X had headaches since receiving a sanction and halted bout 2 weeks prior to his fatal bout." X did not report headaches to the ringside physician during physicals. At autopsy of a 15-year-old reveals a "healing subdural hematoma" from a fight that was stopped two weeks earlier.

38.10.1 The Upper Extremity

Those who compete within the combat arts are virtually stripped of the protective equipment adorned by those within the contact sports such as ice hockey and American football. What they do utilize should be functional, certainly not hand wraps!! A 1000-year-old Egyptian mummy gauze wraps the "tools of the trade" while training in state-of-the-art supportive impact protective running shoes created with modern biomaterials. When interviewing as to why competitive athletes and fitness exercisers still fail to protect their hands with modern materials, they respond, "tradition." Yet the foot, groin, ankles, and knees are allowed enhanced protection options. Are the hands of the boxer less important than her feet?

Especially if boxing serves as a fitness tool for an otherwise employed secretary, dentist, accountant, etc.?

The art of optimally wrapping a hand with these limited materials narrows the elite craftsmen to a small number. Limited materials are further restricted by skill and time! Wet gauze gains weight and is impossible to wash and allows cheating. We, as doctors, should therefore be aware of hand and wrist injuries to susceptible anatomical structures.

The known directional forces of a punch follow three patterns (Fig. 38.5a):

(a) Axial compression—a direct blow.
(b) Angular forces—missed or misdirected punches.
(c) Excess tension—we microscopically subluxated our knuckle joint at impact.

Boxers consolidate injury to:

1. Traumatize MCP joints of index and long fingers.
2. Impact the carpal-metacarpal joints of index and long fingers to cause arthritis called metacarpal-carpal bossing.
3. Catch the thumb in an awkward position spraining the ulnar collateral ligament (gamekeeper's thumb).
4. Suffer a variety of metacarpal fractures.
5. Wrist sprains.
6. When not wearing a full boxing glove, as in martial arts, DIP and PIP joint sprains occur including mallet finger.
7. Flexor and extensor tendon injuries are rare.
8. Review illustration of hand forces to view the proper loading forces within the clenched fist. Each contact loading force should maximize onto the index and long digits. The smaller and less stabile ring and little fingers were not built to absorb the brunt of these quite large and highly repetitive punching forces. Thus, we practitioners often treat "boxer" fractures to the fifth metacarpal

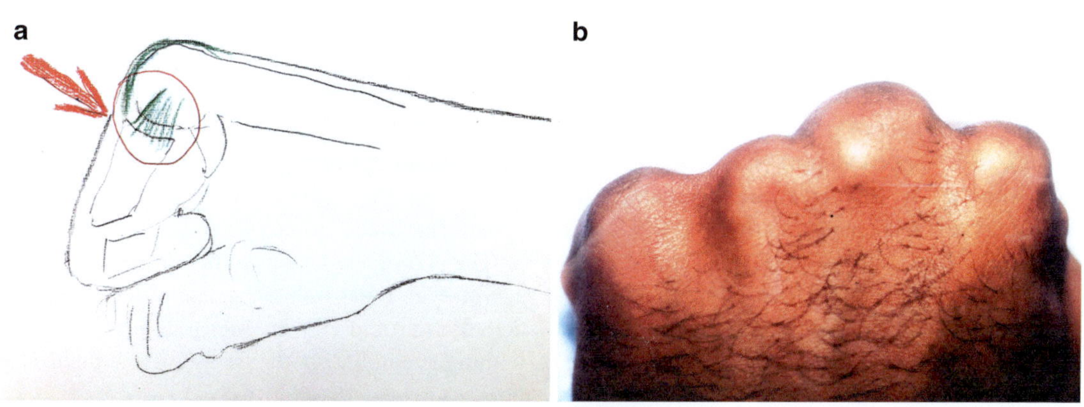

Fig. 38.5 Boxer's knuckle: mechanism (**a**) and clinical appearance (**b**)

which would be more accurately named "lousy boxer" fractures.

9. The "**boxer's knuckle**" results from overloaded compressive forces destabilizing the extensor tendon, capsule, and sagittal bands of the index and long fingers (Fig. 38.5b). Eventually after prolonged swelling and degradation, the extensor tendon becomes destabilized and dislocates.
10. Elbow injury generally results from a missed or blocked punch leading to hyperextension. Coaches holding focus pads/mitts in training can absorb rotational overload injuring the medial ligaments of their elbow. The elbow joint even more than other joints has a "long memory" for that injury mechanism, and that causative force or movement is the last activity to be tolerated during a recovery (see illustration of memory). Smart and knowledgeable rehab is sport specific!
11. Within mixed martial arts and wrestling, elbow joint injury occurs from the hyperextension of a missed spinning backlist blow or the opponent's massive and focused forces of submission elbow locks. I certainly have seen my share of significant ligament/capsular tears and frank dislocations. Be smart; tap out when you are caught!!!
12. Shoulder dislocations/subluxations certainly do occur following missed or misdirected punches in boxing or the planned or unplanned contortions of mixed martial arts submission techniques. All combat sports athletes can damage their glenohumeral or AC joints during a fall from a slip or a knockout. My first suspicion however when called into the ring for this concern centers upon a prior history of instability. Usually, a preexisting mechanism predated that episode within the bout. Although helpful, the bout is usually stopped due to this circumstance. Even if it spontaneously reduces, the Ringside Physician is not allowed to TREAT within a competition, and the fighter's ability to adequately protect themselves is compromised. Rotator cuff tears usually occur in the older athletes being less common at ringside. Acromioclavicular separations do occur as entangled, or knocked out athletes pile drive onto the affected side. Burners/stingers should be suspected with transient single extremity neurological complaint as cervical spine disorders such as hereditary canal stenosis, or disk protrusions are investigated also. Biceps tendinitis and labral traction tears (SLAP lesions) are more common in the course of training or competing.

38.11 Chest and Abdomen Injury

"Go to the body," "work the body," and "take the tires of that truck" all refer to body blows. Direct COMPRESSION forces from a punch or the weight of an opponent's body will produce injury. Miraculously, despite the tonnage of forces hammered onto the torso and abdomen region, rarely does a doctor have to treat. Certainly, rib fractures do occur, and the ultimate worry of a tension pneumothorax must be acknowledged. Costochondral sprains will not show on an X-ray, but their location is a giveaway and they hurt just as much. Occasionally the TORSIONAL forces applied to the rib cage in a wrestling or a ground fighting maneuver will be the causative factor for rib or cartilage stresses. Just this week, I have observed on two separate televised events, bouts ending with a vicious single left-handed punch to the flank and a single front kick to the solar plexus area of the body. This "liver shot" punch and the "solar plexus" kick immediately dropped the opponent to the mat rendering each helpless and ending each bout. Recovery was rather rapid as each downed fighter stood next to the referee as the victor's hand was raised. Locker room follow-up is certainly advised for lingering complications. Punches or kicks to the flank are rarely a cause for stoppage or trouble, but be aware that very often the fighter will demonstrate some hematuria should urinalysis be performed.

The significant causative factor for renal damage or even renal failure relates to the dangerous dehydration and weight loss practices tolerated within the combat sports. Be aware that the loss is not isolated to just water but also electrolytes and glucose. Starvation is also an accomplice of dehydration. Wrestling has significantly and positively improved this scourge by requiring (1) annual euhydrated percent body fat calculation and minimal weight category requirements so that combatants cannot choose an unphysiologic, unsafe lower weight class. (2) Weigh-ins are timed close to the competition so that unfair advantage is not empowered, and each athlete competes fairly.

The creation of weight categories was initiated for fairness, safety, and competitiveness. All wisdom is sacrificed as athletes truly have been allowed to compete after gaining 25 lb within a 24-h period. So much for weight classes! Known body and organ physiology confirm that redistribution of fluids, glucose, and electrolytes require 2–3 days. No consideration for equilibration within the brain and above the blood/brain barrier has been documented.

Does a dehydrated brain fully recover on the same schedule of the kidney of liver? How can a valid middleweight or welterweight champion be declared if the actual competition occurred at two weight classes above the claimed title weight? So much for safety and fairness! The sports of boxing and MMA must follow the leadership of wrestling.

38.12 Mouthpieces

So little equipment is allowed for a boxer. Gloves, hand wraps, no foul cup, shoes, trunks, and mouthpiece complete the list. Little attention, information, and inspection are dedicated to the structure that guards the mouth. Actually, comments should not be limited to the mouth.

Mouthpieces fit over the teeth, should be form fitting, can be professionally created by a dentist or by a home-style boil-and-bite. The structure can be single or dual arch. Noting the biomechanics resulting from a punch, an uppercut or a cross tends to create the most knockout acceleration of the brain within its boney skull. The mandible loosely articulates with the skull housing the brain. This articulation involves the condyle within the temporal fossa, some of the thinnest bone in our body. The temporal lobes of the brain sit nestled adjacent to this temporal-mandibular joint. MRIs of famously afflicted retired boxers demonstrate pathological changes on the inferior surface of this neighboring brain surface. Recall the facial distortion seen on replays of famous knockouts and the distortion of the jaw slamming either side-to-side with a cross or impacted upward with an uppercut, confirming these compressive shockwave forces. Within sports medicine, our goal is to stabilize joints. The innovative thumb-attached boxing glove now stabilizes the thumb MCP joint virtually ending ligamentous injury. An unstable ankle is either prophylactically or therapeutically stabilized by tape. An anterior cruciate-deficient knee is braced. Buddy taping protects injured fingers. The very mobile jaw joint complex should likewise be stabilized to prevent tooth, mandible, TMJ, and brain injury.

A proper fitting mouth piece with proper thickness can create a spacer effect so that the lower jaw (mandible) is not in contact with the base of the skull, actually creating a spacer or cushion. The teeth are also protected both from injury and preventing cuts to the wearer and the opponent. A human bite can initiate a serious infectious condition. Some designs of mouth pieces on X-ray review actually create a protective gap within the TMJ. When studying the mouthpieces worn by fighters, the majority of the wear is always posterior adjacent to the molars. The front tooth area remains totally intact. Very clearly, wear signs confirm the forces delivered to the jaw-TMJ-fossa-brain.

What should the Ringside Physician look for when inspecting the mouthpiece? (Fig. 38.6). First, I require that all fighters bring their mouthpiece to the physical exam [3]. I then view it for:

1. Wear almost always on the posterior molar segment. This is consistently the location where they are "chewed out" with the usage by the veterans.
2. Tooth imprints to confirm that it has been properly boiled or fitted and not out of the box.

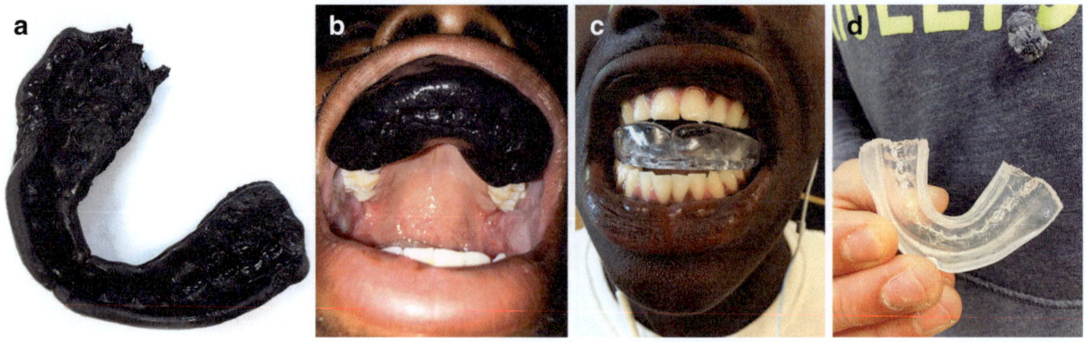

Fig. 38.6 Problems related to mouthpiece: chewed up molar (**a**), chopped of molar area (**b**), not form fitted, loose (**c**), and short and with poor impressions (**d**)

3. Proper length and not cut off short exposing the most critical zone of impact absorption.
4. Hygiene.
5. A true suction fit within the mouth.

Many times, during my exams I request the athlete who has inserted his mouthpiece to open her mouth widely. I often use my cell phone to photograph the mouthpiece within their mouth and confirm with them their picture of a "chopped off" equipment with vulnerable molars exposed. They greatly appreciate this explanation. A well-molded, tooth capturing, suction fit defines a proper fit. The poorly shaped, incompetent mouthpiece will fall down from the upper teeth, and they quickly close their mouth again to replace it. This confirms an incompetent useless mouthpiece. No wonder we see boxers "spitting" their mouthpiece when hit or tired. An athlete has to be able to open their mouth to breathe at times and not loose the protection. A great Olympic-level coach shared his mouthpiece wisdom with me. "If the athlete can remove their mouthpiece with their gloves on, it is too loose. I should have to be the one who removes it." I do prefer the two-sided dual arch design as it more fully stabilizes and braces the jaw while providing more shock-absorbing space within the TMJ. When I discuss price with the athlete and they prefer the low-cost option, I ask if they have a $5 or a $35 brain.

38.12.1 Mouthpiece Menu

- Observe the mouthpiece outside the mouth for a fitted appearance of deep tooth indentations.
- Check inside the mouth for retention and full coverage of the back molars.
- Use your cell phone to photograph inside the mouth for educational purpose.

A survey that I recently performed with the attendees of the annual Association of Boxing Commission and then the international members of the World Boxing Association confirmed a lack of organization for mouthpiece inspection. In fact, there was significant disagreement about the importance of various pieces of safety equipment. Hand wraps, gloves, and mouthpieces seemed to be judged equally important, but more regulation is mandated for hand wrap and glove inspection. As it is clear that no standardized protocol exists for mouthpiece safety check, the doctor must perform this during physicals. This sequence generally allows the competitor time to react and correct. Checkups by the ref entering the ring only prove that "something" is present. No quality control exists for guarding the teeth, gums, jaw, TMJ, and brain. Yet, great pomp and circumstance exist for using ancient technology on the hands. What is the "cost-benefit" analysis for protection of the hand vs. the brain? The current responsibility is highly confusing as there was no statistical conclusion in this survey supporting whether the coach, doctor, referee, or bout inspector should assume responsibility for checking the mouthpiece. By default, I suggest that this duty defaults to the doctor. The doctor has to do this! Note that this discussion applies to all athletes within the contact sports also to include safety for rugby, ice hockey, American football, soccer, and basketball.

38.12.2 Facial and Cuts

Accumulated blows to the face and orbital areas can create macabre swelling for the initial day or two post bout. Most certainly, a trained Ringside Physician should be consulted to confirm that the swelling is superficial only and that no deep structures are compromised. Facial cuts are poorly understood by the boxing/MMA community. They freak out over a cut while also staggering back to their corner. A boxer can be semiconscious, yet a minor facial laceration signals doom and gloom to them. Cuts are readily fixable if understood properly, while head injuries are very unforgiving and dangerous. The Ringside Physician's Manual by USA Boxing clearly classifies the cuts of a boxer (Fig. 38.7a) according to the area of involvement:

- **A**—Rarely lead to long-term disability, do not endanger vision, nor damage significant underlying structures.
- **B**—(Supraorbitial nerve) or **C** in the area of the infraorbital nerve and near the nasal lacrimal duct strongly indicates that a bout should be stopped in these danger zones.
- **D**—In the upper eyelid can endanger the tarsal plate and are also a danger zone.
- **E**—(Vertical cuts) through the vermillion borders of the lip creates the potential for further tearing, and the edges must be precisely sutured to prevent future disfigurement.
- **F**—Near the bridge of the nose requires evaluation for an underlying open nasal fracture or injury to the boney orbit.

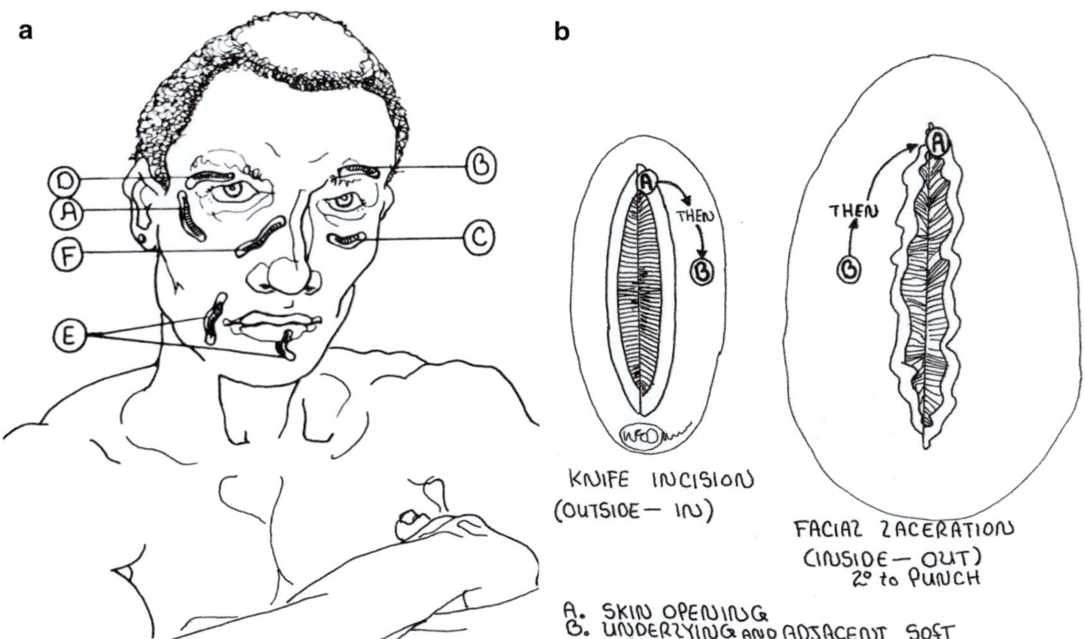

Fig. 38.7 Types of facial cuts (**a**) and type of incision (**b**)

Critical cuts localized near the medial aspect of the eye (orbit) and near the bridge of the nose are dangerous because they can extend into the lacrimal tear duct that lies close to the surface. This area should be only sutured by experts as a deep suture could tie off this duct requiring further extensive reconstruction.

Plenty of misunderstanding of the nature of boxing cuts exists. Cuts to the face of a combatant are not at all similar to lacerations from a sharp object like a knife or surgical scalpel (Fig. 38.7b). The mechanics of these facial cuts are similar to those of a gunshot with a little entrance wound but larger internal cavitation (see Fig. 38.7a). The typical laceration by a sharp object is an outside insult that is extended inward to the underlying tissues. The "punched" facial cut represents a skin-bursting injury that begins with deeply damaged tissues that then extend upwards as a cut. Believe it or not, the cut actually begins against the bone as the skin is forced against those underlying boney ridges. Boxers' cuts are "inside-outside" cuts! The bones of the face are the "sharp" objects that cause the skin to finally split or explode open externally. Thus, most of the damage is truly dealt to the subcutaneous tissues rather than misleadingly apparent in the skin surface. What fans recognize as a cut is only the tip of the iceberg.

This remarkably useful pocket card available on their Association of Ringside Physician website was created by Doctor Larry Lovelace and Daniel O'Donoghue PA-C, PhD. It succinctly and creatively again confirms the dangerous laceration zones (Fig. 38.8b) and on its flip side highlights very useful pressure points to stop bleeding (Fig. 38.8b). If one **imagines the eye covered by a coin or a circle, the inner 1/2 nearest the nose is *the danger zone***. Those on the outer half of the coin are relatively safe zones for the continuance of a fight based on actual size, bleeding that might interfere with vision (hence safety) and age-/skill-appropriate "sliding scale of tolerance."

The basics of repairing cuts in fighters are:

- Don't freak out at a minor cut. A little red blood goes a long way. The face is a very vascular area that heals fast.
- Recognize laceration zones that might become dangerous because of their proximity to underlying important structures (Fig. 38.8a).
- Understand that more tissue is damaged deep to the skin than is first evident. Understand that deep tissues are more extensively damaged than superficial skin: inside-out injury.
- A sutured wound heals faster and stronger than a comparable non-repaired wound.
- The application of buried subcutaneous sutures in combination with skin closure by suture, glue, or tape is the superior method of repair in deeper cuts. That regathered and repaired subcutaneous tissue serves as a cushion against future impacts and serves far better

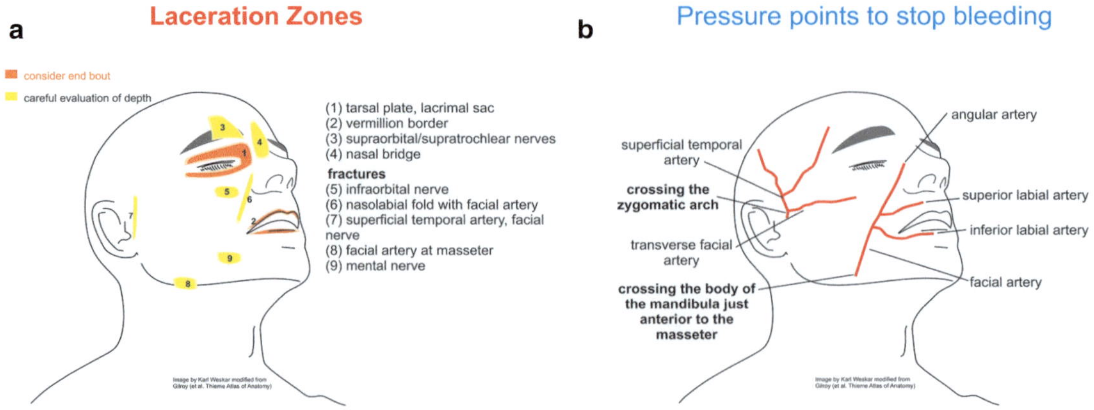

Fig. 38.8 Laceration zones (**a**) and pressure points to stop bleeding (**b**)

than "thin skin" against the future tendency to "cut easily."

- Wound healing times require more weeks than one would guess. It has been estimated that even if a wound is repaired, it takes 3 months just to obtain 60% of pre-injury strength.
- Wound strength for the forces applied within the fighting arts is as follows:
  30 days = 20% of strength
  60 days = 50% of strength
  1 year = 80% of strength

Other frequent facial injuries to be dealt with include ear **tympanic membrane ruptures** from "slaps," an open hand, or broad surface of the glove that creates significant air pressure within the ear canal as the eardrum tears from these shock waves. Avoid water entering this defect when showering. Pain pills, cotton ear plug, and possibly antibiotics are used. Most small tears will repair on their own, but experts need to follow the recovery and intervene as needed.

Speaking of ears, who can't recognize the pugilist, wrestler, or judo player by their ears. **Cauliflower ear** doesn't really have to result as preventative drainage, and **compression** will mitigate this telltale deformity. The ears and the nasal septum are both stiffened by multilayers of cartilage just as layers of mica rock form in nature. A shearing split between layers allows blood to collect and, if not depressurized, to thicken. Under strict sterility, aspirate the hematoma layer and compress, or it will refill.

Punches to the nose can also tear the cartilaginous nasal septum creating a **septal hematoma**, a cousin of the cauliflower ear. They appear upon nasal inspection with a light to be a "blueberry." These also demand mandatory drainage. If left intact, the cartilage will erode, collapse, and create the "saddle nose" sunken in, collapsed nose that stereotypes our image of the old-time boxers.

Epistaxis is so common. Rarely is a fight stopped due to this. But I have stopped bouts when severe bleeding either obstructs vision, grotesquely damages the image of the sport, hinders breathing, swallowing of blood compromises breathing, or a displaced nasal fracture is present. Many times, when requested to mount the apron to examine, I will use a sponge to wipe away blood to visualize, apply compression as I prepare to view, and squeeze to elicit the pain of a fracture. Having been painted by spatters of blood too numerous to count, I now instruct the athlete to "breathe through your mouth only," for my good, not theirs! Most of the bleeding arises from Kiesselbach's plexus where vessels converge. View the back of the throat for excessive bleeding due to a posterior bleed. Most bleeding from the plexus of vessels is amenable to being compressed by the thumb and index finger during the 1-min rest period in their corner or post bout. Often, I will allow the bout to continue, but, if bleeding is not reasonably controlled then, it ends on a reevaluation. I try to give the athlete's corner personnel the opportunity to work on it. Dental sponges shaped like a short cigarette are inserted for compression after the bout PRN. The usual advice is given: tip your head forward, don't stop squeezing your nose, and do not blow out the clot. Send for X-ray if suspicious.

Orbital fractures are definitely seen within the fight game. These "blowout" orbital floor fractures are dangerous and must be recognized and referred for definitive reconstruction. The symptoms of this defect include:

1. Interference with upward gaze
2. Enophthalmos (the entire eyeball sinking inward toward the skull)
3. Double vision
4. Sometimes a fractured medial wall of the ethmoid sinus's (lamina papyracea), a paper-thin bone layer, allows air to travel to the soft tissues of the eye. Blowing the nose will force air quite disturbingly into the now bulging eye region.

A broken jaw will definitely stop a bout. See if the competitor can open their mouth and slide their jaw from side-to-side. Their failure to firmly bite down on several layers of tongue depressors elicits the diagnosis. Also, view their dental alignment. Any step off or misalignment of teeth is confirmatory also.

I have seen the cheek bone or **zygomatic arch** fractured in many ways: punches, head butts, kicks, and elbow strikes. That cheek appears flatter or "stove in" compared to the opposite side.

Localized pain and the inability to fully and comfortably open their mouth occur due to associated muscles trapped under the depressed area. They need to be fixed.

Eye injury occurs from three mechanisms:

- **Direct contact** (coup). A direct blow either creates local injury such as an "eye poke" causing corneal abrasion, conjunctival hemorrhage, hyphema (visible blood in the anterior chamber), or eyelid injury.
- **Contrecoup**. This line of force traveling through the eye with wave-like force creates damage.
- **Globe distortion**. This distortion weakens layers which can tear and buckle the retina, resulting in a retinal tear. In boxers, most of the early ones are far peripheral and only adequately viewed by a dilated exam within an ophthalmologist office setting. This is why office screening eye exams should be periodically required as a matter of licensing.

38.12.3 Skin Lesions

Any infectious skin condition disqualifies one from competing.

If the active, non-crusted lesions of **herpes simplex** are discovered at physical exam, they cannot fight. If active viral lesions of a "cold sore" are transferred from glove to eye, blindness can result. Bacterial IMPETIGO can spread like wildfire through a gym or training camp and is a disqualifying condition. HIV and active hepatitis B and C disqualify. Recent technological advances for the treatment of hepatitis C currently have us reconsidering a lifetime ban, if stated cure rate claims evolve.

Since inclusion within the original Olympics, boxing and wrestling have thrived from within the humblest facilities to arenas and stadiums viewed by millions. The equal application of modern sports medicine advances utilized within other sports must be shared with these highly motivated and dedicated athletes.

References

1. World Boxing Association. http://www.wbaboxing.com/wba-regulations/by-laws.
2. World Boxing Federation. http://www.worldboxing-federation.net.
3. Association of Ringside Physicians. http://www.ringsidearp.org.

Part VI

Different Scenarios in Sports

Indoor Sports

39

Alex Behar, Mark R. Hutchinson, Aimee Bobko, Benjamin Mayo, Garrett Schartzman, Erwin Secretov, Matthew Steffes, and Samantha Tayne

39.1 Introduction

Alex Bejar and Mark R. Hutchinson

Although it is unknown when sports were first played indoors, we know that sports have been around for over 15,000 years, with the first documented event as a footrace between two cavemen. Progress in architecture and technology have allowed for outdoors competition to transition into indoor sporting events. In modern day, indoor sports continue to represent a high proportion of athletic events as many outdoor sports are being played under the confines of an indoor facility. Indoor sports allow for a healthy alternative to playing outdoors all year round. Participation can occur during any time of the year and training has subsequently improved. Indoor sports participation is also on the rise as heat and cold illness awareness has increased. Participating in sports in an indoor environment can place unique demands and challenges on the athlete, coaches, healthcare team, and administration.

The goal of this chapter is to not only outline the epidemiology, etiology, and treatment of common injuries associated with indoor sporting activities but also address the special challenges faced by competing indoors including such environmental factors as playing surface, air quality, temperature, air movement, and lighting as well as architectural design could influence not only actual sports performance but introduce unique safety risks into the equation. Facility design may also influence emergency access within the facility and to the facility. Every event should have a defined plan of how the emergency healthcare team will have access to an injured athlete, where they will be taken on-site for triage or treatment, and how they might be transported and evacuated out of the facility for more catastrophic injuries. While prevention of injury is the physician's goal, this emergency plan is essential to understand every time you care for athletes but particularly when you are in a foreign environment. As indoor sports become more popular, the role of the sports medicine physician will continue to evolve with the expectation to continue injury prevention, diagnosis, and treatment.

A. Behar
Elmhurst Neuroscience Institute, Elmhurst, IL, USA
e-mail: Alex.behar@eehealth.org

M. R. Hutchinson (✉)
University of Illinois at Chicago, Chicago, IL, USA

United States Olympic Committee, Colorado Springs, CO, USA
e-mail: mhutch@uic.edu

A. Bobko · G. Schartzman · E. Secretov · M. Steffes
University of Illinois at Chicago, Chicago, IL, USA

B. Mayo · S. Tayne
Department of Orthopedic Surgery, University of Illinois at Chicago, Chicago, IL, USA

S. Rocha Piedade et al. (eds.), *The Sports Medicine Physician*,
https://doi.org/10.1007/978-3-030-10433-7_39

39.2 Basketball

Erwin Secretov

39.2.1 Introduction

Basketball has become increasingly more popular over the past decade. The National Federation of High Schools reports that approximately one million high school student athletes participate in basketball in the United States on a yearly basis [1]. Traditionally basketball has been perceived as a noncontact sport. However, the modern game of basketball puts great emphasis on maximizing both speed and power. With the increased importance placed on strength and quickness in combination with the rising number of participants globally, injuries tend to occur.

39.2.2 Injury Rates

Research has shown that the adolescent population accounted for the majority of basketball-related injuries (50.7%), and adolescents were three times more likely to sustain injuries to the lower extremity compared to younger children. Younger children, 5–10 years old, were more likely to injure the upper extremity, sustain traumatic brain injuries, or suffer fractures. The male population accounted for three-fourths of the injuries and were more likely to sustain injuries such as laceration, fractures, or dislocations, while females were more likely to sustain traumatic brain injuries and knee injuries [2]. Furthermore, reports have shown that high school basketball players sustain 1.94 injuries per 1000 athlete exposures (AE). Injuries have also been shown to be more prevalent in games versus practice (3.37 vs. 1.40 per 1000 AE) [3]. The most common injuries reported were to the ankle/foot (39.7%), knee (14.7), head/face (13.6%), arm/hand (9.6%), and hip/thigh upper leg (8.4%). The female high school basketball player sustained more injuries than men (2.08 vs. 1.83 per 1000 AE). Females also accounted for a greater portion of concussions and knee injuries, while men had a higher prevalence of fractures and contusions [3].

The National Collegiate Athletic Associated (NCAA) injury surveillance system data has shown that lower extremity injuries accounted for 60% of all game and practice injuries in collegiate basketball players. Furthermore, injury rates during games were two times higher than those in practice. Male basketball players sustained more injuries than female players during the game (9.9 vs. 6.75 per 1000 AE). Male basketball players also sustained more injuries than female players during practice (4.3 vs. 2.84 per 1000 AE) [4, 5].

The injury patterns at the professional level are similar to the collegiate rates. Lower extremity injuries account for 65% of all injuries when looking at professional basketball players. Lateral ankle sprains (13.7%) account for the most common diagnosis in both the NBA and WNBA. Interestingly, WNBA players experienced higher in-game-related injury rates compared to their NBA counterparts (23.9 vs. 19.3 per 1000 AE) [6].

While in the ambulatory setting, the annual visit rate for basketball-related injuries in the adult population was 3.2 per 1000 patient visits. The most common injuries reported were sprains and strains to the lower leg and ankle, as well as fractures and dislocations to the wrist, hand, and fingers [7].

39.2.3 Injury Mechanism

It has been shown that the majority of basketball-related injuries tend to occur to the lower extremity. The most common injuries documented in literature are to the foot and ankle region with ankle sprains and muscle strains dominating the landscape. Lateral ankle sprains predominate when compared to medial ankle sprains [8]. The lateral ankle sprain typically occurs from an inversion/plantar flexion mechanism to the foot and ankle. Typically, this will occur as a player lands on another player's foot, rolling one's ankle inward, or when the player lands awkwardly twisting one's own ankle on the ground. The most common ligament involved in an inversion mechanism would be the anterior talofibular ligament, followed by the calcaneofibular ligament. Eversion/external rotation mechanism of the foot tends to occur at a much lower rate. These injuries tend to affect the deltoid ligament complex, anterior tibiofibular ligament, and interosseous membrane which may potentially disrupt the stability of the ankle mortise [8, 9].

Anterior cruciate ligament (ACL) disruptions is one of the more devastating injuries that a basketball player can experience, many times requiring surgical reconstruction and a lengthy rehabilitation process. Unlike ACL tears in the game of football, ACL injuries in basketball are associated with a noncontact injury. During the game of basketball, there are frequent moments where a player will have to decelerate and perform sudden stops or changes of direction which may cause abnormal rotation of the tibia resulting in ACL injury [10]. A study evaluating the mechanism of ACL tears in basketball players with video analysis found that a majority of ACL tears occurred by a noncontact variety. In addition, female basketball players were found to have a higher mean flexion angle and were more inclined to undergo valgus knee collapse [11]. A meta-analysis studying the incidence of ACL tears as a function of sport and gender found that females were roughly three times more likely to sustain an ACL tear in comparison to male athletes while playing basketball [12].

A study by the International Olympic Committee attributed the increased risk of ACL injury in female athletes to elevated risk in the preovulatory phase of the menstrual cycle, decreased intercondylar notch width, and a predisposition to increased knee abduction on landing in female athletes [13].

39.2.4 Common Injuries

In basketball, lower extremity injuries tend to predominate. The most common injuries seen in Men's Collegiate Basketball were ankle sprains (26.2%), knee internal derangement (7.4%), patellar injuries (2.4%), upper leg contusions (3.9%), and concussions (3.6%) [5]. A prospective study spanning 10 NBA seasons found that ankle sprains are extremely common. The study demonstrates the prevalence of ankle sprains to be 9.4% of all injuries [14]. In addition to acute ankle injuries, overuse injuries to the foot, ankle, and lower leg have been described. The four most common stress injuries that have been frequently described include proximal fifth metatarsal, medial malleolus, navicular, and anterior tibia. Navicular stress fractures make up approximately 14% of stress fractures [15]. Navicular stress fractures typically occur in sports that involve running and jumping. Patients typically present with an insidious onset of pain, and frequently, initially radiographs will be negative. Stress fractures relating to the tibia more commonly involve the posterior medial aspect, which are relative low-risk stress injuries. However, anterior tibial stress fractures are high-risk injuries and are slower to heal with non-operative treatment, potentially requiring prophylactic nailing [16]. Medial malleolus stress fractures are quite rare, accounting for 0.6–4.1% of stress fractures. The repetitive jumping and running makes basketball players more prone to these injuries [17]. The Jones fracture involves the metaphyseal and diaphyseal junction of the proximal fifth metatarsal, which is a watershed area of poor vascularity. These fractures are prone to non-union and will typically require operative treatment in high-level athletes in order to return them to sport [18].

Twelve percent of all injuries in male college athletes occur at the knee, with knee injuries affecting 19% of females in college sports. ACL injuries in basketball players show a strong female tendency. A review of injuries sustained in collegiate women's basketball players at the University of Connecticut found that woman experienced ACL injuries 2–4 times the rate of their male basketball players [19]. Meniscus surgery has been found to be the second most common surgery of college women basketball players entering the WNBA behind ACL reconstruction [20]. Overuse injuries of the knee involve the extensor mechanisms. Patellar tendinopathy or "jumper's knee" has been found to be a common problem in basketball players. It has been reported as high as 7% of high school players suffer from patellar tendinopathy. A 10-year prospective study of injury in the NBA found that patellofemoral inflammation accounted for 8.1% of orthopedic injuries, second only to ankle sprains [14].

The most common upper extremity injuries that a basketball player will sustain involve the wrist, hand, and fingers. Among pediatric basketball injuries presenting to the emergency department, finger sprains and finger fractures were the second and third most common diagnosis [21]. Long-term disability is a possibility when a fracture at the PIP joint goes untreated. X-rays should be considered when a PIP injury is identified.

Back injuries and more specifically lumbar spine injuries account for 6.8% of all injuries sustained by NBA players but represent 11% of all days missed [14]. Predominantly injuries to the back involved muscle strains and disc rupture/herniation being far less prevalent. This is a result of the repetitive extension and hyperextension from rebounding, shooting, or guarding the opponent.

Concussions account for 6.5% of the injuries sustained during games in the WNBA [4]. Concussions are less frequently reported in men's NCAA competition at 3.6% and NBA competition [5, 14]. The most likely etiology is player collision, although concussions can also occur with direct contact with the hardwood floors.

Sudden cardiac death, although rare, is a risk when participating in sport. Basketball has been found to be the highest-risk sport with an overall death rate of 1/11,394. Division 1 male basketball players are at five and half times greater risk than female basketball players. African American basketball players are three times more at risk compared to white athletes [22].Hypertrocphic cardiomyopathy (HCM) accounts for 36% of sudden cardiac deaths in young athletes. HCM has an incidence rate of 1:500 people. A thorough history and physical exam during the pre-participation screening is the best method to prevent sudden death in athletes.

39.3 Combat Sports: Boxing/Martial Arts/MMA

Benjamin Mayo

39.3.1 Introduction

Martial arts are some of the oldest sports still practiced today, with origins dating back as far as ancient Mongolia [23]. Today, as many as 6.4 million kids participate in martial arts in the United States [24]. Worldwide, the World Taekwondo Federation reports as many as 120 million participants across 140 countries [25]. Boxing, though once extremely popular, has lost participation in recent years due to scrutiny from the medical community, as there is a high injury rate, but especially due to the risk of chronic brain injury such as chronic traumatic encephalopathy or dementia pugilistica [26, 27]. Mixed martial arts, more commonly known as MMA, has approximately 1.3 million participants in the United States [28, 29].

39.3.2 Injury Rates

There is a high overall rate of injury in combat sports, with varying risk depending on the type of rules and experience of the athlete. In large studies of professional boxing matches, there was an injury rate between 17.1 and 23.6/100 matches, or 3.4 per 100 boxing rounds [30, 31]. A study by the same group also analyzed professional mixed martial arts competitions and found a significantly higher rate of injury at 12.5/100 rounds [32]. During the 2016 Rio Olympics, boxers sustained the second highest rate of injury at nearly 30% of athletes. This was followed closely by Taekwondo at 24% of athletes. Wrestling and judo were slightly lower at 14% and 12%, respectively [33].

One analysis of injury rates in combat sports at the 2008 Summer Olympics showed the highest injury rate in Taekwondo, with as high as 37% of participating athletes experiencing an injury and 16.2% missing time [34]. Boxing and judo were the next highest with rates between 10 and 15% of athletes experiencing injury. A systematic review of combat sports in the Olympics again demonstrated that Taekwondo had the highest injury rate, with reported values between 19.09 and 69.5 injuries per 1000 athlete exposures. Boxing had a rate of 12.8 injuries per 1000 h in training, while judo was the lowest at 4.2/1000 h [35]. Other studies have reported an injury rate in Taekwondo as high as 139.5/1000 athlete exposures and 4.6 injuries per athlete annually [25]. One 10-year prospective study reported that participants in Taekwondo sustain 4.6 injuries annually, for an overall injury rate of 26.1/1000 athlete exposures [36]. Karate has a reported injury rate of 5.6/100 athletes over a 1-year period [37]. Though less frequently reported on, kickboxers have an exceptionally high injury rate as well, with one large study over 16 years reporting an overall injury rate of 109.7/1000 athlete exposures [38].

Few studies have directly compared injury rates between types of combat events. One such study reported a slightly higher rate of injury in mixed martial arts compared to boxing but a higher rate of minor injuries. Boxing had a higher rate of loss of consciousness, as well as longer medical suspensions by 6 days [39]. In one analysis of professional mixed martial arts fights, 40.3% of the time at least one athlete sustained an injury [32]. Brazilian jiu-jitsu, a form of mixed martial arts focused on grappling and ground fighting, has a relatively low rate of orthopedic injuries compared to other combat sports, with an overall injury rate of 9.2/1000 athlete exposures [40].

39.3.3 Injury Mechanism

The mechanism of injury in combat sports varies based on the rules regarding striking, as well as grappling techniques allowed. In short, a majority of injuries are due to direct blows from the opponent in striking sports, while grappling sports have a higher incidence of injuries due to contact with the mat or pressure applied from submission techniques. In forms of martial arts that allow both striking and grappling, as well as mixed martial arts, there is a wide array of injury patterns.

Injury patterns in amateur boxing have changed secondary to rule changes by the Amateur International Boxing Association in 2013 in which head guards were no longer permitted, and changes were made to both glove specifications and the scoring system. A recent study examining fight characteristics found that fights were less likely to last the full time, a decrease in head-to-body punch ratio, higher percentage of missed punches, and more defensive tactics. They theorized that head protection actually made the head a larger target, limited vision, and combatants were more willing to take a punch to the head due to increased perception of protection. These factors, along with an attenuated force from the padding in the headgear, may lead to an athlete absorbing a larger number of punches over a longer period of time instead of a few heavier punches that may end the fight. However, future research on whether traumatic brain injury is more likely after receiving one heavy punch that results in a knockout, or to be hit with less force several times, will need to be performed before the true benefit of these rule changes can be concluded [41].

When comparing striking (boxing, kendo, taekwondo) versus non-striking (judo, ssireum, wrestling) combat sports, dislocations and injuries to the neck, shoulder, and elbow were more common in non-striking sports, while injuries to the wrist and hands are much more common in striking sports [42]. There is a high rate of sprains and strains in both (approximately 60% of all injuries). There were similar rates of fracture (37.7 vs. 45.3), ligament ruptures (57.1 vs. 43.7), muscle rupture (26 vs. 32%), and herniated discs (26 vs. 32%) in each group. In judo, the most common mechanism of injury has been described as being thrown from a standing position, as then in a defensive position, and may lose control of being able to land appropriately and safely [43].

Two separate analyses of youth karate participants demonstrated an overall injury incidence of 41.4–45.3/1000 athlete exposures [44]. However, only 10% of such injuries resulted in time loss from participation. Older youth participants (12–17 years old) were at nearly double the risk of injury compared to younger athletes, likely due to the increased strength and force of striking. There is a bimodal injury rate in terms of experience, with the lowest belt ranks and highest belt ranks experiencing the highest [45]. These results have been corroborated in other studies, with older age and beginners being associated with a higher injury risk [32, 46]. Other analyses have failed to find a correlation between age or weight and a higher injury risk [30, 38, 47].

Many studies have analyzed other risk factors for injury. Intuitively, the loser in a fight has demonstrated to have twice the injury risk as the winner. Additionally, participating in more than three bouts per year was associated with a higher risk of injury [48]. Though most sports have a higher rate of injury in competition, Taekwondo athletes have a relatively high percentage of injuries sustained during training as well [33, 34]. In mixed martial arts, a video analysis found common takedown moves are a high risk for cervical spine injuries and whiplash mechanisms [28].

A majority (up to 82.8%) of injuries reported in combat sports are acute versus recurrent [49]. One study demonstrated that females are more likely to be injured than males at the lower weight classes of martial arts, but at the larger weights, this difference disappears [36]. In youth karate tournaments, females had a lower relative risk of injury at 0.63 [50].

39.3.4 Common Injuries

The common body locations and types of injuries in each combat sport is variable based on the type of striking or grappling that is allowed. Although there is a high overall injury rate, fortunately a majority of injuries sustained in each of these sports are mild, with the most frequently reported injuries being sprains, strains, tendinosis, and contusions with a rate of nearly 80% of all injuries in some studies [36, 51, 45, 47]. In addition to these injuries, striking sports also have a high rate of lacerations and abrasions. Wrestling, discussed in a different portion of this chapter, has the highest rates of sprains and strains. This is logical, as sports with a lower emphasis on striking compared to grappling, throws, and submissions are more likely to overstrain a joint compared to more strike focused sports which will have a high rate of fractures and contusions. In striking sport such as boxing and mixed martial arts, fractures have been reported to be between 8.4 and 43.3% of all injuries [31, 47].

In boxing, the highest number of injuries occurs to the head, face, and hand, depending on the skill level of the boxer. These injuries have reported rates as high as 71% of all injuries [33, 35, 48, 52]. Professional boxers have a higher rate of head injury, with a reported 24% of fights overall demonstrating an injury to these areas, though a majority were lacerations [30]. One analysis demonstrated that 23.6% of boxing-related injuries presenting to emergency departments are to the head and face, compared with 11.1% of martial arts-related injuries [53]. Other studies have reported that close to two-thirds of boxing injuries are to the upper extremity, while only 23% are to the head and face [54]. Similarly, a large analysis of kickboxing injuries reported that injuries to the head and neck were the most common at over 50% of injuries [38]. In kickboxing, head injuries are the second most common in both professional and amateurs rates between 31% and 4.5% [46].

In mixed martial arts, injury location has a more equal distribution, with injuries to the head and neck, upper extremities, and lower extremities having a much closer rate than other sports due to the fact that there is no one particular focus or technique that can be used [45]. For head and neck injuries, up to 64% of injuries have been reported to be facial lacerations, while concussions are up to 33% of all injuries and 47% of head injuries [31, 32, 54].

Approximately 5–10% of injuries in boxing and mixed martial arts are concussions [48]. Some studies have reported that martial arts has significantly fewer concussions than boxing or wrestling, likely due to the wide variation in martial arts techniques that do not focus on head striking [39]. A 2016 study of the World Karate Championships reported an overall concussion rate of 0.43/1000 athlete exposures. There are fewer knockouts in mixed martial arts compared with boxing, likely due to the multiple ways of winning, whereas boxing is more focused on winning by knockout [53]. Despite this, the reported rates of head and neck injuries in martial arts have been reported as high as 80% of all injuries [47]. In amateur kickboxers, nearly 31% of matches were stopped due to injury in one analysis, of those, 65.2% were from traumatic brain injury, while 17.4% were from musculoskeletal orthopedic trauma [55]. There is a high rate of non-specific lower back pain in martial arts competitors. One review of judo participants reported a rate of 35.4%, with radiologic abnormalities of the spine in 81.7% [43].

39.3.4.1 Upper Extremity

The most common injury location in nearly all forms of striking combat sports is to the upper extremity, most notably the hands and wrists. In an analysis of emergency department visits by combat sport, upper extremity injuries account for 63.7% of boxing visits compared to 32% of martial arts visits [53]. In Taekwondo, the overall rate of upper extremity injuries is between 11.2 and 15.1 per 1000 athlete exposures [36]. The hand and wrist is the most common location of injury to the upper extremity with up to 53% of all upper extremity injuries [32, 48]. Mixed martial arts reports an overall upper extremity injury rate between 11.8 and 22.8%, with 6–12% being injuries to the hand and wrist. Most commonly these injuries are dislocations or sprains [47]. Hand and arm injuries account for nearly 50% of fractures, followed by the fractures of the face between 30 and 40% of injuries [56]. One study has reported an overall hand injury rate of 302 injuries per 1000 training hours [39]. Boxing has a high rate of hand and wrist injuries incidences between 20 and 35% of all injuries in amateurs [49]. Up to 70% of boxing injuries to the hand and wrist were in training versus competition. This may be due to the high number of hours spent training and frequent contact with heavy bags while fatigued [33]. This is more common in amateurs who may have worse form, as one study demonstrated that professional boxers had an injury rate of 347/1000 h of competition compared to <0.5 injuries/1000 h in training [27]. In professionals, head and face injuries are more common, with injuries to the hand and wrist being second overall [49]. Taekwondo has a high rate of injuries to the fingers due to a focus on grappling, with as many as 23% of injuries occurring to the hand or finger [57]. Judo also has a high rate of injuries to the finger, as they can get caught in opponents uniform during grappling maneuvers [43]. Repeated injuries to the same joint can commonly lead to finger joint osteoarthritis in these athletes.

Sprains and ligament injuries were the most common type of injury to the upper extremity [57]. The most common of these injuries include CMC instability (21.7%), UCL injury (14.6%), and MCP sprain/extensor hood injury, also known as boxer's knuckle (15.8%), and wrist sprains (13.5%) [49]. Hand and wrist injuries had a high rate of serious injury; mean duration of days lost was 50.7 for the hand [35].

The shoulder is typically the second most commonly injured area of the upper extremity, at up to 27% of combat sport-related injuries, followed closely by the elbow at 19% [33, 35, 43, 56, 57],. Glenohumeral dislocations, AC and SC joint separations, and clavicle fractures all have been reported, with the usually mechanism being resisting a fall [35, 43].

Judo has a relatively high rate of elbow injuries with a rate near 25% of all injuries. Elbow injuries also have a high incidence of severity with up to 73% of athletes missing significant time [58]. Brazilian jiu-jitsu demonstrated the highest injury rate to the elbow, as a common submission technique is the arm bar in which the opponent's elbow is forced in to hyperextension [40]. During these arm lock maneuvers, poor defensive technique often leads to medial collateral ligament injuries [43]. Boxers have been known to develop both anterior and posterior elbow impingement, with the lead arm more likely to develop the condition, and can often be effectively treated with debridement [49, 59].

39.3.4.2 Lower Extremity

Lower extremity injuries occur at a relatively lower rate than injuries to the upper extremity in most martial arts specialties; however there is still a high overall injury rate. In mixed martial arts there is a comparatively higher rate of lower extremity injuries due to the variability in techniques used, with injuries to the lower extremities reported as high as 30% of all injuries [47]. Judo also has demonstrated a high rate of lower extremity injuries, with nearly 28% of injuries being sprains, strains, or contusions of the knee, while ankle sprains occur at a slightly lower rate [43]. Around the knee, the MCL and ACL are the most commonly injured ligaments [43]. Taekwondo has also been reported to have a high rate of injuries to the lower extremities, with injuries to the knee and ankle occurring at a rate of 13% and 20% overall, respectively. In a review of emergency department visits due to martial arts-related injuries, the lower extremity was the site of injury in 41.6% of injuries, while only 32% were injuries to the upper extremity. Many of these injuries were sprains and strains, but nearly 25% were fractures [56]. Another large study reported that the knee was the most commonly injured area at 21.3% of all taekwondo injuries, followed by the foot at 17% [53]. Other studies have corroborated these findings, with as high as 65.5% of reported injuries occurring to the lower extremities in Taekwondo [36].

Boxing logically has a low rate of lower extremity injuries, with less than 10% of injuries reported [53]. Conversely, kickboxing has a relatively high rate of injuries to the lower leg where a majority of the striking is performed [38]. In professional kickboxing, lower extremity injuries have been reported as up to 53.4% of injuries, while this rate increases to nearly 75% for amateurs [46].

39.3.5 Catastrophic Injuries

Unfortunately, all combat sports have a high potential for catastrophic injury. Typically this is due to acute trauma to the head or spine [43]. Baird et al. reviewed all reported fatalities in boxing from 1950 to 2007, in which there were 339 mortalities over the time period. Sixty-four percent of them were decided by knockout, 15% by TKO. The preterminal event was noticed in the ring in 61% of such cases [60]. The rate of mortality significantly decreased after 1983, likely due to rule changes, increased medical oversight, and an overall reduction in career length and number of fights. It was noted that a higher percentage of mortalities were in the lower weight classes [25]. Some rule changes have been made. However, a recent study out of Japan examined mortalities before and after rule changes and noted that prohibiting 6 ounce gloves and changing the weigh-in day may not result in reduced mortality [60]. High rate of catastrophic head injury secondary to the force when being punched is more rotational as opposed to translational acceleration as seen in other sports. This is thought to create a higher tension on blood vessels and a risk of injury [61]. In martial arts, nearly 70% of catastrophic injuries are to the brain and cervical spine, which are secondary to being thrown and landing incorrectly [43]. These are more likely to occur in younger participants less than 20 years old and those who are new to the sport and practicing less than 3 years [43].

39.4 Diving

Samantha Tayne

39.4.1 Introduction

Diving is an ancient sport with the earliest documentation found in Naples, Italy, in the Tomba del Tuffatore (the Tomb of the Diver). In the seventeenth century, diving began to evolve as Swedish and German gymnasts began to perform acrobatics over water at the beach, also known as "fancy diving." The first modern diving competition was held in England in 1880, and in 1904 the first men's springboard dive competition was introduced at Olympics. Four years later, in 1908 platform diving was introduced, and in 1912 women's diving was added. The number of dives and complexity of the dives has increased over the years. In the early 1900s, there were 14 platform and 20 springboard dives; now there are close to 100 dives with vastly increased complexity [62–65].

39.4.2 Injury Rates

It is important to recognize the differences between recreational diving and competitive diving. Most notably, recreational diving is associated with much higher rates of acute spinal and catastrophic injury. In fact, 10–20% of hospital admissions for a spinal cord injury are associated with recreational diving accidents [65]. Meanwhile there has not been a reported acute fracture or dislocation of the cervical spine in competitive diving [64]. And there have only been two fatalities noted worldwide in competitive diving, both reported outside of the United States. Catastrophic diving accidents involving the cervical spine are seen more commonly among male patients, under 25 years old, diving into a shallow pool of water [65, 66].

Though competitive divers rarely suffer cervical spine injuries, they do demonstrate a slew of other injuries. Competitive divers train on average 40 h per week with one study suggesting about 200 dives per week [64] and another with an even higher estimate of 100–150 dives per day for springboard and 50–100 dives per day for platform [63]. Injury risk has found to be increased for platform over springboard diving. Haase et al. explain the increased risk of injury through the physics of diving, with a diver falling from a 10 m platform accelerating to about 14.1 m/s or 31.5 mph before hitting the water, leading to an impact force of between 2.0 and 2.4 g (1 g 5 9.8 m/s^2) at the surface of the water, which is a significant force [64]. Training also occurs both in the pool and on dryland, though the incidence of injury during training is higher for the pool than on land [62].

One study in the Netherlands followed divers prospectively for about 3 months and found an injury rate of 8.8 injuries per 1000 training hours. The USA Diving Injury Surveillance Program estimates an injury rate of 6.5 injuries per 100 divers per year [64]. Another study looking at the NCAA swimming and diving injuries from 2009 to 2014 found an injury rate of 1.94 injuries per 1000 athlete exposures for males and 2.49 injuries per 1000 athlete exposures for females [63, 67]. The majority of dive injuries, about 89%, were found to occur during practice and the remaining during competition [64].

39.4.3 Common Injuries

The majority of diving injuries involve the upper extremities, likely due to the force of impacting the water, typically performed hands first. Additionally, the way in which divers maneuver when impacting the water to limit their splash and improve their score, also known as a rip entry, can lead to injury. Importantly, there have been differences found between male and female divers as the most common injured areas. About 32.0% of men's diving injuries were associated with the shoulder, while hand and wrist accounted for 8.0% of injuries. In women, the shoulder accounted for just 5.4% of injuries, whereas 16.2% of injuries involved the hand and wrist [64].

The best way to evaluate injuries is by breaking down the aspects of a dive: takeoff, flight, and entry. Each of these portions of a dive is associated with various injury patterns. The takeoff involves the approach, which on a springboard includes a hurdle or an upward jump to the end of the board, and the press or the depression of the board leading to an upward acceleration of the body. For platform dives the takeoff may begin from standing or from a handstand position. Common injuries during the takeoff include knee extensor mechanism injuries, including patellar tendon or quadriceps tendon injuries, as well as Achilles tendon and posterior tibial tendon injuries. Handstand dives may result in more wrist, elbow, or shoulder overuse injuries [62–65].

The next stage of the dive is the flight, from the moment of leaving the board or platform to the initial contact with the water, during which time the diver performs a midair maneuver. To initiate the motion in the air, the diver must throw his or her arms in the direction of spin, which may cause issues with shoulder instability or irritation of the long head of the biceps. Additionally, the rapid and forced flexion of the trunk can cause increased loads in the anterior segment of the spinal column, leading to disc pathology and thoracic or lumbar strains. There is also the possibility of a poor takeoff leading the diver to make contact with the board or platform, which could result in any number of acute injuries [62–65].

Entry, the final phase, occurs upon entry into the water. This is the phase involving the majority of injuries. The diver is attempted to dissipate the impact force, up to 2.4 g as mentioned previously, while limiting the splash, performing a rip entry. Divers often hyperflex their shoulders in an effort to "save" a dive, leading to increased risk of anterior glenohumeral subluxation. Scapular position and motion is essential for divers to achieve a well-executed entry. Malposition of the scapula due to weakness of the serratus anterior, lower trapezius, and rhomboids may impair energy dissipation upon water entry and therefore increase the demands on the soft tissue, leading to injury, to ligament laxity, and many times to shoulder instability [64, 65]. A study of the United States National Team in the 1990s indicated that about 80% of athletes were found to have had shoulder injuries kept them out of training for at least 1 week [62].

The diver requires a stable shoulder for water entry but also needs to maintain flexibility in the shoulders to minimize forces in the spine. Divers often create hyperextension in their back during entry leading to injury of the posterior elements of the spine. However, they may also hyperflex, especially at the neck. One case report illustrates a 19-year-old female collegiate diver who suffered from C5–C6 instability due to the hyperflexion, presenting with symptoms of neck pain and upper extremity paresthesias. Most commonly, injury involves soreness or spasm of the thoracic or lumbar musculature or strains of the ligaments within the spine. Less commonly, there are bony injuries or apparent instability. Young divers are more susceptible to discogenic problems and have potentially accelerated degenerative process [65]. Overall, diving does place high demands on the spinal column, but the incidence of processes such as spondylolysis, spondylolisthesis, and lumbar facet arthropathy have been observed less frequently than in gymnasts [62].

There are two main techniques divers utilize to hold their hands when entering the water – the thumb-in-fist and the flat-hand grab. The flat-hand grab is a new technique, which creates a larger, flatter surface to enter the water [64]. The deceleration forces at the water surface may cause forced dorsiflexion at the wrist and forced flexion of the elbow, leading to stress fractures, sprains, and strains of the wrist and triceps strains [62]. A case study of a 14-year-old male diver was reported with an olecranon stress fracture [65]. Wrist injuries include carpal instability, dorsal impaction syndrome, dorsal ganglion cysts, flexor carpi ulnaris tendinopathy, and scaphoid fractures. There may also be hyperextension at the elbow leading to injury of the medial collateral ligament and possible ulnar neuritis due to continued instability.

Divers are susceptible to several non-orthopedic injuries that are important to mention. Perforations of the tympanic membrane may occur from the pressure upon entering the water, either from landing directly on one side of the head or even during well-executed dives. More common and less severe divers may experience otitis externa or swimmer's ear. Microdefects on the corneal epithelium can occur, again due to repetitive microtrauma upon entering the water [64]. There has been a case report on hemoptysis due to pulmonary contusion due to trauma from water entry [68]. And as mentioned previously, there have been two fatalities in competitive diving, both from severe head injuries after striking their head on the platform in the attempt of a reverse dive [62].

Fact Box

In competitive diving, the majority of injuries are due to the impact at the water's surface and the maneuvering to "save" a dive. Scapular stabilization is important in maintaining shoulder stability and flexibility. Recreational diving carries a far greater risk of spinal or catastrophic injury than competitive diving, often involving the cervical spine. In competitive divers, lumbar strains are often self-limited in competitive diving and can be treated with conservative measures.

39.5 Fencing

Alex Behar

39.5.1 Introduction

Fencing is an open-skilled asymmetric combat sport. It consists of three different weapons: the foil, the saber, and the epee. In comparison to most other sports, direct physical contact in fencing is forbidden and the two athletes fight indirectly using their weapons [69]. There are limited studies reporting on injuries occurring while fencing, and although rare, serious injury in fencing may still occur.

39.5.2 Injury Rate

In a 5-year prospective study, Harmer et al. looked at 78,223 male and female competitors ranging in age from 8 to >70. He reported 184 time-loss injuries among 78,223 competitors, 60% of which consisted of males and 39.3% females, for an overall rate of 0.3 per 1000 athletic exposures (AE) [70]. In another study involving 1356 fencers, only 3 injuries resulted in athlete withdrawal from competition [71]. Women suffered from a significantly higher risk of time-loss injury compared to men (RR = 1.35, 95% CI = 1.01–1.81) [70].

39.5.3 Mechanism of Injuries

The majority of injuries leading to time loss in fencing are due to rapid change in direction and stop-start actions resulting in strains, sprains, and ligament ruptures. Injuries from an opponent's weapon are rare but may result in serious injuries. Heat exhaustion has also been reported as a result of the heaviness protective gear's weight and material [72].

39.5.4 Common Injuries

Fencing injuries mostly occur in the lower extremity (63%). While the knee was the most commonly reported injured body part, thigh and ankle sprains were the most frequently injured [73]. The lumbar region (9.2%) and fingers (7.6%) are the most commonly injured sites above the hips. Interestingly, penetrating puncture wounds accounted for only 2.7% of injuries with two resulting in serious injuries (one penetrating the forearm and one penetrated the lateral neck) [72].

39.5.5 Treatment Principles

Given that fencing is an asymmetric sport, overuse injuries are common. Prevention strategies should include appropriate warm-up, stretching, physical conditioning, and improvement in technique of the athlete. The athlete should wear fencing protective gear to prevent significant penetrating injuries. Broken blades are the most common cause of serious penetrating injuries and it is mandatory for fencers to check their weapon regularly.

39.6 Gymnastics

Matthew Steffes

39.6.1 Introduction

The origin of gymnastics dates back to ancient civilizations from the Far East and the Mediterranean, with the word gymnastics stemming from the ancient Greek word *gymnaziem*, meaning "to exercise naked" [74]. Ancient forms of gymnastics encompassed many different athletic events, from track and field to wrestling. This has evolved over time to encompass both artistic and rhythmic gymnastics events, in addition to trampoline and tumbling. The artistic events currently include vault, floor exercise, balance beam, uneven bars, parallel bars, horizontal bar, pommel horse, and still rings. Rhythmic events include ring, ball, ribbon, club, rope, and group. There is much overlap in the maneuvers required for these events, yet some involve very unique maneuvers or use of an apparatus. Additionally, the population participating these acrobatic events is distinct, with the overwhelming majority of athletes being adolescent females. USA Gymnastics reported 67,626 female members, more than 5 times as many male members (12, 120), and nearly all female members (99%) were 18 years or younger [75]. For these reasons, injury is frequent and unique injury patterns are encountered.

39.6.2 Injury Rates

Most injuries occur upon contact with the ground surface. This is best demonstrated by the 16-year review of NCAA female gymnasts by Marshall and associates. Floor exercise was the most common event for injury at 31.1%, followed by the vault (27.3%), parallel bars (21.4%), and balance beam (12.1%) [76]. The floor event is associated with the highest frequency of injury during international competition [91] with the majority of all knee and ankle injuries occurring during this event [92]. During these events, injuries were incurred specifically during floor exercise routine and upon dismount/landing for the vault, parallel bars, and balance beam. Overall injury rate was more than twice as frequent during competition compared with practice (15.2 vs 6.1 injuries per 1000 exposure hours). Of note, however, back and upper extremity injuries were more common during practice, whereas lower extremity injuries were more frequent during competition. No difference in injury rate has been demonstrated between genders [77].

Saluan and colleagues examined injury characteristics among precollegiate female gymnasts of varying competition level. The authors reported elite and high-level gymnasts sustained significantly higher rates of injury (2.86 and 2.82 injuries per 1000 exposure hours), compared to novice gymnasts (0.69 injuries per 1000 exposure hours), pointing toward a directly proportional relationship between activity time and injury risk [78].

39.6.3 Common Injuries

Gymnastics is a unique sport that often requires using all four extremities as weight-bearing limbs and contortion of the spine to create dynamic and acrobatic displays. This leads to all areas of the body being affected by injury.

The lower extremity accounts for the majority of injuries in both male and female gymnast, followed by the spine and the upper extremity [78]. This trend has been consistently demonstrated by multiple studies [79–82]. The foot and ankle are injured at a rate of 33.3%, the highest of all precollegiate gymnastics injuries [78]. These are often inversion sprains, Achilles tendonitis, or stress fractures. The knee is the next most common area injured. The top diagnoses are patellar tendinosis, patellofemoral syndrome, and nondescript sprains. The knee, foot, and ankle account for the most injuries requiring over 10 days of missed sporting activity [83].

Many gymnastic events require the upper extremity to bear full body weight, while others require to maintain the body in a hanging position. This leads to many wrist injuries, with wrist sprains leading as the most common upper extremity injury pattern for both genders. Chronic wrist pain affects 46–87% of young gymnast [93, 94]. Following wrist injuries, shoulder injuries predominate for male gymnasts, while elbow pathology is more common among females [84]. Given most gymnasts are skeletally immature during prime competitive years, growth plate injury is of particular concern. Early and intense gymnastics participation has long been suspected to cause damage to the distal radial physis and positive ulnar variance. Though there seems to be a positive correlation, no study to date shows a clear causal relationship [85, 86]. A high index of suspicion should be maintained when presented with dorsal-sided wrist pain without a clear injury. A rare type of injury, usually only described in gymnastics, are clavicular stress fractures. The repetitive forces to which the upper extremity is exposed to in tumbling and vaulting are the cause of these stress injuries [90].

The lower back is involved in all maneuvers and is a common source of disability. Muscular strains, stress reactions, and spondylolysis of the L5 vertebrae are common sources of pain, followed by sacralization of the L5 vertebrae and scoliosis [87]. The prevalence of spondylolysis is higher in gymnasts (5.9–33%) than the general population (5–6%) [84].

Catastrophic spinal cord injuries are devastating and injuries encountered in gymnastics. In a case series by Schmitt and Gerner, gymnastics injuries accounted for 15.9% of all sporting spinal cord injuries and were from neck hyperflexion injuries. Forty-five percent of these were during trampoline events and led to cervical level spinal cord injuries with paraplegia [88].

39.6.4 Injury Mechanisms

The overwhelming majority of injuries occur as the gymnast contacts the hard ground surface. This is obvious for floor exercise and rhythmic events but also includes events requiring use of an apparatus [76]. For these apparatus events, dismount and landing requires an abrupt halt of the body's momentum and tremendous energy transfer, to either the lower or upper extremity. Kerr and colleagues reported injury mechanisms among NCAA female gymnasts, noting contact with the surface was the most frequent cause of injury in both practice and competition, followed by overuse injuries (29.8%) and direct contact with the apparatus (16.5%) [83]. This trend was re-demonstrated with no difference between practice and competition by Marshall et al. [76].

Chronic, overuse-type injuries are commonly attributed to many of the injuries seen in gymnastics [86]. It has been proposed that chronic concentric loading through tendons and soft tissues is the underlying cause of attritional losses, chronic inflammatory changes, and apophysitis in the young gymnast.

39.6.5 Treatment Principles

Given the frequency and severity of injuries faced by the gymnast, much effort should be channeled at preventing injury occurrence. Joint immobilization and bracing often restrict motions necessary to properly execute required event maneuvers and are rarely feasible. Therefore, preseason physical conditioning programs emphasizing joint stabilization and core stability would prove beneficial in prevention of common injuries about the ankle and wrist. Maintenance training programs would also likely be of benefit to this extent.

Injury incidence appears to be directly correlated with amount of time spent in sport and level of competition. This, combined with the repetitive nature of gymnastics training, is likely a large contributor to chronic overuse injuries. Periodization and increased variety of training activities may also be of benefit and such methods have found acceptance abroad [89].

Additionally, Kolt and Kirkby allude to a high recurrence rate for gymnastics injuries [80, 84]. Whether this is truly a recurrence or merely undertreatment of acute injuries, proper rest and recovery time should be allotted to the gymnast without outside pressure to return prior to satisfactory resolution of symptoms.

Age requirements for event participation have not been implemented in the United States but are a possible avenue for injury reduction. In Germany, trampoline events were eliminated from grade school competition with the aim to eliminate catastrophic injuries, yet no data is currently available regarding outcome [88]. This would be a drastic measure and would need great consideration of necessity prior to introduction.

In the event of traumatic neck and spine injuries, proper Advanced Trauma Life Support protocol and C-spine immobilization precautions should be followed at all times. Coordination with event officials and emergency medical services prior to the start of an event is paramount to avoid delays in transport to higher levels of care. Figure 39.1 outlines ATLS guidelines with respect to spine immobilization and examination.

Fact Box

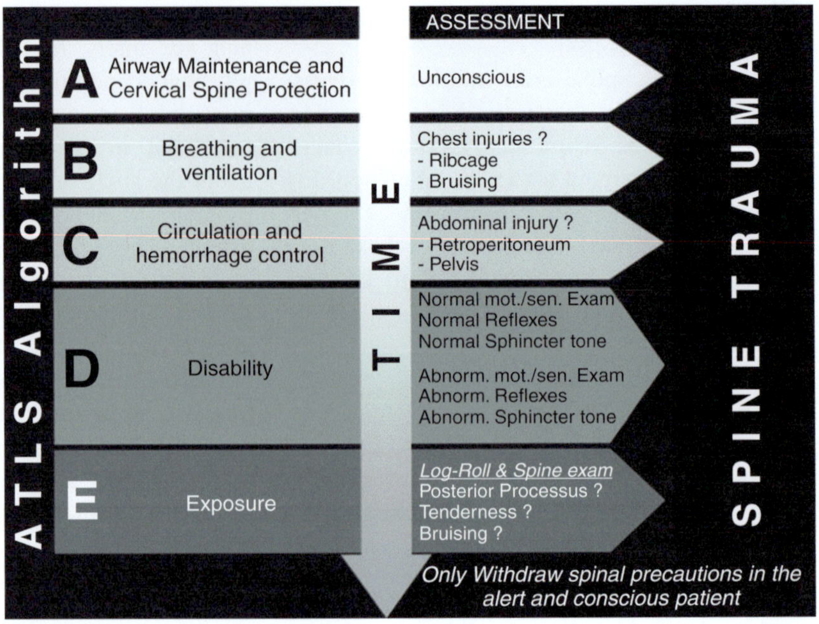

Fig. 39.1 ATLS algorithm and spine assessment in the trauma patient. Schmidt OI et al. ATLS and damage control in spine trauma. *World J Emerg Surg WJES*. 2009;4:9. doi:10.1186/1749-7922-4-9

39.7 Racquet and Wall Sports

Garrett Schartzman

39.7.1 Introduction

Indoor racquet sports are a very popular form of physical exercise. Sports such as badminton and table tennis are also commonly played in countries such as China and India [95]. This category of sports also includes racquetball, handball, and squash. Given the unique aspects of these sports such as running into a wall, projectiles coming toward the player very quickly, and being within close proximities of another player swinging a racquet, injuries are common. They are also at times unique from other racquet sports such as tennis given the nature of the games.

39.7.2 Injury Rates

Given the niche nature of these sports, injury data is difficult to find. From small case studies, extrapolations can be made into the injury rates sustained by athletes competing in these sports [95, 96]. Lower extremity injuries are the most common encountered by these athletes. Whether it be ligamentous or bony in nature, these injuries are similar to any running or cutting athlete. Wall sports such as squash and racquetball also encounter a high rate of eye injuries, necessitating the use of eye protection. A large retrospective study of patients regarding injuries during badminton and squash found the incidence rates at 20% and 59%, respectively [96]. These were attributed to the constant contact with the wall and the opposing player.

39.7.3 Injury Mechanism

As with other cutting and running sports, indoor racquet athletes sustain lower extremity sprains and ligamentous injuries. Appropriate shoe wear and ankle protection can help with these injuries. A unique aspect again is the wall encountered in some of these sports. This creates a contact that other racquet sports do not encounter. This has been attributed to injuries such as fractures and eye injuries from deflections [96, 97]. Indoor racquet athletes also encounter injuries from the overhead swinging nature of the sports and may incur rotator cuff and shoulder injuries. Badminton in particular sees a high rate of wrist injuries due to the snapping nature of the movement. Proper racquet weight for the athlete can help to prevent this from occurring.

39.7.4 Common Injuries

Injuries among indoor racquet sport players encompass the entire body. Most commonly seen are lower extremity injuries from cutting or lunging. However, in squash or racquetball, lower extremity trauma, such as fractures or contusions, is also seen from interactions with the wall. Upper extremity injuries from repetitive overhead motion are also seen and include rotator cuff tears, AC impingement, De Quervain's tenosynovitis, and wrist sprains. Finally, eye injuries are also seen in indoor racquet sports. All athletes are highly recommended to use eye protection. There are multiple reports of eye contusions and retinal damage from deflections [95–97].

39.8 Swimming

Erwin Secretov

39.8.1 Introduction

Swimming is one of the most popular sports around the world and is the second largest sport based on total athlete participation in the Olympic Games [98]. On average 27.5 million prime-time viewers tuned into the 2016 Olympic Games with swimming being one of the marquee events [99]. Swimming is a unique sport as it takes place in the water, which results in different gravitational and resistive forces. These forces will predispose the aquatic athlete to primarily overuse injuries to the shoulder, knee, and lower back.

39.8.2 Injury Rate

It has been reported by the National Collegiate Athletic Association (NCAA) injury surveillance program that the 5-year injury rates for men and women's swimming and diving teams are 1.54 and 1.74 per 1000 AE. The majority of injuries were secondary to overuse and involved the shoulder. The female swimmers had a 58% higher rate of overuse injury in comparison to male swimmers (1.04 vs. 0.66 per 1000 AE) [100]. A survey of Division 1 NCAA competitive swimmers showed that injury rates of 4.0 per 1000 training hours for men and 3.78 per 1000 training hours for women. In addition, underclassmen were prone to more injuries than their upperclassmen teammates. The survey also showed that different strokes contributed to the injury risk with non-free style specialist experiencing more injuries with a relative risk of 1.33 [101]. During the 2013 FINA World Championships, the incidences of injury were 8.3 per 100 registered aquatic athletes [102].

39.8.3 Mechanisms of Injury

The sport of swimming is specifically dependent on the upper extremity for propulsions through the water. The body type of a successful swimmer is characterized by having large upper and middle body muscle masses. The swimmer is also usually lean and quite tall with long limbs and wide shoulders. This body type allows the swimmer to develop significant amount of power to drive the body forward, overcoming the resistance from water drag [103]. The majority of injuries seen in swimming have to do with overuse. The shoulder is fundamentally an unstable joint that requires firm scapular base and coordinated pattern of muscle forces to maintain stability, motion, and function. Anatomically, the shoulder joint is stabilized by static stabilizers (labrum and capsular ligaments), as well as dynamic stabilizers (rotator cuff muscles and scapular muscles). With intact shoulder kinematics, the humeral head should maintain balance forces with the glenoid fossa [104]. Swimmers, however, frequently will have increased shoulder laxity as their careers progress [105]. The enhanced shoulder laxity may provide a competitive advantage by allowing swimmers to achieve ideal body positions to reduce drag and generate larger stroke lengths. Consequently, the increased shoulder laxity leaves them more prone to relying on the dynamic stabilizers of the shoulder to control the improper translation and ultimately producing instability, impingement, and shoulder pain [106]. The main propulsive mechanism of swimming is the upper extremity, generated by powerful pectoralis major and latissimus dorsi muscles. With the development of muscle fatigue, the potential strength imbalance of opposing musculature is intensified, leading to further destabilization of the humeral head, scapular dyskinesis, and rotator cuff tendinopathy [106]. Scapular dyskinesis has been thought to predispose patients to impingement by placing the scapula in a relative abducted, protracted, and lateral displaced position during activity [107]. Another common overuse injury in swimmers is the "breaststroker's knee" which causes anterior and medial knee pain. These can potentially be attributed to recurrent medial collateral ligament sprains, patellofemoral pain syndrome, patellar tendinopathy, medial plica syndrome, and pes anserine bursitis [103, 108–110]. The mechanism of injury is thought to involve repetitive valgus load of the breaststroke kick, which causes medial distraction and lateral compression to the compartments of the knee [111]. In order to maintain proper streamlined body position in the water, swimmers will frequently be forced into a hyperextension of their lumbar spine. This position predisposes the swimmer to both lumbosacral and ligament injuries [112].

39.8.4 Common Injuries

The most common complaint in competitive swimming is shoulder pain [101], with overuse injuries being more common than acute injuries. Competitive swimmers will frequently complete more than 2500 shoulder revolutions and train up to 9 miles per day [113]. The term "swimmers' shoulder" has been described as anterior shoulder pain that frequently will occur during or after training due to repetitive impingement of the rotator cuff tendons under the coracoacromial arch. It can also be caused by scapular dyskinesis, overuse-related fatigue, and relative shoulder instability [103, 114]. Knee pain is the second most common musculoskeletal injury in competitive swimmers and has been called "breaststroker's knee" [109]. The documented incidence of knee pain in Olympic athletes has been reported to be as high as 34%. Interestingly, non-breaststroking specialties report 48% knee pain, while 73–86% of breaststroke swimmers reports knee pain [109, 110, 115]. Furthermore, groin pain is also frequently seen in the swimming populations. Hip adductors injury is common in the breaststroke specialty of swimmers. A survey of US swimmers found that groin pain affects 41% of breaststroke swimmers, 21% of individual medley swimmers, and only 6% of non-breaststroke/nonindividual medley swimmers [116]. Most cases of hip adductor/flexor strain injuries occur after repetitive hip adduction and squeezing of the legs during the breaststroke kick [41]. Also, lumbar spine pain is commonly reported in the swimming population, affecting 33–50% of butterfly specialist and 22–47% of breaststrokers [117]. Radiographic studies have shown that lumbar spine MRI in elite-level swimmers will frequently identify high grade of degenerative disc disease, most commonly at the L5/S1 level compared to controls [118]. With hyperextension of the lumbar spine in swimming being commonplace, the stresses on the lower back, specifically in the butterfly and breaststroke, can produce excessive posterior spine loads that may eventually lead to spondylolysis and spondylolisthesis [112].

39.9 Tennis

Samantha Tayne

39.9.1 Introduction

Tennis is a very popular recreational and competitive sport with 17.9 million players in the United States [119] and over 75 million people playing throughout 200 countries worldwide [120]. There continues to be growth in youth tennis, as well. Though tennis is played on varied surface types, indoor tennis is most often played on a hard court. This type of court has the highest coefficient of friction and lowest shock absorption. Due to the physics of playing on a hard court, sliding is difficult with short stopping distances and therefore high peak loads on the ankles and knees [119]. Additionally, the high velocities with which players hit the ball and the various positions of the racquet may cause the transfer of large loads to the joints of the upper extremities. As racquets have evolved over the past 30 years from heavy, wood models to the lighter graphite composite models, they have also been made to have a larger head with stiffer material [121]. The player must make efficient use of the kinetic chain in order to minimize the force transferred to each joint from the racquet or the court surface. Overall, high aerobic and anaerobic demands over the course of a match on a hard, indoor tennis court may lead to overuse and acute traumatic injuries.

39.9.2 Injury Rates

Several studies have been published observing the injury rate among various populations of tennis players, including recreational players, juniors, college athletes, and the professional circuit. Most of these studies, especially among the elite-level athletes, measure injuries as a physical complaint during training or a match, which interrupts the training or match for a period of time. The incidence of injuries can be recorded in several ways: per 1000 match hours, per 1000 exposure hours, or simply per number of athlete exposures (either match or training). One comprehensive meta-analysis by Pluim et al., which includes all levels of players, reported an overall injury incidence of 0.04–3.0 injuries per 1000 h of play [122].

One study observing elite junior tennis players in Australia found no difference in the incidence of injury between male and female players; however it found that male players tend to have more severe injuries, with severity defined as number of days off from training and/or matches. Injury incidence increased with age, with an incidence of 2 injuries per 1000 h for 13-year-olds and 2.9 injuries per 1000 h for 18-year-olds [122]. The National Collegiate Athletic Association (NCAA) had an Injury Surveillance Program (ISP) from 2009 to 2015, which found a higher injury rate of 4.9 injuries per 1000 exposures in a sample of 19 men's and 25 women's varsity tennis program. Here exposure was defined as participation in official NCAA practice or match [119, 124]. Another study on NCAA athletes showed that 67% of players had at least one musculoskeletal condition during the season. Importantly, they also found that all of the injuries sustained during match play were acute, while 69.6% of injuries sustained during training were gradual onset. Almost one-third of the NCAA players had at least one chronic condition during the season [119, 125].

Professional athletes were evaluated in a study analyzing injury trends from the US Open Tennis Championships from 1994 to 2009, demonstrating a comparably very high injury rate of 48.1 injuries per 1000 match exposures. This study also showed a significantly higher rate of acute injuries at 27.7 per 1000 match exposures than chronic overuse injuries 19.5 per 1000 match exposures [119, 126]. A study performed with participation of the Women's Tennis Association (WTA) showed similarly high injury incidence rates of 56.6 per 1000 h of match play or 62.7 per 1000 match exposures. Greater ranking of the athlete typically resulted in increased number of matches and match hours per season and was associated with a greater number of injuries per season [120].

A study in the Netherlands performed via telephone survey on participation on recreational sport found an injury rate of 9.6 injuries in 10,000 h played. This study identified tennis as one that should be targeted for injury prevention for male and female recreational athletes, especially within the 35–54-year-old age group [127].

39.9.3 Common Injuries

The kinetic chain, from the feet interacting with the court surface through the trunk to the shoulder and down the arm controlling the racket, allows tennis players to transfer energy from the racket to the ball. Any break or malfunction within this kinetic chain may lead to injury, either acute or chronic. Serving is the most strenuous stroke in tennis, with high forces generated through the trunk, shoulder, and into the forearm and wrist. The serve is characterized similarly to pitching in baseball with a windup, early cocking, late cocking, acceleration, and follow through. Ground strokes, though they may not generate as much force, also are characterized in a similar fashion with the racket preparation, acceleration, and follow through [128]. The most common chronic, overuse injuries are related to the repetitive motion of the upper extremities in these strokes and may also lead to abdominal muscle strains, lumbar strains, or discogenic injuries. The lower extremities are more susceptible to acute injuries such as ankle sprains, meniscal knee injuries, and hip injuries, during quick directional changes and sliding on a hard court, as the body compensates for the change in direction or velocity [121].

As described previously, upper extremity injuries tend to be less prevalent than lower extremity injuries; however a study of NCAA men's and women's tennis injuries suggested that tennis has a higher proportion of upper extremity injuries than other NCAA sports [128]. Maladaptive motion of overhead athletes such as tennis players, including glenohumeral internal rotation deficit (GIRD) and SICK scapula (scapula malposition, inferior medial border prominence, coracoid pain and malposition, and dyskinesis of scapular movement), may lead to further injury [129, 130]. Such injuries may include internal impingement and superior labrum anterior-to-posterior (SLAP) tears in the shoulder, tendinopathy at the medial or lateral elbow, tendinopathy or subluxation of the extensor carpi ulnaris tendon at the wrist, valgus extension overload of the elbow, and TFCC sprains. These injuries are all affected by the inefficiency of the transfer of force and may be related to muscle weakness or imbalance, all the way down to the grip on the racket.

A study of 184 elite tennis players between 11 years old and 24 years old were evaluated in terms of their shoulder range of motion. This study found that reduced internal range of motion and increased external range of motion were common in the dominant arm of these players. Additionally, GIRD increased with age. The players under 14 years old had significantly more internal rotation than those over 14 years old [129]. In SICK scapula syndrome, there is weakness of the muscles stabilizing the scapula, including the serratus anterior, infraspinatus, deltoid, and lower and middle trapezius. Meanwhile the increased tension of opposing scapular stabilizers, which includes the levator scapulae, upper trapezius, and pectoralis, leads to abnormal motions of the scapula, causing increase in the angulation of the humerus on the glenoid, and increased injury risk [130].

Lateral elbow epicondylitis, also known as tennis elbow, is commonly associated with tennis injuries. The torque of the racquet as it makes contact with the ball is opposed by eccentric loading of the forearm muscles, which can cause microtrauma and lead to tendinopathy [121]. However, 5-year injury data from the Association of Tennis Professionals and the WTA the world tour actually found that medial epicondylitis was three times more likely than lateral epicondylitis. Fu et al. comment that this may be due to the repetitive loads of forehand groundstrokes and serve loading in modern tennis that stress the medial flexor-pronator mass [119]. Similarly, valgus extension overload is caused by a combination of valgus forces along with rapid extension, leading to tensile forces on the medial side of the elbow, compression on the lateral portion of the elbow, and shear forces in the posterior compartment. Valgus extension overload may result in injury to the UCL (ulnar collateral ligament), posterior impingement of the elbow, ulnar neuritis, or even osteochondritis dessicans [131].

Acute injuries to the lower extremities are the most frequent in adult professional athletes and

NCAA athletes. Dakic studied professional women in the WTA and found that lower limb injuries were most common and occur twice the rate of upper limb injuries and three times the rate of trunk injuries [120]. It is important to note that this study looked per match exposure, so likely more acute injuries were taking place during a competitive match rather than chronic injuries, which may have prevented the athlete from competing altogether or was adequately controlled and treated prior to match play. A study mentioned previously, looking at data from 19 men's NCAA programs and 25 women's NCAA programs, found that the lower extremities were the most commonly injured; however they did also have high rates of trunk injuries, 16.6% of injuries for the men and 17.6% for the women [124].

Lower extremity injuries may include a variety of injuries to the knee and ankle, often from rapid change of direction on the tennis court surface. The ankle is the most common location of acute injuries in professional and elite-level athletes, specifically inversion ankle sprains, though knee injuries to the anterior cruciate ligament and collateral ligaments are also seen [119, 121, 124, 126]. In recreational tennis players, tennis toe and tennis leg are common lower extremity injuries. Tennis toe is due to repetitive stress of the toe against the front of the shoe, most commonly to the big toe, leading to a subungual hematoma and a painful toe. Tennis leg, first described in 1883, has historically thought to be related to a tear of the plantaris tendon. However, more recently it has been shown to be a tear of the medial head of the gastrocnemius or disruption of the gastrocnemius-soleus aponeurosis, due to extension at the knee with forced dorsiflexion of the ankle, often in middle aged athletes [132, 133].

Trunk injuries, including lumbar spine, abdominal, and groin strains, are unique to tennis or overhead serving sports. The forced flexion of the trunk is initiated by the rectus abdominis and supported by the internal and external obliques and the iliopsoas; meanwhile the gluteal muscles help drive the core and relieve some of the load. Poor core strength or poor coordination of these muscle groups may lead to strains or tears, which can be debilitating injuries. Athletes may also suffer muscular strains or inflammation of structures around the hip joint, as well as labral tears due to similar stresses [121]. In Gescheit's study on elite junior-level players, the lumbar spine was both the most commonly injured and the most severely injured area, especially among 14–18-year-olds [123]. Another 1-year prospective study on elite junior players found that overuse injuries made up 47% of the health problems experienced by this cohort over the year and the lower back was a common site of injury [134]. Athletes suffering from an abdominal or lumbar strain typically require at least 1–2 weeks off from any strenuous activity, and initially even walking may be difficult. Core strengthening may help prevent these and other injuries, throughout the kinetic chain [121].

> **Fact Box**
> It is important to consider the equipment and surface type when treating a tennis injury. Acute injuries are more common in the lower extremities, while chronic, overuse injuries tend to involve the upper extremities. Preventative measures should include evaluation of the kinetic chain and addressing any muscle imbalances.

39.10 Volleyball

Matthew Steffes

39.10.1 Introduction

Volleyball, originally termed *mintonette*, was created by William G Morgan in a New England YMCA in 1896. He intended to create a game that incorporated elements from badminton, tennis, handball, and the popular new game of basketball. The game found new popularity abroad among Allied countries during World War I. This popularity led to becoming an official Olympic Summer sport in 1964, while the outdoor version played on sand was officially added in 1996. It is estimated that global volleyball participation rates are second only to soccer [135]. In the United States, participation rates are higher among females and are reflected in the disparity of varsity Division 1 collegiate volleyball programs [136].

39.10.2 Injury Rates

Several case series have been reported regarding injury incidence at various levels of competition. Pastor et al. reported a mean of 2.58 injuries per player among the German Men's National Team over a 6-year period. These athletes were 3 times more likely to sustain an acute injury versus a chronic injury (3.3 vs. 1.08/1000 h) and averaged fewer injuries in the second season of competition compared to first season (1.92 vs. 3.25 injuries/year). These injuries caused the athlete to miss on average 16.9 participation days [137].

The lower extremity is the most commonly affected area, accounting for over 58% of all injuries, compared to the upper extremity at 21%. The majority of these injuries occurred in the attack zone, which is the area nearest the net when related to the backline defensive position players. Collegiate athletes showed a 6.19 injury rate per 1000 exposures during preseason practice as compared to 4.52 injury rate per 1000 exposures during in-season competition [138]. There is a lack of studies reporting differences in injury prevalence or incidence between genders. Agel et al. presented 16 years of data on female collegiate volleyball players, showing similar rates of shoulder injuries incurred during competition and practice (21.4% and 18.7%), whereas spine injuries were more common in practice compared with competition (10.8 vs. 17.4%) [139].

39.10.3 Common Injuries

Volleyball requires high demands on both the upper and lower extremities, in addition to the trunk and spine. At all levels of play, ankle sprains are the most prevalent injury. In a prospective series by Verhagen et al., ankle sprains accounted for 41% of all injuries incurred during one season among an Olympic National Team. Additionally, ankle sprains were the most common injury leading to at least 10 days of missed time from activity among collegiate athletes [140].

The next most common acute injuries are ACL ruptures, most prevalent among females landing from a jump. Among high school females, ACL ruptures are 5 times more likely during competition compared to practice [141]. Incidence of ACL ruptures has been rising among women collegiate players, with a mean 0.06 injury rate per 1000 game and practice exposures per season [139].

In contrast, injuries to the shoulder and lumbar spine are mostly due to overuse. We also see significant overuse injuries in the knee. Patellar tendinosis, or jumper's knee, is the most common chronic injury overall, approaching nearly 50% among high amateur athletes [142]. Ferretti et al. demonstrated the development of patellar tendinosis is directly associated with the amount of participation and that participating in practice or a game more than 4 times per week for at least 2 years was the highest risk factor [143].

Shoulder impingement and rotator cuff tendonitis, suprascapular neuropathy, glenohumeral internal rotation deficit, and shoulder instability are all common pathologies leading to shoulder pain and disability in the volleyball athlete. Among amateur and recreational athletes, shoulder impingement predominates, whereas suprascapular neuropathy is the most common shoulder pathology seen at the elite level. Lumbar muscle strains and herniated lumbar discs are the most common spine injuries seen, with strains more prevalent among elite-level athletes and disc pathology higher among amateurs [144].

39.10.4 Injury Mechanism

Ankle sprains account for the majority of acute injuries encountered and many studies have been done involving the circumstances and mechanism of these injuries. Bahr et al. showed that these injuries occur when an offensive player charging the net lands on a teammate's or opposing player's foot at the centerline, inverting the ankle [145]. Many studies have shown fewer ankle sprains in beach volleyball, pointing toward the role the hard playing surface contributes [146].

The ACL is often injured as the landing attacker strikes the surface with the lower extremity in a valgus and internally rotated position, placing undue stress on the ACL. The majorities of these injuries are noncontact injuries and involve other intra-articular structures [138]. Zahradnik et al. compared the biomechanics of two differing methods of landing after a block maneuver. By landing on both feet simultaneously, each extremity is loaded evenly, as opposed to using one foot to quickly step backward in a staggered stance. The latter places an increased valgus moment at the knee causing increased tension of the ACL [147].

Many volleyball-related injuries can be attributed to repetition and overuse. Kugler et al. reported that the elite volleyball player will perform 41,000 overhead spikes and serves per season [148]. The overhead spike, standing serve, and jump-serve maneuvers all require maximum abduction and external rotation of the shoulder to fully "cock" the arm prior to forward acceleration and ball strike. This position may lead to stretching of the glenohumeral capsule in addition to inflammation or attrition of the rotator cuff muscles.

The overhead spike and jump-serve maneuvers also involve extremes of motion in the lower spine. During both actions the lumbar spine rotates and hyperextends to increase the "cocked" position and maximize the torque generated. This produces both compressive load on the posterior elements and stresses through the intervertebral disc and is suspected to lead to muscle strains, disc disease, pars interarticularis stress reactions, or overt fractures.

39.10.5 Treatment Principles

Injury prevention has been the focus of many efforts over the last 30 years, involving changes to rules, rehabilitation, and training approach. A rule change was previously proposed to penalize any violation of the centerline to avoid player collisions in the attack zone. This greatly impeded the game and was removed in favor of allowing players to completely cross the line. Curiously this leniency did not lead to expected increase in ankle sprains and has been incorporated into the current game regulations [149].

The use of ankle bracing was originally embraced as a successful method at reducing ankle sprains, by Pedowitz et al. showing a rate of 0.07 ankle sprains per 1000 exposures with use of a double-supported ankle brace. This was significantly lower than the national average of 0.98 sprains per 1000 exposures [150]. However, Stasinopoulos et al. showed that bracing was as effective as proprioceptive training and technical training in reducing ankle sprains [151]. While debate remains, this points to the importance of incorporating some modality to address ankle stability prior to injury.

Ankle sprains carry a significant risk of recurrence, with rates approximating 42% within 6 months of index injury [152]. Rehabilitation programs aimed at reducing this rate share many similarities with preventive programs. Many different protocols varying in length, amount of guided therapy, and the use of supportive devices have been developed, but all emphasize proprioceptive training under the supervision of a physical therapist or athletic trainer. These have yielded good results at restoring general ankle strength and proprioception as well as lowering reinjury rate [153].

Fact Box

See Table 39.1.

Table 39.1 Classification of acute lateral ankle sprains

Classification of acute lateral ankle sprains [154]	
Grade	Description
I	The ATFL is stretched and some of the ligament fibers are torn. No frank ligamentous disruption is present. Mild swelling, little or no ecchymosis on the lateral aspect of the ankle, point tenderness on the ATFL, and no or mild restriction of active ROM. Difficulty with full weight bearing is sometimes seen. No laxity on examination
II	Moderate injury to the lateral ligamentous complex, frequently with a complete tear of the ATFL ± partial tear of the CFL. Restricted ROM with localized swelling, ecchymosis, hemorrhage, and tenderness of the anterolateral aspect of the ankle. Abnormal laxity may be mild or absent. May be indistinguishable from a grade III injury in the acute setting.
III	Complete disruption of the ATFL and the CFL ± capsular tear ± PTFL tear. Diffuse swelling, ecchymosis on the lateral side of the ankle and heel, and tenderness over the anterolateral capsule, ATFL, and CFL

Adapted from Maffulli N, Ferran NA. Management of acute and chronic ankle instability. *J Am Acad Orthop Surg*. 2008;16 (10):608–615

39.11 Water Polo

Aimee Bobko

39.11.1 Introduction

Water polo is a unique sport that combines features of swimming, throwing, and wrestling [155]. In addition to the injuries commonly seen with swimming and overhead sports, water polo has a high rate of acute traumatic injuries secondary to physical contact. Water polo has the highest rate of injuries of aquatic sports [156].

39.11.2 Injury Rate and Epidemiology

There were 15.3 injuries/100 water polo athletes in the FINA World Championships 2009/2013 [157]. A majority of the injuries were the result of physical contact, including lacerations and contusions [155]. The next most common are upper extremity injuries, a majority involving the shoulder. Reported shoulder injury rates in the sport vary from 24 to 51% [158]. Other reports have documented an incidence of 67% of shoulder soreness or swimmer's shoulder by the time players are at the collegiate or postcollegiate level. The incidence of shoulder pain in water polo has been directly correlated to the number of years a player has participated in the sport [161]. Elite women's water polo players have been shown to have a higher rate of shoulder soreness with increased shooting volume [163].

39.11.3 Common Injuries and Mechanism of Injury

The most common mechanism of injury results from physical contact. The only protective equipment is ear covering and mouth guards, which are not required [159]. "Nail checks" are performed prior to each match to assess finger and toenails of players. However, many types of lacerations including facial lacerations and corneal abrasions still occur. Another contact injury includes concussions; goalies are specifically at risk from other players as well as from the water polo ball from shots or rebounds [160]. Another traumatic injury from being slapped on the side of the head with a cupped palm includes a tympanic membrane perforation (perforated eardrum). The spine is at risk for degenerative changes due to repeated rotation and extension activities with swimming and throwing [160]. Shoulder injuries often occur from repetitive movements and sustained microtrauma, which include swimmer's shoulder, rotator cuff injury, and labral tears [160]. Shoulder dislocations are also a potential injury, especially when in possession of the water polo ball and being pulled by a defender [161]. A result from the aquatic environment includes otitis externa, also known as swimmer's ear, as well as ocular conjunctivitis. Blocking and catching movements put players at risk for finger dislocations and lacerations. The most common finger laceration is the web space tear [161]. This injury will occur during forced abduction with the ball between neighboring fingers. This injury can be superficial or complex with involvement of collateral ligament tears [161]. Elbow injuries can also occur, including thrower's elbow, ulnar collateral ligament injury, and osteochondritis dissecans of the capitellum [162]. Without the solid foundation of land to generate power from, a greater amount of force is generated from the upper extremity, placing greater tension on structures including the UCL [161].

39.11.4 Treatment Principles

Education regarding injury prevention and treatment is crucial. Currently, it is up to the player's discretion whether they wear a mouth guard. In fact, it's reported that only 7.7% of players wear mouth guards [159]. Smaller lacerations can be treated with Steri-Strips or a plastic-based waterproof spray; larger lacerations may require sutures [160]. Corneal abrasions include topical analgesics, topical antibiotics, and oral analgesics [164]. Overuse injuries can be treated by adjustments to swimming/throwing form, decreased training intervals, and rest [161]. Thrower's elbow can be treated conservatively with rest, ice, immobilization, and extension block splinting [161]. Web space tears range in severity and can be treated with simple wound care or could require surgical treatment for associated instability [161]. Finger dislocations can be treated with reduction. If there is an associated articular fracture of a greater percentage, surgical fixation may be required [161]. For a ruptured tympanic membrane, players should be kept out of the water until healed. There are options available with customized ear plugs if necessary to play [165]. In addition, as with all aquatic sports, all pools should be equipped with a spine board and cervical collars with a plan in place where a player needs to be extracted from the water [155].

39.12 Weight Lifting

Aimee Bobko

39.12.1 Introduction

Weight lifting as a competitive sport involves attempting to lift maximum weight loads [166]. It's an activity that presents extreme forces and may produce the greatest power the human body can generate [167]. Weight lifting was included as its own Olympic event in 1920. Current modern competition consists of two exercises: the snatch and the clean and jerk. Besides Olympic lifting, weight lifting in the community and the development of activities such as CrossFit have continued to rise in popularity and the subsequent associated injuries [168].

39.12.2 Injury Rate and Epidemiology

An incidence of one to two injuries/lifter/year has been reported [166]. Another study reports an injury incidence in weight lifting of 2.4–3.3 injuries/1000 hours of training [169]. Prevalence varies throughout the literature, widely from 16 to 90% of lifters sustaining injuries [166]. Shoulder injuries are the most prevalent, 6–36% [166]. Knee injuries are the next most common with a prevalence of 10–32% [166].

Elite lifters have lower rate of injuries (3.6 vs. 5.8 injuries per 1000 h) and acute injuries (50 vs. 72%) than novice lifters [168]. Elite lifters have more thigh injuries and less chest and shoulder injuries compared to novice lifters [171]. When looking at children versus adult lifters, children are more likely to sustain accidental injuries from dropping or pinching weights, specifically to the hand and foot regions [172].

39.12.3 Common Injuries and Mechanism of Injury

Acute injuries include spontaneous pneumothorax, myocardial infarction, fractures, dislocations, tendon ruptures, meniscus tears, and acute herniated discs [170]. Tendon ruptures most often seen in weight lifting include bicep tendon, Achilles tendon, pec major tendon, patellar tendon, quadriceps tendon, and triceps tendon. Tendon ruptures are associated to occur more frequently in those who use anabolic steroids, older age, and fluoroquinolone [170]. Dislocations seen include glenohumeral joint, elbow joint, acromioclavicular joint, patella femoral joint, and ankle joint. Injuries such as these have been seen to occur in high rates when in the overhead position such as in the snatch and a portion of the clean and jerk [170]. More common injuries are strains, sprains, and tendinitis of the upper extremity, spine, and lower extremity. Chronic injuries result mainly from overuse and account for approximately 30% of injuries in strength training [170]. Specifically patellar tendonitis from deep flexion in squatting has been reported. Spondylolysis from excessive repetitive forces on the lumbar spine have been seen [170].

39.12.4 Treatment Principles

Using equipment safely and learning proper lifting technique can help decrease the rate or severity of injuries [173]. Athletes looking to start using supplements or change their body weight should consult with a professional nutritionist, dietician, physician, etc. [170]. For injury management, emergent treatment is warranted for medical conditions such as subarachnoid hemorrhage, MI, and spontaneous pneumothorax. Dislocations should be treated immediately as well. Surgical fixation is recommended for many of the acute tendon ruptures. Chronic injuries can be first treated conservatively with training modifications, rest, physical therapy, and potential role of corticosteroid injections and may progress to surgical intervention.

39.13 Wrestling

Benjamin Mayo

39.13.1 Introduction

Wrestling is one of the oldest known sports, with origins dating back to the ancient Sumerians in 5000 BC and the first recorded wrestling competitions in 708 BC in Greece. Rules and equipment have developed over time, but the modern iteration of wrestling was noted to be the Olympics in the 1896 Athens games [174]. Today, two predominant styles prevail – Greco-Roman wrestling in which touching of the lower extremities is forbidden, and freestyle, in which there are no restrictions on leg contact. In the United States, there are an estimated 2.5 million participants per year, and wrestling was the sixth most popular high school sport in 2006 [175, 176]. However, there is a significant risk of injury secondary to the combative nature of the sport.

39.13.2 Injury Rates

There is a significant risk of injury in wrestling that has been reported in the literature. A recent prospective study by Argarwal in 2016 demonstrated injury rates of 5.13 injuries per 1000 exposures [177]. In multiple analysis of injury rates among high school sports, wrestling was consistently second behind football with an injury rate between 7.3 and 30.7 injuries per 1000 athlete exposures [178–180]. Although the overall injury rate is high, some studies have reported that nearly two-thirds of injuries are deemed minor [179]. However, a significant portion of wrestling injuries is severe and has been reported to have the highest severe injury rate in the NCAA at 1.73/1000 athlete exposures [181]. Additional studies have reported that up to 37.6% of injuries required at least a week off from competition and up to 14.8% being classified as major [179–182]. Notably, more elite athletes appear to be at higher risk of injury, as in an analysis of wrestling matches in the 2008 Olympics demonstrated an injury rate of 9.3/100 athletes and 7.88 injuries per 100 matches [183].

39.13.3 Injury Mechanism

Several studies have reported on the most common injury mechanisms. As expected, most injuries occur from contact with other athletes or with the playing surface from throws and grappling maneuvers. A significantly higher percentage of injuries occur during live competition, with as high as 93.3% of all injuries occurring during matches. The reported incidence of injury during matches has been as high as 8.2/1000 athlete exposures, with an odds ratio of 8.66 compared to training sessions [179, 181, 183]. Additionally, a high percentage of injuries that do occur during training sessions are a result of live-match training. This relationship appears true for both minor and major injuries. Nearly 80% of catastrophic injuries occurred during competition versus training, and the rate of elbow dislocations was nearly three times lower in training compared to competition [185, 186].

Injuries to the legs occur more often in freestyle, with nearly 57% of injuries occurring to the lower extremities [176]. Because of this, freestyle wrestling has been reported to have a higher overall injury rate (10.1% or 7.0 injuries per 1000 exposures) in Olympic athletes compared to the Greco-Roman style, with knee injuries being four times more prevalent [176]. Conversely, injuries to the upper extremity are more often noted in Greco-Roman style, up to 55% of injuries to the arms, hands, or wrists [176, 187]. Greco-Roman has also demonstrated to have a higher risk of concussion and other injuries to the head and face, largely from being driven to the mat [176].

Numerous studies have reported that a wrestler is more likely to be injured in the defensive position while being taken down from standing, and as high as 81.3% of injuries in elite athletes occurs from the standing position [180, 188, 189]. This is intuitive, as the process of being taken down may put the competitor in a vulnerable position and high probability to land without adequately protecting them self. For catastrophic injuries, it has been reported as many as 74% of occur as a result of a takedown [185]. Similarly, a study focusing on elbow dislocations reported that 63.3% of elbow dislocations occurred during takedown with the athlete landing on an outstretched arm, while only 10% occurred during an escape [190]. When analyzing emergency department visits for wrestling injuries, approximately 34% of injuries were from being struck by or against the opponent, with another 22% as a result from a fall or takedown, while the remaining majority had a diagnosis of overexertion [175].

Few studies have attempted to analyze maneuvers that may be more risky for injury and have had typically failed to demonstrate any pattern leading to injury [185, 188]. However, it is consistently found that player contact is the most common cause in up to 56.6% of injuries, with contact to the surface the second most common cause [181]. A majority of injuries are acute in nature instead of chronic or recurrent injuries [188]. In one study of Olympic athletes, only 21.9% of all injuries were recurrent [182], while one study of high school athletes demonstrated that 39% were re-aggravated injuries [191].

39.13.4 Common Injuries

The most commonly reported injuries in the literature are sprains, strains, and contusions, which account for up to 65% of injuries [179, 180, 182]. Fractures do occur, though at a lower rate than soft tissue injuries. Fractures are more common in children under 18 years old. An analysis of emergency department visits reported fractures were the second most common diagnosis at 22.1–25.9% of injuries, led only by sprains and strains at 36.6–38.7% [175]. In more elite older athletes, the fracture rate has been reported to be 6.3% [179]. One study of Olympic wrestlers demonstrated a rate of 0.8/10,000 athlete exposures in freestyle wrestlers and 0.3/10,000 in Greco-Roman [192].

Although all body parts are commonly injured in wrestling, the knee and shoulder are the most frequently injured [180]. However, when included in analysis, injuries to the skin occur at an exceptionally high rate and should be noted. In one study, as many as 62% of reported injuries were classified as skin abrasions or contusions [187]. Though not an injury per se, skin infections are a common reason a wrestler may be held from participating in the sport. Skin infections in wrestlers are reported at a rate as high as 14.23/10,000 adverse events, 74% of which caused athletes to miss more than 24 h of training. Importantly, these infections are highly communicable and are frequently recurrent (22%), highlighting the importance of diligently disinfecting facilities using bleach as well as frequent skin checks of athletes [193].

39.13.5 Head, Neck, and Face

Head and neck injuries account for 14.5% of emergency department visits in youth wrestlers, with 4.5–6.2% due to traumatic brain injury [175]. The most commonly reported injury to the head and face are minor lacerations, abrasions, and contusions from contact with the mat or other athlete body parts, with a rate 69.9% of all injuries when included [188]. One extremely common injury is perichondrial hematoma, more commonly known as cauliflower ear in which the cartilage in the ear is damaged after trauma and leads to deformity. In a review of the NCAA injury surveillance system, Chorney et al. demonstrated a maxillofacial injury rate of 7.02 injuries/1000 athlete exposures. Most frequently this was an injury to the nasal bone, followed by mandible and dental injury. However, these rarely needed surgery with a rate of 0.50/10,000 [194].

An increasing focus on concussion diagnosis and prevention has raised the importance of understanding risks and incidence in all sports but particularly in sports like wrestling where the head is frequently contacted. Concussions are one of the more frequent injuries of the head and have been reported between 1 and 8% of all injuries, with a higher rate in older age groups [180, 195]. A recent survey of NCAA wrestling coaches reported that their knowledge of concussions was lacking, and they were more likely to believe it was ok to keep playing after a concussion in a playoff-type event compared to an early season competition. This highlights the importance of a need for continued concussion education even at the higher levels [196].

Neck injuries have a reported incidence of 0.8–14.9% of wrestling injuries, depending on the level of severity recorded. Most commonly, neck injuries are minor cervical strains [195, 197, 198]. Less frequently, neuropraxias can occur typically from a forced hyperextension mechanism while shooting in. The neck is also a potential site of catastrophic injury, which will be discussed later.

39.13.6 Upper Extremity

Upper extremity injuries are extremely common in wrestlers, with a reported incidence between 9.3 and 42% of all injuries [188]. The shoulder is frequently reported as the most commonly injured part of the upper extremity and occasionally as the most common injury overall with rates as high as 24% [175, 180]. Wrestling has also been noted to have the second most frequent dislocation injuries, only behind football, with 1.99/10,000 dislocations per athlete exposures, and 7.2% of all wresting injuries were reported as dislocation – most commonly in the shoulder (24–54%), elbow (14.2%), and knee (13.5%) [180]. Recurrent shoulder dislocations were to be at a rate of 17.3% and 12.8% eventually required surgery [199].

Elbow injuries, though less common than shoulder injuries with an incidence of 1.0–7.9% of injuries, are often more severe [175]. Most commonly the mechanism is from a hyperextension abduction motion, resulting in a sprain of the

UCL and anterior capsule. However, if continued pressure is applied, it can result in an elbow dislocation. Elbow dislocations have commonly been reported in the literature for wrestlers. Recent studies examining high school and NCAA athletes revealed that wrestling had the highest rate of elbow dislocations across both age categories, with an injury rate of 6.63–10.8/100,000 athlete exposures during competition [190]. Younger wrestlers are more susceptible to avulsion fractures of the elbow including the olecranon and medial condyle [200, 201].

Though frequently not reported due to the low severity, injuries to the wrist, hand, and fingers are also common and account for 18.5% of wrestling-related emergency department visits [175]. Sprains of the metacarpophalangeal and interphalangeal joints are the most common injuries to the hand [182, 188]. Less common upper extremity injuries that have also been described in the literature include ruptures of the pectoralis major, avulsion fractures of the scapula, avulsions of the lesser tuberosity, subscapularis injuries, and suprascapular nerve injuries [202–205].

39.13.7 Torso and Spine

Injuries to the torso are relatively common in wrestlers, with a reported incidence between 1.2 and 18.6% of injuries. A majority of these are rib and chest injuries such as costochondral sprains and rib fractures [188]. Wrestlers have also been identified as a group with a high rate of spondylosis or spondylolisthesis, with as many as 25% of athletes demonstrating these changes on radiographs and up to 30% of wrestlers with back pain [206, 207].

39.13.8 Lower Extremity

Injuries to the lower extremity are extremely common in both types of wrestling but more so in the Greco-Roman style. The knee is often reported as the most frequently injured body area, with rates between 7.6 and 44% of all injuries [188, 190]. Ligament sprains of the MCL, LCL, ACL, and PCL are the most common knee injuries reported with an incidence near 40% and fortunately are often mild. Despite being a very common injury, only 6.7–8.4% of wrestling-related emergency department visits were for knee complaints [175, 206]. A recent study focusing on knee injuries reported that 18% of all knee injuries are strains or sprains, while another 17% were prepatellar bursitis and 24% as effusions or bone contusion [177]. However, when they are more severe, they often require surgery and account for up to 44% of season-ending injuries in high school athletes [180]. Many of these are for ACL injuries, which have been reported to be approximately 10% of all knee injuries. There are mixed reports about whether the medial or lateral side of the knee is more frequently injured, but wrestling has demonstrated a relatively higher rate of lateral meniscus injuries compared to other sports [178]. Although a majority of knee injuries are minor, the knee is one of the most common sites of significant injury. One study has reported that nearly 40% of significant injuries were of the knee, while another demonstrated that the knee accounted for 65% of injuries requiring surgery [181, 206].

One unique knee injury to wrestling is prepatellar bursitis. While it is a relatively rare injury in most sports, however, it is one of the more common knee injuries in wrestlers due to the amount of time spent kneeling [190]. A study by Mysnyk et al. reported that 21% of all new knee injuries were prepatellar bursitis and often would reoccur [184].

39.13.8.1 Catastrophic Injuries

Unfortunately, catastrophic injuries have been reported in the literature [208]. Though rare overall, with a reported rate of 0.97/100,000 in wrestlers, 50% of these injuries affecting the cervical vertebral column, head, or spinal cord resulting from rotational or axial blows to the region [188]. The other 50% are attributed to cardiac dysfunction [188]. A large review by Boden et al. in 2002 reported 54 catastrophic injuries over an 18-year period. Fifteen of such injuries were attributed to indirect causes such as heart failure and weight loss-related systemic failure. Overall there was a rate of 2.11 direct catastrophic injuries per year or

1/100,000 participants [185]. These included 27 cervical fractures or injury to major cervical ligaments, 4 spinal cord contusions w/transient quadriparesis, and 3 severe head injuries. Quadriplegia was present in 11 cases, with residual neurologic deficits in 6 athletes and 1 death in a head-related injury from head-to-head contact in a practice [185]. They did determine that 11 of such injuries were preventable, as there were rules infractions or instances of poor officiating that resulted in a delayed call that may have stopped play before injury. Other studies have reported wrestling as having the second highest rate of cervical spine injuries in high school athletes, with a rate of 7.42/100,000 athlete exposures [209]. One study of catastrophic cervical spine injuries found that 50% were permanent, while 50% had full recovery [210].

Non-axial catastrophic injuries have also been reported, with an example being brachial artery disruption following elbow dislocation [211, 212]. Overall, it has been reported that less experienced athletes were more likely to experience a catastrophic injury, as they are more likely to get themselves in to dangerous situations [185].

Fact Box: Medical Issues

There is a relatively high incidence of medical issues to be aware of for wrestlers. The process of cutting weight can have profoundly negative impacts on the athlete's health and have deleterious effects on performance, strength, and aerobic capacity. While maintaining a low body percentage is expected, weight loss is often achieved through unhealthy methods such as fluid and calorie restriction and less commonly diuretics and laxatives leading up to a match. Both the NCAA and NFHS have placed restrictions on the amount of weight loss athletes can achieve during season based on a preseason assessment and body fat assessment. It is important for physicians to be familiar with their local protocols to ensure their athletes are eligible and safe for participation.

39.14 Universal Challenges to Consider When Caring for any Indoor Sport

Alex Behar and Mark R. Hutchinson

39.14.1 Playing Surfaces and Environment

Playing surface is a key controllable factor when targeting prevention of injuries in indoor sports. Certain flooring materials such as concrete may be more unforgiving and lead to increased risk of overuse injuries. If a more rigid surface is necessary and is different than the athlete is used to, consideration of modifying shoe wear with increased shock absorption can work to balance out the increased risk. Many events will install some sort of temporary playing surface or court made of wood or synthetic. These surfaces may be raised and include some additional structural shock absorption. It is a good idea for the healthcare provider or athletic trainer to walk the floor before competition looking for flaws in structure or installation that might increase the risk of athlete tripping. There should be no sharp, raised edges, gaps, valleys, or defects. The surface finish should be consistent so that one area does not provide more or less traction than another. The playing surface should be dry with no evidence of prior leaks. If the surface has been recently refinished or treated the athletes should be allowed time to acclimate to the new playing surface to get a feel for traction and shock absorption. Certain playing surfaces may also introduce an increased risk of certain types of injuries such as rug burns, road rash, abrasions, and splinters that the healthcare provider should be prepared to address.

Alternative playing surfaces such as water and ice will introduce additional unique injury risks that should be considered and planned for. For temporary swimming events, leakages outside of the pool deck may increase the risk of slipping and all electrical devices need to be carefully grounded and kept away from standing water. Indoor swimming, diving, and water polo also introduce the presence of chlorine into the air that may trigger bronchospasm or asthma attacks in select athletes who are at risk. Optimizing ventilation systems may minimize the risk. For indoor ice sports such as ice hockey, figure skating, curling, and speed skating, the potential risk of slipping on the playing surface is obvious; however, the maintenance of an indoor ice introduces unique risks that should be considered when caring for athletes. Electrical ice resurfacing "Zamboni" machines can produce ultrafine particulate debris that in combination with the cold environment can place an athlete at risk for exercise-induced bronchospasm secondary to airway inflammation and hyperactivity. A study by Rundell in 2006 demonstrated an 18-fold particulate matter in ice arenas, which was caused by the combustion of ice resurfacing machines [213].

39.14.2 Structural Issues and Access

In addition to the playing surface, careful inspection of the venue should be done before competition to assure a clear field of play and that no structural obstacles place the competitors at risk. Adequate lighting to allow appropriate visualization of targets and goals should also be assured. If air conditioning is not present, temperature monitoring should be assessed as if the competition was outdoors to reduce risk of heat-related illnesses.

Emergencies can occur at any time during a sporting event. It is important to have an emergency action plan within the participating facility and to the nearest healthcare facility in order to provide the best possible medical care. Designated leadership should be promptly identified in addition to delineating responsibilities including emergency equipment retrieval, directing the emergency medical system to the scene, and transportation of the individual. Access to the athletic training room from the playing field should be direct and uncomplicated. The most qualified individual on the emergency response team should make the decision as to how and where the patient should be treated. In the case of catastrophic events, an exit strategy should be carefully mapped. Is there a ramp to the playing surface? How close can emergency transport get to the facility and to the playing surface? What is the quickest and safest route for emergency transport to get the nearest hospital? While such emergency plans are necessary for all competitions whether indoors or outdoors, the unique limitations regarding access to an indoor venue must be accounted for.

Take-Home Message
The sports medicine physician covering an indoor sporting event is required to know the intricacies of such event by understanding how to prevent, diagnose, and treat injuries involved with the sport. One must also consider the layout of the facility to develop an appropriate emergency action plan and appropriately manage an injury. Performing a walk-through of the facility prior to an event is highly recommended to prepare for any unforeseen incidents. The goal is to limit risk and prepare for catastrophic injuries with an appropriate emergency action plan in consideration of the sporting event complex's geographical and architectural limitations.

References

Basketball

1. Participation Statics. http://www.nfhs.org/ParticipationStatics/ParticipationStatics.aspx/. Accessed 13 Aug 2018.
2. Randazzo C, Nelson NG, McKenzie LB. Basketball-related injuries in school-aged children and adolescents in 1997-2007. Pediatrics. 2010;126(4):727–33. https://doi.org/10.1542/peds.2009-2497.
3. Borowski LA, Yard EE, Fields SK, Comstock RD. The epidemiology of US high school basketball injuries, 2005-2007. Am J Sports Med. 2008;36(12):2328–35. https://doi.org/10.1177/0363546508322893.
4. Agel J, Olson DE, Dick R, Arendt EA, Marshall SW, Sikka RS. Descriptive epidemiology of collegiate women's basketball injuries: National Collegiate Athletic Association Injury Surveillance System, 1988-1989 through 2003-2004. J Athl Train. 2007;42(2):202–10.
5. Dick R, Hertel J, Agel J, Grossman J, Marshall SW. Descriptive epidemiology of collegiate men's basketball injuries: National Collegiate Athletic Association Injury Surveillance System, 1988-1989 through 2003-2004. J Athl Train. 2007;42(2):194–201.

6. Deitch JR, Starkey C, Walters SL, Moseley JB. Injury risk in professional basketball players: a comparison of Women's National Basketball Association and National Basketball Association athletes. Am J Sports Med. 2006;34(7):1077–83. https://doi.org/10.1177/0363546505285383.
7. Hammig BJ, Yang H, Bensema B. Epidemiology of basketball injuries among adults presenting to ambulatory care settings in the United States. Clin J Sport Med. 2007;17(6):446–51. https://doi.org/10.1097/JSM.0b013e31815aed13.
8. Johnson KA, Teasdall RD. Sprained ankles as they relate to the basketball player. Clin Sports Med. 1993;12(2):363–71.
9. Newman JS, Newberg AH. Basketball injuries. Radiol Clin N Am. 2010;48(6):1095–111. https://doi.org/10.1016/j.rcl.2010.07.007.
10. Emerson RJ. Basketball knee injuries and the anterior cruciate ligament. Clin Sports Med. 1993;12(2):317–28.
11. Krosshaug T, Nakamae A, Boden BP, et al. Mechanisms of anterior cruciate ligament injury in basketball: video analysis of 39 cases. Am J Sports Med. 2007;35(3):359–67. https://doi.org/10.1177/0363546506293899.
12. Prodromos CC, Han Y, Rogowski J, Joyce B, Shi K. A meta-analysis of the incidence of anterior cruciate ligament tears as a function of gender, sport, and a knee injury-reduction regimen. Arthroscopy. 2007;23(12):1320–1325.e6. https://doi.org/10.1016/j.arthro.2007.07.003.
13. Renstrom P, Ljungqvist A, Arendt E, et al. Non-contact ACL injuries in female athletes: an International Olympic Committee current concepts statement. Br J Sports Med. 2008;42(6):394–412. https://doi.org/10.1136/bjsm.2008.048934.
14. Starkey C. Injuries and illnesses in the national basketball association: a 10-year perspective. J Athl Train. 2000;35(2):161–7.
15. Torg JS, Moyer J, Gaughan JP, Boden BP. Management of tarsal navicular stress fractures: conservative versus surgical treatment: a meta-analysis. Am J Sports Med. 2010;38(5):1048–53. https://doi.org/10.1177/0363546509355408.
16. Varner KE, Younas SA, Lintner DM, Marymont JV. Chronic anterior midtibial stress fractures in athletes treated with reamed intramedullary nailing. Am J Sports Med. 2005;33(7):1071–6. https://doi.org/10.1177/0363546504271968.
17. Lempainen L, Liimatainen E, Heikkilä J, et al. Medial malleolar stress fracture in athletes: diagnosis and operative treatment. Scand J Surg. 2012;101(4):261–4. https://doi.org/10.1177/145749691210100407.
18. Frankel DZ, DiFiori JP. Stress reaction of the fifth metatarsal head in a college basketball player. Curr Sports Med Rep. 2007;6(5):285–7.
19. Trojian TH, Ragle RB. Injuries in women's basketball. Conn Med. 2008;72(3):147–50.
20. McCarthy J, Mc MS. Arthroscopy of the hip: factors affecting outcome. Orthop Clin North Am. 2013;44(4):489–98. https://doi.org/10.1016/j.ocl.2013.06.002.
21. Pappas E, Zazulak BT, Yard EE, Hewett TE. The epidemiology of pediatric basketball injuries presenting to US emergency departments: 2000-2006. Sports Health. 2011;3(4):331–5. https://doi.org/10.1177/1941738111409861.
22. Harmon KG, Asif IM, Klossner D, Drezner JA. Incidence of sudden cardiac death in National Collegiate Athletic Association athletes. Circulation. 2011;123(15):1594–600. https://doi.org/10.1161/CIRCULATIONAHA.110.004622.

Combat Sports

23. Rudgley R. The lost civilizations of the stone age. 1st ed. New York: Touchstone; 2000.
24. Yard EE, Knox CL, Smith GA, et al. Pediatric martial arts injuries presenting to emergency departments, United States 1990-2003. J Sci Med Sport. 2007;10:219–26.
25. Altarriba-Bartes A, Drobnic F, Til L, et al. Epidemiology of injuries in elite taekwondo athletes: two Olympic periods cross-sectional retrospective study. BMJ Open. 2014;4:e004605.
26. American Academy of Pediatrics CoSM, Fitness, Canadian Paediatric Society HAL, et al. Policy statement-boxing participation by children and adolescents. Pediatrics. 2011;128:617–23.
27. Purcell LK, Leblanc CM, Canadian Paediatric Society HAL, et al. Boxing participation by children and adolescents: a joint statement with the American Academy of Pediatrics. Paediatr Child Health. 2012;17:39–40.
28. Kochhar T, Back DL, Mann B, et al. Risk of cervical injuries in mixed martial arts. Br J Sports Med. 2005;39:444–7.
29. Association SFI. Mixed Martial Arts (Competition) Participation Report 2017], 2017. https://www.sfia.org/reports/553_Mixed-Martial-Arts-%28Competition%29-Participation-Report-2017. Accessed on 2018.
30. Bledsoe GH, Li G, Levy F. Injury risk in professional boxing. South Med J. 2005;98:994–8.
31. Zazryn TR, McCrory PR, Cameron PA. Injury rates and risk factors in competitive professional boxing. Clin J Sport Med. 2009;19:20–5.
32. Bledsoe GH, Hsu EB, Grabowski JG, et al. Incidence of injury in professional mixed martial arts competitions. J Sports Sci Med. 2006;5:136–42.
33. Soligard T, Steffen K, Palmer D, et al. Sports injury and illness incidence in the Rio de Janeiro 2016 Olympic summer games: a prospective study of 11274 athletes from 207 countries. Br J Sports Med. 2017;51:1265–71.
34. Junge A, Engebretsen L, Mountjoy ML, et al. Sports injuries during the summer Olympic games 2008. Am J Sports Med. 2009;37:2165–72.

35. Bromley SJ, Drew MK, Talpey S, et al. A systematic review of prospective epidemiological research into injury and illness in Olympic combat sport. Br J Sports Med. 2018;52:8–16.
36. Park KJ, Song BB. Injuries in female and male elite taekwondo athletes: a 10-year prospective, epidemiological study of 1466 injuries sustained during 250 000 training hours. Br J Sports Med. 2018;52:735–40.
37. Demorest RA, Koutures C, Council On Sports M, et al. Youth participation and injury risk in martial arts. Pediatrics. 2016;138:e20163022.
38. Zazryn TR, Finch CF, McCrory P. A 16 year study of injuries to professional kickboxers in the state of Victoria, Australia. Br J Sports Med. 2003;37:448–51.
39. Karpman S, Reid P, Phillips L, et al. Combative sports injuries: an Edmonton retrospective. Clin J Sport Med. 2016;26:332–4.
40. Scoggin JF 3rd, Brusovanik G, Izuka BH, et al. Assessment of injuries during Brazilian Jiu-Jitsu competition. Orthop J Sports Med. 2014;2:2325967114522184.
41. Davis P, Waldock R, Connorton A, et al. Comparison of amateur boxing before and after the 2013 rules change and the impact on boxers' safety. Br J Sports Med. 2018;52:741–6.
42. Noh JW, Park BS, Kim MY, et al. Analysis of combat sports players' injuries according to playing style for sports physiotherapy research. J Phys Ther Sci. 2015;27:2425–30.
43. Pocecco E, Ruedl G, Stankovic N, et al. Injuries in judo: a systematic literature review including suggestions for prevention. Br J Sports Med. 2013;47:1139–43.
44. Cierna D, Lystad RP. Epidemiology of competition injuries in youth karate athletes: a prospective cohort study. Br J Sports Med. 2017;51:1285–8.
45. Rainey CE. Determining the prevalence and assessing the severity of injuries in mixed martial arts athletes. N Am J Sports Phys Ther. 2009;4:190–9.
46. Gartland S, Malik MH, Lovell ME. Injury and injury rates in Muay Thai kick boxing. Br J Sports Med. 2001;35:308–13.
47. Lystad RP, Gregory K, Wilson J. The epidemiology of injuries in mixed martial arts: a systematic review and meta-analysis. Orthop J Sports Med. 2014;2:2325967113518492.
48. Siewe J, Rudat J, Zarghooni K, et al. Injuries in competitive boxing. A prospective study. Int J Sports Med. 2015;36:249–53.
49. Loosemore M, Lightfoot J, Palmer-Green D, et al. Boxing injury epidemiology in the Great Britain team: a 5-year surveillance study of medically diagnosed injury incidence and outcome. Br J Sports Med. 2015;49:1100–7.
50. Cierna D, Barrientos M, Agrasar C, et al. Epidemiology of injuries in juniors participating in top-level karate competition: a prospective cohort study. Br J Sports Med. 2018;52:730–4.
51. Slimani M, Chaabene H, Miarka B, et al. Kickboxing review: anthropometric, psychophysiological and activity profiles and injury epidemiology. Biol Sport. 2017;34:185–96.
52. Porter M, O'Brien M. Incidence and severity of injuries resulting from amateur boxing in Ireland. Clin J Sport Med. 1996;6:97–101.
53. Pappas E. Boxing, wrestling, and martial arts related injuries treated in emergency departments in the United States, 2002-2005. J Sports Sci Med. 2007;6:58–61.
54. Zazryn T, Cameron P, McCrory P. A prospective cohort study of injury in amateur and professional boxing. Br J Sports Med. 2006;40:670–4.
55. Buse GJ, Wood RM. Safety profile of amateur kickboxing among military and civilian competitors. Mil Med. 2006;171:443–7.
56. Drury BT, Lehman TP, Rayan G. Hand and wrist injuries in boxing and the martial arts. Hand Clin. 2017;33:97–106.
57. Loosemore M, Lightfoot J, Gatt I, et al. Hand and wrist injuries in elite boxing: a longitudinal prospective study (2005-2012) of the Great Britain Olympic boxing squad. Hand (N Y). 2017;12:181–7.
58. Valkering KP, van der Hoeven H, Pijnenburg BC. Posterolateral elbow impingement in professional boxers. Am J Sports Med. 2008;36:328–32.
59. Robinson PM, Loosemore M, Watts AC. Boxer's elbow: internal impingement of the coronoid and olecranon process. A report of seven cases. J Shoulder Elb Surg. 2017;26:376–81.
60. Baird LC, Newman CB, Volk H, et al. Mortality resulting from head injury in professional boxing: case report. Neurosurgery. 2010;67:E519–20.
61. Teramoto M, Cross CL, Cushman DM, et al. Boxing fatalities in relation to rule changes in Japan: secondary data analysis. Phys Sportsmed. 2018:1–6.

Diving

62. Rubin BD. The basics of competitive diving and its injuries. Clin Sports Med. 1999;18(2):293–303.
63. Jones NS. Competitive diving principles and injuries. Curr Sports Med Rep. 2017;16(5):351–6.
64. Haase SC. Management of upper extremity injury in divers. Hand Clin. 2017;33:73–80.
65. Badman BL, Rechtine GR. Spinal injury considerations in the competitive diver: a case report and review of the literature. Spine J. 2004;4:584–90.
66. Day C, Stolz U, Mehan TJ, Smith GA, McKenzie LB. Diving-related injuries in children<20 years old treated in emergency departments in the United States: 1990–2006. Pediatrics. 2008;122(2):e388–94.
67. Kerr ZY, Baugh C, Hibberd E, et al. Epidemiology of National Collegiate Athletic Association men's and women's swimming and diving injuries from 2009/2010 to 2013/2014. Br J Sports Med. 2015; 49:465Y71.

68. Chan JS, Wee JC, Ponampalam R, Wong E. Pulmonary contusion and traumatic pneumatoceles in a platform diver with hemoptysis. J Emerg Med. 2017;52(2):205–7.

Fencing

69. Roi GS, Bianchedi D. The science of fencing. Sports Med. 2008 Jun 1;38(6):465–81.
70. Harmer PA. Incidence and characteristics of time-loss injuries in competitive fencing: a prospective, 5-year study of national competitions. Clin J Sport Med. 2008;18(2):137–42.
71. Roi GS, Fasci A. Indagine sulle richieste di intervento del medico durante le gare di scherma. Ital J Sport Traumatol. 1988;10:55–62.
72. Naghavi H. A study of traumatic events in junior fencing competitions. Med Sci Sports Exerc. 2002;34(5):56.
73. Harmer PA. Minimal risk of time-loss injury in masters fencing: USA National and World Championships Data 2002–2006. Med Sci Sports Exerc. 2007;39(Supplement):S412.

Gymnastics

74. Weiker GG. Introduction and history of gymnastics. Clin Sports Med. 1985;4(1):3–5.
75. USA Gymnastics. USAG Membership Statistics. https://usagym.org/pages/index.html. Accessed 1 Mar 2007.
76. Marshall SW, Covassin T, Dick R, Nassar LG, Agel J. Descriptive epidemiology of collegiate women's gymnastics injuries: National Collegiate Athletic Association Injury Surveillance System, 1988-1989 through 2003-2004. J Athl Train. 2007;42(2):234–40.
77. Westermann RW, Giblin M, Vaske A, Grosso K, Wolf BR. Evaluation of Men's and Women's Gymnastics injuries: a 10-year observational study. Sports Health. 2015;7(2):161–5. https://doi.org/10.1177/1941738114559705.
78. Saluan P, Styron J, Ackley JF, Prinzbach A, Billow D. Injury types and incidence rates in Precollegiate female gymnasts: a 21-year experience at a single training facility. Orthop J Sports Med. 2015;3(4):2325967115577596. https://doi.org/10.1177/2325967115577596.
79. Singh S, Smith GA, Fields SK, McKenzie LB. Gymnastics-related injuries to children treated in emergency departments in the United States, 1990-2005. Pediatrics. 2008;121(4):e954–60. https://doi.org/10.1542/peds.2007-0767.
80. Kolt GS, Kirkby RJ. Epidemiology of injury in elite and subelite female gymnasts: a comparison of retrospective and prospective findings. Br J Sports Med. 1999;33(5):312–8.
81. Cupisti A, D'Alessandro C, Evangelisti I, et al. Injury survey in competitive sub-elite rhythmic gymnasts: results from a prospective controlled study. J Sports Med Phys Fitness. 2007;47(2):203–7.
82. Edouard P, Steffen K, Junge A, Leglise M, Soligard T, Engebretsen L. Gymnastics injury incidence during the 2008, 2012 and 2016 Olympic games: analysis of prospectively collected surveillance data from 963 registered gymnasts during Olympic games. Br J Sports Med. 2018;52(7):475–81. https://doi.org/10.1136/bjsports-2017-097972.
83. Kerr ZY, Hayden R, Barr M, Klossner DA, Dompier TP. Epidemiology of National Collegiate Athletic Association Women's Gymnastics injuries, 2009-2010 through 2013-2014. J Athl Train. 2015;50(8):870–8. https://doi.org/10.4085/1062-6050-50.7.02.
84. Caine DJ, Nassar L. Gymnastics injuries. Med Sport Sci. 2005;48:18–58. https://doi.org/10.1159/000084282.
85. DiFiori JP, Caine DJ, Malina RM. Wrist pain, distal radial physeal injury, and ulnar variance in the young gymnast. Am J Sports Med. 2006;34(5):840–9. https://doi.org/10.1177/0363546505284848.
86. Malina RM, Baxter-Jones ADG, Armstrong N, et al. Role of intensive training in the growth and maturation of artistic gymnasts. Sports Med Auckl NZ. 2013;43(9):783–802. https://doi.org/10.1007/s40279-013-0058-5.
87. PubMed Entry. http://www.ncbi.nlm.nih.gov/pubmed/26665051. Accessed 10 Aug 2018.
88. Schmitt H, Gerner HJ. Paralysis from sport and diving accidents. Clin J Sport Med. 2001;11(1):17–22.
89. Burt L, Naughton G, HIgbam D, Landeo R. Training load in pre-pubertal female artistic gymnastics. Sci Gymn J. 2010;2:5–14.
90. Fallon KE, Fricker PA. Stress fracture of the clavicle in a young female gymnast. Br J Sports Med. 2001;35(6):448–9.
91. Caine D. Injury and growth. In: Sands WA, Caine DJ, Borms J, editors. Scientific aspects of women's gymnastics, vol. 45. Basel: Karger; 2003. p. 46–71.
92. Kirialanis P, Malliou P, Beneka A, Giannakopoulos K. Occurance of acute lower limb injuries in artistic gymnast in relation to event and exercise phase. Br J Sports Med. 2003;37(2):121–6.
93. Caine D, Roy S, Singer KM, Broekhoff K. Stress changes in distal radial groth plate. A radiographic survey and review of the related literature. Am J Sports Med. 1992;20(3):290–8.
94. Difiori JP, Puffer JC, Mandelbaum BR, Mar S. Factors associated with wrist pain in the young gymnast. Am J Sports Med. 1996;24(1):9–14.

Racquet and Wall Sports

95. Silko GJ, Cullen PT. Indoor racquet sports injuries. Am Fam Physician. 1994;50(2):374–80.

96. Chard MD, Lachmann SM. Racquet sports—patterns of injury presenting to a sports injury clinic. Br J Sports Med. 1987;21(4):150–3.
97. Jones NP. One year of severe eye injuries in sport. Eye. 1988;2(5):484.

Swimming

98. Mountjoy M, Junge A, Alonso JM, et al. Consensus statement on the methodology of injury and illness surveillance in FINA (aquatic sports). Br J Sports Med. 2016;50(10):590–6. https://doi.org/10.1136/bjsports-2015-095686.
99. Rio 2016: Daily viewership figures | statistic. Statista. https://www.statista.com/statistics/589506/olympics-daily-viewership/. Accessed 14 Aug 2018.
100. Kerr ZY, Baugh CM, Hibberd EE, Snook EM, Hayden R, Dompier TP. Epidemiology of National Collegiate Athletic Association men's and women's swimming and diving injuries from 2009/2010 to 2013/2014. Br J Sports Med. 2015;49(7):465–71. https://doi.org/10.1136/bjsports-2014-094423.
101. Wolf BR, Ebinger AE, Lawler MP, Britton CL. Injury patterns in division I collegiate swimming. Am J Sports Med. 2009;37(10):2037–42. https://doi.org/10.1177/0363546509339364.
102. Mountjoy M, Junge A, Benjamen S, et al. Competing with injuries: injuries prior to and during the 15th FINA world championships 2013 (aquatics). Br J Sports Med. 2015;49(1):37–43. https://doi.org/10.1136/bjsports-2014-093991.
103. Nichols AW. Medical Care of the Aquatics Athlete. Curr Sports Med Rep. 2015;14(5):389–96. https://doi.org/10.1249/JSR.0000000000000194.
104. Burkhart SS, Morgan CD, Kibler WB. The disabled throwing shoulder: spectrum of pathology part I: pathoanatomy and biomechanics. Arthroscopy. 2003;19(4):404–20. https://doi.org/10.1053/jars.2003.50128.
105. Rupp S, Berninger K, Hopf T. Shoulder problems in high level swimmers--impingement, anterior instability, muscular imbalance? Int J Sports Med. 1995;16(8):557–62. https://doi.org/10.1055/s-2007-973054.
106. Bak K. The practical management of swimmer's painful shoulder: etiology, diagnosis, and treatment. Clin J Sport Med. 2010;20(5):386–90. https://doi.org/10.1097/JSM.0b013e3181f205fa.
107. Myers JB, Laudner KG, Pasquale MR, Bradley JP, Lephart SM. Scapular position and orientation in throwing athletes. Am J Sports Med. 2005;33(2):263–71. https://doi.org/10.1177/0363546504268138.
108. Scovazzo ML, Browne A, Pink M, Jobe FW, Kerrigan J. The painful shoulder during freestyle swimming. An electromyographic cinematographic analysis of twelve muscles. Am J Sports Med. 1991;19(6):577–82. https://doi.org/10.1177/036354659101900604.
109. Vizsolyi P, Taunton J, Robertson G, et al. Breaststroker's knee. An analysis of epidemiological and biomechanical factors. Am J Sports Med. 1987;15(1):63–71. https://doi.org/10.1177/036354658701500109.
110. Kennedy JC, Hawkins R, Krissoff WB. Orthopaedic manifestations of swimming. Am J Sports Med. 1978;6(6):309–22. https://doi.org/10.1177/036354657800600602.
111. Richardson AB. Orthopedic aspects of competitive swimming. Clin Sports Med. 1987;6(3):639–45.
112. Nyska M, Constantini N, Calé-Benzoor M, Back Z, Kahn G, Mann G. Spondylolysis as a cause of low back pain in swimmers. Int J Sports Med. 2000;21(5):375–9. https://doi.org/10.1055/s-2000-3780.
113. Pink MM, Tibone JE. The painful shoulder in the swimming athlete. Orthop Clin North Am. 2000;31(2):247–61.
114. Kibler WB, Ludewig PM, McClure PW, Michener LA, Bak K, Sciascia AD. Clinical implications of scapular dyskinesis in shoulder injury: the 2013 consensus statement from the "Scapular Summit." Br J Sports Med 2013;47(14):877–885. doi:https://doi.org/10.1136/bjsports-2013-092425.
115. Rovere GD, Nichols AW. Frequency, associated factors, and treatment of breaststroker's knee in competitive swimmers. Am J Sports Med. 1985;13(2):99–104. https://doi.org/10.1177/036354658501300204.
116. Grote K, Lincoln TL, Gamble JG. Hip adductor injury in competitive swimmers. Am J Sports Med. 2004;32(1):104–8. https://doi.org/10.1177/0363546503258905.
117. Capaci K, Ozcaldiran B, Durmaz B. Musculoskeletal pain in elite competitive male swimmers. The Pain Clinic. 2002;14(3):229–34. https://doi.org/10.1163/156856902320761432.
118. Hangai M, Kaneoka K, Hinotsu S, et al. Lumbar intervertebral disk degeneration in athletes. Am J Sports Med. 2009;37(1):149–55. https://doi.org/10.1177/0363546508323252.

Tennis

119. Fu MC, Ellenbecker TS, Renstrom PA, Windler GS, Dines DM. Epidemiology of injury in tennis players. Curr Rev Musculoskelet Med. 2018;11:1–5.
120. Dakic JG, Smith B, Gosling CM, Perraton LG. Musculoskeletal injury profiles in professional Women's tennis association players. Br J Sports Med. 2018;52:723–9.
121. Dines JS, Bedi A, Williams PN, Dodson CC, Ellenbecker TS, Altchek DW, et al. Tennis injuries: epidemiology, pathophysiology, and treatment. J Am Acad Orthop Surg. 2015;23(3):181–9.

122. Pluim BM, Staal JB, Windler GE, Jayanthi N. Tennis injuries: occurrence, aetiology, and prevention. Br J Sports Med. 2006;40(5):415–23.
123. Gescheit DT, Cormack SJ, Duffield R, Kovalchik S, Wood TO, Omizzolo M, Reid M. A multi-year injury epidemiology analysis of an elite national junior tennis program. J Sci Med Sport. 2018;22:11. https://doi.org/10.1016/j.jsams.2018.06.006.
124. Lynall RC, Kerr ZY, Djoko A, Pluim BM, Hainline B, Dompier TP. Epidemiology of National Collegiate Athletic Association men's and women's tennis injuries, 2009/2010–2014/2015. Br J Sports Med. 2016;50(19):1211–6.
125. Colberg R, Aune K, Choi A, Fleisig G. Incidence and prevalence of musculoskeletal conditions in collegiate tennis athletes. J Med Sci Tennis. 2015;20(3):137–44.
126. Sell K, Hainline B, Yorio M, Kovacs M. Injury trend analysis from the US open tennis championships between 1994 and 2009. Br J Sports Med. 2014;48(7):546–51.
127. Schmikli SL, Backx FJG, Kemler HJ, van Mechelen M. National Survey on sports injuries in the Netherlands: target populations for sports injury prevention programs. Clin J Sports Med. 2009;19(2):101–6.
128. Chung KC, Lark ME. Upper extremity injuries in tennis players: diagnosis, treatment, and management. Hand Clin. 2017;33(1):175–86.
129. Nutt C, Mirkovic M, Hill R, Ranson C, Cooper SM. Reference values for glenohumeral joint rotational range of motion in elite tennis players. International Journal of Sport Physical Therapy. 2018;13(3):501–10.
130. Edmonds EW, Dengerink DD. Common conditions in the overhead athlete. Am Fam Physician. 2014;89(7):537–41.
131. Eygendaal D, Rahussen FTG, Diercks RL. Biomechanics of the elbow joint in tennis players and relation to pathology. Br J Sports Med. 2007;41:820–3.
132. Harwin JR, Richardson ML. "Tennis leg;" a gastrocnemius injury is far more common than plantaris rupture. Radiology Case Reports. 2017;12:120–3.
133. Delgado GJ, Chung CB, Lektrakul N, et al. Tennis leg: clinical US study of 141 patient and anatomic investigation of four cadavers with MR imaging and US. Radiology. 2002;224:112e9.
134. Pluim BM, Loeffen FG, Clarsen B, Bahr R, Verhagen EA. A one- season prospective study of injuries and illness in elite junior tennis. Scand J Med Sci Sports. 2016;26(5):564–71.

Vollleyball

135. Briner WW, Kacmar L. Common injuries in volleyball. Mechanisms of injury, prevention and rehabilitation. Sports Med Auckl NZ. 1997;24(1):65–71.
136. Boys' and Mens' Volleyball Participation Continues to Lag - Athletic Business. https://www.athleticbusiness.com/College/boys-and-mens-volleyball-participation-continues-to-lag.html. Accessed 12 Aug 2018.
137. Pastor MF, Ezechieli M, Classen L, Kieffer O, Miltner O. Prospective study of injury in volleyball players: 6 year results. Technol Health Care. 2015;23(5):637–43. https://doi.org/10.3233/THC-151009.
138. Agel J, Palmieri-Smith RM, Dick R, Wojtys EM, Marshall SW. Descriptive epidemiology of collegiate women's volleyball injuries: National Collegiate Athletic Association Injury Surveillance System, 1988-1989 through 2003-2004. J Athl Train. 2007;42(2):295–302.
139. Agel J, Rockwood T, Klossner D. Collegiate ACL injury rates across 15 sports: National Collegiate Athletic Association Injury Surveillance System Data Update (2004-2005 through 2012-2013). Clin J Sport Med. 2016;26(6):518–23. https://doi.org/10.1097/JSM.0000000000000290.
140. Verhagen EALM, Van der Beek AJ, Bouter LM, Bahr RM, Van Mechelen W. A one season prospective cohort study of volleyball injuries. Br J Sports Med 2004;38(4):477–481. doi:https://doi.org/10.1136/bjsm.2003.005785.
141. Joseph AM, Collins CL, Henke NM, Yard EE, Fields SK, Comstock RD. A multisport epidemiologic comparison of anterior cruciate ligament injuries in high school athletics. J Athl Train. 2013;48(6):810–7. https://doi.org/10.4085/1062-6050-48.6.03.
142. Lian O, Engebretsen L, Ovrebø RV, Bahr R. Characteristics of the leg extensors in male volleyball players with jumper's knee. Am J Sports Med. 1996;24(3):380–5. https://doi.org/10.1177/036354659602400322.
143. Ferretti A, Papandrea P, Conteduca F, Mariani PP. Knee ligament injuries in volleyball players. Am J Sports Med. 1992;20(2):203–7. https://doi.org/10.1177/036354659202000219.
144. Seminati E, Minetti AE. Overuse in volleyball training/practice: a review on shoulder and spine-related injuries. Eur J Sport Sci. 2013;13(6):732–43. https://doi.org/10.1080/17461391.2013.773090.
145. Bahr R, Karlsen R, Lian O, Ovrebø RV. Incidence and mechanisms of acute ankle inversion injuries in volleyball. A retrospective cohort study. Am J Sports Med. 1994;22(5):595–600. https://doi.org/10.1177/036354659402200505.
146. Bahr R, Reeser JC. Fédération Internationale de Volleyball. Injuries among world-class professional beach volleyball players. The Fédération Internationale de Volleyball beach volleyball injury study. Am J Sports Med. 2003;31(1):119–25. https://doi.org/10.1177/03635465030310010401.
147. Zahradnik D, Jandacka D, Uchytil J, Farana R, Hamill J. Lower extremity mechanics during landing after a volleyball block as a risk factor for anterior cruciate

ligament injury. Phys Ther Sport. 2015;16(1):53–8. https://doi.org/10.1016/j.ptsp.2014.04.003.
148. Kugler A, Krüger-Franke M, Reininger S, Trouillier HH, Rosemeyer B. Muscular imbalance and shoulder pain in volleyball attackers. Br J Sports Med. 1996;30(3):256–9.
149. Reeser JC. Strategies for the prevention of volleyball related injuries * Commentary 1 * Commentary 2. Br J Sports Med. 2006;40(7):594–600. https://doi.org/10.1136/bjsm.2005.018234.
150. Pedowitz DI, Reddy S, Parekh SG, Huffman GR, Sennett BJ. Prophylactic bracing decreases ankle injuries in collegiate female volleyball players. Am J Sports Med. 2008;36(2):324–7. https://doi.org/10.1177/0363546507308358.
151. Stasinopoulos D. Comparison of three preventive methods in order to reduce the incidence of ankle inversion sprains among female volleyball players. Br J Sports Med. 2004;38(2):182–5.
152. Bahr R, Lian O, Bahr IA. A twofold reduction in the incidence of acute ankle sprains in volleyball after the introduction of an injury prevention program: a prospective cohort study. Scand J Med Sci Sports. 1997;7(3):172–7.
153. Holme E, Magnusson SP, Becher K, Bieler T, Aagaard P, Kjaer M. The effect of supervised rehabilitation on strength, postural sway, position sense and re-injury risk after acute ankle ligament sprain. Scand J Med Sci Sports. 1999;9(2): 104–9.
154. Maffulli N, Ferran NA. Management of acute and chronic ankle instability. J Am Acad Orthop Surg. 2008;16(10):608–15.

Water Polo

155. Spittler J, et al. Water polo injuries and training methods. Curr Sports Med Rep. 2016;15(6):410–6.
156. Stromberg JD. Care of water polo players. Curr Sports Med Rep. 2017;16(5):363–9.
157. Prien A, et al. Injury and illness in aquatic sport: how high is the risk? A comparison of results from three FINA World Championships. Br J Sports Med. 2017;51(4):277–82.
158. Miller AH, et al. Shoulder injury in water polo: A systematic review of incidence and intrinsic risk factors. J Sci Med Sport. 2018;21(4):368–77.
159. Herberger S, et al. Dental injuries in water polo, a survey of players in Switzerland. Dent Traumatol. 2012;28(4):287–90.
160. Brooks JM. Injuries in water polo. Clin Sports Med. 1999 Apr;18(2):313–9.
161. Colville JM, Markman BS. Competitive water polo: upper extremity injuries. Clin Sports Med. 1999;18(2):305–12.
162. Dugas J, et al. Ulnar collateral ligament in the overhead athlete: a current review. Sports Med Arthrosc Rev. 2014;22(3):169–82.
163. Wheeler K, et al. The volume of goal shootig during training can predict shoulder soreness in elite female water polo players. J Sci Med Sport. 2013 May;16(3):255–8.
164. Wilson SA. And a. last. Management of corneal abrasions. Am Fam Physician. 2004;70(1):123–8.
165. Franic M, et al. Injuries in water polo. Croat Med J. 2007;48(3):281–8.

Weight Lifting

166. Keogh JW, Winwood PW. The epidemiology of injuries across the weight-training sports. Sports Med. 2017 Mar;47(3):479–501.
167. Chlewicki J, et al. Lumbar spine loads during the lifting of extremely heavy weights. Med Sci Sports Exerc. 1991;23(10):1179–86.
168. Mazur LJ, et al. Weight-training injuries. Common injuries and preventative methods. Sports Med. 1993 Jul;16(1):57–63.
169. Aasa U, et al. Injuries among weightlifters and powerlifters: a systematic review. Br J Sports Med. 2017;51(4):211–9.
170. Lavallee ME, Balam T. An overview of strength training injuries: acute and chronic. Curr Sports Med Rep. 2010;9(5):307–13.
171. Keogh J, et al. Retrospective injury epidemiology of one hundred one competitive Oceania power lifters: the effects of age, body mass, competitive standard, and gender. J Strength Cond Res. 2006;20(3):672–81.
172. Myer GD, et al. Youth versus adult "weightlifting" injuries presenting to United States emergency rooms: accidental versus nonaccidental injury mechanisms. J Strength Cond Res. 2009;23(7): 2054–60.
173. Kulund, et al. Olympic weight-lifting injuries. Phys Sportsmed 1978; 6(11):111–119.

Wrestling

174. Associates FW-FIdL. Roots and History of Olympic Wrestling], 2009. http://www.fila-official.com/index.php?option=com_content&view=article&id=12&Itemid=100152&lang=en.
175. Myers RJ, Linakis SW, Mello MJ, et al. Competitive wrestling-related injuries in school aged athletes in U.S. emergency departments. West J Emerg Med. 2010;11:442–9.
176. Yard EE, Comstock RD. A comparison of pediatric freestyle and Greco-Roman wrestling injuries sustained during a 2006 US national tournament. Scand J Med Sci Sports. 2008;18:491–7.
177. Agarwal S, Mann E. Knee injuries in wrestlers: a prospective study from the Indian subcontinent. Asian J Sports Med. 2016;7:e35000.

178. Baker BE, Peckham AC, Pupparo F, et al. Review of meniscal injury and associated sports. Am J Sports Med. 1985;13:1–4.
179. Powell JW, Barber-Foss KD. Injury patterns in selected high school sports: a review of the 1995-1997 seasons. J Athl Train. 1999;34:277–84.
180. Pasque CB, Hewett TE. A prospective study of high school wrestling injuries. Am J Sports Med. 2000;28:509–15.
181. Jarret GJ, Orwin JF, Dick RW. Injuries in collegiate wrestling. Am J Sports Med. 1998;26:674–80.
182. Kay MC, Register-Mihalik JK, Gray AD, et al. The epidemiology of severe injuries sustained by National Collegiate Athletic Association Student-Athletes, 2009-2010 through 2014-2015. J Athl Train. 2017;52:117–28.
183. Shadgan B, Feldman BJ, Jafari S. Wrestling injuries during the 2008 Beijing Olympic games. Am J Sports Med. 2010;38:1870–6.
184. Mysnyk MC, Wroble RR, Foster DT, et al. Prepatellar bursitis in wrestlers. Am J Sports Med. 1986;14:46–54.
185. Boden BP, Lin W, Young M, et al. Catastrophic injuries in wrestlers. Am J Sports Med. 2002;30:791–5.
186. Dizdarevic I, Low S, Currie DW, et al. Epidemiology of elbow dislocations in high school athletes. Am J Sports Med. 2016;44:202–8.
187. Akbarnejad A, Sayyah M. Frequency of sports trauma in elite national level greco-roman wrestling competitions. Arch Trauma Res. 2012;1:51–3.
188. Hewett TE, Pasque C, Heyl R, et al. Wrestling injuries. Med Sport Sci. 2005;48:152–78.
189. Snook GA. Injuries in intercollegiate wrestling. A 5-year study. Am J Sports Med. 1982;10:142–4.
190. Strauss RH, Lanese RR. Injuries among wrestlers in school and college tournaments. JAMA. 1982;248:2016–9.
191. Kordi R, Heidarpour B, Shafiei M, et al. Incidence, nature, and causes of fractures and dislocations in olympic styles of wrestling in Iran: a 1-year prospective study. Sports Health. 2012;4:217–21.
192. Herzog MM, Fraser MA, Register-Mihalik JK, et al. Epidemiology of skin infections in men's wrestling: analysis of 2009-2010 through 2013-2014 National Collegiate Athletic Association Surveillance Data. J Athl Train. 2017;52:457–63.
193. Lorish TR, Rizzo TD Jr, Ilstrup DM, et al. Injuries in adolescent and preadolescent boys at two large wrestling tournaments. Am J Sports Med. 1992;20:199–202.
194. Kroshus E, Kerr ZY, DeFreese JD, et al. Concussion knowledge and communication behaviors of collegiate wrestling coaches. Health Commun. 2017;32:963–9.
195. Lok V, Yuceturk G. Injuries of wrestling. J Sports Med. 1974;2:324–8.
196. Snook GA. A survey of wrestling injuries. Am J Sports Med. 1980;8:450–3.
197. Kerr ZY, Collins CL, Pommering TL, et al. Dislocation/separation injuries among US high school athletes in 9 selected sports: 2005-2009. Clin J Sport Med. 2011;21:101–8.
198. Banas MP, Lewis RA. Nonunion of an olecranon epiphyseal plate stress fracture in an adolescent. Orthopedics. 1995;18:1111–2.
199. Weiss CB Jr, Sauers RJ. Avulsion fracture of the olecranon process. Phys Sportsmed. 1990;18:110–6.
200. Pavlik A, Csepai D, Berkes I. Surgical treatment of pectoralis major rupture in athletes. Knee Surg Sports Traumatol Arthrosc. 1998;6:129–33.
201. Berry H, Kong K, Hudson AR, et al. Isolated suprascapular nerve palsy: a review of nine cases. Can J Neurol Sci. 1995;22:301–4.
202. Brindle TJ, Coen M. Scapular avulsion fracture of a high school wrestler. J Orthop Sports Phys Ther. 1998;27:444–7.
203. Swischuk LE. Pain and decreased movement of left arm. Pediatr Emerg Care. 1991;7:169–70.
204. Estwanik JJ 3rd, Bergfeld JA, Collins HR, et al. Injuries in interscholastic wrestling. Phys Sportsmed. 1980;8:111–21.
205. Rossi F, Dragoni S. Lumbar spondylolysis: occurrence in competitive athletes. Updated achievements in a series of 390 cases. J Sports Med Phys Fitness. 1990;30:450–2.
206. Wroble RR, Mysnyk MC, Foster DT, et al. Patterns of knee injuries in wrestling: a six year study. Am J Sports Med. 1986;14:55–66.
207. Chorney SR, Sobin L, Goyal P, et al. Maxillofacial injuries among National Collegiate Athletic Association athletes: 2004-2014. Laryngoscope. 2017;127:1296–301.
208. Narayana Kurup JK, Jampani R, Mohanty SP. Catastrophic cervical spinal injury in an amateur college wrestler. BMJ Case Rep. 2017;2017
209. Meron A, McMullen C, Laker SR, et al. Epidemiology of cervical spine injuries in high school athletes over a ten-year period. PM R. 2018;10:365–72.
210. Bailes JE, Maroon JC. Management of cervical spine injuries in athletes. Clin Sports Med. 1989;8: 43–58.
211. Schaefer WW, Voight SJ. Rupture of the brachial artery from closed posterior dislocation of the elbow in a wrestler. Orthopedics. 1993;16:820–2.
212. Thomas PJ, Noellert RC. Brachial artery disruption after closed posterior dislocation of the elbow. Am J Orthop (Belle Mead NJ). 1995;24:558–60.

Indoor Surfaces

213. Rundell KW. High levels of airborne ultrafine and fine particulate matter in indoor ice arenas. Inhal Toxicol. 2003;15(3):237–50. https://doi.org/10.1080/08958370304502.

40 Outdoor Sports: Winter

R. Kyle Martin, Mitchell I. Kennedy, J. P. Begly, Rob LaPrade, and Lars Engebretsen

40.1 Introduction

Outdoor winter sports present unique challenges for the sports medicine physician. Not only are athletes pushed to their physical limits in sports that often involve high speeds, but the additional influence of environmental factors can increase their injury risk and impede prompt medical care. Weather can change quickly, impacting visibility, the frictional properties of snow and ice, and jumping trajectory. Athletes that travel great distances from start to finish may experience delays in receiving on-scene medical attention in the event of an injury midway through their event. Events that take place in remote locations pose a further challenge of achieving timely evacuation to hospital in emergency situations, especially in poor weather conditions. Medical staff and event organizers must be aware of all these factors ahead of time in order to optimize athlete safety.

Comprehensive injury surveillance systems have been implemented across various sporting events. The goals are to identify factors associated with increased injury risk and subsequently to mitigate injuries through preventative measures. The introduction of these surveillance systems to the Olympic Games and the International Ski Federation (FIS) events has vastly increased our knowledge and understanding of injuries associated with winter sports [1–5]. Sport-specific injury prevention initiatives and improved athlete safety are the next steps, and their efficacy can be monitored through ongoing surveillance. This chapter outlines the epidemiology, etiology, and treatment of common injuries associated with alpine skiing, freestyle skiing, snowboarding, ice hockey, and the sliding sports (bobsleigh, luge, and skeleton). Comprehensive knowledge in these areas is essential for team physicians of winter sports athletes.

This chapter will provide clinically useful and evidence-based information regarding medical coverage of common outdoor winter sports.

R. K. Martin · L. Engebretsen (✉)
Department of Orthopaedic Surgery, Oslo University Hospital, Oslo, Norway

Faculty of Medicine, University of Oslo, Oslo, Norway

OSTRC, The Norwegian School of Sports Sciences, Oslo, Norway
e-mail: ummart36@myumanitoba.ca; lars.engebretsen@medisin.uio.no

M. I. Kennedy · R. LaPrade
Steadman Philippon Research Institute, Vail, CO, USA

The Steadman Clinic, Vail, CO, USA
e-mail: mkennedy@sprivail.org; rlaprade@thesteadmanclinic.com

J. P. Begly
The Steadman Clinic, Vail, CO, USA
e-mail: jbegly@thesteadmanclinic.com

S. Rocha Piedade et al. (eds.), *The Sports Medicine Physician*,
https://doi.org/10.1007/978-3-030-10433-7_40

40.2 Alpine Skiing (Figs. 40.1 and 40.2)

The origins of skiing date back approximately 5000 years, and formal alpine skiing was established in 1767 in Norway [6]. Since this time, alpine skiing has evolved into the most popular winter sports in the world [7], attracting over 40 million participants across the world [8]. Despite significant advancements in equipment, technique, and safety protocols, alpine skiing continues to be a pastime associated with substantial injury risk.

40.2.1 Injury Rates

Alpine skiing carries a significant risk of injury. A recent study involving a large American ski resort reported an overall rate of persons injured between 206.7 and 233.8 per 100,000 mountain visit [9]. The incidence of injuries to the lower leg and ankle has decreased over the past several decades; however, the rate of injuries to the knee continues to rise [10, 11]. Ten percent of all snow-related accidents involve the anterior cruciate ligament (ACL), and 45–60% of knee injuries sustained while alpine skiing are ACL tears [12]. In a study of 7155 professional skiers over a 6-year period, Viola and colleagues reported an ACL tear rate of 4.2 per 100,000 skier days in men and 4.4 per 100,000 skier days in females [13]. Pujol et al. examined the rate of ACL injuries among 379 athletes on elite French National ski teams. They reported an ACL tear rate of 28.2% in males and 27.2% in females; overall, ACL tear incidence was 8.5 tears per 100 skier seasons [7]. Reinjury incidence was 19% for the ipsilateral knee, and bilateral injuries occurred in 30.5% of athletes. The level of skiing was associated with an increased risk of injury, because more tears were identified in skiers ranked in the world top 30.

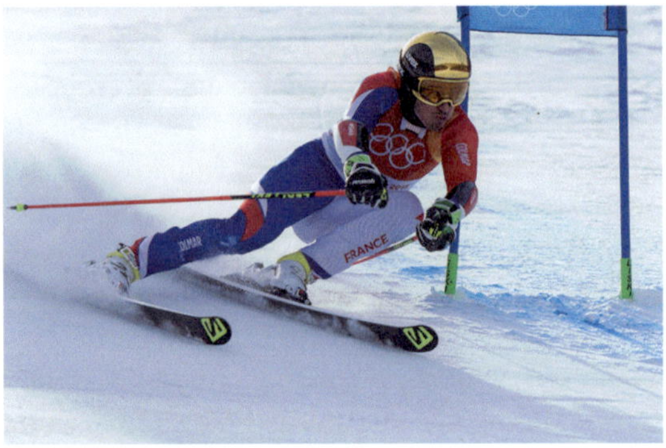

Fig. 40.1 An alpine skier maintains control through a high-speed turn

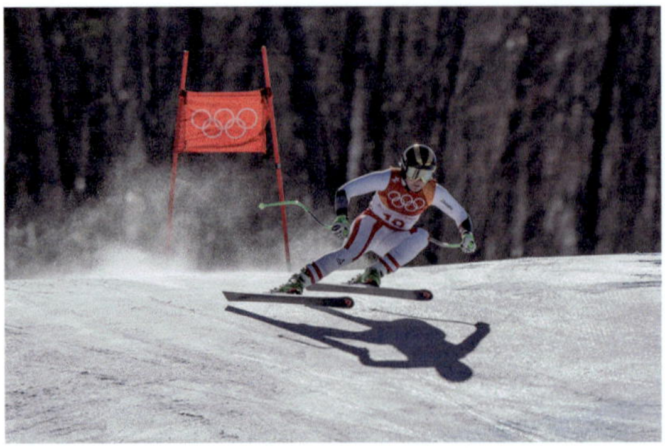

Fig. 40.2 The combination of high speeds, turns, jumps, and icy terrain places athletes at risk of injury

Bere and colleagues examined FIS ACL injury rates over a 6-year period and found no significant differences between genders [14]. The authors reported that the strongest risk factor for ligament injury was participation in speed events. While there appears to be no gender-related differences in tear rate among adult alpine skiers, Raschner et al. demonstrated that female skiers aged 14–19 are at increased risk for injury compared to their male counterparts [15]. In this age group, knee injuries were the most common type of injury among ski racers, and inadequate core strength was identified as a significant risk factor for injury in the adolescent age group.

40.2.2 Injury Mechanism

The use of video replay from event television coverage yields valuable information for the study of injury mechanisms [16]. Overall, falls account for the majority of shoulder injuries sustained during alpine skiing [6]. Possible mechanisms of upper extremity injury include falls onto an outstretched hand, direct trauma to the shoulder region, and eccentric forces as the skier attempts to resist forced abduction. Additionally, direct collisions with other skiers and/or stationary obstacles such as trees represent additional mechanism for injury. Pole planting during a fall increases external rotation forces on the shoulder and upper extremity. A planted pole essentially lengthens the lever arm of the upper extremity and increases the risk of glenohumeral instability. The use of wrist straps may additionally exacerbate the risk inherent with these mechanisms.

Ligamentous disruption may occur via several mechanisms. In elite alpine athletes skiing at high speeds, ACL tears typically occur during jumping/landing activities [11]. As the athlete lands under significant force, a boot-induced anterior drawer mechanism occurs by which the tibia is driven anterior with respect to the femur, increasing ACL strain that is not compensated by surrounding musculature. Gerritsen et al. performed video analysis of knee injuries sustained during the 1994 Lillehammer Olympic downhill event and identified high external rotation forces on the knee during landing [17]. Gilgien and colleagues compared ACL injury rates between the race disciplines of downhill, super-G, giant slalom, and slalom and reported that while forces and speed differed between the disciplines, the ACL injury risk was equal when injury rate was corrected for race times [18]. Landing, higher speeds, and crashes accounted for the majority of injuries in downhill and super-G, while turning speeds, turn radius, and high loading and torque forces were associated with injury in the technical events. Recreational skiers are more likely to sustain an ACL tear due to valgus and internal rotation forces, typical of noncontact ACL injuries. While functional bracing has not been demonstrated to improve long-term patient-reported outcomes following ACL reconstruction, bracing has been shown to reduce injury rates during skiing in both ACL-deficient and ACL-reconstructed knees [19].

40.2.3 Common Injuries

Upper extremity injuries are common among alpine skiers. The true incidence of these injuries is likely underreported. Shoulder injuries comprise 4–11% of all alpine skiing injuries and account for up to 34% of all injuries to the upper extremity [6]. Kocher and colleagues examined the incidence of specific shoulder-related ski injuries and found that rotator cuff pathology (24%), anterior glenohumeral instability (22%), acromioclavicular separations (20%), and clavicle fractures (11%) were the most common injuries [20]. Unlike snowboarding, there does not appear to be a predominant laterality component to skiing-related upper extremity injuries. The most common upper extremity injury in skiers is a sprain of the ulnar collateral ligament of the thumb at the metacarpal-phalangeal joint, appropriately known as "skier's thumb" [6].

The majority of skiing-related injuries are orthopedic in nature; however, injuries to the head and spinal cord are particularly dangerous and may be life-threatening. Ackery et al. performed a systematic review of head and spinal cord injuries in 2007 and reported an overall increasing incidence among skiers and snowboarders [21]. Head injury and traumatic brain injury are the most common causes of death among skiers, highlighting the importance of helmet compliance [5, 21]. At the World Cup level among FIS athletes, injuries to the head and face accounted for 10–13% of all injuries [5]. Eighty-two percent of these injuries were concussions, and 24% of injuries lead to an absence from sports of over 28 days. Steenstrup et al. performed a video analysis of 29 skiing-related head injuries over 10 World Cup seasons [22]. They found that alpine skiers were most likely to fall backward or sideways and impact the back or side of their helmet respectfully. A high percentage of head injuries occurred due to collisions with racing gates, and 10% of events resulted in helmet ejection.

Fact Box
Head injury is the most common cause of death and catastrophic injury associated with alpine skiing [21]. Several studies have demonstrated the importance of helmet use in reducing the rate of head injuries [23–27]. While helmet use among skiers has increased over the past several years, approximately 30% of adult skiers continue to ski without a helmet [28, 29]. Sports medicine physicians can play an important role in the prevention of these injuries through education and encouragement of proper helmet use for all ski and snowboard athletes.

40.3 Freestyle Skiing

Aerials, moguls, half-pipe, slopestyle, and ski-cross are the five disciplines of freestyle skiing. What sets them apart from other FIS events is the acrobatic element that accompanies the high speeds and big jumps (Fig. 40.3). Inherent in all of these exciting displays of athleticism is the risk of injury, which can be significant (Fig. 40.4).

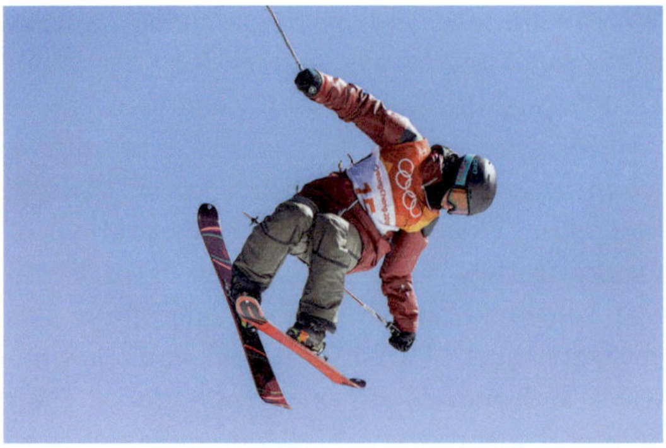

Fig. 40.3 A freestyle skier soars through the air while performing acrobatic maneuvers

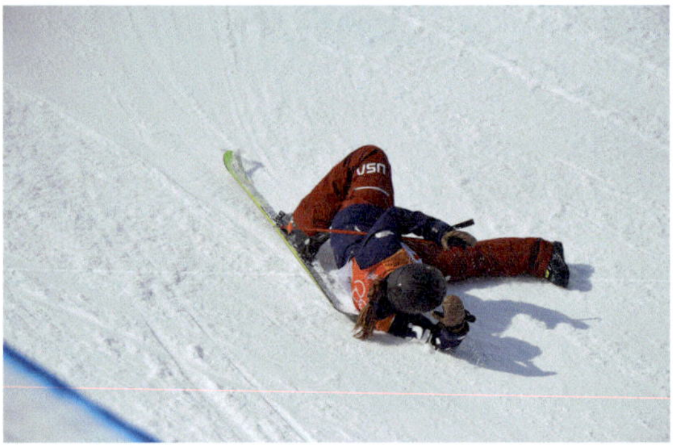

Fig. 40.4 Big jumps can mean hard landings and possible injuries

40.3.1 Injury Rates

Flørenes et al. reported injury rates for freestyle skiers competing in the World Cup over three winter seasons (aerials, moguls, half-pipe, and ski-cross). They found a high rate of injuries, and a large proportion of these were classified as severe, defined as precluding participation in training or competition for more than 28 days. Across all disciplines, the injury rate was 44.0 per 100 skiers per season. When only injuries that resulted in 1 or more days absence from skiing were considered, the incidence was 31.9 per 100 skiers per season. Severe injuries accounted for 44% of all time-loss injuries. Moguls had a lower rate of total injuries than the other disciplines, but no difference was seen in the rate of severe injuries. No differences in injury rates were seen between men's and women's competitions [30]. Injury surveillance studies from the 2010 and 2014 Winter Olympics also demonstrated high overall and severe injury rates among freestyle skiers [1, 2].

40.3.2 Injury Mechanism

The majority of injuries result from skier contact with the ground, often when landing from a jump. The most common reasons skiers experience uncontrolled flight and an unbalanced landing are technical error at takeoff or contact with another athlete in the case of ski-cross [1, 2, 31]. Overrotation in the air causing a slapback episode upon landing has been proposed as a typical mechanism of head injury in disciplines involving aerials [5, 22]. As outdoor events, the weather conditions can also play a factor with wind gusts and snow conditions influencing skier coordination.

40.3.3 Common Injuries

The lower extremity is the most commonly injured body region in freestyle skiing, followed by the head/face. The knee is the most frequently injured body part overall, accounting for approximately 25% of all injuries, of which half are classified as severe. Up to 40% of freestyle skiing injuries involve the anterior cruciate ligament [1, 4, 30]. Freestyle skiing has been reported to have the highest rate of head and face injuries of all FIS ski events, and two of these injuries have recently resulted in fatalities [5]. Injuries to the head and face account for approximately 13% of all freestyle skiing injuries, of which 80% are concussions. Up to a quarter of these are severe injuries. There is also increasing evidence to suggest that women may be at higher risk for head injuries than their male counterparts [5, 30].

40.4 Snowboarding

Slalom, half-pipe, snowboard cross, slopestyle, and big air are the five disciplines of snowboard competition included in the Winter Olympic Games (Fig. 40.5). Due to the nature of these events requiring extreme acrobatic displays of athleticism and highly difficult tricks, injuries are common.

40.4.1 Injury Rates

The incidence of injuries has been reported across various snowboarding competitions.

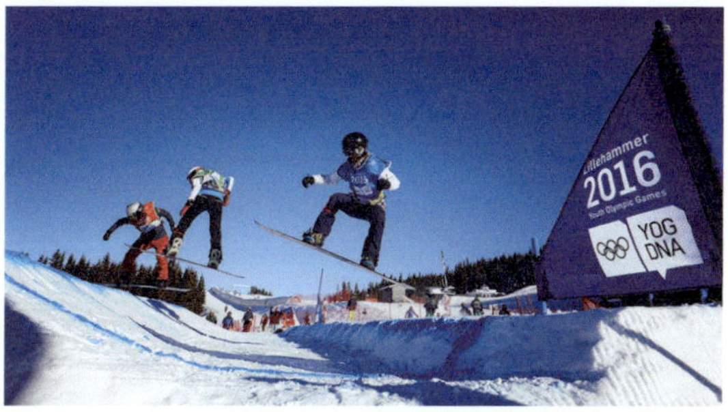

Fig. 40.5 Athletes compete against each other during a snowboard cross event

In snowboarding national cup events, the overall incidence during competition is reported to range from 3.4 to 4.0 per 1000 runs. This is further divided into incidences of 1.9–2.1 for half-pipe, 2.1–5.8 for cross, and 0.6–6.6 for slalom disciplines [32, 33]. From the 2010 to 2014 Winter Olympic Games, there was an increase in the number of athletes sustaining snowboard injuries in the slalom and half-pipe disciplines (7% to 14% and 13% to 18%, respectively), while the snowboard cross-discipline was unchanged (35% to 34%). Slopestyle snowboarding was introduced to the 2014 Winter Olympics, and an injury rate of 37% was reported [1, 2].

A significant proportion of snowboarding injuries occur during training. In the 2010 Winter Olympics, Engebretsen et al. reported that training injuries accounted for 75%, 89%, and 79% of the total injuries in slalom, half-pipe, and snowboard cross, respectively. Of these injuries, a large proportion resulted in time loss from competition [1]. Soligard et al. similarly reported high rates of training injuries at the 2014 Winter Olympics [2].

40.4.2 Injury Mechanism

The most common mechanism of injury is contact made with the ground during a fall [2, 34]. Falls, occurring from either slopes or jumps, generate 80–90% of all snowboarding injuries. Collisions account for the rest, but relative to skiing this is a less common mechanism of injury [35–42]. Skill level also influences the incidence of injuries occurring by isolated falls or upon landing from jumps. Expert riders generally sustain higher-impact injuries due to the expert-level tricks they attempt during training and competition [4, 36, 43, 44].

40.4.3 Common Injuries

Injury rates of snowboarding have been reported to be two to three times higher than that of skiing, ranging from 1.16 to 4.20 per 1000 snowboard days. A large proportion of these injuries are to the upper extremities (45%), while lower extremity injuries occur approximately half as often (23%) [34]. The wrist is the most common area affected by injury, with the head, face, and neck also frequently injured [35–37, 40, 45–51]. In contrast to skiing where most lower extremity injuries are focused about the knee, snowboarding injuries more often affect the ankle. These are most common in the form of sprains and fractures [35, 37, 45, 47–50, 52, 53].

Fractures to the lateral process of the talus (LPT), also known as "snowboarder's fracture," frequently occur from landing after jumps. The usual mechanism is sudden ankle dorsiflexion with concomitant hindfoot inversion and axial loading [54]. Treatment guidelines are tailored according to the classification of the fracture pattern [55]. Type 1 fractures denote a small avulsion without extension to the talofibular joint and are managed nonsurgically with a 4–6 week non-weight-bearing protocol and immobilization. Type 2 fractures involve a single large fragment, which may be displaced. Non-displaced fractures are treated similarly to type 1, while displaced fractures >2 mm should undergo open reduction and internal fixation. A type 3 injury describes a comminuted fracture and is best treated by surgical excision of the small displaced fragments.

In elite snowboarding athletes, the injury distribution is different, with wrist injuries seen far less often (5–6%) and elevated rates of knee injuries [4, 34, 56]. The knee (16–18%) and back (13–22%) are the most commonly injured body parts, while shoulder injuries also occur frequently (10–13%) [32, 33]. Elite athletes also experience a high rate of head and neck injuries [32, 33, 47].

40.5 Ice Hockey

Ice hockey requires high levels of athleticism, but the fast pace and aggressive nature of the sport means injuries are common. Sticks, pucks, skates, boards, and other players are all potential sources of injury, and the severity of these injuries can be variable. Healthcare providers should be familiar with common injury patterns, rules governing play, and current return-to-play protocols if engaged in hockey medical coverage.

40.5.1 Injury Rates

Several studies have investigated the incidence of injury among ice hockey players. Risk of injury has been shown to increase with age and with increasing levels of competition. Emery and Meeuwisse reported injury rates of 4.13 injuries per 1000 player-hours among minor hockey players in Canada. A similar study of US Junior A hockey injuries identified a rate of 9.4/1000 player-hours. Both of these studies included time spent in practice and games in the rate calculations and found that injuries were far more likely to occur during games versus practices [57, 58].

Other studies have focused on the rate of injuries during game competition, excluding time spent in practice. Tuominen et al. published on the injury rates at World Championship and Winter Olympic ice hockey tournaments over a 7-year period. Injuries at the men's junior hockey world championship tournament occurred at a rate of 39.8/1000 player-game-hours. At the adult level, injuries were more frequent with a rate of 52.1/1000 player-game-hours overall and

59.6/1000 player-game-hours. International women's hockey had much lower rates of injury, averaging 22.0/1000 player-game-hours over an 8-year study period [59–61].

There are several explanations for the different injury rates seen at different ages and levels of competition. At the minor hockey level, the initiation of body checking results in a sharp increase in observed injuries. Recent rule changes in North America have raised the age at which body checking is first introduced in response to studies highlighting this association [57, 62, 63]. As players progress to higher levels of competition, the size and speed of the players also increase which can lead to more injuries during game play. Finally, the lack of facial protection worn by players competing at the junior hockey level and higher leads to more injuries of the head, face, and neck [64]. In women's hockey, body checking is prohibited and players wear full facial protection, two factors that contribute to the lower rate of injuries among these players [61].

40.5.2 Injury Mechanism

The most common causes of injuries to hockey players are body contact (intentional or incidental), stick contact, or puck contact. Overuse injuries and fighting are other less common etiologies [1, 2, 58–61, 65].

40.5.3 Common Injuries

The most common anatomic regions affected by injury across all levels of ice hockey are the head and face, followed by the lower extremities (knee and hip) and upper extremities (shoulder). In men's hockey, lacerations occur most frequently, while in women's hockey and minor hockey, sprains, contusions, and concussions are most commonly encountered. Most injuries are considered minor with players returning within 1 week, but moderate and severe injuries also regularly occur [57–61, 66].

In hockey, all players must wear a helmet, but the level of facial protection worn can vary greatly. Mandatory full facial protection is enforced for all minor and women's hockey. Junior and professional men's hockey often allow players to wear half-visors that leave the lower part of the face exposed. Several players in the National Hockey League and recreational leagues still choose to wear no facial protection attached to their helmets. The rate of head and face injuries has been shown to be directly related to the amount of facial protection worn, with full facial shields significantly reducing the frequency of these injuries [64].

The face and neck are the only fully exposed parts of the body and injuries can range from simple lacerations to catastrophic airway emergencies. Ocular and dental injuries frequently occur, requiring prompt evaluation and access to specialist care. Medical personnel should be familiar with the management of these injuries and have an emergency action plan should rapid evacuation to a medical facility be required.

Concussions are the most common injury reported in women's hockey and are of increasing concern for both men and women at all levels of hockey competition [66, 67]. Recognition of concussion symptoms and prompt removal from play is the most important step in concussion management. At the professional level, players may undergo an evaluation, and a decision can be made regarding their return to play in the same game. For all other levels, return to play in the same game is contraindicated, and the general approach is: "When in doubt, sit them out." The Sports Concussion Assessment Tool version 5 (SCAT5) and the Child SCAT5 are the most widely used sideline assessment tools [68, 69]. Physicians must be familiar with the SCAT5, and players should be assessed promptly following a suspected concussion. This should be performed in a quiet setting away from distractions. Further, vigilance on the part of the medical staff is imperative, as players may under report symptoms in an attempt to return to competition [70–73].

Fact Box

Players sustaining a concussion should follow a graduated return-to-play protocol [69]. Players should be symptom-free at each stage for at least 24 h before progressing to the next level. If symptoms reoccur, players should revert back to the previous stage until symptom-free for 24 h. Clearance from a sports medicine professional must be obtained before progressing to Stage 5. Symptoms persisting for longer than 10–14 days in adults and >4 weeks in children warrant referral to a specialist experienced with sports-related concussions.

- Stage 1: No activity, complete rest
- Stage 2: Light aerobic activity such as walking or stationary bicycle
- Stage 3: Sports-specific training (skating)
- Stage 4: Noncontact advanced training drills and progressive resistance training
- Stage 5: Full-contact training drills
- Stage 6: Return to full competition

The knee is the most common site of lower extremity injury among hockey players. Injury to the medial collateral ligament is the most frequent diagnosis secondary to the risk of valgus force from collision with other players while the skate is caught in the ice. Meniscus and anterior cruciate ligament injuries also occur but at a lower rate [59, 60].

The ankle and hip are the next most common lower body regions to sustain injury. High ankle sprains and Maisonneuve fractures can occur with rotational injuries because of the high skate boot, and foot fractures and contusions are commonly the result of contact with the puck during shot blocking [59, 60, 73].

Injuries to the hip can be extra- or intra-articular and are common in hockey players due to the repetitive complex skating motion. Extra-articular injuries include adductor tendon strains, flexor tendon strains, hip pointers, and core muscle injuries. History and clinical examination often clarify the diagnosis, and magnetic resonance imaging (MRI) or ultrasound may also be useful. Treatment of these injuries is primarily non-operative in the acute setting with adductor tenotomy utilized for refractory or chronic cases of adductor tendinopathy. The exception to this is the core muscle injury, which has shown good results with surgical treatment in hockey players [74–77].

Intra-articular hip pathology includes femoroacetabular impingement (FAI), labral tears, and chondral injury. Diagnosis is based on the patient history, clinical signs of impingement (in the case of FAI), and radiographic evidence of pathology. Non-operative treatment consists of physiotherapy, activity modification, nonsteroidal anti-inflammatory medication, and intra-articular injection of corticosteroids. If symptoms persist, surgical management can be pursued and generally yields good outcomes with most players returning to the ice around 4 months [73, 74, 78–80].

Upper extremity injuries most often involve the shoulder and are usually acromioclavicular (AC) or glenohumeral joint related. Type I–II AC separations are managed non-operatively, while types IV–VI are treated surgically. Treatment of type III AC separations remains controversial, but there is an increasing trend toward non-operative treatment of these injuries. Players who sustain one glenohumeral dislocation can often be managed with brief immobilization followed by strength rehabilitation and a gradual return to play. If recurrent instability or a significant bony defect is present, operative stabilization is recommended. The timing of surgical intervention can be individualized to each player, and the use of a brace to prevent recurrent dislocation can sometimes delay the need for surgery until the end of the season. Injuries to the upper extremity also frequently affect the hand and wrist [59, 60, 73].

40.5.4 Catastrophic Injuries

Catastrophic injuries can and do occur during ice hockey participation. These include but are not limited to airway compromise, cervical spine injury, commotio cordis, major lacerations, and eye injury.

Upper airway injuries can result from direct blows to the neck, foreign body obstruction, and cervical spine injury. Advanced Trauma Life Support (ATLS) principles should be followed.

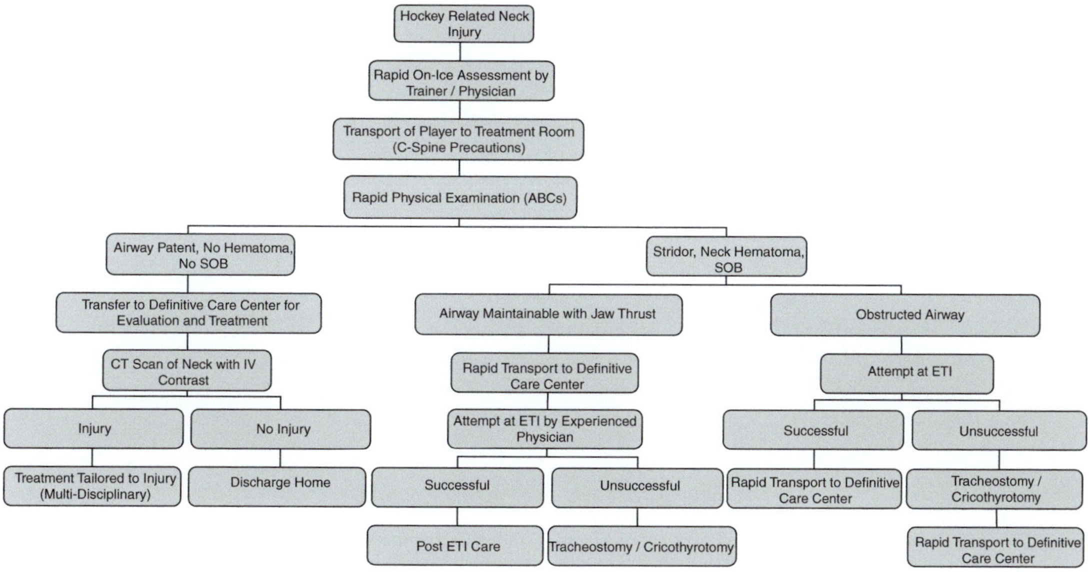

Fig. 40.6 Airway Injury Management Algorithm. Adapted with permission from: Liberman and Mulder (2007). Airway Injuries in the Professional Ice Hockey Player. *Clin J Sport Med.* 17(1):61–67. https://journals-lww-com.uml.idm.oclc.org/cjsportsmed/pages/default.aspx

A jaw-thrust or chin-lift is often sufficient to keep a patent airway, but endotracheal intubation or a surgical airway may be necessary. On-site medical personnel should be familiar with the equipment available and possess the skills needed to secure the airway. Due to the possibility of delayed airway compromise, there should be a low threshold to transfer any player with a suspected airway injury to a definitive care center [81]. An airway management algorithm is presented in Fig. 40.6.

Cervical spine injuries include fractures and dislocations. The rate of these injuries has been decreasing over the past several years, in part due to increased awareness and preventative strategies. However, cervical spine injuries do still occur and are frequently associated with neurologic injury. The most common mechanism is headfirst contact with the boards while the torso remains in motion. This creates an axial compression load to the cervical spine which manifests as injury most commonly between C5 and C7. Players should be immobilized on a spine board, and prehospital ATLS care should quickly precede transfer to hospital [82, 83].

Commotio cordis is a rare event that can cause sudden death in athletes. The proposed mechanism is a blunt trauma to the chest as may occur when blocking a shot with the torso. If the impact is timed just before the T-wave peaks, it can initiate ventricular fibrillation. Immediate treatment consists of a precordial thump or the use of an automated external defibrillator [83].

The combination of high speeds, body contact, and sharp hockey skates puts players at risk of major lacerations (Fig. 40.7). These may involve neurovascular structures and can result in the loss of a significant amount of blood in a short amount of time. Immediate care consists of direct pressure and emergent transfer to a definitive care center. A tourniquet can be used if direct control of bleeding cannot be achieved in the prehospital setting.

In leagues that allow partial or no facial protection, eye injuries regularly occur. These are most often caused by contact with a stick or puck or during a hockey fight [65]. Possible serious eye injuries include corneal abrasion, traumatic hyphema, traumatic cataract, retinal detachment, vitreous hemorrhage, open globe lacerations, and globe ruptures. Evaluation of the injured athlete involves determining the mechanism of injury, reviewing symptoms, and performing a physical

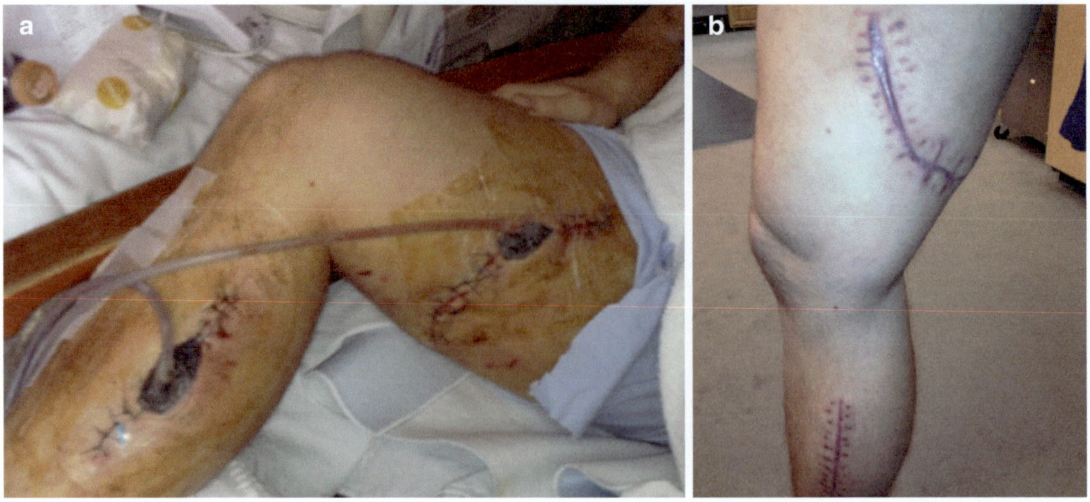

Fig. 40.7 (**a**) Postoperative photograph of a skate blade laceration in a professional hockey player. The femoral artery and vein were lacerated, and the player was transferred to the hospital in unstable condition. He underwent emergent repair, vein grafting, and fasciotomies. (**b**) Six weeks after the injury, the player returned to light skating

Table 40.1 Symptoms and physical examination findings that necessitate urgent evaluation by an ophthalmologist [84]

Symptom	Examination finding
Total vision loss	Asymmetric visual acuity
Partial vision loss (visual field defect)	Asymmetric pupils
Vision changes (diplopia, flashes, floaters)	Restricted extraocular movement
Foreign body	Photophobia with penlight
Ocular pain with nausea/vomiting	Poor visualization of the iris

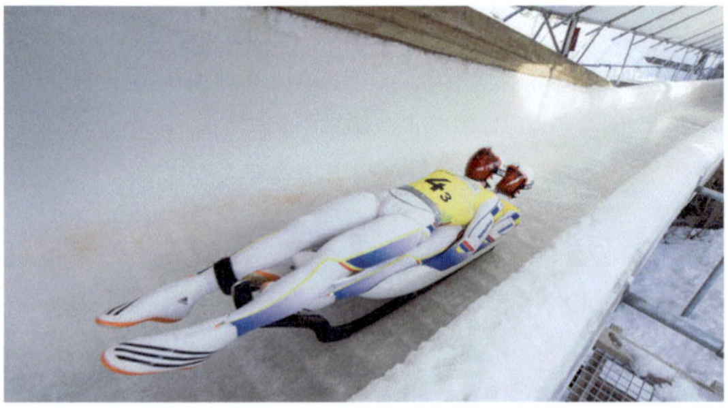

Fig. 40.8 Two athletes race feet-first down the track during a luge competition

examination including assessment of visual acuity, pupils, extraocular movement, and the globe. Table 40.1 highlights symptoms and physical examination findings that warrant urgent referral to an ophthalmologist [84].

40.6 Sliding Sports

The sliding sports include bobsleigh, luge, and skeleton. All of these events are performed on an ice track and involve the risk of significant injury owing to the high speeds achieved by the competitors. In bobsleigh, one, two, or four-person teams compete in a seated-position sled. Smaller sleds designed for lying flat are used for luge and skeleton competitions. In luge, one or two persons lie in a supine position and proceed down the track in a feet-first direction (Fig. 40.8). In contrast, skeleton is an individual sport, whereby the athletes lie prone and race headfirst down the track (Fig. 40.9). Top speeds for each of these events can exceed 120 km/h.

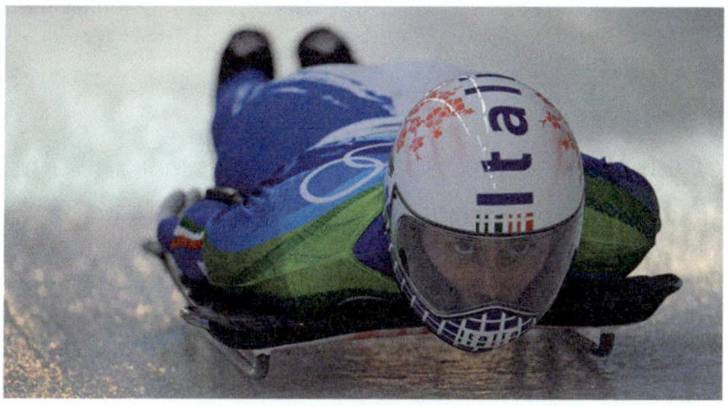

Fig. 40.9 A skeleton athlete slides headfirst toward the finish line

40.6.1 Injury Rates

Injury epidemiology publications from the Winter Olympics provide some information regarding the injury incidence of the sliding sports. At the 2002 Olympic Games in Salt Lake City, sliding sports athletes accounted for 19.6% of all polyclinic visits [85]. At subsequent Olympic Games, 14.7% (Torino 2006), 11.5% (Vancouver 2010), and 13.8% (Sochi 2014) of all registered sliding sports athletes sustained an injury. The potential for severe injury on the ice track must be acknowledged as there was one luge fatality at the Vancouver Olympics following ejection from the track during training [1, 2, 85, 86].

A review of injuries sustained at the Whistler Sliding Centre over a 4-year period was performed by Stuart et al., and an incidence of 0.5% per run was reported. Severe injuries occurred at a rate of 0.1% per run. The authors also reported an association between experience and injury rate, finding a higher incidence of injury among athletes with less experience [87].

40.6.2 Injury Mechanism

Despite the high incidence of injuries to sliding sports athletes, there is a paucity of information regarding the mechanism of these injuries. Cummings et al. published a review of all luge injuries occurring over a 7-year period. The authors reported that crashes were responsible for 64% of all injuries, while 24% could not be attributed to a specific incident. Moderate and severe injuries were usually caused by crashes [88].

40.6.3 Common Injuries

Abrasions, contusion, strains, and lacerations are the most common injuries sustained by sliding sports athletes. Fractures and head injuries also occur at a significant rate [87, 88].

40.7 Treatment Principles

40.7.1 Skiing and Snowboarding

Although modern orthopedic surgical techniques allow athletes to return to competition and function at a high rate, continued efforts to improve prevention of alpine skiing injuries are of great importance. Equipment characteristics such as side-cut radius, length, bindings, and stiffness all contribute to the risk of knee injury in skiers [89]. Longer skis are more stable at higher speeds, and a small side-cut radius has been demonstrated to decrease the self-steering effect of a ski, which allows for increased ski control and subsequently less risk of aberrant rotational forces acting on the knee. Modern bindings feature multidirectional release characteristics which help protect against lower extremity injuries such as tibial fractures and ligamentous tears [7, 11]. Environmental conditions and skier fatigue, both physical and mental, can also contribute to injury risk [90]. Programs aimed at increasing awareness regarding the risk factors surrounding alpine skiing-related injuries have been demonstrated to decrease injury risk by 62% in specific studies [91]. More future work and effort are necessary to continue to develop and advance both the prevention and treatment of alpine skiing-related injury.

Injury prevention of snowboarders through additional protection gear is heavily advocated, being primarily focused on wrist guards, back protectors, and helmets [54]. Due to the frequent falling that snowboarders endure, this gear acts to reduce the injury occurrence resultant from excessive contact forces with the ground. The less experienced snowboard population is at most risk for these types of injuries and therefore benefits most from utilizing such preventative measures.

Alpine ski, freestyle ski, and snowboarding events can involve high speeds and large jumps, which place athletes at risk for high-energy injuries. Physicians providing care to these athletes must be prepared for the various injuries that can occur on the slopes. Following ATLS principles will guide the prehospital care. Since these events often take place in remote locations, physicians must be familiar with the local emergency action plan should the athlete require evacuation to the hospital. Prior to large events, on-site training of involved medical personnel is imperative. This may involve walk-throughs or simulation-based activities to optimize the efficiency of the team and ensure safety for the athletes. Roles should be clearly defined and the team leader(s) identified.

40.7.2 Ice Hockey

Hockey is a contact sport and injuries occur frequently. An understanding of the most common injuries is essential for sports medicine physicians who care for these athletes. The vast majority of hockey-related injuries are minor, and players can often return to play following functional rehabilitation. Other injuries may require surgical management for resolution. Thankfully, catastrophic injuries are rare in ice hockey, but those engaged in rink-side coverage must be prepared to act quickly and effectively should they arise.

Injury prevention can also play a central role in the provision of care for hockey players. This can be accomplished through encouraging the optimal use of protective equipment such as mouth-guards and face protection or by educating players and coaching staff regarding concussion awareness. Physicians should also engage in discussions about possible rule changes that could reduce injury incidence and/or severity. These preventative strategies have proven successful in the past, but there is a need for more research and science surrounding hockey injuries in the future [62, 63, 73].

40.7.3 Sliding Sports

Owing to the potential for severe injury, medical providers must maintain vigilance and ensure all medical team members are familiar with the emergency action plan. Using an ATLS approach with protection of the cervical spine is the standard. Close collaboration with track officials regarding track conditions and design, specifically to avoid slider ejection from the track, is also important to optimize the safety of the athletes.

Take-Home Message
Sports medicine physicians engaged in coverage of winter sports must be familiar with the unique characteristics of each event. This includes the common injury patterns, treatment modalities, and return-to-play guidelines. Weather and venue location are additional variables that must be considered when devising event-specific emergency action plans. Physicians should also take an active role in injury prevention through encouraging safe behavior and the proper use of protective equipment.

References

1. Engebretsen L, Steffen K, Alonso JM, Aubry M, Dvorak J, Junge A, Meeuwisse W, Mountjoy M, Renstrom P, Wilkinson M. Sports injuries and illnesses during the Winter Olympic Games 2010. Br J Sports Med. 2010;44:772–80. https://doi.org/10.1136/bjsm.2010.076992.
2. Soligard T, Steffen K, Palmer-Green D, Aubry M, Grant M-E, Meeuwisse W, Mountjoy M, Budgett R, Engebretsen L. Sports injuries and illnesses in the Sochi 2014 Olympic Winter Games. Br J Sports Med. 2015;49:441–7. https://doi.org/10.1136/bjsports-2014-094538.
3. Flørenes TW, Nordsletten L, Heir S, Bahr R. Recording injuries among World Cup skiers and snowboarders: a methodological study. Scand

J Med Sci Sports. 2011;21:196–205. https://doi.org/10.1111/j.1600-0838.2009.01048.x.
4. Flørenes TW, Nordsletten L, Heir S, Bahr R. Injuries among World Cup ski and snowboard athletes. Scand J Med Sci Sports. 2012;22:58–66. https://doi.org/10.1111/j.1600-0838.2010.01147.x.
5. Steenstrup SE, Bere T, Bahr R. Head injuries among FIS World Cup alpine and freestyle skiers and snowboarders: a 7-year cohort study. Br J Sports Med. 2014;48:41–5. https://doi.org/10.1136/bjsports-2013-093145.
6. McCall D, Safran MR. Injuries about the shoulder in skiing and snowboarding. Br J Sports Med. 2009;43:987–92. https://doi.org/10.1136/bjsm.2009.068767.
7. Pujol N, Blanchi MPR, Chambat P. The incidence of anterior cruciate ligament injuries among competitive Alpine skiers: a 25-year investigation. Am J Sports Med. 2007;35:1070–4. https://doi.org/10.1177/0363546507301083.
8. Lund M. A short history of skiing: from telemark to today. Skiing Heritage. 1996;8:5–19.
9. Rust DA, Gilmore CJ, Treme G. Injury patterns at a large Western United States ski resort with and without snowboarders: the Taos experience. Am J Sports Med. 2013;41:652–6. https://doi.org/10.1177/0363546512472045.
10. Deibert MC, Aronsson DD, Johnson RJ, Ettlinger CF, Shealy JE. Skiing injuries in children, adolescents, and adults. J Bone Joint Surg Am. 1998;80:25–32.
11. Natri A, Beynnon BD, Ettlinger CF, Johnson RJ, Shealy JE. Alpine ski bindings and injuries. Current findings. Sports Med. 1999;28:35–48.
12. Johnson R, Mote C, Zelcer J. Skiing trauma and safety: Ninth international symposium. West Conshohocken: ASTM International; 1993.
13. Viola RW, Steadman JR, Mair SD, Briggs KK, Sterett WI. Anterior cruciate ligament injury incidence among male and female professional alpine skiers. Am J Sports Med. 1999;27:792–5. https://doi.org/10.1177/03635465990270061701.
14. Bere T, Flørenes TW, Nordsletten L, Bahr R. Sex differences in the risk of injury in World Cup alpine skiers: a 6-year cohort study. Br J Sports Med. 2014;48:36–40. https://doi.org/10.1136/bjsports-2013-092206.
15. Raschner C, Platzer H-P, Patterson C, Werner I, Huber R, Hildebrandt C. The relationship between ACL injuries and physical fitness in young competitive ski racers: a 10-year longitudinal study. Br J Sports Med. 2012;46:1065–71. https://doi.org/10.1136/bjsports-2012-091050.
16. Steenstrup SE, Mok K-M, McIntosh AS, Bahr R, Krosshaug T. Reconstruction of head impacts in FIS World Cup alpine skiing. Br J Sports Med. 2017. https://doi.org/10.1136/bjsports-2017-098050.
17. Gerritsen KG, Nachbauer W, van den Bogert AJ. Computer simulation of landing movement in downhill skiing: anterior cruciate ligament injuries. J Biomech. 1996;29:845–54.
18. Gilgien M, Spörri J, Kröll J, Crivelli P, Müller E. Mechanics of turning and jumping and skier speed are associated with injury risk in men's World Cup alpine skiing: a comparison between the competition disciplines. Br J Sports Med. 2014;48:742–7. https://doi.org/10.1136/bjsports-2013-092994.
19. Smith SD, Laprade RF, Jansson KS, Arøen A, Wijdicks CA. Functional bracing of ACL injuries: current state and future directions. Knee Surg Sports Traumatol Arthrosc Off J ESSKA. 2014;22:1131–41. https://doi.org/10.1007/s00167-013-2514-z.
20. Kocher MS, Dupré MM, Feagin JA. Shoulder injuries from alpine skiing and snowboarding. Aetiology, treatment and prevention. Sports Med. 1998;25:201–11.
21. Ackery A, Hagel BE, Provvidenza C, Tator CH. An international review of head and spinal cord injuries in alpine skiing and snowboarding. Inj Prev J Int Soc Child Adolesc Inj Prev. 2007;13:368–75. https://doi.org/10.1136/ip.2007.017285.
22. Steenstrup SE, Bakken A, Bere T, Patton DA, Bahr R. Head injury mechanisms in FIS World Cup alpine and freestyle skiers and snowboarders. Br J Sports Med. 2018;52:61–9. https://doi.org/10.1136/bjsports-2017-098240.
23. Hagel BE, Pless IB, Goulet C, Platt RW, Robitaille Y. Effectiveness of helmets in skiers and snowboarders: case-control and case crossover study. BMJ. 2005;330:281. https://doi.org/10.1136/bmj.38314.480035.7C.
24. Macnab AJ, Smith T, Gagnon FA, Macnab M. Effect of helmet wear on the incidence of head/face and cervical spine injuries in young skiers and snowboarders. Inj Prev J Int Soc Child Adolesc Inj Prev. 2002;8:324–7.
25. Mueller BA, Cummings P, Rivara FP, Brooks MA, Terasaki RD. Injuries of the head, face, and neck in relation to ski helmet use. Epidemiol Camb Mass. 2008;19:270–6. https://doi.org/10.1097/EDE.0b013e318163567c.
26. Russell K, Christie J, Hagel BE. The effect of helmets on the risk of head and neck injuries among skiers and snowboarders: a meta-analysis. CMAJ Can Med Assoc J J Assoc Medicale Can. 2010;182:333–40. https://doi.org/10.1503/cmaj.091080.
27. Sulheim S, Ekeland A, Holme I, Bahr R. Helmet use and risk of head injuries in alpine skiers and snowboarders: changes after an interval of one decade. Br J Sports Med. 2017;51:44–50. https://doi.org/10.1136/bjsports-2015-095798.
28. de Montagne M. The accidentology of winter sports season. Chambéry: Maison des Parcs et de la Montagne; 2018. p. 2016–7.
29. Bailly N, Laporte J-D, Afquir S, Masson C, Donnadieu T, Delay J-B, Arnoux P-J. Effect of helmet use on traumatic brain injuries and other head injuries in alpine sport. Wilderness Environ Med. 2018;29(2):151–8. https://doi.org/10.1016/j.wem.2017.11.007.
30. Flørenes TW, Heir S, Nordsletten L, Bahr R. Injuries among World Cup freestyle skiers. Br J Sports

Med. 2010;44:803–8. https://doi.org/10.1136/bjsm.2009.071159.

31. Randjelovic S, Heir S, Nordsletten L, Bere T, Bahr R. Injury situations in Freestyle Ski Cross (SX): a video analysis of 33 cases. Br J Sports Med. 2014;48:29–35. https://doi.org/10.1136/bjsports-2012-091999.
32. Torjussen J, Bahr R. Injuries among competitive snowboarders at the national elite level. Am J Sports Med. 2005;33:370–7. https://doi.org/10.1177/0363546504268043.
33. Torjussen J, Bahr R. Injuries among elite snowboarders (FIS Snowboard World Cup). Br J Sports Med. 2006;40:230–4. https://doi.org/10.1136/bjsm.2005.021329.
34. Wijdicks CA, Rosenbach BS, Flanagan TR, Bower GE, Newman KE, Clanton TO, Engebretsen L, LaPrade RF, Hackett TR. Injuries in elite and recreational snowboarders. Br J Sports Med. 2014;48:11–7. https://doi.org/10.1136/bjsports-2013-093019.
35. Yamagami T, Ishihara H, Kimura T. Clinical features of snowboarding injuries. J Orthop Sci. 2004;9:225–9. https://doi.org/10.1007/s00776-004-0776-5.
36. Idzikowski JR, Janes PC, Abbott PJ. Upper extremity snowboarding injuries: ten-year results from the Colorado Snowboard Injury Survey. Am J Sports Med. 2000;28:825–32. https://doi.org/10.1177/03635465000280061001.
37. Machold W, Kwasny O, Gässler P, Kolonja A, Reddy B, Bauer E, Lehr S. Risk of injury through snowboarding. J Trauma. 2000;48:1109–14.
38. Pino EC, Colville MR. Snowboard injuries. Am J Sports Med. 1989;17:778–81. https://doi.org/10.1177/036354658901700610.
39. Matsumoto K, Miyamoto K, Sumi H, Sumi Y, Shimizu K. Upper extremity injuries in snowboarding and skiing: a comparative study. Clin J Sport Med. 2002;12:354–9.
40. Dickson TJ, Terwiel FA. Snowboarding injuries in Australia: investigating risk factors in wrist fractures to enhance injury prevention strategies. Wilderness Environ Med. 2011;22:228–35. https://doi.org/10.1016/j.wem.2011.04.002.
41. Hagel BE, Goulet C, Platt RW, Pless IB. Injuries among skiers and snowboarders in Quebec. Epidemiology. 2004;15:279–86. https://doi.org/10.1097/01.ede.0000120044.62029.b4.
42. Machida T, Hanazaki K, Ishizaka K, Nakamura M, Kobayashi O, Shibata H, Nakafuji H, Amano J. Snowboarding injuries of the chest: comparison with skiing injuries. J Trauma. 1999;46:1062–5.
43. Goulet C, Hagel BE, Hamel D, Légaré G. Self-reported skill level and injury severity in skiers and snowboarders. J Sci Med Sport. 2010;13:39–41. https://doi.org/10.1016/j.jsams.2008.10.002.
44. Girardi P, Braggion M, Sacco G, De Giorgi F, Corra S. Factors affecting injury severity among recreational skiers and snowboarders: an epidemiology study. Knee Surg Sports Traumatol Arthrosc. 2010;18:1804–9. https://doi.org/10.1007/s00167-010-1133-1.
45. Sasaki K, Takagi M, Ida H, Yamakawa M, Ogino T. Severity of upper limb injuries in snowboarding. Arch Orthop Trauma Surg. 1999;119:292–5. https://doi.org/10.1007/s004020050413.
46. Langran M. Snow sports injuries in Scotland: a case-control study. Br J Sports Med. 2002;36:135–40. https://doi.org/10.1136/bjsm.36.2.135.
47. Made C, Elmqvist L-G. A 10-year study of snowboard injuries in Lapland Sweden. Scand J Med Sci Sports. 2004;14:128–33. https://doi.org/10.1111/j.1600-0838.2003.00342.x.
48. Sulheim S, Holme I, Rodven A, Ekeland A, Bahr R. Risk factors for injuries in alpine skiing, telemark skiing and snowboarding—case-control study. Br J Sports Med. 2011;45:1303–9. https://doi.org/10.1136/bjsports-2011-090407.
49. Davidson TM, Laliotis AT. Snowboarding injuries, a four-year study with comparison with alpine ski injuries. West J Med. 1996;164:231–7.
50. Xiang H, Kelleher K, Shields BJ, Brown KJ, Smith GA. Skiing- and snowboarding-related injuries treated in U.S. emergency departments, 2002. J Trauma. 2005;58:112–8.
51. Wasden CC, McIntosh SE, Keith DS, McCowan C. An analysis of skiing and snowboarding injuries on Utah slopes. J Trauma Inj Infect Crit Care. 2009;67:1022–6. https://doi.org/10.1097/TA.0b013e3181b0d559.
52. Sutherland AG, Holmes JD, Myers S. Differing injury patterns in snowboarding and alpine skiing. Injury. 1996;27:423–5. https://doi.org/10.1016/0020-1383(96)00026-5.
53. Pigozzi F, Santori N, Di Salvo V, Parisi A, Di-Luigi L. Snowboard traumatology: an epidemiological study. Orthopedics. 1997;20:505–9.
54. Sachtleben TR. Snowboarding injuries. Curr Sports Med Rep. 2011;10:340–4. https://doi.org/10.1249/JSR.0b013e318237be2a.
55. McCrory P, Bladin C. Fractures of the lateral process of the talus: a clinical review "Snowboarder's ankle". Clin J Sport Med. 1996;6:124–8.
56. Major DH, Steenstrup SE, Bere T, Bahr R, Nordsletten L. Injury rate and injury pattern among elite World Cup snowboarders: a 6-year cohort study. Br J Sports Med. 2014;48:18–22. https://doi.org/10.1136/bjsports-2013-092573.
57. Emery CA, Meeuwisse WH. Injury rates, risk factors, and mechanisms of injury in minor hockey. Am J Sports Med. 2006;34:1960–9. https://doi.org/10.1177/0363546506290061.
58. Stuart MJ, Smith A. Injuries in Junior A ice hockey. A three-year prospective study. Am J Sports Med. 1995;23:458–61. https://doi.org/10.1177/036354659502300415.
59. Tuominen M, Stuart MJ, Aubry M, Kannus P, Parkkari J. Injuries in world junior ice hockey championships between 2006 and 2015. Br J Sports Med. 2017;51:36–43. https://doi.org/10.1136/bjsports-2016-095992.
60. Tuominen M, Stuart MJ, Aubry M, Kannus P, Parkkari J. Injuries in men's international ice hockey: a 7-year study of the International Ice Hockey Federation Adult

World Championship Tournaments and Olympic Winter Games. Br J Sports Med. 2015;49:30–6. https://doi.org/10.1136/bjsports-2014-093688.
61. Tuominen M, Stuart MJ, Aubry M, Kannus P, Tokola K, Parkkari J. Injuries in women's international ice hockey: an 8-year study of the World Championship tournaments and Olympic Winter Games. Br J Sports Med. 2016;50:1406–12. https://doi.org/10.1136/bjsports-2015-094647.
62. Black AM, Macpherson AK, Hagel BE, Romiti MA, Palacios-Derflingher L, Kang J, Meeuwisse WH, Emery CA. Policy change eliminating body checking in non-elite ice hockey leads to a threefold reduction in injury and concussion risk in 11- and 12-year-old players. Br J Sports Med. 2016;50:55–61. https://doi.org/10.1136/bjsports-2015-095103.
63. Black AM, Hagel BE, Palacios-Derflingher L, Schneider KJ, Emery CA. The risk of injury associated with body checking among Pee Wee ice hockey players: an evaluation of Hockey Canada's national body checking policy change. Br J Sports Med. 2017;51:1767–72. https://doi.org/10.1136/bjsports-2016-097392.
64. Stuart MJ, Smith AM, Malo-Ortiguera SA, Fischer TL, Larson DR. A comparison of facial protection and the incidence of head, neck, and facial injuries in Junior A hockey players. A function of individual playing time. Am J Sports Med. 2002;30:39–44. https://doi.org/10.1177/03635465020300012001.
65. Black AM, Eliason PH, Patton DA, Emery CA. Epidemiology of facial injuries in sport. Clin Sports Med. 2017;36:237–55. https://doi.org/10.1016/j.csm.2016.11.001.
66. Abbott K. Injuries in women's ice hockey: special considerations. Curr Sports Med Rep. 2014;13:377–82. https://doi.org/10.1249/JSR.0000000000000102.
67. Agel J, Harvey EJ. A 7-year review of men's and women's ice hockey injuries in the NCAA. Can J Surg J Can Chir. 2010;53:319–23.
68. Echemendia RJ, Meeuwisse W, McCrory P, Davis GA, Putukian M, Leddy J, Makdissi M, Sullivan SJ, Broglio SP, Raftery M, Schneider K, Kissick J, McCrea M, Dvořák J, Sills AK, Aubry M, Engebretsen L, Loosemore M, Fuller G, Kutcher J, Ellenbogen R, Guskiewicz K, Patricios J, Herring S. The Concussion Recognition Tool 5th Edition (CRT5): background and rationale. Br J Sports Med. 2017;51:870–1. https://doi.org/10.1136/bjsports-2017-097508.
69. McCrory P, Meeuwisse W, Dvorak J, Aubry M, Bailes J, Broglio S, Cantu RC, Cassidy D, Echemendia RJ, Castellani RJ, Davis GA, Ellenbogen R, Emery C, Engebretsen L, Feddermann-Demont N, Giza CC, Guskiewicz KM, Herring S, Iverson GL, Johnston KM, Kissick J, Kutcher J, Leddy JJ, Maddocks D, Makdissi M, Manley GT, McCrea M, Meehan WP, Nagahiro S, Patricios J, Putukian M, Schneider KJ, Sills A, Tator CH, Turner M, Vos PE. Consensus statement on concussion in sport—the 5th international conference on concussion in sport held in Berlin, October 2016. Br J Sports Med. 2017;51(11):838–47. https://doi.org/10.1136/bjsports-2017-097699.
70. Harmon KG, Drezner JA, Gammons M, Guskiewicz KM, Halstead M, Herring SA, Kutcher JS, Pana A, Putukian M, Roberts WO. American Medical Society for Sports Medicine position statement: concussion in sport. Br J Sports Med. 2013;47:15–26. https://doi.org/10.1136/bjsports-2012-091941.
71. Mrazik M, Perra A, Brooks BL, Naidu D. Exploring minor hockey players' knowledge and attitudes toward concussion: implications for prevention. J Head Trauma Rehabil. 2015;30:219–27. https://doi.org/10.1097/HTR.0000000000000018.
72. Delaney JS, Lamfookon C, Bloom GA, Al-Kashmiri A, Correa JA. Why university athletes choose not to reveal their concussion symptoms during a practice or game. Clin J Sport Med. 2015;25:113–25. https://doi.org/10.1097/JSM.0000000000000112.
73. LaPrade RF, Surowiec RK, Sochanska AN, Hentkowski BS, Martin BM, Engebretsen L, Wijdicks CA. Epidemiology, identification, treatment and return to play of musculoskeletal-based ice hockey injuries. Br J Sports Med. 2014;48:4–10. https://doi.org/10.1136/bjsports-2013-093020.
74. Kuhn AW, Noonan BC, Kelly BT, Larson CM, Bedi A. The hip in ice hockey: a current concepts review. Arthrosc J Arthrosc Relat Surg. 2016;32:1928–38. https://doi.org/10.1016/j.arthro.2016.04.029.
75. Irshad K, Feldman LS, Lavoie C, Lacroix VJ, Mulder DS, Brown RA. Operative management of "hockey groin syndrome": 12 years of experience in National Hockey League players. Surgery. 2001;130:759–66. https://doi.org/10.1067/msy.2001.118093.
76. Brown RA, Mascia A, Kinnear DG, Lacroix V, Feldman L, Mulder DS. An 18-year review of sports groin injuries in the elite hockey player: clinical presentation, new diagnostic imaging, treatment, and results. Clin J Sport Med. 2008;18:221–6. https://doi.org/10.1097/JSM.0b013e318172831a.
77. Jakoi A, O'Neill C, Damsgaard C, Fehring K, Tom J. Sports hernia in National Hockey League players: does surgery affect performance? Am J Sports Med. 2013;41:107–10. https://doi.org/10.1177/0363546512462679.
78. Griffin DR, Dickenson EJ, O'Donnell J, Agricola R, Awan T, Beck M, Clohisy JC, Dijkstra HP, Falvey E, Gimpel M, Hinman RS, Hölmich P, Kassarjian A, Martin HD, Martin R, Mather RC, Philippon MJ, Reiman MP, Takla A, Thorborg K, Walker S, Weir A, Bennell KL. The Warwick Agreement on femoroacetabular impingement syndrome (FAI syndrome): an international consensus statement. Br J Sports Med. 2016;50:1169–76. https://doi.org/10.1136/bjsports-2016-096743.
79. Philippon MJ, Weiss DR, Kuppersmith DA, Briggs KK, Hay CJ. Arthroscopic labral repair and treatment of femoroacetabular impingement in professional hockey players. Am J Sports Med. 2010;38:99–104. https://doi.org/10.1177/0363546509346393.

80. McDonald JE, Herzog MM, Philippon MJ. Performance outcomes in professional hockey players following arthroscopic treatment of FAI and microfracture of the hip. Knee Surg Sports Traumatol Arthrosc. 2014;22:915–9. https://doi.org/10.1007/s00167-013-2691-9.
81. Liberman M, Mulder DS. Airway injuries in the professional ice hockey player. Clin J Sport Med. 2007;17:61–7. https://doi.org/10.1097/01.jsm.0000168072.44003.98.
82. Tator CH, Provvidenza C, Cassidy JD. Spinal injuries in Canadian Ice Hockey: an update to 2005. Clin J Sport Med. 2009;19:451–6. https://doi.org/10.1097/JSM.0b013e3181bd0db6.
83. Boden BP. Direct catastrophic injury in sports. J Am Acad Orthop Surg. 2005;13:445–54.
84. Micieli JA, Easterbrook M. Eye and orbital injuries in sports. Clin Sports Med. 2017;36:299–314. https://doi.org/10.1016/j.csm.2016.11.006.
85. Reeser JC, Willick S, Elstad M. Medical services provided at the Olympic Village polyclinic during the 2002 Salt Lake City Winter Games. WMJ. 2003;102:20–5.
86. Piat SC, Minniti D, Traversi D, Gianino MM, Massazza G, Siliquini R. Torino 2006 Winter Olympic Games: highlight on Health Services Organization. J Emerg Med. 2010;39:454–61. https://doi.org/10.1016/j.jemermed.2009.08.028.
87. Stuart CA, Richards D, Cripton PA. Injuries at the Whistler Sliding Center: a 4-year retrospective study. Br J Sports Med. 2016;50:62–70. https://doi.org/10.1136/bjsports-2015-095006.
88. Cummings RS, Shurland AT, Prodoehl JA, Moody K, Sherk HH. Injuries in the sport of luge. Epidemiology and analysis. Am J Sports Med. 1997;25:508–13. https://doi.org/10.1177/036354659702500414.
89. Jordan MJ, Aagaard P, Herzog W. Anterior cruciate ligament injury/reinjury in alpine ski racing: a narrative review. Open Access J Sports Med. 2017;8:71–83. https://doi.org/10.2147/OAJSM.S106699.
90. Bere T, Flørenes TW, Krosshaug T, Nordsletten L, Bahr R. Events leading to anterior cruciate ligament injury in World Cup Alpine Skiing: a systematic video analysis of 20 cases. Br J Sports Med. 2011;45:1294–302. https://doi.org/10.1136/bjsports-2011-090517.
91. Ettlinger CF, Johnson RJ, Shealy JE. A method to help reduce the risk of serious knee sprains incurred in alpine skiing. Am J Sports Med. 1995;23:531–7. https://doi.org/10.1177/036354659502300503.

Part VII

Sports Equipment

Sports Footwear: Problems and Advances

41

Marcelo Pires Prado and Guilherme Honda Saito

41.1 Background

During the early Greek games, athletes used to compete barefoot. As the Greek empire expanded and many athletes from different regions came to compete, runners wearing sandals started to appear, since it supposedly improved traction and running efficiency [1–3]. But it was not until the second half of the nineteenth century that specific sports footwear became available. Crocket sandals made with a rubber sole, a canvas upper, and laces were designed and became known as sneakers [2]. Since then, a wide variety of specific sports footwear for different modalities was developed, culminating in the multibillion-dollar sports shoe industry. Every year a number of sports footwear with new designs and technologies are released in the market. The benefits and risks of these different footwear concepts are debatable, but it is undeniable that footwear innovations throughout the years allowed an inestimable development on sports, enhancing performance both for the amateur and professional athlete.

The knowledge regarding sports footwear is constantly evolving, and the amount of information may be overwhelming for the general physician. However, the demand for the most appropriate sports footwear is no longer restricted to the professional athlete. The number of the so-called weekend warriors is increasing every year, and the sports professional must be capable of prescribing the most suitable shoe in order to provide comfort while preventing injuries. In this chapter, we summarize the main aspects of footwear anatomy and the current topics of debate in the literature. Moreover, we describe the rationale behind the choice of an athletic shoe.

41.2 Athletic Shoe Anatomy

To fully understand the biomechanics involved in an athletic shoe, it is essential to understand its anatomy first. The footwear is made of two main elements: the upper and the bottom (Fig. 41.1). The bottom can be divided into three main components: outsole, midsole, and wedge [1, 2, 4]. Here we will briefly describe each of these components.

41.2.1 Upper

The upper covers the sides and top of the foot, being directly exposed to dirt and water. Therefore, the choice of materials is important in order to provide comfort and protection to the

M. P. Prado (✉) · G. H. Saito
Hospital Israelita Albert Einstein, São Paulo, Brazil
e-mail: mpprado@einstein.br

S. Rocha Piedade et al. (eds.), *The Sports Medicine Physician*,
https://doi.org/10.1007/978-3-030-10433-7_41

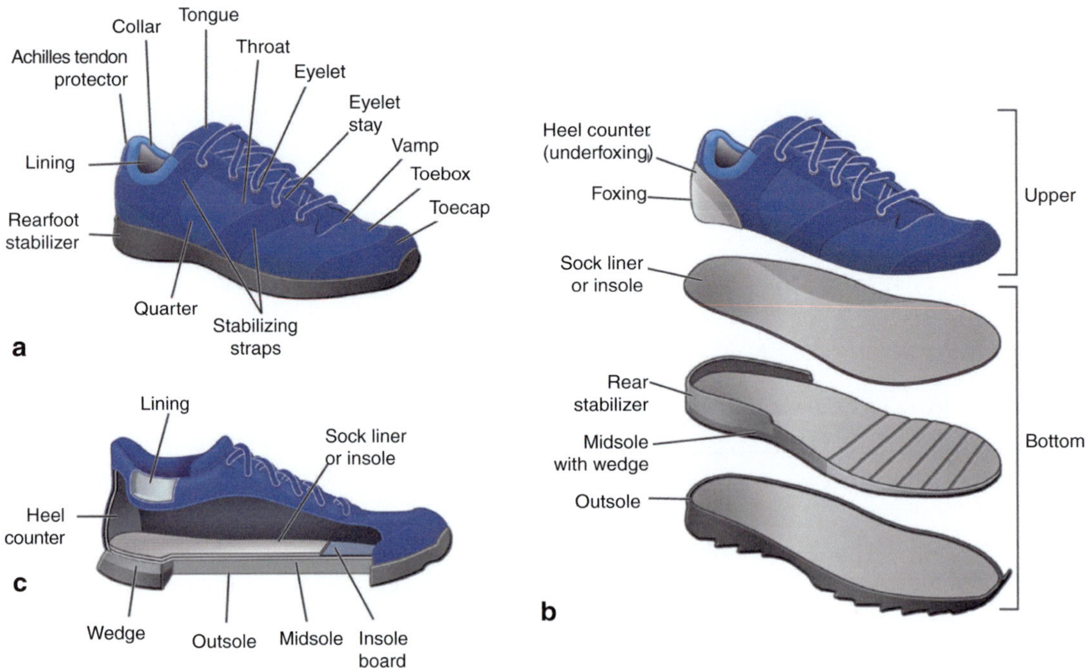

Fig. 41.1 Illustrations of athletic shoes. (**a**) An overview of the external appearance. (**b**) Separation of shoe into its component parts. (**c**) A sectional view of the interior of a shoe. **(From LeCursi N. Sports shoes and orthoses. In: *DeLee & Drez's Orthopaedic Sports Medicine*. 4th ed. Saunders, 2014:1389)**

foot while maintaining the material's properties after exposure to external conditions. The upper should be made from a material that is breathable, washable, resistant to deformation, and yet comfortable. Nylon is usually the material of choice in athletic footwear.

41.2.2 Bottom

41.2.2.1 Midsole

The midsole is considered the most important part of the shoe, located between the outsole and the upper. The midsole provides stability, cushioning, and shock absorption. It is usually made of foam, the most common being the ethylene-vinyl acetate (EVA). The polyurethane is more resistant and stiffer than the EVA and is also commonly used in athletic footwear. The stiffer the midsole, the more stability is provided, at the expense of cushioning. Therefore, a balance must be obtained among these variables according to the patient's profile. Different materials with different densities may be used to achieve an optimal balance.

41.2.2.2 Outsole

The outsole is the part of the shoe that contacts the ground, thus providing traction, shock absorption, and flexibility. The outsole is made from different types of rubber. Several properties are taken into consideration when choosing the most appropriate type of rubber for the footwear, such as durability, weight, softness, and traction. Different types of rubber can be used at different locations of the shoe according to the athlete's needs.

41.2.2.3 Wedges

The wedges are located at the rear of the footwear, between the midsole and the outsole. Its main function is to provide medial stability against overpronation. The wedges are made from a stiff material, capable of providing adequate stability and shock attenuation.

41.3 Choosing the Correct Footwear

Shoes act like interfaces between the foot and ground, protecting the foot sole, providing shock absorption against repetitive impact, stabilizing the rear foot by protecting it from uneven ground and inclined surfaces. Moreover, they allow flexibility to prevent overuse injuries related to muscle and tendon tension forces. The combination of these properties must be balanced to provide adequate foot motion control, comfort, and physiologic function.

The choice on which sports footwear is more appropriate for each athlete should always be made on an individual basis. No footwear is suitable for all individuals since each person has their own characteristics regarding foot shape, foot size, gait pattern, level of activity, type of activity, and previous pathologies, among others [2, 5]. All these variables should be analyzed by the professional in order to prescribe the most appropriate shoe. Still, each person and each foot is so unique that it is hard to predict whether an individual will adapt to a specific shoe. Ultimately, the athlete is the best person to evaluate the footwear, according to the subjective experience while wearing it. Physicians should use their best judgment by analyzing the multiple factors and suggesting a shoe that will most likely suit the person's needs and expectations.

First, the type of activity should be taken into consideration. Sports footwear evolved significantly in the past decades, and now shoes for different modalities are completely unique. A running shoe that is designed for a straightforward motion will have a different structure than a high-top basketball shoe, which is more supportive and provides additional stability for multidirectional movements.

An essential factor to be considered is the athlete's fitness level. An elite athlete will have a different demand when compared to an amateur. Their type and level of training, body structure, body self-awareness, and muscle strength will be distinct. Thus, different types of footwear will be required for each. In addition, a balance among performance, comfort, and injury prevention should be achieved, since these variables do not necessarily come together. While an elite athlete cannot afford giving up performance, a recreational athlete does not need a sports shoe that provides performance at the expense of comfort or one that puts him under the unnecessary risk of injuries. For example, previous studies [6, 7] have shown that climbing shoes can cause several types of foot injuries. This type of shoe is designed to provide an extremely close fit, which allows the climber to stand on small holds. Some climbing shoes present with more aggressive characteristics, having a more downward pointing toe box. This type of footwear is usually worn by professional climbers and conceivably leads to higher rates of injuries and foot deformities. Thereby, the amateur climber does not need it to fulfill their purpose.

Foot size, type, and function during gait should also be assessed. The examiner must assure that the length and width of the shoe are correct. The end of the toes should not be in contact with the toe box. Meanwhile, the footwear should be tight enough in order to prevent the foot from sliding within the shoe. Foot type is also evaluated. A pes planus behaves differently from a pes cavus, thus requiring specific footwear. When considering a certain type of foot, one must keep in mind that there are several degrees of foot deformity. Therefore, there is no recipe, and the choice of footwear should be made on an individual basis. Insoles are useful in these cases and may be used as a complement to make fine adjustments.

Regarding foot type, it is important to understand that specific foot alignment changes foot biomechanics and interferes with foot response to load. In the pronated foot, the mechanical axes of the rearfoot (talonavicular and calcaneocuboid joints) remain parallel, resulting in a more flexible foot. As a consequence, an increased muscle effort is required to maintain the same level of activity compared with other types of foot. On the contrary, the supinated foot has an oblique rearfoot joint axis alignment, resulting in a stiffer foot [8]. Consequently, a high incidence of ankle sprains, tendinopathies (mainly of the peroneal tendons), and overload lesions is observed.

Specific shoe design can mitigate these functional peculiarities by increasing stiffness and medial support for the pronated foot and flexibility for the supinated foot.

Despite these concepts, Knapik et al. [9] prospectively compared a large group of Marine Corps recruits, who received different shoe models depending on the shape of the foot (low, medium, or high arches, receiving, respectively, motion control, stability, or cushioned shoes), to a group who received a stability shoe regardless of plantar shape, showing little influence on injury risk.

41.4 Pathologic Conditions

Foot pathologies play an important role during footwear selection. Feet with distinct pathologies benefit from shoes with specific characteristics.

41.4.1 Forefoot Conditions

The forefoot is commonly affected by stress lesions, mainly stress fractures, and metatarsal injuries. They are normally caused by an increment in mechanical demand, which is above the body ability to heal and adapt after an overload. Sportive shoes proper adaptation is important to prevent and treat these injuries.

Patients with hallux valgus should wear shoes with a wide toe box and more rigid soles in the forefoot in order to increase space for the widened foot, to decrease friction and mechanical solicitation on the metatarsophalangeal joint, and to protect the joint from wearing associated with valgus misalignment. Due to the decreased capacity to bear weight on the first ray, lesser toe overload and deformities are common in hallux valgus patients. As a consequence, lesions of the plantar plate and progressive claw toe deformities may occur. Instability of the lesser toe metatarsophalangeal joint can be decreased by less flexible shoes, in order to protect these joints from direct load. Toe claw deformity can be handled by the use of extra deep toe box shoes.

Overload lesions as sesamoiditis and stress fractures may affect the sesamoid bones. In these conditions, sportive shoes with midfoot support, cushioning under the toes, and less flexible soles are recommended, in an attempt to decrease pressure under these bones.

A previous study [10] showed that the use of rigid rockers restricts toe dorsiflexion and decreases plantar pressure under the lesser toe metatarsophalangeal joints. Higher plantar pressures on the first metatarsophalangeal joint are expected following the restriction of toe dorsiflexion in this joint in comparison to rockers that do not restrict this motion.

41.4.2 Midfoot Conditions

Patients with midfoot pathologies, such as arthritic conditions affecting the Lisfranc joints, may need a rigid and supportive shoe to reduce the load and stress in these joints, as well the use of insoles to aid treatment.

41.4.3 Rearfoot Conditions

The rearfoot is frequently affected by overload problems. Patients with plantar fasciitis, the most common issue affecting the rearfoot in recreational and professional athletes, will probably benefit from shoes with stiffer and cushioned soles.

Achilles tendinopathy is also common in athletes. This pathology is associated with overload caused by rearfoot misalignments (valgus and varus hindfoot), muscle imbalance, and excessive training. Patients suffering from this problem may need medial supportive shoes, with elevation under the rearfoot.

The posterior tibial tendon is an important dynamic stabilizer of the medial arch of the foot. Tendinopathies affecting this tendon may be related to trauma, overload, and degenerative conditions, decreasing the medial arch support power. As a consequence, overload of static supporters of the arch, such as the deltoid ligament and spring ligament, may occur, with subsequent acquired flat foot deformities. In the early stages of the disease, athletes must be advised to decrease the intensity of exercises and wear medial arch supportive shoes. Peroneal tendon issues may be associated with varus hindfoot. In this situation, a flexible shoe without medial support is helpful.

41.4.3.1 Patients with Special Needs

In many cases, only footwear correction is not enough. When an orthotic or insole is required, it is necessary to fit them in the specific sportive shoe. Many of sportive shoes already have some medial arch support, which should be taken into account during the manufacturing process.

Injury history and previous pathologies should also be discussed with the athlete, as they may predict structures that are subject to overload. Deformities and pathologies from the back, hip, and knee must also be assessed.

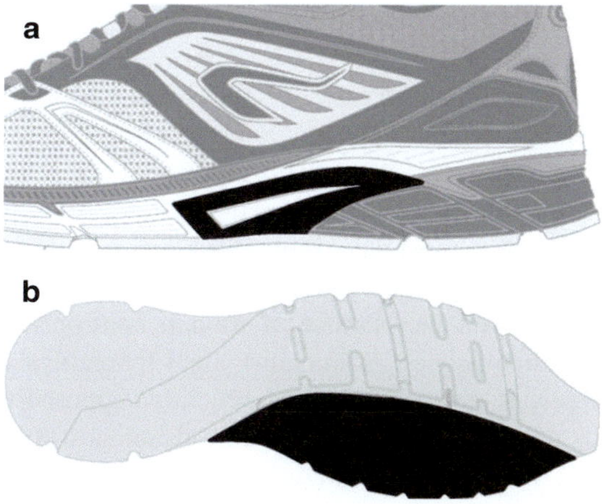

Fig. 41.2 Illustration of technical features designed to prevent overpronation of the feet in runners. (**a**) Polyurethane used in the medial side at the midsole. (**b**) EVA (ethylene-vinyl acetate) foam used at the midsole. **(From Malisoux L et al. Injury risk in runners using standard or motion control shoes: a randomised controlled trial with participant and assessor blinding. *Br J Sports Med.* 2016;50(8):481–487)**

41.5 Types of Running Shoes

Previous reports demonstrated that almost all recreational shod runners are rearfoot strikers [11]. Based on that knowledge, during many years running shoes were developed to relieve rearfoot impact and decrease the chance of lesions related to physical activities.

41.6 Regular Running Shoes

Regular running shoes provide shock absorption properties and support to rearfoot motion during activities. The use of cushioning in running shoes is based on the following assumptions: (1) impact forces while running are a significant cause of injury, (2) running on hard surfaces is a cause of high impact forces, (3) a cushioned shoe can reduce impact forces to a less injurious level, and (4) the potential of the cushioning itself to cause injury is minimal.

The protective effect of normalizing the subtalar joint motion is built on the following assumptions: (1) overpronation and supination are causally linked to overuse injuries, and (2) promoting limited pronation reduces this risk [12].

The use of shoes that provide support and stability to the rearfoot is supported by the fact that motion control shoes correct foot pronation (Fig. 41.2) in the transverse and sagittal planes during stance when compared to neutral shoes and barefoot conditions, decreasing the incidence of injuries in recreational runners, mainly flat feet runners [13, 14]. On the other hand, some studies suggest that the use of stable shoes with medial support to decrease lesions in running athletes is not supported by the literature [15].

Unstable running shoes are related to an increase in lumbar stress and incidence of low back pain in athletes because they intensify lumbar spine muscle solicitation and lumbar spine motion [16].

Another interesting topic is that shoelace closure techniques have been associated with an influence on plantar foot pressures and are a factor that could collaborate on forefoot overload problems in athletes and healthy subjects [17].

41.7 Minimalist Shoes

In recent years, the use of minimalist shoes for running has emerged as a topic of great interest. Esculier et al. [18] defined minimalist shoes as "footwear providing minimal interference with the natural movement of the foot due to its high flexibility, low heel to toe drop, weight and stack height, and the absence of motion control and stability devices." Minimalist shoes theoretically replicate barefoot running, which is supposedly associated with biomechanical advantages [19–21]. However, the literature regarding this matter is controversial.

As previously mentioned, the functional definition of a minimalist shoe is one that promotes kinematic similarities to that of running barefoot. A previous report [22] has determined the maximal specifications that constitute a minimalist shoe (Fig. 41.3):

Mass: ≤200 g
Heel stack height: ≤20 mm
Heel-toe differential: ≤7 mm

Therefore, only shoes with values equal to or lower than these proposed thresholds could be defined as minimalist footwear. Furthermore, a minimalist shoe cannot present any other device that is intended to control the motion of the shoe, such as medial support, a stiff carbon fiber plate, or any structure that alters the interaction of the shoe with the ground.

Some authors advocate that improvements in running economy can be achieved with the use of minimalist shoes. Cheung et al. [20] suggested that running in minimalist shoes requires lower utilization of oxygen, possibly leading to improved performance. Furthermore, previous reports [23] demonstrated an increase in leg and foot muscle volume with the use of minimalist shoes, which could be a protective factor against injuries. However, some studies [24–26] associated the use of minimalist shoes with an increased risk of injury. Firminger et al. [24] observed significant increases in metatarsal strains in recreational runners acutely transitioning to minimalist shoes.

There is evidence in the literature showing that both cushioned running shoes and minimalistic shoes increase ground contact time during walking and running, compared to barefoot conditions. However, this increase is higher with the use of cushioned shoes when compared to minimalist shoes [27].

In a previous report [28], 32% of runners showed a rearfoot strike pattern at the first attempt running barefoot. This led to increased muscle activation and impact accelerations and thereby to a potentially higher risk of injury compared to running shod.

Despite the controversies, most authors [25, 29–31] agree that the transition from traditional to minimalist shoes must be done with caution since runners who are not used to minimalist shoes or barefoot running are more prone to injury during this period. However, there is no standardized protocol in the literature regarding the methods that should be employed during the transition. Fuller et al. [29] suggested that runners should limit their weekly training distance in order to prevent running-related pain. Future studies should look at the efficacy of minimalist shoes in pro-

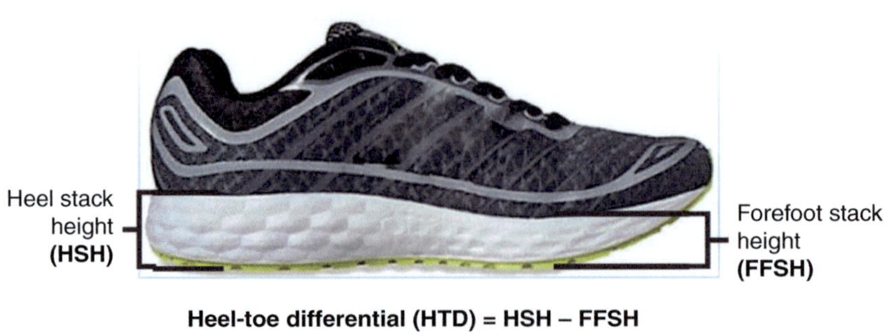

Fig. 41.3 Illustration showing the structure of a running shoe and its specifications. **(From Coetzee DR et al. Conceptualizing minimalist footwear: an objective definition. *J Sports Sci.* 2018;36(8):949–954)**

moting kinematic adaptations in terms of reducing the risk of running-related injury, rather than drawing conclusions on minimalist footwear by grouping runners that adapt biomechanically and those that do not [22]. The literature regarding minimalist shoes is controversial, and there is insufficient evidence either to promote or to demote its use. The physician should be cautious when prescribing minimalist shoes, especially for amateur athletes who are not well adapted.

Further studies are needed in order to clarify the effects of minimalist shoes on running biomechanics and injury rate. Nevertheless, this topic brought to light an important debate, motivating investigations regarding running efficiency and intrinsic muscle strengthening. Ultimately, this knowledge may lead to improvements in running performance and a decreased risk of injury among athletes.

Take-Home Message

The demand for the most appropriate sports footwear is no longer restricted to the professional athlete. The sports health professionals must be capable of prescribing an appropriate shoe, by analyzing the multiple factors involved in the decision. Knowledge regarding foot anatomy, gait biomechanics, and footwear characteristics are essential during this process. Nevertheless, each athlete is unique, and it is hard to predict whether a specific shoe will suit his or her needs. Therefore, the choice should be made on an individual basis, considering the athlete's characteristics and needs.

Fact Box 1

The midsole is considered the most important part of the shoe, providing stability, cushioning, and shock absorption. Distinct materials with different densities are used in an attempt to achieve an optimal balance with respect to these characteristics.

Fact Box 2

The risks and benefits regarding minimalist footwear are still controversial in the literature. When opting for a minimalist shoe, most authors agree that the transition should be made with caution, respecting the adaptation period.

References

1. Khan MN, Jacobs BC, Ashbaugh S. Considerations in footwear and orthotics. Prim Care Clin Office Pract. 2013;40(4):1001–12. https://doi.org/10.1016/j.pop.2013.08.013.
2. LeCursi N. Sports shoes and orthoses. In: DeLee & Drez's orthopaedic sports medicine. 4th ed. Philadelphia: Saunders; 2014. p. 1384–91. https://doi.org/10.1016/B978-1-4557-4376-6.00115-3.
3. Subotnick S. Evolution of athletic footwear. In: Werd MB, Knight EL, Langer PR, editors. Athletic footwear and orthoses in sports medicine. 2nd ed. Cham: Springer; 2017. p. 3–18. https://doi.org/10.1007/978-3-319-52136-7.
4. Blazer MM, Jamrog LB, Schnack LL. Does the shoe fit? Considerations for proper shoe fitting. Orthop Nurs. 2018;37(3):169–74. https://doi.org/10.1097/NOR.0000000000000447.
5. Werd M, Knight E. Insights on prescribing athletic footwear and orthoses: the game plan. In: Werd MB, Knight EL, Langer PR, editors. Athletic footwear and orthoses in sports medicine. 2nd ed. Cham: Springer; 2017. p. 165–80. https://doi.org/10.1007/978-3-319-52136-7.
6. Jones G, Asghar A, Llewellyn DJ. The epidemiology of rock-climbing injuries. Br J Sports Med. 2008;42(9):773–8. https://doi.org/10.1136/bjsm.2007.037978.
7. McHenry RD, Arnold GP, Wang W, Abboud RJ. Footwear in rock climbing: current practice. Foot (Edinb). 2015;25(3):152–8. https://doi.org/10.1016/j.foot.2015.07.007.
8. Elftman H. The transverse tarsal joint and its control. Clin Orthop. 1960;16:41–6. http://www.ncbi.nlm.nih.gov/pubmed/13819895.
9. Knapik JJ, Trone DW, Swedler DI, et al. Injury reduction effectiveness of assigning running shoes based on plantar shape in marine corps basic training. Am J Sports Med. 2010;38(9):1759–67. https://doi.org/10.1177/0363546510369548.
10. Reints R, Hijmans JM, Burgerhof JGM, Postema K, Verkerke GJ. Effects of flexible and rigid rocker profiles on in-shoe pressure. Gait Posture.

2017;58:287–93. https://doi.org/10.1016/j.gaitpost.2017.08.008.

11. de Almeida MO, Saragiotto BT, Yamato TP, Lopes AD. Is the rearfoot pattern the most frequently foot strike pattern among recreational shod distance runners? Phys Ther Sport. 2015;16(1):29–33. https://doi.org/10.1016/j.ptsp.2014.02.005.
12. Richards CE, Magin PJ, Callister R. Is your prescription of distance running shoes evidence-based? Br J Sports Med. 2009;43(3):159–62. https://doi.org/10.1136/bjsm.2008.046680.
13. Anselmo DS, Skolnik J, Keeter E, El-Sayed AM, Love E. Comparative evaluation of radiographic parameters of foot pronation in two different conditions versus barefoot. J Am Podiatr Med Assoc. 2018;108(4):285–91. https://doi.org/10.7547/16-144.
14. Malisoux L, Chambon N, Delattre N, Gueguen N, Urhausen A, Theisen D. Injury risk in runners using standard or motion control shoes: a randomised controlled trial with participant and assessor blinding. Br J Sports Med. 2016;50(8):481–7. https://doi.org/10.1136/bjsports-2015-095031.
15. Van Gent RN, Siem D, Van Middeloop M, Van Os AG, Bierma-Zeinstra SMA, Koes BW. Incidence and determinants of lower extremity running injuries in long distance runners: a systematic review. Sport Geneeskd. 2007;40(4):16–29. https://doi.org/10.1136/bjsm.2006.033548.
16. Lisón JF, Ortega-Santana B, Antón-Nogués Á, et al. Effects and underlying mechanisms of unstable shoes on chronic low back pain: a randomized controlled trial. Clin Rehabil. 2018;32(5):654–62. https://doi.org/10.1177/0269215517753972.
17. Rahemi H, Armstrong DG, Enriquez A, Owl J, Talal TK, Najafi B. Lace up for healthy feet: the impact of shoe closure on plantar stress response. J Diabetes Sci Technol. 2017;11(4):678–84. https://doi.org/10.1177/1932296817703669.
18. Esculier JF, Dubois B, Dionne CE, Leblond J, Roy JS. A consensus definition and rating scale for minimalist shoes. J Foot Ankle Res. 2015;8(1):1–9. https://doi.org/10.1186/s13047-015-0094-5.
19. Barcellona MG, Buckley L, Palmer LJM, et al. The effect of minimalist footwear and instruction on running: an observational study. BMJ Open Sport Exerc Med. 2017;3(1):e000160. https://doi.org/10.1136/bmjsem-2016-000160.
20. Cheung RT, Ngai SP. Effects of footwear on running economy in distance runners: a meta-analytical review. J Sci Med Sport. 2016;19(3):260–6. https://doi.org/10.1016/j.jsams.2015.03.002.
21. Fuller JT, Thewlis D, Tsiros MD, Brown NAT, Buckley JD. Effects of a minimalist shoe on running economy and 5-km running performance. J Sports Sci. 2016;34(18):1740–5. https://doi.org/10.1080/02640414.2015.1136071.
22. Coetzee DR, Albertus Y, Tam N, Tucker R. Conceptualizing minimalist footwear: an objective definition. J Sports Sci. 2018;36(8):949–54. https://doi.org/10.1080/02640414.2017.1346816.
23. Chen TLW, Sze LKY, Davis IS, Cheung RTH. Effects of training in minimalist shoes on the intrinsic and extrinsic foot muscle volume. Clin Biomech. 2016;36:8–13. https://doi.org/10.1016/j.clinbiomech.2016.05.010.
24. Firminger CR, Fung A, Loundagin LL, Edwards WB. Effects of footwear and stride length on metatarsal strains and failure in running. Clin Biomech. 2017;49:8–15. https://doi.org/10.1016/j.clinbiomech.2017.08.006.
25. Fuller JT, Thewlis D, Buckley JD, Brown NAT, Hamill J, Tsiros MD. Body mass and weekly training distance influence the pain and injuries experienced by runners using minimalist shoes: a randomized controlled trial. Am J Sports Med. 2017;45(5):1162–70. https://doi.org/10.1177/0363546516682497.
26. Salzler MJ, Bluman EM, Noonan S, Chiodo CP, de Asla RJ. Injuries observed in minimalist runners. Foot Ankle Int. 2012;33(4):262–6. https://doi.org/10.3113/FAI.2012.0262.
27. Roca-Dols A, Losa-Iglesias ME, Sánchez-Gómez R, et al. Effect of the cushioning running shoes in ground contact time of phases of gait. J Mech Behav Biomed Mater. 2018;88:196–200. https://doi.org/10.1016/j.jmbbm.2018.08.032.
28. Lucas-Cuevas AG, Priego Quesada JI, Giménez JV, Aparicio I, Jimenez-Perez I, Pérez-Soriano P. Initiating running barefoot: effects on muscle activation and impact accelerations in habitually rearfoot shod runners. Eur J Sport Sci. 2016;16(8):1145–52. https://doi.org/10.1080/17461391.2016.1197317.
29. Fuller JT, Thewlis D, Tsiros MD, Brown NAT, Buckley JD. Six-week transition to minimalist shoes improves running economy and time-trial performance. J Sci Med Sport. 2017;20(12):1117–22. https://doi.org/10.1016/j.jsams.2017.04.013.
30. Salzler MJ, Kirwan HJ, Scarborough DM, Walker JT, Guarino AJ, Berkson EM. Injuries observed in a prospective transition from traditional to minimalist footwear: correlation of high impact transient forces and lower injury severity. Phys Sportsmed. 2016;44(4):373–9. https://doi.org/10.1080/00913847.2016.1238282.
31. Warne JP, Gruber AH. Transitioning to minimal footwear: a systematic review of methods and future clinical recommendations. Sport Med Open. 2017;3(1):33. https://doi.org/10.1186/s40798-017-0096-x.

Part VIII

Biologics in Sports Injuries

Biologic Treatment in Tendon and Muscle Injuries

42

Moises Cohen, Gustavo Gonçalves Arliani, and Camila Cohen Kaleka

42.1 Introduction

In the last decades, we have observed a great increase in the number of people practicing sports around the world. Much of this increase is due to widespread media coverage of the health benefits of regular physical exercise, such as improved quality of life and reduced risk of various diseases [1].

However, these beneficial effects must be balanced with injuries that are to some extent unavoidable [2]. The estimated number of sports-related injuries annually in the UK is 10 million [3]. In Sweden the incidence of sports injuries is approximately 22.5 per 1000 inhabitants per year [4].

These numbers show not only the enormous medical but also the social and economic importance of the problem. Most of these injuries are not serious but are usually painful and lead to a temporary withdrawal from work and sports activities [5].

M. Cohen (✉) · G. G. Arliani
Department of Orthopedics and Traumatology, UNIFESP, São Paulo, Brazil

C. C. Kaleka
Cohen Institute, São Paulo, São Paulo, Brazil

Hospital Israelista Albert Einstein, São Paulo, Brazil
e-mail: camilacohen@kaleka.com.br

42.2 Muscle Injury

In this context, muscle injuries are among the most common, accounting for approximately 10–55% of all sports injuries. Muscle injuries can be caused by contusion, stretching, lacerations, and other mechanisms [6]. These injuries correspond to approximately 40% of all soccer injuries and 25% of all injury-time withdrawals. And 15–20% of these muscular injuries are recurrences of previous injuries [7].

Woods et al. have described that 12% of injuries in professional soccer players affect hamstring muscles, and the financial burden of these injuries is estimated at 74.7 million pounds sterling [8].

Despite the enormous advances in medicine in recent decades, the treatment of muscle injuries has changed little and still consists of the use of the PRICE protocol (protection, rest, ice, compression, and elevation of the affected limb), medications, and physiotherapy for analgesia, muscular stretching, and strengthening [9]. In the case of mild muscle injuries, these treatment modalities are satisfactory. However, moderate and severe muscle injuries usually lead to prolonged absence and tend to form large areas of fibrotic tissue at the site of the injury that can lead to loss of strength and function as well as increase chances of a new injury [10].

S. Rocha Piedade et al. (eds.), *The Sports Medicine Physician*,
https://doi.org/10.1007/978-3-030-10433-7_42

Another key factor is that none of these treatments addresses the major problems of muscle injury that are cell loss and scar tissue formation. In addition, routine treatments do not improve the number, proliferation, and differentiation of satellite cells [11]. Therefore, the efforts to develop new treatments that promote a faster and more complete recovery after muscle injuries with improved function and lower incidence of reinjuries are fundamental.

In recent years, some biological treatments have been studied with promising initial results: platelet-rich plasma (PRP), mesenchymal cells, and losartan and gene therapy.

42.2.1 Platelet-Rich Plasma

Platelet-rich plasma (PRP) can be defined as a blood derivative with higher platelet concentration than blood [12]. PRP is prepared from an initial volume of blood of the patient that is processed and centrifuged to separate the various blood components [13]. This type of treatment has been investigated due to promising initial results, low costs, and minimally invasive form of application. The concept of the use of this technique in the treatment of muscular lesions is that after the injection of PRP in the injured muscle, the local development of the platelet-rich fibrin structure provides hemostasis and allows the slow delivery of growth factors and cytokines from platelets and plasma, with anti-inflammatory and regenerative effects. PRP was effective in stimulating the proliferation and migration of mesenchymal cells in response to the release of some specific growth factors by platelets. Another possible action of PRP is the stimulation of proliferation of fibroblasts in the muscle [14, 15]. However, excessive deposition of type 1 collagen by fibroblasts can lead to the formation of large areas of fibrosis. The control of this process is done by TGF-β1, which may be present in great concentration in the platelet α granules, and we know that the formation of large areas of fibrosis in the muscle can lead to lesion recurrence as well as a decrease in functional capacity.

There are many protocols for preparation of platelet-rich plasma (open and closed systems, number of different centrifugation processes), so the products obtained differ in terms of cellular and molecular compositions. Distinct clinical findings are attributed both to variability in PRP formulations and to variability in application protocols. The perception that PRP was not a unique and similar product led some authors to classify the PRPs. The initial classification is still the easiest and most intuitive and divides PRPS into pure PRP (pPRP) and PRP with leukocytes (L-PRP) [16]. However, there are other widely used classifications such as PAW which is based on absolute number of platelets (P), platelet activation (A), and the presence or absence of leukocytes (W) [17].

Currently PRP is used in the definitive or coadjuvant treatment of many musculoskeletal and tendinous disorders. However, the results and outcomes in the treatment of muscle injuries are still controversial. Numerous doubts exist regarding the best preparation, ideal concentration of platelets and specific growth factors, and a better time to start treatment with PRP after a muscle injury.

Delos et al., in a study with rats, performed PRP applications acutely (2 h) and late (1 and 3 days) after gastrocnemius injury. The authors did not find functional and histological differences independent of the moment of application (early or late) [18]. A randomized clinical trial, however, showed improvement in pain and less time to return to sports after a single application of PRP (3 mL) after acute grade 2 hamstring injury (<7 days). In this study, patients treated with PRP associated with rehabilitation returned to sports on average 26.7 days after injury, whereas the control group treated only with physical therapy took, on average, 42.5 days [19].

On the other hand, a similar study did not find differences in time for complete recovery of patients with gastrocnemius or rectus femoris injury after PRP application (4–8 mL) with drainage of the hematoma when compared to the control group (isolated drainage). The authors also found no differences in pain improvement [20].

Some systematic reviews on the subject have concluded that despite the promising concept, animal and clinical studies with good results, effective treatment of muscle injuries with PRP has not yet been confirmed by recent randomized clinical trials. Therefore, there is still insufficient support in the literature for any benefit in terms of pain, function, return to sports, and recurrence of injuries using PRP applications in the treatment of muscle injuries [21, 22]. One way forward would be the customization and individualization of PRP formulations according to the patient and type of lesion. In this way, we would guarantee the beneficial effects of PRP in certain types of tissues avoiding their potential deleterious effects.

42.2.2 Mesenchymal cells

Muscle injuries and their reinjuries are a great challenge for sports medicine, as they cause great problems in sports, economic, and social areas. Despite the great capacity of healing and regeneration of muscles, a fully injured muscle regains only part of its function and around 50% of its strength [23]. The main treatments used today do not address the main problem of muscle injuries that is the cellular loss. Mesenchymal cell transplantation meets this requirement and has been tested in the treatment of muscle damage.

Mesenchymal cells are found in large numbers in adipose tissue and bone marrow. The Mesenchymal Stem Cell Committee of the International Society for Cell Therapy proposed three criteria for defining mesenchymal cells: (1) they should be adherent when maintained in standard culture; (2) must express CD105, CD73, and CD90 and exhibit poor expression of CD34, CD45, CD14 or CD11b, CD79a or CD19, and HLA-DR in culture; and (3) must have the potential to differentiate into osteoblasts, adipocytes, and chondrocytes in vitro [24].

Mesenchymal cells have multiple effects on the body that include anti-inflammatory and immunomodulatory action. Previous studies have reported that mesenchymal cells contain several vascular and multipotent cells. These cells would be responsible for the secretion of cytokines and growth factors, such as vascular endothelial growth factor (VEGF) and hepatocyte growth factor (HGF) [25, 26]. Andrade et al. tested in mice the use of mesenchymal cells in the treatment of muscle injuries and reinjuries. After 14 and 28 days of application, the authors observed a faster recovery and improved muscle function. However, they didn't observe any improvement in the scar formation tissue (fibrosis) in the injured area [11].

The application of mesenchymal cells derived from adipose tissue accelerates muscle repair and improves the function of the injured muscle with the promotion of angiogenesis and myogenesis and the prevention of fibrosis formation through the secretion of growth factors. The authors also believe that this mechanism of action is more important in faster muscle regeneration than the proliferation and differentiation of mesenchymal cells injected into the tissue. Recent studies have shown that direct cell differentiation is not always essential, as it is unlikely that these cells differentiate over such a short time in the setting of an acute muscle injury.

Despite the great prospect and hope in the success of mesenchymal cells in the treatment of muscular injuries, more studies are required, with larger samples and longer follow-up in order to have more safety and confidence in this treatment modality [26].

42.2.3 Losartan

Losartan is classically an antihypertensive drug that acts by blocking the angiotensin II receptor and is used in the treatment of patients with systemic arterial hypertension, congestive heart failure, and sequelae of these diseases [27, 28]. The use of angiotensin-converting enzyme inhibitors and angiotensin II receptor blockers in patients with renal, hepatic, and pulmonary diseases caused a decrease in fibrotic tissue formation and an improvement in the function of these organs [29, 30].

The development of fibrosis after muscle injuries is a major concern of physicians involved in the treatment of athletes due to the increased risk of reinjury and functional loss caused by scar formation in the injured muscle. The promising results in previous research incentivated new lines of research.

Bedair et al. [31] demonstrated a reduction in fibrosis area and increase in the number of fibers in the gastrocnemius muscle of rats after acute muscle injury and administration of losartan. The authors concluded that the use of losartan is safe and can aid not only in the treatment of sports-related injuries but also in muscular dystrophies, trauma, and postoperative injuries.

However, the optimal timing for administration of the drug is still controversial. Kobayashi et al. [32] investigated the dose and the best time to initiate treatment with losartan after acute muscle injury. The authors concluded that the standard dose of 10 mg/kg/day, used for hypertensive patients, started 3 or 7 days after the injury, led to a significant increase in muscle regeneration, a decrease in local fibrosis, and improvement of function.

Other studies have sought to evaluate the association of losartan with other substances such as platelet-rich plasma and mesenchymal cells. The concept is to take advantage of the strengths of PRP therapy and to use losartan to inhibit TGFβ and consequently the formation of fibrosis. Combination therapy of PRP and losartan improved muscle healing, increasing angiogenesis and follistatin expression and reducing Smad2/3 expression and fibrosis development. These results suggest that blocking TGFβ expression with losartan improves the effect of PRP therapy on muscle healing [33].

A similar study was conducted in rats comparing the isolated use of mesenchymal cells and combined with losartan in the treatment of muscle injuries. The simultaneous treatment of muscle contusions with mesenchymal cells and losartan significantly reduced fibrotic scar formation, increased fiber numbers, and improved muscle functional recovery. These effects would have been caused, at least in part, by the regulation of Smad7 and MyoD with the inhibition of TGFβ [34].

However, despite promising results, quality studies in humans are still needed to assess the safety and efficacy of this medication in the musculoskeletal system. However, these studies are fundamental for the development of biological treatments that aim to accelerate and improve muscle healing after injury.

42.2.4 Gene Therapy

Another promising treatment modality for muscle injuries is gene therapy. The principle of treatment is based on the transfer of genes to provide genetic products at the site where the tissue damage occurred [35].

The transfer of the genetic material is performed by a vector that transports the genes of interest to the host cells. Viruses are widely used as vectors because of their inherent ability to efficiently translocate their own genetic material. In order to create a vector for gene therapy, viral genome sequences that contribute to virulence and disease are usually removed and replaced with genes of interest. However, this method still has some safety and cost-benefit concerns [36].

Some alternatives have been tested in an attempt to improve and accelerate the process of muscle healing after injury. Schertzer et al. [37] carried out the transfer of IGF-1 gene using adenovirus as vector to improve angiogenesis and muscle regeneration. The authors concluded that gene transfer was superior to systemic administration of IGF-1 but that both methods were effective in the treatment of muscle injuries. Other authors promoted gene transfer of decorin in order to decrease the expression of TGFβ and formation of fibrotic tissue [38].

Currently, there is extensive literature supporting the concept of the use of gene therapy in the repair and regeneration of lesions of the musculoskeletal system; however the first clinical trials in humans are still ongoing [39]. Therefore, we must await the results of the studies already in progress and develop new quality studies in humans in order to confirm the safety, economic viability, and efficiency of this treatment modality.

Best Evidence

- Huard J, Lu A, Mu X, Guo P, Li Y. Muscle injuries and repair: what's new on the horizon! Cells Tissues Organs. 2016;202(3–4):227–36.
- Grassi A, Napoli F, Romandini I, Samuelsson K, Zaffagnini S, Candrian C, et al. Is platelet-rich plasma (PRP) effective in the treatment of acute muscle injuries? A Systematic review and meta-analysis. Sports Med. 2018;48(4):971–89.
- Kobayashi M, Ota S, Terada S, Kawakami Y, Otsuka T, Fu FH, et al. The combined use of losartan and muscle-derived stem cells significantly improves the functional recovery of muscle in a young mouse model of contusion injuries. Am J Sports Med. 2016;44(12):3252–61.

42.3 Tendon Injuries

Acute and chronic tendon injuries affect millions of people in both occupational and athletic settings each year. With the increasing popularity of sports activities, the frequency of sports-related lesions, such as tendon injuries, is rapidly increasing [40]. Tendon problems are one of the main causes of musculoskeletal morbidity, and it has been reported that 30–50% of all sports lesions are painful tendon injuries [41]. Tendon lesions may be caused by traumatic events or chronic degenerative changes, making tendon weaker and more prone to ruptures.

Healing of acute injuries results in the formation of scar tissue in tendons, which have inferior mechanical strength that makes them susceptible to reinjury. On the other hand, the current treatment of chronic tendon injury (or tendinopathy) is largely palliative because of the incomplete understanding of the tendon disorder [41]. The tendon healing process is slow, and multiple phases are well-defined, from inflammatory cytokine recruitment to growth factors and reparative cell involvement [42].

In recent years, new treatment option involving biologic has been used in orthopedic surgery and sports medicine to treat tendon injuries [43]. Nowadays, the aim of the treatment is the clinical application of biologically derived materials to stimulate the repair or regeneration of musculoskeletal tissues. The orthobiologic approaches include the administration of hyaluronic acid or biological factors, such as platelet-rich plasma (PRP) or growth factors. With the advent of those, several options exist for increasing the strength and ability of the repair, as well as decreasing the length of the recovery period [42].

Regenerative medicine approaches may be indicated in the case of tissue healing significantly impaired due to aging, disease, or the presence of an extended lesion [44].

42.3.1 Platelet-Rich Plasma (PRP)

PRPs can be used in the management of tendinopathy if we improve our understanding of pathophysiology and to integrate molecular knowledge about PRP participation in healing mechanisms [42].

Development of PRP treatments is challenging because a typical group of patients with tendinopathy does not exist, as it affects multiple segments of the population. Moreover, the pathophysiology and origin of pain are not elucidated yet. Although some degree of success has been achieved, PRP is not considered standard medical treatment, and it is largely not paid nor reimbursed by insurance companies. However, the arguments for using PRP in tendinopathy are increasing, and its potential to rebalance inflammation merits further research. Moreover, PRP contains tendoinductive factors that can drive the fate of stem cells. Tailoring PRPs to the specific needs of the host tendon has not been possible to date, because unanswered questions remain about the characteristics of tendinopathy within the different stages of progression [45].

There is still no consensus as to whether PRP confers a beneficial effect, as not all trials have failed to demonstrate a positive benefit. Six systematic reviews published between 2010 and 2014 assess the effectiveness of PRP in tendinopathy [46–51]. Despite analyzing the same data, they reported contrasting conclusions, from concluding that PRP is efficacious to finding that there is "strong evidence against platelet-rich plasma" [46–49]. The majority of comments stated that there is great difficulty reaching a conclusion because of the variance of the type of PRP produced. In a Cochrane review of PRP in soft tissue injuries, Moraes et al. [51] indicated that "there is need for standardization of PRP preparation methods." However most of the authors state that "it would be better to break out the results by specific study design and PRP type" [49].

One critical component that affects PRP preparations is the presence or absence of white blood cells (WBCs) or leukocytes (neutrophils, monocytes, macrophages, and lymphocytes), which can be beneficial because they stimulate the immune response against infections; promote chemotaxis, proliferation, and differentiation of cells; and induce extracellular matrix production and angiogenesis. Owing to these properties, PRP-containing leukocytes (L-PRP) are often used to treat traumatic injuries [40].

Thus, a meta-analysis was performed and published in 2016 to assess the comparative effectiveness of PRP types in tendinopathy [42]. A total of 18 studies (1066 participants) were included, and all treatments consisted of intratendinous injections with a prior administration of 1–2 mL of local anesthetic (7 studies with autologous blood injection, 10 studies with leukocyte-rich PRP produced from the buffy coat layer, and 1 with leukocyte-poor PRP) [42]. The meta-analysis showed that the outcome of PRP is different depending on the method of preparation of PRP and the injection technique; for that reason, both informations should always be included to evaluate the study results. Nevertheless, this meta-analysis found strong evidence that leukocyte-rich PRP can improve outcome in tendinopathy [42].

A study conducted with tenocytes isolated from patellar tendons of rabbits indicates that the use of L-PRP to treat injured tendons may lead to scar formation in healing tendons [40]. Moreover, L-PRP induces extensive catabolic responses in differentiated tenocytes, which may delay the repair of acutely damaged tendon matrix and new matrix formation, thus slowing the healing of injured tendons. Last, because L-PRP induces inflammatory responses in tenocytes, its use to treat the already-inflamed tendinopathic tendons may only exacerbate the tendon disorder by prolonging the inflammatory phase, thus impairing the healing process and leading to increased pain in patients. Caution should therefore be exercised when using PRP.

Based on the data from this study, the authors suggest the use of pure PRP to augment the repair of tendinopathic tendons because of its anabolic properties and low inflammatory effects [40]. On the other hand, it is plausible that the strong anabolic effects of pure PRP may cause fibrosis/scar tissue formation in acutely injured tendons simply because tenocytes differentiated from stem cells after pure PRP treatment produce too much collagen in the wound areas. Therefore, they suggest that whether to use L-PRP or pure PRP depends on the type of tendon injury (acute vs. chronic) and treatment phase (early- or late-stage healing) in clinical settings [40].

42.3.2 Mesenchymal Stem Cells (MSC)

A growing field of research has explored tendon, bone, and cartilage regeneration using mesenchymal stem cells (MSCs), because of their multipotency and because they are relatively easy to harvest. Great expectations arose from the use of MSCs in regenerative medicine in the last decade, although both the potential and the drawbacks of this method remain under reflection [52].

Stem cells are cells with the capacity to differentiate into multiple types of tissues and able to self-renew. They are able to establish daughter-cell lines for tissue generation [53]. They have three main characteristics: multipotency, capacity to adhere to plastic, and the presence of stem cell-specific antigens on their surface with the absence of *negative markers* that are used to identify other cell lineages, such as hematopoietic endothelial cells (e.g., CD 14, 31, 34, and 35) [54, 55]. A common source of MSCs is the bone marrow, especially from the iliac crest. The cells harvested from the bone marrow are called

BMDSCs. Another common source of MSCs is the adipose tissue. In that case, they are commonly called ADSCs. They have an advantage: they are more readily accessible than BMDSCs. The poor regenerative capacity of tendons has greatly encouraged the research in finding new ways to aid in their repair after a tear. The good results found in animal models are encouraging, but there is lack of clinical studies supporting the use of stem cells in clinical practice. So, a recommendation for the routine use of stem cells cannot be made as yet [55].

Further research is needed to determine whether MSCs are an effective treatment option in augmentation of tendon healing. Also, the long-term safety of these cells and the best scaffold for their seeding and growth have to be demonstrated with larger animal model studies and randomized clinical trials with a longer follow-up period [56].

Nowadays there are only a few orthopedic studies that investigate the use of MSCs in the clinical practice. Some studies showed good results in terms of outcome scores, ultrasound appearance, pain, and mechanical performances in the treatment of lateral epicondylitis of the elbow [57, 58]. A study was performed even regarding patellar tendinopathy on a population on 60 patients that were treated alternative with skin-derived tenocyte-like cells (N = 33) or plasma (N = 27) [59]. There was an improvement in clinical scores in the group treated with the stem cells (VISA score) with a concomitant significant reduction of the thickness of the tendon. Ultrasonography demonstrated improvements in tendon hypoechogenicity and tear size in both groups.

The progress achieved with the rapid development of biomaterial-based strategies for tendon regeneration has not yielded broad benefits to clinical patients. In addition to the interplay between stem cells and biomaterials, the innate immune response to biomaterials also plays a determinant role in tissue regeneration. One of the principles for biomaterial development in tendon regeneration is to stimulate tenogenic differentiation of stem cells. However, recent progress indicated that innate immune cells, especially macrophages, can also respond to the material cues and undergo phenotypical changes, which will either facilitate or hinder tissue regeneration. This process has been, to some extent, neglected by traditional strategies and may partially explain the unsatisfactory outcomes of previous studies; thus, more researchers have turned their focus on developing immunoregenerative biomaterials to enhance tendon regeneration [60].

42.3.3 Growth Factors

The use of growth factors for healing of musculoskeletal injuries is relatively recent. Recombinant growth factors were first considered and proposed, but the high costs gradually reduced their use, in favor of autologous blood products. Several growth factors are expressed as tendons heal, but it remains unknown whether their combined application enhances the healing process. In an animal study, the authors concluded that the implantation of a GF-loaded collagen sponge at the time of surgery could provide a promising treatment, especially in high-performance athletes and revision cases prone to re-rupture. For conservative treatment, tiered percutaneous GF application could be an option for improving clinical outcome [61].

42.3.4 Prolotherapy

Prolotherapy, also called proliferation therapy, is an injection-based treatment used in chronic musculoskeletal conditions. It has been characterized as an alternative medicine practice [62]. It consists by rehabilitation of an incompetent structure, such as ligament or tendon, by the induced proliferation of new cells. Prolotherapy is differentiated from other regenerative injection therapies, such as platelet-rich plasma (PRP) and stem cell injection by the absence of a biologic agent. The most commonly used prolotherapy solution reported in current literature is hypertonic dextrose, a simple monosaccharide synonymous with glucose [62]. The mechanism of action hypothesized of dextrose prolotherapy is that injection of dextrose causes a small amount of cell irritation or necrosis that results from osmotic shock [63]. This method of intentional small-scale cell trauma at the injection site initiates the body's wound healing cascade of inflammation, granulation tissue formation, and matrix formation and remodeling, promoting local healing of chronically injured tissues [63].

The use of prolotherapy injections for chronic, painful tendon and fascia overuse conditions has been predominantly guided by anecdotal clinical success [64]. Randomized controlled trial studies have demonstrated Level I–III evidence for injection of 10–25% dextrose in areas of damaged tendon to manage Achilles tendinosis, plantar fasciitis rotator cuff tendinopathy, and lateral epicondylitis [65–69].

Best Evidence

- Fitzpatrick J, Bulsara M, Zheng MH. The effectiveness of platelet-rich plasma in the treatment of tendinopathy: a meta-analysis of randomized controlled clinical trials. Am J Sports Med. 2016;45(1):226–33.
- Moraes VY, Lenza M, Tamaoki MJ, Faloppa F, Belloti JC. Platelet- rich therapies for musculoskeletal soft tissue injuries. Cochrane Database Syst Rev. 2014;4:CD010071.
- Krogh TP, Bartels EM, Ellingsen T, et al. Comparative effectiveness of injection therapies in lateral epicondylitis: a systematic review and network meta-analysis of randomized controlled trials. Am J Sports Med. 2013;41(6):1435–46.

Take-Home Message

Muscle and tendon injuries are very common, and to better approach those injuries, more medical research are warranted to advance in the treatment and to enhance tissue healing. New therapies are emerging with promising results, but further investigations are required to better define indications techniques, modalities, safety, and cost-effectiveness.

References

1. Arliani GG, Astur DC, Yamada RK, Yamada AF, da Rocha Correa Fernandes A, Ejnisman B, et al. Professional football can be considered a healthy sport? Knee Surg Sports Traumatol Arthrosc. 2016;24(12):3907–11.
2. Maffulli N, Longo UG, Gougoulias N, Caine D, Denaro V. Sport injuries: a review of outcomes. Br Med Bull. 2011;97:47–80.
3. Nicholl JP, Coleman P, Williams BT. The epidemiology of sports and exercise related injury in the United Kingdom. Br J Sports Med. 1995;29(4):232–8.
4. Lindqvist KS, Timpka T, Bjurulf P. Injuries during leisure physical activity in a Swedish municipality. Scand J Soc Med. 1996;24(4):282–92.
5. Galer BS, Rowbotham M, Perander J, Devers A, Friedman E. Topical diclofenac patch relieves minor sports injury pain: results of a multicenter controlled clinical trial. J Pain Symptom Manage. 2000;19(4):287–94.
6. Jarvinen TA, Jarvinen TL, Kaariainen M, Aarimaa V, Vaittinen S, Kalimo H, et al. Muscle injuries: optimising recovery. Best Pract Res Clin Rheumatol. 2007;21(2):317–31.
7. Ekstrand J, Hagglund M, Walden M. Epidemiology of muscle injuries in professional football (soccer). Am J Sports Med. 2011;39(6):1226–32.
8. Woods C, Hawkins R, Hulse M, Hodson A. The Football Association Medical Research Programme: an audit of injuries in professional football-analysis of preseason injuries. Br J Sports Med. 2002;36(6):436–41; discussion 41.
9. Manning MR, Levy RS. Soccer. Phys Med Rehabil Clin N Am. 2006;17(3):677–95, vii.
10. Huard J, Lu A, Mu X, Guo P, Li Y. Muscle injuries and repair: what's new on the horizon! Cells Tissues Organs. 2016;202(3–4):227–36.
11. Andrade BM, Baldanza MR, Ribeiro KC, Porto A, Pecanha R, Fortes FS, et al. Bone marrow mesenchymal cells improve muscle function in a skeletal muscle re-injury model. PLoS One. 2015;10(6):e0127561.
12. Filardo G, Kon E, Roffi A, Di Matteo B, Merli ML, Marcacci M. Platelet-rich plasma: why intra-articular? A systematic review of preclinical studies and clinical evidence on PRP for joint degeneration. Knee Surg Sports Traumatol Arthrosc. 2015;23(9):2459–74.
13. Malanga G, Abdelshahed D, Jayaram P. Orthobiologic interventions using ultrasound guidance. Phys Med Rehabil Clin N Am. 2016;27(3):717–31.
14. Andia I, Abate M. Platelet-rich plasma in the treatment of skeletal muscle injuries. Expert Opin Biol Ther. 2015;15(7):987–99.
15. Vidal B, Serrano AL, Tjwa M, Suelves M, Ardite E, De Mori R, et al. Fibrinogen drives dystrophic muscle fibrosis via a TGFbeta/alternative macrophage activation pathway. Genes Dev. 2008;22(13):1747–52.
16. Dohan Ehrenfest DM, Rasmusson L, Albrektsson T. Classification of platelet concentrates: from pure

platelet-rich plasma (P-PRP) to leucocyte- and platelet-rich fibrin (L-PRF). Trends Biotechnol. 2009;27(3):158–67.
17. DeLong JM, Russell RP, Mazzocca AD. Platelet-rich plasma: the PAW classification system. Arthroscopy. 2012;28(7):998–1009.
18. Delos D, Leineweber MJ, Chaudhury S, Alzoobaee S, Gao Y, Rodeo SA. The effect of platelet-rich plasma on muscle contusion healing in a rat model. Am J Sports Med. 2014;42(9):2067–74.
19. MS AH, Mohamed Ali MR, Yusof A, George J, Lee LP. Platelet-rich plasma injections for the treatment of hamstring injuries: a randomized controlled trial. Am J Sports Med. 2014;42(10):2410–8.
20. Martinez-Zapata MJ, Orozco L, Balius R, Soler R, Bosch A, Rodas G, et al. Efficacy of autologous platelet-rich plasma for the treatment of muscle rupture with haematoma: a multicentre, randomised, double-blind, placebo-controlled clinical trial. Blood Transfus. 2016;14(2):245–54.
21. Grassi A, Napoli F, Romandini I, Samuelsson K, Zaffagnini S, Candrian C, et al. Is platelet-rich plasma (PRP) effective in the treatment of acute muscle injuries? A systematic review and meta-analysis. Sports Med. 2018;48(4):971–89.
22. Andia I, Maffulli N. Muscle and tendon injuries: the role of biological interventions to promote and assist healing and recovery. Arthroscopy. 2015;31(5):999–1015.
23. Noonan TJ, Garrett WE Jr. Muscle strain injury: diagnosis and treatment. J Am Acad Orthop Surg. 1999;7(4):262–9.
24. Dominici M, Le Blanc K, Mueller I, Slaper-Cortenbach I, Marini F, Krause D, et al. Minimal criteria for defining multipotent mesenchymal stromal cells. The International Society for Cellular Therapy position statement. Cytotherapy. 2006;8(4):315–7.
25. Iyer SS, Rojas M. Anti-inflammatory effects of mesenchymal stem cells: novel concept for future therapies. Expert Opin Biol Ther. 2008;8(5):569–81.
26. Uccelli A, Moretta L, Pistoia V. Mesenchymal stem cells in health and disease. Nat Rev Immunol. 2008;8(9):726–36.
27. Mori R, Kamei N, Okawa S, Nakabayashi A, Yokota K, Higashi Y, et al. Promotion of skeletal muscle repair in a rat skeletal muscle injury model by local injection of human adipose tissue-derived regenerative cells. J Tissue Eng Regen Med. 2015;9(10):1150–60.
28. Lim DS, Lutucuta S, Bachireddy P, Youker K, Evans A, Entman M, et al. Angiotensin II blockade reverses myocardial fibrosis in a transgenic mouse model of human hypertrophic cardiomyopathy. Circulation. 2001;103(6):789–91.
29. Paizis G, Gilbert RE, Cooper ME, Murthi P, Schembri JM, Wu LL, et al. Effect of angiotensin II type 1 receptor blockade on experimental hepatic fibrogenesis. J Hepatol. 2001;35(3):376–85.
30. Suga S, Mazzali M, Ray PE, Kang DH, Johnson RJ. Angiotensin II type 1 receptor blockade ameliorates tubulointerstitial injury induced by chronic potassium deficiency. Kidney Int. 2002;61(3):951–8.
31. Bedair HS, Karthikeyan T, Quintero A, Li Y, Huard J. Angiotensin II receptor blockade administered after injury improves muscle regeneration and decreases fibrosis in normal skeletal muscle. Am J Sports Med. 2008;36(8):1548–54.
32. Kobayashi T, Uehara K, Ota S, Tobita K, Ambrosio F, Cummins JH, et al. The timing of administration of a clinically relevant dose of losartan influences the healing process after contusion induced muscle injury. J Appl Physiol (1985). 2013;114(2):262–73.
33. Terada S, Ota S, Kobayashi M, Kobayashi T, Mifune Y, Takayama K, et al. Use of an antifibrotic agent improves the effect of platelet-rich plasma on muscle healing after injury. J Bone Joint Surg Am. 2013;95(11):980–8.
34. Kobayashi M, Ota S, Terada S, Kawakami Y, Otsuka T, Fu FH, et al. The combined use of losartan and muscle-derived stem cells significantly improves the functional recovery of muscle in a young mouse model of contusion injuries. Am J Sports Med. 2016;44(12):3252–61.
35. Evans C. Using genes to facilitate the endogenous repair and regeneration of orthopaedic tissues. Int Orthop. 2014;38(9):1761–9.
36. Ginn SL, Alexander IE, Edelstein ML, Abedi MR, Wixon J. Gene therapy clinical trials worldwide to 2012—an update. J Gene Med. 2013;15(2):65–77.
37. Schertzer JD, Lynch GS. Comparative evaluation of IGF-I gene transfer and IGF-I protein administration for enhancing skeletal muscle regeneration after injury. Gene Ther. 2006;13(23):1657–64.
38. Li Y, Li J, Zhu J, Sun B, Branca M, Tang Y, et al. Decorin gene transfer promotes muscle cell differentiation and muscle regeneration. Mol Ther. 2007;15(9):1616–22.
39. Evans CH, Huard J. Gene therapy approaches to regenerating the musculoskeletal system. Nat Rev Rheumatol. 2015;11(4):234–42.
40. Zhou Y, Zhang J, Wu H, Hogan MV, Wang JH-C. The differential effects os leukocyte-containing and pure platelet-rich plasma (PRP) on tendon stem/progenitor cells—implication of PRP application for the clinical treatment of tendon injuries. Stem Cell Res Ther. 2015;6:173.
41. Kannus P, Natri A. Etiology and patophysiology of tendon ruptures in sports. Scand J Med Sci Sports. 1997;7:107–12.
42. Fitzpatrick J, Bulsara M, Zheng MH. The effectiveness of platelet-rich plasma in the treatment of tendinopathy: a meta-analysis of randomized controlled clinical trials. Am J Sports Med. 2016;45(1):226–33.
43. Docheva D, Müller SA, Majewski M, et al. Biologics for tendon repair. Adv Drug Deliv Rev. 2015;84:222–39.
44. Ambrosio F, Wolf SL, Delitto A, et al. The emerging relationship between regenerative medicine and physical therapeutics. Phys Ther. 2010;90(12):1807–14.

45. Andia I, Martin JI, Maffulli N. Advances with platelet rich plasma therapies for tendon regeneration. Expert Opin Biol Ther. 2018;18(4):389–98.
46. Ahmad Z, Brooks R, Kang SN, et al. The effect of platelet-rich plasma on clinical outcomes in lateral epicondylitis. Arthroscopy. 2013;29(11):1851–62.
47. Baksh N, Hannon CP, Murawski CD, Smyth NA, Kennedy JG. Platelet-rich plasma in tendon models: a systematic review of basic science literature. Arthroscopy. 2013;29(3):596–607.
48. de Vos RJ, van Veldhoven PL, Moen MH, Weir A, Tol JL, Maffulli N. Autologous growth factor injections in chronic tendinopathy: a systematic review. Br Med Bull. 2010;95:63–77.
49. de Vos RJ, Windt J, Weir A. Strong evidence against platelet-rich plasma injections for chronic lateral epicondylar tendinopathy: a systematic review. Br J Sports Med. 2014;48(12):952–6.
50. Krogh TP, Bartels EM, Ellingsen T, et al. Comparative effectiveness of injection therapies in lateral epicondylitis: a systematic review and network meta-analysis of randomized controlled trials. Am J Sports Med. 2013;41(6):1435–46.
51. Moraes VY, Lenza M, Tamaoki MJ, Faloppa F, Belloti JC. Platelet- rich therapies for musculoskeletal soft tissue injuries. Cochrane Database Syst Rev. 2014;4:CD010071.
52. Giai Via A, McCarthy MB, de Girolamo L, Ragni E, Oliva F, Maffulli N. Making them commit: strategies to influence phenotypic differentiation in mesenchymal stem cells. Sports Med Arthrosc Rev. 2018;26(2):64–9.
53. Leo AJ, Grande DA. Mesenchymal stem cells in tissue engineering. Cells Tissues Organs. 2006;183:112–22.
54. Rosenbaum AJ, Grande DA, Dines JS. The use of mesenchymal stem cells in tissue engineering: a global assessment. Organogenesis. 2008;4:23–7.
55. Chaudhury S. Mesenchymal stem cell applications to tendon healing. Muscles Ligaments Tendons J. 2012;2(3):222–9.
56. Liu L, Hindieh J, Leong DJ, Sun HB. Advances of stem cell based-therapeutic approaches for tendon repair. J Orthop Translat. 2017;9:69–75.
57. Lee SY, Kim W, Lim C, et al. Treatment of lateral epicondylosis by using allogeneic adipose-derived mesenchymal stem cells: a pilot study. Stem Cells. 2015;33:2995–3005.
58. Connell D, Datir A, Alyas F, et al. Treatment of lateral epicondylitis using skin-derived tenocyte-like cells. Br J Sports Med. 2009;43:293–8.
59. Clarke AW, Alyas F, Morris T, et al. Skin-derived tenocyte-like cells for the treatment of patellar tendinopathy. Am J Sports Med. 2011;39:614–23.
60. Lin J, Zhou W, Han S, Bunpetch V, Zhao K, Yin Z, Ouyang H. Cell-materail interactions in tendon tissue engineering. Acta Biomater. 2018;70:1–11.
61. Majewski M, Heisterbach P, Jaquiéry C, et al. Improved tendon healing using bFGF, BMP-12 and TGFβ1 in a rat model. Eur Cell Mater. 2018;35:318–34.
62. Rabago D, Slattengren A, Zgierska A. Prolotherapy in primary care practice. Prim Care. 2010;37:65–80.
63. Freeman J, Empson Y, Ekwueme E, Paynter D, Bsolinson P. Effect of prolotherapy on cellular proliferation and collagen deposition in MC3T3-E1 and patellar tendon fibroblast populations. Transl Res. 2011;158:132–9.
64. Rabago D, Best T, Beamsley M, Patterson J. A systematic review of prolotherapy for chronic musculoskeletal pain. Clin Sports Med. 2005;15(5):376–80.
65. Yelland M, Sweeting K, Lyftogt J, Ng SK, Scuffham P, Evans K. Prolotherapy injections and eccentric loading exercises for painful Achilles tendinosis: a randomized trial. Br J Sports Med. 2011;45:421–8.
66. Kim E, Lee J. Autologous platelet rich plasma versus dextrose prolotherapy for the treatment of chronic recalcitrant plantar fasciitis. Phys Med Rehabil Int. 2014;6:152–8.
67. Ryan M, Wong A, Gillies J, Wong J, Taunton J. Sonographically guided intratendinous injections of hyperosmolar dextrose/lidocaine: a pilot study for the treatment of chronic plantar fasciitis. Br J Sports Med. 2009;43:303–68.
68. Scarpone M, Rabago DP, Zgierska A, Arbogast G, Snell E. The efficacy of prolotherapy for lateral epicondylosis: a pilot study. Clin Sports Med. 2008;18(3):248–54.
69. Bertrand H, Reeves KD, Bennett CJ, et al. Dextrose prolotherapy versus control injections in painful rotator cuff tendinopathy. Arch Phys Med Rehabil. 2016;97:17–25.

43 Biologic Treatment of Ligament Injuries by the Sports Physician

Jonas Pogorzelski, Mitchell Kennedy, and Robert F. LaPrade

43.1 Background

Ligament injuries are one of the most frequent injuries in athletes. The annual incidence of an injury to the anterior cruciate ligament (ACL) is about 0.1% in the United States, and ACL reconstructions are among the most frequently performed surgeries [9]. Although the short-term success rate of an ACL reconstruction is generally excellent, these calculations fail to account for a significant proportion of athletes who fail to return to their previous level of sports and continue to show symptoms of rapidly progressing osteoarthritis due to persistent instability [6, 7, 11, 12]. The vast majority of these failures in athletes occur from new injuries to ACL grafts that have not fully matured, even after technically well-performed reconstruction procedures. In today's society with a significant commercial interest in sports, athletes sometimes become pressured to return to their sports before the implanted graft has fully matured, leading to potential graft elongation and re-rupture, which are both known to contribute to persistent knee instability [12]. In fact, it is known that an implanted ACL graft is in its weakest state approximately 3–6 months after surgery, which often corresponds to the time at which patients return to sporting activities [17]. This disturbance has triggered the search for possible strategies of accelerating graft healing. Because currently accepted surgical techniques are essentially fully developed, a drastic acceleration of graft healing is an unrealistic expectation due to the adjustment of the surgical technique. Thus, biologic augmentation methods have recently gained attention in the realm of the orthopedic community, because they are theorized to potentially accelerate ligamentous healing.

The purpose of this chapter is to (1) summarize and explain commonly used biologics and their mode of action in ligament injuries, (2) present a rationale for the use of biologics in ligament injuries, (3) provide an overview of how to use biologics in daily practice, and (4) present published results of the use of biologics following ligament injuries in the literature.

J. Pogorzelski
Department of Orthopaedic Sports Medicine, Hospital Rechts der Isar, Technical University of Munich, Munich, Germany
e-mail: jonas.pogorzelski@tum.de

M. Kennedy
Steadman Philippon Research Institute, Vail, CO, USA
e-mail: mkennedy@sprivail.org

R. F. LaPrade (✉)
Twin Cities Orthopaedics, Minneapolis, MN, USA
e-mail: drlaprade@sprivail.org; rlaprade@thesteadmanclinic.com

S. Rocha Piedade et al. (eds.), *The Sports Medicine Physician*,
https://doi.org/10.1007/978-3-030-10433-7_43

43.2 Biologics: Growth Factor Therapy and Cell Therapy

Biologics is a widely used term for a subset of endogenous substances, which have shown hypothetical therapeutic potential for modulating the biologic microenvironment at the site of injury [20]. In order to better categorize biologics, they are commonly divided into the two subgroups: growth factors and cells.

43.2.1 Growth Factor Therapy

The most commonly used growth factor therapy contains the use of autologous platelet-rich plasma (PRP), due to its easy preparation and high availability [12]. Autologous PRP consists of platelets, plasma, and varying amounts of leukocytes; it is made by obtaining blood from a patient and processing by centrifugation into a concentrated platelet substance above baseline levels [2, 15]. In general, platelets are the first responders to soft tissue injuries and house a large number of alpha granules, which contain more than 1000 bioactive molecules such as cytokines and growth factors [13]. The rationale for the therapeutic application of PRP is based from delivery of supraphysiologic concentrations of platelets into the injured area, with the potential for improving the quality of the repair while also reducing the time of regeneration by functioning as chemoattractants and stimulators of cell proliferation [2, 13]. Examples of growth factors that have been identified to exist in PRP and trigger the aforementioned processes include transforming growth factor-β (TGF-β), platelet-derived growth factors (PDGF), insulin-like growth factor-1 (IGF-1), morphogenetic proteins (BMPs), matrix metalloproteinases (MMPs), fibroblastic growth factor (FGF), and vascular endothelial growth factor (VEGF). However, until today only a small subset of molecules and their mode of action are known, thus leading to a change of strategy. Rather than identifying and characterizing each of the many thousands of bioactive molecules, current research proposes to inhibit growth factors known to be detrimental to certain types of tissue regeneration—so-called second-generation PRP [14, 23]. A typical example for the preparation of second-generation PRP is the use of losartan, an angiotensin II receptor blocker known to prevent the action of TGF-β1 and inhibit scar formation. That is why this drug can be added to PRP in cases where scar formation is unintended, such as muscular injuries. On the other side, TGF-β is known to be an important growth factor in the healing process of ligament and cartilage injuries; thus the application of losartan should be avoided in these cases [14].

43.2.2 Cell Therapy

In addition to having similar levels of growth factors to those found in PRP, bone marrow aspirate concentrate (BMAC) contains an increased amount of mesenchymal stem cells (MSCs) [5]. Generally, MSCs have the ability to differentiate into different types of tissues such as muscle, bone, cartilage, tendon, or ligament, dependent on the local environment, and thus are considered beneficial in the healing process of injuries. They can be harvested from numerous places in the human body, including the periosteum, bone marrow, and adipose tissue (being the most common) [11]. The rationale of the transplantation of stem cells is that the delivery of the isolated MSCs directly into the healing zone of ACL grafts or partially torn ACLs may provide a more organized and functional transition zone—thus leading to more rapid and enhanced bony ingrowth. While the theoretical advantages are obvious, there exist a lot of practical barriers translating basic science into daily practice [12]. In order to separate MSCs from other cell types, a laboratory culture is most commonly used. Besides the high costs of such an institution, it has been reported that the cell phenotype might temporally change during the separation process, thus affecting cell behavior and therapeutic efficacy [12]. In addition, the Food and Drug Administration (FDA) does not allow biologics to be manipulated and used in patients. That is why most of the time whole bone marrow cell suspensions (e.g., BMAC) or stromal vascular fractions (from lipoaspirates) are directly used to harness the potential of the contained stem cells and growth factors. However, these highly heterogeneous cell populations demonstrate poor tissue formation combined with a lower regenerative potential compared to isolated MSCs [11]. More recently, flow cytometry has shown promising results in separating MSCs from stromal vascular fractions, potentially allowing for the extraction of a sufficient number of isolated stem cells without needing a laboratory culture [11]. Although this facilitates the use of stem cells in daily practice, the clinical effect of the high purity of MSC remains unclear.

43.3 Ligament Healing and Rationale for the Use of Biologics in Ligament Injuries

While ligaments such as the MCL have a high healing capacity and usually do not need to be augmented with biologics, the ACL does not heal in most cases [12]. This is even more surprising considering the fact that the fibroblasts of both ligaments show comparable rates of proliferation and collagen production [17]. Possible explanations for this poor healing response by the ACL may be found in the altered environments surrounding the ligament. While the ACL is surrounded by synovial fluid and is poorly vascularized, all extra-articular ligaments, such as the MCL, are not covered by synovial fluid and are better vascularized, allowing a more effective healing environment [17]. More precisely, synovial fluid prevents the two ends of the torn ligament to rejoin by washing out a fibrin clot that consists of important extracellular matrix proteins and cytokines. The lack of this provisional scaffold explains why a completely torn ACL has a poor healing response, making an ACL reconstruction necessary [17]. This is contrasted by some types of partial ACL tears. For partial femoral-based ACL tears, if a sufficient amount of ACL fibers are still intact, thus a scaffold for a healing response exists, and an ACL reconstruction might not be necessary [7].

In general, biologic approaches to the treatment of partial ACL injuries aim to optimize clinical outcomes by improving tissue healing. More precisely, multiple recent studies suggest a possibility for partial ACL tears to heal following primary suture repairs augmented with the use of biologics [7]. Therefore, biologics such as PRP, may be applied directly into the torn fibers during an arthroscopic procedure, sometimes utilizing and augmenting artificial extracellular matrix (ECM) scaffold, which is wrapped around the ligament and soaked in PRP or a stem cell solution [17].

The intended goal for the use of biologics in ACL reconstruction is more geared toward the improvement of graft ingrowth while also minimizing the risk of graft failure; thereby the graft incorporation and maturation processes are of particular interest. After ACL reconstruction, the incorporation of a soft tissue grafts within bone tunnels takes about 12 weeks or longer to complete [11, 12]. During this time period, a process of multiple microbiologic reactions involving granulation tissue, chondrogenic progenitors, and type II collagen takes place, finally ending in endochondral ossification of the graft into the bone tunnels [17]. Simultaneously, the intra-articular soft tissue graft is gradually decellularized by macrophages before the resulting ECM scaffold is repopulated with infiltrating progenitor cells. Activated by the progenitor cells, fibroblasts begin to migrate into the tendon and deposit type III collagen, which is later transformed into type I collagen and thus ending the maturation process. In contrast to soft tissue grafts, bone-tendon-bone (BTB) grafts rely upon bony union, which only takes about 6 weeks [11]. However, intra-articular graft maturation undergoes the same remodeling process as described before, therefore it seemingly requires a similar overall length of rehabilitation. There exist multiple strategies to enhance and accelerate healing by the use of biologics, including direct application into the graft and bone tunnels, biologics-impregnated scaffolds out of ECM, silk, or poly-L-lactic acid, among others [21].

43.4 Biologics in Daily Practice for Treatment of (Partial) Anterior Cruciate Ligament Tears

43.4.1 Preparation and Processing of PRP

With a temporary elastic tourniquet used to accentuate the peripheral veins, approximately 60 mL of blood is draw from the arm of the patient. This peripheral blood is then processed in the laboratory, first by dividing the blood into two 50 mL conical tubes where they are spun at 2600 rotations per minute (rpm) for 10 min; before centrifugation, assure that a 1 mL sample has undergone hematology analysis, and the amounts of platelets, erythrocytes, leukocytes, and differentials including neutrophils, lymphocytes, monocytes, eosinophils, and basophils are quantified. The resultant top fraction, consisting of platelet-poor plasma (PPP), is extracted and added to a separate 50 mL conical tube. The remaining buffy layer (white blood cell layer) and erythrocyte layer are consolidated into another 50 mL conical tube. This is then centrifuged once more at 3400 rpm for 6 min. A final PRP product is then acquired once the remaining PPP layer has been extracted following the final centrifugation, and 1 mL of the final product is again analyzed for hematology.

43.4.2 Preparation and Processing of BMAC

Patient positioning is carried out in the prone position, with the resultant BMAC being harvested under sterile conditions from the posterosuperior iliac crest region [3]. A bone marrow aspiration kit is opened, and the BMAC aspiration device is sterilely draped. Bony landmarks of the posterior iliac crest and sacroiliac joint are palpated, and 1% lidocaine without epinephrine is injected down to the periosteum. Through the skin and subcutaneous tissue, the trochar of the bone marrow aspiration is percutaneously inserted until reaching the posterior iliac crest, followed by the manual positioning of the trochar, with pressure, upon dense cortical bone; one's aim should be directed centrally between the middle of the posterior crest cortical walls, with the trajectory of the needle parallel to the iliac crest or perpendicular to the anterior superior iliac spine or posterior superior iliac spine. The trochar and needle are then drilled into the medullary cavity of the posterior iliac crest with the battery-powered instrument. Prior to aspiration, 1 mL of heparin should be preloaded into the syringe (to reduce clot formation and coagulation and maximize the potential yield). Upon completion, the aspiration will have yielded 60 mL of bone marrow using two 30 mL syringes. The bone marrow aspirate is first transferred into 50 mL conical tubes through a 200 μm mesh filter. A sample of 1–1.5 mL of filtered bone marrow aspirate is processed for hemanalysis, and the remaining is transferred into two 50 mL conical tubes and centrifuged at 2400 rpm for 10 min. The buffy coat and platelet-poor plasma layers are then extracted and discarded, leaving behind red blood cell layers which are combined and centrifuged for an additional 6 min at 3400 rpm. This yields a BMAC/white cell pellet, which is resuspended in platelet-poor plasma, which undergoes one final hemanalysis to obtain the final product to inject.

43.4.3 Application

The optimal timing to deliver PRP or BMAC and the perfect concentration during application remain largely unexplored [11]. Generally speaking, biologics can be applied preoperatively, intraoperatively, or postoperatively. As platelets are released almost immediately after any type of trauma to the human body (e.g., during surgery) and subsequently activate growth factors which only have a limited lifespan of minutes to hours, the authors believe that the intraoperative application of biologics seems to be the best solution [11, 12]. The optimal technique of application also remains vague. In principle, PRP and BMAC can either be applied directly into the graft or tissue and simply applied into the knee joint, or finally a scaffold can be impregnated with PRP or BMAC solution and subsequently wrapped around the graft or partially torn ACL. While the current literature fails to show a superior technique, the authors believe that a combination of direct application and application into the joint is the most promising technique.

In summary, there exists a need for well-defined studies evaluating the kinetics according to the activation process of cytokines or methods of localization within a tissue.

43.5 Outcomes of Biologics in Ligament Injuries

In general, the current literature lacks high-level studies on the use of biologics in ligament injuries [11, 12]. Even more problematic is the fact that the limited number of existing studies is hardly comparable among each other due to the lack of standardized preparation of biologics [2, 16]. The only two FDA-approved biologics, namely, PRP and BMAC, suffer from many inconsistencies during their harvest and preparation [2, 11, 12]. While the harvest of a sufficient number of stem cells from BMAC without ex vivo expansion is generally difficult, the possible pitfalls of PRP are more complex. It is known that the growth factor concentration in PRP, even within the same person, is influenced by donor-specific factors such as age, gender, time of day, or nutritional status [11]. Moreover, different processing techniques and methods of delivery make PRP a highly individual product with generally low comparability. However, even though there is a need for more high-level studies in the future, there exist some studies with interesting findings about biologic augmentation in ligament injuries, which are worth being mentioned.

43.5.1 Growth Factor Therapy

As the application of isolated growth factors is so far not approved by national board authorities, most trials involving growth factor therapy deal with the application of PRP. In general, numerous preclinical and clinical trials have been performed to evaluate the impact of PRP application on histological and clinical outcomes following ACL repair or reconstruction. Unfortunately, many of them are ex vivo studies with a low level of evidence. Dallo et al. [7] summarized the results of added growth factor therapy in partial ACL tears in a systematic review. They reported multiple in vitro and animal studies using specific growth factors, which may demonstrate enhanced cell proliferation and ECM synthesis. Moreover, when taking a closer look at studies dealing with PRP augmentation in the treatment of partial ACL tears, the literature demonstrates ambiguous results. For example, Cheng et al. [4] reported that there are age-dependent differences in ACL cell metabolism, collagen gene expression, and the ability of the cells to respond to growth factors in PRP. They obtained ACL cells from skeletally immature, adolescent, and adult pigs and cultured them in a collagen type I hydrogel with or without PRP for 14 days. As a result, the addition of PRP to the collagen hydrogel resulted in a significantly increased cellular metabolic activity, reduced apoptotic rate, and stimulation of collagen production in cells from both the immature and adolescent animals ($p < 0.05$ for all comparisons), but the adult cells were affected less. In contrast to these findings, a similar animal model by Murray et al. [18] reported on the outcome after application of clotted PRP in the gap of a transected ACL. They concluded that there was no beneficial effect of adding PRP in ACL injuries. The results of multiple clinical trials involving the application of PRP during ACL reconstruction summarized by Figueroa et al. in a recent systematic review of the literature are equivocal [8]. While they could show promising evidence that the maturation of the graft was enhanced and happened more quickly by the addition of PRP, they failed to show superior clinical results after the use of PRP.

43.5.2 Cell Therapy

There is a general paucity of trials involving the application of BMAC following ligament injuries, even when compared to the literature dealing with PRP-augmented ACL reconstructions. Several animal model studies could show beneficial effects of the application of MSCs into a (partially) torn ACL [10, 19]. Animals that were treated with additional MSCs following a partial ACL tear showed superior histological scores, greater load-to-failure, and almost normal histology with more mature spindle cells [10, 19]. Dallo et al. summarized the existing knowledge about biologic augmentation of partial ACL tears in a recent systematic review [7]. They concluded that preclinical and short-term results are promising, but further research is required to better define the role of biologic augmentation in partial ACL tears for long-term settings. Concerning MSC augmentation for patients that underwent ACL reconstruction, Silva et al. [22] compared the radiological tendon-to-bone healing in 43 patients with and without augmentation, finding no significant differences between the two groups. In a further study, Centeno et al. [1] reported on ten patients suffering from ACL tears with less than 1 cm retraction of the tendon stumps and treated with an percutaneous intraligamentous injection of BMAC. A total of seven out of ten patients showed improved radiological results on postoperative magnetic resonance imaging, which lead them to the conclusion that augmentation with BMAC is promising, but further high-level studies are required to draw final conclusions.

In summary, it appears that the translation of basic science data into clinical application is a challenging endeavor. Although promising results in preclinical studies exist, there is currently insufficient evidence to suggest that biologic augmentation using any of the currently available techniques provides any clinical benefit, and the ongoing efforts of basic and clinical research should accelerate the development of effective biologic therapies (Figs. 43.1, 43.2, 43.3, and 43.4).

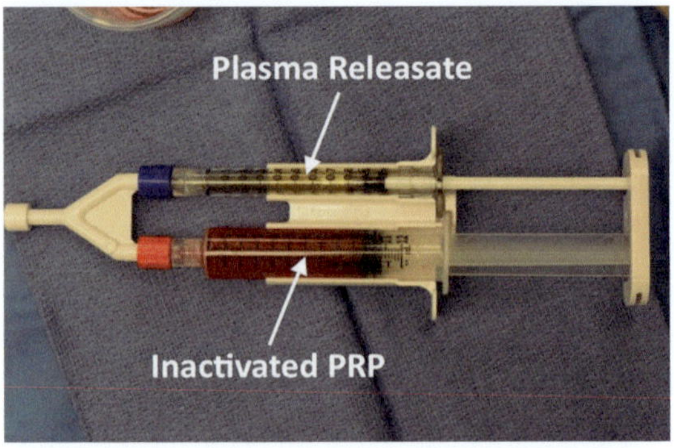

Fig. 43.1 A 10–12 mL platelet-rich plasma (PRP) product is formulated from an original sample of approximately 60 mL of blood, in which the platelet-poor plasma (PPP) composition has been removed following a differentiation process of PPP and PRP via dual centrifugation. A diluted plasma releasate is then combined with inactivated PRP to activate the injected growth factors over time

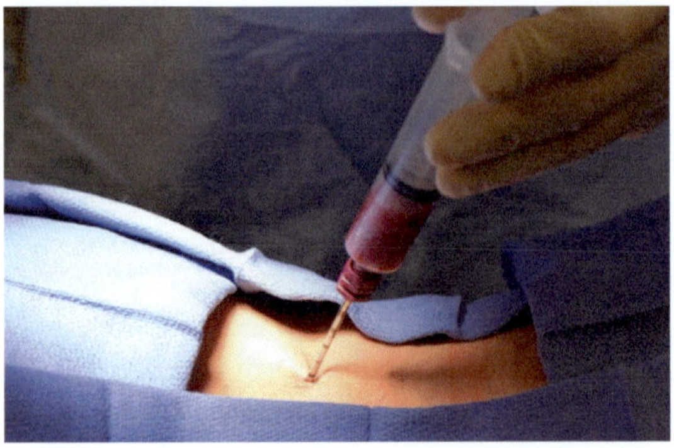

Fig. 43.2 With the patient in prone positioning, bone marrow aspiration is performed under sterile conditions on the posterior superior iliac spine; the cortex is penetrated, and approximately 60 mL of bone marrow is extracted using two 30 mL syringes

Take-Home Messages

- Biologics can be divided into growth factor therapy and cell therapy with PRP and BMAC being the most commonly used. While PRP belongs to the growth factor therapy, BMAC belongs to the cell therapy because it contains stem cells.
- While the vast majority of ligaments are located extra-articular and have a high healing capacity and thus don't need to be augmented with biologics, the ACL does not heal in most

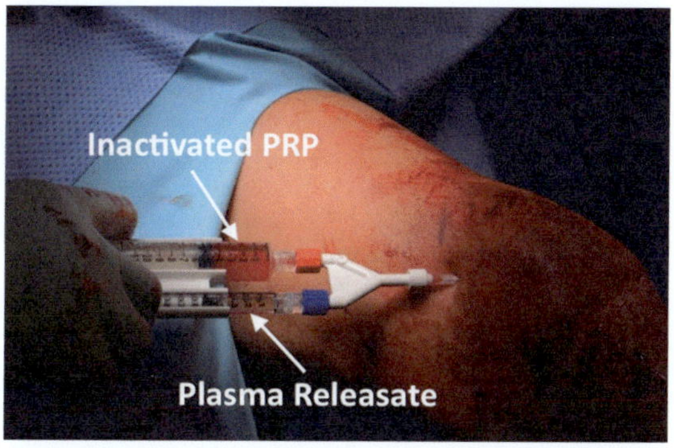

Fig. 43.3 Although there is a lack of valid information, injection of platelets for activation of growth factors is believed to yield the most optimal results during the time period of intraoperative injection. The application can be directly into the targeted tissue as well as into the joint in which the tissue of interest is encompassed

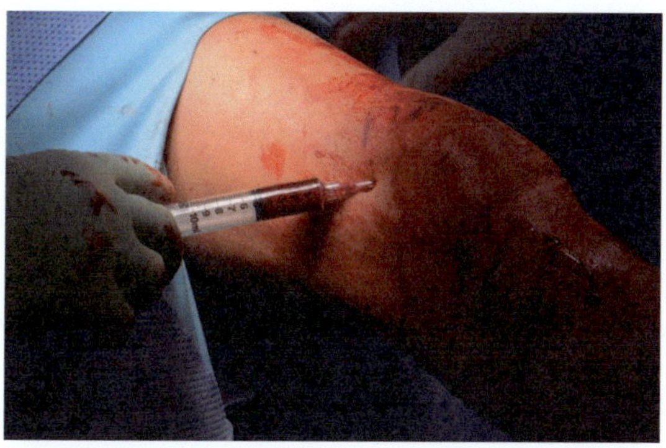

Fig. 43.4 The final product of bone marrow aspirate concentrate (BMAC) is formulated by a dual centrifugation process with each subsequent removal of platelet-poor plasma (PPP) and buffy coat layers, leaving behind the red blood cell layer; for this case, injection is performed directly throughout the joint of interest

of the cases making it an appropriate target for biologic augmentation in the future.

- The intended goals for the use of biologics in ACL injuries are primarily geared toward accelerating healing while at the same time minimizing the risks of reinjury.
- Although there exist promising results in preclinical studies, there is currently insufficient evidence to suggest that biologic augmentation using any of the currently available techniques provides any significant clinical benefit.

References

1. Centeno CJ, Pitts J, Al-Sayegh H, et al. Anterior cruciate ligament tears treated with percutaneous injection of autologous bone marrow nucleated cells: a case series. J Pain Res. 2015;8:437–47.
2. Chahla J, Cinque ME, Piuzzi NS, et al. A call for standardization in platelet-rich plasma preparation protocols and composition reporting: a systematic review of the clinical orthopaedic literature. J Bone Joint Surg Am. 2017;99:1769–79.
3. Chahla J, Mannava S, Cinque ME, et al. Bone marrow aspirate concentrate harvesting and processing technique. Arthrosc Tech. 2017;6:e441–5.
4. Cheng M, Johnson VM, Murray MM. Effects of age and platelet-rich plasma on ACL cell viability and collagen gene expression. J Orthop Res. 2012;30:79–85.
5. Cheng MT, Liu CL, Chen TH, et al. Comparison of potentials between stem cells isolated from human anterior cruciate ligament and bone marrow for ligament tissue engineering. Tissue Eng Part A. 2010;16:2237–53.
6. Cinque ME, Dornan GJ, Chahla J, et al. High rates of osteoarthritis develop after anterior cruciate ligament surgery: an analysis of 4108 patients. Am J Sports Med. 2017;46(8):2011–9. https://doi.org/10.1177/0363546517730072.
7. Dallo I, Chahla J, Mitchell JJ, et al. Biologic approaches for the treatment of partial tears of the anterior cruciate ligament: a current concepts review. Orthop J Sports Med. 2017;5:2325967116681724.
8. Figueroa D, Figueroa F, Calvo R, et al. Platelet-rich plasma use in anterior cruciate ligament surgery: systematic review of the literature. Arthroscopy. 2015;31:981–8.
9. Frobell RB, Lohmander LS, Roos HP. Acute rotational trauma to the knee: poor agreement between clinical assessment and magnetic resonance imaging findings. Scand J Med Sci Sports. 2007;17:109–14.
10. Kanaya A, Deie M, Adachi N, et al. Intra-articular injection of mesenchymal stromal cells in partially torn anterior cruciate ligaments in a rat model. Arthroscopy. 2007;23:610–7.
11. Laprade RF, Dragoo JL, Koh JL, et al. AAOS research symposium updates and consensus: biologic treatment of orthopaedic injuries. J Am Acad Orthop Surg. 2016;24:e62–78.
12. Laprade RF, Geeslin AG, Murray IR, et al. Biologic treatments for sports injuries II think tank-current concepts, future research, and barriers to advancement, part 1: biologics overview, ligament injury, tendinopathy. Am J Sports Med. 2016;44:3270–83.
13. Leslie M. Cell biology. Beyond clotting: the powers of platelets. Science. 2010;328:562–4.
14. Li H, Hicks JJ, Wang L, et al. Customized platelet-rich plasma with transforming growth factor beta1 neutralization antibody to reduce fibrosis in skeletal muscle. Biomaterials. 2016;87:147–56.

15. Moatshe G, Morris ER, Cinque ME, et al. Biological treatment of the knee with platelet-rich plasma or bone marrow aspirate concentrates. Acta Orthop. 2017;88:670–4.
16. Murray IR, Geeslin AG, Goudie EB, et al. Minimum information for studies evaluating biologics in orthopaedics (MIBO): platelet-rich plasma and mesenchymal stem cells. J Bone Joint Surg Am. 2017;99:809–19.
17. Murray MM, Fleming BC. Biology of anterior cruciate ligament injury and repair: kappa delta ann doner Vaughn award paper 2013. J Orthop Res. 2013;31:1501–6.
18. Murray MM, Palmer M, Abreu E, et al. Platelet-rich plasma alone is not sufficient to enhance suture repair of the ACL in skeletally immature animals: an in vivo study. J Orthop Res. 2009;27:639–45.
19. Oe K, Kushida T, Okamoto N, et al. New strategies for anterior cruciate ligament partial rupture using bone marrow transplantation in rats. Stem Cells Dev. 2011;20:671–9.
20. Pogorzelski J, Godin JA, Fritz EM, et al. The use of biological approaches in the treatment of shoulder pathology: a critical analysis review. JBJS Rev. 2017;e5:5.
21. Richmond JC, Weitzel PP. Bioresorbable scaffolds for anterior cruciate ligament reconstruction: do we need an off-the-shelf ACL substitute? Sports Med Arthrosc. 2010;18:40–2.
22. Silva A, Sampaio R, Fernandes R, et al. Is there a role for adult non-cultivated bone marrow stem cells in ACL reconstruction? Knee Surg Sports Traumatol Arthrosc. 2014;22:66–71.
23. Terada S, Ota S, Kobayashi M, et al. Use of an antifibrotic agent improves the effect of platelet-rich plasma on muscle healing after injury. J Bone Joint Surg Am. 2013;95:980–8.

Biological Treatment in Cartilage Injuries

44

Elizaveta Kon, Berardo Di Matteo, Francesco Iacono, Filippo Vandenbulcke, Nicolò Danilo Vitale, and Maurilio Marcacci

44.1 Background

Cartilage injuries are common, and their incidence is getting higher due to the greater emphasis on physical activity with an increase in sports participation in all age groups [1]. Different authors [2–4] found cartilage lesions in about 60% of the patients who undergone a knee arthroscopy, with defects ranging from 0.5 to 12 cm. It has also been estimated that between 5 and 10% of young active subjects affected by traumatic hemarthrosis of the knee have a focal chondral injury [5].

Although a significant number of such injuries may remain asymptomatic, patients frequently present complaining of pain, recurrent effusions, and loss of function.

Concomitantly with the increasing incidence, the expectations of patients about function restore have risen as well. In an attempt to fulfill patients' expectations and successfully treat this pathology, various techniques have been proposed over the years, but none has shown a tissue healing with biomechanical properties that match the physiologic condition.

Hyaline cartilage has a complex and unique architecture allowing it to provide a low-friction surface and to distribute the load. Chondrocytes are sparsely distributed within the surrounding matrix with minimal cell-to-cell contact. The interaction between cells, collagen framework, aggrecan, and fluid constitutes a complex biomechanical feature making hyaline cartilage difficult to replace or reproduce [6]. Moreover, none of the inflammatory processes are available for its repair, and unlike other tissues chondrocytes cannot migrate to the site of injury from an intact, healthy site [7]. This poor intrinsic regenerative capacity of articular cartilage increases the importance of obtaining effective treatment options for symptomatic lesions of this tissue.

Another important problem concerning cartilage injuries is that they represent a risk factor for more extensive joint damage. Even small isolated defects may cause further degeneration, due to higher mechanical stress on the lesion's edge. Tissue near a defect experiences increased overall compression, and excessive strains may contribute to cell death, matrix damage, or accelerated wear. The degenerative process leading to unicompartimental osteoarthritis following an isolated critical-sized defects has been clearly demonstrated in the animal model [8, 9].

Several therapeutic strategies have been developed, both conservative and surgical.

E. Kon · B. Di Matteo · F. Iacono · F. Vandenbulcke
N. D. Vitale (✉) · M. Marcacci
Department of Biomedical Sciences, Humanitas University, Milan, Italy

Humanitas Clinical and Research Center, Milan, Italy
e-mail: elizaveta.kon@humanitas.it; francesco.iacono@humanitas.it; maurilio.marcacci@humanitas.it

S. Rocha Piedade et al. (eds.), *The Sports Medicine Physician*,
https://doi.org/10.1007/978-3-030-10433-7_44

The latter include simple arthroscopic debridement, bone marrow stimulation techniques (microfractures), transplantation of autologous tissue (e.g., mosaicplasty), implantation of cultured autologous cells, implantation of allograft tissue, and prosthetic options.

Nowadays the conservative approach is gaining constant increasing attention, and authors struggle to find the better biological therapy capable of restoring the cartilaginous tissue and relieving clinical symptoms.

Among them, infiltrative therapies, such as platelet-rich plasma (PRP) and mesenchymal stem cells (MSCs), stand out as the most conservative and suitable for different types of cartilage lesions.

A more surgical biological approach is represented by the bioengineered scaffold, used to treat osteochondral defects.

44.2 Platelet-Rich Plasma (PRP)

Platelet-rich plasma (PRP) is among current biologic interventions used in medical conditions that necessitate tissue healing [10]. It is a concentrate obtained from autologous blood containing high concentrations of human platelets and platelet-derived growth factors.

Inside platelets indeed lies a powerful reservoir of factors capable of providing clinical benefits by modulating the early healing response through secretion of an array of signaling cytokines that influence inflammation, angiogenesis, and cell migration [11–14].

Among them the most relevant is platelet-derived growth factor (PDGF), transforming growth factor beta (TGF-beta), fibroblast growth factor (FGF), insulin-like growth factor 1 (IGF-1), connective tissue growth factor (CTGF), epidermal growth factor (EGF), and hepatocyte growth factor (HFG) [10, 15]. Moreover, the anti-inflammatory properties of PRP have been investigated as an associate effect in promoting tissue repair. Lowering the inflammation in the synovial tissue would lead to a reduction of matrix metalloproteinases, which are cartilage-matrix degrading enzymes [16].

PRP also contains different plasma proteins, which are critical components in the healing mechanism of connective tissues [17]. In contrast with serum, plasma contains clotting factors and fibrogen, which can be activated to form a provisional fibrin scaffold for cells to adhere, migrate, and proliferate [18].

Articular hyaline cartilage contains no blood vessels and is thus unable to initiate the same healing process as other tissues with good regenerative potential. The three-dimensional scaffold created with the infiltration of PRP may mimic the initial stage of wound healing and tissue repair.

Different authors demonstrated in vitro that PRP has a strong positive effect on chondrocyte proliferation [19–24].

This is the rationale that led to the development of several clinical studies and the subsequent use of PRP as a novel biological treatment for articular cartilage lesions.

Some problems came out during the in vivo study of PRP and its effects. Firstly, many variables have to be considered when making comparisons, and it is not possible to establish a univocal definition of PRP. There are several PRP formulations, whose comparison in terms of potentials and limits is very difficult to test due to the large inter-product variability [25]. A good starting point might be to clarify what the essential features are to define a blood product as PRP. It is generally regarded as a blood derivate with a higher concentration of platelets compared to basal level. It has been proposed that platelet concentration should be at least 200% of the peripheral blood PLT count [26, 27] even if in the literature PRP concentrations have been reported to range widely, up to eight times that of basal levels [26]. Therefore, just concerning the definition of PRP, it is possible to understand the first variable involved in the comparison of different types of PRP [28]: the platelet count that can vary in such a significant way that the possible correlation between platelet concentration and clinical outcome could be a critical aspect. However, with regard to the scientific evidence available up to now, good clinical outcome can be obtained even with lower platelet concentration. Some studies also report correlations between outcome and platelet count [27, 29], but further investigations are needed to fully explore this topic.

The platelet count is strictly linked to the procedures employed: there are two main preparation methods used in clinical practice [28]. The first one is by using a laboratory centrifuge, and the second one a density gradient cell separator. In the first case several variables, such as a number of centrifugations, their speed, and timing, might influence the final product in terms of concentration of different cellular types. Furthermore, this preparation method is more technician-dependent, and therefore its reproducibility is biased. Concerning cell separators, they are closed-circuit devices that allow PRP preparation without excessive manipulation of the blood. A large and constantly increasing number of these devices are available on the market, each with its **own** features and specifications, so it is impossible to obtain the same products, and again the comparison is very difficult.

Furthermore, we have to consider the overall cell types contained in PRP: even in this case, the preparation method is a key factor. In fact, some PRP preparations, besides plasma and platelets, also contain leukocytes and residual blood cells. With regard to this, some disagreement has emerged among authors. In fact, whereas the antimicrobial effect of leukocyte-rich PRP has been underlined, some authors highlight the fact that leukocytes can release matrix metalloproteinases and reactive oxygen species capable of damaging articular tissues and determining a catabolic effect. Concerning the presence of residual blood cells, it has been reported in some studies that even erythrocytes have a pro-inflammatory effect in the joint [30].

Storage procedure is also a hot topic: in fact, freeze-thawing is one method, but it is thought to impair platelet function and lifespan and alter the GFs' release pattern negatively, besides favoring the accumulation of pyrogenic cytokines and increasing the risk of bacterial proliferation. For these reasons, some authors prefer fresh administration of PRP immediately after its preparation (thus requiring blood harvesting for each injection, in case of multiple treatments) [31].

Another issue is the activation method. Several options are available even in this case: from no activation, counting on the in vivo activating effect of endogenous collagen, to the use of chemical agents or biomaterials or even physical agents. Calcium chloride and thrombin are the most commonly used substances, whereas batroxobin is less often employed. These molecules contribute to PRP clot formation and increase overall GF release even if their effect on single GF kinetic is controversial and needs further studies. In particular, thrombin, besides being a strong activator of platelets, has its own biological properties that might influence the interpretation of the effect of PRP [32].

Beyond the intrinsic differences among PRP preparations due to all the aforementioned factors, applicative variables should also be taken into account. Individual authors apply their own therapeutic protocol: the amount of PRP used for each injection, the number of the injections, and the time intervals can vary widely, so study comparison is even harder than just comparing product differences. Standardization has not yet been proposed on this issue. Thus the different protocols of each author introduce further confounding factors.

Another variable regards the application of PRP in the treatment of cartilage lesions. It can be used as an augmentation procedure in different types of surgeries or alone as a conservative method. Looking at the surgical application, it is not possible to draw definite conclusions about the efficacy of this approach. It is a consequence of this particular kind of treatment: it is very difficult to identify how much PRP might contribute to determine the clinical outcome with respect to the surgical treatment performed alone. Comparative studies aimed at assessing the specific role of PRP are needed.

Furthermore, in many cases, PRP is administered together with other biological augmentation methods, such as mesenchymal stem cells [33–35] or bioengineered scaffolds [36, 37], so it is even more difficult to determine the contribution of PRP. The studies available are just case series treating disparate conditions in biomechanically very different joints (knee and ankle). Maximum follow-up evaluation is 24 months, so further studies are needed to determine the persistence of the good clinical outcome of these particular procedures. In the near future, PRP will be more and more widely used in regenerative cartilage techniques, but, despite being safe, according to the present evidence, there is still no recommendation for using PRP in such procedures.

Considering PRP as conservative management, things look a bit different, especially when treating the knee region. In fact, whereas a few studies have been published both on hip and ankle cartilage lesions, several trials focus on knee treatment. As a consequence, few indications can be proposed for hip and talar osteochondral lesions. For what regards talar osteochondral lesions, only one comparative quasi-randomized trial has been published [38]: despite presenting statistically superior results for the PRP group, the low number of patients treated and the short follow-up evaluation do not allow, even in this case, the use of PRP to be endorsed.

For the knee, it is possible to have more detailed indications. A lot certainly still needs to be clarified, but the considerable amount of studies published allows us to draw some conclusions. The first consideration regards the safety of the procedure, which was confirmed by all the different trials present in literature. They reported only minor adverse events with just some differences linked to the particular PRP formulation used: in fact, leukocyte-rich PRP seems to determine increased pain and swelling reaction when compared to leukocyte-poor PRP. With regard to the clinical outcome, it can be said that this kind of conservative approach is time-dependent since a gradual worsening occurs over time.

Analyzing efficacy, the encouraging results reported in case series cannot be the backbone to support the clinical application of PRP since each study faces an important bias related essentially to the lack of a control group. All the randomized controlled trials available compared the efficacy of PRP versus HA. Actually it should be pointed out that each trial employed a different type of PRP. Two out of three studies [39, 40] revealed better results in the PRP group at 6 months of follow-up. The third one [41], which had the longest follow-up evaluation (1 year), reports no overall difference between PRP and HA in terms of clinical outcome. Just a tendency toward better results in patients affected by a lower degree of cartilage degeneration was found. Therefore, in the case of more advanced signs of OA, PRP does not seem to be superior to viscosupplementation, a conclusion that was also reached in the study by Sanchez et al. Surprisingly, Cerza et al. reported significantly better results for ACP even in grade III OA: worthy of consideration is the fact that they used a different blood-derived product with evaluation limited up to 6 months of follow-up.

All the randomized trials deal with the application of PRP in patients affected by very different stages of the disease, from chondropathy to severe OA. Therefore no conclusions can be drawn about the possibility of applying this approach to a specific phase of degenerative cartilage pathology: subgroup analysis does not allow, in any of the trials published, sufficient statistical strength to provide a real clinical indication. What emerges can be considered just a suggestion to avoid the indiscriminate use of PRP, which seems to offer a clinical benefit but cannot yet be considered a first-line treatment for this pathology. Moreover, its use should be limited to those patients who can take most advantage from this approach, such as young patients with less articular degeneration or those not responsive to other more traditional treatments.

44.3 Mesenchymal Stem Cells (MSCs)

Another powerful tool for cartilage repair emerging in recent years is a mesenchymal stem cell (MSC). They have the marked ability to differentiate into a variety of connective tissues including cartilage, bone, fat, tendon, ligament, marrow stroma, and others [42]. The regenerative effects of MSCs are due to their structural contribution to tissue repair and their immunomodulatory and anti-inflammatory action, through direct cell-cell interaction or secretion of bioactive factors [43]. MSCs have a capacity for self-renewal, stemness maintenance, and a potential for differentiation into cells forming multiple mesodermal tissues (plasticity). They can migrate toward injured tissues (homing) where they display trophic effects (synthesis of proliferative, proangiogenic, and regenerative molecules). Most remarkably, MSCs exert a suppressive effect on components of the immune system by inhibiting T and B lymphocyte activation and proliferation, suppressing NK cell activation, escaping CTL-mediated lysis, and modulating the secretion profiles of dendritic cells/macrophages [44]. The Mesenchymal and Tissue Stem Cell Committee of the International Society for Cellular Therapy has established the following minimal set of standard criteria to provide a uniform characterization of such cells [45]: (1) They must be plastic-adherent when maintained in standard culture conditions; (2) they must express CD105, CD73, and CD90 and lack surface expression of CD45, CD34, CD14 (or CD11b), CD79a (or CD19), and HLA-DR; (3) and they must be capable of differentiating to chondrocytes, osteoblasts, and adipocytes in vitro. MSCs were first identified by Friedenstein et al. [46] in 1966 in bone marrow (BMSCs). Subsequently, in 1970, Caplan's group [47] provided the first evidence of chondrogenic, osteogenic, and muscular differentiation potential of these cells and introduced the term "mesenchymal stem cells" in the early 1990s [48]. Another important study performed by Wakitani et al. [49] first showed the efficacy of autologous MSC implantation in rabbit osteochondral defect healing, and finally, in 2001, Quarto et al. [50] described the first successful clinical application of cultured MSCs by focusing on bone healing in humans. Nowadays, MSCs can be isolated from human sources other than the bone marrow, such as adipose tissue, umbilical cord blood, synovial membrane, synovial fluid, periosteum, dermis, trabecular bone, infrapatellar fat pad, and muscle, with similar phenotypic characteristics but different propensities in proliferation and differentiation potentials [51]. Numerous studies have described the success of different MSC application modalities, through injection [52] or scaffold implantation [34], involving different biomaterials and sometimes combined with growth or transcription factors (such as recombinant molecules or even in the form of genetic sequences), such as TGF-b, BMP-7, FGF-2, or SOX9, hyaluronic acid, or magnetic devices. Some researchers have investigated the possibility of predifferentiating MSCs into the chondrogenic lineage before implantation [53] to provide better-targeted tissue regeneration. However, the optimal strategy has not yet been identified. Peripheral blood is another possible source of MSCs (PBMSCs), but current knowledge is still very limited, with poor results, a low number of patients, and shorter follow-up [54]. They cannot be easily isolated, and their number is very low, especially in adult humans; moreover, a previous patient stimulation is required to increase their number, making this procedure more complicated.

Knowledge about the use of MSCs in the treatment of cartilage defects is still preliminary, as shown by the prevalence in the literature of preclinical studies and, among the clinical findings, by the presence of studies of low quality due to weak methodology, a small number of patients, and short-term follow-up. Nonetheless, the studies available suggest a potential for these cell-based treatments to be developed and to represent a promising new approach with preliminary interesting findings ranging from focal chondral defects to articular OA degeneration. However, many aspects are still controversial, and they have to be clarified. Firstly, the optimal MSC source has not yet been identified. The yield of cells obtained by extraction might also be a limiting factor and contributes to the choice of cell source for the clinical application. The continually emerging field of experimental stem cell research and cartilage repair, particularly with the help of preclinical large animal models, will provide some new solutions to this issue. The most appropriate cell source is not the only controversial aspect. For example, many important biological pathways that determine the fate of transplanted MSCs in cartilage defects, particularly with the view of hypertrophic differentiation, are unknown. Controlling the chondrogenesis of MSCs in this environment is not understood. The interplay of MSCs with the adjacent osteochondral unit has not yet been clarified. Another aspect that has to be considered is the potential risks in MSCs use: one possibility is, besides cancer or immunological disease, the differentiation of these cells into unwanted tissue, as reported by Breitbach et al. [55] who described the calcification of MSCs injected into infarcted rat hearts. For the treatment of articular cartilage defects, this implies, in theory, the risk of such MSC-mediated endochondral ossification to occur at least in some parts of the repair tissue, thus jeopardizing the formation of good-quality tissue and the clinical outcome. Improvement in noninvasive imaging of the cartilaginous repair tissue will help to detect with high-resolution early signs of such unwanted ossifications and to understand the real dimension of this problematic aspect.

Conversely, Wakitani et al. [56] demonstrated the safeness of using BMSCs in cartilage repair in 41 patients followed up 5–137 months after transplantation: neither tumors nor infection were observed. The debate is still ongoing and warrants close scrutiny, since such stem cell therapies are far from being accepted in the field of clinical articular cartilage repair, nor has their long-term safety been convincingly proven. Moreover, reliable clinical data based on long-term, randomized, double-blind, controlled, multicenter studies with systematic follow-up are largely lacking. Such information is needed, as it might determine the true value of MSC therapy for articular cartilage defects and help to identify the best indications for it. This cell-based treatment for cartilage regeneration is still in its infancy, and many aspects remain to be clarified and optimized. Among these, one of the most clearly missing elements is the knowledge of the proper cell dosage to be administered. The dose-response relationship of MSC transplantation for clinical cartilage repair has not yet been established. The current literature shows the variety in quantity of transplanted cells into the defect site, making clinical outcome comparison very difficult. As the number of cells per defect volume that would be required for successful articular cartilage regeneration remains unclear, identification of such an effective quantity of MSCs represents another key point.

44.4 The Osteochondral Unit and Bioengineered Scaffolds

The osteochondral junction is the interface between bone and cartilage, where the subchondral bone form the layer of transition between the two different histotypes [57]. Cartilage damage may lead to subchondral degeneration: in particular, certain defects, such as consequences of osteochondritis dissecans (OCD), osteonecrosis, and traumas, may involve primarily the subchondral bone [58, 59].

Moreover, in the case of large cartilage lesions, as well as untreated focal defects, the subchondral bone is often secondarily involved in the degenerative process of the articular surface. Thus, the defect size can increase over time, and concomitant changes can appear, such as osteophytes and bone resorption [60–62].

The treatment of osteochondral defects is particularly challenging because of the involvement of two tissues (bone and cartilage) with a different intrinsic regenerative potential. Traditional surgical techniques for such lesions mainly concern an autograft or allograft implantation of the entire osteochondral unit. Thanks to recent achievements in the field of tissue engineering, in the last years, new bioengineered scaffolds specific for these defects have been developed, able to induce an in situ cartilage regeneration.

The implantation of biomaterials directly into the lesion site aims at restoring a tissue as conform as possible to the native hyaline cartilage, with physiological properties similar to those of the entire osteochondral unit and durable over time, thus providing a valid therapeutic alternative to the orthopedic surgeon.

44.4.1 Indications

- Grade III–IV chondral or osteochondral defects, symptomatic.
- Etiology: Traumatic, degenerative, and osteochondritis dissecans (OCD).
- Defect size: Depending on the kind of scaffold applied.
- Age: Less than 60 years is recommended (this approach represents an evolution of bone marrow stimulation, and, as for this latter technique, better results have been reported for young patients, despite an established cutoff has not been defined yet).
- Body mass index (BMI): Less or equal to 30.

44.4.2 Contraindications

- Medium or advanced osteoarthritis (OA).
- Misalignment and ligamentous instability.

Currently, different scaffolds used for osteochondral regeneration are commercialized for clinical application.

44.5 Matrix-Associated Chondrocyte Transplantation (MACT)

This procedure belongs to second-generation autologous chondrocyte implantation (ACI), and it is based on the use of temporary and biodegradable polymeric scaffolds as a growth site for viable cells in vitro; these cells are then implanted in the site of the lesion.

Chondrocytes kept in monolayer culture at low density eventually change from a polygonal or round to a flattened, amoeboid-like shape, and instead of cartilage collagen (type II collagen), they synthesize the genetically different type I collagen [63]; on the other side, it was demonstrated that the use of 3D scaffolds favors the retainment of their original phenotype [64].

Some essential features of these scaffolds are biocompatibility and biodegradability through safe biochemical processes and adequate time spans. Solid scaffolds have a substrate to which cells can adhere. Differently, gel scaffolds physically entrap the cells. Many different scaffolds have been used while trying to create new cartilage tissue, from natural to synthetic, many different shapes and compositions.

The most used synthetic materials are polylactides like polylactic acid (PLA) and polyglycolic (PGA).

Mechanical properties and synthetic biomaterials degradation are more easily modified with respect to natural fibers, but degradations of their components can be harmful to the native tissue and implanted cells.

Natural materials used to produce scaffolds are agarose, alginate, hyaluronic acid, gel, and fibrin glue, all coming from collagen and acellular collagen matrix. Matrices that are commonly used in the clinical practice in Europe include collagen or hyaluronic acid.

The use of 3D scaffolds for cellular cultures in open surgery allows a reduction in the time of the joint exposition because we can avoid the periosteal patch and so the suture.

Moreover, in some scaffolds, arthroscopic techniques for implantation have been developed.

Hyaluronan is an important component of extracellular matrix [65]: it is a glycosaminoglycan, a linear polymer made by a dimer that is regularly repeated; it is a soluble molecule, whose molecular weight varies from 4000 and 8000 Da; in water it forms a viscous solution. This polysaccharide is not just a spacer; it has many functions in determining cartilage structure and functionality.

Hyaluronic acid is important in maintaining the structure of the tissue and to hydrate it, thanks to its hydrophilic properties; it can influence cellular movements regulating osmotic pressure.

It actively interacts with proteoglycans and growth factors stimulating the production of ECM and acts as a scavenger of free radicals. Furthermore, it was recently discovered that hyaluronic acid contains some receptors like CD-44, through which it can regulate cellular adhesion, growth, and differentiation.

Considering all its properties, it seems the ideal candidate for tissue engineering procedures.

Unfortunately, its rapid water solubility and the quick reabsorption make it not usable in purified form, so it has to be processed in a different form.

HYAFF is a scaffold derived from the total esterification of sodium hyaluronate with different alcohol, and according to the esterification percentage, we can obtain different polymers, different in duration and consistency.

The most used is HYAFF-11, entirely based on the benzylic ester of hyaluronic acid; it consists of a network of 20-lm-thick fibers with interstices of variable sizes and has been demonstrated to be an optimal physical support to allow cell-cell contacts, cluster formation, and extracellular matrix deposition. It has a weight of 120 g/m^2 and thickness of 2 mm.

Degradation mechanism of these biomaterials is very important; de-esterification in water causes the release of molecules that are not toxic [66].

This tridimensional structure presents interstitial spaces of different dimensions that act as physical support for cells, allowing contact among them, and cluster formation maintaining phenotypical differentiation.

The cells harvested from the patient are expanded and then seeded onto the scaffold to create the tissue-engineered product Hyalograft C® (Fig. 44.1). Seeded on the scaffold, the cells are able to redifferentiate and retain a chondrocytic phenotype even after a long period of in vitro expansion in monolayer culture [67].

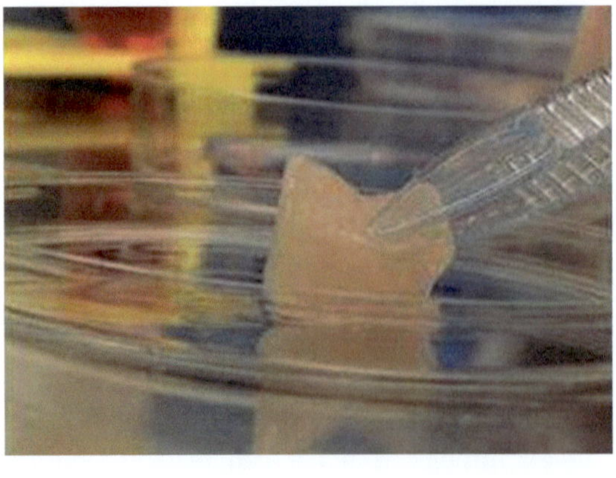

Fig. 44.1 Hyalograft C®

Properties of HYAFF-11 to favor the growth of human chondrocytes and maintain the original phenotype have been demonstrated in vitro, and the efficacy of the cell-scaffold construct was also proven by in vivo implantation in an animal model.

One of these studies has evaluated reparation tissue in chicks: chondrocytes attached to the support fibers tend to aggregate and produce those molecules typical of hyaline cartilage: collagen type I and II and glycosaminoglycans.

Another study based on Hyalograft C® transplantation with human cells in athymic mice has documented the formation of a tissue similar to hyaline cartilage: the implant was white, nonvascularized, and well attached to the articular surface. Histological examination showed cells with round nuclei inside structures similar to lacunae and surrounded by abundant ECM whose composition was based on collagen and glycosaminoglycans.

According to the good results, obtained in vitro and on animals, this technique seemed promising, and study on humans started. After some positive results, HYAFF started to be used for the treatment of symptomatic chondral lesions. Cells harvested from the patient are expanded and then seeded on the HYAFF-11 scaffold to create Hyalograft C®.

At the beginning the patch was fixed at the site of the lesion with fibrin glue; later, it was seen that thanks to hydrophilic properties of the matrix, if the graft is well positioned, the tenso-active pression is enough to fix it.

The press-fit technique is enough because of the shape and the properties of the graft. Another advantage is that it can be inserted through an arthroscopic procedure with less morbidity for the patient, shorter surgical time, shorter stay in the hospital, and fewer complications related to open surgery.

Implantation arthroscopic technique was first invented to treat localized lesions of the medial or lateral femoral condyle. Nowadays it is used for almost all the lesions of the femoral condyles, even if very big. Lesions of the patellar cartilage and the tibial plate are an exception, and they need open surgery.

Sometimes, when the lesion is very big, we can add fibrin glue in order to increase stability.

Medium-long-term results showed good results at 2-year follow-up and the maintenance of stable values at 7 years [68].

This assumption is also reinforced by the fact that second-look arthroscopy [69] and histological [70] examination showed a normal appearance of the newly formed cartilage in six and an abnormal appearance in two patients.

In the past a study comparing microfractures and implant of autologous chondrocytes was performed; it took into consideration 80 patients [71] with defects grades III–IV on the femoral condyle and the trochlea; these patients were admitted to the study and divided into two groups. Both groups showed a significant improvement at 5 years from surgery; however, the ACI group showed greater improvements in the objective-subjective scores of the International Knee Documentation Committee.

Even more interesting is the return to sports activity; it was the same up to 2 years of follow-up. Later on, it remained stable in the ACI group, while it decreased in the microfractures group; this is a sign of the bigger reliability of the Hyalograft C®.

44.6 New "One-Step" Regenerative Treatments

Recently, new solutions have been proposed in order to overcome problems correlated to second-generation ACI that were high costs and the two-step surgery, needed because of the cellular culture.

Experimental studies have demonstrated the growth and migration of chondrocytes coming from healthy cartilage of the ipsilateral knee of the patient; these fragments are then put into a polymeric, tridimensional scaffold which is implanted at the site of the defect of articular cartilage.

Results demonstrate a redistribution of chondrocytes inside the scaffold reproducing a hyaline-like reparative tissue after 6 months [72].

Among the one-step techniques for cartilage reconstruction, the use of bone marrow concentrate added to the scaffold instead of chondrocyte has been introduced.

Using a kit to concentrate bone marrow-derived cells in the operating room, collagen powder or hyaluronic acid membrane (as scaffolds for cell support), and platelet gel, a one-step arthroscopic technique was developed by Giannini et al. [33]

The evaluation of 48 patients treated for talar osteochondral lesions at 24 months of follow-up documented a significant clinical improvement and histologic and immunohistologic results obtained confirmed the presence of new cartilaginous tissues with various degrees of tissue remodeling toward hyaline cartilage. These data suggest the one-step technique is an alternative for cartilage repair, permitting improved functional scores and overcoming the drawbacks of previous techniques.

Progress made in material science, cellular biology, and nanotechnology allowed the realization of TEC (tissue engineering constructs) for lesions repair. The ultimate goal is to obtain a complete integration of the TEC with the host tissue, up to the complete remodeling of the implantation site.

Musculoskeletal tissue, bone, and cartilage are under extensive investigation in tissue engineering research. A number of biodegradable and bioresorbable materials, as well as scaffold designs, have been experimentally and/or clinically studied. Ideally, a scaffold should have the following characteristics such as:

- Three-dimensional and highly porous with an interconnected pore network for cell growth and flow transport of nutrients and metabolic waste.
- Biocompatible and bioresorbable with a controllable degradation and resorption rate to match cell/tissue growth in vitro and/or in vivo.
- Suitable surface chemistry for cell attachment, proliferation, and differentiation and mechanical properties to match those of the tissues at the site of implantation.

Lately, the awareness of the involvement of the subchondral bone in many of these lesions resulted in the need to develop cell-free treatment strategies focused on the entire osteochondral unit. Currently, heterogeneous scaffolds have been proposed that combine distinct but integrated layers corresponding to the cartilage and bone regions to regenerate both components of the osteochondral unit to restore the articular surface [73].

The "cell-free" osteochondral grafts have been developed with the aim to give specific regenerative signals to mesenchymal cells coming from the bone marrow [74, 75].

An ideal graft would be an off-the-shelf product from both a surgical and commercial standpoint, so many biomaterials have been proposed in the last years to induce cartilage "regeneration" in situ, directly in the site of the lesion.

Among them MaioRegen® and, more recently, Agili-C® have shown some of the most promising results.

44.7 MaioRegen®

MaioRegen® is a nanostructured biomimetic and bioresorbable implant with a porous composite structure, mimicking the whole osteochondral anatomy with three different layers [76] (Fig. 44.2):

- Superficial (100% type I collagen): Has a smooth surface to reproduce the articular surface.
- Intermediate (60% type I collagen and 40% hydroxyapatite): Tidemark—Like a layer.
- Lower (30% type I collagen and 70% hydroxyapatite): Reproducing the subchondral bone composition.

Promising results in terms of both cartilage and bone tissue formation have been published in a preclinical study. Even if similar macroscopic, histological, and radiographic results are obtained implanting scaffold loaded with autologous chondrocytes or scaffold alone; given that, this scaffold has been introduced into clinical practice as a cell-free approach, trying to take advantage from an in situ regeneration induced by stem cells coming from the surrounding bone marrow [77].

The surgical technique needed to implant MaioRegen® requires the following steps:

- Position: Supine position, tourniquet at the proximal extremity of the lower leg.
- Access approach: Classical arthroscopic or arthrotomic (medial or lateral) to expose lesions.
- Procedure: Identification of the lesion site and confirmation of indications.
- Preparation of the defect with an adequate osteotome.
- Excision of subchondral sclerotic bone: 8 mm depth.

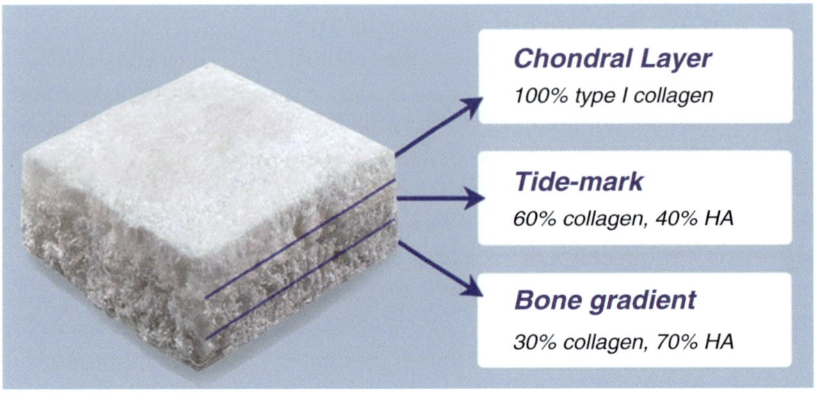

Fig. 44.2 MaioRegen®

- Preparation of the scaffold based on the shape and size of the defect.
- Press-fit implantation, the addition of fibrin glue is recommended to improve the early stability of the implant.
- The continuous passive of motion before and after tourniquet removal.

It is important to have a well-prepared defect area and stable vertical shoulders to implant scaffold correctly.

Promising preliminary results of a pilot study on 28 patients affected by chondral and osteochondral lesions have been recently reported. A slower recovery was observed in older, less active patients who experienced adverse events or in patellar lesions. However, at 2-year follow-up, good results were reported in all patients with both clinical and MRI evaluations, showing the potential of this osteochondral one-step procedure also for the treatment of complex salvage lesions [78].

44.8 Agili-C™: A Novel Biphasic Aragonite-Based Scaffold

Agili-C™ is a coral-based scaffold; the coralline skeletal material is composed of calcium carbonate in the crystalline form of aragonite.

Coral exoskeletons (aragonite) are a remarkably similar biological material to human bone including its 3D structure and pore interconnections and crystalline form of calcium carbonate (CaCO3). These characteristics are thought to confer its osteoconductive ability and make it a suitable material for bone repair. Corals are marine invertebrates from the Anthozoa class that include over 7000 species with a wide variety of skeletal topologies, different morphologies, and crystalline structures. Corals used for medical applications are limited to a select number of species: Porites, Acropora, Lobophyllia, Goniopora, Polyphyllia, and Pocillopora [79].

These biomaterials provide a three-dimensional (3D) structure with mechanical properties and high interconnected macroporosity (between 100 and 200 μm) required for vascular tissue ingrowth. These characteristics are thought to confer aragonite its osteoconductive ability and make it suitable for bone repair. The calcium carbonate structures are gradually resorbed and replaced by functional bone tissue. Coral derivatives are commonly used as a bone graft substitute and bone void fillers.

Agili-C™ is a porous scaffold designed for the treatment of knee-joint surface lesions. Agili-C™ consists of a porous, interconnected calcium carbonate (aragonite) structure, derived from purified coral (Fig. 44.3).

The lower part of the implant is composed of inorganic aragonite, while a square grid pattern of 2-mm deep-drilled channels are made in the top part, where HA is added (Fig. 44.4).

Histology performed by an independent laboratory in a series of preclinical studies confirmed the regeneration of hyaline cartilage, as demonstrated by the presence of collagen type II and aggrecan, and the lack of collagen type I in the repaired tissue, alongside the reconstruction of the subchondral bone (Fig. 44.5).

The basic scaffold consists of coralline aragonite. Following a machining process, a square grid pattern of 1- to 2-mm-deep-drilled channels is made, in the chondral phase or the bone phase, using Bungard CCD, a CNC drilling and routing machine, and an appropriate drill bit. This scaffold configuration is used and developed in the shape of cylinders for the treatment of both chon-

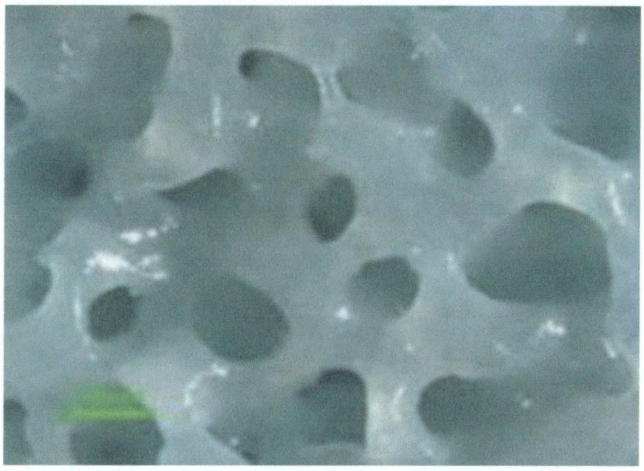

Fig. 44.3 Porous structure of Agili-C™

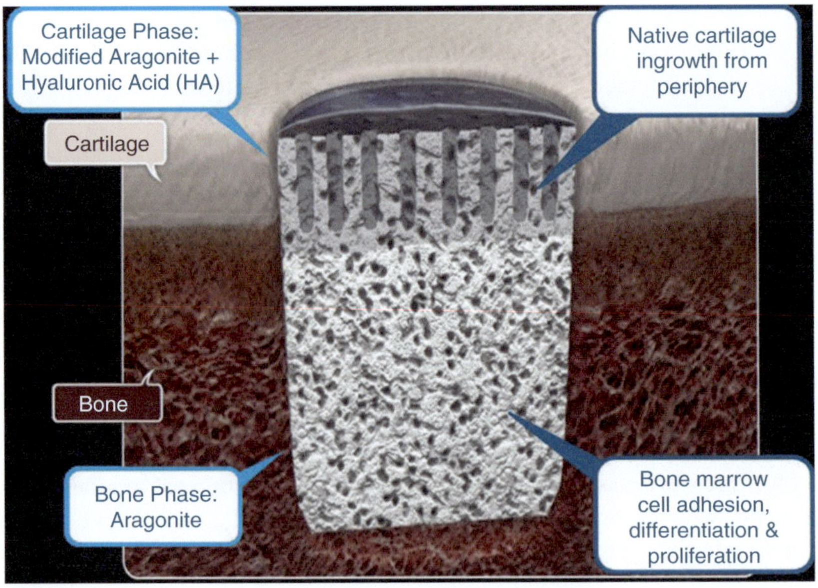

Fig. 44.4 Different layers of Agili-C™

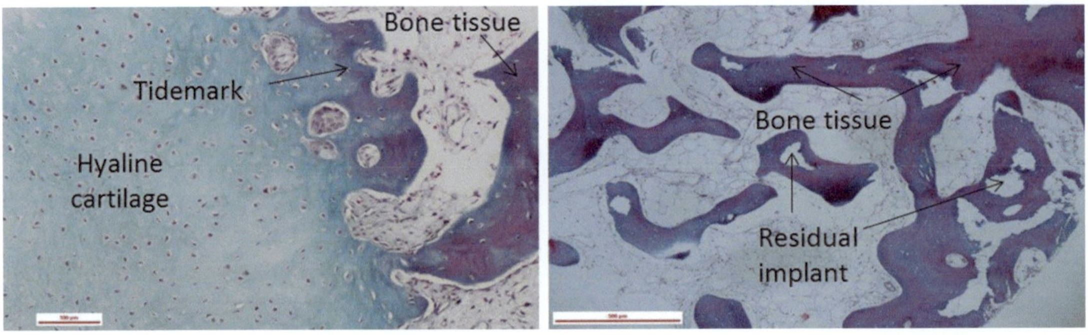

Fig. 44.5 Hystological demonstration of the cartilage regeneration process

dral and osteochondral defects in humans. It is 10 mm high with a variable diameter available, from 7.5 to 20 mm according to the lesion size.

Recently, a tapered version of the implants, with an angle of 2° from the longitudinal axis, has been designed to improve the press-fit implantation. After extensive purification processes, needed to treat and remove trapped particles, debris and organic remnants, the implants are sterilized by 25 kGy gamma radiation. Further modifications leads to different prototypes. The implants are then impregnated with HA homogenously in the chondral phase of the implant.

The surgical technique is carried out with the patient lying in the supine position in general or spinal anesthesia. A pneumatic tourniquet is applied at the proximal level of the thigh in order to block the vascular supply to the lower limb for a limited time span. According to the size and the location of the lesion, a mini-arthrotomy is performed using medial or lateral parapatellar approach in order to expose the lesions. The medial parapatellar incision is preferred for lesions of the MFC and the patellar cartilage, while the lateral parapatellar incision is preferred for the lesions of the lateral compartment.

It is fundamental to have a complete vision of the lesion of the defects are exposed.

The site of the lesion is then prepared using a proprietary surgical toolset.

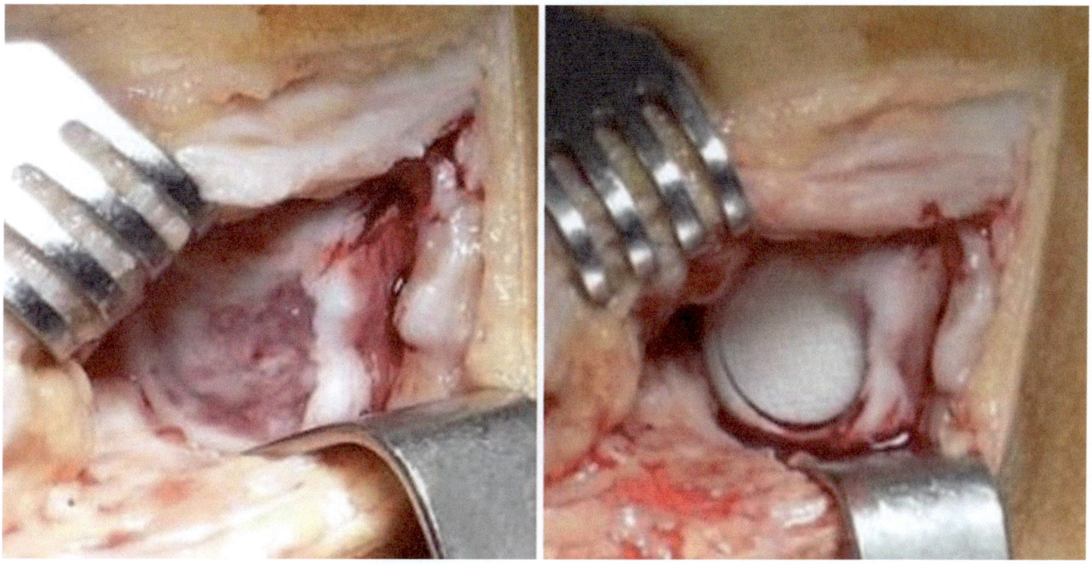

Fig. 44.6 Surgical implant of Agili-C™ scaffold

A perpendicular aligner is positioned in the center of the lesion upon verification that it is perpendicular to the articular surface. The aligner is used to place a K-wire, which is used to correctly position a drill sleeve where a motorized drill is inserted to prepare the defect up to the desired depth. A reamer is then inserted to ensure the correct depth is obtained, and a shaper is introduced to finalize the lesion with the correct wall inclination.

A lodge 12-mm deep with perpendicular shoulders is created to allow press-fit fixation of the implant, which is 10 mm long (Fig. 44.6).

The shaper and the K-wire are removed; the hole is appropriately cleaned with saline solution to wash out any debris.

The peripheral cartilage is regularized using a specific cartilage cutter or a scalpel to ensure smooth edges and to avoid invagination during implant insertion.

The Agili-C™ implant is manually inserted into the hole, firmly pushed with the thumb and subsequently gently impacted to a position 2 mm below the surface of the articular cartilage through a silicone-covered tamper.

When multiple Agili-C™ implants are used, it is important to keep a bone bridge of at least 5 mm between the implants to avoid impingement.

The stability of the implant is visually tested by cyclic bending of the knee while the graft is under direct vision, both before and after tourniquet removal.

Following promising results obtained in animal models [80], recently, clinical studies with Agili-C™ have been developed. Significant improvements at 12 months follow-up were documented in all clinical scores considered after the implantation of the aragonite-based scaffold [81]. Moreover, MRI findings revealed graft integration with good bone and cartilage formation.

References

1. Marcacci M, Filardo G, Kon E. Treatment of cartilage lesions: what works and why? Injury. 2013;44(Suppl 1):S11–5.
2. Widuchowski W, Widuchowski J, Trzaska T. Articular cartilage defects: study of 25,124 knee arthroscopies. Knee. 2007;14(3):177–82.
3. Arøen A, Løken S, Heir S, et al. Articular cartilage lesions in 993 consecutive knee arthroscopies. Am J Sports Med. 2004;32(1):211–5.
4. Hjelle K, Solheim E, Strand T, et al. Articular cartilage defects in 1,000 knee arthroscopies. Arthroscopy. 2002;18(7):730–4.
5. Noyes FR, Bassett RW, Grood ES, Butler DL. Arthroscopy in acute traumatic hemarthrosis of

the knee: incidence of anterior cruciate tears and other injuries. J Bone Joint Surg Am. 1980;62:687–95.
6. Buckwalter JA, Mankin HJ. Articular cartilage: tissue design and chondrocyte–matrix interactions. Instr Course Lect. 1998;47:477–86.
7. Buckwalter JA. Articular cartilage: injuries and potential for healing. J Orthop Sports Phys Ther. 1998;28(4):192–202.
8. Gratz KR, Wong BL, Bae WC, Sah RL. The effects of focal articular defects on intra-tissue strains in the surrounding and opposing cartilage. Biorheology. 2008;45(3–4):193–207.
9. Schinhan M, Gruber M, Vavken P, et al. Critical-size defect induces unicompartmental osteoarthritis in a stable ovine knee. J Orthop Res. 2012;30(2):214–20.
10. Andia I, Abate M. Platelet-rich plasma: underlying biology and clinical correlates. Regen Med. 2013;8:645–58.
11. Andia I, Sanchez M, Maffulli N. Tendon healing and platelet-rich plasma therapies. Expert Opin Biol Ther. 2010;10:1415–26.
12. Bosch G, Moleman M, Barneveld A, van Weeren PR, van Schie HT. The effect of platelet-rich plasma on the neovascularization of surgically created equine superficial digital flexor tendon lesions. Scand J Med Sci Sports. 2011;21:554–61.
13. Lyras D, Kazakos K, Verettas D, Polychronidis A, Simopoulos C, Botaitis S, Agrogiannis G, Kokka A, Patsouris E. Immunohistochemical study of angiogenesis after local administration of platelet-rich plasma in a patellar tendon defect. Int Orthop. 2010;34:143–8.
14. Lyras DN, Kazakos K, Verettas D, Polychronidis A, Tryfonidis M, Botaitis S, Agrogiannis G, Simopoulos C, Kokka A, Patsouris E. The influence of platelet-rich plasma on angiogenesis during the early phase of tendon healing. Foot Ankle Int. 2009;30:1101–6.
15. Alvarez P, Green PG, Levine JD. Role for monocyte chemoattractant protein-1 in the induction of chronic muscle pain in the rat. Pain. 2014;155:1161–7.
16. Andia I, Rubio-Azpeitia E, Maffulli N. Platelet-rich plasma modulates the secretion of inflammatory/angiogenic proteins by inflamed tenocytes. Clin Orthop Relat Res. 2015;473(5):1624–34.
17. Mann KG. Biochemistry and physiology of blood coagulation. Thromb Haemost. 1999;82:165–74.
18. Xie X, Wang Y, Zhao C, Guo S, Liu S, Jia W, Tuan RS, Zhang C. Comparative evaluation of MSCs from bone marrow and adipose tissue seeded in PRP-derived scaffold for cartilage regeneration. Biomaterials. 2012;33:7008–18.
19. Akeda K, An HS, Okuma M, Attawia M, Miyamoto K, Thonar EJ, Lenz ME, Sah RL, Masuda K. Platelet-rich plasma stimulates porcine articular chondrocyte proliferation and matrix biosynthesis. Osteoarthr Cartil. 2006;14:1272–80.
20. Chien CS, Ho HO, Liang YC, Ko PH, Sheu MT, Chen CH. Incorporation of exudates of human platelet-rich fibrin gel in biodegradable fibrin scaffolds for tissue engineering of cartilage. J Biomed Mater Res B Appl Biomater. 2012;100:948–55.
21. Spreafico A, Chellini F, Frediani B, Bernardini G, Niccolini S, Serchi T, Collodel G, Paffetti A, Fossombroni V, Galeazzi M, Marcolongo R, Santucci A. Biochemical investigation of the effects of human platelet releasates on human articular chondrocytes. J Cell Biochem. 2009;108:1153–65.
22. Kaps C, Loch A, Haisch A, Smolian H, Burmester GR, Haupl T, Sittinger M. Human platelet supernatant promotes proliferation but not differentiation of articular chondrocytes. Med Biol Eng Comput. 2002;40:485–90.
23. Gaissmaier C, Fritz J, Krackhardt T, Flesch I, Aicher WK, Ashammakhi N. Effect of human platelet supernatant on proliferation and matrix synthesis of human articular chondrocytes in monolayer and three-dimensional alginate cultures. Biomaterials. 2005;26:1953–60.
24. Drengk A, Zapf A, Sturmer EK, Sturmer KM, Frosch KH. Influence of platelet-rich plasma on chondrogenic differentiation and proliferation of chondrocytes and mesenchymal stem cells. Cells Tissues Organs. 2009;189:317–26.
25. Kon E, Filardo G, Di Matteo B, Marcacci M. PRP for the treatment of cartilage pathology. Open Orthop J. 2013;7:120–8.
26. Marx R. Platelet rich plasma (PRP): what is PRP and what is not PRP? Implant Dent. 2001;10:225–8.
27. Dohan Ehrenfest DM, Rasmuson L, Albrektsson T. Classification of platelet concentrates: from pure platelet-rich plasma (P-PRP) to leucocyte- and platelet-rich fibrin (LPRF). Trends Biotechnol. 2009;27(3):158–67.
28. Tschon M, Fini M, Giardino R, et al. Lights and shadows concerning platelet products for musculoskeletal regeneration. Front Biosci. 2011;3:96–107.
29. Torricelli P, Fini M, Filardo G, et al. Regenerative medicine for the treatment of musculoskeletal overuse injuries in competition horses. Int Orthop. 2011;35(10):1569–76.
30. Boswell SG, Cole BJ, Sundman EA, Karas V, Fortier LA. Platelet-rich plasma: a milieu of bioactive factors. Arthroscopy. 2012;28(3):429–39.
31. Wasterlain A, Braun HJ, Dragoo JL. Contents and formulations of platelet-rich plasma. Oper Tech Orthop. 2012;22(1):33–42.
32. Arnoczky S, Delos D, Rodeo S. What is platelet-rich plasma? Oper Tech Sports Med. 2011;19(3):142–8.
33. Giannini S, Buda R, Vannini F, Cavallo M, Grigolo B. One-step bone marrow-derived cell transplantation in talar osteochondral lesions. Clin Orthop Relat Res. 2009;467(12):3307–20.
34. Giannini S, Buda R, Cavallo M, et al. Cartilage repair evolution in post-traumatic osteochondral lesions of the talus: from open field autologous chondrocyte to bone-marrow-derived cells transplantation. Injury. 2010;41(11):1196–203.
35. Buda R, Vannini F, Cavallo M, Grigolo B, Cenacchi A, Giannini S. Osteochondral lesions of the knee: a

new one-step repair technique with bone-marrow-derived cells. J Bone Joint Surg Am. 2010;92(Suppl 2):2–11.
36. Dhollander AA, De Neve F, Almqvist KF, et al. Autologous matrix-induced chondrogenesis combined with platelet-rich plasma gel technical description and a five pilot patients report. Knee Surg Sports Traumatol Arthrosc. 2011;19(4):536–42.
37. Siclari A, Mascaro G, Gentili C, Cancedda R, Boux E. A cell-free scaffold-based cartilage repair provides improved function hyaline-like repair at one year. Clin Orthop Relat Res. 2012;470(3):910–9.
38. Mei-Dan O, Carmont MR, Laver L, Mann G, Maffulli N, Nyska M. Platelet-rich plasma or hyaluronate in the management of osteochondral lesions of the talus. Am J Sports Med. 2012;40(3):534–41.
39. Filardo G, Kon E, Pereira Ruiz MT, et al. Platelet-rich plasma intra-articular injections for cartilage degeneration and osteoarthritis: single- versus double-spinning approach. Knee Surg Sports Traumatol Arthrosc. 2012;20(10):2082–91.
40. Spaková T, Rosocha J, Lacko M, Harvanová D, Gharaibeh A. Treatment of knee joint osteoarthritis with autologous platelet-rich plasma in comparison with hyaluronic acid. Am J Phys Med Rehabil. 2012;91(5):411–7.
41. Sánchez M, Fiz N, Azofra J, et al. A randomized clinical trial evaluating plasma rich in growth factors (PRGF-Endoret) versus hyaluronic acid in the short-term treatment of symptomatic knee osteoarthritis. Arthroscopy. 2012;28(8):1070–8.
42. Filardo G, Madry H, Jelic M, Roffi A, Cucchiarini M, Kon E. Mesenchymal stem cells for the treatment of cartilage lesions: from preclinical findings to clinical application in orthopaedics. Knee Surg Sports Traumatol Arthrosc. 2013;21(8):1717–29.
43. Caplan AI. Mesenchymal stem cells: cell-based reconstructive therapy in orthopedics. Tissue Eng. 2005;11(7–8):1198–211.
44. Singer NG, Caplan AI. Mesenchymal stem cells: mechanisms of inflammation. Annu Rev Pathol. 2011;6:457–78.
45. Dominici M, Le Blanc K, Mueller I, Slaper-Cortenbach I, Marini F, Krause D, Deans R, Keating A, Dj P, Horwitz E. Minimal criteria for defining multipotent mesenchymal stromal cells. The International Society for Cellular Therapy position statement. Cytotherapy. 2006;8(4):315–7.
46. Friedenstein AJ, Piatetzky-Shapiro II, Petrakova KV. Osteogenesis in transplants of bone marrow cells. J Embryol Exp Morphol. 1966;6(3):381–90.
47. Caplan AI, Koutroupas S. The control of muscle and cartilage development in the chick limb: the role of differential vascularization. J Embryol Exp Morphol. 1973;29(3):571–83.
48. Spencer ND, Gimble JM, Lopez MJ. Mesenchymal stromal cells: past, present, and future. Vet Surg. 2011;40(2):129–39.
49. Wakitani S, Goto T, Pineda SJ, Young RG, Mansour JM, Caplan AI, Goldberg VM. Mesenchymal cell-based repair of large, full-thickness defects of articular cartilage. J Bone Joint Surg Am. 1994;76(4):579–92.
50. Quarto R, Mastrogiacomo M, Cancedda R, Kutepov SM, Mukhachev V, Lavroukov A, Kon E, Marcacci M. Repair of large bone defects with the use of autologous bone marrow stromal cells. N Engl J Med. 2011;344(5):385–6.
51. Lodi D, Iannitti T, Palmieri B. Stem cells in clinical practice: applications and warnings. J Exp Clin Cancer Res. 2011;30:9.
52. Davatchi F, Abdollahi BS, Mohyeddin M, Shahram F, Nikbin B. Mesenchymal stem cell therapy for knee osteoarthritis. Preliminary report of four patients. Int J Rheum Dis. 2011;14(2):211–5.
53. Chang CH, Kuo TF, Lin FH, Wang JH, Hsu YM, Huang HT, Loo ST, Fang HW, Liu HC, Wang WC. Tissue engineering based cartilage repair with mesenchymal stem cells in a porcine model. J Orthop Res. 2011;29(12):1874–80.
54. Saw KY, Anz A, Merican S, Tay YG, Ragavanaidu K, Jee CSY, McGuire DA. Articular cartilage regeneration with autologous peripheral blood progenitor cells and hyaluronic acid after arthroscopic subchondral drilling: a report of 5 cases with histology. Arthroscopy. 2011;27(4):493–506.
55. Breitbach M, Bostani T, Roell W, Xia Y, Dewald O, Nygren JM, Fries JW, Tiemann K, Bohlen H, Hescheler J, Welz A, Bloch W, Jacobsen SE, Fleischmann BK. Potential risks of bone marrow cell transplantation into infarcted hearts. Blood. 2007;110(4):1362–9.
56. Wakitani S, Okabe T, Horibe S, Mitsuoka T, Saito M, Koyama T, Nawata M, Tensho K, Kato H, Uematsu K, Kuroda R, Kurosaka M, Yoshiya S, Hattori K, Ohgushi H. Safety of autologous bone marrow-derived mesenchymal stem cell transplantation for cartilage repair in 41 patients with 45 joints followed for up to 11 years and 5 months. J Tissue Eng Regen Med. 2011;5(2):146–50.
57. Keeney M, Pandit A. The osteochondral junction and its repair via bi-phasic tissue engineering scaffolds. Tissue Eng Part B Rev. 2009;15(1):55–73.
58. Kocher MS, Tucker R, Ganley TJ, Flynn JM. Management of osteochondritis dissecans of the knee: current concepts review. Am J Sports Med. 2006;34(7):1181–91.
59. Pape D, Filardo G, Kon E, Van Dijk CN, Madry H. Disease-specific clinical problems associated with the subchondral bone. Knee Surg Sports Traumatol Arthrosc. 2010;18(4):448–62.
60. Gomoll AH, Madry H. The subchondral bone in articular cartilage repair : current problems in the surgical management. Knee Surg Sports Traumatol Arthrosc. 2010;18(4):434–47.
61. Gratz KR, Wong BL, Bae WC, Sah RL. The effects of focal articular defects on cartilage contact mechanics. J Orthop Res. 2009;27(5):584–92.
62. Wong BL, Kim SHC, Antonacci JM, Mcilwraith CW, Sah RL. Cartilage shear dynamics during tibio-femoral articulation: effect of acute joint injury and

tribosupplementation on synovial fluid lubrication. Osteoarthr Cartil. 2010;18(3):464–71.
63. Von Der Mark K, Gauss V, Von Der Marl H, Muller P. Relationship between cell shape and type of collagen synthesised as chondrocytes lose their cartilage phenotype in culture. Nature. 1977;267(5611):531–2.
64. Freed L, Marquis J, Nohria A. Neocartilage formation in vitro and in vivo using cells cultured on synthetic biodegradable polymers. J Biomed Mater Res. 1993;27(1):11–23.
65. Gricolo B, Lisignoli G, Piacentini A, Fiorini M, Gobbi P, Mazzotti G, Duca M, Pavesio A, Facchini A. Evidence for redifferentiation of human chondrocytes grown on a hyaluronan-based biomaterial (HYAFF11): melocular, immunohistochemical and ultrastructural analysis. Biomaterials. 2002;23(4):1187–95.
66. Caterson EJ, Nesti LJ, Li WJ, Danielson KG, Albert TJ, Vaccaro AR, Tuan RS. Three-dimensional cartilage formation by bone marrow-derived cells seed in polyactide/alginate amalgam. J Biomed Mater Res. 2001;57(3):394–403.
67. Marcacci M, Kon E, Zaffagnini S, Filardo G, Delcogliano M, Neri MP, Iacono F, Hollander AP. Arthroscopic second generation autologous chondrocyte implantation. Knee Surg Sports Traumatol Arthrosc. 2007;15(5):610–9.
68. Filardo G, Kon E, Di Martino A, Iacono F, Marcacci M. Arthroscopic second-generation autologous chondrocyte implantation: a prospective 7-year follow-up study. Am J Sports Med. 2011;39(10):2153–60.
69. Podskubka A, Povysil C, Kubes R, Sprindrich J, Sedlacek R. Treatment of deep cartilage defects of the knee with autologous chondrocyte transplantation on a hyaluronic acid ester scaffolds (Hyalograft C). Acta Chir Orthop Traumatol Cech. 2006;73(4):251–63.
70. Hollander AP, Dickinson SC, Sims TJ, Brun P, Cortivo R, Kon E, Marcacci M, Zanasi S, Borrione A, De Luca C, Pavesio A, Soranzo C, Abatangelo G. Maturation of tissue engineered cartilage implanted in injured and osteoarthritic human knees. Tissue Eng. 2006;12(7):1787–98.
71. Kon E, Di Martino A, Filardo G, Tetta C, Busacca M, Iacono F, Delcogliano M, Albisinni U, Marcacci M. Second-generation autologous chondrocyte transplantation: MRI findings and clinical correlations at a minimum 5-year follow-up. Eur J Radiol. 2011;79(3):382–8.
72. Lu Y, Dhanaraj S, Wang Z, et al. Minced cartilage without cell culture serves as an effective cell source for cartilage repair. J Orthop Res. 2006;24(6):1261–70.
73. Kon E, Robinson D, Verdonk P, Drobnic M, Patrascu J, Dulic O. A novel aragonite-based scaffold for osteochondral regeneration: early experience on human implants and technical developments. Injury. 2016;47(Suppl 6):S27–32.
74. Wang X, Grogan SP, Rieser F, Winkelmann V, Maquet V, La Berge M. Tissue engineering of biphasic cartilage constructs using various biodegradable scaffolds: an in vitro study. Biomaterials. 2004;25(17):3681–8.
75. Woodfield TB, Malda J, De Wijn J, Peters F, Riesle J, Van Blitterswijk CA. Design of porous scaffolds for cartilage tissue engineering using a three-dimensional fiber-deposition technique. Biomaterials. 2004;25(18):4149–61.
76. Kon E, Delcogliano M, Filardo G, et al. A novel nano-composite multi-layered biomaterial for treatment of osteochondral lesions: technique note and an early stability pilot clinical trial. Injury. 2010;41(7):693–701.
77. Kon E, Delcogliano M, Filardo G, et al. Orderly osteochondral regeneration in a sheep model using a novel nano-composite multilayered biomaterial. J Orthop Res. 2010;28(1):116–24.
78. Kon E, Delcogliano M, Filardo G, Busacca M, Di Martino A, Marcacci M. Novel nano-composite multilayered biomaterial for osteochondral regeneration a pilot clinical trial. Am J Sports Med. 2011;39(6):1180–90.
79. Demers C, Hamdy C, Corsi K, Chellat F, Tabrizian M, Yahia L. Natural coral exoskeleton as a bone graft substitute: a review. Biomed Mater Eng. 2002;12(1):15–35.
80. Kon E, Filardo G, Shani J, Altschuler N, Levy A, Zaslav K, Eisman JE, Robinson D. Osteochondral regeneration with a novel aragonite-hyaluronate biphasic scaffold: up to 12-month follow-up study in a goat model. J Orthop Surg Res. 2015;10:81.
81. Kon E, Robinson D, Verdonk P, Drobnic M, Patrascu JM, Dulic O, Gavrilovic G, Filardo G. A novel aragonite-based scaffold for osteochondral regeneration: early experience on human implants and technical developments. Injury. 2016;47(Suppl 6):S27–32.

Part IX

Major Events in Sports

Olympic Games: Special Considerations—Medical Care for Olympians

45

David J. Pohl, Garrett Schwartzman, Mark R. Hutchinson, William Moreau, Roald Bahr, Robert McCormack, Juan-Manuel Alonzo, Andre Pedrenelli, and Roberto Nahon

45.1 Introduction

The purpose of this chapter is to present and review the unique challenges that the sports medicine clinician may face regarding the Olympic Games and Olympic-level athletes. Specific anatomic injuries as well as sports-specific injuries have been covered elsewhere in the text. Several factors make the Olympic Games a unique event regarding sports medicine care. It is not only one of the largest mass sporting events in the world; it often represents the penultimate competition of an athlete's career. Unique challenges include acclimatization to a new country, travel, geography, foods, and language. The athlete not only has pressure from their coach and the fans of that particular sport but also a global audience and the pressures coming from stress related to representing their country. From the medical planning and organization perspective, the Olympic Games is a multisport, international, and mass sporting event. For the host country, the organization must provide optimal communication, transportation, and facilities to care for thousands of elite-level athletes. For national organizations, preparations can begin years in advance of the games and include planning how dependent they wish to be on the host country's medical plan; which facilities may be used in case of emergencies; what equipment, staff, and medications will be necessary to retain independent care of their own athletes; and arranging local licensure, contacts, and training facilities for its athletes throughout the course of competition.

D. J. Pohl · G. Schwartzman
University of Illinois at Chicago, Chicago, IL, USA

M. R. Hutchinson (✉)
University of Illinois at Chicago, Chicago, IL, USA

United States Olympic Committee,
Colorado Springs, CO, USA
e-mail: mhutch@uic.edu

W. Moreau
United States Olympic Committee,
Colorado Springs, CO, USA
e-mail: Bill.Moreau@usoc.org

R. Bahr
Department of Sports Medicine, Olympiatoppen,
Norwegian Olympic Training Center, Oslo, Norway
e-mail: Roald.bahr@nih.no

R. McCormack
Canadian Olympic Team, Toronto, ON, Canada

J.-M. Alonzo
Qatar Olympic Team, Doha, Qatar

Past Medical Team for Spanish Olympic and Track and Field Teams, Barcelona, Spain
e-mail: Juan-Manuel.Alonzo@aspetar.com

A. Pedrenelli
Team Physician Brazilian Olympic Team and National Men's Soccer Team, Rio de Janeiro, Brazil

R. Nahon
Brazilian Olympic Medical Services,
Rio de Janeiro, Brazil

S. Rocha Piedade et al. (eds.), *The Sports Medicine Physician*,
https://doi.org/10.1007/978-3-030-10433-7_45

45.2 Brief History

The modern Olympic Games began in Athens, Greece, in 1896, and encompassed 241 male athletes competing for 14 countries across 43 events in 9 sports [1]. These first sports included athletics, cycling, fencing, gymnastics, shooting, swimming, tennis, weightlifting, and wrestling. The Summer Olympics have been held in 18 different countries and grown significantly since that time. During the 2016 Summer Olympic Games, hosted in Rio de Janeiro, Brazil, over 11,238 athletes (6179 men and 5059 women) competed for 207 nations in 306 events in 28 sports [2] (Fig 45.1).

While initially part of the Summer Olympics, snow and ice sports split into a different Olympic Games, forming the Olympic Winter Games. The first Winter Olympic Games were held in 1924 in Chamonix, France. During those Games 258 athletes (245 men and 13 women) from 16 nations competed in 16 events across 5 sports that included bobsleigh, curling, ice hockey, skating, and Nordic skiing [3]. The Winter Olympics have grown in size and scope along with their Summer counterparts. The 2018 Winter Games in Pyeongchang, South Korea, featured 2922 athletes (1680 men and 1242 women) competing for 92 nations in 102 events in 15 sports [4] (Table 45.1).

Until 1992 the Summer and Winter Olympic Games were held in the same years, after which the Winter Games were switched to the even years between Summer Olympics to help with planning the two massive events. The International Olympic Committee (IOC) is the organization responsible for planning and putting on the Olympic Games. Established in 1894, the IOC is

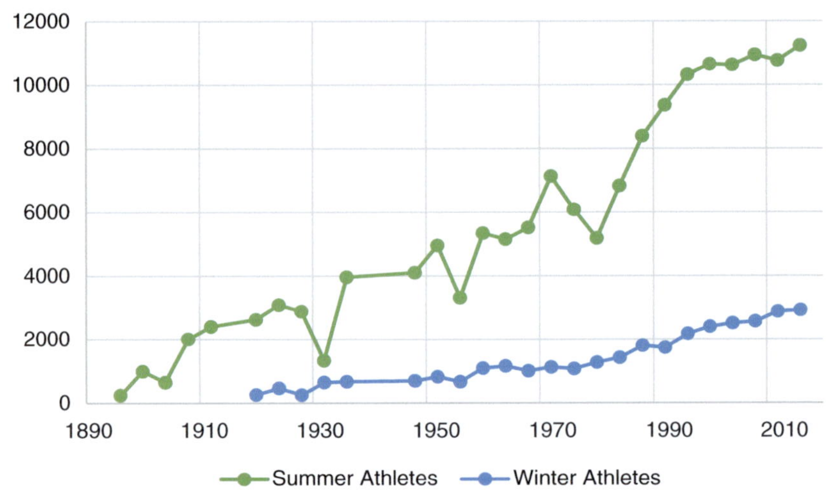

Fig. 45.1 Athletes participating in Olympic Games by year

Table 45.1 2016–2018 Olympic sports

2016 Summer sports			2018 Winter sports	
Aquatics	Field hockey	Shooting	Alpine skiing	Luge
Archery	Football	Table tennis	Biathlon	Nordic combined
Athletics	Golf	Taekwondo	Bobsleigh	Short track speed Skating
Badminton	Gymnastics	Tennis	Cross-country skiing	
Basketball	Handball	Triathlon	Curling	Skeleton
Boxing	Judo	Volleyball	Figure skating	Ski jumping
Canoeing	Modern pentathlon	Weightlifting	Freestyle skiing	Snowboarding
Cycling	Rowing	Wrestling	Ice hockey	Speed skating
Equestrian	Rugby sevens			
Fencing	Sailing			

an international, not-for-profit organization who's stated goal is "to ensures the regular celebration of the Olympic Games, supports all affiliated member organizations[sic] of the Olympic Movement and strongly encourages, by appropriate means, the promotion of the Olympic values" [5]. As of 2018 the IOC consisted of 100 active members, 41 honorary (or past) members, and 1 honorary president, all of who's role is to represent and promote the interests of the IOC and of the Olympic Movement.

Several of these members serve as chairpersons of one of the 27 IOC commissions. One such group, the Medical and Scientific Commission, is tasked with providing "a guiding reference for all other sports organizations on matters relating to the protection of the health of athletes" [6]. To this end, the Medical and Scientific Commission has worked to increase research on, and dissemination of, relevant educational topics. Since 2011 the IOC has sponsored triennial meetings to discuss and spread information on injury prevention. The IOC World Conference on Prevention of Injury and Illness in Sport focuses on the clinical aspects of sports and exercise medicine. These goals have also led the publication of 25 IOC consensus statements since 2004. Topics are wide-ranging and have included Sudden Cardiovascular Death in Sport (2004), Sexual Harassment and Abuse in Sport (2007), Asthma in Elite Athletes (2008), Sports Nutrition (2010), Concussion in Sport (2013), Relative Energy Deficiency in Sport (2015), Sex Reassignment and Hyperandrogenism (2015), and Dietary Supplements (2017).

Similarly, the Medical and Scientific Commission has published several educational tools available for athletes, coaches, and physicians. These tools range from articles and brochures to videos to the "Get Set—Train Smarter" smartphone/tablet application, and topics include injury prevention, harassment and abuse in sport, female athlete health, safeguarding athletes, and healthy body image. As of this book's publishing, these resources are available on the IOC's website at https://www.olympic.org/educational-tools.

As part of their commitment to promotion of the health of athletes and protection of clean athletes, the Medical and Scientific Committee is intimately involved in detecting and preventing doping. The IOC has established a zero-tolerance policy toward doping to combat cheating and works in conjunction with the World Anti-Doping Agency (WADA) to monitor and detect athletes in violation of this policy. Further discussion of WADA and doping is presented later in this chapter.

45.3 Pathways to Serve at Olympic Games

There are numerous pathways to become part of the healthcare team at the Olympic Games, and those paths vary from country to country and from games to games. The host country carries the responsibility of providing services to all residents of the Olympic Village, usually through establishment of a polyclinic. Each national organization will also decide to what extent to provide their own medical care to their athletes and how much to rely on the host country's services. Specific application processes will vary for each national organization, and those wishing to serve should contact their national organization or the host country's organization committee.

45.4 Host Country/City Organizing Committee

Planning for medical care during the Olympic Games begins years before the opening ceremonies. Facilities, transportation, and supplies must be obtained to account for any potential injury or illness that an athlete may suffer. Additionally, organizers must also plan for illnesses and injuries with coaches, national delegates, officials, members of the media, spectators, and members of the Olympic workforce.

As part of a larger network of medical care, the host country establishes one or more polyclinics for athletes and their support staff. These centers are typically capable of managing most medical complaints and, as the name implies, offer a variety of medical specialties including primary care, sports medicine, physiotherapy, chiropractic, podiatry, optometry, ophthalmology, and dentistry. There are typically additional specialists on call, including orthopedic surgery, cardiology, otolaryngology, obstetrics and gynecology, dermatology, neurology, psychiatry, and gastroenterology. There is a pharmacy, laboratory, and advanced radiology suite including X-ray, ultrasound, and MRI scanners. The polyclinics are aimed at making an accurate diagnosis quickly to allow for competent treatment of the athletes so that they may return to their competition as soon and as safely as possible [7].

The polyclinics are typically located in the Olympic Villages where a majority of the athletes stay and are staffed by a variety of expert, yet volunteer, medical professionals including physicians, nurses, physiotherapists, masseurs, technicians, and administrative staff. The polyclinic runs in conjunction with the Olympic Village: opening several days before the start of the Olympic Games, operating 24 h per day, and finally shutting their doors after the closing ceremony.

For the first time, the polyclinic at Rio 2016 also utilized an electronic medical record (EMR) during the treatment of their patients [8]. This allowed for better communication among the treatment team and also assisted with injury and illness data collection. Since 2008 the IOC has sought to establish an injury and illness surveillance system to better track, study, and hopefully prevent the various maladies afflicting the top athletes in the world. The IOC used the 2008 Beijing Summer Olympics as a model. The IOC injury surveillance system standardized injury definition, as well as methods and forms for reporting such injuries. This system ensured the comparability of results and thereby provided important epidemiological information, directions for injury prevention, and the ability to monitor long-term trends in the frequency and circumstances of injury [9]. This system was then expanded in 2010 for the Vancouver Winter Olympics to include illnesses [10]. This injury and illness surveillance system asks the medical teams of each National Olympic Committee (NOC) to report the daily occurrence (or nonoccurrence) of any injuries or illnesses suffered by their constituent athletes on standardized report forms. The same information is also obtained from the polyclinic and other medical facilities associated with the Olympic Games and cross-referenced.

The total incidence of injury in the Rio Games (8%) was the lowest reported since implementation of the IOC surveillance system [8]. Previously, the reported injury rates had been above 10%, specifically 10% in Beijing 2008 [9], 11% in Vancouver 2010 [10], 11% in London 2012 [11], and 12% in Sochi 2014 [12]. Specific injuries, sport-specific injury rates, and severity of injuries vary from year to year and, while beyond the scope of this chapter, are reported and discussed after each Olympic Games [8–12].

Services at the polyclinic are provided free of charge to athletes and members of their national delegations, and many individuals seek elective care during the Games from the expert staff and utilizing the advanced healthcare technology available to them [13]. For scale, the Rio 2016 polyclinic was staffed by 180 medical professional who covered 3500 square meters and 160 rooms [7]. In total, 1015 radiologic examinations were performed, including 607 MRI scans (59.8% of total studies) [14]. The previous record of 650 patient consultations in 1 day during the London 2012 Olympic Games was easily surpassed by the Rio 2016 polyclinic when it treated 900 patients in 1 day [15].

But polyclinics are just one part of the medical care offered at the Olympic Games. During the 2016 Rio Olympic Games, over 3000 volunteers were utilized across all aspects of the medical care team [16]. The importance of early planning and effective communication among the numerous groups and agencies involved has been well established [17]. First aid and appropriate medical care must be provided at the various Olympic sites, including the training and sporting venues and any affiliated hotels. Specific levels of services provided will vary by year and location. Most medical needs are addressed within the Olympic system and rarely result in transfer to outside hospitals [17]. However, consideration should be made for any medical need, from simple first aid up to and including mass casualty incidents and emergency transfers. Organizers should establish individualized emergency plans for each specific venue based on anticipated staff and supplies on site and proximity and transport to other resources. Organizers should therefore coordinate with local hospitals, off-site medical facilities, ambulance, and emergency responders to facilitate transfers, referrals, or other necessary services.

45.5 Caring for the National Team

In addition to providing local service during the Olympic Games, the International Olympic Committee empowers each National Olympic Committee to either take advantage of host country services or establish and develop their own healthcare team or, more commonly, a blend of their own team balanced with host equipment and providers. All providers are subject to the rules and licensure regulation of the host country which are usually liberalized for visiting physicians and healthcare providers during the Olympic Games and restricted to the care of the team's athletes and entourage. In general, you have to get a temporary medical license within the host country to serve as a medical provider.

Approaches to creating a healthcare team vary from country to country based on a myriad of factors ranging from size and specific needs of delegation, past history, and organizational history of the individual national governing body, with occasional political influence. Fundamentally, the core goals and missions are the same regardless structure and include fielding a healthy team, safely optimizing athletic performance, and efficient and effective response to injury and illness. Another key factor in the success of a healthcare team is their ability to work together across specialties and skill sets with the singular focus on athlete wellness and performance.

Ideally organizational planning to address the core goals and missions begins years before the Olympic Games and includes a national reporting structure that optimizes communication between healthcare professionals, athletes, and administrative leadership. Such structure can define expected roles and responsibilities of healthcare providers, design a health support system for athletes long before the games that can optimize their health and performance, provide access to necessary therapeutic and diagnostic equipment and treatments prior to and during the Games, and establish a chain of command that optimizes communication between athletes, coaches, healthcare providers, and administrators. Establishing a unified system of medical record keeping (ideally via an electronic medical record) is essential for continuity of care, communication between healthcare professionals, and can be used for medical research and future optimization of performance.

For Team USA, the healthcare team at the Olympic Games is brought together and led by a chief medical officer who is formally employed by the United States Olympic Committee and head team physician, who is a volunteer physician, with a long history expertise in sports medicine and established service to elite Olympic-level athletes. They, with other professional staff, begin years in advance of the games to develop programming to preserve athletes' health for national-level athletes and optimizing collaborative sports medicine programming with individual national sports governing bodies. It is their responsibility to create plans for medical emergency responses and review of athletes' periodic health evaluations, staff education (e.g., anti-doping and safe sport), staff selection, background checks, medical equipment, and medication requirements for their team at the Games. Team USA has several national training sites where national-level athletes can receive treatment, become educated about their health, and optimize high performance outcomes throughout the Olympic quadrennium. The actual medical team at an Olympic Games is a blend of USOC professionals, volunteer healthcare providers, and nominated national governing body healthcare providers who are credentialed with approval of the United States Olympic Committee. Regarding professional qualifications, the sports medicine team for Team USA at the Olympic Games includes primary care physicians, orthopedic surgeons, chiropractic physicians, physical therapists, athletic trainers, massage therapists, as well as nutritionists, exercise physiologists, and sports psychologists. The USOC leadership strives to create a positive athlete-centric environment within the collaborative multispecialty healthcare team that focuses on the preservation of athlete health while supporting high performance outcomes.

For Team Canada the organization is similar, with a chief medical officer who works with a head physician and a head therapist. As noted above planning for the games starts years in advance, and the medical team leads will perform site visits to determine the needs and specific challenges for the Games. Along with the National Sports Organizations, strategies are developed to prepare the teams for optimal performance at the Games. These plans need to include management of a variety of potential stressors including heat, nutrition, local health risks, travel fatigue, and jet lag. Experts are engaged to help develop specific protocols, so recommendations can be made to the athletes, coaches, and their support team.

Between games, the athlete's health is managed directly by the national sports organization or through regional Canadian Sports Institutes. Our goal is to have an integrated support team for each sport that includes physicians, therapists, strength and conditioning, sports scientists, nutritionists, and sports psychologists. This group (integrated support team) is responsible for optimization of athlete health. This includes performing an annual health examination, anti-doping education (including medication and supplement reviews), and making sure the athletes have an optimized dental care, appropriate physiologic monitoring, vaccinations, baseline concussions testing (high-risk sports), cardiac screening, etc. The goal is to not only care for injuries and illnesses that present but to also monitor the athletes, to ensure optimal health.

All physicians working with the Canadian national teams are required to hold the Diploma in Sport Medicine. The Canadian Academy of Sports and Exercise Medicine developed this "certificate of qualification," in cooperation with the Royal College of Physicians and Surgeons of Canada. It consists of a validated, OSCE-based examination. There are similar qualifications required for each of the other expert provider groups including the Diploma in Sports Physiotherapy, certification by the Canadian Sports Massage Therapy Association, Fellowship of the Royal College Chiropractic Sports Sciences, etc. Canada brings a large team of health professionals to the games. This reflects the fact that athletes have prioritized the healthcare team to optimize their performance (rated most important group after coaches). The larger sports will nominate their own practitioners, and the Canadian Olympic Committee tries to ensure continuity of care as much as possible (within the constraints of limited accreditation). There is also a small "core" team that supports smaller sports and rounds out the skill set of the overall Canadian Health Services Team.

The Olympic Games present special challenges, and it is not always the best athletes that wins, but the one that is best prepared to handle the Olympic environment. To help our health team prepare for this unique, high-pressure environment, we organize workshops and team preparation seminars in the lead up to the Games. At these sessions we not only table top scenarios but also stress the importance of communication and value/importance of working as one Canadian team at the games. Post Games debriefs are also carried out, as we constantly strive to improve our healthcare delivery and plan for the next quadrennial.

For Team Norway, Olympiatoppen, the national training site, serves as the hub for all athlete support, including healthcare. Although preparations for each Games are intensified toward the end of each Olympic cycle, the goal is to ensure that there is continuous, optimal medical care during the 4-year period. Olympiatoppen is set up with a sports medicine department with full- or part-time doctors and physical therapists specialized in sports medicine, orthopedics, rehabilitation, psychiatry, and allergy/asthma, serving all types of national team athletes, senior or junior, as well as students at elite sports schools. Day-to-day care is also provided by the medical teams of each national federation, in close collaboration with the Olympiatoppen team. Specific pre-Olympic preparations begin with the appointment of a chief medical officer and chief physical therapist 2–3 years before each Olympic Games and the formation of a large medical team consisting of all Olympiatoppen and national federation physicians and physical therapists engaged in the care of candidate athletes and their teams. Except for a few smaller federations with less resources, the medical teams are under contract. At the same time, candidate athletes are offered an extensive screening examination organized by Olympiatoppen to establish their health status and develop a specific plan of preventive initiatives. The screening examination is thought to represent a key event, establishing a close relationship between the athlete and his/her medical team. This is also the starting point for weekly, continuous health monitoring using a smartphone app as a communication and surveillance tool for the athlete and his/her medical team. In Norway, the focus is less on the selection of the smaller medical team going to the Olympic Games to provide on-site care and more on the large team working between Games ensuring that athletes are healthy on the night of the opening ceremony.

For Team Brazil, the planning of the medical department of the Brazilian delegation, known in Brazil as Team Brazil, begins long before the Olympic year. Besides all knowledge accumulated in the history of the Brazilian Olympic Committee (COB) in South American, Pan-American, and Olympic (summer and winter) games, there is an effort to remodel all medical services during the 4-year period that preceded the Games, culminating in the available service not only to athletes but also to all of those in Team Brazil (coach, technical commission, and staff). Two main principles are used for the medical department for the Games. First is the highest number of follow-ups possible of athletes, not only during missions but for the whole period. The second principle was to standardize assessment and team training in sports events that preceded the Games, including briefing and debriefing for the events.

The entire process of planning the medical team is a result of building a risk matrix for each sport, where the COB MD is able to optimize the use and avoid waste of financial and human resources. A preselection of professionals that would be responsible for each sport allows the possibility to enhance knowledge because of interactions with original team staff, such as physicians, physiotherapists, psychologists, and coaches, making work with athletes easier and enhancing doctor-patient relation. Furthermore, this improves knowledge in sports that Brazil is competing in for the first time, such as in Rio the sports of badminton, golf, field hockey, and rugby, representing a total of 46 athletes. For the Rio Games, this planning allowed thorough assessment and planning for the largest Olympic Team Brazil has ever fielded, indeed, larger than any other sports event. The COB supplied and staffed all official athletes in the village as well as two exclusive training centers for COB athletes, covering over 1000 people, 465 of these being athletes, and 342 events, considering official training sessions and competitions.

Assessments were divided into two categories: disease (26% of total assessments) and orthopedic and trauma (74% of total assessments). The most common complaint for diseases was upper airway infection, comprising of 25% of complaints, and diarrhea, 7% of complaints. Among orthopedic cases, the main diagnosis was muscle soreness, comprising of 37% of assessments, followed by back pain with 11% of complaints. Several key lessons were learned in medical team development for the games but particularly from the Rio Games. One that stands out is the importance of previous integration with each sport and its multidisciplinary teams. A legacy outcome of the Rio Games was the inauguration of the Olympic Laboratory of Brazil, where sports teams have direct access to lab and performance evaluations, making possible to assess health in a more individualized way related to high performance.

For Team Qatar, the healthcare team is appointed by the Qatar Olympic Committee among health practitioners working at Aspetar Hospital (the national sports medicine hospital), usually by choosing those professionals with larger experience at previous Olympic Games.

The chief medical officers (CMOs) who were sports medicine physicians formally employed by Aspetar usually are appointed some months in advance. The Qatar CMOs put together medical teams of sports physicians, sports physiotherapists, and massage therapists working with national federations qualified to Olympics. The Qatar CMOs were responsible to assist medical team members to get adequate licensing and accreditations, provision of medications and medical equipment, as well as getting the necessary permit for importing all equipment and medication. The vision of the Qatar medical team has been to create a focused group of sports health practitioners with good internal coordination and communication to deal with a small Olympic team of 30–40 athletes.

For Team Spain, the chief medical officer is appointed more than 1 year in advance by the Spanish Olympic Committee among the members of its Medical and Scientific Commission. The CMO is a sport physician, orthopedic surgeon, or medical doctor with extended experience related to the Olympic Games, management of health for elite athletes, as well as appropriate language skills. The Spanish CMO assembles a medical team of sports physicians, sports physiotherapists, and other health allied professionals that are especially knowledgeable and skilled within their relevant national federations to accompany their individual sports teams. These health professionals know their athletes very well and take care of their athletes' health during the competitive and training seasons prior to and during the Olympic Games. Additionally, some sports physicians and sports physiotherapists are usually appointed to support athletes from individual team sports that do not meet the Olympic quota to bring health team accompanying persons. The Spanish CMO traditionally organizes informative workshops and coordination meetings during the mission preparation to assure all medical team members are aware of important logistic aspects (such required vaccinations, jet-lag preparations, acclimatization camps, etc.) and to review communication pathways and guidelines. The Spanish CMO is responsible for assisting medical team members to get adequate licensing and accreditations, provision of medications and medical equipment, as well as getting the necessary permit for importing all equipment and medications. At the Rio Olympic Games, the Spanish medical team included 25–30 sports health practitioners to care for its Olympic team of 300–400 athletes and fulfilled its goal of being internally well-coordinated and communicated assuring optimized health of its athletes to provide a foundation that they could excel in performance.

45.6 Specific Lessons Learned

Each Olympic Games is a unique experience that offers various learning points for future events. Multiple variables affect an Olympic Games. Some are more obvious, such as the host city and current world events; but others are less apparent, such as the climate and athlete security. By reflecting on, and learning from, previous Games' shortcomings, future competitions can continue to produce outstanding events.

The first major event that provided serious lessons to future Olympic Games occurred during the Munich 1972 Games. On the morning of September 5, 1972, 8 Palestinian terrorists took 11 Israeli Olympic athletes and coaches hostage. The attack eventually ended in the death of all 11 Israeli Olympic athletes and 5 of the terrorists. The security at these Games was intentionally meant to be out of sight as a "care-free" game [18]. Security personnel were primarily equipped to handle unarmed conflicts and not large-scale terrorist attacks. What evolved out of these events was a change in tactics into a noticeable security presence at the Olympic Games. It has now become standard protocol to make well-armed security personnel visible to all who attend the Games. There are also demonstrations and numerous sweeps of the venues prior to events occurring to ensure the safety of the athletes and spectators [18, 19]. This single event at the Munich 1972 Games may have had the most profound and lasting impact on all future Olympic Games.

With the continued global spread of the Games, and more countries participating and hosting, new challenges have arisen with various Games [20–23]. An example of this is the air or water pollution at various host cities, with the 2008 Beijing and 2016 Rio Games being prime examples. Prior to, and during, the Beijing Games, one of the major concerns was the air quality and pollution that athletes would be facing. Beijing has been consistently ranked as one of the cities with the worst air quality in the world. A number of factors contribute to this, including industrialization, climate, as well as geography (the mountains around Beijing help to trap the already poor air in the valley) [24]. Prior to the Olympics, organizers took numerous steps in order to attempt to alleviate the dense pollution, including closing factories and restricting driving. However, studies conducted during the 2008 Games suggested that the particulate matter in the air was still "2.9, 3.5, and 1.9 times higher than those in Atlanta, Sydney, and Athens" [24–26]. Double the amount of pollutants in the air can have profound effects on the respiratory system. Research has shown that this amount of particulate matter in the airways can lead to substantial inflammation and smooth muscle dysfunction. Given the extremely strenuous nature of most Olympic events, this does not provide an ideal environment for athletes to perform at their optimal levels [27]. Although very few negative effects were reported due to the poor air quality in Beijing, athletes should still be aware of the potential effects of pollution and take appropriate steps to protect themselves in future Games. The steps taken by Beijing to decrease air pollution did have a lasting effect on the host country itself. Samples taken from individuals following the Beijing Games continued to show lower levels of inflammatory markers in the airways than prior to the Olympic Games [27].

The 2016 Rio Games presented another pollution challenge for the International Olympic Committee, water pollution. The poor water quality was highly publicized prior to the Rio games. An article published prior to the Games stated that the athletes "will be swimming and boating in waters so contaminated with human faeces that they risk becoming violently ill and unable to compete" [28]. There were multiple reports of athletes becoming sick prior to the Games during Olympic test events, including rowing and sailing. An estimated 1400 athletes came in direct contact with the contaminated water due to the nature of their sporting events [8]. The main issue with Rio was the failure to handle waste effectively, as most sewage in the city was not treated. The same Associated Press report found dangerously high viral loads throughout the city just days before the Olympic Games began [28]. Despite efforts by the city to improve water quality, viral and bacterial loads were similar during the Games as they had been at previous testing times. This underlines the difficulty of solving the problem. Despite the concern prior to the games, there were only a minimal number of athletes who became sick from the water [29]. Given the persistent poor quality of the water, these low infection rates are likely more due to awareness and preventative measures taken by individual athletes and teams than the attempted cleanup by the host country. In the end, whether the issue is air or water pollution, the IOC and individual organizing committees must be aware of these specific challenges that face a possible host city and work to correct or reduce the potential exposure to ensure the safety and optimal performance of the athletes. Additionally, team doctor must also be aware of the potential threats from environmental pollution and may wish to take their own measures to reduce their athletes' exposure. In the above examples, this could include bringing bottled water or respirator masks for their contingents.

Finally, given the mass numbers of people and athletes crowding into a city during the games, it is inevitable that various communicable diseases should be a worry of IOC organizers and team physicians. The London 2012 and Rio 2016 Games gave Olympic physicians helpful yet hard-earned lessons to ensure that athletes stay healthy and are able to compete at their optimal levels. According to data collected by the IOC Injury and Illness Surveillance System, the incidence of illness during the Rio Games (5%) was the lowest reported since illnesses began being recorded in 2010 [8]. London 2012 and Vancouver 2010 each showed a 7% illness rate [10, 11], while Sochi 2014 reported an 8% illness rate [12]. Respiratory and gastrointestinal diseases account for a majority (68–75%) of the reported illnesses [8, 12, 17]. The ability to identify the most common illnesses and possible causes can help keep athletes at their optimal levels in future Games.

Given the diversity of host cities around the world, it is necessary to consider the variety of local infections that may not affect athletes while in their home countries. A unique infectious aspect of the Rio Games that required physician awareness was the Zika virus outbreak. With the prevalent mosquito as a vector for human transmission, the cases of Zika infection increased prior to the games [30]. Research into the virus found that it caused minimal affects in the infected individual, at the most a severe upper respiratory infection, but the real concern was the devastating birth defects, especially microcephaly, found in newborns of infected mothers. This caused grave concern among many athletes and spectators, especially due to the childbearing age of many Olympians. The world community took extensive action and was able to learn about the virus prior to the games. This information helped with prevention techniques, especially encouraging anti-mosquito and safer sex precautions [31, 32]. As a result, there was not an increase in cases during the Games. Rio 2016 helps demonstrate how local disease or infections must be studied ahead of the Games and thus may be prevented in the future. Team physicians should also consider specific precautions for their athletes and delegations based on the potential infections and vectors they may encounter. With the mosquito-borne Zika virus, physicians employed mosquito nets and bug spray to help prevent infection. By considering previous examples and studying the upcoming environment, team physicians can gain the tools to handle most any future geographic infectious diseases they may encounter [33].

45.7 Doping

Doping is an unfortunate reality that affects every Olympic Games. Although the first doping tests were instituted at the 1968 Winter Olympic Games in Grenoble, France, the World Anti-Doping Agency (WADA) was not established until 1999 [34]. The organization's mission is "to lead a collaborative worldwide movement for doping free sport." The organization publishes a code that 660 international sports organizations and government bodies must adhere to when competing in sanctioned sporting events. The code provides a coordinated approach to anti-doping strategies and research activities for the participating organizations [35].

For the 2018 PyeongChang Games, the entire Russian Olympic Committee was suspended due to evidence of state-sponsored doping, cover-up, and manipulation extending back to the 2014 Sochi Games. With this renewed emphasis placed on catching and example of punishing cheaters, it is even more important for physicians to be aware of, and compliant with, the rules of WADA. The list of banned substances and methods is easily obtainable from the WADA website as a downloadable file. An example is shown below in Fig. 45.2. It is important to note that there are unique substances banned for each sport, as well as for inside and outside of competition season. One specific example is the prohibition of beta blockers in shooting sports, as they help to slow heart rate and steady the hand while shooting.

WADA does offer exemptions for certain medications based on athlete medical conditions. This is called a Therapeutic Use Exemption (TUE) and must be applied for by the medical team. The TUE is narrow and specific in scope, and a documented medical condition must be present prior to any exemption being granted. There are specific sets of criteria regarding diagnostic testing, documentation, and alternative medications that vary for each medication and medical condition. These guidelines must be followed to ensure the exemption is granted. It is important for the treating physician to be aware of any chronic or acute medical condition that may require a TUE, as failure to apply and receive an exemption can result in a positive test for the athlete and subsequent disqualification from competition and possible forfeiture of previous results.

Physicians and athletes must also be compliant with WADA monitoring and testing policies.

SUBSTANCES PROHIBITED IN PARTICULAR SPORTS

P1 **BETA-BLOCKERS**

Beta-blockers are prohibited *In-Competition* only, in the following sports, and also prohibited *Out-of-Competition* where indicated.

- Archery (WA)*
- Automobile (FIA)
- Billiards (all disciplines) (WCBS)
- Darts (WDF)
- Golf (IGF)
- Shooting (ISSF, IPC)*
- Skiing/Snowboarding (FIS) in ski jumping, freestyle aerials/halfpipe and snowboard halfpipe/big air
- Underwater sports (CMAS) in constant-weight apnoea with or without fins, dynamic apnoea with and without fins, free immersion apnoea, Jump Blue apnoea, spearfishing, static apnoea, target shooting, and variable weight apnoea.

*Also prohibited *Out-of-Competition*

Including, but not limited to:

Acebutolol;	Labetalol;
Alprenolol;	Levobunolol;
Atenolol;	Metipranolol;
Betaxolol;	Metoprolol;
Bisoprolol;	Nadolol;
Bunolol;	Oxprenolol;
Carteolol;	Pindolol;
Carvedilol;	Propranolol;
Celiprolol;	Sotalol;
Esmolol;	Timolol.

Fig. 45.2 Taken from the World Anti-Doping Code, International Standard, Prohibited List January 2018

This includes random and timed drug tests, both inside and outside of competition. Therefore, athletes and physicians must be aware of any substances that the athlete is ingesting or utilizing, including supposedly allowed dietary supplements such as creatine and protein. Survey data from 2012 to 2016 showed 57% of US high school teenagers used protein supplementation and 34% used creatine supplementation. It was also shown that a high percentage of these supplements were contaminated with banned substances, including steroids [36]. While there are several third-party companies that will test and certify supplements against WADA standards, athletes are still ultimately responsible for everything they ingest and should exercise caution when choosing and using supplements [37, 38].

Overall, it is the responsibility of the physician and the athlete to have an open and candid conversation regarding doping and the rules that WADA has provided. If there is any question as to the legality of a substance, multiple resources exist to ensure that the athlete is not in violation of any anti-doping rules. In the event that an exemption is required, there is also a clearly defined means for providing this to the athlete. There should be minimal hurdles or difficulty in the partnership between the physician and athlete to keep Olympic sports free from doping.

45.8 Caring for Olympic-Level Athletes Outside of Olympic Games

As discussed above, detecting and preventing doping is a point of emphasis for the IOC and WADA. It is vital that physicians working with Olympic athletes know these doping rules and the specific medication statutes of the athlete's sport. Physicians should also be familiar with the specific terminology, in-game rules, and biomechanical requirements of their athletes' sports. Not only does this allow for improved communication regarding injuries, it also provides additional credibility for the physician with the athletes, fostering an improved doctor-patient relationship.

An additional, and sometimes only, opportunity to establish a doctor-patient relationship with the Olympic-level athlete is during the preparticipation physical examination (PPE) or periodic health evaluation (PHE). While not mandated by the IOC, the PHE is recommended by the IOC's 2009 consensus statement [39]. The main purpose of the PHE is to screen for injuries or medical conditions that place the athlete at higher risk during competition. Therefore, the

PHE should be based on scientific evidence and established criteria and tailored to the athlete's specific sport, age, gender, and race when appropriate. If a condition is detected or suspected, additional workup and management should be performed as necessary. In addition to screening for conditions and establishing medical care, the PHE can also serve to ensure proper diagnosis and management of some silent conditions that still affect performance, such as mild iron deficiency or astigmatism [39]. The PHE should be part of an ongoing process for elite athletes and ideally performed far in advance of any major competitions to allow for adequate treatment of any identified conditions.

Throughout the years and months leading up to the Olympic Games, a national team physician may be called upon to perform other preliminary services for the teams and athletes of their nation. These can range from performing the PHE to working national competitions or Olympic Trials. Throughout this process communication with not only the athletes but also the training staff, coaches, and national organizers is crucial to helping the Olympic athletes become or remain healthy enough to compete at the highest level.

45.9 Unique Challenges at Olympic Games

45.9.1 Licensure and Access in Foreign Country

National team physicians and other healthcare practitioners will need to obtain licensure or accreditation in the host country for the duration of their visit, including any time before or after the Olympic Games. This process will vary based on the home country's laws and regulations but will, at the very least, require registration of each national team healthcare provider with the host country. After registration, the process has varied from simply allowing registrants to practice within their usual scopes of practice without further licensure or certification from the host country [40] to granting accredited physicians a temporary license to practice during the duration of the operation of the Olympic Village [16]. The licensure or accreditation will allow NOC team doctors to treat only members of their own national delegation, unless specific permission is granted by another national organization. The registration will also allow the NOC team physicians to request physiotherapy, medications, imaging, or other diagnostic services from the polyclinic, but not outside facilities or hospitals.

Care should also be taken to ensure proper malpractice insurance, as the host country usually does not provide coverage for NOC team physicians. National team physicians should inform their insurance companies of the travel abroad with a sports team and confirm that they have adequate coverage for that role. The host country will provide malpractice insurance for the healthcare practitioners and services provided under their auspices, such as those offered at the polyclinic or at specific venues.

45.9.2 Language Barriers/Communication

The official languages of the IOC and thus the Olympic Games are French and English, and all official communications and signage must contain both translations [41]. If different from those two, the dominant language of the host country will also be prevalent throughout each Olympic Games. However, with over 200 nations participating in the Games, there are a myriad of other languages spoken by athletes, national organization members, and spectators alike. As national team physicians are often restricted to treating their country's own athletes and committee members, communication and language barriers should be a relative nonissue. In the instances where discussion or coordination is necessary with the host nation's medical services, or for physicians and medical staff who will be treating patients from a variety of countries, effective communication is paramount. Therefore, translation services should be made readily available to facilitate accurate and timely medical care. Such services can be in person, over the phone or telecommunication, or, as technology continues to advance, via smartphone or computer applications. The 2016 Rio Games employed over 8000 professional translators fluent in over 30 languages to assist throughout all aspects of the Games [42].

45.9.3 Qualification/Disqualification: RTP Decisions

If an injury occurs during competition, each sport has their own rules and medical structure that dictates who is the first to respond to the athlete, whether that be the national team doctor, physiotherapist, or a physician from the sport-specific international federation [43]. The medical providers of the host country are available to assist and advise throughout the diagnosis and treatment process, but the ultimate return-to-play decision rests with the NOC team doctor and IOC Medical Commission if necessary [40].

Take-Home Messages

- When caring for Olympic athletes, the healthcare professional must be aware of the unique demands and pressures of this often once in a lifetime experience for athletes.
- Injury and illness prevention is the key to optimal team performance at any Olympic Games.
- Special planning and preparation is necessary to manage a national team in a foreign country including travel, nutrition, and access to healthcare.

References

1. International Olympic Committee. Athens—1896. 2017. https://www.olympic.org/athens-1896. Accessed 7 Mar 2018.
2. International Olympic Committee. Rio 2016. 2018. https://www.olympic.org/rio-2016. Accessed 7 Mar 2018.
3. International Olympic Committee. Chamonix—1924. 2017. https://www.olympic.org/chamonix-1924. Accessed 7 Mar 2018.
4. International Olympic Committee. PyeongChang—2018. 2018. https://www.olympic.org/pyeongchang-2018. Accessed 7 Mar 2018.
5. International Olympic Committee. The IOC—What We Do. 2018. http://www.olympic.org/the-ioc/what-we-do. Accessed 7 Mar 2018.
6. International Olympic Committee. Medical and Scientific Commission. 2018. http://www.olympic.org/medical-and-scientific-commission. Accessed 7 Mar 2018.
7. Budgett R. On call for Olympic athletes: MRIs, ultrasounds and digital X-rays. 2016. https://www.ge.com/reports/call-olympic-athletes-mris-ultrasounds-digital-x-rays/. Accessed 7 Mar 2018.
8. Soligard T, Steffen K, Palmer-Green D, et al. Sports injury and illness incidence in the Rio de Janeiro 2016 Olympic Summer Games: a prospective study of 11 274 athletes from 207 countries. Br J Sports Med. 2017;51(17):1265–71.
9. Junge A, Engebretsen L, Alonso JM, et al. Injury surveillance in multi-sport events: the International Olympic Committee approach. Br J Sports Med. 2008;42(6):413–21.
10. Engebretsen L, Steffen K, Alonso JM, et al. Sports injuries and illnesses during the Winter Olympic Games 2010. Br J Sports Med. 2010;44(11):772–80.
11. Engebretsen L, Soligard T, Steffen K, et al. Sports injuries and illnesses during the London Summer Olympic Games 2012. Br J Sports Med. 2013;47(7):407–14.
12. Soligard T, Steffen K, Palmer-Green D, et al. Sports injuries and illnesses in the Sochi 2014 Olympic Winter Games. Br J Sports Med. 2015;49(7):441–7.
13. Reeser JC, Willick SE, Elstad MR. Medical services provided at the Olympic Village polyclinic during the 2002 Salt Lake City Winter Games. WMJ. 2003;102(4):20.
14. Guermazi A, Hayashi D, Jarraya M, et al. Sports injuries at the Rio de Janeiro 2016 Summer Olympics: use of diagnostic imaging services. Radiology. 2018;287(3):922–32. https://doi.org/10.1148/radiol.2018171510.
15. GE Healthcare. How a healthcare olympic record was broken in Rio. 2018. http://newsroom.gehealthcare.com/how-a-healthcare-olympic-record-was-broken-in-rio-2/. Accessed 7 Mar 2018.
16. Olympic Games Healthcare Guide. 2016. http://medsport.by/sites/default/files/custom/rio_2016_healthcare_guide_for_the_olympic_games.pdf. Accessed 7 Mar 2018.
17. Kononovas K, Black G, Taylor J, Raine R. Improving Olympic Health Services: what are the common health care planning issues? Prehosp Disaster Med. 2014;29(6):623.
18. Wolff AD. When the terror began. 2002. http://content.time.com/time/world/article/0,8599,2051168,00.html. Accessed 26 Mar 2018.
19. Boyle P, Haggert KD. Planning for the worst: risk, uncertainty and the Olympic Games. Br J Sociol. 2012;63(2):241–59.
20. Enock K, Jacobs J. The Olympic and Paralympic Games 2012: literature review of the logistical planning and operational challenges for public health. Public Health. 2008;122(11):1229–38.

21. Streets DG, Fu JS, Jang C, et al. Air quality during the 2008 Beijing Olympic Games. Atmos Environ. 2007;41(3):480–92.
22. Black G, Kononovas K, Taylor J, Raine R. Healthcare planning for the Olympics in London: a qualitative evaluation. PLoS One. 2014;9(3):e92338.
23. Greenhalgh T. The Olympics are over. What have we learned about organizing and delivering healthcare? J Roy Soc Med. 2012;105(19):373–6.
24. Wang W, Primbs T, Tao S, Massey Simonich SL. Atmospheric particulate matter pollution during the 2008 Beijing Olympics. Environ Sci Technol. 2009;43(14):5314–20.
25. Jamieson A. Beijing Olympics were the most polluted games ever, researchers say. The Telegraph. 2009.
26. Fitch K. Air pollution, athletic health and performance at the Olympic Games. J Sports Med Phys Fitness. 2016;56:922–32.
27. Gao J, Xu X, Ying Z, et al. Post-effect of air quality improvement on biomarkers for systemic inflammation and microparticles in asthma patients after the 2008 Beijing Olympic Games: a pilot study. Inflammation. 2017;40(4):1214–24.
28. Diseases TLI. Concerns raised over water quality at the Rio Olympics. Lancet Infect Dis. 2015;15(9):987.
29. Barchfield J. Rio 2016: swimmers need to ingest only three teaspoons of water to be almost certain of contracting a virus. Independent. Aug 2016;1:2016.
30. Warnke K, Paul J. Zika virus-impact on the 2016 Olympic Games in Rio de Janeiro. Sportverletz Sportschaden. 2016;30(3):154–6.
31. Grills A. Projected Zika virus importation and subsequent ongoing transmission after travel to the 2016 Olympic and Paralympic Games—country-specific assessment, July 2016. MMWR Morb Mortal Wkly Rep. 2016;65(28):711–5.
32. Shadgan B, Pakravan A, Zaeimkohan H, et al. Zika and Rio Olympic Games. Curr Sports Med Rep. 2016;15(4):298–300.
33. Burattini MN, Coutinho FAB, Lopez LF, et al. Potential exposure to Zika virus for foreign tourists during the 2016 Carnival and Olympic Games in Rio de Janeiro, Brazil. Epidemiol Infect. 2016;144(9):1904–6.
34. Fraser AD. Doping control from a global and national perspective. Ther Drug Monitor. 2004;26(2): 171–4.
35. Mountjoy M, Akef N, Budgett R, et al. A novel anti-doping and medical care delivery model at the 2nd Summer Youth Olympic Games (2014), Nanjing China. Br J Sports Med. 2015;49(13):887–92.
36. LaBotz M, Griesemer BA. Use of performance enhancing substances. Pediatrics. 2009;138(1) https://doi.org/10.1542/peds.2016-1300.
37. Barroso O, Schamasch P, Rabin O. Detection of GH abuse in sport: past, present and future. Growth Horm IGF Res. 2009;19(4):369–74.
38. Catlin DH, Fitch KD, Ljungqvist A. Medicine and science in the fight against doping in sport. J Intern Med. 2008;264(2):99–114.
39. Ljungqvist A, Jenoure P, Engebretsen L, et al. The International Olympic Committee (IOC) Consensus Statement on periodic health evaluation of elite athletes March 2009. Br J Sports Med. 2009;43(9):631–43.
40. Sochi 2014 Healthcare Guide. 2014. https://library.olympic.org/Default/doc/SYRACUSE/44832/health-care-guide-sochi-2014-organizing-committee-of-the-xxii-olympic-winter-games-and-paralympic-win. Accessed 10 Mar 2018.
41. Internation Olympic Committee. Olympic charter in force as from 2 August 2015. 2015. https://stillmed.olympic.org/Documents/olympic_charter_en.pdf. Accessed 10 Mar 2018.
42. Internation Olympic Committee. Rio 2016 looking for 8000 volunteers with language skills to be voice of the games. 2014. https://www.rio2016.com/en/news/rio-2016-looking-for-8-000-volunteers-with-language-skills-to-be-voice-of-the-games. Accessed 10 Mar 2018.
43. Budgett R. Healthcare challenges at an Olympic Games. Br J Sports Med. 2013;47:401.

Paralympic Sport

46

Yetsa A. Tuakli-Wosornu, Fiona Doolan, and Jan Lexell

Take-Home Message

For 70 years, organized Para sport has offered individuals with impairment enhanced health and improved quality of life, while the pinnacle event of Para sport, the Paralympic Games, continues to inspire and excite the world.

46.1 History and Structure of the Paralympic Games

Prior to the conclusion of World War II, even the most progressive clinicians viewed severe spinal injuries as fatal due to the severe attendant secondary complications such as septicemia, renal failure, major depression, and others. Approximately 80% of British and American spinally injured World War I veterans did not survive [1], and those who did "dragged out their lives as useless and hopeless cripples, unemployable and unwanted…with no incentive or encouragement to return to a useful life" [2].

Toward the end of World War II, a young Jewish neurosurgeon, Dr. Ludwig Guttmann, challenged the prevailing notion that spinal cord injury was akin to invalidism. Refuting that spinal cord injury inevitably portended a short life with little meaning, Guttmann created an intensive, dynamic clinical rehabilitation program when he became head of the National Spinal Injuries Unit at the Ministry of Pensions Hospital, Stoke Mandeville, in 1943 [3, 4]. Under his direction, multidisciplinary care teams implemented rigorous rehabilitation programs, engaged patients in community recreation, and established prevocational work programs, helping to facilitate health, happiness, confidence, and independence (Fig. 46.1) [5, 6].

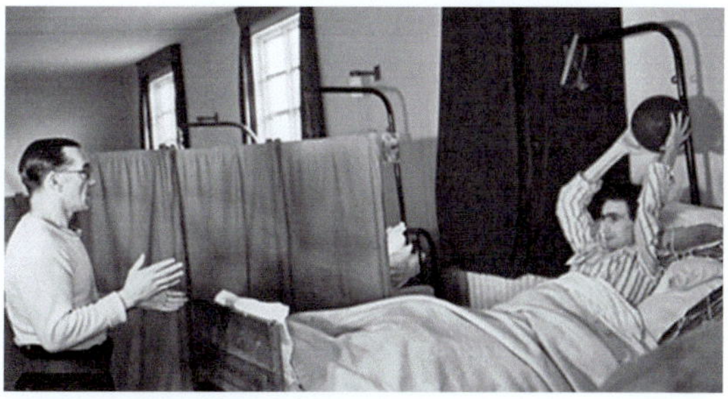

Fig. 46.1 "Q" Hill, Remedial Gymnast, using a medicine ball to strengthen a patient's upper body at Stoke Mandeville Hospital. Image reproduced with permission care of Professor Ian Brittain © International Wheelchair and Amputee Sports Federation (IWAS), Aylesbury College, Buckinghamshire, United Kingdom

Y. A. Tuakli-Wosornu (✉)
Department of Chronic Disease Epidemiology, Yale School of Public Health, New Haven, CT, USA
e-mail: yetsa.tuakli-wosornu@yale.edu

F. Doolan
Trinity College Dublin School of Medicine, Dublin 2, Ireland
e-mail: fcdoolan@bu.edu

J. Lexell
Department of Neuroscience, Rehabilitation Medicine, Uppsala University and Uppsala University Hospital, Uppsala, Sweden
e-mail: jan.lexell@neuro.uu.se

S. Rocha Piedade et al. (eds.), *The Sports Medicine Physician*,
https://doi.org/10.1007/978-3-030-10433-7_46

Uniquely, Guttmann's program incorporated competitive sport, one of the most social and spirited therapeutic modalities. He described sport as "the most natural form of remedial exercise" and saw it as a powerful tool to restore physical strength, cardiorespiratory fitness, and coordination while also repairing psychological health [6].

Guttmann's aim was to "not only give hope and a sense of self-worth to the patients, but to change the attitudes of society towards the spinally injured by demonstrating to them that they could not only continue to be useful members of society, but could take part in activities and complete tasks most of the nondisabled society would struggle with" [7]. Indeed, Guttmann would take patients into nondisabled community archery clubs, engaging nondisabled persons in competitions with Stoke Mandeville teams, further eroding barriers between the community and paraplegic persons [7]. In 1948, Guttmann organized a small archery competition among 16 paralyzed British war veterans from two hospitals, the Stoke Mandeville Games (later the "International Stoke Mandeville Games") (Fig. 46.2) [8].

What started as a modest contest between Stoke Mandeville and the Star and Garter Home for Injured War Veterans evolved in name and scope over the next 12 years, featuring an increasing number of sports, athletes, and nations every year. By 1960, the International Stoke Mandeville Games had evolved into the first large international Para sport festival, held in Rome, Italy, using the same venue as the Rome Olympic Games [1]. The event featured 400 athletes, all of whom were spinally injured, representing 23 countries.

Out of the spirit embodied by Guttmann's pioneering sporting initiatives and transformative notions about injury and ability, the Paralympic Movement has steadily become one of the most successful sporting initiatives in history. What started as a grassroots effort to restore war-wounded citizens to physical, mental, and social health has evolved into a global campaign for unification and empowerment through sport [9].

The contemporary Paralympic Movement is currently enjoying unprecedented growth in both

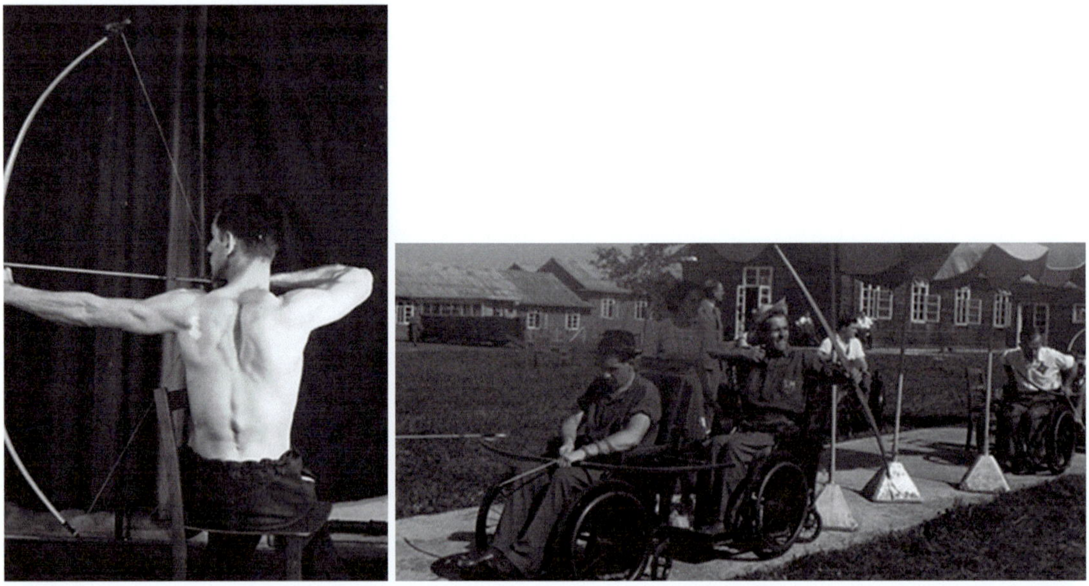

Fig. 46.2 Archery. In Image 2, Roy Jennings (Stoke Mandeville team) releases his arrow watched by his fiancée, Effie Wright. "Old Bill," the specially adapted bus, can be seen in the background. Images reproduced with permission care of Professor Ian Brittain © International Wheelchair and Amputee Sports Federation (IWAS), Aylesbury College, Buckinghamshire, United Kingdom

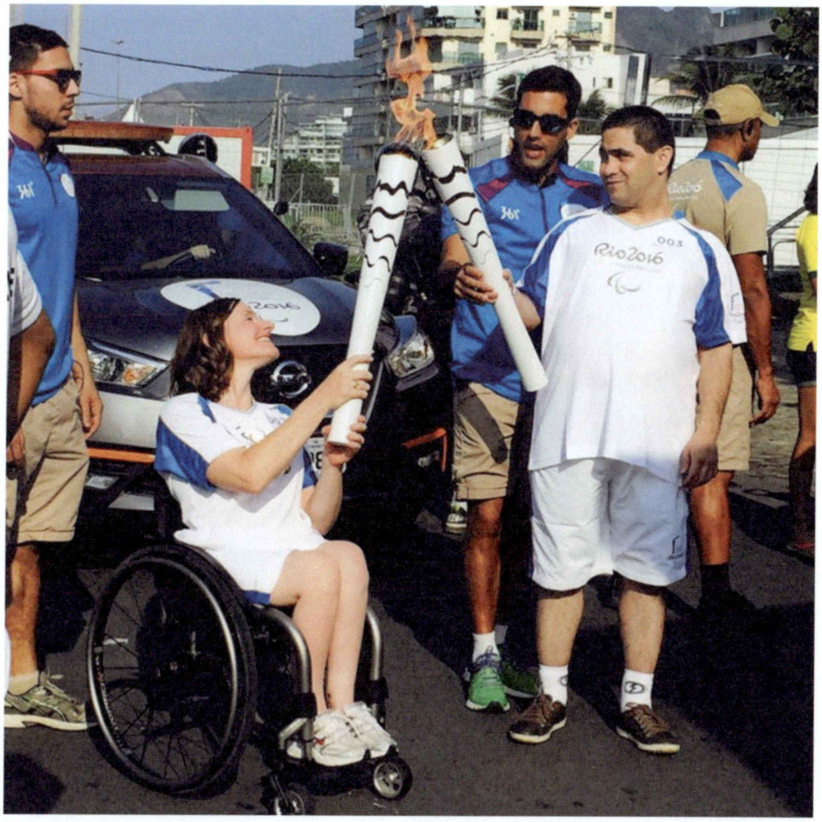

Fig. 46.3 Two Paralympic ambassadors, a wheelchair athlete and a visually impaired athlete, participate in the 2016 Rio Paralympic Games torch relay in Rio de Janeiro, Brazil. Photo reproduced with permission © Yetsa A. Tuakli-Wosornu, MD, MPH, New Haven, Connecticut, USA

size and exposure. In 2016, the 15th meeting of the Paralympic Games was contested in Rio de Janeiro, Brazil. It featured more than 4300 athletes representing 160 countries including a team of Independent Paralympic athletes, competing in 23 sports [10]. The 2016 Summer Games achieved a cumulative global audience of 4.1 billion (Fig. 46.3) [10].

46.2 Classification System

The unique systems of classification used by Para sports carry out two very important functions to uphold the achievement of the Paralympic vision, "to enable para-athletes to achieve sporting excellence and inspire and excite the world" [11]:

1. Defines who is eligible to compete in Para sport and as a result has the opportunity to reach the goal of becoming a Paralympic athlete
2. Group athletes into sport classes which intend to make sure that the impact of impairment is minimized and sporting excellence decides which athlete or team is victorious in the end

Since the early beginnings of Para sport in the 1940s [12], several conceptual models have supported the development and subsequent progression of Para sport classification:

1. Medical
2. Functional sport specific
3. Evidence-based sport specific

Classification initially appeared in the mid-1950s, at which time doctors began to divide competitors based on high or low spinal injury diagnosis to make wheelchair basketball "more fair" [13]. While ostensibly during these early decades classification was based solely on medical diagnosis, a transition was already occurring where athletes with spinal cord injury, poliomyelitis, and spina bifida competed together despite having three separate medical conditions. These conditions resulted in a common impairment in strength. The focus was beginning to shift away from medical diagnosis toward how much impairment impacted upon sport performance [12].

The 1992 Barcelona Paralympic Games advanced the use of sport-specific functional classification models [14]. Decisions for fewer classes, supported by functional classification, were popular with event organizers and accelerated the transition to functional and sport-specific systems, although the science to support an objective, reliable, and valid classification system was immature. A conceptual or theoretical model was looked for to guide classification forward [12].

Evidence-based sport-specific criteria supplanted the variable methods employed by individual physicians to classify athletes by the introduction of three primary documents by the International Paralympic Committee, the global governing body of the Paralympic Movement: the 2003 IPC Classification Strategy, the 2007 IPC Classification Code, and the 2009 IPC Position Stand on Background and Scientific Principles of Classification [15, 16].

The 2007 Code adopted the use of a universal language, the International Classification of Functioning, Disability, and Health (ICF), to interconnect with sport. Each sport governance body was to determine which eligible impairment types would be included in their respective sport. The presence of a permanent verifiable impairment and an underlying health condition was mandated. And sport class decisions were to be based on how the resulting impairment caused activity limitation in the fundamental activities of the sport [16]. Tweedy and Vanlandewijck provided the conceptual clarity that was lacking in the 2007 Code with the 2009 IPC Position Stand on Background and Scientific Principles of Classification.

The contemporary evidence-based model, using a taxonomy perspective, defined the unit of classification as impairment and aligned classification in Para sports with other selective classification systems used in sport, such as age, body mass, and sex. Each sport is required to identify the eligible impairments in that sport, to describe the severity of impairment permitted, known as minimum impairment criteria (MIC), to classify the impairments according to the extent of resulting sport-specific activity limitation, and to develop the evidence to support that the methods used for assigning a sport class achieved the defined purpose of Para classification [15].

An athlete must have an eligible impairment that belongs to one of the ten eligible impairment types to participate. But it is not the only factor; it is the opening to the possibility to participate. Even if the athlete has one of the eligible impairments made available in that specific sport, an athlete may still not be eligible to participate if the athlete does not meet the minimum impairment criteria demonstrating the impairment is severe enough to affect how the athlete does the fundamental activities for the sport (Fig. 46.4) [17].

The sport class an athlete is placed in for competition has a significant effect on accomplishing success in Para sport. Current best practices are informed by advancing research in this field [18–27], but existing systems still lack evidence to support the process and reliability of how athletes are currently grouped in sport classes. To measure impairment, classifiers should have simple,

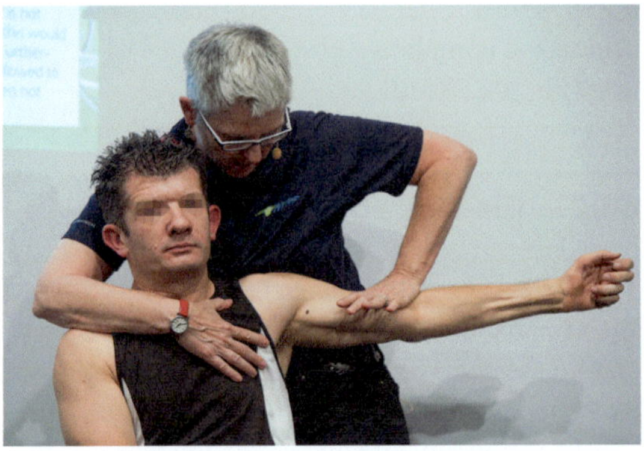

Fig. 46.4 Step 1 of the athlete classification process: a wheelchair rugby athlete and classifier are demonstrating the assessment of impairment in motor power using manual muscle testing. Photo reproduced with permission © Lieven Coudenys, International Paralympic Committee, Bonn, Germany

readily available, affordable, objective, valid, and reliable tests such as manual muscle testing to measure impairment in motor power [28]. Progress is being made all the time, but sport classification continues to have significant challenges. By honoring all past and present contributors, maintaining strong links between medical communities, and engaging scientific and research communities, athlete classification will advance to be the strong cornerstone of the Paralympic Movement into the future.

46.3 Injury in Paralympic Sport

In parallel with the growth of the Paralympic movement, the field of Paralympic sports medicine has emerged as an exciting new frontier of clinical care and scientific exploration [29]. Sports-related injuries in Para athletes, both recreational and elite, show unique features when compared to the general athlete population, and predictably, sports medicine care for Para athletes has grown to accommodate these.

Para sports injury epidemiology research is a growing field of sports medicine research contributing to quality care [30]. Earnest attempts to better understand injury patterns began in multisport events in 2002 when the Paralympic Injury Surveillance System was implemented at the Winter Paralympic Games [31, 32]. Following on this success, an advanced online injury and illness surveillance system was initiated for the London 2012 Paralympic Summer Games—the first to comprehensively capture injury patterns across a wide range of summer Para sports as well as enable the monitoring of both injury and illness [33]. Currently, many countries and sports federations are striving to implement similar systems to enable prospective data collection.

In summer Paralympic sport, the five sports with the highest rates of injury are five-a-side football, powerlifting, goalball, wheelchair fencing, and wheelchair rugby [34]. Additionally, the upper extremity is most frequently injured, particularly involving the shoulder, elbow, and wrist/hand. This pattern varies in comparison to similar data from an Olympic athlete population, for whom the lower limb is more commonly injured. Older athletes and athletes with spinal cord injury are particularly at increased risk for upper limb injuries [35, 36]. Additionally, across all athletes, males and females have similar rates of injury [34].

Recent sport-specific sub-analysis has enabled a more detailed analysis of injury, noting that in the sport of track and field, wheelchair/seated athletes are at higher risk of upper limb injury, which is seen most commonly in the throws events (shot put, discus, and javelin) [37]. Additionally, among ambulant track athletes, those with cerebral palsy are at decreased risk of lower extremity injury when compared to amputees and athletes with visual impairment [37]. This may be due to increased lower extremity muscle tone in athletes with cerebral palsy, which may in fact be protective against injury given the lack of full, forceful eccentric muscle contraction during springs and distance running events.

In the sport of Paralympic football, visually impaired athletes in five-a-side football experience a high incidence of acute injury, particularly to the head/neck and lower limb [38]. Of interest, >60% of these injuries are reported as being attributable to foul play. In Paralympic powerlifting, chronic/overuse injuries are very common, accounting for >60% of all injuries [39]. Of these, the shoulder/clavicle was most commonly involved, and athletes in heavier weight classes were more likely to experience injury.

In winter Paralympic sports, ice sledge hockey and alpine skiing/snowboarding demonstrate a high incidence of injury, while nordic skiing/biathlon and wheelchair curling less so [40]. Of interest, sports such as nordic skiing may be somewhat protective against upper limb injury, given that the nature of propulsion heavily involves scapular retraction, unlike wheelchair court sports which predominantly rely on activation of the anterior chest resulting in overuse injuries, particularly to the rotator cuff. Additionally, concussions, fractures, and contusions are more common in winter Paralympic sport, likely due to the high-speed, high-impact nature of these events [40].

The importance of aforementioned injury research cannot be overstated: it is often inevitable that athletes may incur sports-related injury. In Para sport, sports injuries, incurred at a young age, may result in functional decline later in life. For example, a wheelchair basketball player with spinal cord injury may develop a rotator cuff tear during a game, with immediate onset of symptoms. If left untreated, this tear may progress and ultimately lead to rotator cuff tear arthropathy later in life. Given that the athlete uses his/her shoulder for both sports and functional tasks such as wheelchair transfers and propulsion, this has the potential to cause significant morbidity. Thus, injury prevention in this population is of utmost importance.

46.4 Medical Illnesses in Paralympic Sport

With the advanced online surveillance system implemented during the London 2012 Paralympic Summer Games, our knowledge of illnesses during game time has considerably increased [33]. A medical illness is defined as any newly acquired illness as well as exacerbations of pre-existing illness that occurred during training or competition, either during the games or immediately before. In London 2012, a total of 49,910 athlete days were recorded, with 10,695 athlete days monitored in the pre-competition period and 39,215 athlete days monitored during the competition period.

During the 2012 London Games, the incidence rate of illness was 13.2 illnesses/1000 athlete days [41]. The highest rates of illness were found in equestrian, powerlifting, table tennis, road cycling, and wheelchair tennis. The average age of participating athletes is higher. In some of these sports, this may increase the risk of overall systemic illness within that sport.

The highest proportion of illness was found for the respiratory system, followed by the skin, digestive, nervous, and genitourinary systems. This is similar to the pattern of illness observed in Olympic athletes; illnesses involving the genitourinary system are, however, much more common among Paralympic athletes. The reason is that athletes with a neurologic injury are common in Paralympians, injuries that cause a neurogenic bladder and the need for self-catheterization.

When compared to the Olympic Games (6.7–12.1%), the incidence proportion of illness was higher at the Paralympic Games (14.2%) [41]. As expected, most illnesses were due to infections, and as much as 50% of all respiratory illnesses, 44% of skin and subcutaneous tissue illness, and over 82% of genitourinary illnesses were caused by an infection. Infections involving the skin and subcutaneous tissue infections were most common among athletes with spinal cord injury, those with amputation/limb deficiency and cerebral palsy. The stump-socket interface is also a high-risk area in athletes with amputation. For these conditions, high forces, hot/moist conditions, sweating during exercise, and possible bacterial contamination in the sport setting are likely contributors.

During the 2014 Sochi Winter Paralympic Games, a total of 547 athletes from 45 countries were monitored daily for 12 days over the Sochi 2014 Winter Paralympic Games (6564 athlete days) [40]. The illness data were obtained daily from teams without their own medical support (13 teams, 37 athletes) and teams with their own medical support (32 teams, 510 athletes) through electronic data capturing systems. The total number of illnesses reported was 123, with an illness incidence rate (IR) of 18.7 per 1000 athlete days (95% CI 15.1–23.2%). The highest IR was reported for wheelchair curling (IR of 20.0 (95% CI 10.1–39.6%)). Illnesses in the respiratory system (IR of 5.6 (95% CI 3.8–8.0%)), eye and adnexa (IR of 2.7 (95% CI 1.7–4.4%)), and digestive system (IR of 2.4 (95% CI 1.4–4.2%)) were the most common. Older athletes (35–63 years) had a significantly higher IR than younger athletes (14–25 years, $p = 0.049$). These results confirmed that Paralympic athletes report higher illness incidence rates compared to Olympic athletes at similar competitions.

During the Rio 2016 Summer Paralympic Games, a total of 3657 athletes from 78 countries, representing 83.5% of all athletes at the games, were monitored on the web-based injury and illness surveillance system (WEB-IISS) [42].

Illness data, based on a total of 51,198 athlete days, were obtained daily from teams with their own medical support through the WEB-IISS electronic data capturing systems. The total number of illnesses was 511, with an illness incidence rate (IR) of 10.0 per 1000 athlete days (12.4%). The highest IRs were reported for wheelchair fencing (14.9), para swimming (12.6), and wheelchair basketball (12.5) ($p < 0.05$). Female athletes and older athletes (35–75 years) were also at higher risk of illness (both $p < 0.01$). Illnesses in the respiratory, skin, and subcutaneous and digestive systems were the most common (IRs of 3.3, 1.8, and 1.3, respectively). When compared with the London 2012 Summer Paralympic Games, the rate of illness was lower.

46.5 Controversies in Paralympic Sport

Paralympic athletes may experience various medical issues that can influence their sports participation. These must be well-known to the team that accompany the athletes. Thereby, they can accommodate various preventive measures before, during, and after any games as part of the athlete's sports preparations and medical care [43].

One such issue is autonomic dysreflexia (AD). This is an acute attack of uncontrolled sympathetic activity which leads to a sudden increase in blood pressure that can be life-threatening. Other symptoms are headache, flushing, and sweating. It specifically occurs in persons with a spinal cord injury above the sixth thoracic level. It can be triggered by a noxious stimulus below the lesion, for example, a full bladder or skin wound. Treatment can be both non-pharmacological and pharmacological. A person with AD should be placed in an upright position as this will produce an orthostatic decrease in blood pressure. Moreover, restrictive clothing should be removed, the bladder emptied by CIC and bowel by gently inserting a gloved finger. If the blood pressure remains elevated (above 150 mm/Hg), oral nifedipine, a calcium antagonist, can be used.

AD has also been recognized in Paralympic sports as it can be a way of enhancing sports performance. An athlete with a spinal cord injury may, in AD, be induced, for example, by stimulating a full bladder, and experience an increase in blood pressure, stroke volume, and peak heart rate that can result in a 10% improvement in physical performance. This effect, referred to as "boosting," is prohibited by the International Paralympic Committee (IPC). To enhance our knowledge about AD in Paralympic sports, the IPC Medical Committee has been recording blood pressure in athletes susceptible to AD in certain sports. This work, ongoing since 2008, may improve how to find athletes who may be at risk of developing AD and eventually lead to the prevention of boosting in Paralympic sports.

Other medical factors that need to be addressed are hydration for training, competition, and recovery and the impact of multi-time zone travel. Traveling long distances, boarding and embarking, and many hours spent on an aircraft can affect athletes with an impairment. Athletes with a paralysis, such as spinal cord injury, are particularly susceptible. They have an increased risk of pressure ulcers as well as lower extremity swelling causing deep venous thrombosis (DVT).

Paralympic athletes may, due to their impairment, use specific medications that are prohibited under the guidelines of the World Anti-Doping Agency (WADA) Code and the IPC Anti-Doping Code. This does not exclude them from competing at high levels, as such medication can still be used, pending a Therapeutic Use Exemption (TUE). Examples of such specific medications are desmopressin (antidiuretic hormone) to treat nocturnal bladder overactivity, glucocorticoids, and beta-agonists for upper respiratory tract problems. Of specific concern is beta-blockers used for the treatment of hypertension that are prohibited in precision sports, such as archery and shooting. Finally, some Paralympic athletes may, due to congenital defects, require an anabolic agent, peptide hormone, or growth factor. After careful review, a TUE committee within the specific sports federation or IPC can grant a TUE and thereby allow the athlete to continue to compete at the highest level, despite using potentially performance-enhancing medications.

References

1. Bailey S. Athlete first: a history of the paralympic movement. West Sussex: Wiley; 2008.
2. Guttmann L. Spinal cord injuries: comprehensive management and research. Oxford: Blackwell Scientific Publications; 1973.
3. Goodman S. Spirit of Stoke Mandeville: the story of Sir Ludwig Guttmann. London: Harper Collins Publishing LLC; 1986.
4. Guttmann L. History of the National Spinal Injuries Centre, Stoke Mandeville Hospital, Aylesbury. Paraplegia. 1967;5:115–26.
5. Gallagher M. Athletics. Aylesbury: British Sports Association for the Disabled; 1982.
6. Guttmann L. Textbook of sport for the disabled. Aylesbury: HM & M Publishers; 1976.
7. Brittain I. From Stoke Mandeville to Stratford: a history of the summer paralympic games. Champaign: Common Ground Publishing, LLC; 2012.
8. Guttmann L. The annual Stoke Mandeville games. The Cord. 1949;3:24.
9. Tuakli-Wosornu Y. 'And thereby hangs a tale:' current medical and scientific controversies in paralympic sport. Palaestra. 2016;30(3):9–13.
10. I.P. Committee. http://www.paralympic.org. Accessed 1 Feb 2017.
11. The International Paralympic Committee Strategic Plan 2015 to 2018. I.P. Committee, editor. Bonn; 2015.
12. Tweedy S, Howe PD. Introduction to the paralympic movement. In: Vanlandewijck YC, Thompson WR, editors. The paralympic athlete. West Sussex: Wiley Blackwell; 2011.
13. Van de Vliet P. Paralympic athlete's health. Br J Sports Med. 2012;46(7):458–9.
14. Hart A. Classification: conceptual models. In: International Convention on Science, Education and Medicine in Sport (ICSEMIS). Glasgow; 2012.
15. Tweedy SM, Vanlandewijck YC. International Paralympic Committee position stand—background and scientific principles of classification in Paralympic sport. Br J Sports Med. 2011;45(4):259–69.
16. I.P. Committee. IPC Classification Code and International Standards. Bonn; 2007.
17. I.P. Committee. International Standard for Athlete Evaluation, G.I.P.C. Bonn, editor.
18. Altmann VC, et al. Reliability of the revised wheelchair rugby trunk impairment classification system. Spinal Cord. 2013;51(12):913–8.
19. Altmann VC, et al. Improvement of the classification system for wheelchair rugby: athlete priorities. Adapt Phys Activ Q. 2014;31(4):377–89.
20. Altmann VC, et al. The impact of trunk impairment on performance of wheelchair activities with a focus on wheelchair court sports: a systematic review. Sports Med Open. 2015;1(1):6.
21. Altmann VC, et al. The impact of trunk impairment on performance-determining activities in wheelchair rugby. Scand J Med Sci Sports. 2017;27(9):1005–14.
22. Altmann VC, et al. Construct validity of the trunk impairment classification system in relation to objective measures of trunk impairment. Arch Phys Med Rehabil. 2016;97(3):437–44.
23. Vanlandewijck Y, Theisen D, Daly D. Wheelchair propulsion biomechanics: implications for wheelchair sports. Sports Med. 2001;31(5):339–67.
24. Vanlandewijck YC, Verellen J, Tweedy S. Towards evidence-based classification in wheelchair sports: impact of seating position on wheelchair acceleration. J Sports Sci. 2011;29(10):1089–96.
25. Vanlandewijck YC, et al. Trunk strength effect on track wheelchair start: implications for classification. Med Sci Sports Exerc. 2011;43(12):2344–51.
26. Connick M, Beckman E, Deuble D, et al. Developing tests of impaired coordination for Paralympic classification: normative values and test-retest reliability. Sports Eng. 2016;19:147–54.
27. Deuble RL, et al. Using Fitts' law to detect intentional misrepresentation. J Mot Behav. 2016;48(2):164–71.
28. Tweedy S, Williams G, Bourke J. Selecting and modifying methods of manual muscle testing for classification in Paralympic sport. Euro J Adapt Activ. 2010;3(2):7–16.
29. Blauwet C, Lexell J, Derman W. Paralympic sports medicine. In: Vanlandewijck YC, Thompson WR, editors. IOC handbook of sports medicine and science: training and coaching the paralympic athlete. West Sussex: Wiley Blackwell; 2016. p. 75–95.
30. Ferrara MS, et al. A longitudinal study of injuries to athletes with disabilities. Int J Sports Med. 2000;21(3):221–4.
31. Webborn N, Willick S, Emery CA. The injury experience at the 2010 winter paralympic games. Clin J Sport Med. 2012;22(1):3–9.
32. Webborn N, Willick S, Reeser JC. Injuries among disabled athletes during the 2002 Winter Paralympic Games. Med Sci Sports Exerc. 2006;38(5):811–5.
33. Derman W, et al. Illness and injury in athletes during the competition period at the London 2012 Paralympic Games: development and implementation of a web-based surveillance system (WEB-IISS) for team medical staff. Br J Sports Med. 2013;47(7):420–5.
34. Willick SE, et al. The epidemiology of injuries at the London 2012 Paralympic Games. Br J Sports Med. 2013;47(7):426–32.
35. Tuakli-Wosornu YA, Derman W. Contemporary medical, scientific & social perspectives on para sport. Phys Med Rehabil Clin N Am. 2018;29(2):xvii–xviii.
36. Tuakli-Wosornu Y, Mashkovskiy E, Ottesen T, Gentry M, Jensen D, Webborn N. Acute and chronic musculoskeletal injury in para sport. Phys Med Rehabil Clin N Am. 2018;29(2):205–43.
37. Blauwet CA, et al. Risk of injuries in paralympic track and field differs by impairment and event discipline: a prospective cohort study at the London 2012 Paralympic Games. Am J Sports Med. 2016;44(6):1455–62.

38. Webborn N, et al. The epidemiology of injuries in football at the London 2012 Paralympic Games. PM R. 2016;8(6):545–52.
39. Willick SE, et al. The epidemiology of injuries in powerlifting at the London 2012 Paralympic Games: an analysis of 1411 athlete-days. Scand J Med Sci Sports. 2016;26(10):1233–8.
40. Derman W, et al. High incidence of injury at the Sochi 2014 Winter Paralympic Games: a prospective cohort study of 6564 athlete days. Br J Sports Med. 2016;50(17):1069–74.
41. Schwellnus M, Derman W, Jordaan E, Blauwet CA, Emery C, Pit-Grosheide P, Marques NA, Martinez-Ferrer O, Stomphorst J, Van de Vliet P, Webborn N, Willick SE. Factors associated with illness in athletes participating in the London 2012 Paralympic Games—a prospective cohort study involving 49,910 athlete days. Br J Sports Med. 2013;47:433–40.
42. Derman W, Schwellnus M, Jordaan E, Runciman P, Blauwet CA, Webborn N, Lexell J, Van de Vliet P, Tuakli-Wosornu Y, Kissick J, Stomphorst J. Sport, sex and age increase risk of illness at the Rio 2016 Summer Paralympic Games: a prospective cohort study of 51,198 athlete days. Br J Sports Med. 2018;52:17–23.
43. Vanlandewijck YC, Thompson WR, editors. Training and coaching the paralympic athlete. Handbook of sports medicine and science. Hoboken: Wiley-Blackwell; 2016.

FIFA World Cup

47

Andre Pedrinelli and Caio Senise Drolshagen

47.1 Major Events

Using the example of the 2014 FIFA World Cup (held) in Brazil, we are going to discuss the medical plan of the city of São Paulo with focus to the stadium, conferences, and the logistic involved.

47.2 Mass-Gathering Events

Mass gatherings are events attended by a sufficient number of people to potentially strain the public health resources of community, state, or nation (WHO).

In addition to the large quantity of people attending these events, which by this own is a unique challenge for the health services, there are many other things that increase the complexity of the organization:

- Coordination and cooperation across multiple sectors.
- Some diseases can easily be introduced and spread.
- Communication barriers—language, culture.
- High visibility.

There is a lack of scientific evidence for this emerging area; thus the majority of the information provided here is based in our and other experiences. Despite this, it is a great opportunity for the host place to introduce some good practices and improvements on public health, infrastructure, and education, using it as a legacy for the state/country.

47.3 2014 FIFA World Cup

The *Fédération Internationale de Football Association (FIFA)* World Cup is the biggest football event in the world and the most widely viewed sport event all over the globe [1]. The championship has been awarded every 4 years, and in 2014 it was held in Brazil.

Thirty-two teams entered in the tournament which has a duration of around 30 days. In 2014 this major event took place in Brazil with 12 host cities, including São Paulo with the Itaquera Stadium which hosted 6 games including the opening match and had a capacity of over 63,000 seats at the World Cup. In this chapter, we will discuss the organization of the FIFA Medical Service in São Paulo providing the structural, action plans and challenges involved in that mission.

A. Pedrinelli (✉) · C. S. Drolshagen
Instituto de Ortopedia e Traumatologia—IOT, Faculdade de Medicina da Universidade de São Paulo—USP, São Paulo, Brazil
e-mail: pedrinelli@uol.com.br

S. Rocha Piedade et al. (eds.), *The Sports Medicine Physician*,
https://doi.org/10.1007/978-3-030-10433-7_47

47.4 FIFA Mass-Gathering Medicine

The Local Organizing Committee has started the preparation of the Medical Services of 2014 FIFA World Cup 4 years before, in South Africa (2010 FIFA World Cup). It had included official meetings, visits to the local infrastructure, and planning in conjunction with São Paulo Public Institutions with emphasis in transports, health, and public security institutes.

47.5 FIFA Medical Services: São Paulo

The provision of medical services during the World Cup begins with the arrival of any participating team in the city for training and preparation for the games.

In all places with dignitaries or teams, such as Hotel or Training Camp, there should be a medical team and an ambulance (UCI equipped) for provision if any medical problem occurs. One of the requirements for the organization of medical services for the World Cup was the creation of necessary infrastructure, including number of ambulances, medical equipment available at the stations, and number of personnel available. The checklist of material available at medical stations was developed by LOC and is now used as a reference for FIFA events. In addition, an individual medical care form has been created (Fig. 47.1).

47.6 Medical Duties

FIFA mass-gathering medicine involves provision of medical services in and around the stadium and at the hotels, meetings, and official events for all persons located at the place. Ensuring the well-being of football team, staff, FIFA family, spectators, and dignitaries is the main objective.

All FWC public is divided into three groups:

- Group 01—Players, referees, and team staff
- Group 02—Dignitaries, FIFA managers, and LOC
- Group 03—Spectators, and media

47.7 FWC Medical Services' Main Sites

- Stadium—including 1 km perimeter outside
- Training sites
- Teams' hotels
- FIFA family's hotels
- Chiefs of government's hotels
- Official events

47.8 Stadium Medical Services: Itaquera Stadium—Arena São Paulo

The arrival of the medical team to the Stadium occurred 4 h before the games and finished 2 h

Operations Summary during FIFA World Cup Brasil 2014™								
Structure			Equipes			Operational time	Operational Dates	
Facilities	Unit	MDs	Nurses	Technician	Driver		Start	End
Hotel FIFA Staff	Hotel Medical Room	1	x	1	x	24 hours	10 days before 1st game	2 days after last game
Training Camp A	Ambulance	1	1	×	1	during training	1st training day	last training day
Training Camp B and C	Ambulance	1	1	×	1	during training	1st training day	last training day
Stadium without games	Medical Station	1	×	1	×	Stadium operational time	14 days before 1st game	2 days after last game
Stadium Media Center	Media Medical Station	1	×	1	×	Media Center operational time	5 to 10 days before 1st game	2 days after last game
Match Day - 1	Players Medical Station	2	1	2	×	during training	Match Day - 1	
	Players Ambulance	1	1	×	1	during training	Match Day - 1	

Fig. 47.1 Medical operations summary outside games

after the end. A debriefing was held with the coordinators. In addition to the interior of the stadium, FIFA is responsible for dealing with medical incidents within a perimeter of 1 km outside the stadium.

One of the biggest challenges was the logistics involved in the case of an ambulance removal and assistance to multiple victims. Because of that there were two reference hospitals equipped with heliport for the rapid transportation of emergencies. In addition, in conjunction with the Traffic Engineering Company (CET), the terrestrial ambulance movement was carried out.

47.9 Location

The geographical location of the stadium—address and coordinates are found using Global Positioning System (GPS). It is mandatory to list main roads, nearby highways, and important side roads. During games the road access is restricted for safety, security, and diplomatic purposes. Furthermore, that information will allow emergency rescue to arrive in a short time if necessary.

Because of the efficiency, it is critical that a helicopter landing location is available at the stadium (Fig. 47.2).

47.10 Stadium Major Incident Plan

One of main functions of the medical management is to ensure well-being during the events and prepare, distribute, and train a **major incident plan**. The objective of this plan is to make a rapid and effective response if there is any incident that potentially can produce injury, illness, or death. This includes an evacuation plan. Usually, it takes 8 min to empty 80% of the public from Itaquera Stadium, in normal conditions (Fig. 47.3).

47.11 Staff

47.11.1 Chief Medical Officer (CMO)

Is the individual who has the responsibility of providing appropriate medical services during the World Cup.

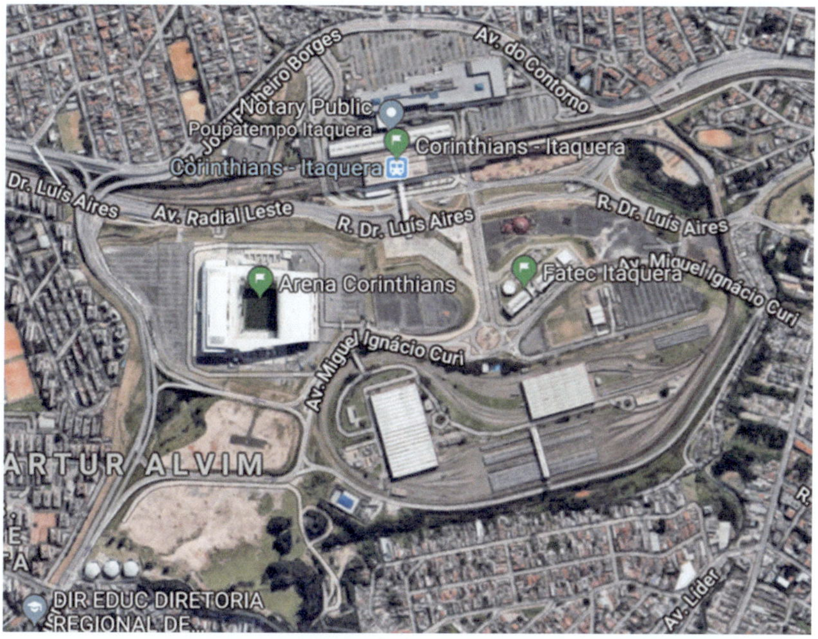

Fig. 47.2 Itaquera Stadium, Itaquera Subway, FAETEC, and nearby highways

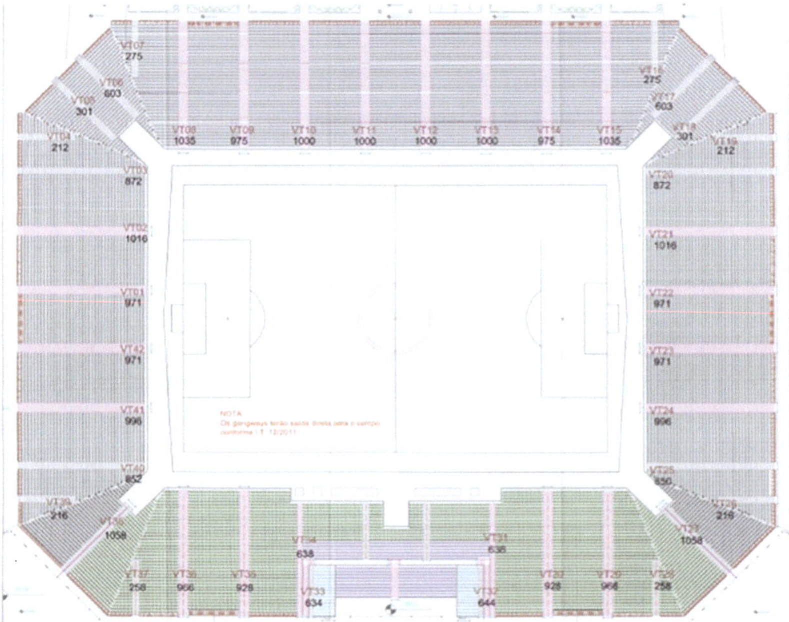

Fig. 47.3 Itaquera Stadium map—main exits and gates

47.11.2 Venue Medical Officer (VMO)

Is responsible for providing efficient and effective medical service in the host city, the equivalent of the CMO regionally. Its main functions are:

- Plan and coordinate the medical service in all locations for each FIFA group.
- Organize, in conjunction with a third-party company, medical care in hotels and the provision of ambulances during events.
- Capture and train the health-care team during the games.
- Inspect medical offices and doping control.

47.11.3 Medical Team

Each medical team consisted of:

- One doctor
- One nurse
- One nurse technician

In addition to the academics prerequisites, each of them had to have knowledge in emergency and football medicine. Besides that, one team of fireman realized initial attendance and removal in case of structural collapse.

47.11.4 Medical Equipment

In addition to hospital medical supplies, each team had a backpack equipped with a first aid kit (Fig. 47.4).

47.11.5 Venue Operations Centre (VOC)

It is the place where the coordinators stayed, with access to the camera closed-circuit and communicate with other members of the team, managing attendances and hospital removals with an ambulance.

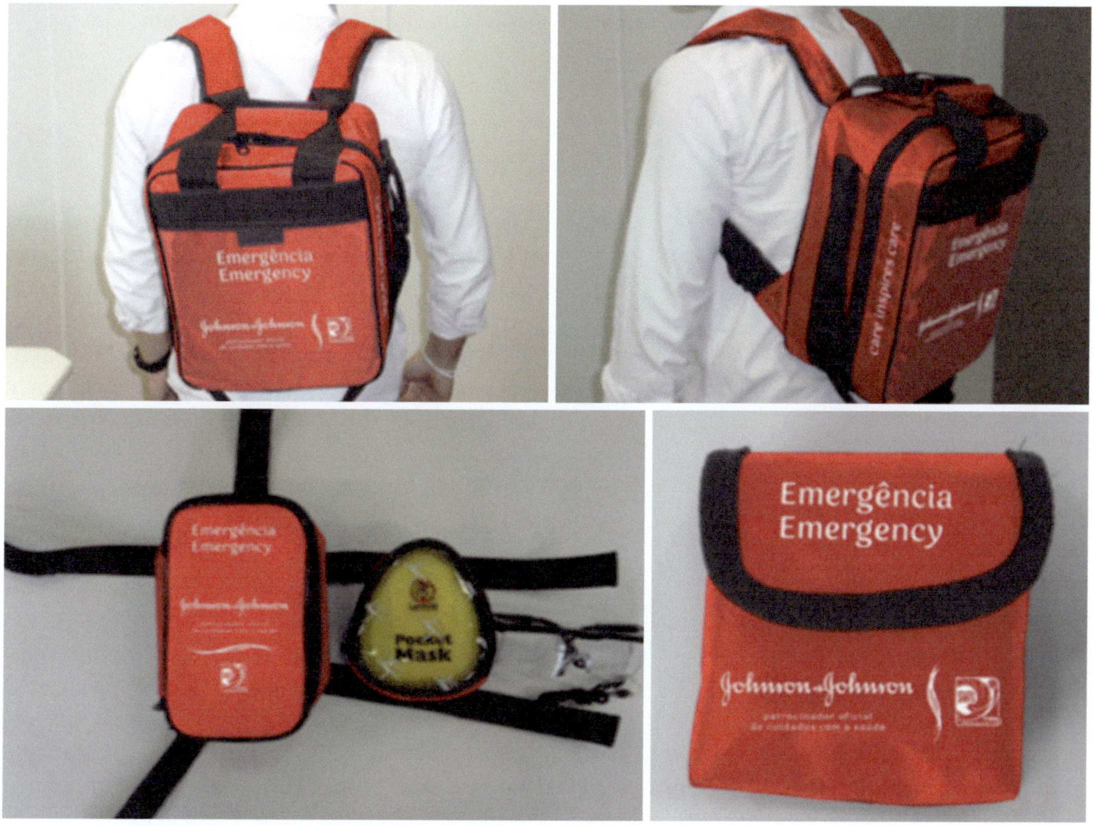

Fig. 47.4 First aid backpack

47.12 Communication

The key to successful medical management is communication. It is mandatory that everyone use the same language. In FWC 2014, telephone, mobile phone and radio with a specific channel was used by everyone working on the medical services.

47.13 Medical Stations

- Players' medical room
  - One medical team of only medical doctors (four)
- Main medical room—the largest service station destined to FIFA group 3
  - Eight beds (four for critical care), five medical doctors, five nurses, and five nurse technicians
  - First choice for patient triage, treatment, and transport if a major casualty occurs
- Secondary medical rooms
  - Five stations
  - One medical team in each one
- VIP medical room
  - One doctor, one nurse, and one nurse technician
- VVIP medical room
  - One doctor, one nurse, and one nurse technician
- Doping control center
- Mobile team
  - Team consisted of paramedics equipped with a "golf car" or bicycle, a radio, first aid kit, and stretcher
- Volunteers

- Four volunteers who know the stadium very well and were used to communicate with the medical teams if any problem occurred with the radio and phone

Medical team—key points
Composition
• One MD
• One nurse
• One nurse technician
Standard uniform
• Medical station—black and white
• Ambulance—white jacket
• Field of play team—blue
Ambulance—12
• One for 10,000 spectators—07
• Two on the field of play
• One for VIP and one for IVIP room
• One for players' medical room

47.14 Ambulances

- An ambulance is required for every 10,000 fans in accordance with current legislation in the city of São Paulo.
- Twelve ambulances, six of them equipped with ICU.
  - Two in the field with one medical team (doctor, nurse, and nursing technician) each.
  - One for players' medical room.
  - One ambulance for VIP room.
  - One ambulance for IVIP room.
  - Seven ambulances for the public.

47.15 Operational Structure

The schematization of a flow of service and hierarchical communication was essential for the success of the operation. The patient arrived in two ways at the medical post: through individuals with or removed from the bleachers or convenience location in the case of an emergency call. For this, the mobile team was available to respond quickly to calls.

From the medical station, the patient could have two ways: stay in the station under the vision or be removed by an ambulance to a hospital of reference.

Otherwise, if he exceeded 20 min of observation, he was transferred to the main post. At the main station, the maximum observation time was 2 h if it exceeded, he/she should be transferred to a hospital. The ambulance coordination followed a hierarchical level too. If the head of the medical station deemed it is necessary to remove a patient, he contacted the VMO who was in contact with an ambulance manager located in the VOC who, together with the reference hospitals, regulated the removal of the patients. This was extremely important in order to keep all the main sites with an ambulance and to not overload the destination Hospital (Figs. 47.5 and 47.6).

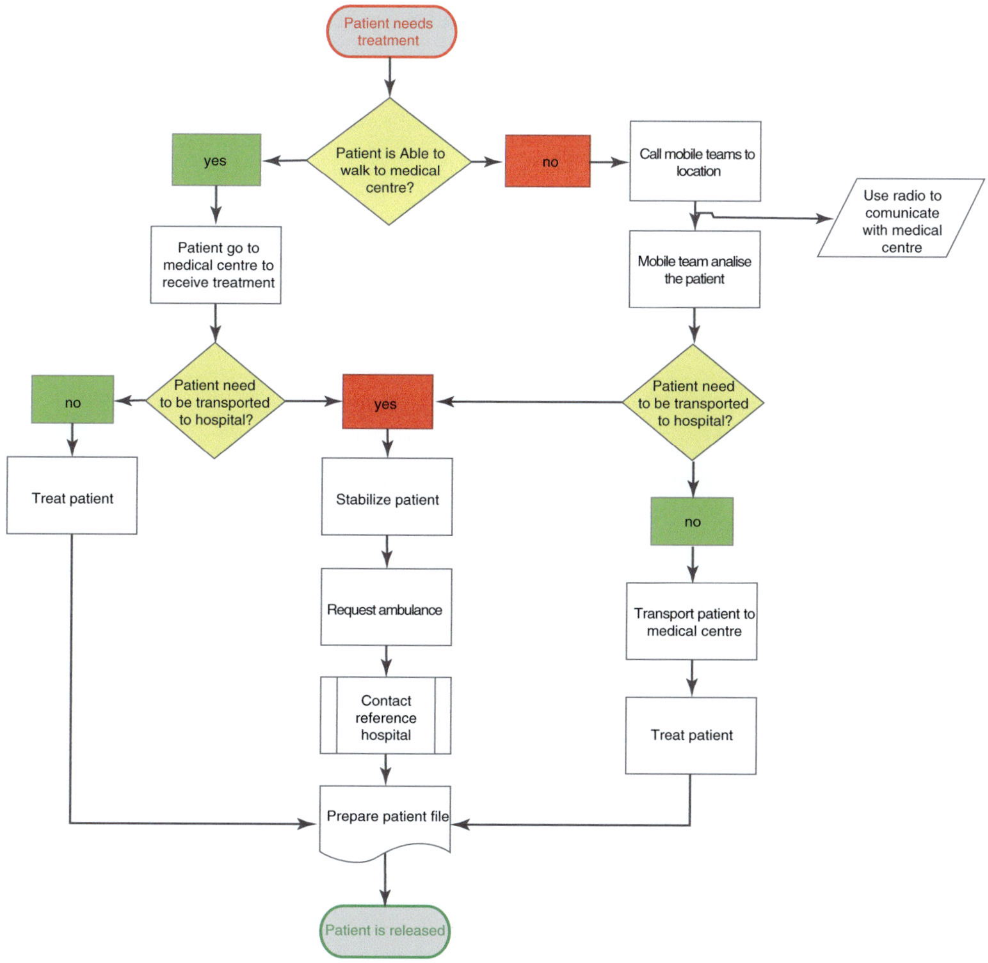

Fig. 47.5 Patient medical station flow

Operations Summary during FIFA World Cup Brasil 2014™									
Structure			Equipes				Operational time		Operational Dates
Facilities		Unit	MDs	Nurses	Technician	Driver			
stadium match day	FIFA Group	Field of play Team	1	×	3	×	ko - 5 hours	fw + 2 hours	Match Days
			1	×	3	×	ko - 5 hours	fw + 2 hours	Match Days
		Players Medical Room	2	1	2	×	ko - 5 hours	fw + 2 hours	Match Days
		VIP Medical Room	2	2	2	×	ko - 5 hours	fw + 2 hours	Match Days
		VVIP Medical Room	1	1	1	×	ko - 5 hours	fw + 2 hours	Match Days
		Field of play Ambulance	1	1	×	1	ko - 5 hours	fw + 2 hours	Match Days
		Players Ambulance	1	1	×	1	ko - 5 hours	fw + 2 hours	Match Days
		VIP Ambulance	1	1	×	1	ko - 5 hours	fw + 2 hours	Match Days
		VVIP Ambulance	1	1	×	1	ko - 5 hours	fw + 2 hours	Match Days
	spectators	Medical Room 1	3	3	6	×	ko - 5 hours	fw + 2 hours	Match Days
		Medical Room 2	2	1	2	×	ko - 5 hours	fw + 2 hours	Match Days
		Medical Room 3	2	1	2	×	ko - 5 hours	fw + 2 hours	Match Days
		Medical Room 4	2	1	2	×	ko - 5 hours	fw + 2 hours	Match Days
		Medical Room 5	2	1	2	×	ko - 5 hours	fw + 2 hours	Match Days
		Medical Room 6	2	1	2	×	ko - 5 hours	fw + 2 hours	Match Days
		Ambulance ICU 1	1	1	×	1	ko - 5 hours	fw + 2 hours	Match Days
		Ambulance ICU 2	1	1	×	1	ko - 5 hours	fw + 2 hours	Match Days
		Ambulance ICU 3	1	1	×	1	ko - 5 hours	fw + 2 hours	Match Days
		Ambulance ICU 4	1	1	×	1	ko - 5 hours	fw + 2 hours	Match Days
		Ambulance ICU 5	1	1	×	1	ko - 5 hours	fw + 2 hours	Match Days
		Ambulance ICU 6	1	1	×	1	ko - 5 hours	fw + 2 hours	Match Days

Fig. 47.6 Operations summary during games

47.16 2014 FIFA Medical Services Statistics

47.16.1 FWC2014: São Paulo (Fig. 47.7)

47.16.2 During Games (Figs. 47.8, 47.9, 47.10, 47.11, 47.12, 47.13, 47.14, 47.15, and 47.16)

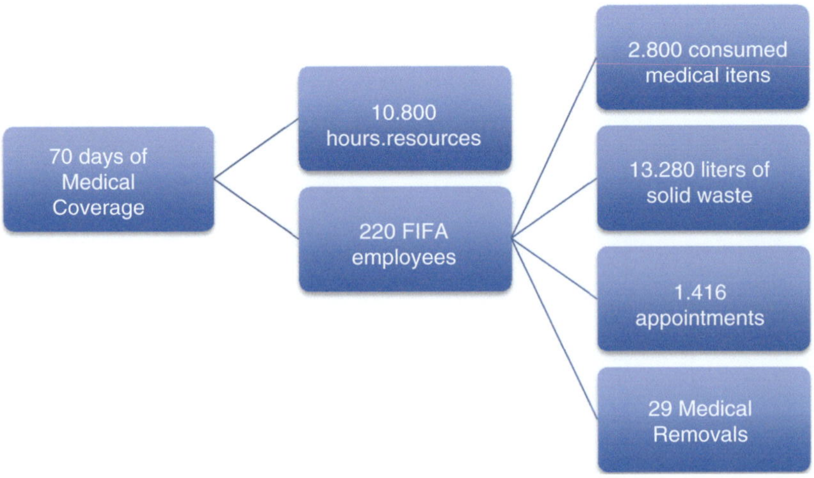

Fig. 47.7 FWC medical services general statistics—from May 21 to July 17

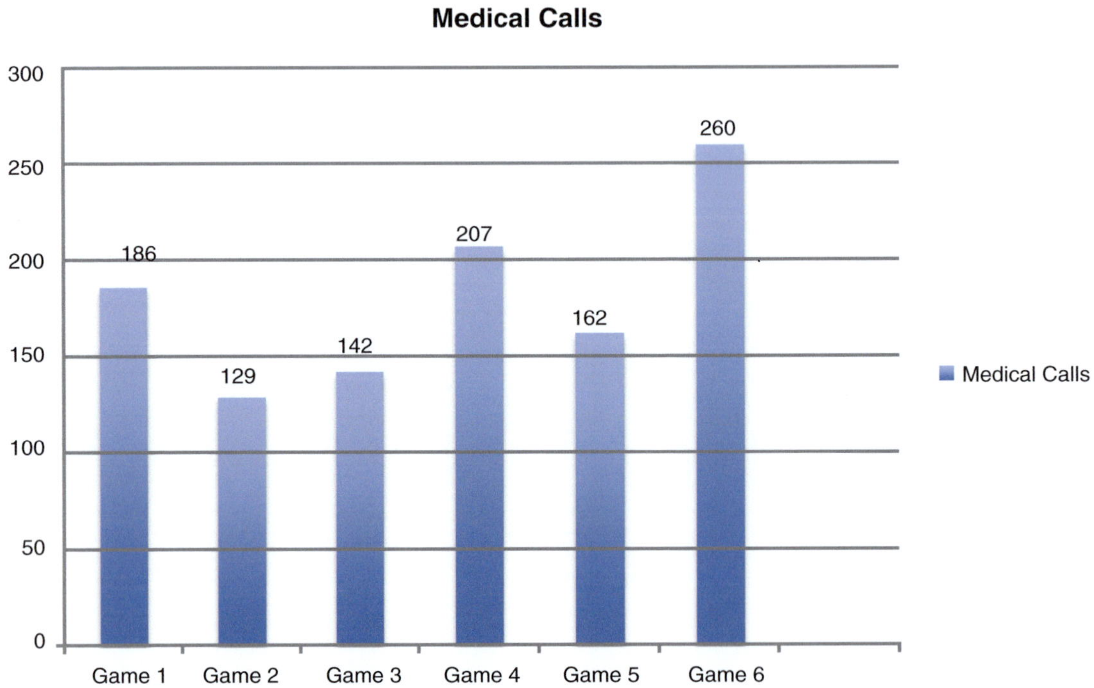

Fig. 47.8 Number of medical calls during Itaquera Stadium Games

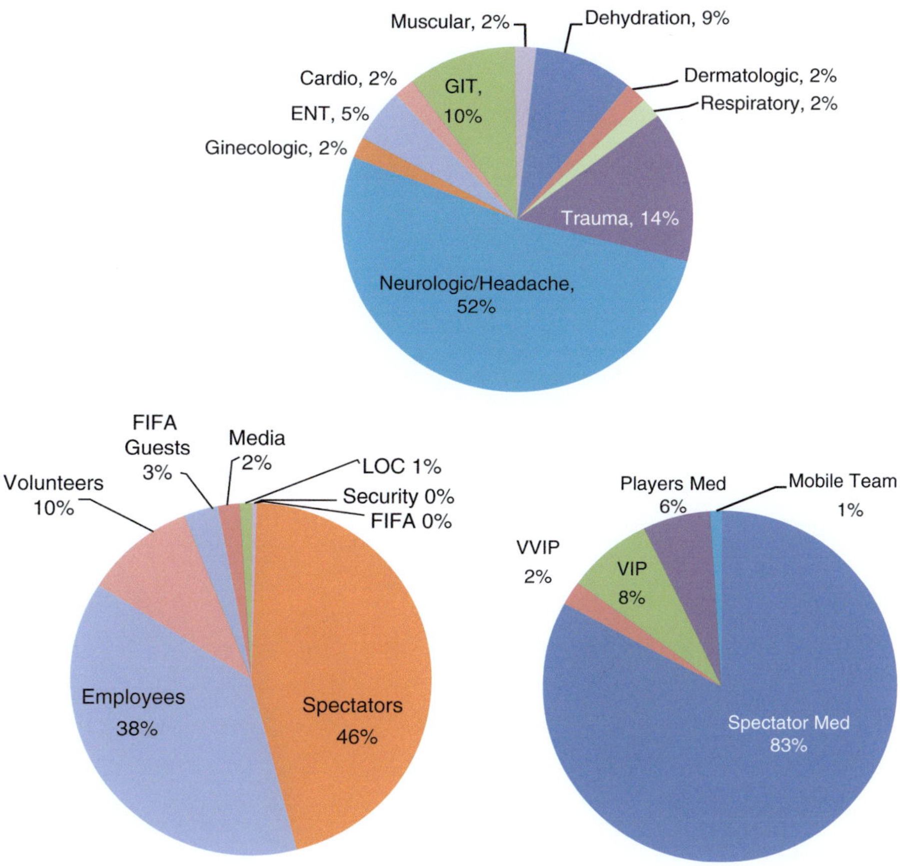

Fig. 47.9 Game 01; June 12; Brazil 3 × 1 Croatia; Spectators: 61,000, Medical Calls: 184, Hospitals Transfer: 4

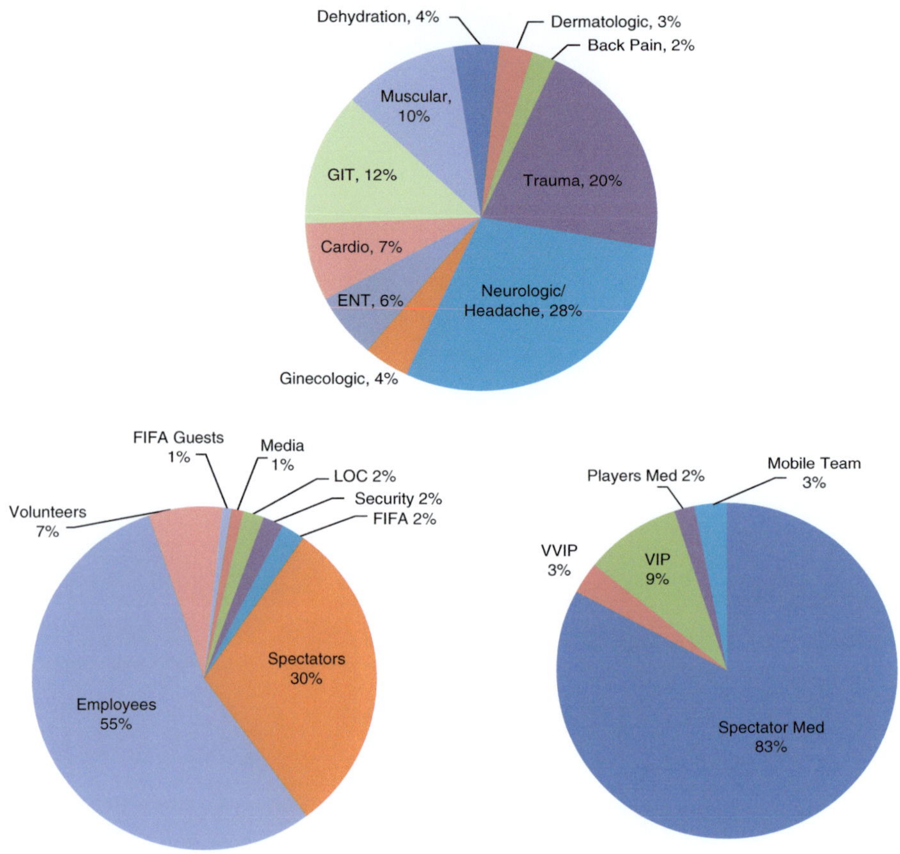

Fig. 47.10 Game 02; June 19; Uruguay 2 × 1 England; Spectators: 62,575, Medical Calls: 129, Hospitals Transfer: 2

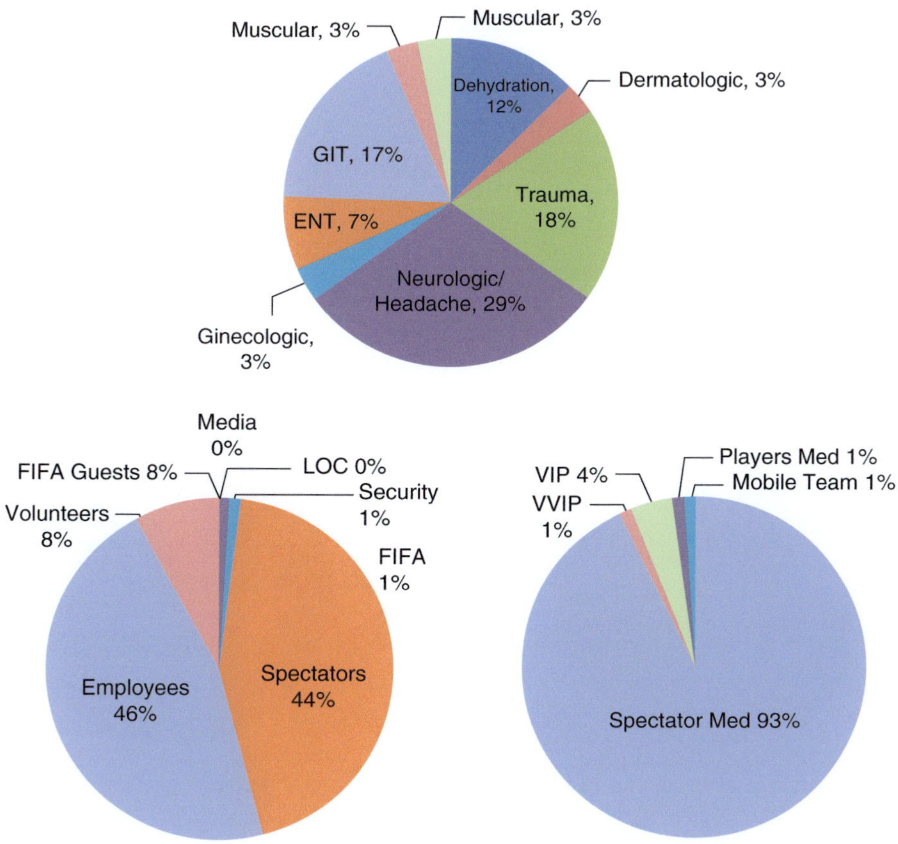

Fig. 47.11 Game 03; June 23; Netherlands 2 × 0 Chile; Spectators: 62,996, Medical Calls: 149, Hospitals Transfer: 2

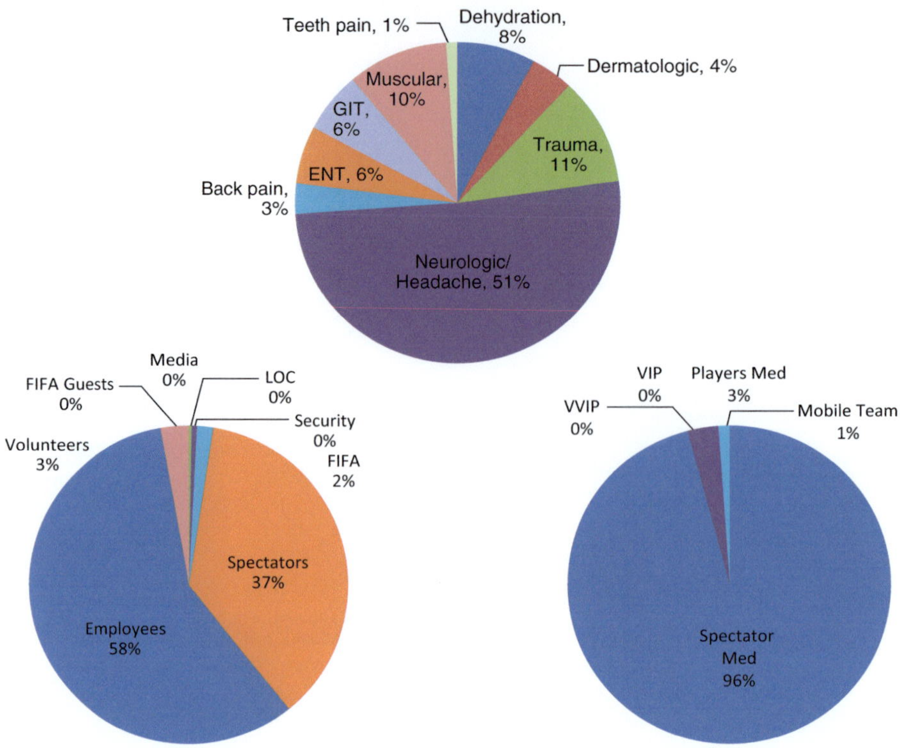

Fig. 47.12 Game 04; June 26; South Korea 2 × 1 Belgium; Spectators: 61,397, Medical Calls: 190, Hospitals Transfer: 3

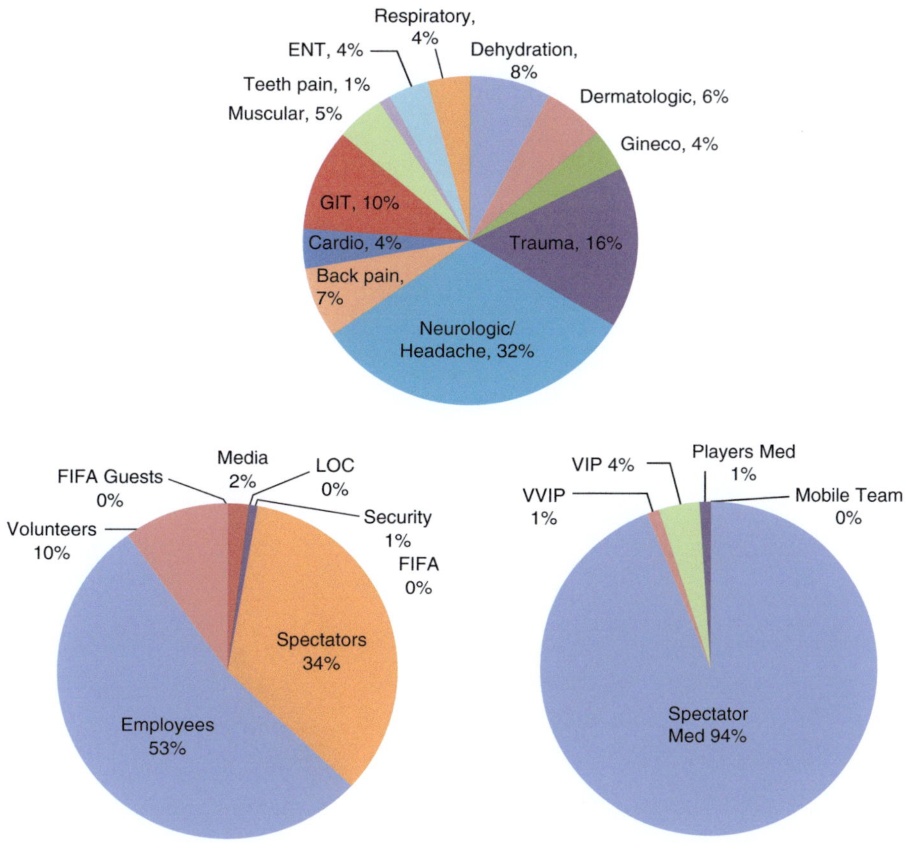

Fig. 47.13 Game 05; July 1; Argentina 1 × 0 Switzerland; Spectators: 63,225, Medical Calls: 134, Hospitals Transfer: 3

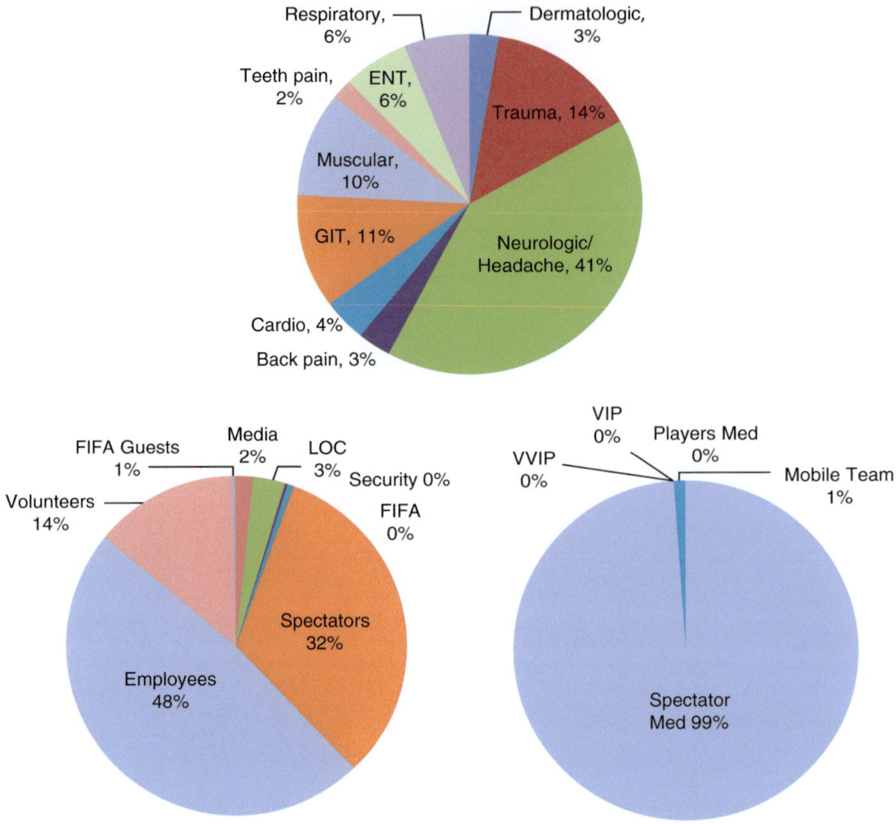

Fig. 47.14 Game 06; July 9; Argentina 0 × 0 Netherlands; Spectators: 63,267, Medical Calls: 222, Hospitals Transfer: 5

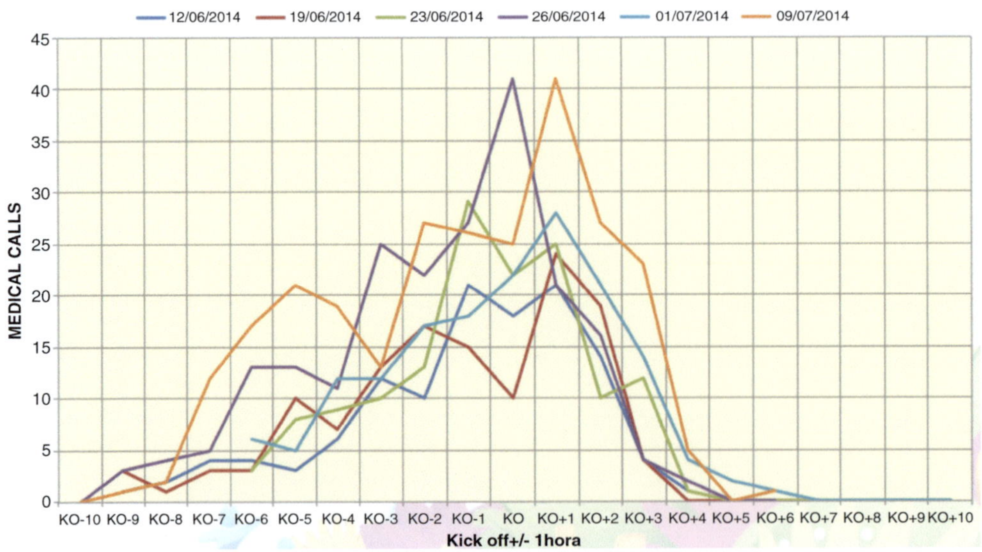

Fig. 47.15 Medical calls in each hour on match day

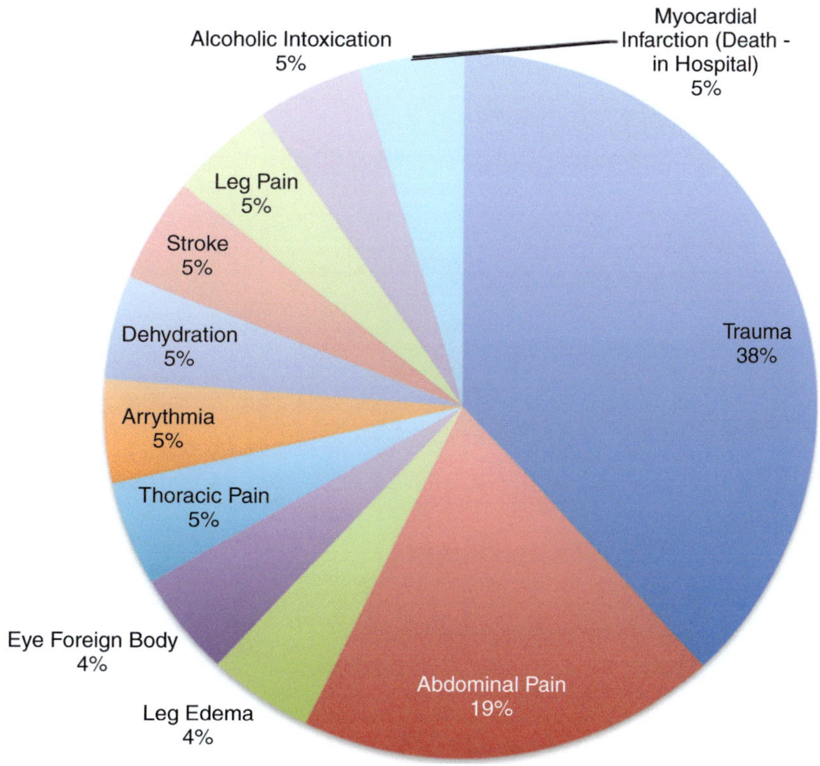

Fig. 47.16 Hospital Transfers – TOTAL from the 06 games

47.17 Outside the Game

47.17.1 Medical Calls (Figs. 47.17 and 47.18)

Take-Home Message

- Mass gatherings are events attended by a sufficient number of people to potentially strain the public health resources of community, state, or nation.
- The complexity of the organization involves coordination and cooperation across multiple sectors, some diseases that can easily be introduced and spread, communication barriers (language, culture), and high visibility.

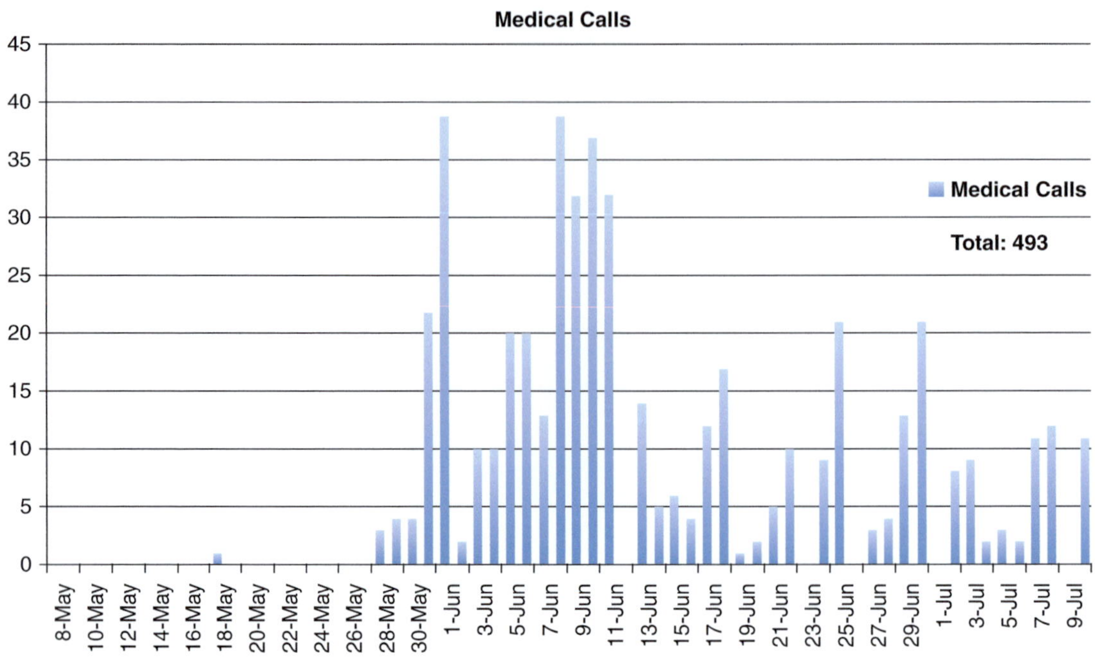

Fig. 47.17 Medical calls outside games

Fig. 47.18 Medical complaints outside game

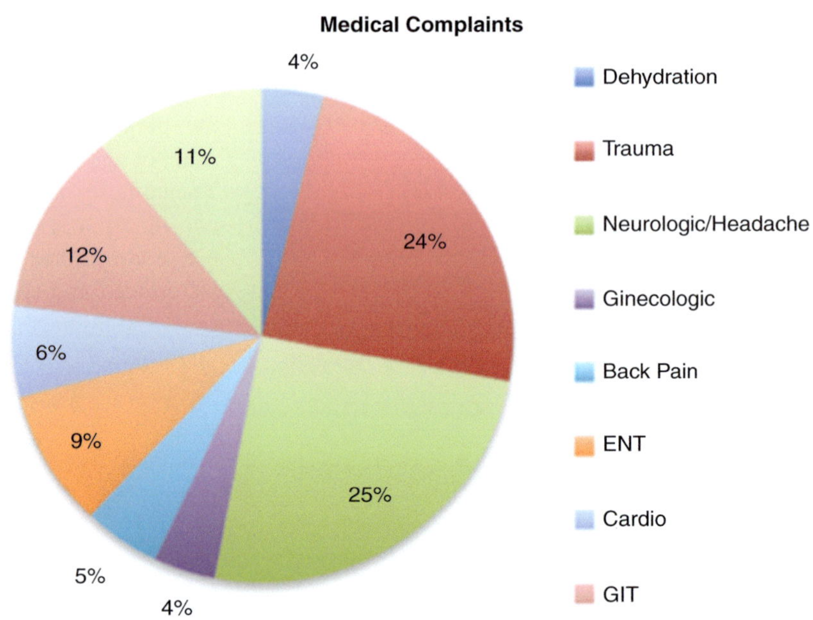

Reference

1. www.fifa.com.

Extreme Sports

48

Torrey Parry, Empryss Tolliver,
and Scott C. Faucett

48.1 Introduction

The popularity of extreme sports has grown dramatically over the past several decades, despite knowledge of the higher risk of injury associated with such activities [1]. There is no specific definition of what categorizes something as extreme versus as a more conventional sport such as baseball, basketball, or football. However, the essential aspects of extreme sports are high speed, extreme height, real or perceived danger, a high level of physical exertion, and highly specialized gear or spectacular stunts. One quality that is universal across all extreme sports is the adrenaline rush involved by the inherent danger in the activity. Whether the athlete is parachuting from the sky, pulling a double backflip off a Moto X freestyle jump, or attempting a frontside double cork 1440 in the halfpipe on a snowboard, part of the appeal appears to be the fact that such activities are not safe. This chapter will explore specific injuries and safety considerations involved in some of the most popular extreme sports.

T. Parry
Department of Orthopedics, George Washington University, Washington, DC, USA

E. Tolliver · S. C. Faucett (✉)
The Centers for Advanced Orthopaedics, Washington, DC, USA

48.2 Surfing

Surfing, as a sport, has grown dramatically since it began to gain widespread appeal in the 1960s. Even since the beginning of the twenty-first century, we have seen an explosion in worldwide participation, with an estimated 37 million surfers in 2013 [2], compared to 13 million in 2002 [3]. With this expansion in total number of surfers, it is important for treating physicians to be aware of the types of injuries that can be expected.

Several factors can contribute to increasing the risk of injury during surfing. Among these are rider experience, size of wave, maneuvers performed, location of wave break, and ocean floor makeup [4]. Some studies have shown that the incidence of moderate to severe injuries in professional surfers is higher than in recreational surfers—4 per 1000 surfing days compared to 3.5 per 1000 surfing days, respectively [5–7]. This is likely related to the larger waves surfed and the riskier maneuvers performed by elite surfers (Fig. 48.1).

In a prospective study looking at injuries sustained during competition surfing, Nathanson et al. [8] found that knee strains and sprains were the most common injury types in competitive events. This is in contrast to multiple studies finding that lacerations are the most common injuries in recreational athletes [3]. Knee injuries most commonly occur during aggressive turning and aerial maneuvers, which are too difficult for less

S. Rocha Piedade et al. (eds.), *The Sports Medicine Physician*,
https://doi.org/10.1007/978-3-030-10433-7_48

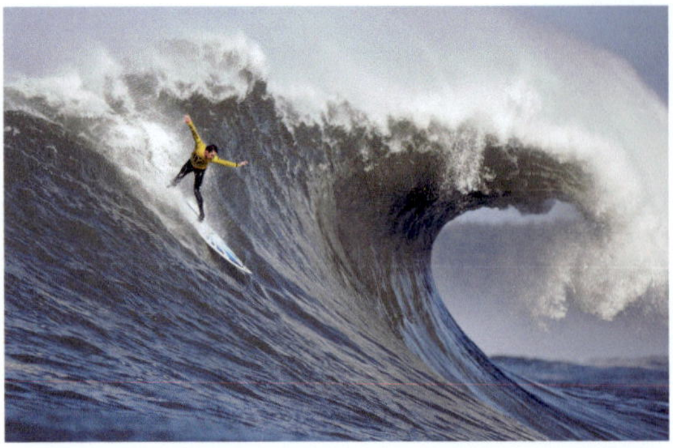

Fig. 48.1 Big Wave surfer riding a wave at the 2010 Mavericks Invitational in Mavericks, California. Mavericks was the site of the deaths of two accomplished Big Wave surfers, Mark Foo and Sion Milosky

experienced surfers to perform. Injuries are significantly more likely to occur when surfing on a hard bottom (e.g., rock or coral) than on a soft sandy bottom. When comparing hard to soft bottom surfing, Nathanson et al. [8] found the odds ratio for sustaining an acute injury to be 2.6. Similarly, the odds ratio for acute injury when comparing large waves—overhead or higher—to small waves was found to be 2.4. Risk of injury is higher when surfing in locations with shore break, where the waves break in shallow water. This makes sense, as the shallow water provides little cushion to falls compared to breaks that are further out in deeper areas [4]. Performing aerial maneuvers—when surfers propel themselves into the air and land back on the wave—is a significant risk factor for a higher rate of injury. Furness et al. [5] found that 48% of surfers who perform aerial tricks sustained a major injury in a 12-month period, with major injury being defined as either having to take at least one day off from work/surfing or requiring treatment from a health professional. This was found to be the single greatest risk factor in that study.

Overall, the majority of injuries sustained while surfing are minor and the rate of significant injury in surfing is fairly low when compared to other sports. When looking at professional surfers, the overall injury rate was 13 injuries per 1000 h surfed and only 6.6 significant injuries per 1000 h. This is relatively low when compared to significant injury rates of 69, 33, 18.8, 9, and 5.4 per 1000 h in professional rugby, college football, men's college soccer, men's college basketball, and snowboarding, respectively [8]. It has been estimated that there are approximately 11,000 surfing injuries per year requiring a visit to an emergency room. As surfing is mostly practiced in an unsupervised environment and injuries sustained are minor, the overall incidence of injury is likely higher than what can be documented. Of those that are seen in emergency rooms, 96% are treated and released, while 4% are admitted. The most common injury diagnosis is laceration (41%), followed by strains and sprains (14%), contusions (13%), and fractures (12%). The most common body location of injury is the lower extremity (26%), followed by the face (23%), head and neck (23%), upper extremity (17%), and trunk (9%). Lacerations are most commonly located on the head, neck, and face (63%). Fractures most commonly involve the upper extremity (32%) and lower extremity (31%). Strains and sprains mostly affect the lower extremity (35%) and the neck (29%). Dislocations account for only 4.5% of injuries and primarily involved the upper extremity (85%), predominantly the shoulder. Other reported, though exceedingly rare, injuries include submersion injuries, acute myocardial infarction, finger amputation, and tympanic membrane rupture. Animal attacks (e.g., shark, seal, stingray, and jellyfish) are also reported as being rare, but as these encounters are generally minor, it is likely that patients do not seek medical attention following injury [9].

While surfing does involve some risk, injuries are comparatively less common and often minor. Certain practices do increase the risk of injury, and patients should be counselled on safe behavior such as avoiding reefs and shore breaks, avoiding surfing on crowded waves, and knowing his or her limitations when deciding which waves to surf and what maneuvers to perform.

48.3 Skateboarding

Skateboarding is believed to have started around the end of the 1940s and early 1950s when a group of surfers began exploring ways of pursuing the thrills of surfing in settings away from the ocean. They thought of the idea of attaching wheels to smaller versions of surfboards and "surfing" the city streets and empty pools. The new activity was nicknamed "sidewalk surfing," which later changed to skateboarding [10]. In the early 1960s, companies such as Larry Stevenson's Makaha and Hobart "Hobie" Alter's Hobie began to mass-produce the first true surfing-inspired skateboards [11]. Skateboarding quickly began to grow in popularity. Today skateboards are used for recreation and transportation and in professional skateboarding. In the USA alone, it is estimated that there are between 6 and 15 million people that participate in skateboarding on some level [12].

As the interest in skateboarding grew over the years, so did the risk of injury. While all extreme sports carry some level of risk, skateboarding has been shown to be particularly dangerous. Between 2015 and 2016, there were an estimated 121,400 skateboarding injuries in patients under 18 years of age treated in US emergency departments [13]. The rate of skateboard-associated injuries has been reported as being 9 injuries per 1000 participants [14]. The majority of injuries (55–63%) involve the upper extremity, followed by the lower extremity (17–26%) and the head (3.5–13%). Thoracoabdominal and spine injuries make up only 1.5–3% of injuries. In children, skateboarding is shown to be a significant source of fractures. In a 2005 study, Zalavras et al. [15] found that 8.1% of all pediatric fractures presenting to a fracture clinic at a level 1 trauma center were attributed to skateboarding. Forearm fractures made up 48% of fractures, 94% of these in the distal third. Concerningly, 11% of forearm fractures were open fractures, compared to 0.3% of fractures sustained by other mechanisms of injury [15]. Risk factors for injury that have been described include fatigue, overuse, poor fitness, age >16 years old, and lack of protective equipment [12].

Head injury is one of the most important considerations when caring for skateboard injuries. Skateboarders were found to have by far the highest risk of skull fractures compared with other extreme sports—55 times greater risk than snowboarding, 28 times greater than snow skiing, and 6 times greater than surfing [16]. Given this fact, it's not surprising that skateboarding also has a greater risk of traumatic brain injury (TBI). With regard to patients admitted to a hospital for a skateboarding injury, it has been shown that 36% have some form of TBI, with more than a third of these classified as severe TBI (e.g., subdural/subarachnoid hemorrhage, epidural hemorrhage, or cerebral laceration/contusion). The risk of TBI was shown to be even greater for patients over the age of 16, with an odds ratio of 2.53 for sustaining severe TBI compared to their younger counterparts. This is likely due to several factors including the higher momentum of injuries from increased speed and body size of older riders, in addition to the fact that older riders were significantly less likely to be wearing a helmet (Figs. 48.2 and 48.3).

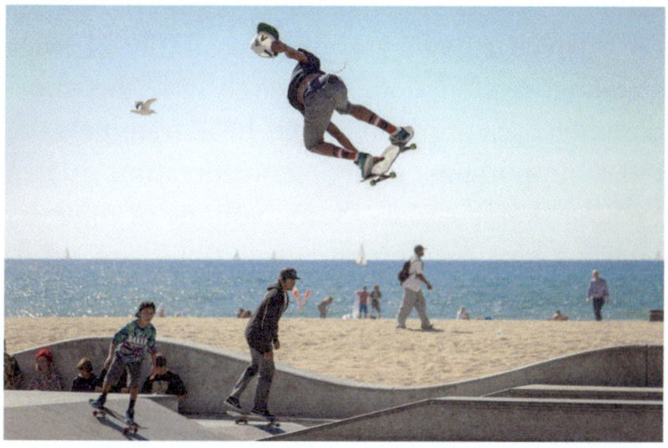

Fig. 48.2 A skateboarder demonstrates the acrobatic heights that put these athletes at risk for head and other bodily injury

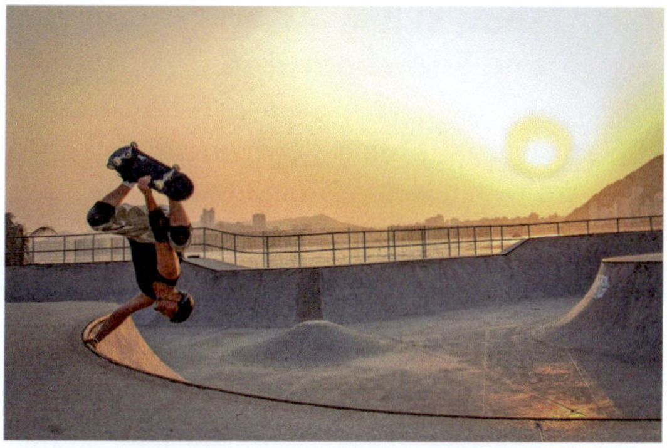

Fig. 48.3 A skateboarder performs a front side invert at an outdoor skate park

Factors that were protective against TBI were the use of a helmet and skating in a skate park, with odds ratios of 0.45 and 0.7, respectively [17]. When major skateboarding injuries, defined as an Injury Severity Scale (ISS) >9, were compared to major injuries sustained during airborne activities (e.g., hang gliding, kiting, and parachuting) and mountain climbing, skateboarding was found to have the highest rate of loss of consciousness (27%), prehospital intubation (33%), and in-hospital mortality (15%) [1]. While admission rate is low in patients presenting to the ED for skateboarding injuries (2.8%) [14], when admission is required it is often due to head trauma and it is often serious.

Skateboarding is one of the most popular extreme sports, particularly among the pediatric population. While most injuries sustained are comparatively minor and treated in the outpatient setting, when hospitalization is required, injuries are often severe and carry the possibility of long-standing dysfunction. Although not the most common area of involvement, head trauma is the most important injury consideration when treating skateboarders. Some volume of injury is unavoidable, but certain precautions can minimize the number of injuries sustained. Patients should be advised to always wear protective equipment including helmets, wrist guards, and elbow and knee pads, skate in skate parks rather than in unregulated street environments, always have appropriate supervision, and receive education on proper safety techniques [17].

48.4 Snow Skiing and Snowboarding

The practice of sliding down a snow-covered mountain with the aid of some form of board or ski beneath the feet is by no means a new concept. In fact, precursors to skis have been found as far back as 2000 BCE in areas of Scandinavia and Siberia. Competitive skiing, however, likely originated in Norway in the mid-eighteenth century. Acceptance slowly propagated around neighboring Scandinavia and, over time, to the rest of the globe [18]. In the 1960s and 1970s, a new form of alpine recreation was developed with the advent of snowboarding. Since its inception, snowboarding has seen an incredible rise in popularity, now rivaling skiing in many countries [19]. At present time, it is estimated that there are several hundred million skiers and snowboarders across the globe [20]. Considering this volume of participation, in addition to the combination of speed, obstacles (both natural and man-made), and aerial maneuvers performed while coming down the mountain, it is not surprising that skiing and snowboarding are a significant source of sports trauma.

Although both sports take place in a similar setting, different injury patterns are observed. Snowboarding appears to cause more frequent injuries than skiing. In a study from a base-lodge clinic in Vermont examining all snowboarder and skier injuries over the course of 18 years, Kim et al. [19] found the mean number of days between injury for snowboarders to be 345, versus 400 for skiers. The most common injury type for snowboarders was involving the wrist—combining sprains, distal radius/ulna fractures, and carpal fractures—whereas for skiers, the most common injury was ACL sprain. When comparing the two sports, snowboarding was more likely to result in wrist injury, ankle injuries, concussions, and clavicle fractures. Skiing, on the other hand, was more likely to result in ACL sprains, MCL sprains, LCL sprains, lower extremity contusions, thumb metacarpophalangeal-ulnar collateral ligament injuries, and tibia fractures.

Differences in types of injuries can be explained by the differences in equipment. During snowboarding, both feet are strapped firmly to a single board. This limits the amount of torsional load applied to the lower extremities, at the expense of balance. Therefore, there are less twisting knee injuries resulting in ligamentous injury, but more falls onto outstretched hands resulting in wrist injury. Interestingly, if a snowboarder gets injured while one of his or her feet detaches from the bindings, then knee ligament injury becomes much more likely to occur [19]. While relatively common in the skiing population, making up 8–10% of all skiing injuries [18], thumb UCL injuries are almost nonexistent in snowboarding. This is likely related to the different factors involved in patients landing on the hand during a fall. In snowboarding, the hand is free, and the thumb tends to hit the ground on the radial side in an abducted and extended position. This puts stress on the radial collateral ligament, if anything. However, when the skier falls with the thumb around a pole, this produces a radial directed force as the pole jams into the ulnar aspect of the thumb, leading to forced adduction and extension and significant stress on the UCL [18, 19]. The differing mechanics and equipment involved between skiing and snowboarding explain the observed differences in expected common injuries.

Any sport involving high speeds and jumps demands special attention toward head and neck injuries. In the 2015 epidemiologic study of head and neck injuries in extreme sports over a 12-year period [16], snowboarding was found to be the number one cause of concussion, accounting for 30% of all reported concussions in that population. Snow skiing followed closely behind snowboarding, accounting for 25% of all concussions in extreme sports. Even after correcting for number of athletes, snowboarding still had the highest incidence rate per person-years, with skateboarding second and snow skiing third. It stands to reason that with this many diagnosed concussions, a substantial number of subclinical head trauma is also taking place. Concussions and repeated mild trauma to the head have been shown to be associated with the development of chronic traumatic encephalopathy (CTE). Symptoms of CTE range from headache, difficulty with concentration, and depression all the way up to dementia, cognitive dysfunction, and explosivity/aggression [21]. Helmet use has been associated with a 60% reduction in the risk for head injury in skiing and snowboarding. Unfortunately, helmet usage has been reported as low as 20% [20]. Neck fractures occur less commonly in skiing and snowboarding. However, they cannot be discounted due to the potential for long-term dysfunction.

In many activities, a participant's rising skill level is often associated with injury risk reduction. Unfortunately, in the world of snowboarding, increased experience does not necessarily translate to increased safety. While it is accurate that the incidence of some injuries decreases with increasing skill level (such as upper extremity injuries, lacerations, contusions, and bruises), other injuries (such as those involving the trunk and multiple body sites) tend to occur more often. In fact, the Injury Severity Score increases significantly with increases in skill level. This trend coincides with injury mechanism. As skill level increases to the intermediate and expert levels, rather than mostly being caused by isolated falls as in novice and beginning snowboarders, injuries are most commonly sustained from jumps [22]. This relationship is further demonstrated when looking at injuries in elite snowboarders that compete on the national level. Torjussen et al. [23] looked at injuries that occurred during snowboarding national cup and championship events in Norway for the 2002 season. The authors found that the most common injury locations were the spine (20%) and knee (16%), both body areas requiring a greater amount of energy to injure. Essentially, as the rider becomes more comfortable on the snowboard, he or she is more likely to attempt more difficult tricks and ride down more difficult slopes, leading to a change in the injury patterns observed (Fig. 48.4).

Skiing and snowboarding are some of the most common recreational sports in the world, with millions of people on the slopes each year. However, recognition must be made of the potential injuries that can occur. It is necessary for treating healthcare professionals to recommend

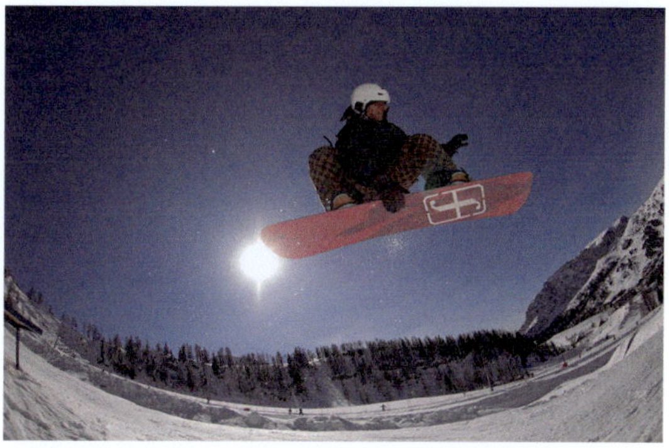

Fig. 48.4 Snowboarder performing a mute grab while snowboarding in Nassfeld, Austria

proper safety measures including helmet use and matching slope style and tricks performed to the rider's skill level. It should also be stressed, however, that more experience does not inexorably result in more safety.

48.5 Motocross

The earliest form of motocross was devised in England in 1924, using small internal combustion engines attached to bicycles. As the sport has evolved over the past century, the bikes have become bigger and more powerful. Currently, bikes weight up to 225 pounds and can generate more than 50 horsepower. While the majority of race time and injuries occur at speeds around 25 miles per hour, this power enables bikes to reach top speeds over 100 miles per hour and careen more than 100 ft in the air off jumps [24]. As one can imagine, this combination of speed, height, distance, and weight of the bike can translate to significant injuries when do crashes occur (Fig. 48.5).

Tomida et al. [25] found the overall injury rate for motocross to be 49.2 per 1000 h. Gobbi [26] reviewed all motocross injuries sustained in the European off-road competition from 1980 to 1981. From this data, the authors calculated an overall annual injury incidence of 9.5%. When separated into indoor and outdoor tracks, the incidence was 15% and 7.6%, respectively. The majority (58%) of injuries are classified as contusions or abrasions, followed by fractures (24%) and dislocations/ligamentous injury (18%). Fractures most frequently involve the upper extremity (51%), followed by the lower extremity (38%) and spine (6%). Interestingly, when the lower extremity was injured, the injury occurred on the left side 60% of the time. This difference has been attributed to the fact that the gear pedal is located on the left side of the bike, both providing less room for the foot to rest and increasing the time when the rider's foot is not secured on the foot peg. This is coupled with the fact that riders often change gears during jumps, leading to shifting on the foot peg right before landing [26].

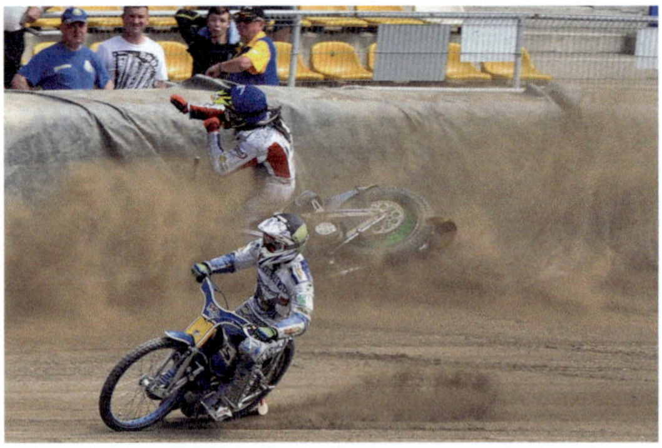

Fig. 48.5 Motocross rider losing control on a turn, crashing into the barrier

Head and neck injuries are of particular concern in motocross. Although the spine is not the most frequent location of fractures, nearly a third of spine fractures sustained in motocross result in permanent neurologic sequelae—paraplegia in 63% and tetraplegia in 37%. Further, since the initiation of indoor tracks, the likelihood of developing permanent neurologic deficits after a spine fracture has increased by 46% [26]. Sharma et al. [16] compared the rates of head and neck injuries across a variety of extreme sports, including skateboarding, snowboarding, snow skiing, mountain biking, surfing, and snowmobiling. It was found that, among these sports, motocross had the highest incidence of neck fractures and the second highest amount of head fractures—skateboarding was number one. On the other hand, when it came to concussion, motocross ranked number four. The rate of head injury in motocross may be higher in the pediatric population. Daniels et al. [27] examined 298 motocross injuries in patients under age 18 and determined that 20% had head injury or TBI. Concerningly, 72% of these patients were wearing helmets at the time of injury. Further, the authors commented that this value likely underestimates the total number of TBIs, as mild TBI is often overlooked. In a prospective study surveying an entire motocross season, 48% of riders self-reported at least one symptom of concussion over the course of the year [28]. With the recent focus on chronic traumatic encephalopathy in other sports, these findings must raise some concerns.

A variety of mechanisms can result in different injuries during a motocross event. Clavicle fractures can occur with direct falls onto the shoulder. Scaphoid and distal radius fractures are more common in indoor stadiums where there are higher triple or double jumps and woops—steep short bumps in close proximity to one another. This allows for less time for riders to adjust and a larger chance for the front wheel to collide directly into face of the jump, driving the handles into the extended wrist. Alternatively, wrist fracture can occur in the more typical mechanism with falls onto outstretched wrists. Metacarpal fractures can occur either indirectly, with forced abduction of the thumb while gripping the handlebars, or directly, with a clenched fist ramming into the ground or an object. Tibial plateau fractures can occur when landing hard on poorly executed jumps or by driving the foot into the ground when using the leg as a pivot. Likewise, meniscal or knee collateral ligament injuries can happen when using the leg as a pivot, putting a large varus or valgus stress on the knee. ACL tears often result from forced hyperextension after the foot slips off the foot peg and drives into the ground when landing. Thoracic spine fractures can occur with sudden and forceful forward flexion after landing from a jump. Cervical spine fractures can result when riders somersault over the handlebars and land directly on the head, causing hyperflexion [26]. This variety of injury patterns emphasizes the small margin of error riders have when landing jumps at high speeds.

Certain considerations need to be in effect when managing injuries at motocross events. Although most injuries sustained during competition involve the extremities, 10% are potentially life-threatening injuries to the head, neck, and other sensitive areas. Therefore, one must always keep these potentially catastrophic injuries in mind when assessing the acutely injured rider. The first assessment must involve scene safety. These injuries occur on an active racetrack with many tight corners and high jumps easily obstructing the view of other riders. Care must be taken to extricate the injured rider as quickly as is safely possible to avoid further injury to the victim, the treatment staff, or other competitors. Riders should be approached face-on to avoid having them inadvertently turning their head to answer questions. Helmet removal is recommended for better assessment of the airway. This must be done with great care by at least two providers—one stabilizes the spine from below and the other removes the helmet from above. Interestingly, loss of consciousness is fairly common in motocross accidents but is not predictive of significant head injury. Generally, riders that lose consciousness recover in 1–2 min without any neurologic deficit. A rapid assessment of whether the patient needs spinal immobilization prior to leaving the track can be made using the acronym FAST—first safety, airway, spine, and thinking. First safety enforces the need for scene awareness. Airway can be assessed by asking the rider "Are you okay?" If able to answer, this confirms a patent and protected airway. The spine can be evaluated by asking if the patient has any neck pain, numbness, tingling, or weakness. Extra care must be taken during this step, however, because of the short duration between time of injury and assessment. At this point, the adrenaline from the crash is still high, and there has not been time for swelling to develop, so neck pain may not be as obvious. Lastly, thinking can be assessed by asking the typical orientation questions, in addition to asking the rider what happened during the crash. Retrograde amnesia of the events of the crash has been shown to be the best predictor of significant head injuries. If the rider fails any of these assessments, they should be placed in full spinal immobilization before being moved from the track and transported to a local ER or trauma center. Patients with less emergent issues, such as extremity injuries, generally also require transport to a local hospital unless appropriate medical staff and imaging capability is available [24].

The speed and aerial spectacle that makes motocross exciting are the same factors that make it a high-risk sport. Protective equipment use is widespread and has been shown to decrease the injury risk. However, safety equipment cannot change the fact that motocross racing is inherently dangerous. Providing care to motocross events requires familiarity with the spectrum of injuries that can occur—both life-threatening and minor.

48.6 All-Terrain Vehicles

The first all-terrain vehicle (ATV) was created by John Plessinger as a graduate project in 1967 [29]. His design involved a rear-mounted engine with the rider sitting more within the vehicle, providing a lower center of gravity compared to today's models. This design was briefly manufactured by Sperry Rand. However, ATVs first became widely available in 1970 with the inception of the ATC 90 model from Honda Motor Company. Originally, the ATV was sold in both three- and four-wheel designs.

Recognition of the high injury rate involving ATV use became widespread in the 1980s. In 1988, ATV manufacturers and dealers agreed to the ATV Final Consent Decree [30]. This agreement pushed manufacturers and dealers to provide sufficient safety information to consumers both at the point of sale and in advertisements. Furthermore, it enacted provisions such as eliminating three-wheeled models, encouraging only single-rider use, offering free safety courses, recommending against use of 70–90cc models to people less than 12 years of age, recommending against use of models greater than 90cc by anyone less than 18 years of age, banning use on roads, requiring helmet use, and not allowing use by children less than 16 without adult supervision. Results following induction of the Consent Decree were encouraging. In 1985, prior to going into effect, the average annual risk for injury while riding an ATV was 2.1% [31]. Contrast this to 1989, just one year after the Consent Decree, when average annual risk fell to less than 1% [32]. The Consent Decree expired in 1998 and was replaced by the ATV Action Plan. The 2008 Consumer Product Safety Improvement Act took regulations a step further and effected an outright ban on importation, manufacture, or sale of three-wheeled models.

While it is important that safety regulations have been put into place, it is essential to recognize the intrinsic risk in operating an ATV. The design of an ATV—with its relatively high center of gravity, narrow wheelbase, and short turning radius—confers an inherent instability that puts the rider at risk for rollover [32]. Operating an ATV involves the rider sitting on top of the vehicle, straddling it like a motorcycle, with no protection in the event of collision or rollover. Furthermore, these vehicles are, by definition, used off-road on uneven terrain with frequent rapid shifts in center of gravity and potential need for swift course correction. Beyond the injuries sustained from simply falling off at high speeds, these are relatively large vehicles with some models weighing up to 600 pounds. This adds to the risk for further injury if the vehicle were to topple onto or run over the ejected rider. The combination of rollover risk, traveling speed, vehicle size, and operating conditions makes ATV riding a particularly dangerous activity (Fig. 48.6) [33]

There is a significant injury risk with ATV use. In 2016 alone, emergency rooms in the USA treated 101,200 injuries associated with ATV use. Approximately 26% of these injuries occurred in children younger than 16. Between 1982 and 2016, there have been an estimated 14,653 ATV-related fatalities. Of the total number of fatalities, 22% occurred in children younger than 16 and 10% occurred in children younger than 12. Injuries predominantly affect the upper extremity, head/neck, lower extremity, and torso—with

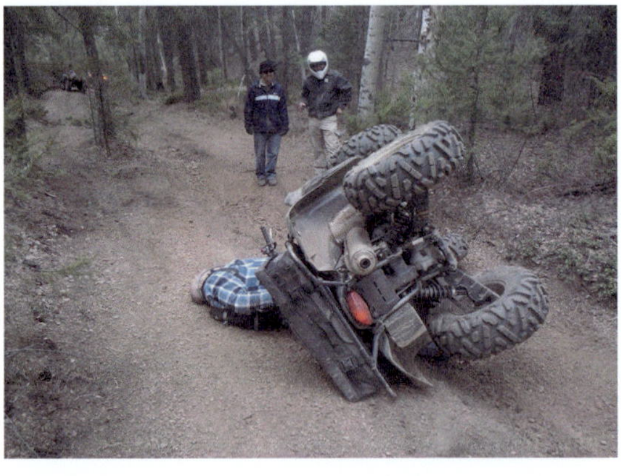

Fig. 48.6 An ATVs due to their short turning radius, high center of gravity, and narrow wheelbase are at high risk for rollover and ejection of the rider

injury rates of 29%, 27%, 22% and 20%, respectively [34]. Around 45% of injuries involve the musculoskeletal system. Fractures and or dislocations account for 30% of all injuries. Pollack et al determined that the most common locations for fractures were the clavicle (24%), forearm (15%), and tibia/fibula (13%) [35].

The rider's age is a substantial risk factor for injury. Although the group only contains 14% of all ATV riders, children aged less than 16 years old account for approximately one third of all injuries [32]. It has been shown that people between the ages of 11 and 15 are up to 10 times more likely to be injured while riding than those over 40 years old [36]. It is thought that lack of both experience and knowledge of the intrinsic danger of ATV riding contributes to the inflated risk in this age group. Additionally, children under the age of 16 have not yet developed the judgment or perceptual ability to safely operate these vehicles. This danger is magnified as the size of the engine and speed of the ATV increase. Because of this, children under the age of 16 require supervision whenever riding and proper safety training prior to use. In the same vein, children in this age group should not ride ATVs with greater than 90cc engines [33].

Other modifiable risk factors include riding with a passenger and helmet usage. Multiple rider usage has been identified as a significant cause of morbidity and mortality. For example, in the USA, there were 1342 pediatric deaths from ATV usage between 1982 and 1998. Of these deaths, 75% were riding as a passenger [37]. It is felt that adding a second passenger increases the likelihood that the vehicle will tip or roll over [33]. Wearing a helmet has been shown to significantly decrease the risk of injury to the head and neck region. Given that 22% of the injuries sustained during ATV use are localized to the head and neck, wearing a helmet has the potential to substantially change outcomes. Despite the effectiveness of helmet usage, actual utilization is worryingly low, with reported usage from 20 to 37% [35, 37].

Given what has been presented here, riding an ATV is an intrinsically dangerous activity with some risks that cannot be eliminated. However, healthcare practitioners should be aware of modifications that can make the activity safer. The AAOS best summarized these recommendations as:

1. ATV drivers should be licensed, demonstrating competence and knowledge of safety hazards.
2. Riders must be at least 12 years old.
3. Children aged 12–16 should have restrictions on usage (supervision, engine size less than 90cc).
4. Safety equipment must be worn (helmet, gloves, boots).
5. ATVs should only be operated during daylight.
6. Only one person should ride at a time.
7. ATVs should not be operated under the influence of drugs and/or alcohol [33].

48.7 Automotive Racing

There are many different varieties of car racing, both on- and off-road, available to competitive drivers. Most types of automotive racing involve maneuvering at high speeds with multiple other drivers sharing the track and, therefore, risk for high-energy collisions and rollover. Despite the popularity of car racing, little studies have investigated the injuries sustained by drivers.

Stock car racing, such as NASCAR, is one of the most popular varieties of car racing. On average, NASCAR viewership is around six million people per race [38]. Average speeds of the winners of these races can range from 190 to 200 miles per hour [39]. The largest study to date examining injuries in stock car racing was performed in 2004 by Minoyama et al. [40], looking at injuries that occurred at races at a single speedway between 1996 and 2000. The investigators separated out single-seat and saloon cars. Single-seat cars are open-roofed with a much smaller cockpit, similar to those used in Formula One racing. Saloon cars are the typical sedan-sized vehicles used in NASCAR. The injury rate in single-seat and saloon cars was found to be 1.2 and 0.9 injuries per 1000 competitors, respec-

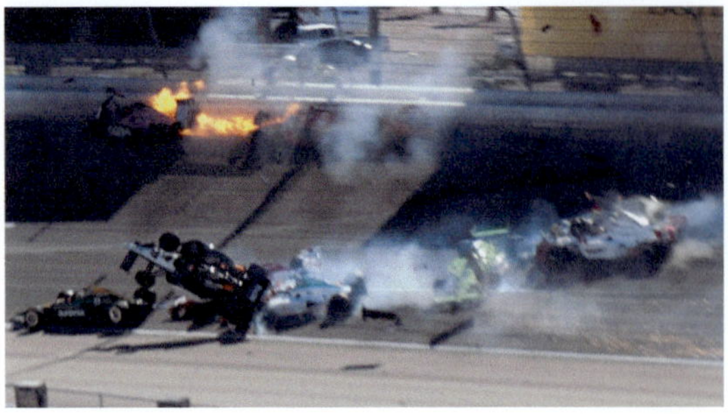

Fig. 48.7 Crash that took place on the 11th lap of the 2011 IZOD IndyCar World Championship. This crash resulted in the death of two-time Indy 500 winner Dan Wheldon. Wheldon was traveling at 220 mph just prior to the crash

tively. The most common injuries in single-seat cars were bruising (58%), neck sprain (34%), and concussion (2%). There was one fatality reported out of 1030 cars participating in 39 races. The most common injuries in saloon cars were neck sprain (53%), bruising (27%), fracture (8%), and concussion (3%). It was felt that the higher rate of bruising in single-seat cars was related to the limited space available in the cockpit, particularly around the legs, with a higher chance for the driver's body to crash into the sides of the car (Fig. 48.7)

This was further evidenced by the fact that most bruises in single-seat cars were in the lower extremity, while most bruises in the saloon cars were in the upper extremity. Neck injury was more common in saloon cars than in single-seat cars, while head/face injury was more common in single-seat cars compared to saloon cars. This is related to the much shorter distance between the driver's head and steering wheel in single-seat vehicles. Because of this, the driver's head is more likely to crash into the steering wheel in single-seat and, thus, cause injury to the head/face. Conversely, since the head is unlikely to contact the steering wheel in saloon cars, the head/face are not injured, but the neck is free to travel through a larger range of motion and become strained. The annual rate of concussion per driver in car racing has been shown to be from 0.67 to 1.64% [41]. This data suggests that the injury rate in professional racecar drivers is surprisingly low; however more research is needed across a broader spectrum of racing environments to have a better understanding of the true injury rate.

Despite the fact that racecar drivers travel at higher speeds than any of the other extreme sports discussed, it has been shown to have the lowest incidence of injury. When injuries do occur, they tend to be mild; however, fatalities do occur. The limited research that does exist has only looked at experienced professional drivers. Likely, if novice drivers attempted to drive at the speeds that these athletes attain, then there would be substantially higher injury and mortality rates. Because of this, automotive racing should only be done by trained professionals in controlled and regulated environments.

48.8 Airborne Sports

Airborne sports are all unified by the high speeds and heights that participants achieve. This being the case, these sports are associated with more severe and, often, fatal injuries. Major injuries from airborne sports trauma—defined as an Injury Severity Score >9—has been shown to be associated with the highest ISS when compared to major injuries from mountain climbing, skating, and contact sports with average scores of 22, 16, 15, and 10, respectively [1]. Because of the small margin of error, when things go wrong in airborne sports they go very wrong.

Skydiving is one of the most popular airborne sports. In the USA in the year 2000, it is estimated that 317,741 people made at least one skydive, adding up to 3.5 million total jumps [42]. The injury rate in skydiving has been shown to be 1.7 injuries for every 1000 jumps. Two thirds of injuries are classified as minor, with simple abrasions, contusions, and lacerations making up 54% of all injuries. The rate of significant injury—requiring treatment at an emergency room—is 0.6/1000 skydives. When patients do require treatment at an emergency department, less than one third require hospital admission. The most common injuries requiring emergency department care were those involving the extremities, making up 47%; 82% of these were to the lower extremity and 18% to the upper extremity. The risk of mortality is fairly low, with one study cataloguing 117,000 skydives reporting only one fatality. Over time, the injury rate in skydiving has been shown to decrease as equipment has become more advanced. Innovations in skydiving include switching from round to rectangular canopies, reserve static line (reserve chutes that automatically deploy if the main canopy is cut away), improved helmet design, and advances in altimeters. Rectangular canopies allow for better steering and braking, giving the skydiver better control [43]. In a study looking at the injury rate in a group of US Reserve Rescue unit skydivers, the injury rate was found to drop from 11 injuries per 1000 jumps down to nearly 0 injuries per 1000 jumps following the switch from round to rectangular parachutes [44]. Overall, the injury rate from skydiving is quite low.

Buildings, Antennas, Spans, and Earth (BASE) jumping is an activity where a person propels him or herself off a fixed, elevated structure and uses a parachute to glide down to the ground below. It has been around for many years, but it became popularized in the 1960s and 1970s by pioneers such as Carl Boenish. Boenish helped coin the term BASE jumping—which is an acronym for buildings, antennas, spans (i.e., bridges), and earth (i.e., cliffs), signifying a collection of the structures from which participants jump (Fig. 48.8)

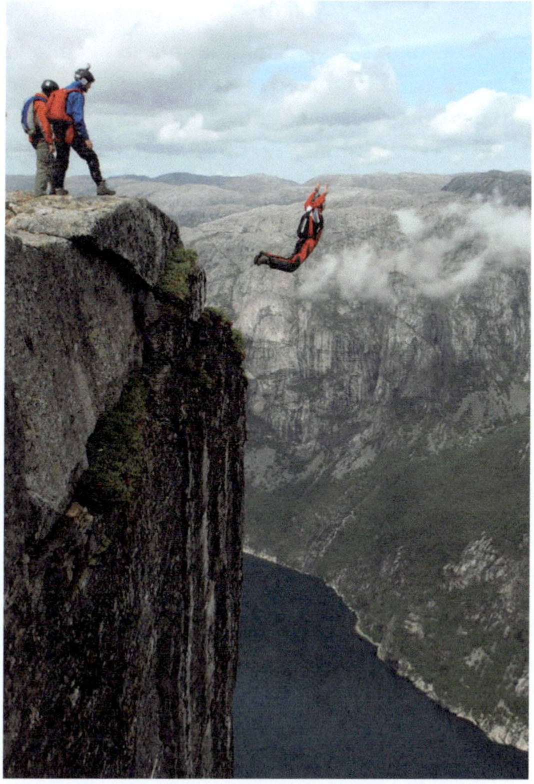

Fig. 48.8 A BASE jumper jumps off of a cliff. The low jump heights give jumpers little time to troubleshoot a complication with their parachute

The fundamental danger of this activity is exemplified by Boenish's unfortunate death during a jump in 1984 [45]. Because of the relatively low height from which jumpers take off, BASE jumpers do not have much time to deploy their chute at a safe altitude. Not surprisingly, then, BASE jumpers have been shown to have a five to eight times increased risk of injury or death when compared to skydiving. Injuries have been reported to occur in 0.4% of all jumps. Most concerningly, the rate of fatal injury has been shown to be 0.4 deaths for every 1000 jumps [46]. During accidents, 72% of injuries involve the lower extremities, 31% involve the spine, 18% involve the upper extremities, and 3% involve a head injury [47]. Typically, accidents occur when the chute opens facing the wrong direction, causing the jumper to collide into the object from which he or she jumped [46]. With the significant speeds that jumpers reach and the small amount of time for course correction, BASE jumping is a high-risk activity with significant chance of major injury or death.

Although the concept behind of skydiving and BASE jumping is similar, the risk profile of the two sports is wildly different. The added dangers of nearby obstacles and limited time available for course correction greatly elevate the risk posed by BASE jumping. In fact, the fatality rate from BASE jumping is just slightly lower than the risk of sustaining an injury requiring treatment at an emergency department while skydiving.

48.9 Conclusion

With the rising pop-culture influence of events like the Winter and Summer X Games, participation in extreme sports is likely to continue to increase over the coming years. More participants will certainly lead to more injuries; therefore, physicians providing care to athletes must be aware of the particular injury considerations for these sports. It is also important to be able to recognize and minimize sport-specific hazards in order to provide counselling for risk reduction. Head and neck injury requires special attention given the relatively high incidence of these injuries in extreme sports, in addition to the potentially devastating consequences if they do occur. Ultimately, the role of the sports physician in caring for the extreme sports athlete is multifaceted. Diligent care requires physicians to serve as educators in injury prevention strategies; as diagnosticians, being careful not to miss injuries that can carry long-term consequences; and, when injuries do occur, as providers of both operative and non-operative treatment modalities.

References

1. Weber CD, Horst K, Nguyen AR, et al. Evaluation of severe and fatal injuries in extreme and contact sports. Arch Orthop Trauma Surg. 2018;138(7):963–70. https://doi.org/10.1007/s00402-018-2935-8.
2. Moran K, Webber J. Surfing injuries requiring first aid in New Zealand, 2007-2012. Int J Aquatic Res Educ. 2013;7:192–203.
3. Nathanson A, Haynes P, Galanis D. Surfing injuries. Am J Emerg Med. 2002;20:155–60.
4. Allen RH, Eiseman B, Straehley CJ, Orloff BG. Surfing injuries at Waikiki. JAMA. 1977;237:668–70.
5. Furness J, Hing W, Walsh J, Abbot A, Sheppard JM, Climstein M. Acute injuries in recreational and competitive surfers. AJSM. 2015;43:1246–54.
6. Lowdon BJ, Pateman NA, Pitman AJ. Surfboard-riding injuries. Med J Aust. 1983;2:613–6.
7. Lowdon BJ, Pitman AJ, Pateman NA, Ross K. Injuries to international competitive surfboard riders. J Sports Med Phys Fitness. 1987;27:57–63.
8. Nathanson A, Bird S, Dao L, Tam-Sing K. Competitive surfing injuries: a prospective study of surfing-related injuries among contest surfers. Am J Sports Med. 2007;35(1):113–7.
9. Klick C, Jones CM, Adler D. Surfing USA: an epidemiological study of surfing injuries presenting to US EDs 2002 to 2013. Am J Emerg Med. 2016;34(8):1491–6.
10. Skateboarding History [Internet]. [cited 2018 May 10]. http://www.skatelog.com/skateboarding/skateboarding-history.htm.
11. Newton DE. Skateboarding. In: Longe JL, editor. The Gale encyclopedia of fitness, vol. 2. Farmington Hills: Gale; 2012. p. 779–83.
12. Shuman KM, Meyers MC. Skateboarding injuries: an updated review. Phys Sportsmed. 2015;43(3):317–23.
13. Bandzar S, Funsch DG, Hermansen R, et al. Pediatric hoverboard and skateboard injuries. Pediatrics. 2018;141(4):1–5.
14. Kyle SB, Nance ML, Rutherford GWJ, Winston FK. Skateboard-associated injuries: participation-based estimates and injury characteristics. J Trauma Acute Care Surg. 2002;53(4):686.
15. Zalavras C, Nikolopoulou G, Essin D, et al. Pediatric fractures during skateboarding, roller skating, and scooter riding. Am J Sports Med. 2005;33(4):568–73.
16. Sharma VK, Rango J, Connaughton AJ, Lombardo DJ, Sabesan VJ. The current state of head and neck injuries in extreme sports. Orthop J Sports Med. 2015;3(1):2325967114564358.
17. Lustenberger T. Skateboard-related injuries: not to be taken lightly. A National Trauma Databank Analysis. J Trauma. 2010;69(4):924–7.
18. Hunter RE. Skiing injuries. Am J Sports Med. 1999;27(3):381–9.
19. Kim S, Endres NK, Johnson RJ, Ettlinger CF, Shealy JE. Snowboarding injuries: trends over time and comparisons with alpine skiing injuries. Am J Sports Med. 2012;40(4):770–6.
20. Sulheim S, Holme I, Ekeland A, Bahr R. Helmet use and risk of head injuries in alpine skiers and snowboarders. JAMA. 2006;296(8):919–24.
21. McKee AC, Stern RA, Nowinski CJ, Stein TD. The spectrum of disease in chronic traumatic encephalopathy. Brain. 2013;136:43–64.
22. Ogawa H, Sumi H, Sumi Y, Shimizu K. Skill level-specific differences in snowboarding-related injuries. Am J Sports Med. 2010;38(3):532–7.
23. Torjusseh J, Bahr R. Injuries among competitive snowboarders at the National Elite Level. Am J Sports Med. 2005;33(3):370–7.
24. Grange JT, Bodnar JA, Corbett SW. Motocross medicine. Curr Sports Med Rep. 2009;8(3):125–30.
25. Tomida Y, Hirata H, Fukuda A, Tsujii M, Kato K, Fujisawa K, Uchida A. Injuries in elite motorcycle racing in Japan. Br J Sports Med. 2005;39(8):508–11.
26. Gobbi A, Tuy B, Panuncialman I. The incidence of motocross injuries: a 12-year investigation. Knee Surg Sports Traumatol Arthrosc. 2004;12(6):574–80.
27. Daniels DJ, Clarke MJ, Puffer R, Luo TD, McIntosh AL, Wetjen NM. High occurrence of head and spine injuries in the pediatric population following motocross accidents. J Neurosurg Pediatr. 2015;15(3):261–5.
28. Luo TD, Clarke MJ, Zimmerman AK, et al. Concussion symptoms in youth motocross riders: a prospective, observational study. J Neurosurg Pediatr. 2015;15:255–60.
29. Pellen J. Who invented the 3-wheel ATV? 2009. http://www.atvscene.com.
30. United States of America vs. Polaris Industries, L.P. Civil Action No. 87-3525. Washington, DC: U.S. District Court for the District of Columbia; 1988.
31. Helmkamp JC. Injuries and deaths and the use of all-terrain vehicles. N Engl J Med. 2000;343:1733–4.

32. Balthrop PM, et al. Risk factors and musculoskeletal injuries associated with all-terrain vehicle accidents. J Emerg Med. 2009;36(2):121–31.
33. Position statement on all-terrain vehicles. American Academy of Orthopaedic Surgeons. Document no. 1101, 2005. Revised September 2015. http://www.aaos.org.
34. 2016 annual report of ATV-related deaths and injuries. U.S. Consumer Product Safety Commission. Washington, DC. December 2017. https://www.cpsc.gov/Safety-Education/Safety-Education-Centers/ATV-Safety-Information-Center
35. Pollack CV Jr, Pollack SB. Injury severity scores in desert recreational all-terrain vehicle trauma. J Trauma. 1990;30:888–92.
36. Rodgers GB. All-terrain vehicle injury risks and the effects of regulation. Accid Anal Prev. 1993;25:335–46.
37. Upperman JS, Shultz B, Gaines BA, et al. All-terrain vehicle rules and regulations: impact on pediatric mortality. J Pediatr Surg. 2003;38(9):1284–6.
38. Wertman G, Gaston RG, Heisel W. Upper extremity injuries in NASCAR drivers and pit screw: an epidemiological study. Orthop J Sports Med. 2016;4(2):1–5.
39. USA Today. Daytona 500: all-time pole winners and speeds in NASCAR's biggest race. 2018. http://www.usatoday.com.
40. Minoyama O, Tsuchida H. Injuries in professional motor car racing drivers at a racing circuit between 1996 and 2000. Br J Sports Med. 2004;38(5):613–6.
41. Deakin ND, Cronin T, Trafford P, Olvey S, Roberts I, Mellor A, Hutchinson PJ. Concussion in motor sport: a medical literature review and engineering perspective. J Concuss. 2017;1:1–11.
42. United States Parachute Association membership statistics, 2000.
43. Barrows TH, Mills TJ, Kassing SD. The epidemiology of skydiving injuries: World Freefall Convention, 2000-2001. J Emerg Med. 2005;28(1):63–8.
44. Baldwin CC. Parachuting injuries and type of parachute in a reserve rescue unit. Aviat Space Environ Med. 1988;5:780–2.
45. Patterson T. Meet the father of BASE jumping. 2016. http://www.cnn.com
46. Soreide K, Ellingsen CL, Knutson V. How dangerous is BASE jumping? An analysis of adverse events in 20,850 jumps from the Kjerag Massif, Norway. J Trauma. 2007;62:1113–7.
47. Monasterio E, Mei-Dan O. Risk and severity of injury in a population of BASE jumpers. N Z Med J. 2008;121:70–5.

49 Judo, Brazilian Jiu-Jitsu, Wrestling, and Mixed Martial Arts

John A. Bergfeld, Jonathan Gelber, Scott A. Lynch, Peter H. Seidenberg, and Sérgio Rocha Piedade

49.1 Judo

Created in 1882, in Japan, judo has in its DNA contributions from various martial arts of samurais and feudal warriors, but mainly from its creator Dr. Jigoro Kano who brought together concepts and techniques of traditional Japanese jujutsu, ancient forms of self-defense and physical concepts of action and reaction. Judo is a sport based on education, hierarchy, humility, and, mainly, respect for others, which are moral values established by its maker. **The philosophy of judo** ("**gentle way**") is present in most of **the sayings of Dr. Kano**, such as "**to give in to win**"; "only those who seek it with constancy, wisdom and above all great humility, comes close to perfection."

J. A. Bergfeld
Cleveland Clinic, Cleveland, OH, USA
e-mail: BERGFEJ@ccf.org

J. Gelber
West Harford, CT, USA
e-mail: jgelber@connecticutchildrens.org

S. A. Lynch · P. H. Seidenberg
Penn State University, Hershey, PA, USA
e-mail: slynch@pennstatehealthpsu.edu; seidenph@slu.edu

S. R. Piedade (✉)
Department of Orthopedics and Traumatology, State University of Campinas – UNICAMP, Exercise and Sports Medicine, Campinas, SP, Brazil
e-mail: piedade@fcm.unicamp.br

The milestone of judo as an Olympic sport occurs when Dr. Jigoro Kano becomes the first Japanese member of the International Olympic Committee (IOC) in 1909, bringing the philosophy of judo and the Olympic principles together. Many years later, judo was introduced to the Olympic Program in Tokyo, Japan, in 1964, during the XVIII Olympic Games, where judo had its first participation with male athletes, and then the female athletes officially joined the Program of the XXV Olympic Games in Barcelona, Spain, in 1992.

With every Olympic cycle, the interest and strength of this sport have been increasing worldwide [1], and this was notably evident during the XXXI Olympic Games in Rio de Janeiro, Brazil, in 2016, when 40 athletes from different countries were awarded medals. Even now, Japan remains a reference in this sport, but countries such as France, Russia, Brazil, Azerbaijan, the Netherlands, Georgia, and the USA have a fantastic history of achievements in world Championship and Olympic Games.

Like other martial arts, judo involves tremendous combat, and, therefore, it is not free from injuries [2]. **The dynamics of judo takes in throwing techniques** (*Nage-waza*) that are performed standing and **control techniques** mainly done on the ground (*Katame-waza*). This martial art is practiced on a square area called dojo, which has a minimum of 64 m^2 or a maximum of 100 m^2. In this space, two athletes fight, gripping

S. Rocha Piedade et al. (eds.), *The Sports Medicine Physician*,
https://doi.org/10.1007/978-3-030-10433-7_49

the judogui (judo uniform) to accomplish leverage body techniques, to change the opponent's center of gravity, making him off balance and, therefore, more vulnerable to fall.

Regarding the injuries, cuts and bruises usually present as minor and superficial injuries, when they are deeper cuts that will need to be stitched or glued to stop blood flow, and the judo combat may be interrupted. The acromioclavicular, elbow, hand, and knee joints are commonly affected, mostly when the opponent tries to avoid his fall to account for ippon (perfect throwing technique) and to lose the combat. Although severe spine injuries are a rare clinical event, the sports medicine physician should keep the eyes open to this possibility, particularly, when, during the combat, the athlete falls hitting his head first on the ground, followed by neck hyperflexion or hyperextension, a potential mechanism for cervical spine injury [3].

49.2 Jiu-Jitsu

Although Japan is recognized as a stage of development and improvement of Jiu-jitsu, the precise origin of this martial art is not clear, as history records the presence of other similar martial arts in other places such as India, China, Egypt, and Persia.

Jiu-jitsu was created to make a samurai able to skillfully defend himself from an enemy, even when he had no weapons (sword). Thus, this "**art of self-defense without the use of weapons**" is based on the application of body leverage and twisting techniques, opposing to martial arts where weapons are used (Kenjutsu). Over the years, new martial arts were derived from the jiu-jitsu, making it temporarily distant and fragmented, until it returned in fullness with the advent of the Brazilian jiu-jitsu.

49.2.1 Brazilian Jiu-Jitsu: Gracie Family's Contribution

The pathway of jiu-jitsu in Brazil started when a Japanese master of jiu-jitsu called Esai Maeda Koma, known as Conde Koma, recognized defender of self-defense techniques, arrived in Belem, state of Para, in 1914. To spread the art, the master challenged fighters of different styles of martial arts around the world. His many and incontestable victories aroused a great interest in learning jiu-jitsu.

The friendship between master Maeda and a member of the Gracie family, Gastao Gracie, was decisive to quickly incorporate this martial art into the life of the Gracie family. Over time, Helio, Gastao's youngest son, improved the techniques and concepts that allowed him to win combats against athletes physically stronger than him from different fighting styles [4]. This incredible trajectory was continued by his sons and grandchildren, with remarkable achievements and victories in the martial arts scene, where many of them are referred to as a legend in this sport.

A key point in the popularity of jiu-jitsu was established by Helio Gracie's oldest son, Rorion Gracie, who created the Ultimate Fighting Championship® (UFC), where seven great fighting athletes were reunited, including his brother, Royce Gracie, who was physically weaker compared to the other competitors. The tournament was broadcast in the USA by the pay-per-view system, and basically, there were no rules, and the fights did not have limit time, except for the elimination of the loser. Royce's fantastic victory over the other opponents further consolidated the respect for Brazilian jiu-jitsu (Gracie's jiu-jitsu) in the universe of fights [4], and, undoubtedly, the event has become the embryo of the current MMA tournaments.

Unlike Judo, where the throwing techniques are prominent in the combat (Fig. 49.1), **jiu-jitsu focuses on techniques developed on the ground**, such as immobilization, strangling, attacks on the joints (Fig. 49.2), which are performed by body leverage, and overtaking, and therefore, skins abrasions, cuts, and contusions to the auricular and mandibular regions are commonly reported [5]. Joint-attack techniques can lead to injuries such as sprains, contusions, dislocation, and fractures. Bottlenecks (mechanical asphyxia) are common combat techniques, and

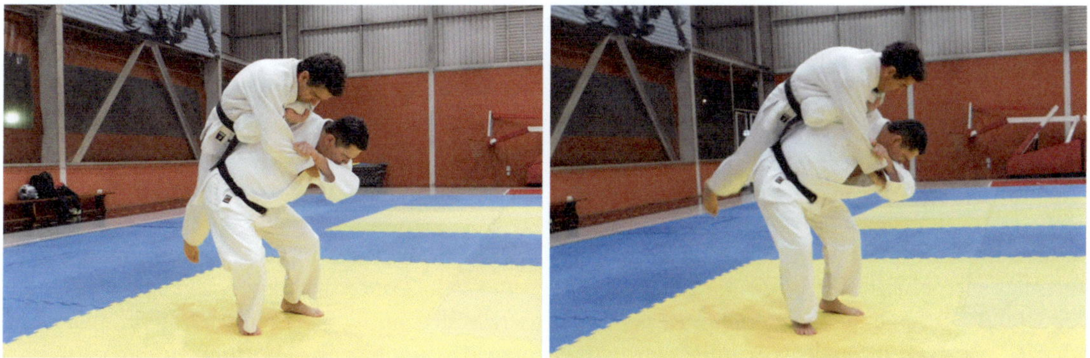

Fig. 49.1 Throwing technique: Nage-waza (Morote Seoi Nague)

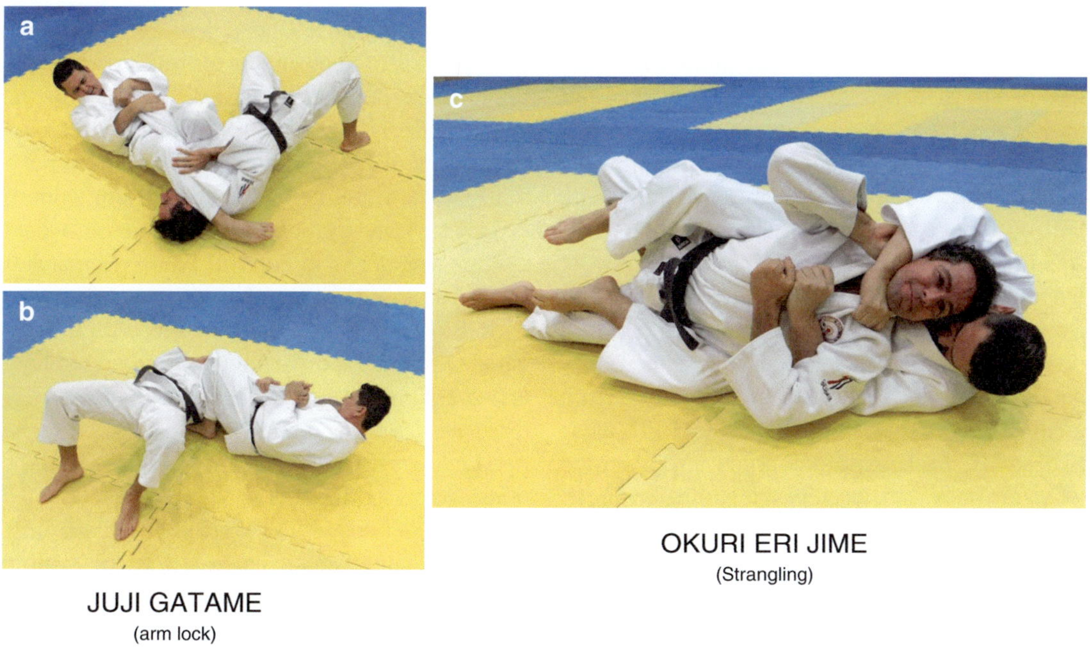

Fig. 49.2 Control techniques (Katame-waza): Juji gatame (**a** and **b**), Okuri eri jime (**c**)

therefore the referee and the sports medicine staff need to closely observe the athlete's response to the attack and avoid the athlete's longtime exposition without adequate oxygenation.

49.3 Wrestling

Wrestling is one of the oldest known sports. It is also among the most physically challenging of all sports. It is unique in many ways, requiring both aerobic and anaerobic conditioning, strength, flexibility, balance, and above all, a keen knowledge of wrestling techniques. For high-level, equally-matched wrestlers, it becomes a physical chess match with small adjustments that often are unrecognized by spectators. The most popular forms of wrestling can be divided into three forms. International wrestling, with its styles that are included in the Olympic Games, consists of Greco-Roman and Freestyle wrestling. The most practiced style in the USA, which is not practiced much elsewhere, is Folkstyle—sometimes called Collegiate or School Boy—wrestling. The ultimate goal in all styles is to pin the opponent's back to the mat with both scapulae touching the surface at the same time. Once this occurs, the match is over, and the pinning wrestler is declared the winner. In each style, points are awarded for dominating moves or penalties for illegal moves. If no pin occurs, the wrestler with the most points at the end of the match is declared the winner. As the rules and point scoring systems of these styles are slightly different, some of the most common injuries are also different as a reflection of the different rules.

Greco-Roman and Freestyle scoring rules are essentially the same, with the only difference being that in Greco-Roman wrestling opponents are not permitted to attack the other wrestlers' legs or use their legs to trip opponents. The pin occurs when both scapulae of the shoulder touch the mat simultaneously, even for an instant. This is sometimes referred to as a "touch fall." The bulk of the wrestling occurs with both opponents standing on their feet, attempting to "takedown" the other wrestler to the mat to gain control. Bonus points can be gained for taking the opponent down to the mat while exposing the opponent's back to the mat or for high amplitude and arching throws to the opponent's back. In these two styles, back exposure points are awarded when the back is exposed past a 90-degree angle, even for an instant. Once the "takedown" occurs, the wrestler on top will have several seconds to attempt to turn the opponent to expose the back. If there is no progress toward turning the opponent over, the referee will stop the match and return the wrestlers to the standing position for a restart. In general, in these two styles of wrestling, there is little attempt by the bottom wrestler to get out or escape. Greco-Roman and Freestyle have two periods of wrestling (3 min each for the higher-level competitions) with a rest between periods (1-min rest period for higher-level competition). If no pin occurs, the wrestler with the most points is declared the winner. There is no overtime in Greco-Roman or Freestyle wrestling; instead, in case of tie-on points, the winner is declared by a tie-breaking criterion.

Folkstyle wrestling is mainly practiced by youth, high school, and collegiate wrestlers in the USA. In this style, the pin occurs when both scapulae are held to the mat for 1 s in collegiate wrestling and 2 s in the high school and youth classes. The match starts with both opponents on their feet; this is called the "neutral" position, and each wrestler attempts to take the opponent to the mat to gain control. One main difference from Greco-Roman and Freestyle rules and Folkstyle rules is that once the "takedown" is awarded, the wrestling continues regardless of time, and the wrestler in the control position (top) tries to turn the defensive opponent (bottom position) to their back. "Back points" are awarded for turning the opponent, with back exposure of 45° or less to the mat, for at least 2 s. No points are awarded for brief periods of exposure or for rolling across the back. Back points can only be earned by the wrestler that is in control. One other main difference is that the defensive wrestler (bottom position) can earn points by either reversing control or getting back to the "neutral" position, where neither wrestler is in control. Folkstyle matches are three periods in length with no rest between periods. Period lengths vary by age, with the collegiate level at 3-2-2 (in minutes) and high school at 2-2-2. The starting position for periods two and three are determined by the choice of each wrestler. One wrestler chooses for period two and the other for period three. The wrestler that chooses for period two is determined by coin flip. Wrestlers can choose neutral, top, or bottom position. If no pin occurs, the wrestler with the most points is declared the winner. Unlike Greco-Roman and Freestyle wrestling, if the regular match ends in a tie, overtime periods will continue until a wrestler outscores the opponent.

49.4 Epidemiology

Unfortunately, there is only limited data on wrestling injuries. The majority of published studies come from the USA and show that injury patterns and severity vary by age and style of wrestling [6–14]. A limitation of this research is that, in the USA, Greco-Roman and Freestyle participation are usually limited to the more skilled group of wrestlers, as nearly all novice wrestling clubs in the USA begin with teaching of Folkstyle wrestling. This may bias the data to a different injury type based on skill level or age, rather than a true difference based on style. Likewise, most of the literature does not account for hours of practice and participation but usually reports the injury data from a particular competition [9, 14, 15]. A few studies, which will be reviewed in more detail later, encompass longer periods of time, from a low of one season to a high of 11 years [7, 10, 11, 13, 16]. These studies are only in high school and collegiate programs in US Folkstyle, so its transference to other styles or age groups is uncertain.

49.4.1 Greco-Roman and Freestyle

Only a few studies address injury patterns for Greco-Roman and Freestyle. Yard and Comstock [14] examined injuries for the pediatric age group (up to 20 years old) at the US National tournament. This tournament was the 2006 ASICS/Vaughan Cadet and Junior National Championships. The authors collected injury data on 3000 male wrestlers. In order to qualify for this tournament, a wrestler must place highly in state and/or regional qualifying tournaments. As such, this data encompasses elite level wrestlers in the Greco-Roman and Freestyle disciplines. In addition, at this age, it is common for wrestlers to be entered into both styles. At the international level, competing in both Greco-Roman and Freestyle is extremely rare. The injury rate at this tournament was 7.0 per 100 matches in freestyle and 4.6 per 100 matches in Greco-Roman. Freestyle had a higher incidence of knee injuries, while Greco-Roman had a higher incidence of elbow and head/face/neck injuries. This is to be expected based on the rules of each discipline, since attacking the legs is not allowed in Greco-Roman wrestling, leading to more upper body contact and attempted throws in Greco-Roman wrestling.

Lorish et al. [9] prospectively examined injury patterns during two youth (6–16-year-old) international Freestyle and Greco-Roman tournaments. The overall injury incidence was 12.7% in the combined cohort of 1742 athletes. The most common locations for injury were upper extremity (34%) followed by the neck and back (24%) and the head and face (15%). Only 4.6% of participants had injuries that were severe enough to warrant removal from competition. Age was positively correlated with injury risk in the study. There were two significant limitations of the study. First, the injuries were not differentiated by wrestling style, which is problematic as the rule differences may result in varying injury patterns. A second limitation is that injury rates could not be calculated as the number of matches in which each athlete competed was not recorded.

Kordi et al. [16] reported on catastrophic injuries sustained during Olympic style wresting, i.e., Freestyle and Greco-Roman, in the county of Iran. Wrestling is the national sport in Iran. This was a retrospective survey of wrestling clubs throughout the country from July 1998 to June 2005. In Iran, as with most countries outside of the USA, sports are not associated with schools, and athletes of all ages participate through clubs. The authors identified 29 catastrophic injuries associated with wrestling (12 fatalities, 11 nonfatal, and 6 serious). Catastrophic injury was defined as "a sport injury that resulted in a brain or spinal cord injury or skull or spinal fracture." Although they do not explain well how they determined the number of wrestlers, the authors estimated a catastrophic injury rate of 1.99 cases per 100,000 wrestlers per year. Most of the injuries occurred during practice during a takedown maneuver and were more frequent in the higher level and more experienced groups.

Shadgan et al. [15] reported on wrestling injuries during the 2008 Beijing Olympic Games. This is one of the only studies that specifically included elite female wrestling. At elementary and high school levels, girls will almost always be competing against boys. There are a limited number of all-women collegiate programs, with the great majority of collegiate wrestling only including men. At the international, including Olympic levels, women and men are in separate tournaments that include only one sex. Women's tournaments are wrestled with Freestyle rules. This study included a total of 343 athletes. Injuries were only considered if they occurred during tournament competition. Any injuries sustained during a practice session during the tournament were excluded. There were 32 injuries sustained during 406 matches (9.3 injuries/100 athletes and 7.88 injuries/100 matches). Men's freestyle wrestling had the highest injury rate, followed by Greco-Roman, with women's wrestling having the lowest rate. These rates were 10.1%, 9.3%, and 7.5%, respectively. However, these were not statistically significant differences. The majority of these injuries were minor, with skin lacerations making up 59.4% of the injuries. There were no major or catastrophic injuries. Eighty-one percent of the injuries occurred in the standing position, which is expected since the majority of the match is wrestled from the standing position for the Freestyle and Greco-Roman disciplines.

49.4.2 Folkstyle (Also Called Collegiate or Schoolboy)

Yard et al. [13] compared high school and collegiate wrestling injury rates and patterns by collecting data at 74 high schools throughout the USA and collecting data from 15 NCAA teams from all NCAA Divisions. The high school data was collected via the High School Reporting Information Online (RIO) system, and the NCAA data was collected via its Injury Surveillance System (ISS). These two systems relied on each school's athletic trainers to input online injury information. This study encompassed one season of competition, using the 2005–2006 academic wrestling season data. The injury rate for high school wrestlers was 2.33 injuries per 1000 athlete-exposures. The injury rate for college wrestlers was 7.25 injuries per 1000 athlete-exposures. This was a statistically significant difference. In addition, in both high school and college wrestlers, there was a statistically significant higher rate of injuries during competition than during practice. This study also collected skin infection data. The rate of skin infections for high school athletes was 0.22 infections per 1000 athlete-exposures, and the rate for college was 1.91 skin infections per 1000 athlete-exposures. This was again a statistically significant difference. Impetigo, herpes simplex and ringworm were the main three types of skin infections, with herpes being more common in the college wrestlers than high school wrestlers. Skin infections accounted for 8.5% of high school and 20.9% of college reported incidents, respectively. Among both the high school and college wrestlers, strains and sprains made up about half of all injuries. The knee and shoulder were the two most common sites of injury in both the high school and college wrestlers. A little less than half of all wrestlers in both high school (44.9%) and college (42.6%) missed less than 1 week of participation time from wrestling. Most injuries occurred with the wrestlers in the standing position or while executing a takedown, 54% in high school and 69% in college. This is not surprising since when the skill gap narrows, as it does in college, wrestlers usually spend more time in the standing positions because it is harder to establish dominance over the other wrestler.

Jarrett et al. [7] reported wrestling injury data over an 11-year period from 1985 to 1996 using the NCAA Injury Surveillance System (ISS). Note, that this data was collected prior to the ISS implementation to the online reporting system. Schools included in the ISS at that time were voluntary contributors collected annually from 15 to 20% of NCAA schools that sponsor a particular sport. A minimum of 15% of school participants were required to come from each of the three NCAA Divisions and 15% from one of each of four geographic regions. The schools participating in the data collection were not the same every year. The average number of wrestling teams that participated each year was 45. This represented approximately 16% of the total number of schools that had wrestling during that time period. During this time, wrestlers had 873,479 athlete-exposures. The definition of athlete-exposure is one athlete participating in one team organized practice or competition. This definition can sometimes be problematic in wrestling or other individual sports, since it is common for wrestlers to work out on their own or with one other wrestler. These exposures are likely not accounted for. Admittedly, it would be extremely difficult to track those types of workouts. The rate of injury for wrestlers was 9.6 injuries per 1000 athlete-exposures. Only 37.6% missed more than a week of time due to injury, and there was only one catastrophic injury, which was nonfatal. Similar to the Yard et al. study [13], the knee and shoulder were the most common locations for injuries, and sprains and strains made up the highest types of injuries. For knee injuries, one of the collateral ligaments was involved 30% of the time and meniscal tears accounted for 15% of the knee injuries, with 6% involving the patellar and/or patellar tendon, and 5% involving the anterior cruciate ligament (ACL). Competition injuries were more common than practice injuries at 30.7 and 7.2 per 1000 athlete-exposures, respectively. These rates were fairly stable throughout each year of the study. Injuries that resulted in more than 1 week of missed time included the knee at 30%, the shoulder at 15%, and the ankle at 8%. When surgery was performed, it was for the knee in 65% of the cases. Only 6.3% of injuries required surgical intervention. Fifty percent of injuries occurred while in the standing positions or during takedowns, which is roughly similar to the Yard et al. study [13]. Injury patterns did not differ between practice and competition or between weight classes. Skin infections accounted for 17.4% of incidences in this study.

Otero's group [10] retrospectively evaluated injuries in 125 NCAA Division I wrestlers from a single institution over 10 years. The combined practice and competition injury rate was 19.6 per 1000 exposures, with 96% of the athletes sustaining an injury. The rate of injuries requiring surgery was 1.4 per 1000 exposures. It should be noted that the authors considered skin infections as injuries, and when this was combined with lacerations, skin injury became the most common site of injury (17.5%) followed by the knee (17.1%). There were no differences in injury rates between weight classes.

Pasque and Hewett's [11] study of injury patterns in high school Folkstyle wrestling prospectively examined 458 athletes over a single season. The cohort included both varsity and junior varsity level athletes. The injury rate was 52 per 100 wrestlers and 6.0 injuries per 1000 exposures. Practice caused 63% of injuries with an injury rate of 5 per 1000 practice-exposures; however, the injury rate was higher during competition with a reported rate of 9 per 1000 match-exposures. The most common locations for injuries were the shoulder (24%) and knee (17%). Most injuries were minor with an average time missed from sport of 5 days. However, 5% of athletes suffered season-ending injuries, with the majority of these due to knee trauma. The authors also reported a skin infection rate of 5%, with impetigo as the most common diagnosis. However, skin infections were not considered injuries in the study. In this cohort, older and more experienced wrestlers were more likely to be injured.

49.4.3 Miscellaneous Issues Specific to Wrestling

Three issues are relatively unique to wrestling and other sports that have either weight categories or close one-on-one infighting, such as mixed martial arts. These include weight management and sometimes severe and rapid weight loss and dehydration, skin infections, and auricular hematoma.

Weight loss and dehydration is common in wrestling. Kraemer et al. [17] looked at the physiologic effects of a simulated Freestyle wrestling tournament. The week prior to the tournament, the wrestlers lost 6% of their body weight. They then wrestled five matches over a 2-day period. The authors found that lower body power and strength decreased significantly as the tournament progressed. After each match, testosterone, lactate levels, cortisol, norepinephrine, and plasma osmolarity significantly increased as compared to pre-match levels. Pre-match concentrations, however, serially lowered throughout the tournament, so that by the end of the tournament, levels were far below age-matched controls and were in the range of prepubescent boys. With such low levels, there may be compromise of testosterone's anabolic properties. Whether weight loss associated with wrestling is a cause of stunted growth has been long debated, but this study might suggest that it is certainly a possibility.

The skin-to-skin contact between wrestlers increases the risk of transmitting skin infections as shown in some of the studies cited previously in this chapter [7, 10, 11, 13], particularly impetigo, herpes simplex, and ringworm. Imai et al. [18] showed that T-cell response to anti-CD3 antibody was comprised, and interferon-gamma production was reduced during rapid weight loss when comparing wrestlers that underwent rapid weight loss as compared to those that didn't. This may be a contributing factor in the high rates of herpes viral infections and outbreaks in wrestlers.

Auricular hematomas, which can cause ear deformity, often called cauliflower ear in layman's terms, is common in wrestlers. In wrestling circles, it is often viewed as a badge of courage and sign of brotherhood. This is a silly concept since the ear deformity can be associated with hearing loss or increased risk of infection due to obstruction of the ear canal. After blunt trauma, blood can form in the subperichondrial space. This leads to formation of abnormal cartilage with fibrosis resulting in a hard and stiff deformed cartilage layer that permanently deforms the ear [19]. Treatments are designed to try to maintain the ear's normal shape, but these are often unsuccessful.

49.4.3.1 Summary Points

There are three styles of wrestling: Greco-Roman, Freestyle, and Folkstyle. The first two are international forms included in the Olympic Games, while the third is most common in the USA. Each style has different rules and, theoretically, injury patterns. In studies comparing Freestyle to Greco-Roman wrestling, Freestyle had higher injury rates with a higher percentage of knee injuries [14, 15]. In the only study to include women's Freestyle wrestling, women had the lowest injury rate [15]. In youth Freestyle and Greco-Roman tournaments, there was a 12.7% injury incidence during two tournaments, though this study did not break out the two different disciplines [9].

The most common injuries reported in the literature on international forms vary among authors, making it difficult to form a consensus. The upper extremity, knee, and skin have been listed as the most commonly injured body parts in different studies [9, 14, 15]. But it seems that lacerations, knee, and shoulder injuries make up the bulk of the injuries, with knee injuries being more common in Freestyle than Greco-Roman wrestling. This is to be expected since in Greco-Roman wrestling, participants are not permitted to grab the opponents' legs or use their legs to trip opponents. Catastrophic injuries are reported by many investigators to be rare [9, 15], although in Iran, the catastrophic injury rate was discovered to be 1.99 per 100,000 wrestlers [16]. Most injuries occur when in the standing position or when executing a takedown [9, 14, 15, 16]. Again, this is to be expected since the majority of the match is spent with both wrestlers in the standing position.

The reported injury rates in Folkstyle are 2.33–6.0 injuries per 1000 exposures [11, 13] for high school and 9.6–19.6 for college [7, 10, 13]. Competition rates are higher than that of practice in all styles and age groups [7, 10, 11, 13]. The most common mechanism of injury for all forms of wrestling is the takedown, but Folkstyle injuries had a higher percentage of knee injuries and more injuries from when the wrestlers were not in the standing position than the international styles [6–15]. Again, this is to be expected since Folkstyle rules create much more time for the wrestlers to be in non-standing positions.

Skin infections are also common in wrestling with an estimated incidence of 5–17.5% and a skin infection rate of 0.22 and 1.91 per 1000 athlete-exposures for high school and collegiate wrestlers [10, 11, 13]. The most common of these are impetigo, herpes gladiatorum, and ringworm. We have not seen rates of auricular hematoma and cauliflower ear reported in the literature, but these appear to be quite high based on anecdotal observations [6, 8, 19].

49.5 Mixed Martial Arts

Mixed martial arts (MMA) is a combination of fighting arts including wrestling, boxing, and jiu-jitsu and **is arguably the world's most rapidly**

growing sport. Although the sport may seem foreign to some doctors and elicit an unsubstantiated negative response, today's MMA competitor is a well-rounded, multidimensional athlete who may need orthopedic care.

49.5.1 Background and Evolution

Although evidence of similar forms of unarmed combat contests can be traced back to the original Olympics, today's **MMA largely evolved from the Brazilian tradition of Vale Tudo** (or "anything goes") **in the early 1900s**. The Japanese fighting form jiu-jitsu was adapted by the Gracie family into a Brazilian form that stressed technique over strength. These ground techniques rely on joint locks and choke holds to make an opponent submit through a verbal or physical "tapout" [20].

The original "Ultimate Fighting Championship" (UFC) was partly an effort to market Gracie jiu-jitsu to North American audiences. In this multifight, single-night tournament, practitioners of different martial arts would face off to prove the superiority of their fighting form. With few rules and no time limits, rounds, or weight classes, the UFC incited a wave of criticism. Detractors called the sport barbaric, comparing it to a human version of cockfighting.

In response, the UFC—along with knowledgeable ringside physicians and referees—began to establish weight classes, rounds, and a point-based judging system. These changes enhanced fighter safety, and states began to regulate the sport. Soon the disciplines of the fighters began to evolve as well. Instead of training in only one discipline, athletes began to train in multiple fighting forms, leading to the term "mixed martial arts" [20].

MMA involves both stand-up and ground work. Stand-up fighting entails punches, kicks, knees, and elbows. (Elbows to the back of the head and kicking/kneeing a downed opponent in the head are illegal.) Ground work is often a combination of wrestling and jiu-jitsu or another submission-based martial art. While on the ground, fighters will attempt to lure their opponents into positions that will allow them to apply a joint lock or choke hold.

An example of ground work during an MMA bout; hyperextension injuries to elbows and knees, shoulder dislocations, and labral tears are commonly sustained.

Today's MMA athlete focuses on a wide variety of martial arts disciplines as well as strength and conditioning. Due to the individual nature of the sport, athletes may not have athletic trainers, physical therapists, or team physicians, although some employ a nutritionist. As a result, MMA athletes may seek advice from fellow fighters, boxing or jiu-jitsu coaches, or health professionals who train at the same gym.

Many MMA athletes have wrestling or other backgrounds that rely on more "holistic" approaches to limit interventions by doctors and avoid surgery. As a result, many of these athletes shun traditional medicine in favor of Eastern medical practitioners. Although alternative treatments may have a role, team physicians need to educate MMA athletes on the value of classic sports medicine.

49.5.2 Common Orthopedic Injuries

MMA athletes are at risk for a wide variety of musculoskeletal injuries. During a fight, an MMA athlete may experience lacerations, orbital fractures, metacarpal fractures, or other striking-related injuries. Because the lightweight gloves are also fingerless, inadvertent eye-pokes may occur. Athletes have also sustained shoulder dislocations and tibial fractures [20].

Many joint locks require hyperextension of the affected joint. Such hyperextension can lead to injury during training or before a referee can stop a fight. Elbows and knees are most at risk for hyperextension injuries although shoulder dislocation or labral tears from cranking the shoulder in an awkward position are also common. In addition, MMA athletes often sustain injuries to the anterior cruciate ligament (ACL) or meniscus.

Knee and shoulder injuries commonly occur during training camp or practice, because the athletes are using grappling and takedown techniques rather than sparring or stand-up striking. These often include meniscal or ligament injuries in the knee and labral, rotator cuff, or acromioclavicular joint injuries in the shoulder. Because many MMA athletes also lift weights for strength and conditioning, overuse injuries may occur [20].

Other injuries include hyperextension injuries of the elbow capsule and ligaments or foot sprains from getting caught on the mat or during a scramble. During competition or in the training camp leading up to the fight, striking becomes a more regular training routine, and metacarpal fractures and finger dislocations tend to occur.

The athlete's needs and the pressures of the sport must be considered when recommending treatment. For example, an ACL allograft may allow a quicker rehabilitation (which the MMA athlete will seek) but increase the risk of re-rupture (given the intense nature of the sport and its training). Similarly, a metacarpal fracture may be immobilized, but the pressure to continue to train may limit the athlete's compliance. Frank discussions about treatments and options to work around the injury are necessary.

Treating physicians must also consider the athlete's schedule. An athlete who misses a scheduled fight will not get paid and may lose the weeks of training he has invested to that point. After the fight, the athlete will have more time for possible surgery and recovery.

Although MMA gloves are lighter, and the fights are shorter than in boxing, MMA fighters are still at significant risk for concussion and long-term mild traumatic brain injury. In fact, most of the accumulated brain injury may occur during training for a fight. Many athletes may not even know that a knockout involves a concussion [20].

Education on the long-term risk of hard sparring as well as on the impact of multiple subconcussive episodes is important, especially for young athletes entering the sport. More research is required to understand the effects of long-term exposure in earlier generations of MMA fighters.

As MMA becomes more popular, we as sports physicians and surgeons will see more of its athletes in our practices. By understanding the athlete's needs and the sport's culture, we can build a bridge between sports medicine and MMA while educating and providing better care for these athletes.

49.6 Responsibility of the Sports Physician Unique to Combat Sports

To adequately treat these athletes, the sports physician must understand the culture of the sport as well as the unique medical issues. These athletes are not part of a team, they participate as individuals. Most do not have medical insurance, and there is no off-season. The governing bodies are often weak and in the USA, each state has different rules of competition. An athlete may suffer a concussion and be prohibited from competition for 3 months in one state yet fight a week later in another state [21].

These athletes often have weight restrictions, and the most weigh-ins occur the day before the competition or often the day of competition. These athletes may also use rapid, unsafe weight controlling techniques resulting in significant kidney dysfunction, cardiovascular strain, and neurocognitive dysfunction. In the USA, the NCAA wrestling federation recognized these issues and has strict rules concerning the athlete's weight competition.

Performance-enhancing drugs are often abused as regulation of their use is often vague in different countries and in the USA by state. Anabolic steroids, human growth hormones, and abuse of the testosterone replacement therapy are significant and are a poorly controlled issue.

Concussion is a significant problem in combat sports. A knockout or a technical knockout is the often the determining factor in winning a bout.

The MMA gloves are significantly light than the classic boxing gloves, therefore able to deliver a significant concussive blow to the head. Many mild concussions may occur while training for a bout where there may be unrecognized significant cumulative mild traumatic brain injury.

Being physicians to these combat athletes is rewarding as there is no sport that needs well-trained culturally savvy physicians to protect the athletes from significant harm yet letting them compete.

In the USA, the Association of Ringside Physicians conducts an annual seminar addressing the problems, issues, and concerns of combat sports, designed for physicians, physicians in training, mid-level practitioners, nurses, physical therapists, and athletic trainers [21].

In association with the American College of Sports Medicine, the Association sponsors a certification examination. More information may be obtained from the Association's website—www.ringsideARP.org.

It is our job not to prevent competition but to do all we can to allow these athletes fulfill their dreams to compete safely.

Take-Home Message

- The dynamics of judo involves throwing techniques (*Nage-waza*) that are performed standing and control techniques mainly done on the ground (*Katame-waza*).
- Jiu-jitsu emphasizes techniques developed on the ground, such as immobilization, strangling, and attacks on the joints, which are performed by body leverage and overtaking.
- Wrestling has a close relationship with weight management and sometimes severe and rapid weight loss and dehydration, skin infections, and auricular hematoma.
- Today, an MMA athlete should have broad knowledge on variety of martial arts disciplines as well as to be strong and conditioned.
- The knowledge of sports dynamics helps the sports physician to approach the injury more adequately and also preserve the athlete's health in the field.

References

1. Akoto R, Lambert C, Balke M, Bouillon B, Frosch KH, Höher J. Epidemiology of injuries in judo: a cross-sectional survey of severe injuries based on time loss and reduction in sporting level. Br J Sports Med. 2018;52(17):1109–15. https://doi.org/10.1136/bjsports-2016-096849. Epub 2017 Apr 26.
2. Pocecco E, Ruedl G, Stankovic N, Sterkowicz S, Del Vecchio FB, Gutiérrez-García C, et al. Injures in judo: a systematic literature review including suggestions for prevention. Br J Sports Med. 2013;47(18):1139–43.
3. Čierna D, Štefanovský M, Matejová L, Lystad RP. Epidemiology of competition injuries in elite European judo athletes: a prospective cohort study. Clin J Sport Med. 2017. https://doi.org/10.1097/JSM.0000000000000526. Epub ahead of print.
4. Scoggin JF III, Brusovanik G, Izuka BH, Zandee van Rilland E, Geling O, Tokumura S. Assessment of injuries during Brazilian jiu-jitsu competition. Orthop J Sports Med. 2014;2(2):2325967114522184. https://doi.org/10.1177/2325967114522184. eCollection 2014 Feb.
5. Ingvaldsen CA, Tønseth KA. Auricular haematoma. Tidsskr Nor Laegeforen. 2017;137(2):105–7. https://doi.org/10.4045/tidsskr.15.1279.
6. Halloran L. Wrestling injuries. Orthop Nurs. 2008;27(3):189–92; quiz 193–4. https://doi.org/10.1097/01.NOR.0000320548.20611.16.
7. Jarrett GJ, Orwin JF, Dick RW. Injuries in collegiate wrestling. Am J Sports Med. 1998;26(5):674–80.
8. Kiningham R, Monseau A. Caring for wrestlers. Curr Sports Med Rep. 2015;14(5):404–12. https://doi.org/10.1249/JSR.0000000000000193.
9. Lorish TR, Rizzo TD Jr, Ilstrup DM, Scott SG. Injuries in adolescent and preadolescent boys at two large wrestling tournaments. Am J Sports Med. 1992;20(2):199–202.
10. Otero JE, Graves CM, Bollier MJ. Injuries in collegiate wrestlers at an elite division I NCAA wrestling program: an epidemiological study. Iowa Orthop J. 2017;37:65–70.
11. Pasque CB, Hewett TE. A prospective study of high school wrestling injuries. Am J Sports Med. 2000;28(4):509–15.
12. Perri BR, Lynch SA. Common injuries in the skilled wrestler. Curr Opin Orthop. 2003;14(2):109–13.
13. Yard EE, Collins CL, Dick RW, Comstock RD. An epidemiologic comparison of high school and college wrestling injuries. Am J Sports Med. 2008;36(1):57–64. Epub 2007 Oct 11.
14. Yard EE, Comstock RD. A comparison of pediatric freestyle and Greco-Roman wrestling injuries sustained during a 2006 US national tournament. Scand J Med Sci Sports. 2008;18(4):491–7. Epub 2007 Dec 7.
15. Shadgan B, Feldma BJ, Jabari S. Wrestling injuries during the 2008 Beijing Olympic. Am J Sports Med. 2010;38(9):1870–6. https://doi.org/10.1177/0363546510369291. Epub 2010 Jun 3.
16. Kordi R, Akbarnejad A, Wallace WA. Catastrophic injuries in the Olympic styles of wrestling in Iran. Br J Sports Med. 2010;44(3):168–74. https://doi.org/10.1136/bjsm.2008.046870. Epub 2008 Jul 4.

17. Kraemer WJ, Fry AC, Rubin MR, Triplett-McBride T, Gordon SE, Koziris LP, et al. Physiological and performance responses to tournament wrestling. Med Sci Sports Exerc. 2001;33(8):1367–78.
18. Imai T, Seki S, Dobashi H, Ohkawa T, Habu Y, Hiraide H. Effect of weight loss on T-cell receptor-mediated T-cell function in elite athletes. Med Sci Sports Exerc. 2002;34(2):245–50.
19. Grewoode JD, Pribitkin DA, Klein H. Management of auricular hematoma and the cauliflower ear. Facial Plast Surg. 2010;26(6):451–5. https://doi.org/10.1055/s-0030-1267719. Epub 2010 Nov 17.
20. Gelber J. The ultimate guide to preventing and treating MMA injuries. Toronto: ECW Press; 2016.
21. Estwanik JJ. Sports medicine for the combat arts. Charlotte: Boxergenics Press; 1996.

Part X

PROMs

50 PROMs in Sports Medicine

Sérgio Rocha Piedade, Mario Ferreti Filho, Daniel Miranda Ferreira, Daniel A. Slullitel, Sarthak Patnaik, Gonzalo Samitier, and Nicola Maffulli

50.1 Background

The interest in performing regular sports activity has been *increasing* every year, and, consequently, the number of people adopting physical activity as a concept of healthy life or even as "a kind of religion" has risen. Moreover, it is not just a lifestyle for recreational athletes or professional athletes but an activity involving happiness, fitness, and economic purposes and, therefore, reflecting physically and psychologically on their daily living and their quality of life.

Compared to the general population, athletes have different expectations and goals that make their lifestyle singular. Sports are not free from injuries, and consequently their practice exposes the muscle, tendon, ligament, bone, and joint to overload, tensile stress, and direct and indirect trauma of high and low energy that could cause tissue damage of different patterns.

While huge progress has come to the sports medicine area, regarding safety measures for sports practice, protective sports equipment, routine, and periodic pre-participation evaluation before permitting the athlete to start sports or return to sports practice, musculoskeletal injuries remain as "part of the game."

Without doubt, these injuries present a common clinical problem that affects the general population but has a noticeable incidence in sports practitioners, recreational or professional ones. Moreover, according to the modality of sports, some anatomical sites and musculoskeletal structures are more exposed to injury than others, for example, the shoulder in judo, the spine and head in football, the ankle and knee in soccer, and the face, hand, and elbow in martial arts.

For many years, the analysis of outcomes focused on different aspects of knowledge regarding sports injuries, biomechanics, biological behavior of living tissues, extension of tissue

S. R. Piedade (✉)
Department of Orthopedics and Traumatology, State University of Campinas—UNICAMP, Exercise and Sports Medicine, Campinas, Sao Paulo, Brazil
e-mail: piedade@fcm.unicamp.br

M. F. Filho
Department of Orthopedics and Traumatology, UNIFESP, Sao Paulo, Brazil

D. M. Ferreira
Department of Radiology, State University of Campinas—UNICAMP, Exercise and Sports Medicine, Campinas, Sao Paulo, Brazil

D. A. Slullitel
Instituto Jaime Sulllitel, Rosário, Argentina

S. Patnaik
Department of Arthroscopy and Sports Surgeon, Sunshine Hospitals, Bhubaneswar, Odisha, India

G. Samitier
Hospital General de Villalba, Madrid, Spain

N. Maffulli
Department of Musculoskeletal Disorders, Faculty of Medicine and Surgery, University of Salerno Baronissi, Salerno, Italy
e-mail: n.maffulli@qmul.ac.uk

S. Rocha Piedade et al. (eds.), *The Sports Medicine Physician*,
https://doi.org/10.1007/978-3-030-10433-7_50

damage, and also in the sports physician and orthopedic surgeon's experience. However, in the last two decades, the analysis of outcomes has paid more attention to patients' perception on the whole process of treatment, medical care, time of recovery, and expectation to return to prior level of physical activity as well as their understanding of the level of injury. In other words, outcome tools have started considering the client's point of view.

50.2 Patient-Reported Outcome Measures

Patient-reported outcome measures (PROMs) are self-completed questionnaires that can measure a variety of global, disease-specific, and joint-specific outcomes and have become the gold standard when quantifying a patient's posttreatment experience. In the era of patient-centered care, there has been a dramatic increase in the number of PROMs within medicine and orthopedics, specifically. However, we have different types of reports focused on each of the joints, such as the shoulder, elbow, knee, and hip but without taking into account the difference in the evaluation of the overall result of the sports' practice and not just of a joint [1]. Regarding the proposed treatments, there are different psychological and physical outcome expectations for high-performing athletes and recreational athletes.

Outcome measures reported by patients (PROMs) are used to assess satisfaction after surgical or clinical treatment and reflect the patient's perspective on their health status. The use of PROMs in clinical practice helps to ensure that the patient's "voice" is present in all aspects of the care, which is essential to guarantee that the therapeutic management remains patient-centered. PROMs capture the patient's own opinions on the impact of their condition, treatment, and life.

Every physical activity itself is a stressful physical or psychological condition since it is more dependent on the psychological condition of how each athlete faces adverse conditions than the level of competition. Many factors that characterize an athletes' health status cannot be observed, measured with a device, or analyzed even by the most sophisticated imaging methods. With the use of PROMs, we can capture the patient's experience. It may provide a measurement of the outcome of an operation or provide clinical treatment, based on the patient's view.

Professional athletes have different physical and psychological overload from the general population. Not only is the athlete's functional recovery often important but also economic and financial aspects are involved. Although PROMs are considered the gold standard when evaluating outcomes in clinical or surgical treatment, in the case of high-performance athletes, they need to evaluate each individual in a global way, taking into consideration all aspects that may change their physical and psychological expectation. PROMs have been increasingly used by clinicians to guide and audit routine care and are already firmly embedded in clinical research. In addition, the routine clinical use of PROMs may allow to track treatment impact more effectively, and, therefore, help the development of optimal management strategies.

The use of PROMs to measure health status in routine practice has some distinct advantages over traditional research-based outcome measures.

The Activities Scale for Kids (ASK) is a self-report measure of childhood physical disability that has excellent reliability. The ASK is a valid and responsive outcome measure designed for children 5–15 years of age who are experiencing limitations in physical activity due to musculoskeletal disorders. The quality of this measure enables clinicians and researchers to measure outcomes in a way that is relevant to patients and also in a way that is sensitive to small amounts of change [2].

When searching for appropriate PROMs, it is important to ask, "what do I want to measure? What is the reason for the assessment? At which level will the measurement take place (group or individual)?" When aiming to benchmark the service performance, it is also important to ask which PROMs are recommended and being used by others [3].

PROMs can assist in the clinical process for diagnosis and treatment, with specific focus on the patient's perspective, identifying problems related to functioning and activities in daily living. Thus, PROMs can assist establishing treatment objectives and monitoring treatment results. Despite the complexity of health measurements, clinicians recognize that the importance of using PROMs to improve the care process by enhancing communication, improving patient's education, allowing shared decision-making, and monitoring treatment response. However, several barriers have been identified in using PROMs, and these could lessen their usefulness in informing important healthcare decisions: (a) the absence of a PROM collection infrastructure and (b) a lack of knowledge and confidence in using outcome measures [3].

50.3 Instruments of Outcome Measures

In the literature, several outcome measure instruments have been developed in order to evaluate different musculoskeletal disorders and surgical treatments. Many of these are clinician-related outcome measures that evaluate from the clinician's perspective, through a physical exam, for instance. However, the patient's perception in judging the treatment efficacy has become increasingly more important in the orthopedic setting.

In recent years, subjective questionnaires have been created with this objective as well as to evaluate the patient's satisfaction. Such instruments have important advantages over traditional clinician-based outcome measures. Its utilization stimulates better communication between physician and patient, besides helping patients' education regarding their health condition. The patients' active participation when filling out the questionnaire helps them better understands the impact of the injury on their life and to be aware of their physical limitations. In order to provide better value in healthcare, it is mandatory to define what constitutes a good outcome.

PROMs are tools in the form of questionnaires that evaluate results subjectively following musculoskeletal injury or surgical intervention. The questionnaires can be used to compare pre- and postoperative periods and monitor changes in function status over the time.

Due to the ease of collecting information, they are used in both research and clinical practice. They can be general health measures, joint-specific measures, or even disease-specific measures. Generally, they are divided into different domains, such as pain, function, and satisfaction. Each domain consists of questions which should be responded by the patient. These questions should be able to capture the patient's actual health condition.

Ideally, a PROM has to be easily understood and answered by a patient as well as easily interpreted and scored by a clinician or researcher. These characteristics are considered important, since they help to reduce the amount of missing data. The choice of the PROM should also be based on its measurement properties and target patient (e.g., age, gender, disease).

A high-quality measure instrument should be reliable, valid, and responsive for the patient of interest. Reliability refers to the precision of an outcome measure to assess and avoid measurement error. Validity is the ability to correctly measure what the instrument intended to. Finally, responsiveness is a measurement property of the instrument that refers to the ability to detect changes over time.

Many of the measure instruments are only validated for specific conditions, and their quality varies considerably. It is also important to know the Minimally Important Change (MIC) of the PROM to be used. MIC value reflects to the smallest measured change score perceived by the patient as clinically important. Therefore, knowing this value helps to decide whether the patient has benefited or not from a treatment. Unfortunately, the MIC value depends on several factors, and, therefore, they are not always reported.

Even though many PROMs commonly contain questions related to the impact of the injury on sport practiced by the patient, *they are generally developed for the general population.* There is no well-established questionnaire to evaluate athletes specifically. One of the main problems with PROMs used in sport-specific population is that even if the patient reaches the roof of the functional domain in the test, it does not mean that the athlete is ready to return to sport. Therefore, other instruments such as physical exam, muscle reaction time, and muscle strength should be used to decide return to sport.

Anyway, PROMs is a valuable tool to access musculoskeletal injuries and disorders approached surgically or conservatively, and the more frequently used ones in each area are listed and discussed below.

50.4 International Knee Documentation Committee (IKDC) Subjective Knee Evaluation Form

The original IKDC form was published for the first time in 1993 with the purpose to be a standard documentation system for knee ligament injuries. It is a one-page form that includes a documentation section, qualification section, and evaluation section. The form can be used not only in pre- and post-operation but also in patient's follow-ups [4]. In 2000, a new IKDC form (IKDC subject knee evaluation form) was published as a revision of the original IKDC. The IKDC subjective knee evaluation form has been shown to be a reliable and valid tool for measurement of subjective outcomes in several knee disorders, including ligament and meniscal injuries, cartilage lesions, and patellofemoral conditions [5].

The IKDC subject knee form contains 18 questions: 7 questions related to symptoms, 2 questions related to general function (1 item for sports activity and 1 item for current knee function), and 9 questions related to daily activities. The score can be calculated if there are responses for at least 16 questions in the form. Following completion of the form, the scores are then transformed to values in a scale that ranges from 0 to 100 [5]. A score of 100 is interpreted to mean no physical limitations and symptoms. A score of 11.5 and 20.5 points in IKDC is a more sensitive and specific minimum value, respectively, to detect a clinically relevant difference in a patient's status. Normative data from male and female patients of different ages are available [6]. Such values help researchers to interpret results and compare different populations [7, 8].

50.5 Disabilities of the Arm, Shoulder, and Hand (DASH) and QuickDASH Outcome Measure

The DASH outcome measure is a self-report, 30-item questionnaire developed, and published by the Upper Extremity Collaborative Group in 1996 [9]. The questionnaire was designed to evaluate symptoms and physical function in patients with any musculoskeletal disorder in the upper extremity. In addition, it serves to capture restrictions for both work and physical activities as well as monitoring changes in functional status over time perceived by the patient [10]. A new DASH questionnaire with only 11 items to respond to (QuickDASH) was published in 2005. The reliability, validity, and responsiveness of the QuickDash have been shown to be comparable to the DASH [11].

The DASH questionnaire contains 30 items, and its response options range from 1 to 5 (1, no difficulty; 2, mild difficulty; 3, moderate difficulty; 4, severe difficulty; 5, unable). The DASH provides a final score ranging from 0 to 100, where 0 indicates no disability and 100 indicates severe disability. Ideally, all questions should be responded, and the DASH score may not be calculated if more than three items are missing (QuickDASH tolerates only one missing item out of 11 to be answered). An exact score in one scale does not correspond to the same score in another scale. However, they are probably close. The questions are about symptoms and abilities to perform daily activities with the upper extremity, and they should be responded based on the patient's condition in the previous week to the responses. There are still two optional four-item modules (Work Module and Sports/Performing Arts Module) in both questionnaires that are calculated separately. The Work Module measures the ability to work, and the Sports/Performing Arts Module measures the impact of the upper limb disorder on playing musical instrument or sport [9–11].

50.6 The Foot and Ankle Outcome Score (FAOS)

The FAOS was developed to evaluate the opinion of patients about symptoms and physical limitations related to foot and ankle disorders, like lateral ankle instability, Achilles tendinosis, hallux valgus, and hallux rigidus [12–15]. It is one of the most commonly used foot- and ankle-specific PROMs; however, there is still limited evidence evaluating its measurement properties [16, 17]. Content validity and reliability of the FAOS was initially confirmed in patients with lateral instability of the ankle, and it has been shown to be highly reproducible both inter and intra-investigator [12, 18].

FAOS is a 42-item questionnaire separated in five subscales: pain (9 items), other symptoms (7 items), activities of daily life (17 items), functional sports and recreational activities (5 items), and foot- and ankle-related quality of life (4 items). Patients should take into account the last week before answering the questionnaire. The score ranges from 0 to 4 for each question, where 0 indicates extreme symptoms or disability and 4 indicates the absence of symptoms or no disability, depending on the question. Regarding missing data, when up to two values are omitted, they are substituted with the average value for that subscale. If more than two items are omitted, the subscale is considered invalid. Each subscale is graded separately on a scale ranging from 0 to 100, where lower scores indicate more severe symptoms. In the end, the subscores can be presented graphically as an FAOS profile. It takes 7–10 min to fill the questionnaire out and can be downloaded online [12, 13].

50.7 Oswestry Disability Index (ODI)

The Oswestry Disability Index (ODI) is a questionnaire which gives a subjective percentage score of the level of function in daily life activities for those rehabilitating from acute or chronic episodes of low back pain. The ODI is a valid, reliable, and responsive condition-specific assessment tool that is suited for use in clinical practice. The minimum clinically important difference (MCID) has been calculated for ODI for LBP patients, ranging from 7 to 15 [19, 20] and can be used as a threshold change to compare the effectiveness of different surgical and nonsurgical procedures for a variety of conditions affecting the spine [21].

The ODI consists of 10 sections, with 6 statements in each one, scoring from 0 to 5. When answering the questionnaire, patients should take into account the present moment. The items are related to the intensity of pain, personal care (washing, dressing, etc.), lifting objects, walking, sitting, standing, sleeping, sexual life, social life, and locomotion. Scores are obtained by the sum of the 10 questions multiplied by 2 which results in a percentage ranging from 0 to 20%, minimal disability; 21–40%, moderate disability; 41–60%, severe disability; 61–80%, crippled; and 81–100%, bed-bound [22].

50.8 *EQ-5D* EUROQOL Health Status Questionnaire

The EuroQol Health Status Questionnaire (EQ-5D) is a measure of health-related quality of life that can be used in a wide range of health conditions and treatments. It generates a representative index of the health status of an individual based on a classification system that uses five dimensions to describe the health state: mobility, self-care, usual activities, pain/discomfort, and anxiety/depression. Each of these dimensions presents three alternatives with associated severity levels, corresponding to "no problems" (level 1), "some problems" (level 2), and "extreme problems" (level 3) experienced or felt by the individual. The scores on these five dimensions can be presented as a health profile or can be converted into a single summary index number (utility) in order to establish comparisons between other health profiles and allow the description of a total of 243 different health states in evaluated individuals [23, 24].

50.9 *SF-12* Short-Form-12 Quality of Life Questionnaire

The SF-12 is one of the most widely used instruments for assessing self-reported health-related quality of life. Originally developed from the 36-item Short-Form Health Survey SF-36, the SF-12 covers the same eight health domains as the SF-36 (General Health, Physical Functioning, Physical, and Body Pain, Vitality, Social Functioning, Emotional, and Mental Health) with substantially fewer questions, making it a more practical research tool [25].

Twelve questions measure eight health domains to assess physical and mental health, and this instrument has been validated across a number of chronic diseases and conditions [26–28]. Physical and mental health scores are computed using the scores of 12 questions and range from 0 to 100, where a 0 score indicates the lowest level of health measured by the scales and 100 indicates the highest level of health.

50.10 *UCLA* University of California Los Angeles Activity Score

The UCLA activity score is a simple patient-reported scale ranging from 1 to 10. The patient indicates their most appropriate activity level, with 1 defined as "no physical activity, dependent on others" and 10 defined as "regular participation in impact sports." The UCLA activity score represents a reliable tool for assessing the level of physical activity and the return to sport with high functional demand after total joint arthroplasty [27, 28].

50.11 Lower Extremity Functional Scale (LEFS)

Created in 1999, Lower Extremity Functional Scale (LEFS) was developed as a self-report condition-specific measure that would validate measurements and is used as clinical and research tool. Compared at first with SF-36, LEFS proved to be more sensitive to change, as indicated by higher correlations with an external prognostic rating of change. The LEFS is used for measuring lower-extremity function in a wide variety of disorders and treatments [29, 30].

The final version of the LEFS consists of 20 items, each with a maximum score of 4. The total possible score of 80 indicates a high functional level. The introductory statement of the questionnaire states: "Today, do you or would you have any difficulty at all with:" followed by a listing of functional items. Items are rated on a 5-point scale, from 0 (extreme difficulty/unable to perform activity) to 4 (no difficulty) [31]. Questions about activities vary from walking between rooms to running on uneven ground.

The scale is one page, can be filled out by most patients in less than 2 min, and is scored by tallying the responses for all of the items. The LEFS is easy to administer, score, and apply to a wide range of disability levels and conditions and all lower-extremity sites. A recent systematic review showed that LEFS scores demonstrated excellent test-retest reliability and had expected relationships with measures assessing similar constructs [32]. The LEFS can be used by clinicians as a measure of a patient's initial function and outcome as well as to set functional goals [33].

50.12 Hip Sports Activity Scale (HSAS)

This scale was developed in 2013 in German and English for patients with femoroacetabular impingement (FAI). The HSAS consisted of nine different sports activity levels ranging from 0 to 8 [34]. Differences in popular sports in Europe and the USA, as well as league specifics (e.g., collegiate leagues), were taken into account. This scale does not substitute traditional self-reported outcome measures, but the HSAS should be considered as an additional instrument. It can be considered a very useful tool for clinicians and researchers to evaluate sports-active FAI patients and to better compare different treatments. HSAS has been applied to cartilage injuries [34, 35]. In a recent systematic review, there was insufficient evidence to recommend HSAS compared to other hip scores [36].

50.13 Hip Outcome Score (HOS)

Created in 2006 for treatment intervention for individuals with acetabular tears who may be functioning throughout a wide range of ability Hip Outcome Score (HOS) consists of two scales. The activities of daily living (ADL), and sports subscales. The ADL subscale contained 19 items pertaining to basic daily activities, and the sports subscale contained 9 items pertaining to higher-level activities, such as those required in athletics. In addition to the five potential responses, ranging from "unable to do" to "no difficulty," a response of "non-applicable" is possible. This allows subjects to elect that something other than their hip problem limits their activity. HOS is a valid measure of self-reported physical function for individuals with acetabular labral tears who are undergoing either arthroscopic surgical treatment or nonsurgical treatment [37].

The HOS was found to have good psychometric properties, including a strong relationship with concurrent measures of physical function. It has high correlations with concurrent measures of physical function and relatively low correlations with concurrent measures of mental health [38]. Since HOS is a PROM, it may be used for follow-up assessment when objective information is not possible to differentiate individuals. Depending on their current activity level, surgical outcome, and age at a follow-up assessment more than 3 years after surgery on average [37]. In 2008, in the continuous improvement of the score, the same authors concluded that HOS could be used for describing outcomes of hip arthroscopy for labral pathology, femoroacetabular impingement, chondral lesions, or capsular laxity [39].

50.14 Knee Injury and Osteoarthritis Outcome Score (KOOS)

KOOS (Knee Injury and Osteoarthritis Outcome Score) is a functional score that evaluates the outcomes for Total Knee Replacement with regard to symptoms (7 items), pain (9 items), daily living activities (17 items), sports and recreation activities (5 items), and quality of life (4 items). It was developed for younger or more active patients with more demanding physical function as an extension of WOMAC. It has been shown as a valid, reliable, and responsive outcome score [40, 41].

The five dimensions are scored separately, and a Likert scale is used, and all items have five possible answer options scored from 0 (No Problems) to 4 (Extreme Problems), and each of the 5 scores is calculated as the sum of the items included. Scores are transformed to a 0–100 scale, with 100 representing no knee problems and 0 representing extreme problems [41, 42].

50.15 Lysholm

Lysholm score was developed in 1982 by Lysholm and Gillquist and modified in 1985 by Lysholm and Tegner and is used to evaluate patients with knee ligament injury [43, 44].

The score consists of the correlation of symptoms and functional criteria such as limping, instability, pain, and swelling, climbing steps, squatting, restraining, and support. For these eight questions are expressed in a final score ranging from 95 to 100 points regarded as "excellent"; 84 to 94 points, "good," 65 to 83 points, "fair," and "poor" when values were equal to or below 64 points.

The Lysholm questionnaire has been shown as a valid and reliable score since the questions are objective and easy to understand [41, 45]. Even though the Lysholm score was developed to assess patients with knee ligament injury, it has been used to assess other patients including TKA [46].

50.16 Kujala Scale

The Kujala scale (Scoring of Patellofemoral Disorders) was published in 1993, and it is used to evaluate subjective symptoms with a focus on anterior knee pain. It is a 13-item screening instrument containing important questions in scoring patellofemoral disorders. The questions are related to limping, support, walking, stairs, squatting, running, jumping, prolonged sitting with the knees flexed, pain, swelling, abnormal painful kneecap movements (patellar subluxations), and atrophy of thigh, and flexion deficiency. For each multiple-choice question, the patients should choose the answer that corresponds to their symptoms. It is recommended that the patient completes the questionnaire independently to exclude investigator bias. The total score is easily calculated and goes from 0 (extreme symptoms and worst function) to 100 (absence of symptoms) [47].

While the Kujala has been found to be effective and reliable in the adult population [48, 49], modifications may be useful to make it easier to understand in the pediatric population, ensuring a proper of functionality of the outcome measure in those patients [50, 51].

50.17 Considerations on PROMs in Sports Medicine

As observed above, all the PROMs focus on a non-specific population and were designed for the general population.

PROMs play a more important role in the clinical reasoning process for diagnosis and treatment, with a specific focus on the patient's perspective, mainly when designed for a specific population. Involving the patient in this way can also help stimulate self-management. PROMs can also be used with the patient to identify the main problems in functioning and activities in their daily life and, also, contribute to establish treatment objectives and monitor treatment results. Those PROMs that have been developed for use at group level in research settings (especially generic tools) may be less reliable at the individual patient level; therefore, PROM measurement should always be used as an adjunct to clinical judgment.

Clinicians widely recognize the potential use of PROMs for improving the process of care by enhancing communication, improving patient's education, shared decision-making, and monitoring response to treatment. However, several barriers to the use of PROMs have been identified, which could lessen their usefulness in informing important healthcare decisions: (a) the absence of a PROM collection infrastructure and (b) a lack of knowledge and confidence about using outcome measures.

50.18 Developing PROMs in Sport Medicine

The development of PROMs in sports medicine could be a practical tool to analyze the outcomes of different sports injuries in regular sports practitioners, regardless of the involved anatomical site (the shoulder, hip, knee, foot, and ankle). This questionnaire allows a more accurate registering of the patient's perception of their pre-injury status of physical demand in sports, their understanding of injury and expectations of treatment, and their evaluation of received postoperative care and treatment and the "outcomes."

As presented previously, these arguments and stated that PROMs is a valuable tool in clinical practice. Although many questionnaires approaching the knee, shoulder, hip, spine problems, and other anatomical sites have been proposed and validated globally, the focus remains on the general population.

Regarding this approach, the ISAKOS Sports Medicine Committee has developed a systematic review on PROMs in sports medicine that was carried out by Piedade et al. Although the data have not yet been published, this study has shown that there is not a clear approach regarding the subjective evaluation in sports medicine. Moreover, this systematic review has found out that the selected articles had no uniformity on the type of PROMs survey applied for the same joint or surgical procedure, corroborating that there is a void in sports medicine area, and it is our belief that this should be explored!

Other points to be analyzed in this process regarding this particular population are the level of physical demand (athlete's position in the field of play) as well as the stress involved in sports practice according to competition level. Consequently, these points strengthen the need to consider that these individuals have singular expectations and objectives, differing from the general and sedentary population.

In addition, the athlete's psychological status is one of the keys to success in sports competition, mainly in high-level sports, as it affects the athlete's performance directly. It also helps the athlete to face the full process of training and competition better as well as the process of recovery after a sports injury, which reflects on their expectations regarding outcomes.

50.19 ISAKOS Sports Medicine Committee

Regarding this important issue for sports medicine area, the ISAKOS Sports Medicine Committee has been working on PROMs in sports medicine for clinical application. Considering all the main points discussed in the previous sections, the design of this PROMs defines four pillars.

Each one of them represents a specific clinical condition such as pre-injury, post-injury, patient's expectations to the treatment and finally their evaluations of post-operative care and end-results. Each pillar has two questions each, scored from zero to ten. A relevant point of this study is that its intrinsic concept is founded on the athletes' reported baseline of their own pre-injury status of physical and psychological demands and, therefore, allows the registration and comparison of different sports injuries regardless of their anatomical site.

Take-Home Messages

- Sports practitioners and athletes have singular expectations and objectives, differing from the general and sedentary population.
- PROMs in Sports Medicine could be a practical tool to analyze the outcomes of different sports injuries in regular sports practitioners, regardless of the involved anatomical site (shoulder, hip, knee, foot, and ankle).
- PROMs play a more important role in sports, mainly when designed for this specific population.
- The level of physical demand reported as well as the stress involved in sports practice due to competition level should be used as the patient's references.

References

1. Ruzbarsky JJ, Marom N, Marx RG. Measuring quality and outcomes in sports medicine. Clin Sports Med. 2018;37(3):463–82.
2. Young NL, Williams JI, Yoshida KK, Wright JG. Measurement properties of the activities scale for kids. J Clin Epidemiol. 2000;53(2):125–37.
3. Kyte DG, Calvert M, van der Wees PJ, ten Hove R, Tolan S, Hill JC. An introduction to patient-reported outcome measures (PROMs) in physiotherapy. Physiotherapy. 2015;101(2):119–25.
4. Hefti E, Müller W, Jakob RP, Stäubli H-U. Evaluation of knee ligament injuries with the IKDC form. Knee Surg Sports Traumatol Arthrosc. 1993;1:226–34.
5. Irrgang JJ, Anderson AF, Boland AL, Harner CD, Kurosaka M, Neyret P, et al. Development and validation of the International Knee Documentation Committee Subjective Knee Form. Am J Sports Med. 2001;29:600–13.
6. Anderson AF, Irrgang JJ, Kocher MS, Mann BJ, Harrast JJ. The International Knee Documentation Committee Subjective Knee Evaluation Form: normative data. Am J Sports Med. 2006;34:128–35.
7. Irrgang JJ, Anderson AF, Boland AL, Harner CD, Neyret P, Richmond JC, et al. Responsiveness of the International Knee Documentation Committee Subjective Knee Form. Am J Sports Med. 2006;34:1567–73.
8. Greco NJ, Anderson AF, Mann BJ, Cole BJ, Farr J, Nissen CW, et al. Responsiveness of the International Knee Documentation Committee Subjective Knee Form in comparison to the western Ontario and Mcmaster Universities Osteoarthritis Index, Modified Cincinnati Knee Rating System, and Short Form 36 in patients with focal art. Am J Sports Med. 2010;38:891–902.
9. Hudak P, Amadio PC, Bobardier C. UECG. Development of an upper extremity outcome measure: the DASH (disabilities of the arm, shoulder, and hand). Am J Ind Med. 1996;29:602–8.
10. Institute for Work and Health. About the DASH [Internet]. 2006. http://www.dash.iwh.on.ca/about-dash.
11. Beaton DE, Wright JG, Katz JN, Amadio P, Bombardier C, Cole D, et al. Development of the QuickDASH: comparison of three item-reduction approaches. J Bone Joint Surg Am. 2005;87: 1038–46.
12. Roos EM, Brandsson S, Karlsson J. Validation of the foot and ankle outcome score for ankle ligament reconstruction. Foot Ankle Int. 2001;22:788–94.
13. A user's guide to: Foot and Ankle Outcome Score FAOS [Internet]. 2003. http://www.koos.nu.
14. Chen L, Lyman S, Do H. Validation of foot and ankle outcome score for hallux valgus. Foot Ankle Int. 2012;33:1145–55.
15. Hogan MV, Mani S, Chan J, Do H, Deland J, Ellis S. Validation of the foot and ankle outcome score for hallux rigidus. HSS J. 2016;12:44–50.

16. Sierevelt IN, Zwiers R, Schats W, Haverkamp D, Terwee CB, Nolte PA, et al. Measurement properties of the most commonly used foot- and ankle-specific questionnaires: the FFI, FAOS and FAAM. A systematic review. Knee Surg Sport Traumatol Arthrosc. 2018;26(7):2059–73.
17. Jia Y, Huang H, Gagnier JJ. A systematic review of measurement properties of patient-reported outcome measures for use in patients with foot or ankle diseases. Qual Life Res. 2017;26(8):1969–2010.
18. Imote AM, Peccin MS, Rodrigues R, Mizusaki JM. Translation, cultural adaptation and validation of Foot and Ankle Outcome Score (FAOS) questionnaire into Portuguese. Acta Ortop Bras. 2009;17: 232–5.
19. Copay AG, Glassman SD, Subach BR, Berven S, Schuler TC, Carreon L. The minimum clinically important difference in lumbar spine surgery patients. A choice of methods using the Oswestry Disability Index, MOS Short Form 36, and Pain Scales. Spine J. 2008;8(6):968–74.
20. Parker SL, Adogwa O, Paul AR, Anderson WN, Aaronson O, Cheng JS, et al. Utility of minimum clinically important difference in assessing pain, disability, and health state after transforaminal lumbar interbody fusion for degenerative lumbar spondylolisthesis. J Neurosurg Spine. 2011;14(5):598–604.
21. Copay AG, Cher DJ. Is the Oswestry Disability Index a valid measure of response to sacroiliac joint treatment? Qual Life Res. 2016;25:283–92.
22. Fairbank JC, Couper J, Davies JB, O'Brien JP. The Oswestry low back pain disability questionnaire. Physiotherapy. 1980;66(8):271–3.
23. EuroQol Group. EUROQOL—a new facility for the measurement of health-related quality of life. Health Policy. 1990;16(3):199–208.
24. Brooks R. EuroQol: the current state of play. Health Policy. 1996;37(1):53–72.
25. Huo T, Guo Y, Shenkman E, Muller K. Assessing the reliability of the Short Form 12 (SF-12) health survey in adults with mental health conditions: a report from the wellness incentive and navigation (WIN) study. Health Qual Life Outcomes. 2018;16:34.
26. Bohannon RW, Maljanian R, Landes M. Test-retest reliability of Short Form (SF)-12 component scores of patients with stroke. Int J Rehabil Res. 2004;27:149–50.
27. Cheak-Zamora NC, Wyrwich KW, McBride TD. Reliability and validity of the SF-12v2 in the medical expenditure panel survey. Qual Life Res. 2009;18:727–35.
28. Luo X, George ML, Kakouras I, Edwards CL, Pietrobon R, Richardson W, Hey L. Reliability, validity, and responsiveness of the Short Form 12-item Survey (SF-12) in patients with back pain. Spine (Phila Pa 1976). 2003;28(15):1739–45.
29. Mahler E, Cuperus N, Bijlsma J, et al. Responsiveness of four patient-reported outcome measures to assess physical function in patients with knee osteoarthritis. Scand J Rheumatol. 2016;45:518–27.
30. Dingemans SA, Kleipool SC, Mulders MAM, et al. Normative data for the lower extremity functional scale (LEFS). Acta Orthop. 2017;88:422–6.
31. Binkley JM, et al. The lower extremity functional scale (LEFS): scale development, measurement properties, and clinical application. Phys Ther. 1999;79:371–83.
32. Mehta SP, Fulton A, Quach C, et al. Measurement properties of the lower extremity functional scale: a systematic review. J Orthop Sports Phys Ther. 2016;46:200–16.
33. Santos JPM, da Silva RA, Fernandes MTP, et al. Uso do questionário lower extremity functional scale (LEFS-Brasil) em comparação com o Índice Algofuncional de Lequesne para definição de gravidade na osteoartrite de joelho e quadril. Rev Bras Reumatol. 2017;57:274–7.
34. Naal FD, Miozzari HH, Kelly BT, et al. The hip sports activity scale (HSAS) for patients with femoroacetabular impingement. Hip Int. 2013;23:204–11.
35. Lund B, Mygind-Klavsen B, Grønbech Nielsen T, et al. Danish hip arthroscopy registry (DHAR): the outcome of patients with femoroacetabular impingement (FAI). J Hip Preserv Surg. 2017;4:170–7.
36. Thorborg K, Tijssen M, Habets B, et al. Patient-reported outcome (PRO) questionnaires for young to middle-aged adults with hip and groin disability: a systematic review of the clinimetric evidence. Br J Sports Med. 2015;49:812.
37. Martin RL, Kelly BT, Philippon MJ. Evidence of validity for the hip outcome score. Arthroscopy. 2006;22:1304–11.
38. Martin RL, Philippon MJ. Evidence of validity for the hip outcome score in hip arthroscopy. Arthroscopy. 2007;23:822–6.
39. Martin RL, Philippon MJ. Evidence of reliability and responsiveness for the hip outcome score. Arthroscopy. 2008;24:676–82.
40. Roos EM, Toksvig-Larsen S. Knee Injury and Osteoarthritis Outcome Score (KOOS)—validation and comparison to the WOMAC in total knee replacement. Health Qual Life Outcomes. 2003;1:17.
41. Sueyoshi T, Emoto G, Yato T. Correlation between single assessment numerical evaluation score and Lysholm score in primary total knee arthroplasty patients. Arthroplast Today. 2018;4(1):99–102.
42. Faschinbauer M, Kasparek M, Schandler P. Predictive values of WOMAC, KOOS, and SF-12 score for knee arthroplasty: data from OAI. Knee Surg Sports Traumatol Arthrosc. 2017;25:3333–9.
43. Lysholm J, Gillquist J. Evaluation of the knee ligament surgery results with special emphasis on use of a scoring scale. Am J Sports Med. 1982;10:150–3.
44. Tegner Y, Lysholm J. Rating systems in the evaluation of knee ligament injuries. Clin Orthop Relat Res. 1985;(198):43–9.

45. Peccin MS, Ciconelli R, Cohen M. Questionário específico para sintomas do joelho "Lysholm Knee Scoring Scale": tradução e validação para a língua portuguesa. Acta Ortopédica Brasileira. 2006;14(5):268–72.
46. Swanenburg J, Koch PP, Meier N, Wirth B. Function and activity in patients with knee arthroplasty: validity and reliability of a German version of the Lysholm score and the Tegner activity scale. Swiss Med Wkly. 2014;144:w13976.
47. Kujala UM, Jaakkola LH, Koskinen SK, Taimela S, Hurme M, Nelimarkka O. Scoring of patellofemoral disorders. Arthroscopy. 1993;9(2):159–63.
48. Crossley KM, Bennell KL, Cowan SM, Green S. Analysis of outcome measures for persons with patellofemoral pain: which are reliable and valid? Arch Phys Med Rehabil. 2004;85(5):815–22.
49. Green A, Liles C, Rushton A, Kyte DG. Measurement properties of patient-reported outcome measures (PROMS) in patellofemoral pain syndrome: a systematic review. Man Ther. 2014;19(6):517–26.
50. Myer GD, Barber Foss KD, Gupta R, Hewett TE, Ittenbach RF. Analysis of patient-reported anterior knee pain scale: implications for scale development in children and adolescents. Knee Surg Sports Traumatol Arthrosc. 2016;24(3):653–60.
51. Ittenbach RF, Huang G, Barber Foss KD, Hewett TE, Myer GD. Reliability and validity of the anterior knee pain scale: applications for use as an epidemiologic screener. PLoS One. 2016;11(7):e0159204.

MIX
Papier aus verantwortungsvollen Quellen
Paper from responsible sources
FSC® C105338

If you have any concerns about our products,
you can contact us on
ProductSafety@springernature.com

In case Publisher is established outside the EU,
the EU authorized representative is:
Springer Nature Customer Service Center GmbH
Europaplatz 3, 69115 Heidelberg, Germany

Printed by Libri Plureos GmbH
in Hamburg, Germany